Heat packs, neck
Standard terry cover
Neck terry cover
Fluorimethane
Cold spray
Ice bags
Ice bags, Cramer
Kwik-heat pack
Cramer Atomic Rub Down
Flexi-wrap (small, large)
Flexi-wrap handles
Lotion, 1 gal

First Aid
Cotton rolls (nose plugs)
Tongue depressors
Pocket masks
Cotton tip applicators
Cotton tip applicators (sterile)
Sani Cloths
Latex gloves (med., large)
Cotton balls
Skin-preps
Save-A-Tooth
Penlights
Biohazard bags
Safety goggles

Taping Accessories
Heel and lace pads
Tape Adherent Spray
Tape remover

Sharps
Stainless steel prep blades
Scalpel blades, #10, #11 (sterile)
Scissors bandage
Scissors, small
Tweezers
Tweezers (sterile)
Suture sets
Nail clippers (large, small)
Tape cutters
Stethoscopes
Shark refill blades

Inhalants
Afrin

Antiseptics
Triadine
Peroxide
Rubbing alcohol
Betasept, small bottles
Betasept, 1 gal jug
Antimicrobial skin cleaner
Super Quin 9
Zorbicide Spray

Skin Treatments
Polysporin
Bacitracin
1% Tolnaftate Powder
Lamisil
1% Hydrocortisone
Second skin
Collodion
2% Miconazole
10% Hydrocortisone
Baby powder
Tincture of benzoin

Eye Treatment
Dacriose Irrigation
Saline
Eye wash
ReNu contact cleaning agent
Penlights

Teeth Treatment
Blue mouth guards, 25/box
Clear mouth guards, 25/box

Oral Medications
Acetaminophen bottle
Acetaminophen, 2 pk
Cepastat
Chlorpheniramine, 4 mg
Diphenhydramine, 25 mg
Ibuprofen bottle
Ibuprofen, 2 pk
Imodium AD
Pepto-Bismol tabs
Q-fed pkg
Sudodrin, 2 pk
Titralac
Robitussin DM

Crutches
Large
Medium
Small
Large aluminum

Water
Bottle carriers
Water bottles
Coolers (3, 7, 10 gal)
Chest

Other
Stools
Spray bottles
Bucket
Cloth towels

IMPORTANT

HERE IS YOUR REGISTRATION CODE TO ACCESS MCGRAW-HILL PREMIUM CONTENT AND MCGRAW-HILL ONLINE RESOURCES

For key premium online resources you need THIS CODE to gain access. Once the code is entered, you will be able to use the web resources for the length of your course.

Access is provided only if you have purchased a new book.

If the registration code is missing from this book, the registration screen on our website, and within your WebCT or Blackboard course will tell you how to obtain your new code. Your registration code can be used only once to establish access. It is not transferable.

To gain access to these online resources

1. USE your web browser to go to: **www.mhhe.com/esims**
2. CLICK on "First Time User"
3. ENTER the Registration Code printed on the tear-off bookmark on the right
4. After you have entered your registration code, click on "Register"
5. FOLLOW the instructions to setup your personal UserID and Password
6. WRITE your UserID and Password down for future reference. Keep it in a safe place.

If your course is using WebCT or Blackboard, you'll be able to use this code to access the McGraw-Hill content within your instructor's online course.

To gain access to the McGraw-Hill content in your instructor's WebCT or Blackboard course simply log into the course with the user ID and Password provided by your instructor. Enter the registration code exactly as it appears to the right when prompted by the system. You will only need to use this code the first time you click on McGraw-Hill content.

These instructions are specifically for student access. Instructors are not required to register via the above instructions.

20-24

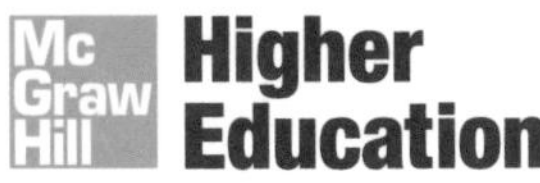

Thank you, and welcome to your McGraw-Hill Online Resources.

0-07-304257-9 t/a
Prentice & Arnheim
Essentials of Athletic Injury Management, 6e

P5N6-5MB2-NH00-D9B1-3DB7

REGISTRATION CODE

REGISTRATION CODE

The McGraw-Hill Companies
Mc Graw Hill Higher Education

arnheim's principles of

Athletic Training

A Competency-Based Approach

twelfth edition

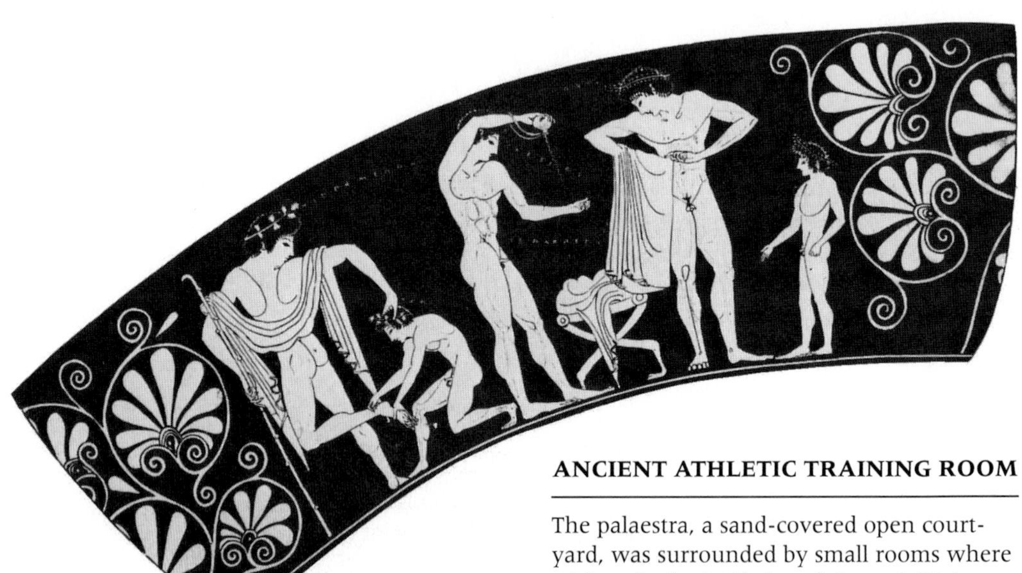

ANCIENT ATHLETIC TRAINING ROOM

The palaestra, a sand-covered open courtyard, was surrounded by small rooms where athletes bathed, oiled, and dressed. Right figure, a youth leaves his outer garment with an attendant; center figure, a competitor oils his body before entering the palaestra; left figure, an attendant removes a thorn from an injured athlete.

arnheim's principles of

Athletic Training

A Competency-Based Approach

twelfth edition

William E. Prentice, Ph.D., A.T.C., P.T.

Professor, Coordinator of Sports Medicine Program
Department of Exercise and Sport Science
The University of North Carolina
Chapel Hill, North Carolina

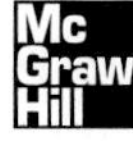

Boston Burr Ridge, IL Dubuque, IA Madison, WI New York San Francisco St. Louis
Bangkok Bogotá Caracas Kuala Lumpur Lisbon London Madrid Mexico City
Milan Montreal New Delhi Santiago Seoul Singapore Sydney Taipei Toronto

The McGraw·Hill Companies

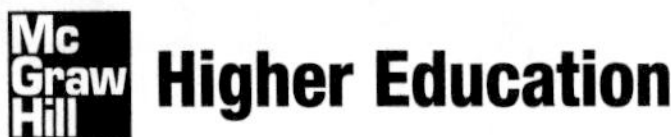

ARNHEIM'S PRINCIPLES OF ATHLETIC TRAINING: A COMPETENCY-BASED APPROACH
Published by McGraw-Hill, a business unit of The McGraw-Hill Companies, Inc., 1221 Avenue of the Americas, New York, NY 10020.

This book is printed on acid-free paper.

1 2 3 4 5 6 7 8 9 0 VNH/VNH 0 9 8 7 6 5

ISBN 0-07-297108-8

Vice president and editor-in-chief: *Emily Barrosse*
Publisher: *William R. Glass*
Executive editor: *Nicholas Barrett*
Executive marketing manager: *Pamela S. Cooper*
Director of development: *Kathleen Engelberg*
Senior developmental editor: *Michelle A. Turenne*
Technology developmental editor: *Julia D. Ersery*
Editorial and marketing coordinator: *Nancy Null*
Managing editor: *Jean Dal Porto*
Senior project manager: *Jill Moline-Eccher*
Manuscript editor: *Jan Nickels (freelance)*
Art director: *Jeanne Schreiber*
Designer: *Preston Thomas*
Text designer: *Adrianne Bosworth*
Cover designer: *Ross Carron*
Art editor: *Emma Ghiselli*
Manager, photo research: *Brian J. Pecko*
Cover credit: © *Taxi/Getty Images*
Senior media project manager: *Ron Nelms*
Associate production supervisor: *Jason I. Huls*
Senior media producer: *Lance Gerhart*
Composition: *10/12 Meridien by Cenveo*
Printer: *PMS Black, 45 # Pub Matte, Von Hoffman Corporation*

Credits: The credits section for this book begins on page C-1 and is considered an extension of the copyright page.

Library of Congress Cataloging-in-Publication Data

Prentice, William E.
Arnheim's principles of athletic training: a competency-based approach / William E. Prentice.—12th ed.
p. cm.
Includes bibliographical references and index.
ISBN 0-07-297108-8 (alk. paper)
1. Athletic trainers. 2. Physical education and training. I. Arnheim, Daniel D. II. Title.
RC1210.P726 2006
617.1′027—dc22

2004066169

The Internet addresses listed in the text were accurate at the time of publication. The inclusion of a website does not indicate an endorsement by the authors of McGraw-Hill, and McGraw-Hill does not guarantee the accuracy of the information presented at these sites.
www.mhhe.com

Remembering a Legacy

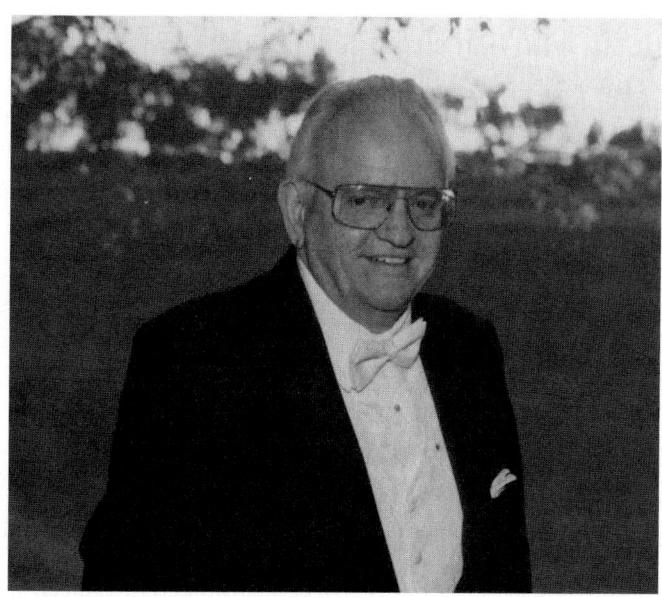

Our longtime author and friend, Daniel D. Arnheim, passed away April 11, 2000. Dr. Arnheim authored numerous textbooks in athletic training, as well as in elementary physical education, motor development, and adapted physical education. Among his most recognizable titles is *Principles of Athletic Training,* which is used by most students going into the field of athletic training, as well as *Essentials of Athletic Training,* which is used by physical education majors and coaching students.

Today, Dr. Arnheim is a legend among men and women who call themselves athletic trainers. For nearly 40 years, anyone who has taken an athletic training course has used one of his textbooks at one time or another. Any of the athletic trainers in the United States as well as throughout the world will recognize his name. He always focused on the needs of students and instructors who would use his books. He cared very much about the professional growth of students, as they hold the keys to the future of his chosen professions—education and athletic training. Dr. Arnheim touched the lives of the thousands of students and athletic trainers through the words in his books and helped to shape the growth and the direction of athletic training as a profession. His impact as an athletic training educator will be missed.

William E. Prentice
The Publishers

A Tribute to a Legend

In 1971, as a college sophomore at the University of Delaware, I took a required course that dealt with athletic injuries. At the time, I was a two-sport athlete who had sustained a couple of injuries and so, unlike many of the courses I had taken to that point in my college experience, I had at least a little interest in this course and in the material being presented. The textbook that we were required to buy for this class was the second edition of a book called *Modern Principles of Athletic Training* written by Karl Klafs and Dan Arnheim. As I sit here writing this, I am holding the copy of that book in my lap. Who would have ever guessed that almost 30 years later I would be coauthoring this textbook with Dan Arnheim?

Dan Arnheim was a living legend among men and women who call themselves athletic trainers. Over the past 30 years just about everyone who has taken an athletic training class has used one of his textbooks. I doubt seriously that there is any one of the 30,000+ athletic trainers in this country and throughout the world—from the youngest students to the old retirees—who would not recognize Dan Arnheim's name. He has literally touched tens of thousands of lives through the words in his books and he has helped to shape the growth and forge the direction of an entire profession. How many of us would love to be able to claim that we had that kind of an impact?

I joined him as coauthor on the *Principles of Athletic Training* book for the 8th edition in 1993. It didn't take me long to realize how incredibly intelligent Dr. Arnheim was. It became readily apparent to me that he had already forgotten more than I knew. Nevertheless, he allowed me to become a part of what had been his passion for more than 20 years, and for that I will always be grateful and indebted to him.

In my last conversations with him before he passed away in April of 2000, he was telling me that his involvement in the next edition of our book would be minimal. I assured him that I would do my best to continue with the high standards that he had set for us in our partnership to which he simply replied, "I know you will." So my charge from Dr. Arnheim is clear. Whether anyone can come close to the standard of excellence he established for us all is debatable. After all how many of us will ever be a "legend"?

William E. Prentice

Preface

Since the first edition of this text was published in 1963, the profession of athletic training has experienced amazing growth, not only in numbers but also in the associated body of knowledge. During those years, the authors of this text have taken it as a personal responsibility to provide the reader with the most current research-based and clinically based information available in athletic training and sports medicine. This text has always been considered by many as the leading text in this field.

In the eleventh edition, the title of this text was changed to *Arnheim's Principles of Athletic Training: A Competency-Based Approach,* to honor the legacy of Dr. Daniel Arnheim, the longtime author of this text. The changes and additions in this twelfth edition are a reflection of my commitment and passion towards continuing Dr. Arnheim's tradition.

The essential philosophy of this edition remains the same as in past editions. The text is designed to lead the student from general foundations to specific concepts relative to injury prevention, evaluation, management, and rehabilitation. As the student progresses from beginning to end, he or she will gradually begin to understand the complexities of the profession of athletic training. As in past editions, a major premise is that the student should be able to apply the appropriate techniques and concepts in the day-to-day performance of his or her job.

ADDRESSING THE ATHLETIC TRAINING EDUCATIONAL COMPETENCIES

Since 1998, the Education Council, established by the National Athletic Trainers' Association, has taken the responsibility for identifying the knowledge and skills that must be included in educational programs preparing students to enter the athletic training profession. The Education Council developed a list of educational competencies and clinical proficiencies categorized according to twelve domains that comprise the role of the athletic trainer. The athletic training educational programs that are accredited by CAAHEP (by the JRC-AT beginning in 2006), as well as those seeking accreditation, must integrate the extensive list of educational competencies and clinical proficiencies into their curriculums. This move toward competency-based athletic training education programs enhanced the need for a comprehensive text for athletic training students. My goal in this twelfth edition, as in the eleventh edition, was to make certain that each and every one of the educational competencies and clinical proficiencies identified by the Education Council is specifically covered at some point in this text.

It was suggested that including in this textbook a complete listing of all the educational competencies and clinical proficiencies and an index of the page number where that specific competency or proficiency is discussed would provide an excellent, logical, and useful resource for both the instructor and the athletic training student. Unfortunately, copyright laws prevented us from reproducing the *Athletic Training Educational Competencies* in this text. However, the McGraw-Hill web site at www.mhhe.com provides an index of where each and every educational competency and clinical proficiency is discussed in this textbook.

WHO IS IT WRITTEN FOR?

Arnheim's Principles of Athletic Training: A Competency-Based Approach should be used by athletic trainers in courses concerned with the scientific and clinical foundations of athletic training and sports medicine. Practicing athletic trainers, physical therapists, and other health care professionals involved with physically active individuals will also find this text valuable.

WHAT IS NEW IN THIS EDITION?

As in previous editions, developing the twelfth edition included serious consideration and incorporation of suggestions made by students, as well as detailed feedback from reviewers and other respected authorities in the field. Consequently, this twelfth edition reflects the major dynamic trends in the field of athletic training and sports medicine. Furthermore, it is my hope that this newest edition will help prepare students to become competent professionals who will continue to enhance the ongoing advancement of the athletic training profession.

In addition to the inclusion of material that addresses specific competencies, this newest edition has undergone extensive changes in content. The changes and additions are reflective of the ever-increasing body of knowledge that is expanding the scope of practice for the athletic trainer.

The chapters have been reorganized into six sections: Professional Development and Responsibilities, Risk Management, Pathology of Sports Injury, Management Skills, Musculoskeletal Conditions, and General Medical Conditions. A detailed listing of new and updated content follows:

Chapter 1: The Athletic Trainer and the Sports Medicine Team

- Expanded discussion of the recent history and development of NATA
- Added addresses of additional sports medicine organizations
- Added new position statements and guidelines for sports medicine organizations
- Added information on the National Academy of Sports Medicine
- Updated the performance domains for the 2004 Role Delineation Study
- Expanded section on dealing with an athlete's parents
- Introduced HIPAA
- Expanded the discussion of a coach's responsibilities on the sports medicine team
- Expanded the list of support personnel
- Added information on the NCAA recommendations for expanding coverage by athletic trainers
- Added information on employment settings in the military and as physician extenders
- Discussed transition of JRC-AT and the move from CAAHEP to CHEA
- Discussed name change from NATABOC to simply BOC
- Added information on specialty certifications (Certificates of Added Qualification)
- Updated requirements for certification post internship route
- Updated information on state-by-state regulation of the athletic trainer
- Expanded the discussion of future directions for the athletic training profession

Chapter 2: Health Care Administration in Athletic Training

- Added new focus box on sections to include in a policies and procedures manual
- Added a new design for a small athletic training room
- Added new information on HIPAA and FERPA and maintaining confidentiality in record keeping
- Expanded section on the use of computers in an athletic training setting
- Updated classification of sports table

Chapter 3: Legal Concerns and Insurance Issues

- Updated language in section on torts
- Expanded section on product liability
- Expanded descriptions of third-party payers
- Updated billing code procedures
- Added new table on numerical billing codes used by athletic trainers
- Added new focus box on guidelines for documentation

Chapter 4: Training and Conditioning Techniques

- Added new information on motion restriction due to tightness of neural tissue
- Redefined and clarified ballistic versus dynamic stretching techniques
- Added new information on stretching of tight neural structures
- Added new information on stretching of fascia
- Added new information on alternative stretching techniques including Pilates and yoga
- Expanded information on improving neuromuscular function in the early stages of weight training
- Revised information on spotting techniques and power lifts
- Added new information on strength training in adolescents

Chapter 5: Nutritional Considerations

- Added new information on transfatty acids
- Added new information on Dietary Reference Intakes
- Updated information on the Food Pyramid
- Added new section on ephedrine
- Added new section on hydrostatic weighing and bioelectrical impedance
- Added new section on low carbohydrate diets and weight loss
- Expanded section on disordered eating
- Added new information on anorexia athletica

Chapter 6: Environmental Considerations

- Added new focus box on factors that influence sweat rate
- Updated information on exertional heat illnesses
- Added new NATA recommendations for preventing heat illness
- Added new focus box on guidelines that should be followed during an electrical storm
- Added new information on lightning detectors

Chapter 7: Protective Gear and Sports Equipment

- Added new focus box on guidelines for selecting, purchasing, and fitting protective sports equipment to help minimize liability
- Added new information on equipment reconditioning and recertification
- Added new information on the Revolution football helmet
- Added new information on soccer headgear
- Updated photos of equipment
- Added new information on shoe lacing techniques

Chapter 9: Mechanisms and Characteristics of Sports Trauma

- Expanded information on myofascial trigger points

Chapter 10: Tissue Response to Injury

- Added new information on unidimensional and multidimensional pain assessment tools

Chapter 11: Psychosocial Intervention for Sports Injuries and Illnesses

- Added new practical suggestions on the athletic trainer's role in providing social support to an injured athlete
- Added new information on the emotional and psychological effects of an athlete's injury upon the athletic trainer

Chapter 12: On-the-Field Acute Care and Emergency Procedures

- Updated and added new information on the emergency action plan

- Added an example of a consent form for medical treatment of minors
- Updated information about equipment removal
- Updated information on CPR techniques
- Expanded information on use of AEDs
- Added information on the ACDU and AVPU level of consciousness scales
- Updated information on pool extraction techniques

Chapter 13: Off-the-Field Injury Evaluation

- Added new information on differential diagnosis
- Added new table on standard abbreviations used in medical documentation
- Added new information on arteriograms, venograms, and Dopplar ultrasonography

Chapter 14: Bloodborne Pathogens

- Added new information on hepatitis C
- Added new information on using nonlatex gloves

Chapter 15: Using Therapeutic Modalities

- Added new information on ensuring athlete privacy
- Updated information on all modalities
- Added new information on Cryo-Cuff and Game Ready systems
- Added new information on extracorporal shock wave therapy

Chapter 16: Using Therapeutic Exercise in Rehabilitation

- Added new information on the RAMP system of rehabilitation
- Added new aquatic therapy workout

Chapter 17: Pharmacology, Drugs, and Sports

- Updated information on new medications throughout
- Updated the NCAA banned substance list
- Added new information on THG

Chapters 18 through 25 cover specific musculoskeletal injuries to regional areas of the body. These chapters have been expanded to include new information and are now as comprehensive as possible within the scope of practice in athletic training. Each body region has been organized to include sections on anatomy, prevention, assessment, management of specific injuries, and rehabilitation (when appropriate). Each injury identified consistently discusses the associated etiology, symptoms and signs, and management. Coverage of rehabilitation techniques includes suggestions for general body reconditioning, joint mobilization, flexibility exercises, muscular strength, neuromuscular control, functional progressions (when appropriate), and guidelines for return to activity.

Chapter 18: The Foot

- Revised and updated information on normal gait patterns
- Added new information on subungual hematoma
- Added new information on incorporating exercise sandals into the rehabilitation program

Chapter 19: The Ankle and Lower Leg

- Incorporated new information on rehabilitation of ankle sprains

Chapter 20: The Knee and Related Structures

- Added new information on modified Lachman tests

Chapter 21: The Thigh, Hip, Groin, and Pelvis

- Revised information on femoral fractures
- Revised information on femoral stress fractures
- Included new photos for femoral retroversion and anteversion

Chapter 22: The Shoulder Complex

- Added new section on O'Brien's active compression test
- Added new focus box on throwing progressions

Chapter 23: The Elbow

- Added new information on Panner's disease
- Updated information on medial and lateral epicondylitis
- Updated information on Volkmann's contracture

Chapter 24: The Forearm, Wrist, Hand, and Fingers

- Added new information on Madelung deformity
- Updated information on triangular fibrocartilage complex

Chapter 25: The Spine

- Corrected information on spinal cord shock and cervical cord neuropraxia
- Added new information on the methods for measuring spinal stenosis
- Updated information about brachial plexus injury

Chapter 26: The Head, Face, Eyes, Ears, Nose, and Throat (formerly Chapter 27)

- Updated and expanded discussions of concussion and mild head injury
- Added new focus box on guidelines for physician referral following concussion
- Added new focus box on home instructions for concussions
- Updated information on malignant brain edema syndrome
- Updated information on subdural hematoma
- Updated information on migraine headaches
- Added new information on Le Fort fractures
- Added new photos for ear examination
- Added new photos for eye examination

Chapter 27: The Thorax and Abdomen (formerly Chapter 26)

- Updated information on bowel sounds in auscultation
- Added new techniques for managing scrotal contusion
- Added new information on commotio cordis

Chapter 28: Skin Disorders

- Added new information on when to use sutures
- Added new information on pityriasis rosea
- Added new information on spider bites
- Added new focus box on wound care
- Added new focus box on managing blisters
- Added new photos of various dermatologic conditions

Chapter 29: Additional General Medical Conditions

- Updated information on hypertension

Critical Thinking Exercises

Critical Thinking Exercises, including 29 new exercises, are presented in every chapter and provide brief case studies that help the student apply the content just studied. Solutions for each case are included at the end of each chapter.

PEDAGOGICAL AIDS

Numerous pedagogical tools are included in this edition:

- *Chapter objectives* Goals begin each chapter to reinforce important key concepts to be learned.
- *Margin information* Key concepts, selected definitions, helpful training tips, and illustrations are placed in the margins throughout the text for added emphasis and ease of reading and studying.
- *Anatomy* Where applicable, extensive discussion of anatomy is presented and illustrated throughout the text.
- *Focus boxes* Important information is highlighted and boxed to make key information easier to find and to enhance the text's flexibility and appearance.
- *Critical Thinking Exercises* 244 brief cases studies are now included that encourage the student to apply the content presented to the clinical setting.
- *Color throughout text* A second color is used throughout the text to accentuate and clarify illustrations and textual material.
- *New photographs and line drawings* Approximately 75 new or replacement photographs and color line drawings have been added.
- *Color illustrations* 24 full-color photographs are included in Chapter 28 to depict common skin disorders.
- *Management plans* In selected chapters, sample management plans are presented as examples of treatment procedures.
- *Chapter summaries* Each chapter's salient points are summarized to reinforce key content.
- *Review questions and class activities* Located at the end of each chapter, review questions and class activities are provided to enhance the learning process.
- *References* References have been extensively updated to provide the most complete and current information available.
- *Annotated bibliography* For students and instructors who want to expand on the information presented in each chapter, an annotated bibliography has been provided.
- *Glossary* An extensive list of key terms and their definitions is presented to reinforce information in one convenient location.
- *Appendixes* The appendixes contain NATA's Code of Ethics, Canada's Food Guide for Healthy Living and the Recommended Nutrient Intake (RNI), Bloodborne Pathogen Guidelines, Helmet Removal Guidelines, Fluid Replacement Guidelines, Lightening Safety Guidelines, Emergency Planning, and a sample resume. New appendixes include NATA position statements on Exertional Heat Illnesses, Management of Sport-Related Concussion, and commotio cordis.
- *End pages* Front and back end pages inside the covers of the text provide helpful lists of suggested supplies for the athletic training room and the athletic trainer's kit, along with charts for metric and celsius conversions.

INSTRUCTOR'S RESOURCE MATERIALS

Course Integrator Guide

Formerly the Instructor's Manual, this guide was prepared by Terri Jo Rucinski, M.A., ATC, P.T. from the University of North Carolina. It includes all the useful features of an Instructor's Manual, including learning objectives, brief chapter overviews, key terminology, discussion questions, class activities, worksheets and the accompanying answer keys, media resources, and Web links. It also integrates the text with image clips and all the health and human performance resources McGraw-Hill offers including the Online Learning Center, The guide also includes references to relevant print and broadcast media.

Test Bank

The test bank includes approximately 2,000 examination questions. Each chapter contains true-false, multiple choice, and completion test questions. The worksheets in each chapter also include a separate test bank of matching, short answer, listing, essay, and personal or injury assessment questions that can be used as self-testing tools for students or as additional sources for examination questions.

Computerized Test Bank CD-ROM

McGraw-Hill's EZ Test is a flexible and easy-to-use electronic testing program. The program allows instructors to create tests from book specific items. It accommodates a wide range of question types and instructors may add their own questions. Multiple versions of the test can be created, and any test can be exported for use with course management systems such as WebCT, BlackBoard or PageOut. The program is available for Windows and Macintosh environments.

PowerPoint Presentation

Developed for the twelfth edition by Jason Scibek, M.A., ATC, of Eastern Michigan University, a comprehensive and extensively illustrated PowerPoint presentation accompanies this text for use in classroom discussion. The PowerPoint presentation may also be converted to outlines and given to students as a handout. You can easily download the PowerPoint presentation from the Online Learning Center at www.mhhe.com/prentice12e. Adopters of the text can obtain the login and password to access this presentation by contacting your local McGraw-Hill sales representative.

Resource Presentation Manager (RPM)

This is a CD-ROM presentation tool of book-specific images designed to engage students and promote critical thinking and dialogue on the most relevant topics in athletic training. Images can be searched by table of contents, key word, or type.

INTERNET RESOURCES

Course Management Systems

www.mhhe.com/support
Now instructors can combine their McGraw-Hill Online Learning Center with today's most popular course-management systems and/or McGraw-Hill's PageOut. The McGraw-Hill Online Learning Center has also been converted into a cartridge that can be used in most course management systems. Our Instructor Advantage program offers customers toll-free telephone support, and unlimited e-mail support. Instructors who use 500 or more copies of a McGraw-Hill textbook can enroll in our Instructor Advantage Plus program, which provides on-campus, hands-on training from a platform specialist. We have also built an interactive support site accessible to anyone with an Internet connection. Located at www.mhhe.com/support, you can ask questions of the prebuilt database, or e-mail a McGraw-Hill specialist. Consult your McGraw-Hill sales representative to learn what other course management systems are easily used with McGraw-Hill online materials.

Online Learning Center

www.mhhe.com/prentice12e
This website offers resources to students and instructors. It includes downloadable ancillaries, Web links, student quizzes, additional information on topics of interest, and more. Resources for the instructor include:

- Downloadable PowerPoint presentations
- Lecture outlines
- Discussion questions
- Concept summaries

Resources for the student include:

- Flashcards
- Online chapter reviews
- Interactive quizzes
- PowerWeb

eSims

www.mhhe.com/esims
eSims is an online assessment tool that provides students with computerized simulation tests with instant feedback that emulate the actual Athletic Training certification exam. eSims is available with each new purchase of *Arnheim's Principles of Athletic Training.* (It is also available for purchase online too!) Check out eSims at the address above.

ACKNOWLEDGMENTS

I would like to express my deepest gratitude to my longtime developmental editor, Michelle Turenne, who, as always, provided invaluable guidance throughout the development of this edition. Her input and dedication to this project have been indispensable. Michelle has left McGraw-Hill, and I cannot thank her enough for her friendship over the years. She will always be an important part of the fabric of this text.

During the revision process for the twelfth edition, we relied heavily on input solicited from our reviewers. My personal thanks are extended to:

Bruce D. Barnhart
California University of Pennsylvania

Jody B. Brucker
Indiana State University

Catherine English
San Jose State University

Leamor Kahanov
San Jose State University

Barry E. McGlumphy
California University of Pennsylvania

Brian G. Ragan
University of Illinois at Urbana-Champaign

Donna M. Ritenour
Western Michigan University

John Storsved
Indiana State University

Karen Straub
The University of West Alabama

Gary Wilkerson
University of Tennessee at Chattanooga

Steven M. Zinder
California State University at Fullerton

I also wish to extend my sincere appreciation to our technical reviewers for their critique of selected chapters. Their input was most valuable to the completion of this edition.

Patsy Huff, Pharm.D.
Student Health Service-Pharmacy
The University of North Carolina at Chapel Hill

Kevin Guskiewicz, Ph.D., A.T.C.
Department of Exercise and Sport Science
The University of North Carolina at Chapel Hill

G. Robert Nugent, M.D.
Adjunct Professor of Neurosurgery
West Virginia University School of Medicine

David Rubenstein, M.D.
Department of Dermatology
The University of North Carolina at Chapel Hill

Finally, I want to thank my wife Tena, and our sons, Brian and Zach, for their enduring support and encouragement. They constantly help me to keep my perspective on both my professional and personal life.

William E. Prentice

Applications at a Glance

The Athletic Trainer and the Sports Medicine Team

Chapter 1

When you finish this chapter you should be able to

- Recognize the historical foundations of athletic training.
- Identify the various professional organizations dedicated to athletic training and sports medicine.
- Differentiate the roles and responsibilities of the athletic trainer, the team physician, and the coach.
- Explain the function of support personnel in sports medicine.
- Identify various employment settings for the athletic trainer.
- Discuss certification and licensure for the athletic trainer.
- Clarify the role of the physical therapist in sports medicine.

An athletic trainer is concerned with the well-being of the athlete and generally assumes the responsibility for overseeing the total health care for the athlete. Participation in sports places the athlete in a situation in which injury is likely to occur. Fortunately, most of the injuries are not serious and lend themselves to rapid rehabilitation, but the athletic trainer must be capable of dealing with any type of trauma or catastrophic injury.

Although millions of individuals participate in organized and recreational sports, there is a relatively low incidence of fatalities and catastrophic injuries among them. A major problem, however, lies with the millions of sports participants who incur injuries or illnesses that could have been prevented and who later, as a consequence, develop more serious chronic conditions. Athletes in organized sports have every right to expect that their health and safety will be kept as the highest of priorities. The field of athletic training, as a specialization, provides a major link between the sports program and the medical community for the implementation of injury prevention, emergency care, and rehabilitative procedures (Figure 1-1).[66]

The certified athletic trainer is a highly educated and skilled professional specializing in athletic health care for the physically active.

HISTORICAL PERSPECTIVES

Early History

The drive to compete was important in many early societies. Sports developed over a period of time as a means of competing in a relatively peaceful and nonharmful way. Early civilizations show little evidence of highly organized sports. Some evidence indicates that in Greek and Roman civilizations there were coaches, trainers (people who helped the athlete reach top physical condition), and physicians to assist the athlete in reaching optimum performance.[51] Many of the roles that emerged during this early period are the same in modern sports.

The history of athletic training draws on the disciplines of exercise, medicine, physical therapy, physical education, and sports.

For many centuries after the fall of the Roman Empire there was a complete lack of interest in sports activities. Not until the beginning of the Renaissance did these activities slowly gain popularity. Athletic training as we know it came into existence during the late nineteenth century with the firm establishment of intercollegiate and interscholastic athletes in the United States. The first athletic trainers of this era were hangers-on who "rubbed down" the athlete. Because they possessed no technical

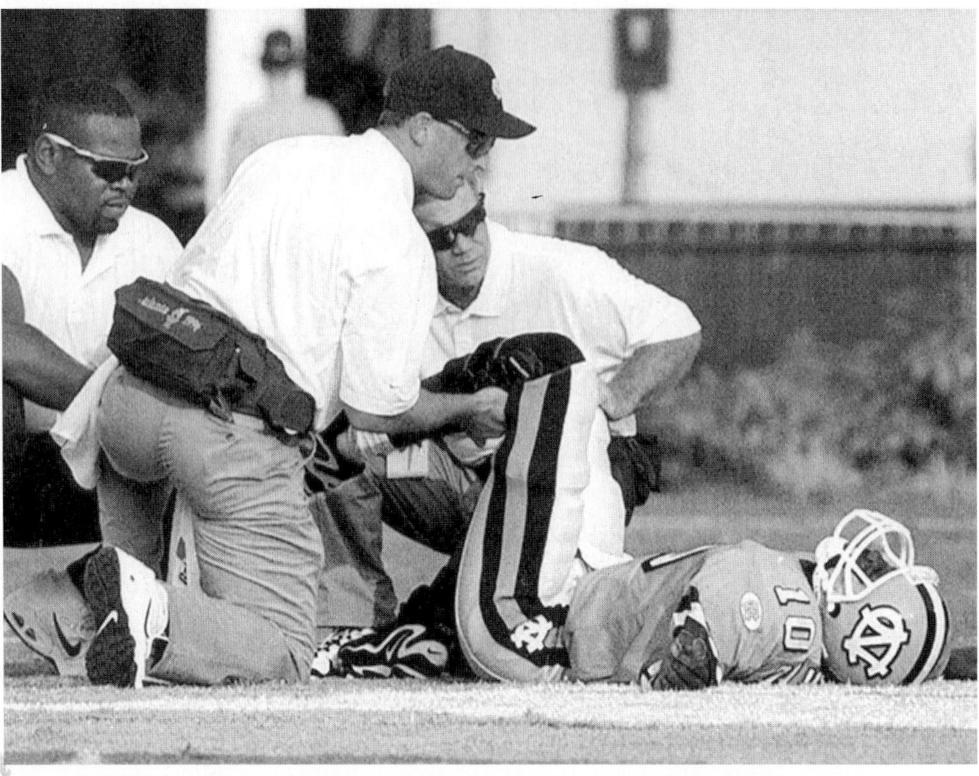

Figure 1-1

The field of athletic training provides a major link between the sports program and the medical community.

knowledge, their athletic training techniques usually consisted of a rub, the application of some type of counterirritant, and occasionally the prescription of various home remedies and poultices. Many of those earlier athletic trainers were persons of questionable background and experience. As a result, it has taken many years for the athletic trainer to attain the status of a well-qualified allied health care professional.[61]

Evolution of the Contemporary Athletic Trainer

A Certified Athletic Trainer provides health care to physically active individuals

The terms *training* and *athletic training, trainer,* and *athletic trainer* are often used interchangeably and are frequently confused with one another. Historically, training implies the act of coaching or teaching. In comparison, athletic training has traditionally been known as the field that is concerned with the athlete's health and safety. A trainer refers to someone who trains dogs or horses or functions in coaching or teaching areas. The *certified athletic trainer* is one who is a specialist in athletic training. Athletic training has evolved over the years to play a major role in the health care of the physically active in general and the athlete in particular. This evolution occurred rapidly after World War I with the appearance of the athletic trainer in intercollegiate athletics. During this period, the major influence in developing the athletic trainer as a specialist in preventing and managing athletic injuries came from the work of Dr. S. E. Bilik, a physician who wrote the first major text on athletic training and the care of athletic injuries, called *The Trainer's Bible,* in 1917.[8]

In the early 1920s the Cramer family in Gardner, Kansas, started a chemical company and began producing a liniment to treat ankle sprains. Over the years, the Cramers realized that there was a market for products to treat injured athletes. In an effort to enhance communication and facilitate an exchange of ideas among coaches, athletic trainers, and athletes, Cramer began publication of the *First Aider* in 1932. The members of this family were instrumental in the early development of the athletic training profession and have always played a prominent role in the education of student athletic trainers.[61]

During the late 1930s an effort was made, primarily by several college and university athletic trainers, to establish a national organization named the National Athletic

Trainers' Association (NATA). After struggling for existence from 1938 to 1944, the association essentially disappeared during the difficult years of World War II.

Between 1947 and 1950 university athletic trainers once again began to organize themselves into separate regional conferences, which would later become district organizations within NATA. In 1950 some 101 athletic trainers from the various conferences met in Kansas City, Missouri, and officially formed the National Athletic Trainers' Association. The primary purpose for its formation was to establish professional standards for the athletic trainer.[61] Since NATA was formed in 1950 many individuals have made contributions to the development of the profession.

After 1950 the growth of the athletic training profession has been remarkable. In 1974 when NATA membership numbers were first tracked there were 4,500 members. Today those numbers have grown to more than 30,000 members. Originally, the traditional settings where athletic trainers worked were in colleges and secondary schools, dealing almost exclusively with the athletic population. Today the contemporary certified athletic trainer can be found not only in schools, but also on the sidelines of professional sports, in hospitals and clinics, in industrial settings, in the military, working as physician extenders, in medical equipment sales and support, and even in NASA and NASCAR, as the profession that began with college sports has expanded its scope to deal with all people involved in physical activity. As the athletic training profession has grown and evolved over the last fifty years, many positive milestones have occurred that have collectively shaped the future direction of the profession, including, among many, recognition of athletic trainers as health care providers; increased diversity of practice settings; the passage of practice acts that regulate athletic trainers in most states; third party reimbursement for athletic training services; and ongoing reevaluation, revision, and reform of athletic training educational programs.

SPORTS MEDICINE AND ATHLETIC TRAINING

The Field of Sports Medicine

The term *sports medicine* refers generically to a broad field of medical practice related to physical activity and sport. The field of sports medicine encompasses under its umbrella a number of more specialized aspects of dealing with the physically active or athletic populations that may be classified as relating either to performance enhancement or to injury care and management (Figure 1-2). Those areas of specialization that are primarily concerned with performance enhancement include exercise physiology, biomechanics, sport psychology, sports nutrition, and strength and conditioning. Areas of specialization that focus more on injury care and management specific to the athlete are the practice of medicine, athletic training, sports physical therapy, sports massage therapy, sports dentistry, osteopathic medicine, orthotists/prosthetists, and chiropractic. The

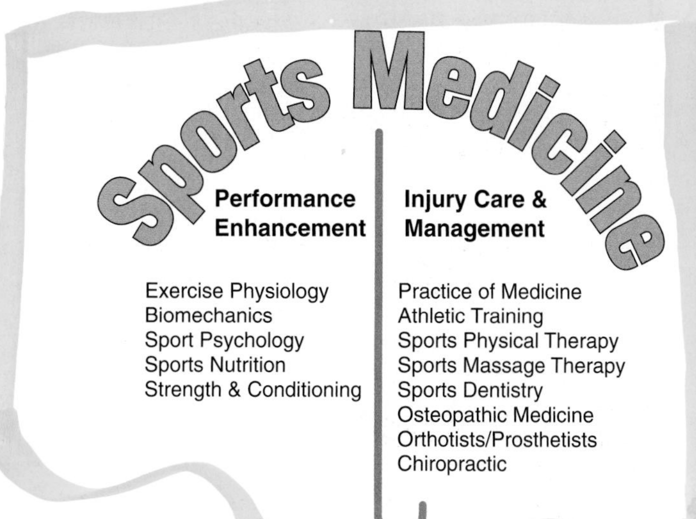

Figure 1-2

Areas of specialization under the sports medicine "umbrella."

American College of Sports Medicine (ACSM) has defined sports medicine as multidisciplinary, including the physiological, biomechanical, psychological, and pathological phenomena associated with exercise and sports.[2] The clinical application of the work of these disciplines is performed to improve and maintain an individual's functional capacities for physical labor, exercise, and sports. It also includes the prevention and treatment of diseases and injuries related to exercise and sports.

Growth of Professional Sports Medicine Organizations

Many professional organizations that are dedicated to achieving health and safety in sports have developed in the twentieth century.

The twentieth century brought with it the development of a number of professional organizations dedicated to athletic training and sports medicine. Professional organizations have many goals: (1) to upgrade the field by devising and maintaining a set of professional standards, including a code of ethics; (2) to bring together professionally competent individuals to exchange ideas, stimulate research, and promote critical thinking; and (3) to give individuals an opportunity to work as a group with a singleness of purpose, thereby making it possible for them to achieve objectives that, separately, they could not accomplish. The organizations in the following list are presented in chronological order according to their year of establishment. Addresses, phone numbers, and/or websites for these and other related sports medicine organizations are in *Focus Box:* "Addresses of professional sports medicine organizations."

Several of these professional organizations also disseminate information to the general public about safe participation in sport activities in the form of guidelines or position statements. *Focus Box:* "Guidelines and position statements" lists the guidelines and position statements that are published by several different organizations.

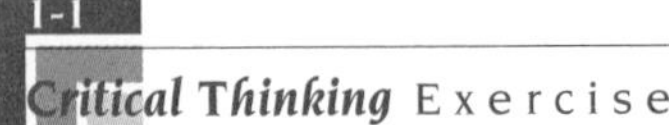

1-1 *Critical Thinking* Exercise

A student athletic trainer has been given a class assignment to put together a list of various sports medicine organizations and to define the missions of those organizations.

? Where can the student find the most information about these organizations?

Focus

Addresses of professional sports medicine organizations

American Academy of Family Physicians, 8880 Ward Parkway, Kansas City, MO 64114. http://home.aafp.org/

American Academy of Ophthalmology Eye Safety and Sports Ophthalmology Committee, 655 Beach St., Box 7424, San Francisco, CA 94120-7424. (415) 561-8500.

American Academy of Orthopaedic Surgeons (AAOS), 6300 N. River Rd., Rosemont, IL 60018-4262. http://www.aaos.org/

American Academy of Pediatrics, Sports Committee, 141 NW Point Boulevard, Elk Grove Village, IL 60007-1098. http://www.aap.org/

American Academy of Physical Medicine and Rehabilitation (AAPMR), Special Interest Group on Sports Medicine, One IBM Plaza, Suite 2500, Chicago, IL 60611-3604. (312) 464-9700.

American Academy of Podiatric Sports Medicine (AAPSM), 1729 Glastonberry Rd., Potomac, MD 20854. http://www.aapsm.org/

American Association of Industrial Sports Medicine, 116 Foxboro Dr., Rochester Hills, MI 48309. (810) 375-9377. www.aaism.org

American Chiropractic Association Council on Sports Injuries and Physical Fitness, ACA Sports Council, 2444 Solomons Island Rd., #218 Annapolis, MD 21401. (410) 266-8285.

American College of Sports Medicine, 401 W. Michigan St., Indianapolis, IN 46202-3233. http://www.acsm.org/

American Massage Therapy Association, 820 Davis St., Evanston, IL 60201. http://www.amtamassage.org/

American Medical Athletic Association (AMAA), 4405 East West Highway, Suite 405, Bethesda, MD 20814. amaasportsmed@aol.com

Continued

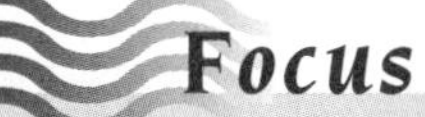

Addresses of professional sports medicine organizations—continued

American Medical Soccer Association (AMSA), 350 Cheshire Dr., Birmingham, AL 35242-3100. (205) 991-6054. www.amsa.org

American Medical Society for Sports Medicine (AMSSM), 7611 Elmwood Ave., Suite 203, Middleton, WI 53562. (608) 831-4484. www.amssm.org

American Medical Tennis Association, 2301 Waleska Rd., Canton, GA 30114. http://www.mdtennis.org/

American Optometric Association (AOA) Sports Vision Section (SVS), 243 N. Lindbergh Blvd., St. Louis, MO 63141-7881. http://www.aoanet.org/

American Orthopaedic Society for Sports Medicine, 6300 N. River Road, Suite 200, Rosemont, IL 60018. http://www.sportsmed.org/

American Osteopathic Academy of Sports Medicine, 7611 Elmwood Ave., Suite 201, Middleton, WI 53562. (608) 831-4400. www.aoasm.org

American Osteopathic Orthopedic Society for Sports Medicine (AOOSSM), RD 3, Clarion, PA 16214. www.aoosm.org

American Physical Therapy Association, 1111 N. Fairfax St., Alexandria, VA 22314. http://apta.edoc.com/

American Physical Therapy Association (APTA), Sports Physical Therapy Section, 505 King St., Suite 115, La Crosse, WI 54601. http://www.apta.org/

American Running Association, 4405 East West Hwy., Suite 405, Bethesda, MD 20814. http://www.americanrunning.org

American Society of Biomechanics (ASB), c/o Joan E. Bechtold, PhD, Secretary/Treasurer, Biomechanics Laboratory, Hennepin County Medical Center, 701 Park Ave., S/860C, Minneapolis, MN 55415. http://www.asb-biomech.org bechto1@attglobal.net

American Sports Medicine Association, 660 W. Duarte Rd, Suite 1, Arcadia, CA 91007. (818) 445-1978.

Association of Volleyball Physicians, 1229 N. North Branch, Suite 122, Chicago, IL 60622. (708) 210-3112.

Canadian Academy of Sport Medicine, Unit 14, 1010 Polytek Street, Suite 100, Ottawa, ON K1J 9H9. (877) 585-2394. http://www.casm-acms.org

Canadian Athletic Therapists Association (CATA), 1600 James Naismith Dr., Suite 507, Gloucester, ON K1B 5N4. (403) 240-7228. jburke@rtm.cdnsport.ca

Canadian Sport Massage Therapists Association (CSMTA), P.O. Box 1330, Unity, SK S0K 4L0. (306) 228-2808.

College Athletic Trainers' Society, Thorp Reed & Armstrong, LLPOne Oxford Centre, 301 Grant Street, 14th Floor, Pittsburgh, PA 15219-1425.

College of Chiropractic Sports Sciences (Canada), c/o Canadian Chiropractic Association, 1396 Eglington Ave. W., Toronto, ON M6C 2E4. (416) 781-5656.

Cooper Institute For Aerobics Research, 12330 Preston Rd., Dallas, TX 75230. (972) 341-3200. www.cooperinst.org

Gatorade Sport Science Institute, 617 W. Main St., Barrington, IL 60010. http://www.gssiweb.com

Institute for Preventative Sports Medicine, P.O. Box 7032, Ann Arbor, MI 48107. (734) 434-3390. www.ipsm.org

International Academy of Sports Vision (IASV), 200 S. Progress Ave., Harrisburg, PA 17109. (717) 652-8080.

International Powerlifting Federation Medical Committee, Box 4160, Opelika, AL 36803. (334) 749-6222.

The International Society for Sport Psychiatry, 316 N. Milwaukee St., Suite 318, Milwaukee, WI 53202. (414) 271-2900.

Joint Commission on Sports Medicine and Science, 90 South Cascade, Suite 1190, Colorado Springs, CO 80903. (719) 475-8609.

Continued

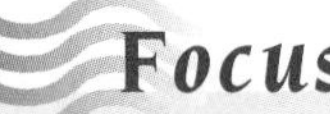

Addresses of professional sports medicine organizations—continued

National Academy of Sports Medicine (NASM), 26632 Agoura Road, Calabascas, CA 91302. (866) 292-6276. www.nasm.org

National Collegiate Athletic Association (NCAA) Injury Surveillance System (ISS), 6201 College Blvd., Overland Park, KS 66211. (913) 339-1906.

National Athletic Trainers' Association, 2952 Stemmons Freeway, Dallas, TX 75247. http://www.nata.org/

National Collegiate Athletic Association, Competitive Safeguards and Medical Aspects of Sports Committee, 6201 College Boulevard, Overland Park, KS 66211-2422. http://www.ncaa.org/

The National Council for Sports Medicine Education (NCSME), P.O. Box 3, Saratoga Springs, NY 12866. (518) 786-1529.

The National Federation of State High School Athletic Associations, 11724 Plaza Circle, P.O. Box 20626, Kansas City, MO 64195. http://nfshsa.org/

National Strength and Conditioning Association, P.O. Box 38909, Colorado Springs, CO 80937-8909. http://www.nsca-lift.org/

North American Society for Pediatric Exercise Medicine (NASPEM), Box 5076, 1607 N. Market St., Champaign, IL 61825-5076. (217) 351-5076.

North American Society for the Psychology of Sport and Physical Activity (NASPSPA), Dept. of Exercise and Sport Science, 254 HHP, UNC Greensboro, Greensboro, NC 27412. (910) 334-3255.

Sports Medicine Council of British Columbia (SMCBC), #3 - 6501 Sprott St., Burnaby, BC V5B 3B8. (604) 473-4850.

United States Rowing Association (USRA) Sports Medicine Society, 201 S. Capitol Ave., Suite 400, Indianapolis, IN 46225-1068. (317) 237-5656.

U.S. Olympic Committee Sports Medicine Society, 1 Olympic Plaza, Colorado Springs, CO 80909-5760. (719) 578-4546.

U.S. Weightlifting Federation Sports Medicine Committee, Box 4160, 2000 Waverly Parkway, Opelika, AL 36803-4160. (334) 749-6222.

Wilderness Medical Society, Box 2463, Indianapolis, IN 46206. (317) 631-1745.

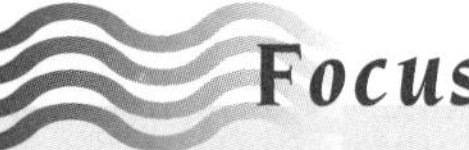

Guidelines and position statements

National Athletic Trainers' Association (NATA)

Position Statements

- Emergency planning in athletics
- Exertional heat illnesses
- Fluid replacement for athletes
- Head down contact and spearing in tackle football
- Lightning safety for athletics and recreation
  - Endorsed by the *American Academy of Pediatrics*
- Management of sport-related concussion

Consensus Statements

- Appropriate medical care for secondary school-age athletes
- Prehospital care of the spine-injured athlete
- Inter-association task force on exertional heat illnesses

Continued

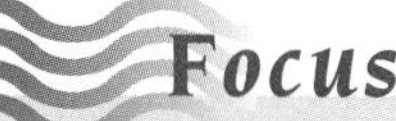

Guidelines and position statements—continued

National Athletic Trainers' Association (NATA)—continued

Official Statements

- Commotio cordis
- Drug and performance enhancement supplement use in athletics
- Full-time, on-site athletic trainer coverage for secondary school athletic programs
- Use of qualified athletic trainers in secondary schools
- Automated external defibrillators
- Community-acquired MRSA infections
- Youth football and heat-related illnesses

Cooperative and Support Statements

- *American Academy of Family Physicians'* support of athletic trainers for high school athletes
- *American Medical Association's* support of athletic trainers in secondary schools
- Appropriate medical care for secondary school-age athletes (Manuscript)
- Endorsement of NATA Lightning Position Statement by the *American Academy of Pediatrics*
- Recommendations and guidelines for appropriate medical coverage of intercollegiate athletics
    - NCAA support of Recommendations and guidelines for appropriate medical coverage of intercollegiate athletics

National Collegiate Athletic Association (NCAA) guidelines

- Sports Medicine Administration
- Medical Evaluations, Immunizations and Records
- Dispensing Prescription Medication
- Lightning Safety
- Institutional Alcohol, Tobacco and Other Drug Education Programs
- Emergency Care and Coverage
- Medical Disqualification of the Student-Athlete
- Skin Infections in Wrestling
- Prevention of Heat Illness
- Weight Loss—Dehydration
- Assessment of Body Composition
- Nutrition and Athletic Performance
- Menstrual-Cycle Dysfunction
- Blood-Borne Pathogens and Intercollegiate Athletics
- Nontherapeutic Drugs
- Nutritional Ergogenic Aids
- The Use of Local Anesthetics in College Athletics
- The Use of Injectable Corticosteroids in Sports Injuries
- Cold Stress
- "Burners" (Bracial Plexus Injuries)
- Concussion and Second-Impact Syndrome
- Participation by the Impaired Student-Athlete
- Participation by the Pregnant Student-Athlete
- The Student-Athlete with Sickle Cell Trait
- Protective Equipment
- Eye Safety in Sports
- Use of Trampoline and Minitramp
- Mouth Guards
- Use of the Head as a Weapon in Football and Other Contact Sports
- Guidelines for Helmet Fitting and Removal in Athletics
- Transparent Eye Shield Exception Procedure for Football

American Academy of Pediatrics (AAP)

- Intensive Training and Sports Specialization in Young Athletes
- Medical Concerns in the Female Athlete
- Human Immunodeficiency Virus and Other Blood-Borne Viral Pathogens in the Athletic Setting
- Promotion of Healthy Weight-Control Practices in Young Athletes
- Adolescents and Anabolic Steroids: A Subject Review
- Protective Eyewear for Young Athletes
- Medical Conditions and Sports Participation

Continued

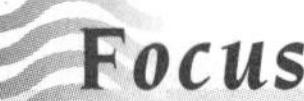

Guidelines and position statements—continued

American Academy of Pediatrics (AAP)—continued

- Amenorrhea in Adolescent Athletes
- Medical Conditions Affecting Sports Participation
- Strength Training, Weight and Power Lifting, and Body Building by Children and Adolescents
- Triathlon Participation by Children and Adolescents
- Cardiac Dysrhythmias and Sports
- Athletic Participation by Children and Adolescents Who Have Systemic Hypertension
- Risks in Distance Running for Children
- Knee Brace Use by Athletes
- Risk of Injury from Baseball and Softball in Children 5 to 14 Years of Age
- Injuries in Youth Soccer: A Subject
- Organized Athletics for Preadolescent Children
- Guidelines for Emergency Medical Care in School
- Climatic Heat Stress and the Exercising Child and Adolescent
- Mitral Valve Prolapse and Athletic Participation in Children and Adolescents
- Participation in Boxing by Children, Adolescents, and Young Adults
- Sports with High Risk of Eye Injury

American College of Sports Medicine (ACSM)

- Nutrition and Athletic Performance
- Exercise and Type 2 Diabetes
- The Recommended Quantity and Quality of Exercise for Developing and Maintaining Cardiorespiratory and Muscular Fitness, and Flexibility in Healthy Adults
- Exercise and Physical Activity for Older Adults
- Recommendations for Cardiovascular Screening, Staffing, and Emergency Policies at Health/Fitness Facilities
- Diabetes Mellitus and Exercise
- The Female Athlete Triad
- Heat & Cold Illnesses During Distance Running
- Exercise and Fluid Replacement
- The Use of Blood Doping as an Ergogenic Aid
- Weight Loss in Wrestlers
- Osteoporosis and Exercise
- Exercise for Patients with Coronary Artery Disease
- Physical Activity, Physical Fitness, and Hypertension
- The Use of Anabolic-Androgenic Steroids in Sports
- Proper and Improper Weight-Loss Programs
- The Use of Alcohol in Sports
- Exercise & Hypertension
- Automated External Defibrillators in Health/Fitness Facilities
- Progression Models in Resistance Training for Healthy Adults
- Appropriate Intervention Strategies for Weight Loss and Prevention of Weight Regain for Adults

International Federation of Sports Medicine

Among the first major organizations was the Federation Internationale de Medecine Sportive (FIMS). It was created in 1928 at the Olympic Winter Games in St. Moritz, Switzerland, by Olympic medical doctors with the principal purpose of promoting the study and development of sports medicine throughout the world. FIMS is made up of the national sports medicine associations of more than 100 countries. This organization is multidisciplinary and includes many disciplines that are concerned with the physically active individual. To some degree the ACSM has patterned itself after this organization.

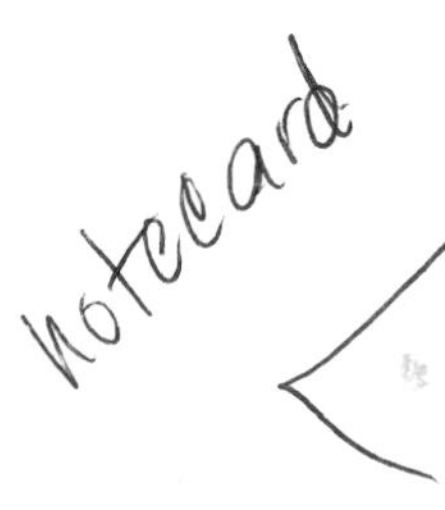

American Academy of Family Physicians

The American Academy of Family Physicians (AAFP) was founded in 1947 to promote and maintain high quality standards for family doctors who are providing continuing comprehensive health care to the public. AAFP is a medical association of more than 93,000 members. Many team physicians are members of this organization. It publishes the *American Family Physician*.

National Athletic Trainers' Association

Before the formation of the National Athletic Trainers' Association, Inc. in 1950, athletic trainers occupied a somewhat insecure place in the athletic program. Since that time, as a result of the raising of professional standards and the establishment of a code of ethics, there has been considerable professional advancement. The stated mission of NATA is:

> To enhance the quality of health care provided by certified athletic trainers and to advance the profession of athletic training.

The association accepts as members only those athletic trainers who are properly qualified and who are prepared to subscribe to a code of ethics and to uphold the standards of the association. NATA currently has more than 30,000 members. It publishes a quarterly journal, *The Journal of Athletic Training,* and holds an annual convention at which members have an opportunity to keep abreast of new developments and to exchange ideas through clinical programs. The organization is constantly working to improve both the quality and the status of athletic training.

American College of Sports Medicine

As discussed previously, the ACSM is interested in the study of all aspects of sports. Established in 1954, ACSM's membership of 18,000 is composed of medical doctors, doctors of philosophy, physical educators, athletic trainers, coaches, exercise physiologists, biomechanists, and others interested in sports. The organization holds national and regional conferences and meetings devoted to exploring the many aspects of sports medicine, and it publishes a quarterly magazine, *Medicine and Science in Sports and Exercise.* This journal includes articles in French, Italian, German, and English and provides complete translations in English of all articles. It reports recent developments in the field of sports medicine on a worldwide basis.

NOTECARDS

American Orthopaedic Society for Sports Medicine

The American Orthopaedic Society for Sports Medicine (AOSSM) was created in 1972 to encourage and support scientific research in orthopedic sports medicine; the organization works to develop methods for safer, more productive, and more enjoyable fitness programs and sports participation. Through programs developed by the AOSSM, members receive specialized training in sports medicine, surgical procedures, injury prevention, and rehabilitation. AOSSM's 1,200 members are orthopedic surgeons and allied health professionals committed to excellence in sports medicine. Its official bimonthly publication is the *American Journal of Sports Medicine.*

National Strength and Conditioning Association

The National Strength and Conditioning Association (NSCA) was formed in 1978 to facilitate a professional exchange of ideas in strength development as it relates to the improvement of athletic performance and fitness and to enhance, enlighten, and advance the field of strength and conditioning.

NSCA has a membership of more than 14,500 professionals, including strength and conditioning coaches, personal trainers, exercise physiologists, athletic trainers, researchers, educators, sport coaches, physical therapists, business owners, exercise instructors, fitness directors, and students training to enter the field. In addition, the NSCA Certification Commission offers two of the finest and the only nationally accredited certification programs: the Certified Strength and Conditioning Specialist (CSCS) and the NSCA Certified Personal Trainer (NSCA-CPT). NSCA publishes both the *Journal of Strength and Conditioning Research* and *Strength and Conditioning.*

American Academy of Pediatrics, Sports Committee

The American Academy of Pediatrics, Sports Committee, was organized in 1979. Its primary goal is to educate all physicians, especially pediatricians, about the special needs of children who participate in sports. Between 1979 and 1983, this committee developed guidelines that were incorporated into a report, *Sports Medicine: Health Care for Young Athletes,* edited by Nathan J. Smith, M.D.

American Physical Therapy Association, Sports Physical Therapy Section

In 1981, the Sports Physical Therapy Section of the American Physical Therapy Association (APTA) was officially established. The mission of the Sports Physical Therapy Section is "to provide a forum to establish collegial relations between physical therapists, physical therapist assistants, and physical therapy students interested in sports physical therapy." The Section and its 9,000 members promote the prevention, recognition, treatment, and rehabilitation of injuries in an athletic and physically active population; provide educational opportunities through sponsorship of continuing education programs and publications; promote the role of the sports physical therapist to other health professionals; and support research to further establish the scientific basis for sports physical therapy. The Section's official journal is the *Journal of Orthopaedic and Sports Physical Therapy.*

NCAA Committee on Competitive Safeguards and Medical Aspects of Sports

The National Collegiate Athletic Association (NCAA) Committee on Competitive Safeguards and Medical Aspects of Sports collects and develops pertinent information about desirable training methods, prevention and treatment of sports injuries, utilization of sound safety measures at the college level, drug education, and drug testing; disseminates information and adopts recommended policies and guidelines designed to further the objectives just listed; and supervises drug-education and drug-testing programs.

National Academy of Sports Medicine

The National Academy of Sports Medicine (NASM) was founded in 1987 by physicians, physical therapists, and fitness professionals and focuses on the development, refinement, and implementation of educational programs for fitness, performance, and sports medicine professionals. According to its mission statement "NASM is dedicated to transforming lives and revolutionizing the health and fitness industry through its unwavering commitment to deliver innovative education, solutions and tools that produce remarkable results." In addition to offering a fitness certification (Certified Personal Trainer) and performance certification (Performance Enhancement Specialist), NASM offers advanced credentials and more than twenty continuing education courses in a variety of disciplines. NATA currently has an agreement whereby NASM offers its Performance Enhancement Specialist and Integrated Flexibility Specialist certifications to NATA members. NASM serves more than 100,000 members and partners in eighty countries.

Other Health-Related Organizations

Many other health-related professions such as dentists, podiatrists, and chiropractors have, over the years, become interested in the health and safety aspects of sports. Besides national organizations that are interested in athletic health and safety, there are state and local associations that are extensions of the larger bodies. National, state, and local sports organizations have all provided extensive support to the reduction of illness and injury risk to the athlete.

Other Sports Medicine Journals

Athletic training must be considered a specialization under the broad field of sports medicine.

Other journals that provide an excellent service to the field of athletic training and sports medicine are *The International Journal of Sports Medicine,* which is published in English by Thieme-Stratton, Inc., New York; *The Journal of Sports Medicine and Physical Fitness,* published by Edizioni Minerva Medica SPA, ADIS Press Ltd., Auckland 10, New Zealand; the *Journal of Sport Rehabilitation and Athletic Therapy Today,* both published by Human Kinetics Publishers, Inc., Champaign, Illinois; the *Physician and Sportsmedicine,* published by McGraw-Hill, Inc., New York; *Physical Therapy* and *Clinical Management,* both published by the American Physical Therapy Association, Fairfax, Virginia; *Physi-*

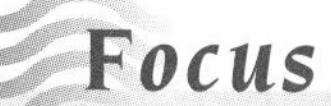

Sports medicine-related journals

Acta Orthopaedica Scandinavica
Adapted Physical Activity Quarterly
Advances in Orthopaedic Surgery
American Journal of Medicine and Sport
American Journal of Orthodontics and Dentofacial Orthopedics
American Journal of Sports Medicine
Archives of Orthopaedic and Trauma Surgery
Archives of Physical Medicine and Rehabilitation
Arthroscopy
Arthroskopie
Athletic Therapy Today
Baillière's Clinical Orthopaedics
Bone
British Journal of Sport Medicine
Canadian Journal of Applied Physiology
Clinical Exercise Physiology
Clinical Journal of Sports Medicine
Clinical Orthopaedics and Related Research
Clinics in Sports Medicine
Complications in Orthopedics
Current Opinion in Orthopedics
Current Orthopaedics
Exercise Immunology Review
European Journal of Orthopaedic Surgery and Traumatology
European Spine Journal
Foot and Ankle
Foot and Ankle Clinics
Hand Clinics
Hand Surgery
International Journal of Sports Medicine
International Journal of Sport Nutrition
International Orthopaedics
Internet Journal of Orthopedic Surgery and related subjects
Journal of Aging and Physical Activity
Journal of the American Academy of Orthopaedic Surgeons
Journal of Athletic Training
Journal of Applied Biomechanics
Journal of Arthroplasty
Journal of Back and Musculoskeletal Rehabilitation
The Journal of Bone and Joint Surgery
Journal of Hand Surgery (American)
Journal of Hand Surgery (British and European Volume)
Journal of Musculoskeletal Research
Journal of Orthopaedic Science
Journal of Orthopaedic Trauma
Journal of Orthopedic and Sports Physical Therapy
Journal of Pediatric Orthopaedics
Journal of Science and Medicine in Sport
Journal of Spinal Disorders
Journal of Sport Rehabilitation
Journal of Sports Chiropractic and Rehabilitation
Journal of Sports Medicine and Physical Fitness
Journal of Strength and Conditioning Research
The Knee
Medicine and Science in Sport and Exercise
Medscape Orthopedics and Sports Medicine
Neuro-Orthopedics
Operative Techniques in Orthopaedics
Operative Techniques in Sports Medicine
Orthopaedic Physical Therapy Clinics
Orthopedic Clinics
Orthopedics
Orthopedics Today
Orthopedic Surgery
Pediatric Exercise Science
Physical Therapy
Physical Therapy in Sport
Physical Medicine and Rehabilitation Clinics
Physician and Sports Medicine
Scandinavian Journal of Medicine and Science in Sports
Seminars in Musculoskeletal Radiology
Skeletal Radiology
Spine
Sports Medicine
Sports Medicine and Arthroscopy Review
Sports Medicine: Health Care for the Young Athlete
Strength and Conditioning
Techniques in Orthopaedics
Training and Conditioning

cal Medicine and Rehabilitation Clinics and *Clinics in Sports Medicine,* both published by W. B. Saunders, Philadelphia; and *Training and Conditioning,* published by MAG, Inc., Ithaca, New York.

There is a significant number of other journals that relate in some way to sports medicine. They are listed in *Focus Box:* "Sports medicine-related journals."

THE SPORTS MEDICINE TEAM

The primary individuals on the sports medicine team consist of the coach, the athletic trainer, and the team physician.

The provision of health care to the athlete requires a group effort to be most effective.[66] The sports medicine team involves a number of individuals, each of whom must perform specific functions relative to caring for the injured athlete.[11] Those people having the closest relationship with the injured athlete are the athletic trainer, the team physician, and the coach.

THE ATHLETIC TRAINER

Of all the professionals charged with injury prevention and health care provision for the athlete, perhaps none is more intimately involved than the athletic trainer.[66] The athletic trainer is the one individual who deals with the athlete throughout the period of rehabilitation, from the time of the initial injury until the athlete's complete, unrestricted return to practice or competition.[66] The athletic trainer is most directly responsible for all phases of health care in an athletic environment, including preventing injuries from occurring, providing initial first aid and injury management, evaluating injuries, and designing and supervising a timely and effective program of rehabilitation that can facilitate the safe and expeditious return of the athlete to activity.

The athletic trainer must be knowledgeable and competent in a variety of specialties encompassed under the umbrella of "sports medicine" if he or she is to be effective in preventing and treating injuries to the athlete.[19] The specific roles and responsibilities of the athletic trainer differ and to a certain extent are defined by the situation in which he or she works.[58]

Roles and Responsibilities of the Athletic Trainer

Board of Certification*

Six performance domains of the athletic trainer:

- Prevention of athletic injuries
- Clinical evaluation and diagnosis
- Immediate care
- Treatment, rehabilitation, and reconditioning
- Organization and administration
- Professional responsibility

Performance Domains In 2004 the Board of Certification (BOC) completed the latest role delineation study,** which defined the profession of athletic training.[10] This study was designed to examine the primary tasks performed by the entry-level athletic trainer and the knowledge and skills required to perform each task. The panel determined that the roles of the practicing athletic trainer could be divided into six major areas, or performance domains: (1) prevention of athletic injuries; (2) clinical evaluation and diagnosis; (3) immediate care of injuries; (4) treatment, rehabilitation, and reconditioning of athletic injuries; (5) organization and administration; and (6) professional responsibilities.

Education Council competencies and clinical proficiencies In 1997, the leadership of NATA established the Education Council to dictate the course of educational preparation for the student athletic trainer.[71] The focus of this Education Council has shifted to competency-based education at the entry level, and thus the Council has significantly expanded and reorganized the educational competencies and clinical proficiencies identified in the NATA's document, the 1999 Athletic Training Educational Competencies.[60] Whereas BOC defined the minimum knowledge base that an entry-level athletic trainer should possess to be able to work in the profession, the Education Council was charged with determining the competencies that should be taught in accredited educational programs.

The twelve domains established by the Education Council include (1) risk management, (2) pathology of injuries and illnesses, (3) orthopedic assessment and evaluation, (4) acute care of injury and illnesses, (5) pharmacology, (6) therapeutic modalities, (7) therapeutic exercise, (8) general medical conditions and disabilities, (9) nutritional aspects of injuries and illnesses, (10) psychosocial intervention and referral, (11) health care administration, and (12) professional development and responsibilities.

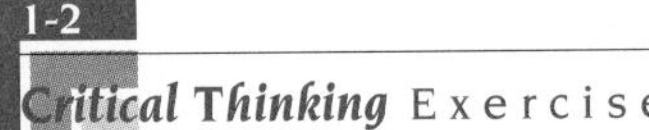

An athletic training student must develop a sound knowledge base in and demonstrate competent performance skills in six major domains: prevention of athletic injuries; clinical evaluation and diagnosis; immediate care of injuries; treatment, rehabilitation, and reconditioning of athletic injuries; health care administration; and professional development and responsibility.

? How can athletic training students best prepare themselves to be competent professional athletic trainers?

*The Board of Certification (BOC) has been responsible for the certification of athletic trainers since 1969. Upon its inception, the BOC was The Certification Committee for NATA, the profession's membership association. However, in 1989, the BOC became an independent nonprofit corporation. Formerly known as the NATABOC, the BOC officially changed its name in 2004.

**The 2004 Role Delineation study goes into effect in 2006.

Focus

Domains and competencies

Six performance domains established by the BOC*

- Prevention
- Clinical evaluation and diagnosis
- Immediate care
- Treatment, rehabilitation, and reconditioning
- Organization and administration
- Professional responsibility

Education competencies content areas established by the Education Council**

- Risk management
- Pathology of injuries and illnesses
- Orthopedic assessment and evaluation
- Acute care of injury and illnesses
- Pharmacology
- Therapeutic modalities
- Therapeutic exercise
- Medical conditions and disabilities
- Nutritional aspects of injuries and illnesses
- Psychosocial intervention and referral
- Health care administration
- Professional development and responsibilities

*Based on the 2004 Role Delineation Study[10]

**Based on the *Athletic training educational competencies,* ed 4. These will take effect in Fall 2006.

These competencies are required for both curriculum development and the education of students enrolled in entry-level athletic training education programs. As can be seen in *Focus Box:* "Domains and competencies," it is obvious that a great deal of overlap exists between the six performance domains identified by the BOC and the twelve competency domains established by the Education Council.[49]

Risk Management

Participation in competitive sports places the athlete in situations in which injuries are possible at any time. One major responsibility of the athletic trainer is to make the competitive environment as safe as possible to minimize the risk of injury. If injury can be prevented initially, there will be no need for first aid and subsequent rehabilitation.

The athletic trainer can minimize the risk of injury by (1) ensuring appropriate training and conditioning of the athlete; (2) monitoring environmental conditions to ensure safe participation; (3) selecting, properly fitting, and maintaining protective equipment; (4) making certain that the athlete is eating properly; and (5) making sure the athlete is using medications appropriately while discouraging substance abuse.

Developing training and conditioning programs Perhaps the most important aspect of injury prevention is making certain that the athlete is fit and thus able to handle the physiological and psychological demands of athletic competition. The athletic trainer works with the coaches to develop and implement an effective training and conditioning program for the athlete (see Chapter 4). It is essential that the athlete maintain a consistently high level of fitness during the preseason, the competitive season, and the off-season. This consistent level of fitness is critical not only for enhancing performance parameters but also for preventing injury and reinjury. An athletic trainer must be knowledgeable in the area of applied physiology of exercise, particularly with regard to strength training, flexibility, improvement of cardiorespiratory fitness, maintenance of body composition, weight control, and nutrition. Many colleges and most professional teams employ full-time strength coaches to oversee this aspect of the total program. The athletic trainer, however, must be acutely aware of any aspect of the program that may have a negative impact on an athlete or group of athletes and must offer constructive

1-3

***Critical Thinking* Exercise**

All American High School is considering hiring an athletic trainer instead of using an emergency medical technician. However, the administrators do not completely understand why an athletic trainer may be more beneficial for their athletes. A group of area athletic trainers will be holding a meeting to discuss the potential change.

? What reasons should the athletic trainers use to persuade the administrators to hire an athletic trainer?

suggestions for alternatives when appropriate. At the high-school level, the athletic trainer may be totally responsible for designing, implementing, and overseeing the fitness and conditioning program for the athletes.

Ensuring a safe playing environment To the best of his or her ability, the athletic trainer must ensure a safe environment for competition. This task may include duties not typically thought to belong to the athletic trainer, such as collecting trash, picking up rocks, or removing objects (e.g., hurdles, gymnastics equipment) from the perimeter of the practice area, all of which might pose potential danger to the athlete. The athletic trainer should call these potential safety hazards to the attention of an administrator. The interaction between the athletic trainer and a concerned and cooperative administrator can greatly enhance the effectiveness of the sports medicine team.

The athletic trainer should also be familiar with potential dangers associated with practicing or competing under inclement weather conditions, such as high heat and humidity, extreme cold, or electrical storms. Practice should be restricted, altered, or canceled if weather conditions threaten the health and safety of the athlete. If the team physician is not present, the athletic trainer must have the authority to curtail practice if the environmental conditions become severe (see Chapter 6).

Selecting, fitting, and maintaining protective equipment The athletic trainer works with coaches and equipment personnel to select protective equipment and is responsible for maintaining its condition and safety (see Chapter 7). Because liability lawsuits have become the rule rather than the exception, the athletic trainer must make certain that high-quality equipment is purchased and that it is constantly being worn, maintained, and reconditioned according to specific guidelines recommended by the manufacturers.

Protective equipment and devices can consume a significant portion of the athletic budget. The person responsible for purchasing protective equipment is usually inundated with marketing literature on a variety of braces, supports, pads, and other types of protective equipment. Decisions on purchasing specific pieces or brands should be based on research data that clearly document effectiveness in reducing or preventing injury (Figure 1-3).

Equipment is expensive, and schools are certainly subject to budgeting restrictions. However, purchasing decisions about protective equipment should always be made in the best interest of the athlete. Most colleges and professional teams hire full-time equipment managers to oversee this area of responsibility, but the athletic trainer must be knowledgeable about and aware of the equipment being worn by each athlete.

The design, building, and fitting of specific protective orthopedic devices are also responsibilities of the athletic trainer. Once the physician has indicated the problem and how it may be corrected, the athletic trainer should be able to construct an orthopedic device to correct it.

Explaining the importance of nutrition Good nutrition can have a substantial impact on health and well-being. Poor nutritional habits can certainly have a negative effect on an athlete's ability to perform at the highest level possible. Yet for all

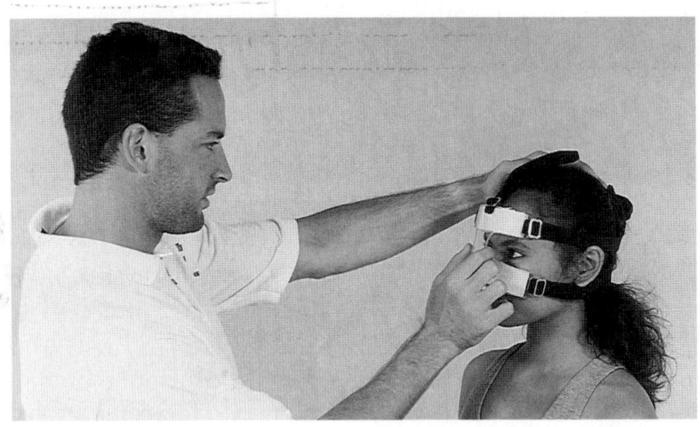

Figure 1-3

The athletic trainer should be responsible for taping and also for fitting of protective devices.

the attention that athletes, coaches, and athletic trainers direct at practicing sound nutritional habits, good nutritional decisions are still subjected to a tremendous amount of misunderstanding, misinformation, and occasionally, quackery. An athletic trainer is often asked for advice about matters related to diet, weight loss, and weight gain, and is occasionally asked about disordered eating. The athletic trainer does not need to be an expert on nutrition but must possess some understanding of the basic principles of nutrition.[79] (See Chapter 5.)

Using medications appropriately The athlete, like anyone else, may benefit greatly from using medications prescribed for various medical conditions by qualified physicians. Under normal circumstances an athlete would be expected to respond to medication just like anyone else would. However, because of the nature of physical activity, the athlete's situation is unique; intense physical activity requires that special consideration be given to the effects of certain types of medication.

For the athletic trainer who is overseeing the health care of the athlete, some knowledge of the potential effects of certain types of drugs on performance is essential. Occasionally, the athletic trainer must make decisions regarding the appropriate use of medications based on knowledge of the indications for use and of the possible side effects in athletes who are involved in training and conditioning as well as in injury rehabilitation programs. The athletic trainer must be cognizant of the potential effects and side effects of over-the-counter and prescription medications on the athlete during rehabilitation as well as during competition. (See Chapter 17.)

In addition, the athletic trainer should also be aware of the problems of substance abuse, both in ergogenic aids that may be used in an effort to enhance performance and in the abuse of so-called recreational or street drugs. The athletic trainer may be involved in drug testing of the athlete and should thus be responsible for educating the athlete in drug use and substance abuse.

Clinical Evaluation and Diagnosis

Frequently, the athletic trainer is the first person to see an athlete who has sustained an injury. The athletic trainer must be skilled in recognizing the nature and extent of an injury through competency in injury evaluation. Once the injury has been evaluated, the athletic trainer must be able to provide the appropriate first aid and then refer the athlete to appropriate medical personnel.

Conducting physical examinations The athletic trainer, in cooperation with the team physician, should obtain a medical history and conduct physical examinations of the athletes before participation as a means of screening for existing or potential problems (see Chapter 2). The medical history should be reviewed closely, and clarification should be sought for any point of concern.

The preparticipation examination should include measurement of height, weight, blood pressure, and body composition. The physician examination should concentrate on cardiovascular, respiratory, abdominal, genital, dermatological, and ear, nose, and throat systems and may include blood work and urinalysis. A brief orthopedic evaluation would include range of motion, muscle strength, and functional tests to assess joint stability. When the athletic trainer knows at the beginning of a season that an athlete has a physical problem that may predispose that athlete to an injury during the course of the season, he or she may immediately implement corrective measures that may significantly reduce the possibility of additional injury.

The athletic trainer must be able to efficiently and accurately evaluate an injury. Information obtained in this initial evaluation may be critical later on when swelling, pain, and guarding mask some of the functional signs of the injury.

It is essential that the athletic trainer be alert and observe, as much as possible, everything that goes on in practice. Invaluable information regarding the nature of an injury can be obtained by seeing the mechanism of the injury.

The subsequent off-the-field examination should include (1) obtaining a brief medical history of exactly what happened, according to the athlete, (2) observation, (3) palpation, (4) special tests that might include range of motion, muscle strength, joint stability, or a brief neurological examination. Information obtained in this initial examination should be documented by the athletic trainer and given to the physician once the athlete is referred. The team physician is ultimately responsible for providing an accurate diagnosis of an injury. The initial evaluation often provides the basis for this diagnosis (see Chapter 13).

Understanding the pathology of injury and illness The athletic trainer must be able to recognize the various types of musculoskeletal and nervous system injuries that can occur in the physically active population. Based on this knowledge of different injuries, the athletic trainer must possess some understanding of both the sequence and time frames for the various phases of healing, realizing that certain physiological events must occur during each of the phases (see Chapter 10). Anything done during training and conditioning or during a rehabilitation program that interferes with this healing process will likely delay a return to full activity. The healing process must have an opportunity to accomplish what it is supposed to. At best the athletic trainer can only try to create an environment that is conducive to the healing process. Little can be done to speed up the process physiologically, but many things may be done both during training and conditioning and during rehabilitation to impede healing.

Referring to medical care After the initial management of an injury, the athletic trainer should routinely refer the athlete to a physician for further evaluation and accurate diagnosis. If an athlete requires treatment from medical personnel other than the team physician, such as a dentist or ophthalmologist, the athletic trainer should arrange appointments as necessary. Referrals should be made after consultation with the team physician.

Referring to support services If needed, the athletic trainer must be familiar with and should have access to a variety of personal, school, and community health service agencies, including community-based psychological and social support services available to the athlete. With assistance and direction from these agencies, the athletic trainer together with the athlete should be able to formulate a plan for appropriate intervention following injury.

Immediate Care of Injury and Illness

The athletic trainer is often responsible for the initial on-the-field injury assessment following acute injury. Once this initial assessment is done, the athletic trainer then must assume responsibility for administering appropriate first aid to the injured athlete and for making correct decisions in the management of acute injury (see Chapter 12). Although the team physician is frequently present at games or competitions, in most cases he or she cannot be at every practice session, where injuries are more likely to occur. Thus the athletic trainer must possess sound skills not only in the initial recognition and evaluation of potentially serious or life-threatening injuries but also in emergency care.

The athletic trainer should be certified in cardiopulmonary resuscitation by the American Red Cross, the American Heart Association, or the National Safety Council. Athletic trainers should also be certified in first aid by the American Red Cross or the National Safety Council. Many athletic trainers have gone beyond these essential basic certifications and have completed emergency medical technician (EMT) requirements.

Emergency care procedures should be established by the athletic trainer in cooperation with local rescue squads and the community hospitals that can provide emergency treatment. Emergency care is expedited and the injured athlete's frustration and concern are lessened if arrangements regarding transportation, logistics, billing procedures, and appropriate contacts are made before an injury occurs.

Treatment, Rehabilitation, and Reconditioning

An athletic trainer must work closely with and under the supervision of the team physician with respect to designing rehabilitation and reconditioning protocols that

1-4 *Critical Thinking* Exercise

A basketball player suffers a grade 2 ankle sprain during midseason of the competitive schedule. After a three-week course of rehabilitation, most of the pain and swelling have been eliminated. The athlete is anxious to get back into practice and competitive games as soon as possible, and subsequent injuries to other players have put pressure on the coach to force the athlete's return. Unfortunately the athlete is still unable to perform functional tasks (cutting and jumping) essential in basketball.

? Who is responsible for making the decision regarding when the athlete can fully return to practice and game situations?

make use of appropriate therapeutic exercise, rehabilitative equipment, manual therapy techniques, or therapeutic modalities. The athletic trainer should then assume the responsibility of overseeing the rehabilitative process, ultimately returning the athlete to full activity (see Chapter 16).

Designing rehabilitation programs Once the team physician has evaluated and diagnosed an injury, the rehabilitation process begins immediately. In most cases, the athletic trainer will design and supervise an injury rehabilitation program, modifying that program based on the healing process. It is critical for an athletic trainer to have a sound background in anatomy. Without this background, an athletic trainer cannot evaluate an injury. And if the athletic trainer cannot evaluate an injury, there is no point in the athletic trainer knowing anything about rehabilitation because he or she will not know at what phase the injury is in the healing process. The athletic trainer must also understand how to incorporate therapeutic modalities and appropriate therapeutic exercise techniques if the rehabilitation program is to be successful.

Supervising rehabilitation programs The athletic trainer is charged with the responsibility of designing, implementing, and supervising the rehabilitation program for the athlete from the time of initial injury until the athlete returns to full activity. It is essential that the athletic trainer has a solid foundation in the various techniques of therapeutic exercise and an understanding of how those techniques can be most effectively incorporated into the rehabilitation program. The athletic trainer must establish both short-term and long-terms goals for the rehabilitation process and then be able to alter and modify the program to most effectively meet those goals.

Incorporating therapeutic modalities Athletic trainers use a wide variety of therapeutic modalities in the treatment and rehabilitation of sport-related injuries. Modality use may involve a relatively simple technique such as using an ice pack as a first-aid treatment for an acute injury or may involve more complex techniques such as the stimulation of nerve and muscle tissue by electrical currents. Certainly, therapeutic modalities are useful tools in injury rehabilitation, and when used appropriately, these modalities can greatly enhance the athlete's chances for a safe and rapid return to athletic competition. It is essential for the athletic trainer to possess knowledge about the scientific basis and the physiologic effects of the various modalities on a specific injury (see Chapter 15). Modalities, though important, are by no means the single most critical factor in injury treatment. Therapeutic exercise that forces the injured anatomic structure to perform its normal function is the key to successful rehabilitation. However, therapeutic modalities play an important role in reducing pain and are extremely useful as an adjunct to therapeutic exercise.

Offering psychosocial intervention The psychological aspect of how the individual athlete deals with an injury is a critical yet often neglected aspect of the rehabilitation process. Injury and illness produce a wide range of emotional reactions. Therefore the athletic trainer needs to develop an understanding of the psyche of each athlete (see Chapter 11). Athletes vary in terms of pain threshold, cooperation and compliance, competitiveness, denial of disability, depression, intrinsic and extrinsic motivation, anger, fear, guilt, and the ability to adjust to injury. Principles of sport psychology may be used to improve total athletic performance through visualization, self-hypnosis, and relaxation techniques. The athletic trainer plays a critical role in social support for the injured athlete.[6]

Organization and Administration

The athletic trainer is responsible for the organization and administration of the training room facility, including the maintenance of health and injury records for each athlete, requisition and inventory of necessary supplies and equipment, the supervision of assistant or student trainers, and the establishment of policies and procedures for day-to-day operation of the athletic training program (see Chapter 2).[82]

Record keeping Accurate and detailed record keeping—including medical histories, preparticipation examinations, injury reports, treatment records, and rehabilitation programs—are critical for the athletic trainer, particularly in light of the number of lawsuits directed toward malpractice in health care. Although record keeping may be difficult and time consuming for the athletic trainer who treats and deals with a large number of patients each day, it is an area that simply cannot be neglected.

Ordering equipment and supplies Although tremendous variations in operating budgets exist, depending on the level and the institution, decisions regarding how available money may best be spent are always critical. The athletic trainer must keep on hand a wide range of supplies to enable him or her to handle whatever situation may arise. At institutions in which severe budgetary restrictions exist, prioritization based on experience and past needs must become the mode of operation. A creative athletic trainer can make do with very little equipment, which should include at least a taping and treatment table, an ice machine, and a few free weights. Like in other professions, the more tools available for use, the more effective the practitioner can be, as long as there is an understanding of how those tools are used most effectively.

Supervising personnel In an athletic training environment, the quality and efficiency of the assistants and athletic training students in carrying out their specific responsibilities is absolutely essential.[17] The person who supervises these assistants has a responsibility to design a reasonable work schedule that is consistent with other commitments and responsibilities they have outside the training room. It is the responsibility of the head athletic trainer to provide an environment in which assistants and athletic training students can continually learn and develop professionally.[3] The supervision of athletic training students necessitates constant visual and auditory interaction and the ability to physically intervene on behalf of the athlete or student.

Establishing policies for the operation of an athletic training program Although the athletic trainer must be able to easily adjust and adapt to a given situation, it is essential that specific policies, procedures, rules, and regulations be established to ensure smooth and consistent day-to-day operation of the athletic training program. A plan should be established for emergency management of injury. Appropriate channels for referral after injury and emergency treatment should be used consistently.

Policies and procedures must be established and implemented that reduce the likelihood of exposure to infectious agents by following universal precautions, which can prevent the transmission of infectious diseases (see Chapter 2).

Professional Responsibilities

The athletic trainer should assume personal responsibility for continuously expanding his or her own knowledge base and expertise within the chosen field. This professional development may be accomplished by attending continuing education programs offered at state, district, and national meetings. Athletic trainers must also routinely review professional journals and consult current textbooks to stay abreast of the most up-to-date techniques. The athletic trainer should also make an effort to be involved professionally with national, regional, or state organizations that are committed to enhancing continued growth and development of the profession.

The athletic trainer as an educator The athletic trainer must take time to help educate athletic training students. The continued success of any profession lies in its ability to educate its students. Education should not simply be a responsibility, it should be a priority.

To be an effective educator, the athletic trainer needs an understanding of the basic principles of learning and methods of classroom instruction. The athletic trainer should seek and develop competence in presenting information to students through the use of a variety of instructional techniques.[33] The athletic training educator should also make an effort to stay informed about the availability of relevant audiovisual aids, multimedia, newsletters, journals, workshops, and seminars that can enhance the breadth of the students' educational experience.[81] The athletic trainer must also be able to evaluate student knowledge and competencies through the development and construction of appropriate tests.[3] The athletic training educator should also assume

1-5

***Critical Thinking* Exercise**

A young athletic trainer has taken his first job at All-American High School. The school administrators are extremely concerned about the number of athletes who get hurt playing various sports. They have charged the athletic trainer with the task of developing an athletic training program that can effectively help prevent the occurrence of injury to athletes in all sports at that school.

? What actions can the athletic trainer take to reduce the number of injuries and to minimize the risk of injury in the competitive athletes at that high school?

some responsibility for helping the students secure a professional position following graduation. Guiding the athletic training student in constructing an appropriate resume will help in this effort (see Appendix G).

Students of athletic training must be given a sound academic background in a curriculum that stresses the competencies that are outlined in this chapter and presented in detail throughout this text. They must be able to translate the theoretical base presented in the classroom into practical application in a clinical setting if they are to be effective in treating patients.[17] The athletic training educator accomplishes this application by organizing appropriate laboratory and/or clinical experiences to evaluate the students' clinical competencies.[18] Certainly the clinical instructor can have a significant impact on the development of the athletic training student.[42]

Promoting the Profession The athletic trainer must also educate the general public, in addition to a large segment of the various allied medical health care professions, as to exactly what athletic trainers are and the scope of their roles and responsibilities. This education is perhaps best accomplished by organizing workshops and clinics in athletic training, holding professional seminars, meeting with local and community organizations, publishing research in scholarly journals, and most important, doing a good and professional job of providing health care to the injured athlete.

The athletic trainer as a counselor The athletic trainer should take responsibility for informing parents and coaches about the nature of a specific injury and how it may affect the ability of the athlete to compete. The athletic trainer should be concerned primarily with counseling and advising the athlete not only with regard to prevention, rehabilitation, and treatment of specific injuries but also on any matter that might be of help to the athlete.[49,50] Perhaps one of the most rewarding aspects of working as an athletic trainer can be found in the relationships that the trainer develops with individual athletes.

During the period of time that athletes are competing, the athletic trainer has the opportunity to get to know them very well on a personal basis because he or she spends a considerable amount of time with them. Athletes often develop a degree of respect and trust in the athletic trainer's judgment that carries over from their athletic life into their personal life. It is not uncommon for an athletic trainer to be asked questions about a number of personal matters, at which point he or she crosses a bridge from athletic trainer to friend and confidant. This considerable responsibility is perhaps best handled by first listening to the problems, presenting several options, and then letting the athlete make his or her own decision. Certainly, the role of counselor and advisor cannot be taken lightly.[69,70]

The athletic trainer as a researcher As the athletic training profession continues to gain credibility as an allied health care profession, it is essential that athletic trainers work to enhance their visibility and credibility by engaging in research and scholarly publication.[75] Certainly not everyone who works as an athletic trainer, in every employment setting, would be expected to engage in research as part of their job responsibilities. Most often, the research that is published in professional journals is conducted by individuals who are program directors, faculty members, or doctoral students employed in colleges and universities.[72] These individuals along with graduate students seeking masters degrees at most NATA-approved graduate athletic training education programs, are required to conduct research either as part of their job description or as a requirement for attaining their degree. It is likely that as the numbers of educators, academicians, and graduate students continue to increase there will be more and more scholarly papers being submitted for publication in professional journals.[76] Regardless of whether an individual possesses the inclination or the ability to conduct research, each certified athletic trainer must at the very least take responsibility for developing some comprehension of basic research design and statistical analysis and thus be able to interpret and evaluate new research. The athletic training profession cannot continue to move forward unless its members generate its own specific body of knowledge.[64]

An athletic trainer's personal qualities:

- Stamina and ability to adapt
- Empathy
- Sense of humor
- Ability to communicate
- Intellectual curiosity
- Ethics

As a member of a helping profession, the athletic trainer is subject to burnout.

informed about their injuries and taught how to listen to what their bodies are telling them to prevent reinjury.

The Athletic Trainer and the Athlete's Parents

In the secondary school setting, the athletic trainer, must also take the time to explain to and inform the parents about injury management and prevention.[28] With an athlete of secondary school age, the parents' decisions regarding health are must be of primary consideration.

In certain situations, particularly at the high school and junior high levels, many parents will insist that their child be seen by their family physician rather than by the individual who may be designated as the team physician. It is also likely that the choice of a physician that the athlete can see will be dictated by the parents' insurance plan (IC, HMO, PPO). This creates a situation in which the athletic trainer must work and communicate with many different "team physicians." The opinion of the family physician must be respected even if the individual has little or no experience with injuries related to sports.

The coach, athletic trainer, and team physician should make certain that the athlete and his or her family are familiar with the Health Insurance Portability and Accountability Act (HIPAA), which regulates how individuals who have health information about an athlete can share that information with others and not be in violation of the privacy rule.[36,37] HIPAA was created to protect a patient's privacy and limit the number of people who could gain access to the athlete's medical records. HIPAA regulations will be discussed in more detail in Chapter 2.

RESPONSIBILITIES OF THE TEAM PHYSICIAN

In most situations, the athletic trainer works primarily under the supervision of the team physician, who is ultimately responsible for directing the total health care of the athlete (Figure 1-4). In cooperation with the team physician, the athletic trainer must make decisions that ultimately have a direct effect on the athlete who has sustained an injury.

From the viewpoint of the athletic trainer, there are a number of roles and responsibilities that the team physician should assume with regard to injury prevention and the health care of the athlete.[45,68] (See *Focus Box:* "Duties of the team physician.")

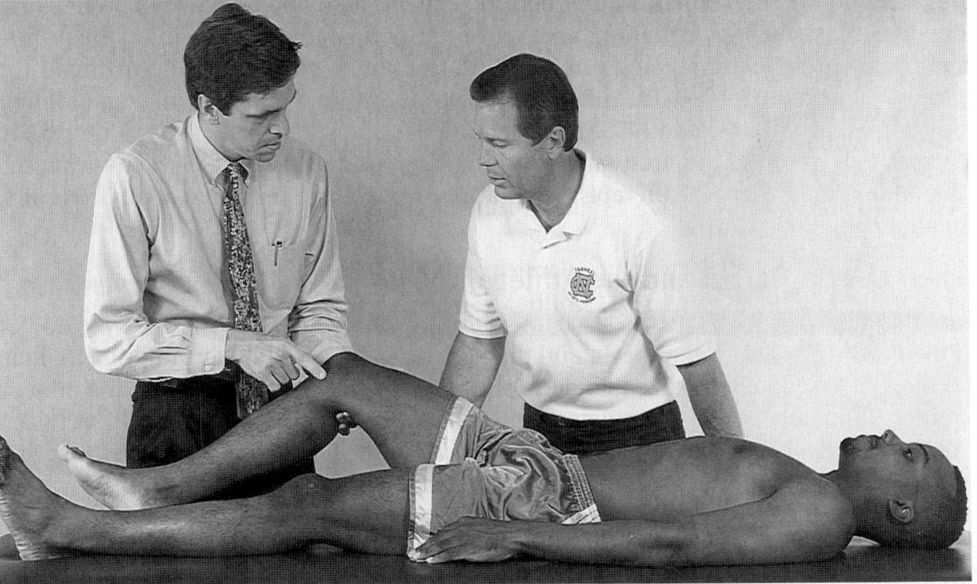

Figure 1-4

In training the athlete, the athletic trainer carries out the directions of the physician.

The Physician and the Athletic Trainer

The physician should be a supervisor and an advisor to the athletic trainer. However, the athletic trainer must be given flexibility to function independently in the decision-making process and must often act without the advice or direction of the physician. Therefore it is critical that the team physician and the athletic trainer share philosophical opinions regarding injury management and rehabilitation programs; this cohesion will help minimize any discrepancies or inconsistencies that may exist. Most athletic trainers would prefer to work with rather than for a team physician.

Compiling Medical Histories

The team physician should be responsible for compiling medical histories and conducting physical examinations for each athlete, both of which can provide critical information that may reduce the possibility of injury. Preparticipation screening done by both the athletic trainer and the physician are important in establishing baseline information to be used for comparison should injury occur during the season.

Diagnosing Injury

The team physician should assume responsibility for diagnosing an injury and should be keenly aware of the program of rehabilitation as designed by the athletic trainer after the diagnosis. Athletic trainers should be capable of doing an accurate initial evaluation after acute injury. Input from that evaluation may be essential to the physician, who may not see the patient for several hours or perhaps days after the injury. However, the physician has been trained specifically to diagnose injuries and to make recommendations to the athletic trainer for treatment based on that diagnosis. The athletic trainer, with a sound background in injury rehabilitation, designs and supervises an effective rehabilitation scheme. The closely related yet distinct roles of the physician and the athletic trainer require both cooperation and close communication if they are to be optimized.

Team physicians must have absolute authority in determining the health status of an athlete who wishes to participate in the sports program.

Deciding on Disqualification and Return to Play

The physician determines when a recommendation should be made that an athlete be disqualified from competition on medical grounds and must have the final say as to

Focus

Duties of the team physician

- Seeing that a complete medical history of each athlete is compiled and is readily available
- Determining through a physical examination the athlete's health status
- Diagnosing and treating injuries and other illnesses
- Directing and advising the athletic trainer about health matters
- Acting, when necessary, as an instructor to the athletic trainer, assistant athletic trainer, and student athletic trainers about special therapeutic methods, therapeutic problems, and related procedures
- If possible, attending all games, athletic contests, scrimmages, and practices
- Deciding when, on medical grounds, athletes should be disqualified from participation and when they may be permitted to reenter competition
- Serving as an advisor to the athletic trainer and the coach and, when necessary, as a counselor to the athlete
- Working closely with the school administrator, school dentist, athletic trainer, coach, and health services personnel to promote and maintain consistently high standards of care for the athlete

when an injured athlete may return to activity.[35] Any decision to allow an athlete to resume activity should be based on recommendations from the athletic trainer. An athletic trainer often has an advantage in that he or she knows the injured athlete well, including how the athlete responds to injury, how the athlete moves, and how hard to push to return the athlete safely to activity. The physician's judgment must be based not only on medical knowledge but also on knowledge of the psychophysiological demands of a particular sport.[74]

Attending Practices and Games

A team physician should make an effort to attend as many practices, scrimmages, and competitions as possible. This attendance obviously becomes difficult at an institution that has twenty or more athletic teams. Thus the physician must be readily available should the athletic trainer (who generally is at most practices and games) require consultation or advice.

If the team physician cannot attend all practice sessions and competitive events or games, it is sometimes possible to establish a plan of rotation involving a number of physicians. In this plan, any one physician needs to be present at only one or two activities a year. The rotation plan has proved practical in situations in which the school district is unable to afford a full-time physician or has so limited a budget that it must ask for volunteer medical coverage. In some instances, the attending physician is paid a per-game stipend.

Commitment to Sports and the Athlete

Most important, the team physician must have a strong love of sports and must be generally interested in and concerned about the young people who compete. Colleges and universities typically employ someone to act as a full-time team physician. High schools most often rely on a local physician who volunteers his or her time. To serve as a team physician for the purpose of enhancing social standing in the community can be a frustrating and potentially dangerous situation for everyone involved in the athletic program.

When a physician is asked to serve as a team physician, arrangements must be made with the employing educational institution about specific required responsibilities. Policies must be established regarding emergency care, legal liability, facilities, personnel relationships, and duties.[23] It is essential that the team physician at all times promotes and maintains consistently high-quality care for the athlete in all phases of the sports medicine program.

Academic Program Medical Director

Accredited athletic training education programs must have a physician medical director who is responsible for the coordination and guidance of the medial aspects of the program. The medical director—who may or may not be the team physician—should provide input to the program's educational content and provide classroom, laboratory, and/or clinical instruction.

RESPONSIBILITIES OF THE COACH

It is critical for the coach to understand the specific roles and responsibilities of each individual who could potentially be involved in the sports medicine team. This becomes even more critical if there is no athletic trainer to oversee the health care and the coach is forced to assume this responsibility. Individual states differ significantly in the laws that govern what nonmedical personnel can and cannot do when providing health care. **It is the responsibility of coaches to clearly understand the limits of their ability to function as health care provider in the state where they are employed.**

All head and assistant coaches should be certified in CPR and first aid.

The coach is directly responsible for preventing injuries by seeing that athletes have undergone a preventive injury conditioning program. The coach must ensure that sports equipment, especially protective equipment, is of the highest quality and is

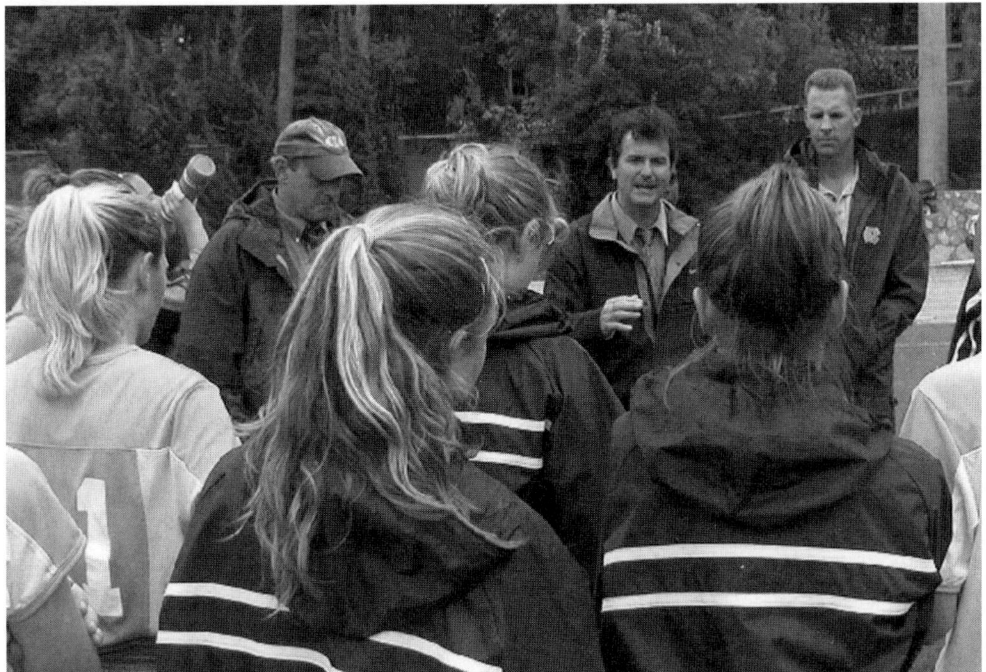

Figure 1-5

The coach is directly responsible for preventing injuries in his or her sport.

properly fitted. The coach must also make sure that protective equipment is properly maintained.[66] A coach must be keenly aware of what produces injuries in his or her particular sport and what measures must be taken to avoid them (Figure 1-5). When necessary, a coach should be able to apply proper first aid. This knowledge is especially important in serious head and spinal injuries. **All coaches (both head and assistants) should be certified in cardiopulmonary resuscitation** (CPR) by either the American Red Cross, the American Heart Association, or the National Safety Council. **Coaches should also be certified in first aid** by the American Red Cross or the National Safety Council.[64] For the coach, obtaining these certifications is important so that he or she is able to provide correct and appropriate health care for the injured athlete. But it is also true that not having these certifications can potentially have some negative legal implications for the coach and his or her employer.

It is essential that a coach have a thorough understanding of the skill techniques and environmental factors that may adversely affect the athlete. Poor biomechanics in skill areas such as throwing and running can lead to overuse injuries of the arms and legs, whereas overexposure to heat and humidity may cause death. Just because a coach is experienced in coaching does not mean that he or she knows proper skill techniques. Coaches must engage in a continual process of education to further their knowledge in their particular sport. When a sports program or specific sport is without an athletic trainer, the coach very often takes over this role.

Coaches work closely with athletic trainers; therefore both must develop an awareness of and an insight into each other's problems so that they can function effectively. The athletic trainer must develop patience and must earn the respect of the coaches so that his or her judgment in all medical matters is fully accepted. In turn, the athletic trainer must avoid questioning the abilities of the coaches in their particular fields and must restrict opinions to athletic training matters. To avoid frustration and hard feelings, the coach must coach, and the athletic trainer must conduct athletic training matters. In terms of the health and well-being of the athlete, the physician and the athletic trainer have the last word. This position must be backed at all times by the athletic director.

This is not to say, however, that the coach should not be involved with the decision-making process. For example, during the time the athlete is rehabilitating an injury, there may be drills or technical instruction sessions that the athlete can participate in that will not exacerbate the existing problem. Thus the coach, the athletic trainer, and the team physician should be able to negotiate what the athlete can and cannot do safely in the course of a practice.

Any personal relationship takes some time to grow and develop. The relationship between the coach and the athletic trainer is no different. The athletic trainer must demonstrate to the coach his or her capability to correctly manage an injury and guide the course of a rehabilitation program. It will take some time for the coach to develop trust and confidence in the athletic trainer. The coach must understand that what the athletic trainer wants for the athlete is exactly the same as what the coach wants—to get an athlete healthy and back to practice as quickly and safely as possible.

REFERRING THE ATHLETE TO OTHER MEDICAL AND NONMEDICAL SUPPORT SERVICES AND PERSONNEL

In certain situations, an athlete may require treatment from or consultation with a variety of both medical and nonmedical services or personnel other than the athletic trainer or team physician. After the athletic trainer consults with the team physician about a particular matter, either the athletic trainer or the team physician can arrange for appointments as necessary. When referring an athlete for evaluation or consultation, the athletic trainer must be aware of the community-based services available and the insurance or managed care plan coverage available for that athlete.

Support personnel concerned with the athlete's health and safety:

- Nurse
- School health services
- Physicians
- Dentist
- Podiatrist
- Physician's assistant
- Biomechanist
- Strength and conditioning coach
- Sport psychologist
- Physical therapist
- Exercise physiologist
- Nutritionist
- Massage Therapist
- Social worker
- Emergency Medical Specialist
- Sports Chiropractors
- Orthotist/Prosthetist
- Equipment Personnel
- Referees

A number of support health services and personnel may be used by a sports program. These services and personnel may include school health services; nurses; physicians including orthopedists, neurologists, internists, family medicine specialists, ophthalmologists, pediatricians, psychiatrists, dermatologists, gynecologists, and osteopaths; dentists; podiatrists; physician's assistants; physical therapists; strength and conditioning specialists; biomechanists; exercise physiologists; nutritionists; sports psychologists; massage therapists; social workers; emergency medical specialists; sports chiropractors; orthotists/prosthetists; equipment personnel; or referees.

School Health Services

Colleges and universities maintain school health services that range from a department operating with one or two nurses and a physician available on a part-time basis to an elaborate setup comprised of a full complement of nursing services with a staff of full-time medical specialists and complete laboratory and hospital facilities. At the secondary-school level, health services are usually organized so that one or two nurses conduct the program under the direction of the school physician, who may serve a number of schools in a given area or district. This organization poses a problem, because it is often difficult to have qualified medical help at hand when it is needed. Local policy determines the procedure for referral for medical care. If such policies are lacking, the athletic trainer should see to it that an effective method is established for handling all athletes requiring medical care or opinion. The ultimate source of health care is the physician. The effectiveness of athletic health care service can be evaluated only to the extent to which it meets the following criteria:

1. Availability at every scheduled practice or contest of a person qualified and delegated to render emergency care to an injured or ill participant
2. Planned access to a physician by phone or nearby presence for prompt medical evaluation of the health care problems that warrant this attention
3. Planned access to a medical facility, including plans for communication and transportation

The Nurse

As a rule, the nurse is not usually responsible for the recognition and management of sports injuries. However, in certain institutions that lack an athletic trainer, the nurse

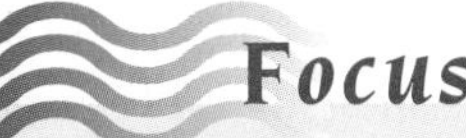

Specializations for physicians

Orthopedist The orthopedist is responsible for treating injuries and disorders of the musculoskeletal system. Many colleges and universities have a team orthopedist on their staff.

Neurologist A neurologist specializes in treating disorders of and injuries to the nervous system. There are common situations in athletics in which consultation with a neurologist would be warranted, such as for head injury or peripheral nerve injury.

Internist An internist is a physician who specializes in the practice of internal medicine. An internist treats diseases of the internal organs by using measures other than surgery.

Family Medicine Physician A physician who specializes in family medicine supervises or provides medical care to all members of a family. Many team physicians in colleges and universities and particularly at the high-school level are engaged in family practice.

Ophthalmologist Physicians who manage and treat injuries to the eye are ophthalmologists. An optometrist evaluates and fits patients with glasses or contact lenses.

Pediatrician A pediatrician cares for or treats injuries and illnesses that occur in young children and adolescents.

Psychiatrist Psychiatry is a medical practice that deals with the diagnosis, treatment, and prevention of mental illness.

Dermatologist A dermatologist should be consulted for problems and lesions occurring on the skin.

Gynecologist A gynecologist is consulted in cases where health issues in the female athlete are of primary concern.

Osteopath An osteopath is a trained medical doctor who uses manual therapy and manipulation of joints extensively in their practice.

may assume the majority of the responsibility in providing health care for the athlete. The nurse works under the direction of the physician and in liaison with the athletic trainer and the school health services.

Physicians

A number of physicians with a variety of specializations can aid the sports medicine team in treating the athlete (see *Focus Box:* "Specializations for physicians").

Dentist

The role of team dentist is somewhat analogous to that of team physician. He or she serves as a dental consultant for the team and should be available for first aid and emergency care. Good communication between the dentist and the athletic trainer should ensure a good dental program. There are three areas of responsibility for the team dentist:

1. Organizing and performing the preseason dental examination
2. Being available to provide emergency care when needed
3. Conducting the fitting of mouth protectors

Podiatrist

Podiatry, the specialized field dealing with the study and care of the foot, has become an integral part of sports health care. Many podiatrists are trained in surgical procedures, foot biomechanics, and the fitting and construction of orthotic devices for the shoe. Like the team dentist, a podiatrist should be available on a consulting basis.

Physician's Assistant

Physician's assistants (PAs) are trained to assume some of the responsibilities for patient care traditionally done by a physician. They assist the physician by conducting preliminary patient evaluations, arranging for various hospital-based diagnostic tests, and dispensing appropriate medications. A number of athletic trainers have also become PAs in recent years.

Physical Therapist

Some athletic trainers use physical therapists to supervise the rehabilitation programs for injured athletes while the athletic trainer concentrates primarily on getting a player ready to practice or compete. In many sports medicine clinics, athletic trainers and physical therapists work in teams, jointly contributing to the supervision of a rehabilitation program. A number of athletic trainers are also physical therapists. A physical therapist can be certified as a Sports Certified Specialist (SCS). The physical therapist is prepared to treat a variety of different patient populations with different types of injuries, while the athletic trainer is focused primarily on treating and working with the physically active population.

Strength and Conditioning Specialist

Many colleges and universities and some high schools employ full-time strength coaches to advise athletes on training and conditioning programs. Athletic trainers should routinely consult with these individuals and advise them about injuries to a particular athlete and exercises that should be avoided or modified relative to a specific injury. A strength coach can be certified by the National Strength and Conditioning Association as a CSCS.

Biomechanist

An individual who possesses some expertise in the analysis of human motion can also be a great aid to the athletic trainer. The biomechanist uses sophisticated video and computer-enhanced digital analysis equipment to study movement. By advising the athlete, coach, and athletic trainer on matters such as faulty gait patterns or improper throwing mechanics, the biomechanist can reduce the likelihood of injury to the athlete.

Exercise Physiologist

The exercise physiologist can significantly influence the athletic training program by giving input to the trainer regarding training and conditioning techniques, body composition analysis, and nutritional considerations.

Nutritionist

Increasingly, individuals in the field of nutrition are becoming interested in athletics. Some large athletic training programs engage a nutritionist as a consultant who plans eating programs that are geared to the needs of a particular sport. He or she also assists individual athletes who need special nutritional counseling.

Sports Psychologist

The sports psychologist can advise the athletic trainer on matters related to the psychological aspects of the rehabilitation process. The way the athlete feels about the injury and how it affects his or her social, emotional, intellectual, and physical dimensions can have a substantial effect on the course of a treatment program and how quickly the athlete may return to competition. The sports psychologist uses different intervention strategies to help the athlete cope with injury. Sport psychologists can seek certification through the Association for the Advancement of Sport Psychology.

Massage Therapist

A qualified sports massage therapist should have training and experience in all areas of sports massage. The American Massage Therapy Association National Sports Massage

Team (NSMT) consists of massage therapists who have passed rigorous written and practical examinations in event sports massage. Team members are qualified to apply their specialized knowledge and skills in the precompetition and post-competition stages of athletic events. Members of the AMTA NSMT are trained to perform the highest level of sports massage therapy techniques while working cooperatively with other health care professionals.

Social Worker

Occasionally, athletes or their families may need a referral for social support services within the community. Social workers can offer counseling and support for a variety of personal or family difficulties, such as substance abuse, family planning, and other social concerns.

Emergency Medical Specialist (EMS)

These individuals are indispensable in providing transport to the injured athlete to a medical care facility.

Sports Chiropractors

Chiropractors make use of spinal extremity manipulation techniques to treat most musculoskeletal conditions.

Orthotist/Prosthetist

These individuals custom fit, design and construct braces, orthotics and support devices based on physician prescriptions.

Equipment Personnel

Sports equipment personnel are becoming specialists in the purchase and proper fitting of protective equipment. They work closely with the coach and the athletic trainer.

Referees

Referees must be highly knowledgeable regarding rules and regulations, especially those that relate to the health and welfare of the athlete. They work cooperatively with the coach and the athletic trainer. They must be capable of checking the playing facility for dangerous situations and equipment that may predispose the athlete to injury. They must routinely check athletes to ensure that they are wearing adequate protective pads.

EMPLOYMENT SETTINGS FOR THE ATHLETIC TRAINER

Opportunities for employment as an athletic trainer have changed dramatically during recent years.[4] Since the 1950s the traditional employment setting for the athletic trainer has been in an athletic training room at the college, university, or professional level. During the 1980s—primarily because of intensive public relations efforts by NATA—the majority of jobs available were at the high-school level.[12] Today the largest percentage of certified athletic trainers are employed in sports medicine clinics or hospitals.

The employment opportunities for athletic trainers continue to become more diverse, expanding to corporate/industrial settings and the military; even NASA and NASCAR employ certified athletic trainers.[39] Other athletic trainers work as physician extenders, and still others are employed in medical supply/equipment sales.

Athletic trainers work in a number of different settings:

- Secondary schools
- School districts
- Colleges and universities
- Professional sports
- Sports medicine clinics
- Corporate/Industrial settings
- The military
- Physician extenders
- Medical supply/equipment sales
- College/university educator
- Researcher
- Administrator

Secondary Schools

It would be ideal to have certified athletic trainers serve every secondary school in the United States.[45] Many of the physical problems that occur later from improperly managed sports injuries could be avoided initially if proper care from an athletic trainer had been provided. Many times a coach does all his or her own athletic training, although in some cases, a coach is assigned additional athletic training responsibilities

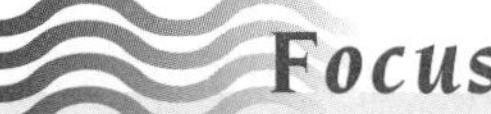

Secondary school official statement

"The National Athletic Trainers' Association, as a leader in health care for the physically active, believes that the prevention and treatment of injuries to student-athletes are a priority. The recognition and treatment of injuries to student-athletes must be immediate. The medical delivery system for injured student-athletes needs a coordinator within the local school community who will facilitate the prevention, recognition, treatment and reconditioning of sports related injuries. Therefore, it is the position of the National Athletic Trainers' Association that all secondary schools should provide the services of a full-time, on-site, certified athletic trainer (ATC) to student athletes."

and is assisted by a student athletic trainer.[7] If a secondary school hires an athletic trainer, it is very often in a faculty-trainer capacity. This individual is usually employed as a teacher in one of the school's classroom disciplines and performs athletic training duties on a part-time or extracurricular basis.[65] Thus, student athletic trainers who hope to find a position in a secondary-school setting should be encouraged to seek teacher certification.[20] In this instance compensation usually is on the basis of released time from teaching, a stipend as a coach, or both.[38] Salaries for the secondary-school athletic trainer are continuing to improve.[5]

Another means of obtaining high-school or community-college athletic training coverage is using a certified graduate student from a nearby college or university. The graduate student receives a graduate assistantship with a stipend paid by the secondary school or community college. In this situation both the graduate student and the school benefit.[26] However, this practice may prevent a school from employing a certified athletic trainer on a full-time basis.

In 1995, the NATA adopted the official statement on hiring athletic trainers in secondary schools that appears in the *Focus Box:* "Secondary school official statement."

Based on a proposal from the American Academy of Pediatrics, in 1998 the American Medical Association adopted a policy calling for certified athletic trainers to be employed in all high-school athletic programs. Although this policy was simply a recommendation and not a requirement, it was a very positive statement supporting the efficacy of athletic trainers in the secondary schools.

Following the adoption of this policy, NATA provided a second official statement on certified athletic trainers in high schools which appears in the *Focus Box:* "Official statement on certified athletic trainers in high schools."

School Districts

Some school districts have found it effective to employ a centrally placed certified athletic trainer. In this case the athletic trainer, who may be full- or part-time, is a nonteacher who serves a number of schools. The advantage is savings; the disadvantage is that one individual cannot provide the level of service usually required by a typical school.

Colleges or Universities

At the college or university level, the athletic training positions vary considerably from institution to institution. In smaller institutions, the athletic trainer may be a half-time teacher in physical education and half-time athletic trainer. In some cases, if the athletic trainer is a physical therapist rather than a teacher, he or she may spend part of the time in the school health center and part of the time in athletic training. Increasingly at the college level, athletic training services are being offered to members of the general student body who participate in intramural and club sports. In most colleges

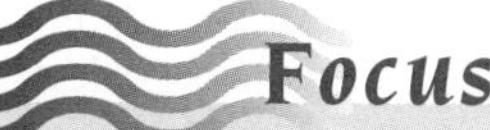

Official statement on certified athletic trainers in high schools

The National Athletic Trainers' Association (NATA) is confident the best way to protect the public is to allow only Board of Certification certified athletic trainers and state licensed athletic trainers to practice as athletic trainers. NATA is not alone in these beliefs. The American Medical Association has stated that certified athletic trainers should be used as part of a high school's medical team. The American Academy of Family Physicians agrees and states on its website, "The AAFP encourages high schools to have, whenever possible, a BOC certified or registered/licensed athletic trainer as an integral part of the high school athletic program."

In states with athletic training regulation, allowing other individuals to continue practicing as athletic trainers without a valid state license or BOC certification places the public at risk. Athletic trainers have unique education and skills that allow them to properly assess and treat acute and traumatic injuries in high school athletics. In coordination with the team physician, they routinely make decisions regarding the return-to-play status of student-athletes. Other allied health professionals are not qualified to perform these tasks. Finally, most situations encountered by athletic trainers should not be left to a coach or layperson who does not have the necessary education and medical and emergency care training.

and universities, the athletic trainer is full-time, does not teach, works in the department of athletics, and is paid by the institution.

In February 1998, the NATA created the Task Force to Establish Appropriate Medical Coverage for Intercollegiate Athletics (AMCIA) to establish recommendations for the extent of appropriate medical coverage to provide the best possible health care for all intercollegiate student-athletes. Essentially the AMCIA task force made recommendations for the number of athletic trainers who should be employed at a college or university based on a mathematical model created by a number of variables existing at that particular institution. These guidelines were revised and updated in 2003. (For directions to determine the recommended number of athletic trainers, consult *Recommendations and Guidelines for Appropriate Medical Coverage for Intercollegiate Athletics.*)[56]

In August 2003, the NCAA Committee on Competitive Safeguards and Medical Aspects of Sports (CSMAS) recommended that NCAA institutions "examine the adequateness of their sports medicine coverage."[46] In particular, whether the increased time demands placed on certified athletic trainers reduces their ability to effectively provide high quality care to all student-athletes. After reviewing the *Recommendations and Guidelines,* the CSMAS "encouraged NCAA institutions to reference the NATA AMCIA in their assessment of the adequateness of their sports medicine coverage . . . and share the responsibility to protect student athlete health and safety through appropriate medical coverage of its sports and supporting activities."

Professional Teams

The athletic trainer for professional sports teams usually performs specific team athletic training duties for six months out of the year; the other six months are spent in off-season conditioning and individual rehabilitation. The athletic trainer working with a professional team is involved with only one sport and is paid according to contract, much like a player. Playoff and championship money may add substantially to the yearly income.

Sports Medicine Clinics

For years, sports medicine clinics have been considered a nontraditional setting for employment as an athletic trainer. Today, more athletic trainers are employed in

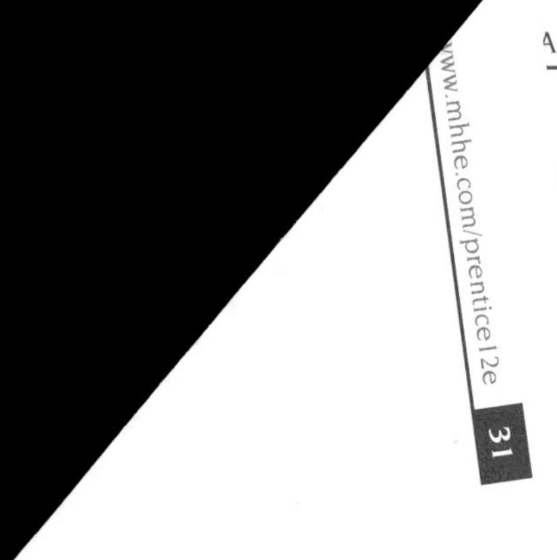

rts medicine clinics than in any other employment setting. The role of the athletic ner varies from one clinic to the next. Most clinical athletic trainers see patients 1 sports-related injuries during the morning hours in the clinic. In the afternoons, etic trainers' services are contracted out to local high schools or small colleges for e or practice coverage. For the most part, private clinics have well-equipped facil- in which to work, and salaries for their trainers are generally somewhat higher in the more traditional settings. In many sports medicine clinics, the athletic r may be responsible for formulating a plan to market or promote athletic train- rvices offered by that clinic throughout the local community.[31]

... as to exactly what role the athletic trainer will play in the function of the clinic.

? How does the role of the athletic trainer working in the clinic differ from the responsibilities of the athletic trainer working in a university setting?

Corporate/Industrial Settings

It is becoming relatively common for corporations or industries to employ athletic trainers to oversee fitness and injury rehabilitation programs for their employees.[1] The athletic trainer working in an industrial setting must have a sound understanding of the principles and concepts of workplace ergonomics, including inspecting, measuring, and observing dimensions of the work space, as well as specific tasks that are performed at the workstation.[24] Once a problem has been identified, the athletic trainer must be able to implement proper adjustments to workplace ergonomics to reduce or minimize possible risks for injury. In addition to these responsibilities, athletic trainers may be assigned to conduct wellness programs and provide education and individual counseling. It is likely that many job opportunities will exist for the athletic trainer in corporate/industrial settings in the next few years.

The Military

The United States military, particularly the Navy, the Marines, and the Army, have demonstrated increased emphasis on injury prevention and health care for the troops.[51] Treatment centers are being developed which closely resemble and, to a great extent, function as athletic training rooms. The centers are staffed by sports medicine physicians, orthopedists, athletic trainers, physical therapists, and support staff. Injured personnel are seen as soon as possible by an athletic trainer, who evaluates an injury, makes decisions on appropriate referral, and begins an immediate rehabilitation program. There are currently over 100 athletic trainers in the military either as active duty or reserve personnel.[51] Occasionally there are some contract positions available. It is likely that the role of the athletic trainer in the military will increase substantially over the next several years.

Physician Extender

While virtually all athletic trainers work under the supervision of a physician, those employed as a physician extender actually work in the physician's office where patients of all ages and backgrounds are being treated. The educational preparation for athletic trainers allows them to function in a variety of domains, including injury prevention, evaluation, management and rehabilitation, health education, nutrition, training and conditioning, organizing preparticipation physicals, and maintaining essential documentation.[52] When working directly in the presence of a physician, the athletic trainer can bill the patient for services provided and expect that they will be reimbursed for their services by third-party payers. While the contact with only the physically active population may not be as great as in other employment settings, the physician extender can expect regular hours, little weekend or evening responsibilities, opportunity for growth, and in general, better pay. All of these factors collectively make physician extender positions attractive for the athletic trainer. Potentially there could be many new jobs created as physicians become more and more aware of the value that an athletic trainer, functioning as a physician extender, can provide to their medical practice.[25]

Treating the Physically Active

In these various employment settings, athletic trainers no longer treat only athletes but instead a physically active population. Physically active individuals may include not only what we have traditionally referred to as athletes in their late teens or twenties, but also both adolescents and older adults who engage in physical activities either recreationally or competitively. *Physically active* individuals engage in athletic, recreational or occupational activities that require physical skills and utilize strength, power, endurance, speed, flexibility, range of motion, or agility. *Physical activity* consists of athletic, recreational or occupational activities that require physical skills and utilize strength, power, endurance, speed, flexibility, range of motion, or agility.

The Adolescent Athlete

Children have always been physically active. But in today's society, playtime or physical activity for many adolescents is focused on organized competition. Certainly many relevant sociological issues arise in answer to questions such as, how old should children be when they begin to compete, or when should a child begin training and conditioning? Skeletally immature adolescent athletes present a particular challenge to the athletic trainer involved in some aspect of their health care. Young athletes cannot be dealt with either physically or emotionally in the same manner as adult athletes. Thus the athletic trainer must be aware of patterns of growth and development and all the special considerations that this process brings with it.

The Aging Athlete

Aging involves a lifelong series of changes in physiological and performance capabilities. These capabilities increase as a function of the growth process throughout adolescence, peak sometime between the ages of eighteen and forty years, then steadily decline with increasing age. However, this decline may be due as much to the sociological constraints of aging as to biological effects. In most cases, after age thirty-five, qualities such as muscular endurance, coordination, and strength tend to decrease. Recovery from vigorous exercise requires a longer amount of time. Regular physical activity, however, tends to delay and in some cases prevent the appearance of certain degenerative processes.

It is possible for individuals to maintain a relatively high level of physiological functioning if they maintain an active lifestyle. Consistent participation in vigorous physical activity can result in improvement of many physiological parameters regardless of age. The effects of exercise on the aging process and the long-term health benefits of exercise have been convincingly documented.

Generally, exercise is considered a safe activity for most individuals. ACSM has recommended that individuals under age forty who are apparently healthy with no significant risks can generally begin an exercise program without further medical evaluation, as long as the exercise program progresses gradually and moderately and no unusual signs or symptoms develop.[1] Individuals who are over age forty or who are at high risk should have a complete medical examination and undergo an exercise test before beginning an exercise program.

RECOGNITION AND ACCREDITATION OF THE ATHLETIC TRAINER AS AN ALLIED HEALTH PROFESSIONAL

In June 1990 the American Medical Association (AMA) officially recognized athletic training as an allied health profession. The primary purpose of this recognition was to have the profession of athletic training recognized in the same context as other allied health professions and to be held to similar professional and educational expectations, as well as to allow for accreditation of educational programs.[45] Once overseen by NATA's Professional Education Committee, overseeing athletic training education programs became the responsibility of the AMA. The AMA's Committee on Allied Health Education and Accreditation (CAHEA) was charged with the responsibility of developing the requirements (Essentials and Guidelines) for the structure and function of academic programs to prepare entry-level athletic trainers. The Joint Review Committee on Athletic Training (JRC-AT) was originally charged with the responsibility of evaluating athletic training educational programs seeking accreditation and making recommendations to CAHEA as to whether those educational programs met the necessary

1-7

***Critical Thinking* Exercise**

A second-semester college sophomore has decided that she is interested in becoming a certified athletic trainer. She happens to be in an institution that offers an advanced master's degree in athletic training yet does not offer an entry-level CAAHEP-approved curriculum.

? How can this student most effectively achieve her goal of becoming a certified athletic trainer?

criteria to become an accredited program in athletic training education. The JRC-AT is made up of representatives from the NATA, the American Academy of Pediatrics, the American Orthopedic Society for Sports Medicine, and the American Academy of Family Physicians. As of 1993, all entry-level athletic training education programs became subject to the CAHEA accreditation process.[18]

In June 1994, CAHEA was dissolved and was replaced immediately by the Commission on Accreditation of Allied Health Education Programs (CAAHEP). The CAAHEP is recognized as an accreditation agency for allied health education programs by the Council for Higher Education Accreditation (CHEA). Entry level bachelors and masters athletic training education programs that were at one time approved by NATA, and subsequently accredited by CAHEA, are now accredited by CAAHEP (through 2005).

In 2003, JRC-AT leadership decided that the profession of athletic training had matured and outgrown the structure and constraints of CAAHEP and that the profession would be better served if the JRC-AT became an independent accrediting agency like those in the other allied health professions. This change meant that instead of the JRC-AT making accreditation recommendations to CAAHEP, the JRC-AT would accredit athletic training education programs. The JRC-AT has begun the transition away from CAAHEP and will seek affiliation with the CHEA once it becomes independent. CHEA is a private, nonprofit national organization that coordinates accreditation activity in the United States. Formed in 1996, its mission is to promote academic quality through formal recognition of higher education accreditation bodies and to work to advance self-regulation through accreditation. Recognition by CHEA affirms that standards and processes of accrediting organizations are consistent with the quality, improvement, and accountability expectations that CHEA has established. Through recognition by CHEA, the JRC-AT will be in the same context/level as is CAAHEP and other national accreditors. CAAHEP accreditation will be discontinued in 2006, at which time the JRC-AT will change its name to the Committee for Accreditation of Athletic Training Education (CAATE). CAATE accreditation will begin at that point and the recognition process from CHEA will commence in 2007.

The JRC-AT also joined the Association of Specialized Professional Accreditors (ASPA), a membership organization. ASPA's members are specialized and professional accreditors. ASPA-member accreditors set national educational standards for entry into more than forty specialized disciplines or defined professions and work with higher education and government officials to enhance education and accreditation.

The effects of CHEA accreditation are not limited to just educational aspects. In the future, this recognition may potentially affect regulatory legislation, the practice of athletic training in nontraditional settings, and insurance considerations. This recognition will continue to be a positive step in the development of the athletic training profession.

Accredited Athletic Training Education Programs

As of February 2005, approximately 300 institutions across the United States offered entry-level athletic training education programs that have been accredited by CAAHEP, while more than 50 others were in the process of seeking CAAHEP accreditation. In addition, thirteen graduate programs in athletic training are accredited by the NATA Graduate Review Committee. The NATA-accredited Advanced Graduate Athletic Training Education Programs are designed to enhance the academic and clinical preparation of individuals who are already certified athletic trainers or those who have completed the requirements for certification.

Specialty Certifications

NATA is in the process of developing specialty certifications to further enhance the professional development of certified athletic trainers by expanding their scope of practice. Entry-level athletic training education programs provide a general educational foundation, whereas specialty certifications build on this foundation. Specialty certifications in athletic training will be voluntary areas of post-graduate study, and certification in areas more advanced than entry level and will ultimately enhance the marketability of certified athletic trainers. Seven specialty certification areas have been proposed: business practice, medical care management, occupational health, wellness, pediatric/adolescent health, adult/geriatric health, and special health populations. Once a specialty certification has been developed and approved, candidates will have to complete experiential requirements and pass a standardized examination.

Other Health Care Organization Accrediting Agencies

Although CAAHEP is the accrediting organization for athletic training, there are other organizations that accredit various health care agencies and organizations.

Joint Commission on Accreditation of Healthcare Organizations

The Joint Commission on Accreditation of Healthcare Organizations (JCAHO) is the nation's largest standards-setting and accrediting body in health care. JCAHO accredits more than 18,000 health care organizations and programs in the United States. Its mission is to improve the quality of care provided to the public through the provision of health care accreditation and related services that support performance improvement in health care organizations.

Commission on Accreditation of Rehabilitation Facilities (CARF)

The Commission on Accreditation of Rehabilitation Facilities (CARF) is an accrediting organization that promotes quality rehabilitation services by establishing standards of quality for organizations to use as guidelines in developing and offering their programs or services to consumers. CARF uses the standards to determine how well an organization is serving its consumers and how it can improve. CARF standards are developed with input from consumers, rehabilitation professionals, state and national organizations, and funders. Every year the standards are reviewed and new ones are developed to keep pace with changing conditions and current consumer needs.

REQUIREMENTS FOR CERTIFICATION AS AN ATHLETIC TRAINER

An athletic trainer who is certified by NATA is a highly qualified paramedical professional educated and experienced in dealing with the injuries that occur with participation in sports. Candidates for certification are required to have an extensive background of both formal academic preparation and supervised practical experience in a clinical setting, according to CAAHEP guidelines.[30] The guidelines listed in *Focus Box:* "Board of Certification requirements for certification as an athletic trainer" have been established by the Board of Certification (BOC).[56] The Board of Certification changed its official name in 2004. Previously the Board of Certification was referred to as the National Athletic Trainers Association Board of Certification. As of 2004 the only way that a candidate can become certified is by completing an entry-level athletic training education program that has been accredited by CAAHEP.

The Certification Examination

Once the requirements have been fulfilled, applicants are eligible to sit for the certification examination.[32] The certification examination has been developed by the BOC in conjunction with an independent examination development and administration company and is currently administered five times each year at various locations throughout the United States.[47,59] The examination consists of three sections: a written portion, a practical portion, and a simulation portion. In 2006 all sections of the certification examination will transition to a computer-based exam (CBE). The examination tests for knowledge and skill in six major domains: (1) prevention of athletic injuries; (2) clinical evaluation and diagnosis; (3) immediate care of injuries; (4) treatment, rehabilitation, and reconditioning of athletic injuries; (5) organization and administration; and (6) professional responsibility. Successful performance on the certification examination leads to BOC certification as an athletic trainer with the credential of **ATC.** (For the latest information on certification requirements, contact the BOC website at www.bocact.org.) BOC certification is a prerequisite for licensure in most states.

ATC
Certified Athletic Trainer

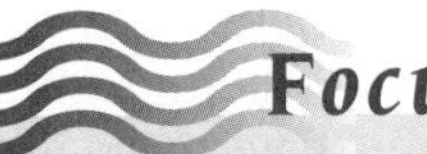

Board of Certification requirements for certification as an athletic trainer

Purpose of Certification

The Board of Certification (BOC) was incorporated in 1989 to provide a certification program for entry-level athletic trainers and recertification standards for certified athletic trainers. The purpose of this entry-level certification program is to establish standards for entry into the profession of athletic training. Additionally, the BOC has established the continuing education requirements that a certified athletic trainer must satisfy to maintain current status as a BOC-certified athletic trainer.

The Process

Annually, the Board of Certification reviews the requirements for certification eligibility and standards for continuing education. Additionally, the Board reviews and revises the certification examination in accordance with the test specifications of the BOC Role Delineation Study that is reviewed and revised every five years. The Board of Certification uses a criterion-referenced passing point for the anchor form of the examination. Each new examination version is equated to the anchor version to ensure that candidates are not rewarded or penalized for taking different versions of the examination.

Procedures for Certification

Requirements for Candidacy for the BOC Certification Examination

1. Candidates must successfully complete an entry-level athletic training program accredited by CAAHEP.*
2. Proof of graduation (an official transcript) at the baccalaureate level from an accredited college or university located in the United States of America. Graduates of foreign universities may petition for a substitution of this degree requirement. Such a request will be evaluated at the candidate's expense by an independent consultant selected by the BOC.

   Students who have begun their last semester or quarter of college are permitted to apply to take the certification examination prior to graduation provided all academic and clinical requirements of the section used for candidacy have been satisfied. A candidate will be permitted to take the examination on the date closest to his or her date of graduation.
3. Endorsement of the examination application by the CAAHEP* Accredited Program Director.
4. Proof of current certification in CPR (Note: CPR certification must be current at the time of initial application and at any subsequent exam retake registration).

*Beginning in 2006 programs will be accredited by CAATE.

Continuing Education Requirements

To ensure the ongoing professional growth and involvement by the certified athletic trainer, BOC has established requirements for continuing education.[9,60]

The purposes of the requirements are to encourage certified athletic trainers to continue to obtain current professional development information, to explore new knowledge in specific content areas, to master new athletic training-related skills and techniques, to expand approaches to effective athletic training, to further develop professional judgment, and to conduct professional practice in an ethical and appropriate manner.

To maintain certification, all certified athletic trainers must document a minimum of eighty continuing education units (CEUs) attained during each three-year recertification term. CEUs may be awarded for attending symposiums, seminars, workshops,

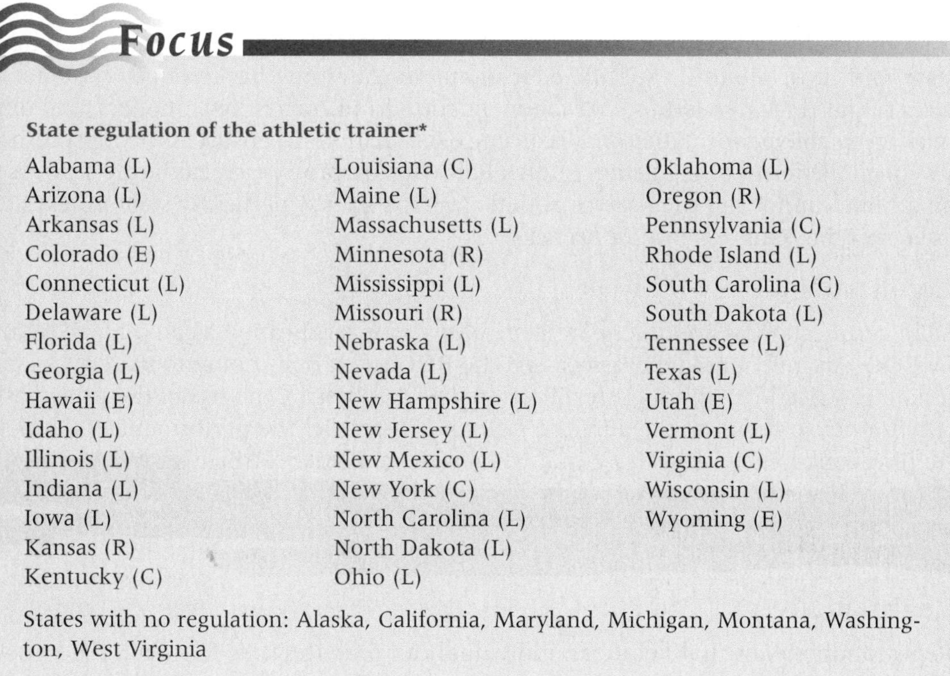

Focus

State regulation of the athletic trainer*

Alabama (L)
Arizona (L)
Arkansas (L)
Colorado (E)
Connecticut (L)
Delaware (L)
Florida (L)
Georgia (L)
Hawaii (E)
Idaho (L)
Illinois (L)
Indiana (L)
Iowa (L)
Kansas (R)
Kentucky (C)
Louisiana (C)
Maine (L)
Massachusetts (L)
Minnesota (R)
Mississippi (L)
Missouri (R)
Nebraska (L)
Nevada (L)
New Hampshire (L)
New Jersey (L)
New Mexico (L)
New York (C)
North Carolina (L)
North Dakota (L)
Ohio (L)
Oklahoma (L)
Oregon (R)
Pennsylvania (C)
Rhode Island (L)
South Carolina (C)
South Dakota (L)
Tennessee (L)
Texas (L)
Utah (E)
Vermont (L)
Virginia (C)
Wisconsin (L)
Wyoming (E)

States with no regulation: Alaska, California, Maryland, Michigan, Montana, Washington, West Virginia

*As of January 2005

E = Exempt from existing licensure standards; C = certification; R = registration; L = licensure. For additional information about individual state regulating boards, contact http://www.nata.org/ on the Web.

or conferences; serving as a speaker, panelist, or certification exam model; participating in the United States Olympic Committee (USOC) program; authoring a research article in a professional journal; authoring or editing a textbook; completing a Journal of Athletic Training quiz; completing postgraduate course work; and obtaining CPR, first aid, or EMT certification. All certified athletic trainers must also demonstrate proof of CPR certification at least once during the three-year term.

STATE REGULATION OF THE ATHLETIC TRAINER

During the early 1970s, the leadership of NATA realized the necessity of obtaining some type of official recognition by other medical allied health organizations of the athletic trainer as a health care professional. Laws and statutes specifically governing the practice of athletic training were nonexistent in most states.

Based on this perceived need, the athletic trainers in many states organized their efforts to secure recognition by seeking some type of regulation of the athletic trainer by state licensing agencies. To date, this ongoing effort has resulted in forty-three of the fifty states enacting some type of regulatory statutes governing the practice of athletic training.[54]

Rules and regulations governing the practice of athletic training vary tremendously from state to state. Regulation may be in the form of certification, registration, licensure, or exemption (see *Focus Box:* "State regulation of the athletic trainer").

For the most part, legislation regulating the practice of athletic training has been positive and to some extent protects the athletic trainer from litigation. However, in some instances, regulation has restricted the limits of practice for the athletic trainer. The leadership of NATA has strongly encouraged athletic trainers in all states to seek licensure.

Licensure

Licensing limits the practice of athletic training to those who have met minimal requirements established by a state licensing board. Through this licensing board the

Forms of state regulation:

- Certification
- Registration
- Licensing
- Exemption

1-8

***Critical Thinking* Exercise**

A certified athletic trainer moves to a different state to take a new job. She discovers that in that state the ATC must be licensed to practice athletic training. Since she was registered as an athletic trainer in the other state, she wonders if she must go through the process of getting a license in her new state.

They have licensing limits

state limits the number of individuals who can perform functions related to athletic training as dictated by the practice act. Requirements for licensure vary from state to state, but most require a specific educational and training background, evidence of good moral character, letters of recommendation from current practitioners, and minimal acceptable performance on a licensing examination. Licensure is the most restrictive of all the forms of regulation. Individuals who are providing health care services to an athlete cannot call themselves athletic trainers in that particular state unless they have met the requirements for licensure.[13]

Certification

State certification as an athletic trainer differs from certification as an athletic trainer by BOC. An individual who has passed the BOC exam does not automatically obtain a state certification. Although certification does not restrict the use of the title of athletic trainer to those certified by the state, it can restrict the performance of athletic training functions to only those individuals who are state certified. State certification indicates that a person possesses the basic knowledge and skills required in the profession and has passed a certification examination. Many states that offer certification use the BOC exam as a criterion for granting state certification.[13]

Registration

Registration means that before an individual can practice athletic training, he or she must register in that state. Registration means that the individual has paid a fee for being placed on an existing list of practitioners. The state may or may not have a mechanism for assessing competency. However, registration does prevent individuals who are not registered with the state from calling themselves athletic trainers.[13]

Exemption

Exemption means that a state recognizes that athletic trainers perform functions similar to those of other licensed professions (e.g., physical therapy) yet still allows them to practice athletic training despite the fact that they do not comply with the practice acts of other regulated professions. Exemption is most often used in those states in which there are not enough practitioners to warrant the formation of a state regulatory board.[13]

THE PHYSICAL THERAPIST AND THE ATHLETIC TRAINER

As the certified athletic trainer continues to gain recognition among health care professionals, interest on the part of many individuals with backgrounds in other health-related professions likewise continues to increase. In particular, it is not unusual to find a physical therapist interested in sports and athletics who is working toward certification as an athletic trainer.[44] Conversely, the certified athletic trainer who is interested in working with patients outside the athletic population is often looking toward licensure as a physical therapist.

Historically, the relationship between athletic trainers and physical therapists has been less than cooperative. Many reasons underlie this lack of cooperation, but the main reason over the years has been failure to clarify the roles of each group in injury rehabilitation.

Athletic trainers have been trained to deal specifically with those injuries that occur in sports, whereas physical therapists have a much broader expertise in injury rehabilitation across many different patient populations. The physical therapist who has not been exposed to the athletic training environment is as inefficient in that setting as is the athletic trainer working with stroke patients in a rehabilitation setting.

The academic curricula required for the athletic trainer and for the physical therapist are similar, particularly in the basic sciences and in the clinical methods courses. The physical therapy curriculum provides a significantly broader background in treating patients of all ages who have a wide variety of physical problems. However, the physical therapist functioning in an athletic training environment must receive additional clinical instruction beyond that which is typically offered in a physical therapy curriculum. Otherwise the period of adjustment and orientation to a nontraditional physical therapy setting is often difficult.

The individual who achieves both certification as an athletic trainer and licensure as a physical therapist is extremely well qualified to function in various sports medicine settings, including both private clinics and colleges and universities. Today, the person who holds a dual credential is in high demand in the job market.

Certification as a Sports Physical Therapist

In the late 1970s the sports physical therapy section of the American Physical Therapy Association (APTA) began identifying competencies specific to the practice of physical therapy in a sports medicine setting. In 1985 the Professional Examination Service was contracted by APTA to develop a specialty examination based on specifically identified competencies.[44]

Candidates for the examination must fulfill the minimal criteria as outlined in the document *Minimal Criteria for Therapist to Sit for the Initial Certification Examination.* These criteria include the completion of a required number of hours of clinical practice in patient care, education, and administration. In addition, written evidence of competency in these areas and research must be submitted.

FUTURE DIRECTIONS FOR THE ATHLETIC TRAINER

The athletic training profession has made remarkable gains during the past decade. Today, certified athletic trainers possess a strong, highly structured academic background in addition to a substantial amount of closely supervised clinical experience in their chosen area of expertise. The athletic trainer continues to gain credibility and recognition as a health care professional trained to deal with injuries that occur in the physically active population. Certainly recognition as an allied health profession by the American Medical Association in 1990 was a major milestone for the profession. In the future, this recognition may potentially affect regulatory legislation, the practice of athletic training in nontraditional settings, and third-party reimbursement. Without question this recognition will continue to be a positive step in the development of the athletic training profession.

Future directions for athletic training will be determined by the efforts of NATA and its membership and will likely include the following:

- Ongoing reevaluation, revision, and reform of athletic training education programs will continue to be a priority.
- The JRC-AT (CAATE in 2006) will become the accrediting agency for entry-level athletic training education programs, and recognition of the JRC-AT by the Council for Higher Education Accreditation will further enhance the credibility of athletic training as an allied health profession.
- Third-party reimbursement for athletic training services provided will gradually become the rule rather than the exception as more and more third-party payers understand what athletic trainers do.
- Eventually every state will regulate the practice of athletic training, and there will be a move to standardize the state practice acts making them more consistent from state to state.
- Athletic trainers will seek and achieve specialty certifications to better assist athletic trainers in expanding their breadth and scope of practice. Initially many will become recognized as Performance Enhancement Specialists for the physically active.
- More and more secondary schools will employ certified athletic trainers.
- While the largest percentage of athletic trainers currently work in clinical settings, there will be an increase in the number of clinics owned and staffed by athletic trainers.

- There will be an increase in the recognition of the athletic trainer as a physician extender who can be incorporated into the daily operations of a physician's office.
- There is great potential for expansion of athletic trainers in the military.
- The potential exists for increasing job opportunities for certified athletic trainers in industrial and corporate settings.
- There will be opportunities for athletic trainers to work with children and teenagers as sport performance specialists.
- There will be increased opportunities for athletic trainers working in fitness and wellness settings.
- As the general population continues to age there will be an increase in opportunities for athletic trainers to work with the elderly physically active population.
- Athletic trainers must continue to enhance their visibility through research efforts and scholarly publication.[28,29,53] Certified athletic trainers must strive to develop some comprehension of basic research design and statistical analysis to be able to interpret new research.[63]
- Athletic trainers should continue to make themselves available for local and community meetings to discuss the health care of the athlete.
- The certified athletic trainer will become recognized internationally as a health care provider and will be found in Canada, South America, Europe, Asia, and Australia.
- Most important, athletic trainers must continue to focus on injury prevention and to provide appropriate, high-quality health care to physically active individuals who are injured while participating in a sport.

SUMMARY

- Athletic training is a specialization within sports medicine, with its major concern being the health and safety of athletes. The primary athletic training team consists of the coach, the athletic trainer, and the team physician. The coach must ensure that both the equipment that is worn and the environment are the safest possible, that all injuries and illnesses are properly cared for, that skills are properly taught, and that conditioning is at the highest level.
- The athletic trainer must be a highly educated, well-trained professional. The athletic trainer must be certified and, if possible, have a state license to practice. The successful athletic trainer loves sports and the competitive environment. He or she must have an abundance of vitality and emotional stability, empathy for people who are in physical or emotional pain, a sense of humor, the ability to communicate, and a desire to learn. All the athletic trainer's actions must follow the highest standards of conduct.
- The team physician can be in varied specializations. Team physicians, depending on their time commitment to a specific sports program, can perform a variety of responsibilities, including conducting the preparticipation health examination; diagnosing and treating illnesses and injuries; advising and teaching the athletic training staff; attending games, scrimmages, and practices; and counseling the athlete about health matters.

Websites

National Athletic Trainers' Association: http://www.nata.org/

This site describes the athletic training profession, how to become involved in athletic training, and the role of an athletic trainer.

American Sports Medicine Institute: http://www.asmi.org/

The American Sports Medicine Institute's mission is to improve through research and education the understanding, prevention, and treatment of sports-related injuries. In addition to stating this mission, the site provides access to current research and journal articles.

American Academy of Orthopaedic Surgeons: http://www. aaos.org/

This site provides some information for the general public as well as information to its members. The public information is in the form of patient education brochures; the site also includes a description of the organization and a definition of orthopedics.

The American Orthopaedic Society for Sports Medicine: http://www.sportmed.org/

This site is dedicated to educating health care professionals and the general public about sports medicine. The site provides access to the American Journal of Sports Medicine *and a wide variety of links to related sites.*

Athletic Trainer.com: http://athletictrainer.com/

This website is specifically designed to give information to athletic trainers, including students, and those interested in athletic training. It provides access to interesting journal articles and links to several informative websites.

NCAA: http://www.ncaa.org/

This site gives general information about the NCAA and the publications that the NCAA circulates. This site may be useful for those working in the collegiate setting.

NATA Education Council: http://www.cewl.com

This site contains information pertaining to the academic preparation of the athletic trainer.

Board of Certification: http://www.bocatc.org

This site provides up-to-date information on requirements for certification as well as a listing of certification test dates and sites.

National Organization for Competency Assurance: http://www.noca.org

This site explains the function of NOCA in getting quality standards for credentialing organizations.

National Commission for Certifying Agencies: http://www.nccaa.org

This site details the function of the NCCA in serving as a national accreditation body for private certification organizations.

Solutions to Critical Thinking EXERCISES

1-1 The student should be able to find all necessary information by simply going to the Internet and contacting these organizations via the World Wide Web.

Know this imp. & review

1-2 Athletic training students must be like sponges, willing to soak up whatever knowledge they can attain to make themselves more efficient in performing their chosen profession. That knowledge may come from attending classes, reading books or journals, attending lectures and conferences, and actively learning the tricks of the trade during the hours spent in the training room and on the field. Students must be able to apply theoretical knowledge to a practical setting if they are to be competent clinicians.

1-3 Although emergency medical technicians are qualified to handle emergency situations, an athletic trainer is able to provide comprehensive health care to the All American High School athletes. An athletic trainer is responsible for the prevention of athletic injuries; the recognition, evaluation, and assessment of injuries; and the treatment and rehabilitation of athletic injuries.

1-4 Ultimately the team physician is responsible for making that decision. However, that decision must be made based on collective input from the athletic trainer, the coach, and the athlete. Remember that everyone on the sports medicine team has the same ultimate goal—to return the athlete to full competitive levels as quickly and safely as possible.

1-5 To help prevent injury, the athletic trainer should (1) arrange for physical examinations and preparticipation screenings to identify conditions that predispose an athlete to injury; (2) ensure appropriate training and conditioning of the athletes; (3) monitor environmental conditions to ensure safe participation; (4) select and maintain properly fitting protective equipment; and (5) educate parents, coaches, and athletes about the risks inherent to sport participation.

1-6 To some extent, the role of the clinical athletic trainer is dictated by that state's regulation of the practice of athletic training. Certainly the clinical and academic preparation of athletic trainers should enable them to effectively evaluate an injured patient and guide that patient through a rehabilitative program. The athletic trainer should treat only those individuals who have sustained injury related to physical activity and not patients with neurological or orthopedic conditions. The athletic trainer may work part-time in the clinic and then cover one or several high schools around the area. The athletic trainer and physical therapist should work as a team to maximize the effectiveness of patient care.

1-7 As of 2004, everyone must graduate from a CAAHEP-accredited program to become a certified athletic trainer. Therefore she must transfer to an institution that offers an entry-level CAAHEP-approved program in which she must complete course work and directly supervised clinical experience.

1-8 The laws regarding regulation of the certified athletic trainer vary from state to state. It is likely that she will have to apply for a license through the athletic training licensing board in her new state to get a new license to practice in that state. It is not likely that there is reciprocity between the two states.

REVIEW QUESTIONS AND CLASS ACTIVITIES

1. How do modern athletic training and sports medicine compare with early Greek and Roman approaches to the care of the athlete?
2. What professional organizations are important to the field of athletic training?

3. Why is athletic training considered a team endeavor? Contrast the coach's, athletic trainer's, and team physician's roles in athletic training.
4. What qualifications should the athletic trainer have in terms of education, certification, and personality?
5. What are the various employment opportunities available to the athletic trainer?
6. Explain the criteria for becoming certified as an athletic trainer.
7. Discuss the methods by which different states regulate the practice of athletic training.

REFERENCES

1. Albensi RJ: The impact of health problems affecting worker productivity in a manufacturing setting. *Athletic Therapy Today* 8(3):13, 2003.
2. American College of Sports Medicine: 1987 annual meeting, Las Vegas, Nev, May 27–30, 1987.
3. Anderson M, Larson G, Luebe J: Student and supervisor perceptions of the quality of supervision in athletic training education, *J Ath Train* 32(4):328, 1997.
4. Arnold B, Gansneder B, VanLunen B: Importance of selected athletic trainer employment characteristics in collegiate, sports medicine clinic, and high school settings, *J Ath Train* 33(3):254, 1998.
5. Arnold B, VanLunen B, Gansneder B: 1994 athletic trainer employment and salary characteristics, *J Ath Train* 31(3):215, 1996.
6. Barefield S, McCallister S: Social supports in the athletic training room: athletes' expectations of staff and student athletic trainers, *J Ath Train* 32(4):333, 1997.
7. Berry J: High school athletic therapy. Part 2, *Athletic Therapy Today* 3(1):47, 1998.
8. Bilik SE: *The trainer's bible,* New York, 1956, Reed (originally published 1917).
9. Board of Certification, Continuing Education Office: *Continuing education file 2003–2005,* Dallas, 2003, BOC.
10. Board of Certification: *Role delineation study,* 5th edition, Raleigh, NC, 2004, Castle Worldwide.
11. Brukner P, Khan, K: Sports medicine: the team approach. In Brukner P, editor: *Clinical sports medicine,* ed 2, Sydney, 2002, McGraw-Hill.
12. Buxton B, Okasaki E, Ho K: Legislative funding of athletic training positions in public secondary schools, *J Ath Train* 30(2):115, 1995.
13. Campbell D, Konin J: Regulation of athletic training. In Konin J: *Clinical athletic training,* Thorofare, NJ, 1997, Slack.
14. Campbell D, Miller M, Robinson W: The prevalence of burnout among athletic trainers, *Ath Train* 20(2):110, 1985.
15. Capel S: Attrition of athletic trainers, *Ath Train* 25(1):34, 1990.
16. Capel S: Psychological and organizational factors related to burnout in athletic trainers, *Ath Train* 21(4):322, 1986.
17. Coker CA: Consistency of learning styles of undergraduate athletic training students in the traditional classroom versus the clinical setting *J Ath Train* 35(4):441, 2000.
18. Committee on Allied Health Education and Accreditation: *Essentials and guidelines for an accredited educational program for athletic trainers,* Chicago, 1992, American Medical Association.
19. Cramer C: A preferred sequence of competencies for athletic training education programs, *Ath Train* 25(2):123, 1990.
20. Cuppett M, Latin R: A survey of physical activity levels of certified athletic trainers, *J Ath Train* 37(3):281, 2002.
21. Curtis N, Helion J, Domsohn M: Student athletic trainer perceptions of clinical supervisor behaviors: a critical incident study, *J Ath Train* 33(3):249, 1998.
22. Curtis N: Teacher certification among athletic training students, *J Ath Train* 30(4):349, 1995.
23. Editorial: The ethics of selecting a team physician. "Show me the money" shouldn't be part of the process, *Sports Med Digest* 23(4):37, 2001.
24. Fícca M: Injury prevention in the occupational setting, *Athletic Therapy Today* 8(3):6, 2003.
25. Finkam S: The athletic trainer or athletic therapist as physician extender, *Athletic Therapy Today* 7(3):50, 2002.
26. Fuller D: Critical thinking in undergraduate athletic training education, *J Ath Train* 32(3):242, 1997.
27. Geick J: Athletic training burnout: a case study, *Ath Train* 21(1):43, 1986.
28. Gould TE: Secondary-school administrators' knowledge and perceptions of athletic training, *Athletic Therapy Today* 8(1):57, 2003.
29. Graber G: Ethics 101, *Athletic Therapy Today* 8(2):6, 2003.
30. Grace P: Milestones in athletic trainer certification, *J Ath Train* 34(3):285, 1999.
31. Gray R: The role of the clinical athletic trainer. In Konin J: *Clinical athletic training,* Thoroughfare, NJ, 1997, Slack.
32. Harrelson G, Gallaspy J, Knight H: Predictors of success on the NATABOC certification examination, *J Ath Train* 32(4):323, 1997.
33. Harrelson GL, Leaver-Dunn D, Wright KE: An assessment of learning styles among undergraduate athletic training students, *J Ath Train* 33(1):50, 1998.
34. Hendrix AE, Acevedo EO, Hebert E: An examination of stress and burnout in certified athletic trainers at division 1-A universities, *J Ath Train* 35(2):139, 2000.
35. Herring SA, Bergfeld J, Boyd J, et al: Sideline preparedness for the team physician: a consensus statement. *Med Sci Sports Exer* 33(5):846, 2001.
36. Hunt V: Meeting clarifies HIPAA regulation, *NATA News,* February: 10, 2003.
37. Jones D: HIPAA: friend or foe to athletic trainers? *Athletic Therapy Today* 8(2):17, 2003.
38. Kahanov L, Andrews L: A survey of athletic training employers' hiring criteria, *J Ath Train* 36(4):408, 2001.
39. Kirkland MK: A case study of athletic training at the Kennedy Space Center, *Athletic Therapy Today* 8(3):9, 2003.
40. Knight KL, Ingersoll CD: Developing scholarship in athletic training, *J Ath Train* 33(3):271, 1998.
41. Knight K: Research in athletic training: a frill or a necessity, *Ath Train* 23(3):212, 1988.
42. Laurent T, Weidner T: Clinical instructors and student athletic trainers' perceptions of helpful clinical instructor characteristics, *J Ath Train* 36(1):58–61, 2001.
43. Lyznicki JM, Riggs JA, Champion HC: Certified athletic trainers in secondary school: report of the Council on Scientific Affairs, American Medical Association, *J Ath Train* 34(3):272, 1999.
44. Malone T: Sports physical therapy specialization, *J Orthop Sports Phys Ther* 7(5):273, 1986.
45. Mathies A, Denegar C, Arnhold R: Changes in athletic training education as a result of changing from NATA-PEC to CAAHEP, *J Ath Train* 30(2):129, 1995.
46. Mitten M: Support for certified athletic trainers in intercollegiate athletics. Memorandum from National Collegiate Athletic Association, August 14, 2003.
47. McLean JL: Does the National Athletic Trainers' Association need a certification examination? *J Ath Train* 34(3):292, 1999.
48. Mellion MB, Walsh WM: The team physician. In Mellion MB, editor: *Sports medicine secrets,* Philadelphia, 1999, Hanley-Balfus.
49. Misasi S, Davis C, Morin G: Academic preparation of athletic trainers as counselors, *J Ath Train* 31(1):39, 1996.
50. Moulton M, Molstad S, Turner A: The role of counseling collegiate athletes, *J Ath Train* 32(2):148, 1997.
51. A closer look at the military setting, *NATA News* 12:30, 2003.
52. National Athletic Trainers' Association: *2001 Standards and Guidelines,* Dallas, 2001, National Athletic Trainers' Association.
53. What is the physician extender?, *NATA News* 1:12, 2004.

54. National Athletic Trainers' Association Governmental Affairs Committee: www.nata.org/members1/committees/gac/statereg boards.htm.
55. National Athletic Trainers' Association: NATA code of ethics, NATA, Dallas, 1995.
56. National Athletic Trainers' Association: *Recommendations and Guidelines for Appropriate Medical Coverage for Intercollegiate Athletics,* Dallas, 2001, National Athletic Trainers' Association.
57. National Athletic Trainers' Association Board of Certification: *Certification Update,* Winter: 5–6, 2000.
58. National Athletic Trainers' Association Board of Certification: *Role delineation study of the entry level athletic trainer certification examination,* Philadelphia, 2004, Davis.
59. National Athletic Trainers' Association Board of Certification: *Study guide for the NATABOC entry level athletic trainer certification examination,* Philadelphia, 1995, Davis.
60. National Athletic Trainers' Association Education Council: Athletic Training Educational Competencies ed 3, Dallas, 2003, National Athletic Trainers' Association.
61. O'Shea M: *A history of the National Athletic Trainers' Association,* Greenville, NC, 1980, National Athletic Trainers' Association.
62. Osternig L: Research in athletic training: the missing ingredient, *Ath Train* 23(3):323, 1988.
63. Pitney WA: Continuing education in athletic training: an alternative approach based on adult learning theory, *J Ath Train* 33(1):72, 1998.
64. Pitney W, Parker J: Qualitative inquiry in athletic training: principles, possibilities, and promises. *J Ath Train* 36(2):, 2001.
65. Prentice W, Mischler B: A national survey of employment opportunities for athletic trainers in the public schools, *Ath Train* 21(3):215, 1986.
66. Prentice W: The athletic trainer. In Mueller F, Ryan A, editors: *Prevention of athletic injuries: the role of the sports medicine team,* Philadelphia, 1991, Davis.
67. Ransone J, Dunn-Bennett L: Assessment of first-aid knowledge and decision making of high school athletic coaches, *J Ath Train* 34(3):267, 1999.
68. Rich BS: All physicians are not created equal: understanding the educational background of the sports medicine physician, *J Ath Train* 28(2):177, 1993.
69. Rock J, Jones M: A preliminary investigation into the use of counseling skills in support of rehabilitation from sport injury, *J Sport Rehabil* 11(4):284, 2002.
70. Shelley GA: Practical counseling skills for athletic therapists, *Athletic Therapy Today* 8(2):57, 2003.
71. Starkey C: Reforming athletic training education, *J Ath Train* 32(2):113, 1997.
72. Starkey C, Ingersoll C: Scholarly productivity of athletic training faculty members, *J Ath Train* 36(2):156, 2001.
73. Staurowsky E, Scriber K: An analysis of selected factors that affect the work lives of athletic trainers employed in accredited educational programs, *J Ath Train* 33(3):244, 1998.
74. Team physician consensus statement. *Med Sci Sports Exer* 32(4):877, 2002.
75. Turocy P: Survey research in athletic training: the scientific method of development and implementation, *J Ath Train* 37(4S):s174, 2002.
76. Turocy P: Overview of athletic training education research publications, *J Ath Train* 37(4S):s162, 2002.
77. Udermann BE: The effect of spirituality on health and healing: a critical review for athletic trainer, *J Ath Train* 35(2):194, 2000.
78. Velasquez BJ: Sexual harassment in the athletic training room: implications for athletic trainers, *Athletic Therapy Today* 8(2):20, 2003.
79. Vinci DM: Nutrition communication and counseling skills, *Athletic Therapy Today* 6(4):34, 2001.
80. Whitehill W, Norton P, Wright K: Navigating the library maze: introductory research and the athletic trainer, *J Ath Train* 31(1):50, 1996.
81. Wiksten D, Spanjer J, LaMaster K: Effective use of multimedia technology in athletic training education, *J Ath Train* 37(4S):s213, 2002.
82. Winterstein A: Organizational commitment among intercollegiate head athletic trainers: examining our work environment, *J Ath Train* 33(1):54, 1998.

ANNOTATED BIBLIOGRAPHY

Bilik SE: *The trainer's bible,* ed 9, New York, 1956, Reed.

A classic book, first published in 1917, by a major pioneer in athletic training and sports medicine.

Cartwright L, Pittney W: *Athletic training for student assistants,* Champaign, IL, 1999, Human Kinetics.

A practical guide for student athletic training assistants, including their roles and responsibilities within the sports medicine team.

Hannum S: *Professional behaviors in athletic training,* Slack, Thorofare, NJ, 2000.

Focuses on essentials of effective career development. Addresses many of skills students will require to build their image as health care professionals, such as communication, critical thinking, networking, interpersonal skills, and recognition of cultural differences.

Mueller F, Ryan A: *Prevention of athletic injuries: the role of the sports medicine team,* Philadelphia, 1991, F.A. Davis.

Provides an in-depth discussion of the various members of the sports medicine team.

National Athletic Trainers' Association Board of Certification: *Role delineation study,* ed 5, Philadelphia, 2004, F.A. Davis.

Contains a complete discussion of the 2003 role delineation study that redefined the responsibilities of the athletic trainer.

National Athletic Trainers' Association: *Code of ethics 1993,* National Athletic Trainers' Association, Dallas, 1993, National Athletic Trainers' Association.

Contains a revision of the previous code of ethics; includes ethical principles, membership standards, and certification standards.

National Athletic Trainers Association: *Far Beyond a Shoe Box: Fifty Years of the National Athletic Trainers' Association,* Dallas, 1999, National Athletic Trainers Association.

An interesting text about the history of NATA that should be read by any student interested in athletic training as a career.

Van Ost L, Manfre K: *Athletic training student guide to success,* Slack, Thorofare, NJ, 2000.

This text emphasizes the roles and responsibilities of the student athletic trainer necessary to make them successful as health care professionals.

Chapter 2 Health Care Administration in Athletic Training

When you finish this chapter you should be able to

- Establish a strategic plan for the athletic training program.
- Plan a functional, well-designed athletic training facility.
- Identify policies and procedures that should be enforced in the athletic training room.
- Explain budgetary concerns for ordering supplies and equipment.
- Explain the importance of the preparticipation physical examination.
- Construct the necessary records that must be maintained by the athletic trainer.
- Describe current systems for gathering data on injuries.

Operating an effective athletic training program requires careful organization and administration regardless of whether the setting is a high school, college, university, professional facility, or a clinical or industrial facility. Besides being a clinical practitioner, the athletic trainer must be an administrator who performs both managerial and supervisory duties. This chapter looks at the administrative tasks required of the athletic trainer for successful operation of the program, including facility design, policies and procedures, budget considerations, personnel management, administration of physical examinations, record keeping, and collecting injury data.

ESTABLISHING A SYSTEM FOR ATHLETIC TRAINING HEALTH CARE

Developing a Strategic Plan

Perhaps the first step in establishing an athletic training program is to determine why there is a need for such a program and what the function of this program should be within the total scope of the athletic program.[35] These two basic questions in the strategic planning process must be answered by administrators, athletic directors, or school boards who, in most cases, will ultimately be responsible for funding and supporting the athletic training program. The depth of the commitment from these decision makers toward providing quality health care will to a large extent determine the size of the staff, the size of the facility, and the scope of operation of the athletic training program. A clearly written mission statement will help focus the direction of the program and should be an outcome of the strategic planning process.[20]

Strategic planning for an athletic training program should involve many individuals including administrators, student-athletes, coaches, physicians, staff athletic trainers, parents, and community-based health leaders. Including many individuals in the planning process will help to secure allies who are committed to seeing the program succeed.[35]

WOTS UP Analysis
- Weaknesses
- Opportunities
- Threats
- Strengths

Strategic planning should be an ongoing process that takes a critical look at the strengths and weaknesses of the program and then takes immediate action to correct deficiencies. The *WOTS UP* analysis—which looks at Weaknesses, Opportunities, Threats, and Strengths underlying planning[38]—is a useful and effective technique in strategic planning for existing athletic training programs.

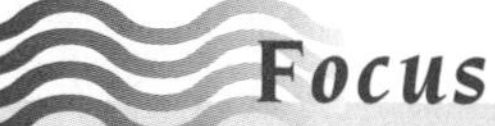

Policies and procedures manual

The following general topics should be addressed in a comprehensive policies and procedures document:

- Scope of the athletic training program (who it will serve)
- Facility use and maintenance
- Risk management plans
- Job descriptions and personnel issues
- Chains of command and supervision
- Use of rehabilitation equipment and modalities

Developing a Policies and Procedures Manual

Once the strategic planning process is complete and some consensus has been reached by those involved in the process, the next step is to create a detailed policies and procedures manual for use by everyone who is involved with providing some aspect of health care for the athlete, including the athletic training staff and student trainers, team physicians, other allied health personnel, coaches, and administrators. *Policies* are clear and accurate written statements that identify the basic rules and principles (the what and why) used to control and expedite decision making. Policies are essential for operating the athletic training room. *Procedures* describe the process by which something is done (the how). The manual should include much of the information presented in the following section titled "Athletic Training Program Operations." In addition, if the institution's budget permits, an abbreviated version of this manual, outlining the rules for using the athletic training room, should be prepared and distributed to the athletes and their parents. *Focus Box:* "Policies and procedures manual" includes recommendations for topics to be included.

Have plan ready for people.

ATHLETIC TRAINING PROGRAM OPERATIONS

It is imperative that every athletic training program develop policies and procedures that carefully delineate the daily routine of the program.

Every athletic training program must develop policies and procedures that carefully delineate the daily routine of the program.

The Scope of the Athletic Training Program

A major consideration in any athletic training program is to determine who is to be served by the athletic training staff. The individual athlete, the institution, and the community are considered.

The Athlete

The athletic trainer must decide the extent to which the athlete will be served. For example, will prevention and care activities be extended to athletes for the entire year, including summer and other vacations, or only during the competitive season? Also, the athletic trainer must decide what care will be rendered. Will it extend to all systemic illnesses or to just musculoskeletal problems?

The Institution

A policy must be established as to who, other than the athletes, will be served by the athletic training program. Often, legal concerns and the school liability insurance dictate who, beyond the athlete, is to be served. A policy should make it clear whether students other than athletes, athletes from other schools, faculty, and staff are to receive care. If so, how are they to be referred and medically directed? Also, it must be decided whether the athletic training program will act as a clinical setting for student athletic trainers.

The Community

A decision must be made as to which, if any, outside group(s) or people in the community will be served by the athletic training staff. Again, legality and the institution's insurance program must be taken into consideration when making this decision. If a policy is not delineated in this matter, outside people may abuse the services of the athletic training facility and staff.

Clinical and Corporate/Industrial Setting Considerations

The athletic trainer working in the clinical or corporate/industrial setting will likely be working with patients other than high school or college athletes. The scope of practice within an individual clinic may include pediatric, work hardening, orthopedic, or even the occasional neurological patient. Athletic trainers in the clinical setting should be assigned to work only with patient populations that may generally be classified as physically active. Clinical administrators should not require athletic trainers to treat other patient populations, because athletic trainers have no formal education or training geared toward those patients' problems.

Athletic trainers in the corporate/industrial setting, in addition to overseeing preventive and rehabilitation programs, are often asked to take on responsibility for employee fitness programs. Therefore a more advanced understanding of the principles of training and conditioning will be necessary (see Chapter 4).

Providing Coverage

Facility Personnel Coverage

A major concern of any athletic department is whether proper personnel coverage is provided for the athletic training facility and specific sports. If a school has a full-time athletic training staff, an athletic training facility could, for example, operate from 7 A.M. to 10 P.M. Mornings are commonly reserved for treatments and exercise rehabilitation; early afternoons are for treatment, exercise rehabilitation, and preparation for practice or a contest; and late afternoons and early evenings are spent in injury management. High schools with limited available supervision may be able to provide athletic training facility coverage only in the afternoons and during vacation periods.

Sports Coverage

Ideally, all sports should have a certified, or at least a student, athletic trainer in attendance at all practices and contests, both at home and away. Many colleges and universities have sufficient personnel to provide coverage to a variety of sports simultaneously. At the secondary-school level, however, only one or occasionally two athletic trainers may be available to cover every sport that the high school offers. Thus it is impossible for the athletic trainer to be in several places at one time. The athletic trainer in this difficult situation must make some decisions about where the greatest need for coverage is, based on the potential risk of a particular sport and the number of athletes involved.

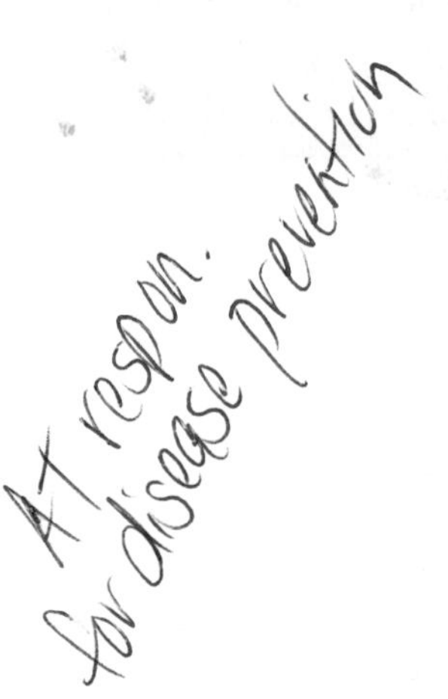

Hygiene and Sanitation

Good hygiene and sanitation are essential for an athletic training program.

The practice of good hygiene and sanitation is of the utmost importance in an athletic training program. The prevention of infectious diseases is a direct responsibility of the athletic trainer, whose duty it is to see that all athletes are surrounded by the most hygienic environment possible and that each individual is practicing sound health habits. Chapter 14 discusses the management of bloodborne pathogens. The athletic trainer must be aware of and adhere to guidelines for the operation of an athletic care facility as dictated by the Occupational Safety and Health Administration (OSHA).

The Athletic Training Facility

The athletic training room should be used only for the prevention and care of sports injuries. Too often the athletic training facility becomes a meeting or club room for the coaches and athletes. Unless definite rules are established and practiced, room cleanliness and sanitation become an impossible chore. Unsanitary practices or conditions must not be tolerated. The following are some important athletic training room policies:

1. No cleated shoes are allowed. Dirt and debris tend to cling to cleated shoes; therefore cleated shoes should be removed before athletes enter the athletic training facility.
2. Game equipment is kept outside. Because game equipment such as balls and bats add to the sanitation problem, they should be kept out of the athletic training room. Coaches and athletes must be continually reminded that the athletic training room is not a storage room for sports equipment.
3. Shoes must be kept off treatment tables. Because of the tendency of shoes to contaminate treatment tables, they must be removed before any care is given to the athlete.
4. Athletes should shower before receiving treatment. The athlete should make it a habit to shower before being treated if the treatment is not an emergency. This procedure helps keep tables and therapeutic modalities sanitary.
5. Roughhousing and profanity should not be allowed. Athletes must be continually reminded that the athletic training facility is for injury care and prevention. Horseplay and foul language lower the basic purpose of the athletic training room.
6. No food or smokeless tobacco should be allowed.

General cleanliness of the athletic training room cannot be stressed enough. Through the athletic trainer's example, the athlete may develop an appreciation for cleanliness and in turn develop wholesome personal health habits. Cleaning responsibilities in most schools are divided between the athletic training staff and the maintenance crew. Care of permanent building structures and trash disposal are usually the responsibilities of maintenance, whereas the upkeep of specialized equipment falls within the province of the training staff.

The division of routine cleaning responsibilities may be organized as follows:

1. Maintenance crew
   a. Sweep floors daily.
   b. Clean and disinfect sinks and built-in tubs daily.
   c. Mop and disinfect hydrotherapy area twice a week.
   d. Refill paper towel and drinking cup dispensers as needed.
   e. Empty wastebaskets and dispose of trash daily.
2. Athletic training staff
   a. Clean and disinfect treatment tables daily.
   b. Clean and disinfect hydrotherapy modalities daily.
   c. Clean and polish other therapeutic modalities weekly.

The Gymnasium

Maintaining a clean environment in sports is a continual battle in the athletic training setting. Practices such as passing a common towel to wipe off perspiration, using common water dispensers, or failing to change dirty clothing for clean are prevalent violations of sanitation in sports. The following is a suggested cleanliness checklist that may be used by the athletic trainer:

1. Facilities cleanliness
   a. Are the gymnasium floors swept daily?
   b. Are drinking fountains, showers, sinks, urinals, and toilets cleaned and disinfected daily?
   c. Are lockers aired and sanitized frequently?
   d. Are mats cleaned routinely (wrestling mats and wall mats cleaned daily)?

2. Equipment and clothing issuance
   a. Are equipment and clothing fitted to the athlete to avoid skin irritations?
   b. Is swapping of equipment and clothes prevented?
   c. Is clothing laundered and changed frequently?
   d. Is wet clothing allowed to dry thoroughly before the athlete wears it again?
   e. Is individual attention given to proper shoe fit and upkeep?
   f. Is protective clothing provided during inclement weather or when the athlete is waiting on the sidelines?
   g. Are clean, dry towels provided each day for each individual athlete?

The Athlete

To promote good health among the athletes, the athletic trainer should encourage sound health habits. The following checklist may be a useful guide for coaches, athletic trainers, and athletes:

1. Are the athletes medically cleared to participate?
2. Is each athlete insured?
3. Does the athlete promptly report injuries, illnesses, and skin disorders to the coach or the athletic trainer?
4. Are good daily living habits of resting, sleeping, and proper nutrition practiced?
5. Do the athletes shower after practice?
6. Do they dry thoroughly and cool off before departing from the gymnasium?
7. Do they avoid drinking from a common water dispenser?
8. Do they avoid using a common towel?
9. Do they avoid exchanging gym clothes with teammates?
10. Do they practice good foot hygiene?
11. Do they avoid contact with teammates who have a contagious disease or infection?

Emergency Telephones

The accessibility of an emergency telephone adjacent to all major activity areas is also essential. It should be possible to use this telephone to call outside for emergency aid and to contact the athletic training facilities when additional assistance is required. Two-way radios or, preferably, cellular or digital telephones provide the greatest flexibility in the communication system and should be bought if the budget permits.

Budgetary Concerns

A major problem often facing athletic trainers is a budget of sufficient size.

One of the major problems faced by athletic trainers is to obtain a budget of sufficient size to permit them to perform a creditable job of athletic training. Most high schools provide only limited budgetary provisions for athletic training except for the purchase of tape, ankle wraps, and an athletic training kit that contains a minimum amount of supplies.[6] Many fail to provide a room and any of the special facilities that are needed to establish an effective athletic training program. Some school boards and administrators fail to recognize that the functions performed in the athletic training facility are an essential component of the athletic program and that even if no specialist is used, the facilities are nonetheless necessary.[6] Colleges and universities are not usually faced with this problem to the extent that high schools are. By and large, athletic training at the college level is recognized as an important aspect of the athletic program.

Budgetary needs vary considerably within programs; some require only a few thousand dollars, whereas others spend hundreds of thousands of dollars. The amount spent on building and equipping a training facility, of course, is entirely a matter of local option. In purchasing equipment, immediate needs and the availability of personnel to operate specialized equipment should be kept in mind.

The budget process should be a continuous process involving prioritizing, planning, documenting and evaluating the goals of the athletic training program, and formulating a plan for how available resources can be utilized and expended during the next budget period.[34]

Budget records should be kept on file so that they are available for use in projecting the following year's budgetary needs. The records present a picture of the distribution of current funds and serve to substantiate future budgetary requests.

Supplies

The supplies that the athletic trainer uses to carry out daily tasks may be classified as either expendable or nonexpendable. Some athletic trainers spend much of their budget on expendable supplies that cannot be reused. Supplies that are expendable are used for injury prevention, first aid, and management. Examples of expendable supplies are adhesive tape, adhesive bandages, and hydrogen peroxide. Nonexpendable supplies are those that can be reused. Examples are compression wraps, scissors, and neoprene sleeves. An annual inventory must be conducted at the end of the year or before the ordering of supplies. Accurate records must be kept to justify future requests.

Supplies may be expendable or nonexpendable.

needed for preven. | dont have to have

Equipment

The term *equipment* refers to items that may be used by the athletic training room for a number of years. Equipment may be further divided into capital and nonconsumable capital equipment. Nonconsumable capital equipment is not usually removed from the athletic training facility. Examples of nonconsumable capital equipment are ice machines, treatment tables, isokinetic machines, and electrical therapeutic modalities. Capital equipment includes things like crutches, coolers, and training kits.

Equipment may be nonconsumable capital or capital.

machines | crutches med. balls training kit

Purchasing Systems

Purchasing of supplies and equipment must be done through either direct buy or competitive bid. For expensive purchases, an institutional purchasing agent is sent out to competing vendors who quote a price on specified supplies or equipment. Orders are generally placed with the lowest bidder. Smaller purchases or emergency purchases may be made directly from a single vendor.[33]

An alternative to purchasing expensive equipment is to lease it. Many manufacturers and distributors are now willing to lease equipment on a monthly or yearly basis. Over the long run, purchasing equipment will be less costly. In the short term, however, if a large capital expenditure is not possible, a leasing agreement should be considered.[34]

Purchasing may be done through direct buy or competitive bid.

expensive = comp. bid

Additional Budget Considerations

In addition to supplies and equipment, the athletic trainer must also consider other costs that may be included in the operation of an athletic training program; these include telephone and postage, utilities, contracts with physicians or clinics for services, professional liability insurance, memberships in professional organizations, the purchase of professional journals or textbooks, travel and expenses for attending professional meetings, and clothing to be worn in the training room.[34,35]

Developing a Risk Management Plan

The athletic trainer, working in conjunction with the appropriate administrative personnel, must be responsible for developing a risk management plan that covers security issues, fire safety, electrical and equipment safety, and developing emergency action plans.[39]

Security Issues

The athletic trainer must decide who will have access to the athletic training room facility. In addition to the staff athletic trainers, the team physician must have keys to access the athletic training room. Student athletic trainers may also be given keys as necessary at the collegiate level; at the high school level, however, student athletic trainers should only be in the athletic training room when directly supervised. At the collegiate level, coaches do not need to have access to the athletic training room; but

2-1

***Critical Thinking* Exercise**

The principal at All-American High School has received a mandate from the school board to develop a risk management plan for the athletic program. The principal asks the athletic trainer to chair a committee to develop this plan.

? What considerations are important for inclusion in this risk management plan?

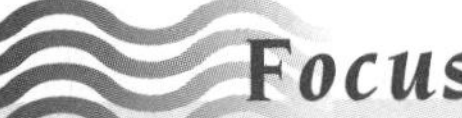

Safety when using electrical equipment

- The entire electrical system of the building or athletic training room should be designed or evaluated by a qualified electrician.
- Problems with the electrical system may exist in older buildings or in situations in which rooms have been modified to accommodate therapeutic devices (e.g., putting a whirlpool in a locker room in which the concrete floor is always wet or damp).
- It should not be assumed that all three-pronged wall outlets are automatically grounded. The ground must be checked. Ground fault interrupters (GFI) should be installed, particularly in those areas in which water may be present (e.g., whirlpools).
- The athletic trainer should become very familiar with the equipment being used and with any potential problems that may exist or develop. Any defective equipment should be immediately removed from the clinic. The plug should not be jerked out of the wall by pulling on the cable.
- Extension cords or multiple adapters should never be used.
- Equipment should be reevaluated on a yearly basis and should conform to National Electrical Code guidelines. A clinic or training room that is not in compliance with this code has no legal protection in a lawsuit.
- Common sense should always be exercised when using electrotherapeutic devices. A situation that appears to be potentially dangerous may in fact result in injury or death.

at the high school level, coaches might need to have a key to get into the facility at times when the athletic trainer may not be available. Access to areas of the building other than the athletic training room should be strictly limited.

Fire Safety

The athletic trainer should establish and have clearly posted a plan for evacuating the athletic training facility should a fire occur. Smoke detectors and fire alarm systems must be periodically tested and inspected to make certain that they are functioning normally.

Electrical and Equipment Safety

Electrical safety in the athletic training setting should be of maximal concern to the athletic trainer. Unnecessary accidents can be avoided by taking some basic precautions and acquiring some understanding of the power distribution system and electrical grounds. *Focus Box:* "Safety when using electrical equipment" lists considerations for electrical safety.

Emergency Action Plan

In cooperation with existing community-based emergency health care delivery systems, the athletic trainer should develop a systematic plan for accessing the emergency medical system and subsequent transportation of injured athletes to an emergency care facility.[5] Meetings should be scheduled periodically with EMTs or paramedics who work in the community to make certain that they understand the role of the athletic trainer as a provider of emergency health care. It is important to communicate the special considerations for dealing with athletic equipment issues before an emergency arises. Chapter 12 discusses the emergency action plan in detail.

Accessing Community-Based Health Services

In addition to the community-based emergency medical services personnel, the athletic trainer should become familiar with existing local and regional community health services and agencies that may be accessed should a need arise to refer an athlete for

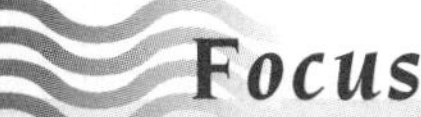

Models of supervision for the head athletic trainer*

Clinical supervision—Involves direct observation of the assistant trainers in the performance of their written job responsibilities, followed by an analysis of strengths and weaknesses and a collaborative effort to correct weaknesses.

Developmental supervision—A mentoring approach in which the head athletic trainer works in a collaborative manner with the assistants, helping them to develop professionally while meeting the needs of the day-to-day athletic training program.

Inspection production supervision—An authoritative management style in which the head athletic trainer demands that lines of authority be strictly maintained to accomplish the stated goals of the athletic training program.

*These models should not be confused with models of clinical supervision established by the Education Council for Students.

psychological or sociological services. Referrals should be made with input and assistance from the team physician. The family of an athlete requiring referral for psychological or sociological counseling must be informed of the existing problems, particularly when the athlete is a minor.

2-2

Critical Thinking Exercise

State University has an opening for an assistant athletic trainer in its Department of Athletics. The athletic director has asked the head athletic trainer to be in charge of the recruitment and hiring process for the new position.

? What factors must be considered in hiring a new employee?

Human Resource and Personnel Issues

The importance of putting together the sports medicine team was discussed in Chapter 1. Any team is only as good as the group of individuals who make up that team. Recruiting, hiring, and retaining the most qualified personnel is essential if the athletic training program is to be effective.

- Specific policies dealing with recruitment, hiring and firing, performance evaluations, and promotions are mandated by federal law.[12] The policies for recruitment and hiring clearly mandate that all qualified applicants should receive equal consideration regardless of their race, gender, religion, or nationality. Athletic trainers who are in a position to hire new staff must strictly adhere to these mandates.
- Once an individual has been hired, it is important for everyone on the sports medicine team to clearly understand what the roles and responsibilities are within that team. Individual job descriptions and job specifications that describe qualifications, accountability, a code of conduct, and the scope of that position should be written. A well-defined organizational chart should be created to show the chain of command.[35]
- The head athletic trainer must serve as a supervisor for the staff assistants, graduate students, and undergraduate student athletic trainers.[22] The supervisor should strive to improve job performance and enhance professional development of those being supervised. *Focus Box:* "Models of supervision for the head athletic trainer" defines supervisory models.[35]
- Performance evaluations should be routinely done at regularly scheduled intervals to analyze the quality of the work being performed. Evaluations should focus first on the positive aspects of job performance and then on any weaknesses.[22]

Each of these policies relative to personnel issues should be included in the policies and procedures manual.

DESIGNING AN ATHLETIC TRAINING FACILITY

The athletic training facility is a multipurpose area used for first aid, therapy and rehabilitation, injury prevention, medical procedures such as the physical examination, and athletic training administration.

Maximizing the use of facilities and effectively using equipment and supplies are essential to the function of any athletic program.[27] The athletic training facility must be specially designed to meet the many requirements of the athletic training program (Figure 2-1).[26,37] The size and the layout of the athletic training facility will depend on

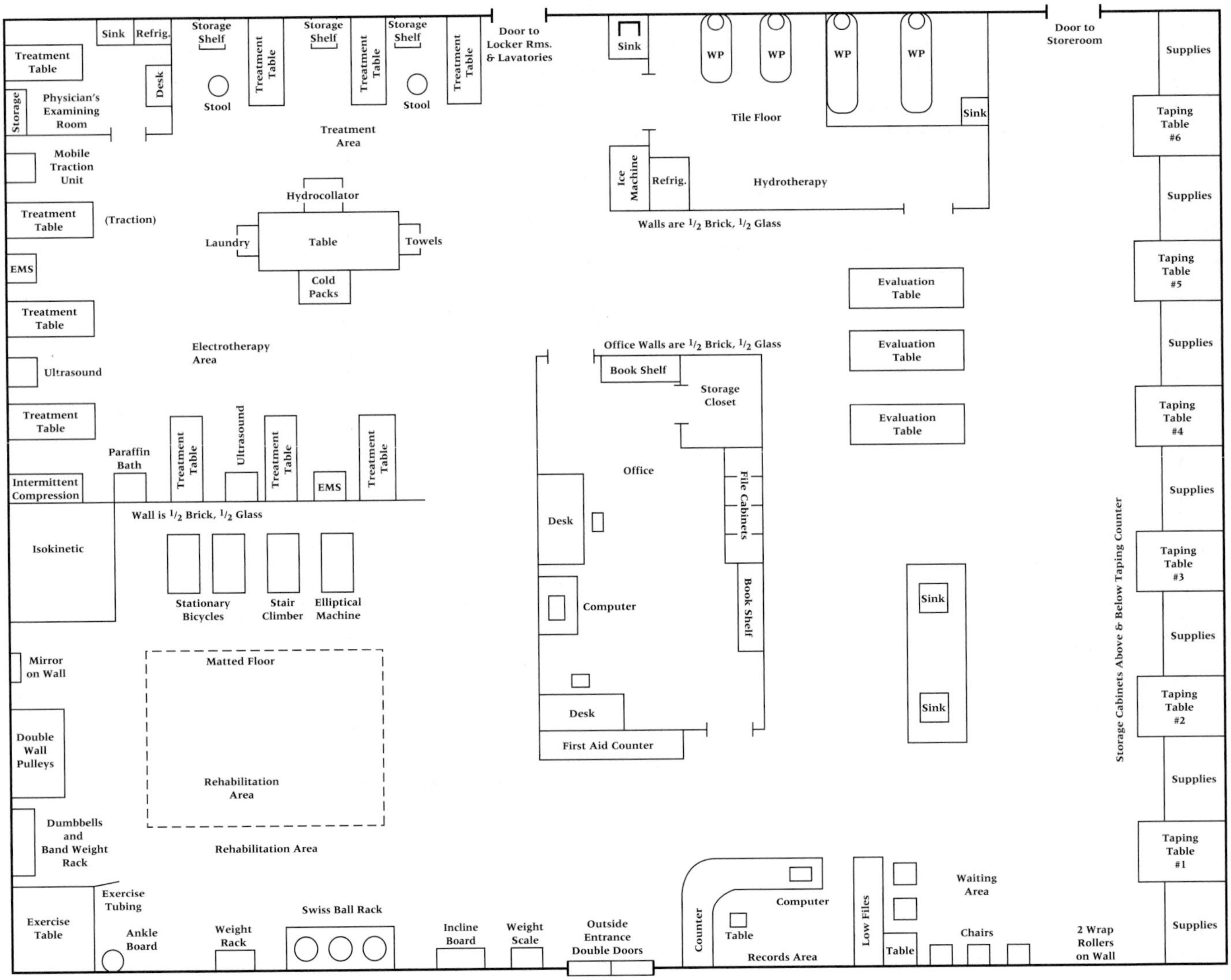

Figure 2-1A

The ideal athletic training room facility should be well designed to maximize its use. **A,** Larger athletic training facility found at a college or university.

Continued

the scope of the athletic training program, including the size and number of teams and athletes and what sports are offered.[29] The clinical setting has a much broader patient population than a school or university program, and thus the requirements for equipment and supplies will be somewhat different.[26] To accommodate the various functions of an athletic training program, the athletic training room must serve as a health care center for athletes.[11,13]

Size

The size of the athletic training room can range anywhere from a large storage closet in some high schools or middle schools to 15,000-square-foot sports medicine complexes in some universities. Certainly the size of the facility can have a major impact on how the athletic training program is managed. But the most important consideration is to organize the athletic training program in a manner that most efficiently takes advantage of the space available. When designing a new athletic training facility, the athletic trainer should work closely with design architects to communicate the specific needs of the institution and the number of athletes who will be served.

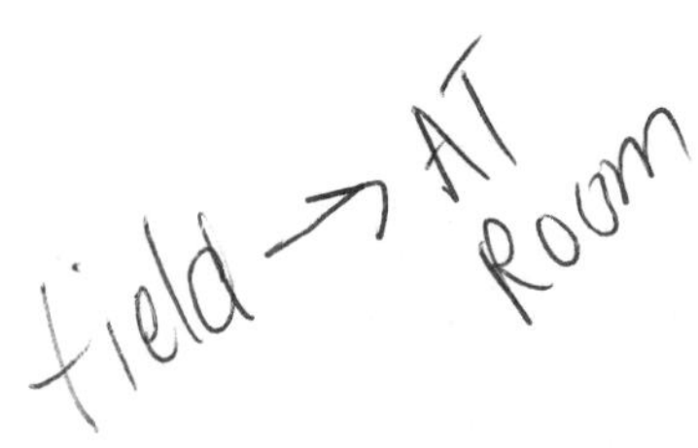

Location

The athletic training facility should have an outside entrance from the athletic field or court. This arrangement makes it unnecessary to bring injured athletes in through the

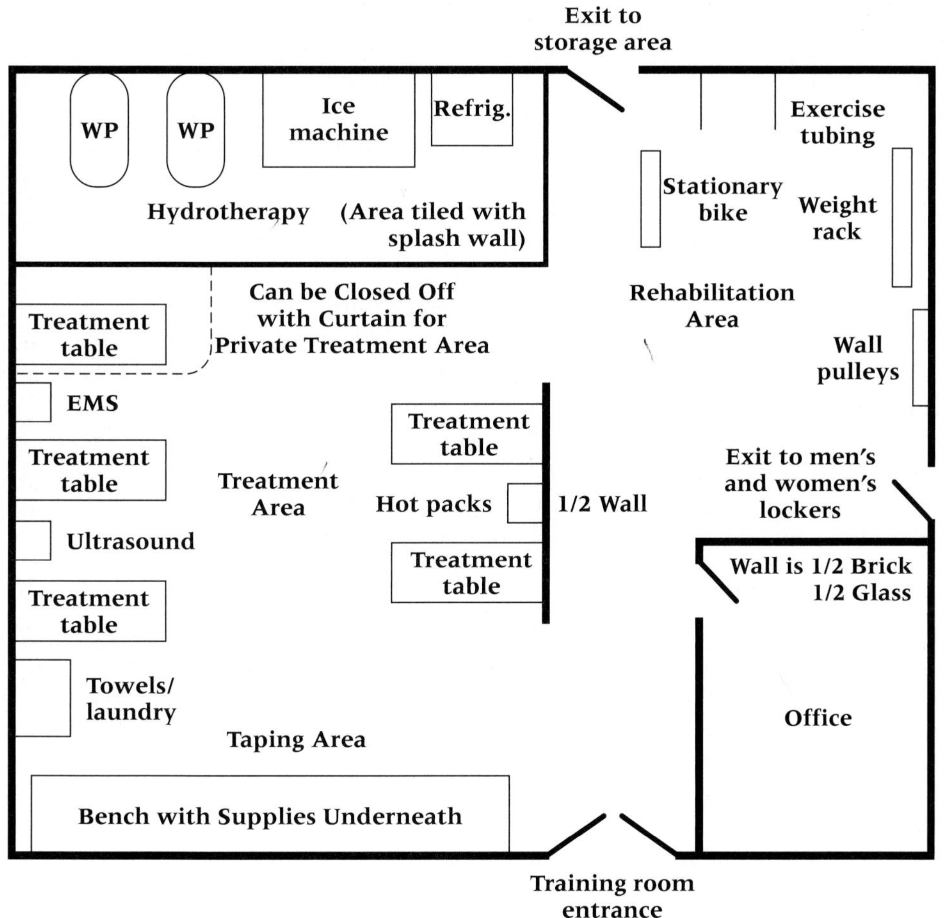

Figure 2-1B—continued

B, Small athletic training facility found at a high school.

building and possibly through several doors; it also permits access when the rest of the building is not in use. A double door at each entrance is preferable to allow easy passage of a wheelchair or a stretcher. A ramp at the outside entrance is safer and far more functional than are stairs.

The athletic training room should be near the locker rooms if possible so that showers are readily available to athletes coming in for treatment following practice. Toilet facilities should be located adjacent to the athletic training room and should be readily accessible through a door in the training room.

Because the athletic training facility is where emergency treatment is given, its light, heat, and water sources should be independent from those for the rest of the building.

Illumination

The athletic training facility should be well lighted throughout. Lighting should be planned with the advice of a technical lighting engineer. Obviously, certain areas need to be better lit than others. For example, the wound care and taping areas need better lighting than is necessary in the rehabilitation area. Ceilings and walls act as reflective surfaces to help provide an equable distribution and balance of light. Natural lighting through windows or skylights can certainly be helpful.

Special Service Areas

Apart from the storage and office space, a portion of the athletic training room should be divided into special sections, preferably by half walls or partial glass walls. Space, however, may not permit a separate area for each service section, and an overlapping of functions may be required.

2-3

***Critical Thinking* Exercise**

The members of the school board at All-American High School voted to allocate \$25,000 to renovate a 25′ × 40′ storage space and to purchase new equipment for an athletic training room. The athletic trainer has been asked to provide the school principal with a wish list of what should be included in this facility. The physical renovation will cost approximately \$17,000.

? How may this space be best used, and what type of equipment should be purchased to maximize the effectiveness of this new facility?

Treatment Area

The treatment area should include four to six treatment tables, preferably of adjustable height, that can be used during the application of ice packs or hydrocollator packs or for manual therapy techniques such as massage, mobilization, or proprioceptive neuromuscular facilitation (PNF). Three or four adjustable stools on rollers should also be readily available. The hydrocollator unit and ice bags should be easily accessible to this area.

Electrotherapy Area

The electrotherapy area is used for treatment by ultrasound, diathermy, or electrical stimulating units. Equipment should include at least two treatment tables, several wooden chairs, one or two dispensing tables for holding supplies, shelves, and a storage cabinet for supplies and equipment. The area should contain a sufficient number of grounded outlets, preferably in the walls and several feet above the floor. It is advisable to place rubber mats or runners on each side of the treatment tables as a precautionary measure. This area must be under supervision at all times, and the storage cabinet should be kept locked when not in use.

Hydrotherapy Area

In the hydrotherapy area, the floor should slope toward a centrally located drain to prevent standing water. Equipment should include two or three whirlpool baths (one permitting complete immersion of the body), several lavatories, and storage shelves. Because some of this equipment is electrically operated, many precautions must be taken. All electrical outlets should be placed four to five feet above the floor and should have spring-locked covers and water spray deflectors. All cords and wires must be kept clear of the floor to eliminate any possibility of electrical shock. To prevent water from entering the other areas, a slightly raised, rounded curb should be built at the entrance to the area. When an athletic training room is planned, ample outlets must be provided; under no circumstances should two or more devices be operated from the same outlet. All outlets must be properly grounded using ground fault interrupters (GFI).[25]

Exercise Rehabilitation Area

Ideally, an athletic training facility should accommodate injury reconditioning under the strict supervision of the athletic trainer. Selected pieces of resistance equipment should be made available. Depending on the existing space, dumbbells and free weights; exercise machines for knee, ankle, shoulder, hip, and so forth; isokinetic equipment; devices for balance and proprioception; and space for using exercise tubing may all be available for use.

Taping, Bandaging, and Orthotics Area

Each athletic training room should provide a place in which taping, bandaging, and applying orthotic devices can be executed. This area should have three or four taping tables adjacent to a sink and a storage cabinet.

Physician's Examination Room

In colleges and universities, the team physician has a special room in which examinations and treatments may be given. This room contains an examining table, sink, locking storage cabinets, refrigerator, and small desk with a telephone. At all times, this facility must be kept locked to outsiders.

Records Area

Some space, either in the office or at the entrance to the training room, should be devoted to record keeping. Record-keeping facilities may range from a filing system to a more sophisticated computer-based system. Records should be accessible to sports medicine personnel only.

NOTECARDS

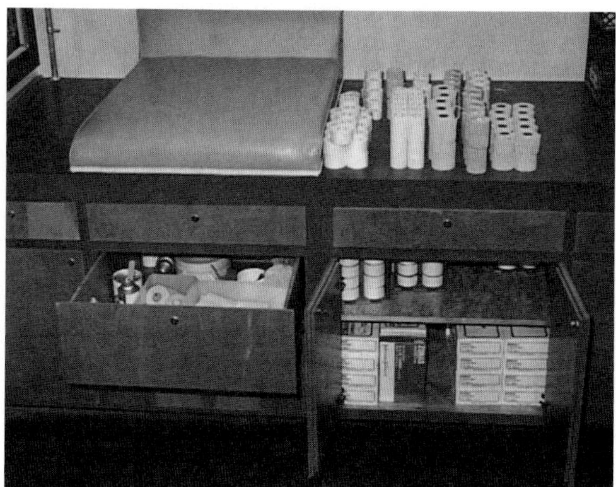

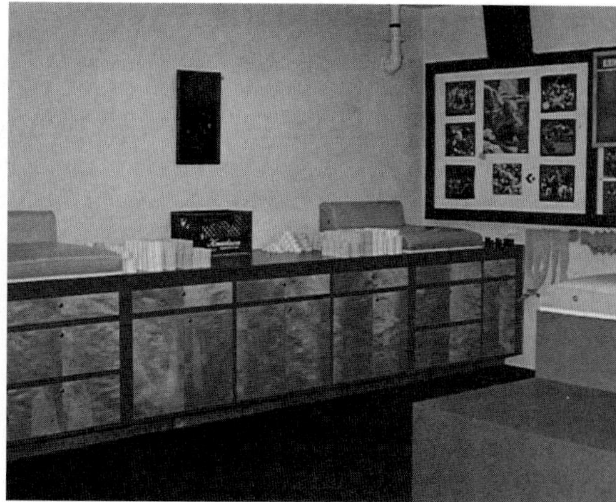

Figure 2-2

An effective athletic training program must have appropriate storage facilities that are highly organized.

Storage Facilities

Many athletic training facilities lack ample storage space. Often, storage facilities are located a considerable distance away, which is extremely inconvenient. In addition to the storage cabinets and shelves provided in each of the three special service areas, a small storage closet should be placed in the athletic trainer's office. All these cabinets should be used for the storage of general supplies as well as for the small, specialized equipment used in the respective areas. A large walk-in closet, 80 to 100 square feet in area, is a necessity for the storage of bulky equipment, medical supplies, adhesive tape, bandages, and protective devices (Figure 2-2). A refrigerator for the storage of frozen water in styrofoam cups for ice massage and other necessities is also an important piece of equipment. Many athletic trainers prefer to place the refrigerator in their office, where it is readily accessible but still under close supervision. In small sports programs, a large refrigerator will probably be sufficient for all ice needs. If at all possible, an ice-making machine should be installed in an auxiliary area to provide an ample and continuous supply of ice for treatment purposes.

It is essential to have adequate storage space available for supplies and equipment.

Athletic Trainer's Office

A space at least ten feet by twelve feet is ample for the athletic trainer's office. The office should be located so that all areas of the training room can be well supervised without the athletic trainer's having to leave the office. Glass partitions on two sides permit the athletic trainer, even while seated at the desk, to observe all activities. A desk, chair, tackboard for clippings and other information, telephones, and record file are the basic equipment. In some cases a computer is also housed in this office. The office should have an independent lock-and-key system so that it is accessible only to authorized personnel.

2-4

***Critical Thinking* Exercise**

A high school athletic trainer is approached by the community recreation department with a request to use the athletic training facility to treat its football and basketball league participants who are injured.

? How should the athletic trainer deal with this request?

Additional Areas

If space is available, several other areas could potentially be included as part of a training room facility.

Pharmacy Area

A separate room that can be secured for storing and administering medications is helpful. All medications, including over-the-counter drugs, should be kept under lock and key. If prescription medications are kept in the training room, only the team physician or pharmacist from a campus health center should have access to the storage cabinet. Records for administering medications to athletes should be kept in this area. It is essential to adhere to individual state regulations regarding the storage and administration of medications (see Chapter 17).

Rehabilitation Pool

It is rare that a pool is located in the training room; however, if the facility has the space and can afford one, a pool can be an extremely useful rehabilitation tool. The pool should be accessible to individuals with various types of injuries. It should have a graduated depth to at least seven feet, the deck should have a nonslip surface, and the filter system should be in a separate room.[34]

X-Ray Room

A separate room for X-ray equipment must have lead shielding in the walls. The X-ray room must be large enough to house all the necessary equipment (X-ray unit, processing unit, etc.).

RECORD KEEPING

Keeping adequate records is of major importance in the athletic training program.

Record keeping is a major responsibility of the athletic training program. Some athletic trainers object to keeping records and filling out forms, stating that they have neither the time nor the inclination to be bookkeepers. Nevertheless, because lawsuits are currently the rule rather than the exception, accurate and up-to-date records are an absolute necessity. Medical records, injury reports, treatment logs, personal information cards, injury evaluations and progress notes, supply and equipment inventories, and annual reports are essential records that should be maintained by the athletic trainer.

Maintaining Confidentiality in Record Keeping

HIPAA Regulations

The Health Insurance Portability and Accountability Act (HIPAA) regulates how coaches, athletic trainers, physicians, or any other member of the sports medicine team who has private health information (PHI) about an athlete can share that information with others.[16] The regulation guarantees that athletes have access to their medical records, gives them more control over how their protected health information is used and disclosed, and provides a clear avenue of recourse if their medical privacy is compromised. Authorization by an athlete to release medical information is not necessary on a per-injury basis. A written blanket authorization signed by the athlete at the beginning of the year will suffice for all injuries and treatments done during the course of participation for that year. These one-time, blanket authorizations must indicate what information may be released, to whom, and for what length of time. *Focus Box:* "HIPAA authorization" is a list of core elements that must be present for the authorization to be valid.

Focus

HIPAA authorization

Below is a list of core elements that must be present for a disclosure authorization to be valid:

- A description of the information to be used or disclosed
- Identification of the persons or class of persons authorized to make use of or disclosure the protected health information
- Identification of the persons or class of persons to whom the covered entity is authorized to provide or disclose to
- A description of each purpose of the use or disclosure
- An expiration date or event
- The individual's signature and date
- If signed by a personal representative, a description of his or her authority to act for the individual

FERPA Regulations

The Family Educational Rights and Privacy Act (FERPA) is a law that protects the privacy of student educational records. It has been suggested that in some instances medical records should be kept along with a student's educational records and thus the right to privacy of medical records would be protected under FERPA instead of HIPAA. FERPA gives parents certain rights with respect to their children's educational records. These rights transfer to the student when he or she reaches the age of 18 or attends a school beyond the high school level. Students to whom the rights have been transferred are "eligible students." Parents or eligible students have the right to inspect and review the student's educational records maintained by the school. Parents or eligible students have the right to request that a school correct records that they believe to be inaccurate or misleading. Schools must have written permission from the parent or eligible student to release any information from a student's educational records.

Administering Preparticipation Examinations

The first piece of information that the athletic trainer should collect on each athlete is obtained from an initial preparticipation examination done prior to the start of practice. The primary purpose of the preparticipation exam is to identify an athlete who may be at risk before he or she participates in a specific sport.[14] The preparticipation examination should consist of a medical history, a physical examination, a brief orthopedic screening, and in some situations, a wellness screening.[30] Information obtained during this examination will establish a baseline to which comparisons may be made after injury. It may also reveal conditions that could warrant disqualification from certain sports.[22] The examination will also satisfy insurance and liability issues. The preparticipation exam may be administered on an individual basis by a personal physician, or it may be done using a station examination system with a team of examiners.[15]

Preparticipation health examination:

- Medical history
- Physical examination
- Maturity assessment
- Orthopedic screening
- Wellness screening

2-5

Critical Thinking **Exercise**

All-American High School offers eighteen sports, six in the fall, six in the winter, and six in the spring. There are a total of approximately 500 athletes, and approximately 200 of them are involved in the fall sports. The athletic trainer is charged with the responsibility of arranging and administering preparticipation examinations so that each athlete can be cleared for competition.

? How can the athletic trainer most efficiently set up the preparticipation exams to clear 200 athletes for competition in the fall sports?

Examination by a Personal Physician

Examination by a personal physician has the advantage of yielding an in-depth history and an ideal physician-patient relationship. A disadvantage of this type of examination is that it may not be directed to the detection of factors that predispose the athlete to a sports injury.[40]

Station Examination

The most thorough and sport-specific type of preparticipation examination is the station examination.[40] This method can provide the athlete with a detailed examination in a short period of time. A team of nine people is needed to examine thirty or more athletes. The team should include two physicians, two medically trained nonphysicians (nurse, athletic trainer, physical therapist, or physician's assistant), and five managers, athletic training students, or assistant coaches (Table 2-1).[40]

Medical History

A medical history form should be completed before the physical examination and orthopedic screening; its purpose is to identify any past or existing medical problems.[1] This form should be updated for each athlete every year. Medical histories should be closely reviewed by both the physician and the athletic trainer so that personnel may be prepared should some medical emergency arise. Necessary participation release forms and insurance information should be collected along with the medical history (Figure 2-3).[18]

Physical Examination

The physical examination should include the assessment of height, weight, body composition, blood pressure, pulse, vision, skin, dental, ear, nose, throat, heart and lung

TABLE 2-1 Suggested Components of Preparticipation Physical Examination

Station	Points Noted	Personnel
1. Individual history (reviewed); height, weight, body composition, body mass index (BMI)	"Yes" answers are probed in depth; height and weight relationships	Physician, nurse, or athletic trainer
2. Snellen test, vision	Upper limits of visual acuity—20/40	Student athletic trainer or manager
3. Oral (mouth), ears, nose, throat	Dental prosthesis or caries, abnormalities of the ears, nose, throat	Physician, nurse, or athletic trainer
4. Chest, heart, lungs	Heart abnormalities, blood pressure, pulse, murmurs, clarity of lungs	Physician
5. Abdomen	Masses, tenderness, organomegaly	Physician or physician's assistant
6. Genitalia (male only)	Abnormalities of genitalia, hernia	Physician or physician's assistant
7. Skin	Suspicious rashes or lesions	Physician or physician's assistant
8. Musculoskeletal	Postural asymmetry, decreased range of motion or strength, abnormal joint laxity	Physician, athletic trainer, physical therapist, or nurse practitioner
9. Urinalysis	After its collection in a plastic cup, urine is tested in a lab for sugar and protein	Athletic training student or manager
10. Blood work	Lab test to determine hematocrit	Nurse or physician
Review	History and physical examination reports are evaluated and the following decisions are made: (a) No sports participation (b) Limited participation (no participation in specific sports such as football or ice hockey) (c) Clearance withheld until certain conditions are met (e.g., additional tests are taken, rehabilitation is completed) (d) Full, unlimited participation is allowed	Physician and athletic trainer

function, abdomen, lymphatics, genitalia, maturation index, urinalysis, and blood work (Figure 2-4).[19]

Cardiovascular Screening

In 1996 the American Heart Association (AHA) published recommendations concerning the cardiovascular component of the preparticipation exam in competitive athletes.[23] The critical task of the preparticipation cardiac examination is identifying life-threatening conditions. Although the cardiac examination needn't involve complex tests, it must permit the recognition of abnormal heart sounds and other signs of pathology.

MEDICAL HISTORY FORM

DATE OF EXAM__________________

Name__________________ **Sex**____ **Age**____ **Date of birth**________

Grade___ **School**__________ **Sport(s)**__________

Address__________________ **Phone**________

Personal physician__________________

In case of emergency, contact

Name__________ **Relationship**________ **Phone (H)**________ **(W)**________

Explain "Yes" answers below.
Circle questions you don't know the answers to.

	Yes	No
1. Has a doctor ever denied or restricted your participation in sports for any reason?	☐	☐
2. Do you have an ongoing medical condition (like diabetes or asthma)?	☐	☐
3. Are you currently taking any prescription or nonprescription (over-the-counter) medicine or pills?	☐	☐
4. Do you have allergies to medicines, pollens, foods, or stinging insects?	☐	☐
5. Have you ever passed out or nearly passed out DURING exercise?	☐	☐
6. Have you ever passed out or nearly passed out AFTER exercise?	☐	☐
7. Have you ever had discomfort, pain, or pressure in your chest during exercise?	☐	☐
8. Does your heart race or skip beats during exercise?	☐	☐
9. Has a doctor ever told you that you have (check all that apply): ☐ High blood pressure ☐ A heart murmur ☐ High cholesterol ☐ A heart infection		
10. Has a doctor ever ordered a test for your heart? (for example, ECG, echocardiogram)	☐	☐
11. Has anyone in your family died for no apparent reason?	☐	☐
12. Does anyone in your family have a heart problem?	☐	☐
13. Has any family member or relative died of heart problems or of sudden death before age 50?	☐	☐
14. Does anyone in your family have Marfan syndrome?	☐	☐
15. Have you ever spent the night in a hospital?	☐	☐
16. Have you ever had surgery?	☐	☐
17. Have you ever had an injury, like a sprain, muscle or ligament tear, or tendonitis, that caused you to miss a practice or game? If yes, circle affected area below:	☐	☐
18. Have you had any broken or fractured bones or dislocated joints? If yes, circle below:	☐	☐
19. Have you had a bone or joint injury that required x-rays, MRI, CT, surgery, injections, rehabilitation, physical therapy, a brace, a cast, or crutches? If yes, circle below:	☐	☐

Head	Neck	Shoulder	Upper arm	Elbow	Forearm	Hand/fingers	Chest
Upper back	Lower back	Hip	Thigh	Knee	Calf/shin	Ankle	Foot/toes

	Yes	No
20. Have you ever had a stress fracture?	☐	☐
21. Have you been told that you have or have you had an x-ray for atlantoaxial (neck) instability?	☐	☐
22. Do you regularly use a brace or assistive device?	☐	☐
23. Has a doctor ever told you that you have asthma or allergies?	☐	☐
24. Do you cough, wheeze, or have difficulty breathing during or after exercise?	☐	☐
25. Is there anyone in your family who has asthma?	☐	☐
26. Have you ever used an inhaler or taken asthma medicine?	☐	☐
27. Were you born without or are you missing a kidney, an eye, a testicle, or any other organ?	☐	☐
28. Have you had infectious mononucleosis (mono) within the last month?	☐	☐
29. Do you have any rashes, pressure sores, or other skin problems?	☐	☐
30. Have you had a herpes skin infection?	☐	☐
31. Have you ever had a head injury or concussion?	☐	☐
32. Have you been hit in the head and been confused or lost your memory?	☐	☐
33. Have you ever had a seizure?	☐	☐
34. Do you have headaches with exercise?	☐	☐
35. Have you ever had numbness, tingling, or weakness in your arms or legs after being hit or falling?	☐	☐
36. Have you ever been unable to move your arms or legs after being hit or falling?	☐	☐
37. When exercising in the heat, do you have severe muscle cramps or become ill?	☐	☐
38. Has a doctor told you that you or someone in your family has sickle cell trait or sickle cell disease?	☐	☐
39. Have you had any problems with your eyes or vision?	☐	☐
40. Do you wear glasses or contact lenses?	☐	☐
41. Do you wear protective eyewear, such as goggles or a face shield?	☐	☐
42. Are you happy with your weight?	☐	☐
43. Are you trying to gain or lose weight?	☐	☐
44. Has anyone recommended you change your weight or eating habits?	☐	☐
45. Do you limit or carefully control what you eat?	☐	☐
46. Do you have any concerns that you would like to discuss with a doctor?	☐	☐
FEMALES ONLY		
47. Have you ever had a menstrual period?	☐	☐
48. How old were you when you had your first menstrual period?____		
49. How many periods have you had in the last 12 months?____		

Explain "Yes" answers here:__________________

I hereby state that, to the best of my knowledge, my answers to the above questions are complete and correct.

Signature of athlete__________ Signature of parent/guardian__________ Date______

Figure 2-3

Sample medical history examination form.

Figure 2-6

The orthopedic screening examination. Equipment that may be needed includes reflex hammer, tape measure, pin, and examining table.

Orthopedic Screening Examination

Activity and Instruction	To Determine
Stand facing examiner	Acromioclavicular joints; general habitus
Look at ceiling, floor, over both shoulders; touch ears to shoulders	Cervical spine motion
Shrug shoulders (examiner resists)	Trapezius strength
Abduct shoulders 90° (examiner resists at 90°)	Deltoid strength
Full external rotation of arms	Shoulder motion
Flex and extend elbows	Elbow motion
Arms at sides, elbows 90° flexed; pronate and supinate wrists	Elbow and wrist motion
Spread fingers; make fist	Hand or finger motion and deformities
Tighten (contract) quadriceps; relax quadriceps	Symmetry and knee effusion; ankle effusion
"Duck walk" four steps (away from examiner with buttocks on heels)	Hip, knee, and ankle motion
Stand with back to examiner	Shoulder symmetry; scoliosis
Knees straight, touch toes	Scoliosis, hip motion, hamstring tightness
Raise up on toes, raise heels	Calf symmetry, leg strength

that potentially warrant disqualification should be identified by a preparticipation examination and noted in the medical history.[28]

Injury Reports and Injury Disposition

An injury report serves as a record for future reference (Figure 2-9, page 66). If the emergency procedures followed are questioned at a later date, an athletic trainer's memory of the details may be somewhat hazy, but a report completed on the spot provides specific information. In a litigation situation, an athletic trainer may be asked questions about an injury that occurred three years in the past. All injury reports should be filed in the athletic trainer's office. One is well advised to make the reports out in triplicate so that one copy may be sent to the school health office, one to the physician, and one retained.

The Treatment Log

Each athletic training facility should have a sign-in log available for the athlete who receives any service. Emphasis is placed on recording the treatments for the athlete who is receiving daily therapy for an injury. Like accident records and injury dispositions, these records often have the status of legal documents and are used to establish certain facts in a civil litigation, an insurance action, or a criminal action after injury.

Personal Information Card

Always on file in the athletic trainer's office is the athlete's personal information card. This card is completed by the athlete at the time of the health examination and serves as a means of contacting the family, personal physician, and insurance company in case of emergency.

Injury Evaluation and Progress Notes

Injuries should be evaluated by the athletic trainer, who must record information obtained in some consistent format. The SOAP format (*S*ubjective, *O*bjective, *A*ssessment, *P*lan for treatment) is a concise method of recording the initial evaluation and progress notes for the injured athlete and is discussed in detail in Chapter 13. The subjective portion of the SOAP note refers to what the athlete tells the athletic

Orthopedic Screening Form

Name: ____________________ SS#: ____________________

FLEXIBILITY Check if Normal

Shoulder:
___ Abduction
___ Adduction
___ Flexion
___ Extension
___ Internal rot.
___ External rot.

Hip:
___ Ext. (flex knee)
___ Flex. (flex knee)
___ Ext. (str. leg)
___ Flex. (str. leg)
___ Abduction
___ Adduction

Knee:
___ Flexion
___ Extension

Ankle:
___ Dorsiflexion
___ Plantar flexion

Trunk:
___ Flexion
___ Extension
___ Rotation
___ Lat. Flexion

Joint Stability

Knee:
___ Lachman
___ Pivot shift
___ Anterior drawer
___ Posterior drawer
___ Valgus
___ Varus
___ McMurray
___ Apley's grind

Ankle:
___ Anterior drawer
___ Talor tilt

Leg Length

Posture:
___ Pelvis height
___ Shoulder height
___ Spine

Previous Injury:

Comments:

Figure 2-7

Sample of a detailed orthopedic screening examination form.

1. Circle the appropriate response for each question.
2. Add the total number of points for each section.

Behavior	Almost Always	Sometimes	Almost Never
Tobacco Use			
If you never smoke or use tobacco products, enter a score of 10 for this section and go to the next section on Alcohol and Drugs.			
1. I avoid smoking cigarettes and chewing tobacco.	2	1	0
2. I smoke only low-tar and low-nicotine cigarettes, or I smoke a pipe or cigars.	2	1	0
Tobacco Use Score: ______			
Alcohol and Drugs			
1. I avoid drinking alcoholic beverages or I drink no more than one or two a day.	4	1	0
2. I avoid using alcohol or other drugs (especially illegal drugs) as a way of handling stressful situations or problems in my life.	2	1	0
3. I am careful not to drink alcohol when taking certain medicines (e.g., medicine for sleeping, pain, colds, and allergies) or when pregnant.	2	1	0
4. I read and follow the label directions when using prescribed and over-the-counter drugs.	2	1	0
Alcohol and Drug Score: ______			
Eating Habits			
1. I eat a variety of foods each day, such as fruits and vegetables, whole grain breads and cereals, lean meats, dairy products, dry peas and beans, and nuts and seeds.	4	1	0
2. I limit my intake of fat, saturated fat, and cholesterol (including fat in meats, eggs, butter, and other dairy products, shortenings, and organ meats such as liver).	2	1	0
3. I limit the amount of salt I eat by cooking with only small amounts, not adding salt at the table, and avoiding salty snacks.	2	1	0
4. I avoid eating too much sugar (especially frequent snacks of sticky candy or soft drinks).	2	1	0
Eating Habits Score: ______			
Exercise/Fitness Habits			
1. I maintain a desired weight, avoiding overweight and underweight.	3	1	0
2. I do vigorous exercises for 15–30 minutes at least three times a week (examples include running, swimming, and brisk walking).	3	1	0
3. I do exercises that enhance my muscle tone for 15–30 minutes at least three times a week (examples include yoga and calisthenics).	2	1	0
4. I use part of my leisure time participating in individual, family, or team activities that increase my level of fitness (such as gardening, bowling, golf, and baseball).	2	1	0
Exercise/Fitness Score: ______			

	Almost Always	Sometimes	Almost Never
Stress Control			
1. I have a job or do other work that I enjoy.	2	1	0
2. I find it easy to relax and to express my feelings freely.	2	1	0
3. I anticipate and prepare for events or situations likely to be stressful for me.	2	1	0
4. I have close friends, relatives, or others with whom I can discuss personal matters and call on for help when needed.	2	1	0
5. I participate in group activities (such as church and community organizations) or hobbies that I enjoy.	2	1	0
Stress Control Score: ______			
Safety			
1. I wear a seat belt when riding in a car.	2	1	0
2. I avoid driving while under the influence of alcohol and other drugs.	2	1	0
3. I obey traffic rules and the speed limit when driving.	2	1	0
4. I am careful when using potentially harmful products or substances (such as household cleaners, poisons, and electrical devices).	2	1	0
5. I avoid smoking in bed.	2	1	0
6. I am not sexually active or I have sex with only one mutually faithful, uninfected partner, or I always engage in safe sex (using condoms), and I do not share needles to inject drugs.	2	1	0
Safety Score: ______			

What your Scores Mean

Scores of 9 and 10: Excellent. Your answers show that you are aware of the importance of this area to your health.

Scores of 6 to 8: Good. Your health practices in this area are good, but there is room for improvement.

Scores of 3 to 5: Fair. Your health risks are showing.

Scores of 0 to 2: Poor. Your answers show that you may be taking serious and unnecessary risks with your health. Perhaps you are not aware of the risks and what to do about them. You can easily get the information and help you need to improve, if you wish.

If you have questions or concerns you should consult your athletic trainers for advice.

Figure 2-8

Wellness screening questionnaire.

trainer about the injury relative to the history or what he or she felt. The objective portion documents information that the athletic trainer gathers during the evaluation, such as range of motion, strength levels, patterns of pain, and so forth. The assessment records the athletic trainer's professional opinion about the injury based on information obtained during the subjective and objective portions. The plan for treatment indicates how the injury will be managed and includes short- and long-term goals for rehabilitation.

TABLE 2-2 Recommendations for Participation in Competitive Sports

	Contact		Noncontact		
	Contact/ Collision	Limited Contact/ Collision	Strenuous	Moderately Strenuous	Nonstrenuous
Atlantoaxial instability	No	No	Yes*	Yes	Yes
*Swimming: no butterfly, breast stroke, or diving starts					
Acute illnesses	*	*	*	*	*
*Needs individual assessment (e.g., contagiousness to others, risk of worsening illness)					
Cardiovascular					
Carditis	No	No	No	No	No
Hypertension					
Mild	Yes	Yes	Yes	Yes	Yes
Moderate	*	*	*	*	*
Severe	*	*	*	*	*
Congenital heart disease	†	†	†	†	†
*Needs individual assessment †Patients with mild forms can be allowed a full range of physical activities; patients with moderate or severe forms or who are postoperative should be evaluated by a cardiologist before athletic participation.					
Eyes					
Absence or loss of function of eye	*	*	*	*	*
Detached retina	†	†	†	†	†
*Availability of American Society for Testing and Materials (ASTM)-approved eye guards may allow competitor to participate in most sports, but this must be judged on an individual basis. †Consult ophthalmologist					
Inguinal hernia	Yes	Yes	Yes	Yes	Yes
Kidney: Absence of one	No	Yes	Yes	Yes	Yes
Liver: Enlarged	No	No	Yes	Yes	Yes
Musculoskeletal disorders	*	*	*	*	*
*Needs individual assessment					
Neurologic status					
History of serious head or spine trauma, repeated concussions, or craniotomy	*	*	Yes	Yes	Yes
Convulsive disorder					
Well controlled	Yes	Yes	Yes	Yes	Yes
Poorly controlled	No	No	Yes†	Yes	Yes††
*Needs individual assessment †No swimming or weight lifting ††No archery or riflery					
Ovary: Absence of one	Yes	Yes	Yes	Yes	Yes
Respiratory status					
Pulmonary insufficiency	*	*	*	*	Yes
Asthma	Yes	Yes	Yes	Yes	Yes
*May be allowed to compete if oxygenation remains satisfactory during a graded stress test					
Sickle cell trait	Yes	Yes	Yes	Yes	Yes
Skin: Boils, herpes, impetigo, scabies	*	*	Yes	Yes	Yes
*No gymnastics with mats, martial arts, wrestling, or contact sports until not contagious					
Spleen: Enlarged	No	No	No	Yes	Yes
Testicle: Absent or undescended	Yes*	Yes*	Yes	Yes	Yes
*Certain sports may require protective cup					

Name ______ Sport ______ Date: __/__/__ Time: ____ Injury number: ______

Player I.D. ______ Age: ____ Location: ______ Intercollegiate—nonintercollegiate

Initial injury Recheck Reinjury Preseason—Practice—Game Incurred while participating in sport: yes ___ no ___

Description: How did it happen? ______

Initial impression: ______

Site of injury
1 Right
2 Left
3 Proximal
4 Distal
5 Anterior
6 Posterior
7 Medial
8 Lateral
9 Other

Site of evaluation
1 SHS
2 Athletic Trn Rm.
3 Site-Competition
4 ______

Procedures
1 Physical exam
2 X-ray
3 Splint
4 Wrap
5 Cast
6 Aspiration
7 Other

Disposition
1 SHS
2 Trainer
3 Hospital
4 H.D.
5 Other

Body part
1 Head
2 Face
3 Eye
4 Nose
5 Ear
6 Mouth
7 Neck
8 Thorax
9 Ribs
10 Sternum
11 Upper back
12 Lower back
13 Shoulder
14 Rotator cuff
15 AC joint
16 Glenohumeral
17 Sternoclavicular
18 Upper arm
19 Elbow
20 Forearm
21 Wrist
22 Hand
23 Thumb
24 Finger
25 MP joint
26 PIP joint
27 Abdomen
28 Hip
29 Thigh
30 Knee
31 Patella
32 Lower leg
33 Ankle
34 Achilles tendon
35 Foot
36 Toes
37 Other

Referral
1 Arthrogram
2 Neurological
3 Int. Med.
4 Orthropedic
5 EENT
6 Dentist
7 Other

Nontraumatic
1 Dermatological
2 Allergy
3 Influenza
4 URI
5 GU
6 Systemic infect.
7 Local infect.
8 Other

Disposition of injury
1 No part.
2 Part part.
3 Full part.

Structure
1 Skin
2 Muscle
3 Fascia
4 Bone
5 Nerve
6 Fat pad
7 Tendon
8 Ligament
9 Cartilage
10 Capsule
11 Compartment
12 Dental
13 ______

Nature of injury
1 Contusion
2 Strain
3 Sprain
4 Fracture
5 Rupture
6 Tendonitis
7 Bursitis
8 Myositis
9 Laceration
10 Concussion
11 Avulsion
12 Abrasion
13 ______

Degree
1° 2° 3°

Treatment ______

Medication ______

Prescription dispensed
1 Antibiotics
2 Antiinflammatory
3 Decongestant
4 Analgesic
5 Muscle relaxant
6 Enzyme
7 ______

Injections
1 Steroids
2 Antibiotics
3 Steriods-xylo
4 ______

Previous injury ______

Figure 2-9

Athletic injury record form.

Supply and Equipment Inventory

A major responsibility of the athletic trainer is to manage a budget, most of which is spent on equipment and supplies. Every year an inventory must be conducted and recorded on such items as new equipment needed, equipment that needs to be replaced or repaired, and the expendable supplies that need replenishing.

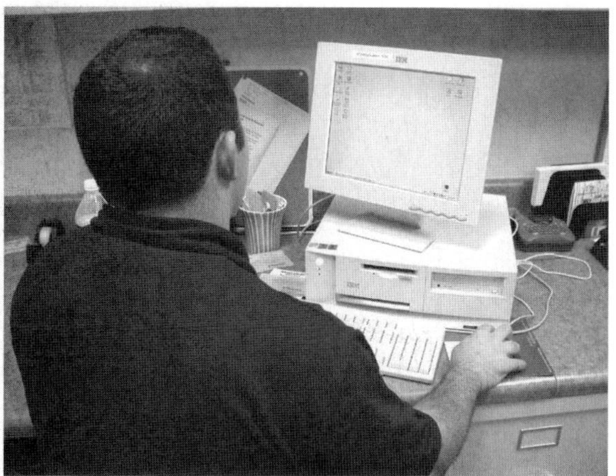

Figure 2-10

Computers are an essential tool in athletic training.

Annual Reports

Most athletic departments require an annual report on the functions of the athletic training program. This report serves as a means for making program changes and improvements. It commonly includes the number of athletes served, a survey of the number and types of injuries, an analysis of the program, and recommendations for future improvements.

Release of Medical Records

The athletic trainer may not release an athlete's medical records to anyone without written consent. If the athlete wishes to have medical records released to professional sports organizations, insurance companies, the news media, or any other group or individual, the athlete must sign a waiver that specifies which information is to be released.

2-6

***Critical Thinking* Exercise**

The athletic trainer has requested that the school purchase a new computer to be housed in the athletic training room. The administrator indicates that funds are tight; however, the athletic trainer is asked to develop a written proposal to justify the purchase.

? What information can the athletic trainer include in the request that could justify purchasing a new computer for the athletic training room?

THE COMPUTER AS A TOOL FOR THE ATHLETIC TRAINER

As is the case in all of our society, computers have become an indispensable tool for the athletic trainer and have completely revolutionized the way information is managed (Figure 2-10). It is becoming rare to find an athletic trainer working in any setting who does not have access to a computer. A great deal of information can be efficiently located and stored for immediate and future use because of constant improvement in storage and retrieval capacities. Software packages are available to help store and retrieve any type of relevant records or information.[21]

Computers facilitate the record-keeping process.

The first step in integrating computers into an athletic training program is to decide exactly how and for what purposes the computer will be used. Most athletic trainers do not have an extensive background or understanding of computer hardware. It is essential to seek advice from expert professionals or consultants prior to purchasing a system to ensure that the hardware and corresponding operating system is capable of supporting the software that will make the computer a useful information management and communication tool. Athletic trainers who work in secondary schools, universities, or in industry may have access to a mainframe computer that can be accessed from a network of connecting terminals. It is more likely that most athletic trainers will use either a desktop or personal computer (PC) or a portable laptop or notebook computer. Many athletic trainers are also using PDAs (personal digital assistants) which are fully functional computers that can be held in one hand. These devices receive, process, and store information and communicate with other computers and PDAs. Their small size and portability makes them always accessible, which is very useful for athletic trainers who don't spend a lot of time in an office.

There are thousands of software programs available that will allow the user to store, manipulate, and retrieve information; create written documents through word processing; analyze data statistically; and communicate with many individuals in a variety of forms.

Record keeping is a time-consuming but essential chore for all athletic trainers regardless of whether they work at a college or university, at a high school, in the clinical setting, or in industry. Several software packages are available specifically for managing injury records in the athletic training setting. A problem that athletic trainers must address is ensuring security and protecting the confidentiality of medical records stored on a computer. Databases that contain such information must only be accessible to the athletic trainer or team physician and must be protected by some type of password required for entry into the database.

Besides record keeping, computer software can also be used for word processing; budgeting; managing a personal schedule or calendar; or creating a database or a spreadsheet from which injury data can be organized, retrieved, or related to specific injury situations or other injury records for statistical analysis. Other software can analyze and provide information about nutrition, body composition, and injury risk profiles based on other anthropometric measures and can be used to record isokinetic evaluation and exercise.[25]

The use of educational software to assist in teaching and the academic preparation of athletic training students has become an integral component in the majority of athletic training educational programs. New instructional and educational software continues to become available, and the use of CD-R and DVD technologies with their interactive capabilities, has made the multimedia presentation of instructional material, and thus learning, more interesting and memorable for the student.

The Internet and the World Wide Web have impacted and changed all of our lives. We live in a world where virtually any kind of information is immediately accessible to anyone who knows how to use the system. The sports medicine community in general and the athletic trainer specifically can access websites that have direct application to our clinical practice, to the education of athletic training students, and to the general base of knowledge that is relevant to our field. The use of e-mail to share information and to communicate immediately with colleagues has created an indispensable tool that has revolutionized our daily lives.

2-7

***Critical Thinking* Exercise**

A basketball coach at All-American High School is concerned about what seems to be an abnormally high frequency of ankle sprains on her varsity team. Her philosophy is to require all her players to wear high-top shoes, yet the budget will not permit all players' ankles to be taped by the athletic trainer for practices and games. Together the coach and athletic trainer decide to purchase a number of lace-up ankle braces in an attempt to reduce the number of ankle sprains.

? How can the athletic trainer determine if the braces are helping decrease the frequency of ankle sprains in these basketball players?

COLLECTING INJURY DATA

Because of the vast number of physically active individuals involved with organized and recreational sports, some knowledge relative to the number and types of injuries sustained during participation in these activities is essential. Although methods are much improved over the past, many weaknesses exist in systematic data collection and analysis of sports injuries.[27]

The Incidence of Injuries

accident
An act that occurs by chance or without intention.

injury
An act that damages or hurts.

The epidemiological approach toward injury data collection provides the most information.

Risk of injury is determined by the type of sport—collision, contact, or noncontact.

An **accident** is defined as an unplanned event capable of resulting in loss of time, property damage, injury, disablement, or even death.[31] An **injury** may be defined as damage to the body that restricts activity or causes disability to such an extent that the athlete is not able to practice or compete the next day.[31] There is little doubt that a *case study* approach, which looks at one single incidence of an injury, can yield some critical information about the cause and subsequent efficacy of treatment for that particular injury. However, an approach that analyzes a large number of similar injuries can provide the greatest amount of information. In general, the incidence of sports injuries can be studied epidemiologically from many points of view—in terms of age at occurrence, gender, body regions that sustain injuries, or the occurrence in different sports. Sports are usually classified according to the risk, or chances, of injuries occurring under similar circumstances and are broadly divided into contact or collision, limited contact, or noncontact[4] (Table 2-3).

Athletes in all sports, recreational and organized, who participate in sports in the span of one year face a 50 percent chance of sustaining some injury. Of the 50 million estimated sports injuries per year, 50 percent require only minor care and no restriction

TABLE 2-3 Classification of Sports*

Contact or Collision	Limited Contact	Noncontact
Basketball	Baseball	Archery
Boxing	Bicycling	Badminton
Diving	Cheerleading	Body building
Field hockey	Canoeing or kayaking (white water)	Bowling
Football (tackle)	Fencing	Canoeing or kayaking (flat water)
Ice hockey	Field events	Crew or rowing
Lacrosse	High jump	Curling
Martial arts	Pole vault	Dancing (ballet, modern, Jazz)
Rodeo	Floor hockey	Field events
Rugby	Football (flag)	Discus
Ski jumping	Gymnastics	Javelin
Soccer	Handball	Shot put
Team handball	Horseback riding	Golf
Water polo	Racquetball	Orienteering
Wrestling	Skating (ice, in-line, roller)	Power lifting
	Skiing (cross-country, downhill, water)	Race walking
	Skateboarding	Riflery
	Snowboarding	Rope jumping
	Softball	Running
	Squash	Sailing
	Ultimate frisbee	Scuba diving
	Volleyball	Swimming
	Windsurfing or surfing	Table tennis
		Tennis
		Track
		Weight lifting

*From the American Academy of Pediatrics Committee on Sports Medicine and Fitness: Medical conditions affecting sports participation, *Pediatrics* 107(5):1205, 2001.

of activity.[9] Approximately 90 percent of injuries are muscle contusions, ligament sprains, and muscle strains; however, 10 percent of these injuries lead to microtrauma complications and eventually to a severe, chronic condition in later life.

Of the sports injuries that must be medically treated, sprains or strains, fractures, dislocations, and contusions are the most common.[8] In terms of the body regions most often injured, the knee has the highest incidence, with the ankle second and the upper limb third. For both males and females the most commonly injured body part is the knee, followed by the ankle; however, males have a much higher incidence of shoulder and upper-arm injuries than do females.

Catastrophic Injuries

Although millions of individuals participate in organized and recreational sports, there is a relatively low incidence of fatalities or catastrophic injuries. Ninety-eight percent of individuals with injuries requiring hospital emergency room medical attention are treated and released.[30] Deaths have been attributed to chest or trunk impact with thrown objects, other players, or nonyielding objects (e.g., goalposts). Deaths have occurred when players were struck in the head by sports implements (bats, golf clubs, hockey sticks) or by missiles (baseballs, soccer balls, golf balls, hockey pucks). Death has also resulted when an individual received a direct blow to the head from another player or the ground. On record are a number of sports deaths in which a playing structure, such as a goalpost or backstop, fell on a participant.

The highest incidence of indirect sports death stems from heatstroke. Less common indirect causes include cardiovascular and respiratory problems or congenital conditions not previously known. Catastrophic injuries leading to cervical injury and quadriplegia are seen mainly in American football. Although the incidence is low for the number of players involved, it could be lowered even further if more precautions were taken.

In most popular organized and recreational sports activities, the legs and arms have the highest risk factor for injury, with the head and face next. Muscle strains, joint sprains, contusions, and abrasions are the most frequent injuries sustained by the active sports participant. The major goal of this text is to provide the reader with the fundamental principles necessary for preventing and managing illnesses and injuries common to the athlete.

Current National Injury Data-Gathering Systems

The state of the art of sports injury surveillance is at this time unsatisfactory.[6] Currently, most local, state, and federal systems are concerned with the accident or injury only after it has happened, and they focus on injuries requiring medical assistance or those that cause time loss or restricted activity.

The ideal system takes an epidemiological approach that studies the relationship of various factors that influence the frequency and distribution of sports injuries.[23] When considering the risks inherent in a particular sport, both extrinsic and intrinsic factors must be studied.[34] Thus information is gleaned from both epidemiological data and the individual measurements of the athlete. The term *extrinsic factor* refers to the type of activity that is performed, the amount of exposure to injury, factors in the environment, and the equipment. The term *intrinsic factor* refers directly to the athlete and includes age, gender, neuromuscular aspects, structural aspects, performance aspects, and mental and psychological aspects.

Over the years, a number of athletic injury surveillance systems have been implemented; most have collected data for a few years and then ceased to exist. The currently active systems that are most often mentioned are the National Safety Council, the Annual Survey of Football Injury Research, the NCAA Injury Surveillance System, the National Center for Catastrophic Sports Injury Research, the National Electronic Injury Surveillance System (NEISS).

National Safety Council

The National Safety Council* is a nongovernmental, nonprofit public service organization. It draws sports injury data from a variety of sources, including educational institutions.

Annual Survey of Football Injury Research

In 1931 the American Football Coaches Association (AFCA) conducted its first Annual Survey of Football Fatalities. Since 1965 this research has been conducted at the University of North Carolina. In 1980 the survey's title was changed to Annual Survey of Football Injury Research. Every year, with the exception of 1942, data have been collected about public school, college, professional, and sandlot football. Information is gathered through personal contact interviews and questionnaires.[20] The sponsoring organizations of this survey are the AFCA, the NCAA, and the National Federation of State High School Athletic Associations (NFSHSAA).

This survey classifies football fatalities as direct or indirect. Direct fatalities are those resulting directly from participation in football. Indirect fatalities are produced by systemic failure caused by the exertion of playing football or by a complication that arose from a nonfatal football injury.

*National Safety Council, 1121 Spring Lake Drive, Itasca, IL 60143-1121.

National Center for Catastrophic Sports Injury Research

In 1977 the NCAA initiated the National Survey of Catastrophic Football Injuries. As a result of the injury data collected from this organization, several significant rule changes have been incorporated into collegiate football. Because of the success of this football project, the research was expanded to all sports for both men and women, and a National Center for Catastrophic Sports Injury Research was established at the University of North Carolina under the direction of Dr. Fred Mueller. With support from the NCAA, the NFSHSAA, the AFCA, and the Section on Sports Medicine of the American Association of Neurological Sciences, this center compiles data on catastrophic injuries at all levels of sport.[27]

NCAA Injury Surveillance System

The NCAA Injury Surveillance System (ISS) was established in 1982 primarily for the purpose of studying the incidence of football injuries so that rule change recommendations could be made to reduce the injury rate. Since that time this system has been greatly expanded and now collects data on most major sports. For the most part, athletic trainers are primarily involved in the collection and transmission of injury data.

The ISS has relied on the willingness of athletic trainers to submit paper forms reporting injuries in various NCAA-sponsored sports. In fall of 2004 the ISS will fully convert to a Web-based data-collection system that can compile far more data than ever before, providing member institutions with a low-cost means of tracking medical information and analyzing injury trends.

National Electronic Injury Surveillance System

In 1972 the federal government established the Consumer Product Safety Act (CPSA), which created and granted broad authority to the Consumer Product Safety Commission to enforce the safety standards for more than 10,000 products that may be risky to the consumer.[8] To perform this mission, the National Electronic Injury Surveillance System (NEISS)** was established. Data on injuries related to consumer products are monitored twenty-four hours a day from a selected sample of 5,000 hospital emergency rooms nationwide. Sports injuries represent 25 percent of all injuries reported by NEISS. It should be noted that a product may be related to an injury but not be the direct cause of that injury.

Once a product is considered hazardous, the commission can seize the product or create standards to decrease the risk.[8] Also, manufacturers and distributors of sports recreational equipment must report to the commission any product that is potentially hazardous or defective.[8] The commission can also research the reasons that a sports or recreational product is hazardous.

2-8

***Critical Thinking* Exercise**

A collegiate athletic trainer is approached by the school administration to determine the potential risk of injury to their football team.

? What approach is best suited to gather this information?

Using Injury Data

Valid, reliable sports injury data can materially help decrease injuries. If properly interpreted, the data can be used to modify rules, assist coaches and players in understanding risks, and help manufacturers evaluate their products against the overall market.[31] The public, especially parents, should understand the risks inherent in a particular sport, and insurance companies that insure athletes must know risks in order to set reasonable costs.

SUMMARY

- The administration of a program of health care for the athlete demands a significant portion of the athletic trainer's time and effort. The efficiency and success of the athletic training program depend in large part on the administrative abilities of the athletic trainer in addition to the clinical skills required to treat the injured athlete.

**National Electronic Injury Surveillance System, U.S. Consumer Product Safety Commission, Directorate for Epidemiology, National Injury Information Clearinghouse, Washington, DC.

- The athletic training program may best serve the athlete, the institution, and the community by establishing specific policies and regulations governing the use of available services.
- Budgets should allow for the purchase of equipment and supplies essential for providing appropriate preventive and rehabilitative care for the athlete.
- The athletic training program can certainly be enhanced by designing or renovating a facility to maximize the potential use of the space available. Space designed for injury treatment, rehabilitation, modality use, office space, physician examination, record keeping, and storage of supplies should be designated within each facility.
- Preparticipation exams must be given to athletes and should include a medical history, a general physical examination, and orthopedic screenings.
- The athletic trainer must maintain accurate and up-to-date medical records in addition to the other paperwork that is necessary for the operation of the athletic training program.
- Computers are extremely useful tools that enable athletic trainers to retrieve and store a variety of records.
- A number of data collection systems tabulate the incidence of sports injuries. The systems mentioned most often are the National Safety Council, the Annual Survey of Football Injury Research, the National Electronic Injury Surveillance System, the NCAA Injury Surveillance System, and the National Center for Catastrophic Sports Injury Research.

Solutions to Critical Thinking EXERCISES

2-1 The athletic trainer should work in conjunction with the appropriate administrative personnel to develop a risk management plan that includes security issues, fire safety, electrical and equipment safety, and emergency injury management.

2-2 Federal law mandates specific policies for recruitment, hiring, and firing. All qualified applicants should receive equal consideration regardless of their race, gender, religion, or nationality. The head athletic trainer must strictly adhere to these mandates.

2-3 The athletic training room should have specific areas designated for taping and preparation, treatment and rehabilitation, and hydrotherapy. It should have an office for the athletic trainer and adequate storage facilities positioned within the space to allow for an efficient traffic flow. Equipment purchases might include four or five treatment tables and two or three taping tables (these could be made in-house, if possible), a large-capacity ice machine, a combination ultrasound/electrical stimulating unit, a whirlpool, and various free weights and exercise tubing.

2-4 It is important that the school principal, the athletic director, and the athletic trainer set policy regarding who may and who may not use the athletic training facility. It would seem that an additional demand created by such a request would be too much for the school to absorb, both in terms of the physical facility and the personnel. It is likely that accommodating this request would interfere with the day-to-day operation of the athletic training program.

2-5 The preparticipation examination should consist of a medical history, a physical examination, and a brief orthopedic screening. The preparticipation physical may be effectively administered using a station examination system with a team of examiners. A station examination can provide the athlete with a detailed examination in a short period of time. A team of people is needed to examine this many athletes. The team should include several physicians, medically trained nonphysicians (nurses, athletic trainers, physical therapists, or physician's assistants), and managers, athletic training students, or assistant coaches.

2-6 The athletic trainer should explain that the computer can be used for maintaining medical records, doing word processing, planning a budget, managing a personal schedule or calendar, and creating a database containing injury data that can be organized, retrieved, or related to specific injury situations or to other injury records for analysis. Additional software can provide the athletic trainer with analysis and information about nutrition, body composition, and injury risk profiles. The computer could also be used for e-mail and for accessing information from the Internet.

2-7 The athletic trainer should do a simple study in which one-half of the players are randomly placed in the ankle braces while the other half continue to play in their high-top shoes. By comparing the number of ankle injuries in the group wearing the braces with those in the group without the braces, the athletic trainer can make some decision as to the effectiveness of the braces in preventing ankle injuries. Collecting and analyzing injury data is helpful in determining the efficacy of many of the techniques used by the athletic trainer.

2-8 The NCAA Injury surveillance system would best suit this purpose. This system of information can also be used to prevent injuries by presenting information to coaches, referees, and administrators to enforce necessary changes to the football program.

REVIEW QUESTIONS AND CLASS ACTIVITIES

1. What are the major administrative functions that an athletic trainer must perform?
2. Design two athletic training facilities—one for a high school and one for a large university.
3. Observe the activities in the athletic training facility. Pick both a slow time and a busy time to observe.
4. Why do hygiene and sanitation play an important role in athletic training? How should the athletic training facility be maintained?
5. Fully equip a new medium-size high school, college, or clinical athletic training facility. Pick equipment from current catalogs.
6. Establish a reasonable budget for a small high school, a large high school, and a large college or university.
7. Identify the groups or individuals to be served in the athletic training facility.
8. Organize a preparticipation health examination for ninety football players.
9. Record keeping is a major function in athletic training. What records are necessary to keep? How can a computer help?
10. Debate what conditions constitute good grounds for medical disqualification from a sport.
11. Discuss the epidemiological approach to recording sports injury data.

REFERENCES

1. Abdenour TE, Weir NJ: Medical assessment of the prospective student athlete, *Ath Train* 21:122, 1986.
2. American Academy of Pediatrics Committee on Sports Medicine and Fitness: Medical conditions affecting sports participation, *Pediatrics* 107(5):1205, 2001.
3. American Academy of Pediatrics Policy Statement: Recommendations for participation in competitive sports, *Physician Sportsmed* 16(5):51, 1988.
4. American Academy of Pediatrics: *Sports medicine: health care for young athletes,* Elk Grove Village, Ill, 1991, American Academy of Pediatrics.
5. Anderson J, Courson R, Kleiner D, McLoda T: National Athletic Trainers Association Position Statement: Emergency planning in athletics. *J Ath Train* 37(1):99, 2002.
6. Bagnall D: Budget planning key in secondary schools, *NATA News.* January, 15, 2001.
7. Caine DJ, Broekhoff J: Maturity assessment: a viable preventive measure against physical and psychological insult to the young athlete? *Physician Sportsmed* 15(3):67, 1987.
8. Damron CF: Injury surveillance systems for sports. In Vinger PF, Hoerner EF, editors: *Sports injuries,* Boston, 1986, Year Book Medical Publishers.
9. Dean CH, Hoerner EF: Injury rates in team sports and individual recreation. In Vinger PF, Hoerner EF, editors: *Sports injuries,* Boston, 1986, Year Book Medical Publishers.
10. Dorsen PJ: Should athletes with one eye, kidney, or testicle play contact sports? *Physician Sportsmed* 14(7):130, 1986.
11. Doyle M: A new dimension for the athletic training room: the spirit of the room. *Athletic Therapy Today* 7(1):34, 2002.
12. Equal Opportunity Commission: *Uniform guidelines on employee selection procedures,* Washington, DC, 1979, Bureau of National Affairs.
13. Forseth EA: Consideration in planning small college athletic training facilities, *Ath Train* 21(1):22, 1986.
14. Herbert D: Professional considerations related to conduct of preparticipation exams, *Sports Med Stand Malpract Report* 6(4):49, 1994.
15. Hunt V: A general look at the preparticipation exam, *NATA News,* May, 15, 2002.
16. Hunt V: Meeting clarifies HIPAA restrictions, *NATA News,* February, 10, 2003.
17. Jones D: HIPAA: friend or foe to athletic trainers? *Athletic Therapy Today* 8(2):17, 2003.
18. Jones R: The preparticipation, sport-specific athletic profile examination, *Semin Adolesc Med* 3:169, 1987.
19. Kibler W: *The sports participation fitness examination,* Champaign, Ill, 1990, Human Kinetics.
20. Knells S: Leadership and management techniques and principles for athletic training, *J Ath Train* 29(4):328, 1994.
21. Koester M, Amundson C: Preparticipation screening of high school athletes: are recommendations enough? *Physician Sportsmed* 31(8): 330, 2003
22. Konin J, Donley P: The athletic trainer as a personnel manager. In Konin J: *The clinical athletic trainer,* Gaithersburg, Md, 1997, Slack.
23. McGrew CA: Insights into the AHA scientific statement concerning cardiovascular preparticipation screening of competitive athletes, *Medicine and science in sports and exercise* 30(10 Suppl.):S351, 1998.
24. McKeag DB: Preseason physical examination for the prevention of sports injuries, *Sports Med* 2:413, 1985.
25. Moss RI: Facilities and foibles. *Athletic Therapy Today* 7(1):22, 2002.
26. Moyer-Knowles J: Planning a new athletic facility. In Konin J: *The clinical athletic trainer,* Gaithersburg, Md, 1997, Slack.
27. Mueller F: Catastrophic sports injuries. In Mueller F, Ryan A: *Prevention of athletic injuries: the role of the sports medicine team,* Philadelphia, 1991, Davis.
28. Myers GC, Garrick JG: The preseason examination of school and college athletes. In Strauss RH, editor: *Sports medicine,* Philadelphia, 1984, Saunders.
29. Peterson E: Insult to injury: feeling understaffed, underequipped and undervalued, athletic trainers say minimum of space and equipment will yield extensive benefits, *Athletic Business* 23(1):57, 1999.
30. Physician and Sportsmedicine: preparticipation physical evaluation monograph, ed 3, New York, 2004, McGraw-Hill.
31. Powell J: Epidemiologic research for injury prevention programs in sports. In Mueller F, Ryan A: *Prevention of athletic injuries: the role of the sports medicine team,* Philadelphia, 1991, Davis.
32. Rankin J: Technology and sports health care administration, *Athletic Therapy Today* 2(5):14, 1997.
33. Rankin J: Financial resources for conducting athletic training programs in the collegiate and high school settings, *J Ath Train* 27(4):344, 1992.
34. Rankin J, Ingersoll C: *Athletic training management: concepts and applications,* St Louis, 2000, Mosby.
35. Ray R: *Management strategies in athletic training,* Champaign, Ill, 2000, Human Kinetics.
36. Sabo J: Athletic training room design and layout, in Proceedings, National Athletic Trainers' Association 50th Annual Meeting and Clinical Symposium, June 16–19, 1999, Kansas City, Mo, Human Kinetics, 1999.
37. Sabo J: Design and construction of an athletic training facility, *NATA News,* May, 10, 2001.
38. Steiner G: *Strategic planning,* New York, 1979, Free Press.
39. Streator S: Risk management in athletic training. *Athletic Therapy Today* 6(2):55, 2001.
40. Swander H: *Preparticipation physical examination,* Kansas City, 1992, American Academy of Family Physicians, American Academy of Pediatrics, American Orthopedic Society for Sports Medicine, American Osteopathic Academy for Sports Medicine.
41. Tanner M: *Growth of adolescence,* ed 2, Oxford, England, 1962, Blackwell Scientific Publications.
42. Thompson PD, Sherman C: Cardiovascular screening: tailoring the preparticipation exam, *Physician Sportsmed* 24(6):47, 1996.
43. Wikston DL et al: The effectiveness of an interactive computer program versus traditional lecture in athletic training education, *J Ath Train* 33(3):238, 1998.

ANNOTATED BIBLIOGRAPHY

Konin J: *The clinical athletic trainer,* Gaithersburg, Md, 1997, Slack.

A unique, practical book that specifically addresses the administration of a health care program for athletic trainers working in a clinical setting.

Konin J, Frederick M: Documentation for Athletic Training, Thoroughfare, NJ, 2005, Slack Incorporated.

This text presents the basic principles of medical documentation, various styles of writing, legal considerations, documentation for reimbursement and many types of written documentation including evaluations, injury reports, medical releases, etc.

Rankin J, Ingersoll C: *Athletic training management: concepts and applications,* St Louis, 2000, Mosby.

Designed for upper-division undergraduate or graduate students interested in all aspects of organization and administration of an athletic training program.

Ray R: *Management strategies in athletic training,* Champaign, Ill, 2000, Human Kinetics.

The first text that covered the principles of organization and administration as they apply to many different employment settings in athletic training; contains many examples and case studies based on principles of administration presented in the text.

Legal Concerns and Insurance Issues

Chapter 3

When you finish this chapter you should be able to

- Analyze the legal considerations for the athletic trainer acting as a health care provider.
- Define the legal concepts of torts, negligence, and assumption of risk.
- Identify measures that can be taken by both the coach and the athletic trainer to minimize the chances of litigation.
- Explain product liability.
- Categorize the essential insurance requirements for the protection of the athlete.
- Classify the types of insurance necessary to protect the athletic trainer who is acting as a health care provider.

LEGAL CONCERNS OF THE COACH AND ATHLETIC TRAINER

In recent years negligence suits against teachers, coaches, athletic trainers, school officials, and physicians arising out of sports injuries have increased both in frequency and in the amount of damages awarded.[10,32] An increasing awareness of the many risk factors present in physical activities has had a major effect on the athletic trainer in particular.[14] **Liability** means being legally responsible for the harm one causes another person.[20] A great deal of care must be taken in following athletic training procedures to reduce the risk of being sued by an athlete and being found liable for negligence.[2,25,26]

liability The state of being legally responsible for the harm one causes another person.

The Standard of Reasonable Care

Negligence is the failure to use ordinary or reasonable care—care that persons would normally exercise to avoid injury to themselves or to others under similar circumstances.[15] The *standard of reasonable care* assumes that an individual is neither exceptionally skillful nor extraordinarily cautious, but is a person of reasonable and ordinary prudence. Put another way, it is expected that an individual will bring a commonsense approach to the situation at hand and will exercise due care in its handling. In most cases in which someone has been sued for negligence, the actions of a hypothetical, reasonably prudent person are compared with the actions of the defendant to ascertain whether the course of action followed by the defendant was in conformity with the judgment exercised by such a reasonably prudent person.[24]

negligence The failure to use ordinary or reasonable care.

The standard of reasonable care requires that an athletic trainer will act according to the standard of care of an individual with similar educational background or training.[12] An athletic trainer who has many years of experience, who is well educated in his or her field, and who is certified or licensed must act in accordance with those qualifications.

To establish negligence, an individual making the complaint must establish three things: (a) a **duty of care** existed between the person injured and the person responsible for that injury, (b) conduct of the defendant fell short of that duty of care, and (c) resultant damages.[22]

duty of care Part of official job description

Torts

torts
Legal wrongs committed against a person.

Torts are legal wrongs committed against the person or property of another.[20] Every person is expected to conduct themselves without injuring others. When they do so, either intentionally or by negligence, they can be required by a court to pay money to the injured party ("damages") so that, ultimately, they will suffer the pain caused by their action. A tort also serves as a deterrent by sending a message to the community as to what is unacceptable conduct.

nonfeasance (or an act of omission)
When an individual fails to perform a legal duty.

malfeasance (or an act of commission)
When an individual commits an act that is not legally his to perform.

misfeasance
When an individual improperly does something they have the legal right to do.

Such wrongs may emanate from **nonfeasance** (also referred to as an *act of omission*), wherein the individual fails to perform a legal duty; from **malfeasance** (also referred to as an *act of commission*), wherein an individual commits an act that is not legally his or hers to perform; or from **misfeasance,** wherein an individual improperly does something that he or she has the legal right to do. In any instance, if injury results, the person can be held liable. In the case of nonfeasance, a coach or athletic trainer may fail to refer a seriously injured athlete for the proper medical attention. In the case of malfeasance, the coach or athletic trainer may perform a medical treatment that is not within his or her legal province and from which serious medical complications develop. In a case of misfeasance, the coach or athletic trainer may incorrectly administer a first aid procedure he or she has been trained to perform.

Negligence

When an athletic trainer is sued by an athlete, the complaint typically is for the tort of negligence. Negligence is alleged when an individual (1) does something that a reasonably prudent person would not do or (2) fails to do something that a reasonably prudent person would do under circumstances similar to those shown by the evidence.[3] To be successful in a suit for negligence, an athlete must prove that the athletic trainer had a *duty* to exercise reasonable care, that the athletic trainer *breached* that duty by failing to use reasonable care, and that there is a reasonable connection between the failure to use reasonable care and the injury suffered by the athlete or that the athletic trainer's action made the injury worse. If the athletic trainer breaches a duty to exercise reasonable care, but there is no reasonable connection between the failure to use reasonable care and the injury suffered by the athlete, the athlete's suit for negligence will not succeed.

3-1 Critical Thinking Exercise

A baseball batter was struck with a pitched ball directly in the orbit of the right eye and fell immediately to the ground. The athletic trainer ran to the player to examine the eye. There was some immediate swelling and discoloration around the orbit, but the eye appeared to be normal. The player insisted that he was fine and told the trainer he could continue to bat. After the game the athletic trainer told the athlete to go back to his room, put ice on his eye, and check in tomorrow. That night the baseball player began to hemorrhage into the anterior chamber of the eye and suffered irreparable damage to his eye. An ophthalmologist stated that if the athlete's eye had been examined immediately after the injury, the bleeding could have been controlled and there would not have been any damage to his vision.

? If the athlete brings a lawsuit against the athletic trainer, what must the athlete prove if he is to win a judgment?

An example of negligence is when an athletic trainer, through improper or careless handling of a therapeutic agent, seriously burns an athlete. Another illustration, occurring all too often in sports, is one in which a coach or an athletic trainer moves a possibly seriously injured athlete from the field of play to permit competition or practice to continue and does so either in an improper manner or before consulting those qualified to know the proper course of action. Should a serious or disabling injury result, the coach or the athletic trainer may be found liable. Liability is the state of being legally responsible for the harm one causes another person.[20]

Athletic trainers employed by an institution have a duty to provide athletic training care to athletes at that institution. An athletic trainer who is employed by the public schools or by a state-funded college or university may be protected by the legal doctrine of **sovereign immunity,** which essentially states that neither the government nor any individual who is employed by the government can be held liable for negligence. However, it should be made clear that the level of protection afforded by sovereign immunity may vary significantly from state to state. Clinical athletic trainers have a greater choice than institutional trainers of whom they may choose to treat as a patient. Once the athletic trainer assumes the duty of caring for an athlete, the athletic trainer has made an obligation to make sure that appropriate care is given. It should be made clear that the athletic trainer, or any other person, is not obligated to provide first aid care for an injured person outside their scope of employment. However, if they choose to become involved as a caregiver for an injured person, they are expected to provide reasonable care consistent with their level of training. The **Good Samaritan law** has been enacted in most states to provide limited protection against legal liability to any individual who voluntarily chooses to provide first aid, should something go wrong. As long as the first aid provider does not overstep the limits of his or her professional training, and exercises what would be considered reasonable care in the situation, the provider will not be held liable.

A person possessing more training in a given field or area is expected to possess a correspondingly higher level of competence than, for example, a student is.[16] An individual will therefore be judged in terms of his or her performance in any situation in which legal liability may be assessed. It must be recognized that liability per se in all its various aspects is not assessed at the same level nationally but varies in interpretation from state to state and from area to area. Athletic trainers therefore should know and acquire the level of competence expected in their particular area. In essence, negligence is conduct that results in the creation of an unreasonable risk of harm to others.[31]

Sovereign immunity
States that neither the government nor any individual who is employed by the government can be held liable for negligence.

Good Samaritan law
Provides limited protection against legal liability to any person who voluntarily chooses to provide first aid.

Statutes of Limitation

A *statute of limitation* sets a specific length of time that individuals may sue for damages from negligence. The length of time to bring suit varies from state to state, but in general plaintiffs have between one and three years to file suit for negligence. The statute of limitations begins to run on a plaintiff's time to file a lawsuit for negligence either from the time of the negligent act or omission that gives rise to the suit or from the time of the discovery of an injury caused by the negligent act or omission. Some states permit an injured minor to file suit up to three years after the minor reaches the age of eighteen. Therefore, an injured minor athlete's cause of action for negligence against an athletic trainer remains valid for many years after the negligent act or omission occurred or after the discovery of an injury caused by the negligent act or omission.

3-2 Critical Thinking Exercise

? How should the first-aid care provided by a certified athletic trainer differ from the care that may be provided by a lay person?

Assumption of Risk

An athlete assumes the risk of participating in an activity when he or she knows of and understands the dangers of that activity and voluntarily chooses to be exposed to those dangers. An assumption of risk can be expressed in the form of a waiver signed by an athlete or his or her parents or guardian or can be implied from the conduct of an athlete under the circumstances of his or her participation in an activity.

Assumption of risk may be asserted as a defense to a negligence suit brought by an injured athlete. The athletic trainer bears the burden of proving that an athlete assumed the risk by producing the document signed by the athlete or his or her parents or guardian or by proving that the athlete knew the risk of the activity and understood and voluntarily accepted that risk.

Assumption of risk, however, is subject to many and varied interpretations by courts, especially when a minor is involved, because he or she is not considered able to render a mature judgment about the risks inherent in the situation. Although athletes participating in a sports program are considered to assume a normal risk, this assumption in no way excuses those in charge from exercising reasonable care and prudence in the conduct of such activities or from foreseeing and taking precautionary measures against accident-provoking circumstances. In general, courts have been fairly consistent in upholding waivers and releases of liability for adults unless there is evidence of fraud, misrepresentation, or duress.[20]

assumption of risk
The individual, through express or implied agreement, assumes that some risk or danger will be involved in the particular undertaking. In other words, a person takes his or her own chances.

Reducing the Risk of Litigation

The coach or athletic trainer can significantly decrease the risk of litigation by paying attention to several key points.[18] The coach should follow these guidelines:

1. Warn athletes of the potential dangers inherent in their sports.[6]
2. Supervise regularly and attentively.
3. Properly prepare and condition athletes.
4. Properly instruct athletes in the skills of their sports.
5. Ensure that proper and safe equipment and facilities are used by athletes at all times.[7]

3-3 Critical Thinking Exercise

A college athletic trainer is cleaning out a filing cabinet and decides to throw some older medical files away. Concern is expressed, however, about how long these files should be maintained for legal purposes.

? What is the statute of limitations for a college-age athlete to file suit?

The athletic trainer should do as follows:

1. Work to establish good personal relationships with athletes, parents, and coworkers.
2. Establish specific policies and guidelines for the operation of an athletic training facility, and maintain qualified and adequate supervision of the training room, its environs, facilities, and equipment at all times.
3. Develop and carefully follow an emergency plan.
4. Become familiar with the health status and medical history of the athletes under his or her care so as to be aware of problems that could present a need for additional care or caution.
5. Keep factually accurate and timely records that document all injuries and rehabilitation steps, and set up a record retention policy that allows records to be kept and used in defense of litigation that may be brought by athletes. A record retention system needs to keep records for long enough to defend against suits brought by athletes after they reach the age of eighteen.
6. Document efforts to create a safe playing environment.
7. Have a detailed job description in writing.
8. Obtain, from athletes and from parents or guardians when minors are involved, written consent for providing health care.
9. Maintain the confidentiality of medical records.
10. Exercise extreme caution in the administration, if allowed by law, of nonprescription medications; athletic trainers may not dispense prescription drugs.
11. Use only those therapeutic methods that he or she is qualified to use and that the law states may be used.
12. Not use or permit the presence of faulty or hazardous equipment.
13. Work cooperatively with the coach and the team physician in the selection and use of sports protective equipment, and insist that the best equipment be obtained, properly fitted, and properly maintained.
14. Not permit injured players to participate unless cleared by the team physician. Players suffering a head injury should not be permitted to reenter the game. In some states a player who has suffered a concussion may not continue in the sport for the balance of the season.
15. Develop an understanding with the coaches that an injured athlete will not be allowed to reenter competition until, in the opinion of the team physician or the athletic trainer, he or she is psychologically and physically able. Athletic trainers should not allow themselves to be pressured to clear an athlete until he or she is fully cleared by the physician.
16. Follow the express orders of the team physician at all times.
17. Purchase professional liability insurance that provides adequate financial coverage and be aware of the limitations of the policy.
18. Know the limitations of his or her expertise as well as the applicable state regulations and restrictions that limit the athletic trainer's scope of practice.
19. Use common sense in making decisions about an athlete's health and safety.

In the case of an injury, the athletic trainer must use reasonable care to prevent additional injury until further medical care is obtained.[19] (See Chapter 12 for additional comments.)

Product Liability

Product liability refers to the liability of any or all parties along the chain of manufacture of any product for damage caused by that product.[17] This includes the manufacturer of component parts, an assembling manufacturer, the wholesaler, and the retail store owner. Products containing inherent defects that cause harm to a consumer of the product, or someone to whom the product was loaned, given, etc., are the subjects of product liability suits. Product liability claims can be based on negligence, strict liability, or breach of warranty of fitness, depending on the jurisdiction within which the claim is based. Many states have enacted comprehensive product liability statutes and these statutory provisions can be very diverse. There is no federal product liability law.

Manufacturers of athletic equipment have a duty to design and produce equipment that will not cause injury as long as it is used as intended. Manufacturers are strictly liable for defects in the design and production of equipment that produces injury. This does not excuse the athletic trainer who misuses the equipment, only equipment that is faulty. An athletic trainer must not alter the equipment in any way. To do so invalidates the manufacturer's warranty and places liability solely on the athletic trainer. An express warranty is the manufacturer's written statement that a product is safe. For example warning labels on football helmets inform the player of possible dangers inherent in using the product. Athletes must read and sign a form indicating that they have read and understand the warning. The National Operating Committee on Standards for Athletic Equipment (NOCSAE) establishes minimum standards for football helmets that must be met to ensure its safety.

INSURANCE CONSIDERATIONS

During the past forty years the insurance industry has undergone a significant evolutionary process. Health care reform initiated in the 1990s has focused on the concept of *managed care,* in which the costs of a health care provider's medical care are closely monitored and scrutinized by insurance carriers. Often preapproval is required prior to health care delivery.

Since 1971 there has been a significant increase in the number of lawsuits filed, caused in part by the steady increase in the number of individuals who have become active in sports. The costs of insurance have also significantly increased during this period. More lawsuits and much higher medical costs are causing a crisis in the insurance industry.[9] Medical insurance is a contract between an insurance company and a policyholder in which the insurance company agrees to reimburse a portion of the total medical bill after some deductible has been paid by the policyholder. The major types of insurance about which individuals concerned with athletic training and sports medicine should have some understanding are general health insurance, accident insurance, professional liability insurance, and catastrophic insurance as well as insurance for errors and omissions. There is a need to protect adequately all who are concerned with sports health and safety. *Focus Box:* "Common insurance terminology" lists some of the more common insurance terms.

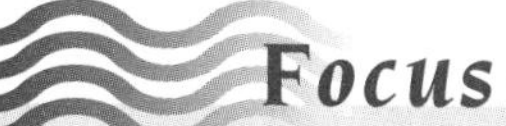

Common insurance terminology

Allowable Charge: The maximum amount, according to the individual policy, that insurance will pay for each procedure or service performed.

Beneficiary: A person eligible to receive the benefits of a specific policy or program.

Benefits: Services that an insurer, government agency, or health care plan offers to pay for an insured individual.

Case Management Services: The process in which the attending physician or agent coordinates the care given to a patient by other health care providers and/or community organizations.

Claim: A form sent to an insurance company requesting payment for covered medical expenses. Information includes the insured's name and address, procedure codes, diagnostic codes, charges, and date of service.

Continued

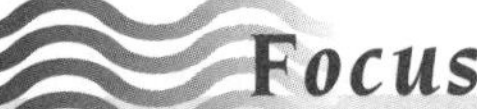

Common insurance terminology—continued

Clean Claim: A filed claim with all the necessary information that may be immediately processed.

Contract: A legally binding agreement between an insurance company and a physician describing the duties of both parties.

Copayment: A provision in an insurance policy requiring the policyholder to pay a specified percentage of each medical claim.

Customary Fees: The average fee charged for a specified service or procedure in a defined geographic area.

Deductible: The amount owed by the insured on a yearly basis before the insurance company will begin to pay for services rendered.

Dependent: A person legally eligible for benefits based on his or her relationship with the policyholder.

Exclusions: Specified medical services, disorders, treatments, diseases, and durable medical equipment that is listed as uncovered or not reimbursable in an insurance policy.

Explanation of Benefits (EOB): An insurance report accompanying all claim payments that explains how the insurance company processed a claim.

Fee Schedule: A comprehensive listing of the maximum payment amount that an insurance company will allow for specified medical procedures performed on a beneficiary of the plan.

Gatekeeper: The primary care physician assigned by the insurer that oversees the medical care rendered to a patient and initiates all specialty and ancillary services.

Participating Provider: A health care provider who has entered into a contract with an insurance company to provide medical services to the beneficiaries of a plan. The provider agrees to accept the insurance company's approved fee and will only bill the patient for the deductible, copayment, and uncovered services.

Policyholder: The person who takes out the medical insurance policy.

Premium: A periodic payment made to an insurance company by an individual policy.

Third Party Administrator: An independent organization that collects premiums, pays claims, and provides administrative services within a health care plan.

UCR Allowable Charge: Usual, customary, and reasonable charge that represents the maximum amount an insurance company will pay for a given service based on geographical averages.

General Health Insurance

Every athlete should have a *general health insurance* policy that covers illness, hospitalization, and emergency care. Some institutions offer primary insurance coverage in which all medical expenses are paid for by the athletic department. The institutions pay an extremely high premium for this type of coverage. Most institutions offer *secondary insurance* coverage, which pays the athlete's remaining medical bills once the athlete's personal insurance company has made its payment. Secondary insurance always includes a deductible that will not be covered by the plan.

Every athlete should have a general health insurance policy that covers illness, hospitalization, and emergency care.

Many athletes are covered under some type of *family health insurance* policy. However, the school or university must make certain that personal health insurance is arranged for or purchased by athletes not covered under family policies.[28] A form letter directed to the parents of all athletes should be completed and returned to the institution to make certain that appropriate coverage is provided (Figure 3-1). Some so-called comprehensive plans do not cover every health need. For example, they may cover physicians' care but not hospital charges. Many of these plans require large prepayments before the insurance takes effect. Supplemental policies such as accident insurance and catastrophic insurance are designed to take over where general health insurance stops.

Emergency and Insurance Information on Student Athletes

Student's Name ______________ Date of Birth ________ Sport ______________

Home Address ____

Home Phone ____

Social Security or Student ID Number ____________________ Sex: M ___ F ___

Family Doctor ____________________ Phone ______________

Address ____

Policy Holder ____________________ Relation to Student ______________

Employer ____

Address ____

Home Phone ____________________ Work Phone ______________

Names of Insurance Companies ______________________________

Address of Insurance Company ______________________________

Certificate Number ______________ Group ________ Type ______________

Should my son/daughter require services beyond those covered by the Sports Medicine Program, I give permission to the Division of Sports Medicine to file a claim for such services with the above health insurer.

I understand that any insurance payments I receive must be returned to be placed on my child's account.

Parent's Signature ______________________________ Date ______________

Figure 3-1

Sample emergency and insurance information form

Accident Insurance

Besides general health insurance, low-cost *accident insurance* is available to the student. It often covers accidents on school grounds while the student is in attendance. The purpose of this insurance is to protect against financial loss from medical and hospital bills, encourage an injured student to receive prompt medical care, encourage prompt reporting of injuries, and relieve a school of financial responsibility.

The school's general insurance may be limited; thus accident insurance for a specific activity such as sports may be needed to provide additional protection.[9] This type of coverage is limited and does not require knowledge of fault, and the amount it pays is limited. For serious sport injuries requiring surgery and lengthy rehabilitation, accident insurance is usually not adequate. This inadequacy can put families with limited budgets into a real financial bind. Of particular concern is insurance that does not adequately cover catastrophic injuries.

3-4

***Critical Thinking* Exercise**

An athletic trainer who recently became certified is planning on working summer camps for an area high school before he starts his full-time employment in the fall.

? What should the athletic trainer do to protect himself from liability?

Professional Liability Insurance

Most individual schools and school districts have general liability insurance to protect against damages that may arise from injuries occurring on school property. Liability insurance covers claims of negligence on the part of individuals.[11] Its major concern is whether supervision was reasonable and if unreasonable risk of harm was perceived by the sports participant.[28]

Because of the amount of litigation based on alleged negligence, premiums have become almost prohibitive for some schools. Typically, a victim's lawsuit has taken a shotgun approach, suing the coach, athletic trainer, physician, school administrator, and school district. If a protective piece of equipment is involved, the product manufacturer is also sued.

Because of the amount of litigation for alleged negligence, all professionals involved with the sports program must be fully protected by professional liability insurance.

All athletic trainers should carry *professional liability insurance* and must clearly understand the limits of its coverage. Liability insurance typically covers negligence in a civil case. If a criminal complaint is filed, however, liability insurance will not cover the athletic trainer.

Catastrophic Insurance

Although catastrophic injuries in sports participation are relatively uncommon, when they do occur the consequences to the athlete, family, and institution, as well as to society, can be staggering.[27] In the past when available funds have been completely diminished, the family was forced to seek funding elsewhere, usually through a lawsuit. Organizations such as the National Collegiate Athletic Association (NCAA) and National Association of Intercollegiate Athletics (NAIA) provide plans that deal with the problem of a lifetime that requires extensive medical and rehabilitative care because of a permanent disability.[5]

Benefits begin when expenses have reached $25,000 and are then extended for a lifetime. A program at the secondary-school level is offered to districts by the National Federation of State High School Associations (NFSHSA). This plan provides medical, rehabilitation, and transportation costs in excess of $10,000 not covered by other insurance benefits.[28] Costs for catastrophic insurance are based on the number of sports and the number of hazardous sports offered by the institution.

To offset the shotgun approach of lawsuits and to cover what is not covered by a general liability policy, *errors and omissions liability insurance* has evolved. It is designed to cover school employees, officers, and the district against suits claiming malpractice, wrongful actions, errors and omissions, and acts of negligence.[28] Even when working in a program that has good liability coverage, each person within that program who works directly with students must have his or her own personal liability insurance.

Insurance that covers the athlete's health and safety can be complex. The athletic trainer must ensure that every athlete is adequately covered by a reliable insurance company. In some athletic programs the filing of claims becomes the responsibility of the athletic trainer. This task can be highly time consuming, taking the athletic trainer away from his or her major role of working directly with the athlete. Because of the intricacies and time involved with claim filing and follow-up communications with parents, doctors, and vendors, a staff person other than the athletic trainer should be assigned this responsibility.

3-5 *Critical Thinking* Exercise

During a high school gymnastics meet, a gymnast fell off the uneven parallel bars and landed on her forearm. The athletic trainer suspected a fracture and decided an X ray was needed. The gymnast's parents had general health insurance through a PPO, but because the gymnast was in severe pain, she was sent to the nearest emergency room to be treated. Unfortunately, the emergency facility was not on the list of preferred providers, and the insurance company denied the claim. The athletic trainer assured the parents that the school would take care of whatever medical costs were not covered by their insurance policy.

? Because the PPO denied the claim, what type of insurance policy should the school carry to cover the medical costs?

THIRD-PARTY REIMBURSEMENT

Third-party reimbursement is the primary mechanism of payment for medical services in the United States.[29] The policyholder's insurance company reimburses health care professionals for services performed. Medical insurance companies may provide group and individual coverage for employees and dependents. Managed care involves a prearranged system for delivering health care that is designed to control costs while continuing to provide quality care. To cut payout costs, many insurance companies pay for preventive care (to reduce the need for hospitalization) and limit where the individual can go for care. A number of different health care systems have been developed to contain costs.[21]

Third-party reimbursement involves reimbursement by the policyholder's insurance company for services performed by health care professionals.

Third-party payers:
- HMOs
- PPOs
- POS
- EPOs
- PHOs
- TPA
- Medicare
- Medicaid
- Worker Compensation
- Indemnity Plans
- Capitation

Health Maintenance Organizations

Health maintenance organizations (HMOs) provide preventive measures and limit where the individual can receive care. Except in emergencies, permission must be obtained before the individual can go to another provider. HMOs generally pay 100 percent of the medical costs as long as care is rendered at an HMO facility. Many supplemental policies do not cover the medical costs that would normally be paid by the general policy. Therefore an athlete treated outside the HMO may be ineligible for any insurance benefits. Many HMOs determine fees using a capitation system, which limits the amount that will be reimbursed for a specific service. It is essential for the athletic trainer to understand the limits of and restrictions on coverage at his or her institution.

Preferred Provider Organizations

Preferred provider organizations (PPOs) provide discount health care but also limit where a person can go for treatment of an illness. The athletic trainer must be apprised in advance as to where the ill athlete should be sent. Athletes sent to a facility that is not on the approved list may be required to pay for care, whereas if they are sent to a preferred facility, all costs are paid.[9] PPOs may provide added services, such as physical therapy, more easily and at no cost or at a much lower cost than would another insurance policy. PPOs pay on a fee-for-service basis.

Point of Service Plan

The point of service (POS) plan is a combination of the HMO and PPO plans. It is based on an HMO structure, yet it allows members to go outside the HMO to obtain services. This flexibility is allowed only with certain conditions and under special circumstances.

Exclusive Provider Organizations

Exclusive provider organizations (EPOs) are also a combination of the HMO and PPO plans. They are restrictive in the number and types of providers they have and consequently are more like an HMO. Most will not pay anything if you use out-of-network providers.

Physician Hospital Organization

Physician hospital organizations (PHOs) involve a major hospital or hospital chain and its physicians. A PHO organization contracts directly with employers to provide services and/or contracts with a managed care organization.

Third Party Administrators

Third party administrators (TPAs) are frequently used to administer services and to pay claims for self-insured group plans thus function as pseudo insurance companies. They perform member services such as enrollment and billing and assist with controlling utilization without the financial risk.

Medicare

Medicare is the federal health insurance program for the aged and disabled. Most people at retirement age qualify for Medicare benefits. There are two parts or sections to Medicare. Part A, the hospital portion, is normally premium-free at retirement to the beneficiary. Part B, the physician portion, has a monthly premium charge to the beneficiary.

Medicaid

Medicaid is a health insurance program for people with low incomes and limited resources. Medicaid is funded by both the federal government and individual states, with the state responsible for handling the administration of the program. Individual states administer Medicaid and thus benefits vary by state.

Workers Compensation

Workers compensation laws and benefits for injured workers are mandated by the states. Employers pay the premiums and the claims are settled by workers compensation insurance carriers whose goal is to return injured workers to the work force as soon as possible.

Indemnity Plans

An indemnity plan is the most traditional form of billing for health care. It is a fee-for-service plan that allows the insured party to seek medical care without restrictions on utilization or cost. The provider charges the patient or a third-party payer for services provided. Charges are based on a set fee schedule.

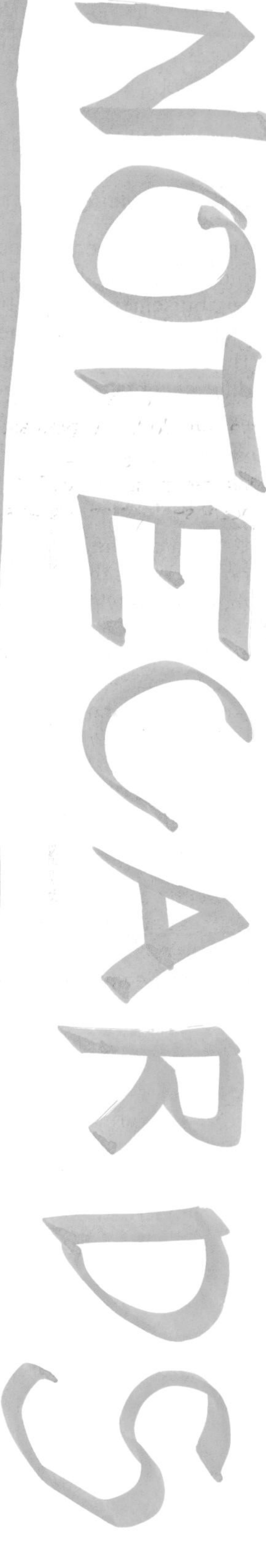

Capitation

Capitation is a form of reimbursement used by managed care providers in which members make a standard payment each month regardless of how much service is rendered to the member by the provider.

Third-Party Reimbursement for Athletic Trainers

3-6

Critical Thinking Exercise

An athletic trainer working in a clinic is seeking third-party reimbursement for athletic training services performed. The trainer is experiencing difficulty obtaining reimbursement from certain payers because of uncertainty about the effectiveness of the treatment program.

? What can the athletic trainer do to address the concerns of the third-party payers?

Athletic trainers have always been able to bill third-party payers for services rendered. Unfortunately in the past, most insurers refused to reimburse the athletic trainer. However over the last few years there has been a significant increase in reimbursement from third-party payers for athletic trainers working in a variety of settings, including hospitals, physicians' offices, sports rehabilitation clinics, and college and university settings.[24] Reimbursement for as much as 85 percent of billings has been reported by some athletic trainers. Some have fared less favorably. There is no question that licensure is key to successful reimbursement from third-party payers. In the case of insurance/managed care contracts, the state ultimately decides who the company will reimburse for services. Most third-party payers view "licensed health care professionals" as the only reimbursable entities. Fortunately in most states this includes certified athletic trainers. Certainly, securing third-party reimbursement for athletic training services must continue to be a priority, especially for the clinical athletic trainer.[29]

In 1995 NATA established the Reimbursement Advisory Group to monitor managed care changes and to help the athletic trainer secure a place as a health care provider. Specifically this group was charged with the responsibility of developing a model for approaching third-party payers for the reimbursement of athletic training services, of educating athletic trainers on issues related to reimbursement, and perhaps most important, of designing and implementing a data-based clinical outcomes study.[8] In 1996 NATA initiated the Athletic Training Outcomes Assessment project designed to present supporting data that measures the results of interventions involving athletic training procedures. This three-year study was designed to provide data that focused on functional outcomes, including assessing the patients' perceptions of their functional capabilities and their overall satisfaction with their treatment program; assessing the physical, emotional, and social well-being of patients; assessing health care cost effectiveness relative to time lost from activity due to injury; and assessing the number of treatments.[12] The results of this study were critical in securing reimbursement for athletic training services, because the majority of third-party payers currently require outcomes research when evaluating a contract.[4,19]

Insurance Billing

The athletic trainer must file insurance claims immediately and correctly.[29] Athletic trainers working in educational settings can facilitate this process by collecting insurance information on every athlete at the beginning of the year. Letters should be drafted to the parents of all athletes explaining the limits of the school insurance policy and what the parents must do to process a claim if injury does occur. Schools with secondary policies should stress that the parents must submit all bills to their insurance company before they submit the remainder to the school. In educational institutions, most claims will be filed with a single insurance company, which will pay for medical services provided by individual health care providers.

Filing an Insurance Claim

When filing an insurance claim to submit for reimbursement, athletic trainers will find that a standard form labeled HCFA-1500/HCFA-1450. is accepted by most carriers (Blue Cross/Blue Shield uses Form UB-92). These forms must be completed in detail with as much information as possible. Experience dictates that the more accurately and thoroughly these forms are completed, the quicker and higher the rate of reimbursement.

TABLE 3-1 Description of Billing Codes Used by Athletic Trainers

The following is a guide to procedure billing codes that may be used by athletic trainers when billing for athletic training services:

Code	Description
97005/97006	Athletic trainer evaluation and reevaluation (per visit)
97750	Physical performance test (each 15 minutes) treatment charges:
97116	Gait training (each 15 minutes)
97110	Therapeutic exercise (each 15 minutes)
97112	Neuromuscular reeducation (each 15 minutes)
97530	Therapeutic activities (each 15 minutes)
97113	Aquatic therapeutic exercise (each 15 minutes)
97124	Massage (each 15 minutes)
97530	Body mechanics training (each 15 minutes)
97140	Manual therapy (each 15 minutes)
97504	Orthotics fitting and training (each 15 minutes)
97150	Therapeutic procedures—group (each visit)
97150	Supervised exercise (each visit)
11040	Debridement (each visit)
97139	Wound care (each 15 minutes)
97139	Taping (each visit)
95831	Manual muscle testing—extremity/trunk
95851	Range of Motion (ROM) measurements
95852	ROM measurements of hand, with or without comparison with normal side
97545	Work hardening/conditioning (initial 2 hours)
97035	Ultrasound (each 15 minutes)
97035	Phonophoresis (each 15 minutes) (Must bill for ultrasound if billing for this service.)
97032	Electrical stimulation (each 15 minutes)
97033	Iontophoresis (each 15 minutes)
97032	Constant electrical stimulation (each 15 minutes)
97034	Contrast baths (each 15 minutes)
97014	Electric stimulation (application to one or more areas)
97022	Whirlpool (application to one or more areas)
97010	Hot packs (application to one or more areas)
97010	Cold packs/ice massage (application to one or more areas)
97012	Traction, mechanical (not time-based)
97016	Compression pump (application to one or more areas)

Athletic trainers working in the clinical setting should understand that the clinic must be able to collect reimbursement from third-party payers for services provided. The athletic trainer should request approval from insurance companies before treating patients.

There are two types of billing codes which must be filed when submitting a claim on standard HFCA-1500 or UB-92 forms to third-party payers, one is a *diagnostic code*, and the other is a *procedural code*.[30] A diagnostic code is required for all procedural billing, and can be found in a book called the *International Classification of Diseases* (ICD-9-CM). This is a five-digit code that specifies the condition or injury that the athletic trainer or any other health care provider is treating. For example code 845.02 indicates that the patient has a sprain of the calcaneofibular ligament in the ankle.

The *Current Procedure Terminology Code* (CPT) was first developed by the American Medical Association in 1966. Each year, an annual publication is prepared, that makes changes corresponding to significant updates in medical technology and practice. The CPT code is used to identify specific medical procedures used in treating a patient. Table 3-1 lists the current CPT codes most often used by the athletic trainer.

Focus

Guidelines for documentation*

When billing for and receiving reimbursement the following points should be documented:

- Initial evaluation, including plan of treatment and goals (SOAP notes)
- Appropriate patient medical history
- Patient examination results
- Functional assessment
- Type of treatment and body parts to be treated
- Expected frequency and number of treatments
- Prognosis
- Functional, measurable, and time-based goals
- Precautions and contraindications
- A statement that the treatment plan and goals were discussed and understood by the patient and possibly by the guardian
- Daily treatment records
- A record of any changes in physical status, physician orders or treatment plan, or goals
- Weekly progress notes, especially on goals (SOAP or function-based)
- Copies of notes to or from the referring physician's office, whether by fax, e-mail, U.S. mail, or phone
- A prescription or other state-mandated documentation from a physician

*From the NATA Committee on Reimbursement

3-7 Critical Thinking Exercise

? When filing an insurance claim for an athlete following injury, what can an athletic trainer do to improve the reimbursement rate as well as to speed up the process?

3-8 Critical Thinking Exercise

A sports medicine clinic is considering hiring an athletic trainer. However, the clinic administrator is concerned that the athletic trainer cannot bill third-party payers for services provided.

? What does the administrator need to be told about third-party reimbursement for athletic training services?

Athletic trainers should never release medical records to third-party payers unless written authorization has been obtained from the patient according to HIPAA guidelines. It is also essential when billing for and receiving reimbursement that the athletic trainer keeps meticulous, accurate, and detailed documentation of all procedures, charges submitted, and payments received for services. *Focus Box:* "Guidelines for documentation" identifies criteria that should be routinely followed when billing for charges.

SUMMARY

- A great deal of care must be taken in following coaching and athletic training procedures that conform to the legal guidelines governing liability for negligence.
- Liability is the state of being legally responsible for the harm one causes another person. It assumes that an athletic trainer would act according to the standard of care of any individual with similar educational background and training.
- An athletic trainer who fails to use reasonable care—care that persons would normally exercise to avoid injury to themselves or to others under similar circumstances—may be found liable for negligence.
- Although athletes participating in a sports program are considered to assume a normal risk, this assumption in no way exempts those in charge from exercising reasonable care.
- Athletic trainers can significantly decrease the risk of litigation by making certain that they have done everything possible to provide a reasonable degree of care to the injured athlete.
- The major types of insurance about which athletic trainers should have some understanding are general health insurance, accident insurance, professional liability insurance, catastrophic insurance, and insurance for errors and omissions.
- Third-party reimbursement is the primary mechanism of payment for medical services in the United States. A number of different health care systems have been developed to contain costs.
- It is essential that the athletic trainer file insurance claims immediately and correctly using appropriate forms and billing codes.

Websites

Legal Information Institute at Cornell: http://www.law.cornell.edu/topics/sports.html

This website is part of a series of legal information and specifically addresses law in sport; the information is rather technical in nature. The area relevant to sports medicine is addressed in the section titled "Torts."

Cramer First Aider: http://www.cramersportsmed.com/firstaider.jsp

The Cramer First Aider is a newsletter published by Cramer that provides information about current topics in sports medicine. For information relevant to this chapter, go to the section titled "Legal Issues."

Sports Lawyers Journal: http://www.law.tulane.edu

Specialized academic and professional publication on legal aspects of sports.

The Center for Sports Law & Policy: http://www.law.duke.edu/sportscenter/

Duke University School of Law.

Health Insurance Association of America: http://www.hiaa.org

The nation's most prominent trade association representing the private health care system. It is the nation's premier provider of self-study courses on health insurance and managed care.

Duhaime & Co. Legal Dictionary: http://www.duhaime.org/dictionary

This is a site that has put together an extensive list of legal terms with clear definitions and explanations.

National Athletic Trainers Association Committee on Reimbursement: http://www.nata.org/members1/committees/cor/rag.cfm

Designed to enhance the reimbursement interests and efforts of NATABOC certified athletic trainers.

Solutions to Critical Thinking EXERCISES

3-1 An athletic trainer who assumes the duty of caring for an athlete has an obligation to make sure that appropriate care is given. If the athletic trainer fails to provide an acceptable standard of care, there is a breach of duty on the part of the athletic trainer, and the athlete must then prove that this breach caused the injury or made the injury worse.

3-2 A person possessing more training in a given field or area is expected to possess a correspondingly higher level of competence than a lay person is. A certified athletic trainer will therefore be judged in terms of his or her performance in any situation in which legal liability may be assessed.

3-3 The athlete would typically have between one and three years to file suit for negligence. The statute of limitations begins to run on a plaintiff's time to file a lawsuit for negligence either from the time of the negligent act or omission that gives rise to the suit or from the time of the discovery of an injury caused by the negligent act or omission.

3-4 The athletic trainer should purchase private professional liability insurance. In addition, the athletic trainer should keep proper records of injuries and keep those records in his possession.

3-5 Besides general health insurance, low-cost accident insurance often covers accidents on school grounds while the athlete is competing. The purpose of this insurance is to protect against financial loss from medical and hospital bills, encourage an injured athlete to receive prompt medical care, encourage prompt reporting of injuries, and relieve a school of financial responsibility.

3-6 The athletic trainer could initiate an outcomes research project designed to present supporting data that measures the results of interventions involving athletic training procedures. This research project would assess the athletes' perceptions of their functional capabilities and overall satisfaction with their treatment program, the cost-effectiveness of the health care relative to time lost from activity due to injury, and the number of treatments. The majority of third-party payers currently require outcomes research when evaluating a contract.

3-7 The athletic trainer should file an insurance claim for reimbursement using the standard form labeled HCFA-1500. The form should be completed in detail with as much information as possible. The athletic trainer who completes these forms accurately and thoroughly probably experiences a quicker and higher rate of reimbursement.

3-8 It should be pointed out that athletic trainers can bill third-party payers for services rendered to a patient. Whether the insurance company will reimburse the athletic trainer for services is up to the individual third-party payer. With the approval of the uniform billing code for athletic training services, it is more likely that the athletic trainer will be successfully reimbursed for treating patients.

REVIEW QUESTIONS AND CLASS ACTIVITIES

1. What are the athletic trainer's major legal concerns for negligence and for assumption of risk?
2. What measures can an athletic trainer take to minimize the chances of litigation should an athlete be injured?
3. Invite an attorney who is familiar with sports litigation to class to discuss how athletic trainers can protect themselves from lawsuits.
4. Discuss what the athletic trainer must do to provide reasonable and prudent care in dealing with an injured athlete.
5. Why is it necessary for an athlete to have both general health insurance and accident insurance?
6. Briefly discuss the various methods of third-party reimbursement.
7. Why should an athletic trainer carry individual liability insurance?
8. What are the critical considerations for filing insurance claims?

REFERENCES

1. Albolm M, Campbell D, Konin J: *Reimbursement for athletic trainers,* Thoroughfare, NJ, 2001, Slack.
2. Appenzeller H: *Safe at first: a guide to help sports administrators reduce their liability,* Chapel Hill, NC, 1999, Carolina Academic Press.
3. Appenzeller H: *Sports and the law: contemporary issues,* Charlottesville, Va, 1985, Michie.
4. Benjamin K: Outcomes research and the allied health professional, *J Allied Health* 24:3, 1995.
5. Berg R: Catastrophic injury insurance, an end to costly litigation, *Ath J* 8:10, 1987.
6. Borkowski RP: Coaches and the courts, *First Aider* 54:1, 1985.
7. Borkowski RP: Lawsuit less likely if safety comes first, *First Aider* 55:11, 1985.
8. Campbell D: Workshop on third party reimbursement, *NATA News* 3:34, 1996.
9. Chambers RL: Insurance types and coverage: knowledge to plan for the future (with a focus on motor skill activities and athletics), *Phys Educ* 44:233, 1986.

10. Clement A: Patterns of litigation in physical education instruction. Paper presented at the American Association of Health, Physical Education, and Dance, National Convention and Exposition, Cincinnati, April 1986.
11. Cotton DJ: What is covered by your liability insurance policy? A risk management essential, *Exercise Standard and Malpractice Reporter* 15(4):54, 2001.
12. De Carlo M: Reimbursement for health care services. In Konin J: *Clinical athletic training,* Thoroughfare, NJ, 1997, Slack.
13. Drowatzky JN: Legal duties and liability in athletic training, *Ath Train* 20:11, 1985.
14. Eickhoff-Shemek JAM, Evans JA: An investigation of law and legal liability content in masters academic programs in sports medicine and exercise science. *Journal of Legal Aspects of Sport* 10(3):172, 2000.
15. Frenkel DA: Medico-legal aspects in sport (abstract), *Exercise & Society Journal of Sport Science* (28):90, 2001.
16. Gallup E: *Law and the team physician,* Champaign, 1995, Human Kinetics.
17. Gorman L: Product liability in sports medicine. *Athletic Therapy Today* 4(4):36, 1999.
18. Graham L: Ten ways to dodge the malpractice bullet, *Ath Train* 20(2):117, 1985.
19. Harada N, Sofaer S, Kominski G: Functional status outcomes in rehabilitation: implications for prospective payment, *Medical Care* 31:345, 1993.
20. Hawkins J, Appenzeller H: Legal aspects of sports medicine. In Mueller F, Ryan A: *Prevention of athletic injuries: the role of the sports medicine team,* Philadelphia, 1991, FA Davis.
21. Health Insurance Association of America: *Fundamentals of health insurance,* Washington DC, 1997, HIAA.
22. Herbert DL, Herbert WG: Legal aspects of preventive, rehabilitative and recreational exercise programs. ed 4, Canton, Ohio, 2002, PRC Publishing.
23. Herbert D: *Legal aspects of sports medicine,* Canton, Ohio, 1995, Professional Reports Corporation.
24. Hunt V: Reimbursement efforts continue steady progress, *NATA News,* October:10–12, 2002.
25. Leverenz L, Helms L: Suing athletic trainers, parts I and II, *Ath Train* 25(3):212, 1990.
26. Mitten M, Mitten R: Legal considerations in treating the injured athlete, *J Orthop Sports Phys Ther* 21(1):38, 1995.
27. Mueller F: Catastrophic sports injuries. In Mueller F, Ryan A: *Prevention of athletic injuries: the role of the sports medicine team,* Philadelphia, 1991, FA Davis.
28. Rankin J, Ingersoll C: *Athletic training management: concepts and applications,* New York, 2000, McGraw-Hill.
29. Ray R: *Management strategies in athletic training,* Champaign, Ill, 2000, Human Kinetics.
30. Ray R: *Uniform billing code takes effect for ATCs, NATA News,* Winter: 20–12, 2000.
31. Yasser R: Calculating risk, *Sports Med Digest* 9(2):5, 1987.
32. Wong G: *Essentials of amateur sports law,* Westport, Conn, 1994, Praeger.

ANNOTATED BIBLIOGRAPHY

Albolm M, Campbell D, Konin J: *Reimbursement for athletic trainers,* Thoroughfare, NJ, 2001, Slack.

Presents a "how to" approach for filing claims, appealing denials, and approaching payers. Covers all current trends in health care reimbursement as well as future directions for reimbursement.

Appenzeller H: *Youth sports and the law: a guide to legal issues,* Chapel Hill, NC, 2000, Carolina Academic Press.

Studies various court cases to understand the legal principles involved in sport participation. The objective of the book is to provide better and safer sporting experiences for today's children.

Gayson E: *Ethics injury and the law in sports medicine,* New York, 1999, Heinemann-Butterworth.

Provides an up-to-date review of the status of sports medicine and the law. Addresses the key legal and ethical issues in sports and exercise medicine. For practitioners and students preparing for sport and exercise medicine exams.

Herbert D: *Legal aspects of sports medicine,* Canton, OH, 1995, Professional Reports Corporation.

A discussion of sports medicine, policies, procedures, responsibilities of the sports medicine team, informed consent, negligence, insurance and risk management, medication, drug testing, and other topics.

Rowell JC: *Understanding medical insurance: a step-by-step guide,* Albany, NY, 1994, Delmar Publishers.

Provides a comprehensive resource for dealing with issues related to insurance.

Training and Conditioning Techniques

Chapter 4

When you finish this chapter you should be able to

- Examine the roles of the athletic trainer and the strength and conditioning coach in getting an athlete fit.
- Identify the principles of conditioning.
- Defend the importance of the warm-up and cooldown periods.
- Evaluate the importance of flexibility, strength, and cardiorespiratory endurance for both athletic performance and injury prevention.
- Analyze specific techniques and principles for improving flexibility, muscular strength, and cardiorespiratory endurance.
- Discuss fitness testing and identify specific tests to assess various fitness parameters.
- Apply the concept of periodization and identify the various training periods in each phase.

Preventing injury to the athlete is one of the primary functions of the athletic trainer. To compete successfully at a high level, the athlete must be fit. An athlete who is not fit is more likely to sustain an injury. Both coaches and athletic trainers recognize that improper conditioning is one of the major causes of sports injuries (Figure 4-1). Thus coaches and athletic trainers should work cooperatively to supervise training and conditioning programs that minimize the possibility of injury and maximize performance.[49]

Lack of physical fitness is one of the primary causes of sports injury.

It takes time and careful preparation to bring an athlete into competition at a level of fitness that will preclude early-season injury. The athletic trainer must possess sound understanding of the principles of training and conditioning relative to flexibility, strength, and cardiorespiratory endurance.

THE RELATIONSHIP BETWEEN ATHLETIC TRAINERS AND STRENGTH AND CONDITIONING COACHES

The responsibility for making certain that an athlete is fit for competition depends on the personnel who are available to oversee this aspect of the athletic program. At the professional level and at most colleges and universities, a full-time strength and conditioning coach is employed to conduct both team and individual training sessions. Many, but not all, strength coaches are certified by the National Strength and Conditioning Association. If a strength coach is involved, it is essential that both the athletic trainers and the team coaches communicate freely and work in close cooperation with the strength coach to ensure that the athletes achieve an optimal level of fitness.

The specific role of the athletic trainer is to critically review the training and conditioning program designed by the strength and conditioning coach and to be extremely familiar with what is expected of the athletes on a daily basis. The athletic trainer should feel free to offer suggestions and make recommendations that are in the best interest of the athletes' health and well-being. If it becomes apparent that a particular exercise or a specific training session seems to be causing an inordinate number of

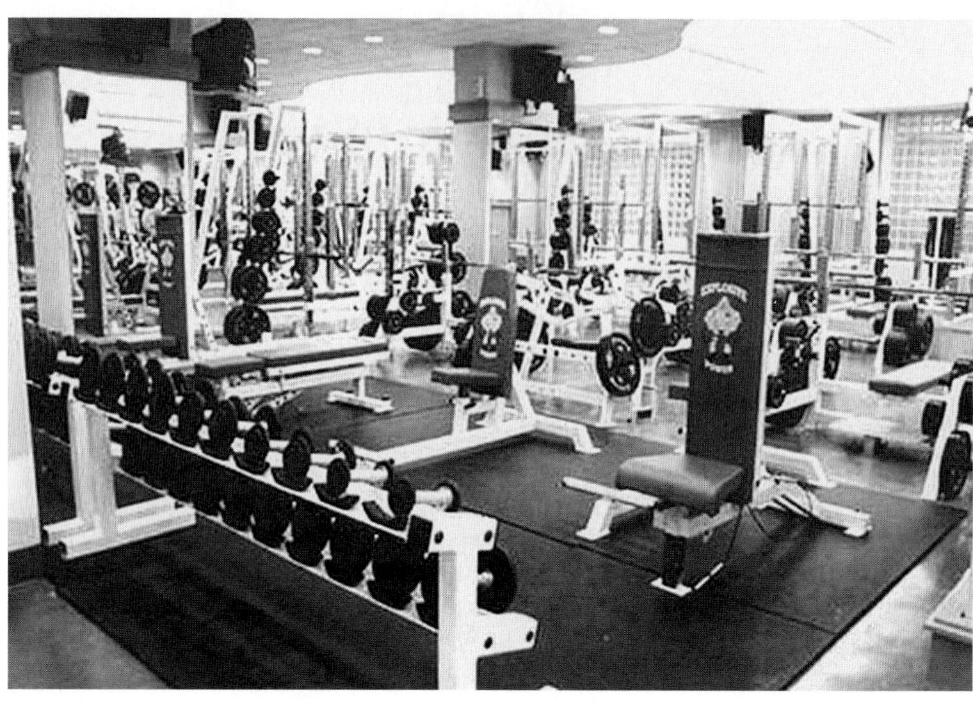

Figure 4-1

Athletic programs often provide elaborate strength and conditioning facilities.

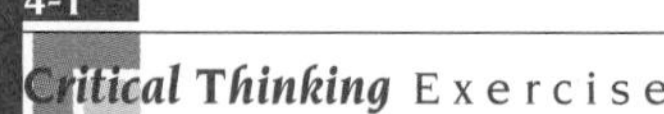

4-1 **Critical Thinking** Exercise

A professional football player sustained a grade 2 hamstring strain during the sixth week of the season. Just before the playoffs he reinjured the muscle while doing some slow-speed cutting drills. Unfortunately, he was forced to remain on the injured reserve list for the duration of the season despite his best efforts to return. He has lost a great deal of cardiorespiratory fitness because he has been unable to run, and he exhibits weakness in lower extremity muscular strength because lifting has been difficult.

? Given that he will be required to attend two minicamps during the spring and early summer and that preseason practice officially begins in July, what should his conditioning plan be during the postseason and the off-season?

The SAID principle indicates that the body will gradually adapt to the specific demands imposed on it.

injuries, the athletic trainer should inform the strength and conditioning coach of the problem so that some alternative exercise can be substituted.

If an athlete is injured and is undergoing a rehabilitation program, it should be the athletic trainer's responsibility to communicate to the strength and conditioning coach how the conditioning program should be limited and/or modified. The athletic trainer must respect the role of the strength and conditioning coach in getting the athlete fit. However, the responsibility for rehabilitating an injured athlete clearly belongs to the athletic trainer.

In the majority of high school settings, a strength and conditioning coach is not available; the responsibility for ensuring that the athlete gets fit lies with the athletic trainer and the team coaches. In this situation the athletic trainer very often assumes the role of a strength and conditioning coach in addition to his or her athletic training responsibilities. The athletic trainer frequently finds it necessary not only to design training and conditioning programs but also to oversee the weight room and to educate young, inexperienced athletes about getting themselves fit to compete. The athletic trainer must demand the cooperation of the team coaches in supervising the training and conditioning program.

PRINCIPLES OF CONDITIONING

The following principles should be applied in all programs of training and conditioning to minimize the likelihood of injury:

1. *Warm-up/cooldown.* Take time to do an appropriate warm-up before engaging in any activity. Do not neglect the cooldown period after a training bout.
2. *Motivation.* Athletes are generally highly motivated to work hard because they want to be successful in their sport. Varying the training program and incorporating techniques of periodization can keep the program enjoyable rather than routine and boring. (See the discussion of periodization at the end of this chapter.)
3. *Overload.* To improve in any physiological component, the athlete must work harder than he or she is accustomed to working. Logan and Wallis identified the **SAID principle,** which directly relates to the principle of overload.[48] SAID is an acronym for specific adaptation to imposed demands. The SAID principle states that *when the body is subjected to stresses and overloads of varying intensities, it will gradually*

adapt over time to overcome whatever demands are placed on it. Although overload is a critical factor in training and conditioning, the stress must not be great enough to produce damage or injury before the body has had a chance to adjust specifically to the increased demands.

4. *Consistency.* The athlete must engage in a training and conditioning program on a consistent, regularly scheduled basis if it is to be effective.
5. *Progression.* Increase the intensity of the conditioning program gradually and within the individual athlete's ability to adapt to increasing workloads.
6. *Intensity.* Stress the intensity of the work rather than the quantity. Coaches and athletic trainers too often confuse working hard with working for long periods of time. They make the mistake of prolonging the workout rather than increasing tempo or workload. The tired athlete is prone to injury.
7. *Specificity.* Identifying specific goals for the training program. The program must be designed to address specific components of fitness (i.e., strength, flexibility, cardiorespiratory endurance) relative to the sport in which the athlete is competing.
8. *Individuality.* The needs of individual athletes vary considerably. The successful coach is one who recognizes these individual differences and adjusts or alters the training and conditioning program accordingly to best accommodate the athlete.
9. *Minimize stress.* Expect that athletes will train as close to their physiological limits as they can. Push the athletes as far as possible but consider other stressful aspects of their lives and allow them time to be away from the conditioning demands of their sport.
10. *Safety.* Make the training environment safe. Take time to educate athletes regarding proper techniques, how they should feel during the workout, and when they should push harder or back off.[38]

SAID principle Specific adaptation to imposed demands.

WARM-UP AND COOLDOWN

Warm-Up

It is generally accepted that a period of warm-up exercises should take place before a training session begins, although a review of the literature reveals little data-based research to support the efficacy of a warm-up. Nevertheless, most athletic trainers would agree empirically that a warm-up period is a precaution against unnecessary musculoskeletal injuries and possible muscle soreness.[22] A good warm-up may also improve certain aspects of performance.[3,68]

The function of the warm-up is to prepare the body physiologically for some upcoming physical work. The purpose is to gradually stimulate the cardiorespiratory system to a moderate degree to increase the blood flow to working skeletal muscles and increase muscle temperature.

Moderate activity speeds up the metabolic processes that produce an increase in core body temperature. An increase in the temperature of skeletal muscle alters the mechanical properties of the muscle. The elasticity of the muscle (the length to which the muscle can be stretched) is increased, and the viscosity (the rate at which the muscle can change shape) is decreased.

The warm-up should begin with two to three minutes of whole body activities that use large muscle groups (e.g., light jogging, riding an exercise bike) to elevate the metabolic rate and raise core temperature.[68] Once the athlete breaks into a light sweat, which indicates that core temperature has been increased, a period of stretching exercises should follow. Stretching exercises should be sport-specific and related to the activity to be performed. For example, a soccer player uses the upper extremity considerably less than the lower extremity, so his or her stretching exercises should be directed more toward the lower extremity.

After stretching, the intensity of the warm-up should be increased gradually by performing sport-specific skills related to the activity in which the athlete is going to participate. For example, a basketball player should warm up by shooting layups and jump shots and by dribbling; a tennis player should hit forehand and backhand shots and serves.

4-2 Critical Thinking Exercise

A track athlete constantly complains of feeling tightness in her lower extremity during workouts. She states that she has a difficult time during her warm-up and cannot seem to "get loose" until her workout is almost complete. She feels that she is always on the verge of pulling a muscle.

? What should the athletic trainer recommend as a specific warm-up routine that this athlete should consistently do before beginning her workout?

Warming up involves general body warming and warming specific body areas for the demands of the sport.

The warm-up should last approximately ten to fifteen minutes. The athlete should not wait longer than fifteen minutes to begin the main sports activity after the warm-up, although the effects will generally last up to about forty-five minutes. Thus the third-string football player who warms up before the game and then does nothing more than stand around until he gets into the game during the fourth quarter is running a much higher risk of injury. This player should be encouraged to stay warmed up and ready to play throughout the course of a game. In general, continued sweating is a good indication that the body has been sufficiently warmed up and is ready for more strenuous activity.[59]

Cooldown

Proper cooling down decreases blood and muscle lactic acid levels more rapidly.

Following a workout or training session, a cooldown period is essential. The cooldown period enables the body to cool and return to a resting state. Such a period should last about five to ten minutes.

Conditioning should be performed gradually, with work added in small increments.

Although the value of warm-up and workout periods is well accepted, the importance of a cooldown period afterward is often ignored. Again, experience and observation indicate that persons who stretch during the cooldown period tend to have fewer problems with muscle soreness after strenuous activity.[54]

IMPROVING AND MAINTAINING FLEXIBILITY

The "tight," or inflexible, athlete performs with a considerable handicap in terms of movement.

Flexibility is the ability to move a joint or series of joints smoothly and easily throughout a full range of motion.[4] Flexibility can be discussed in relation to movement involving only one joint, such as the knees, or movement involving a whole series of joints, such as the spinal vertebral joints, which must all move together to allow smooth bending or rotation of the trunk.

An athlete who has a restricted range of motion will have decreased performance capabilities. For example, a sprinter with tight, inelastic hamstring muscles loses some speed because the hamstring muscles restrict the ability to flex the hip joint, thus shortening stride length.

Lack of flexibility results in uncoordinated or awkward movements and predisposes the athlete to muscle strain.[13] Low back pain is frequently associated with tightness of the musculature in the lower spine and also of the hamstring muscles. Most activities require relatively normal amounts of flexibility.[4] However, some activities, such as gymnastics, ballet, diving, karate, and yoga, require increased flexibility for superior performance (Figure 4-2).

Good flexibility is essential to successful physical performance.[6] Most athletic trainers feel that maintaining good flexibility is important in prevention of injury to the musculotendinous unit, and they will generally insist that stretching exercises be included as part of the warm-up before the athlete engages in strenuous activity.

Factors That Limit Flexibility

A number of factors may limit the ability of a joint to move through a full, unrestricted range of motion. The *bony structure* may restrict the endpoint in the range. An elbow that has been fractured through the joint may deposit excess calcium in the joint space, causing the joint to lose its ability to fully extend. However, in many instances bony prominences stop movements at normal endpoints in the range.

Excessive *fat* may also limit the ability to move through a full range of motion. An athlete who has a large amount of fat on the abdomen may have severely restricted trunk flexion when asked to bend forward and touch the toes. The fat may act as a wedge between two lever arms, restricting movement wherever it is found. *Skin* might also be responsible for limiting movement. For example, an athlete who has had some type of injury or surgery involving a tearing incision or laceration of the skin, particularly over a joint, will have inelastic scar tissue formed at that site. This scar tissue is incapable of stretching with joint movement. *Muscles and their tendons,* along with their surrounding fascial sheaths, are most often responsible for limiting

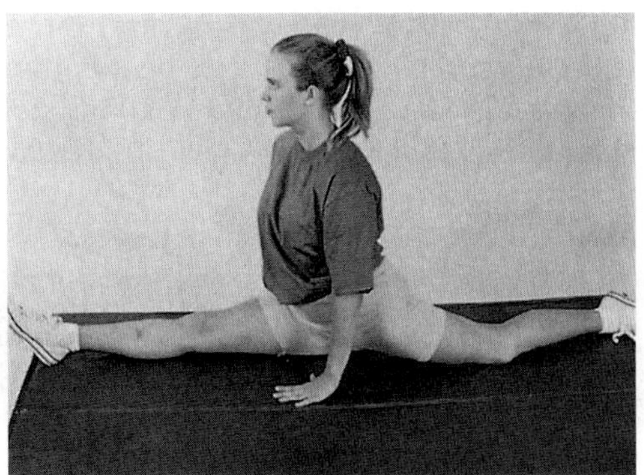

Figure 4-2

Flexibility can be an important factor in decreasing sports injuries.

range of motion. An athlete who performs stretching exercises to improving flexibility about a particular joint is attempting to take advantage of the highly elastic properties of a muscle. Over time it is possible to increase the elasticity, or the length that a given muscle can be stretched.[62] Athletes who have a good deal of movement at a particular joint tend to have highly elastic and flexible muscles. *Connective tissue* surrounding the joint, such as ligaments on the joint capsule, may be subject to contractures. Ligaments and joint capsules do have some elasticity; however, if a joint is immobilized for a period of time, these structures tend to lose some elasticity and shorten. This condition is most commonly seen after surgical repair of an unstable joint, but it can also result from long periods of inactivity.

Neural tissue tightness resulting from acute compression, chronic repetitive microtrauma, muscle imbalances, joint dysfunction, or poor posture can create morphological changes in neural tissues that may result in irritation, inflammation, and pain. Pain causes muscle guarding to protect inflamed and irritated neural structures, and this alters normal movement patterns. Over time neural fibrosis results which decreases the elasticity of neural tissue and prevents normal movement of surrounding tissues.

It is also possible for an athlete to have relatively slack ligaments and joint capsules. These individuals are generally referred to as being loose-jointed. Examples of loose-jointedness would be an elbow or knee that hyperextends beyond 180 degrees (Figure 4-3). Frequently the instability associated with loose-jointedness may present as great a problem in movement as ligamentous or capsular contractures.

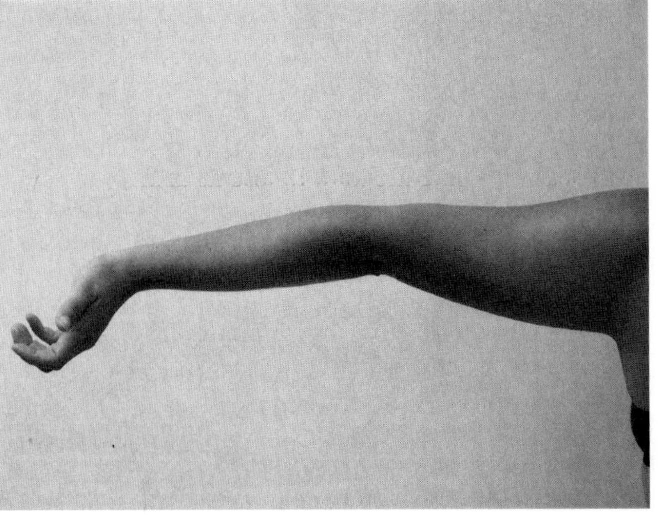

Figure 4-3

Excessive joint motion can predispose to injury.

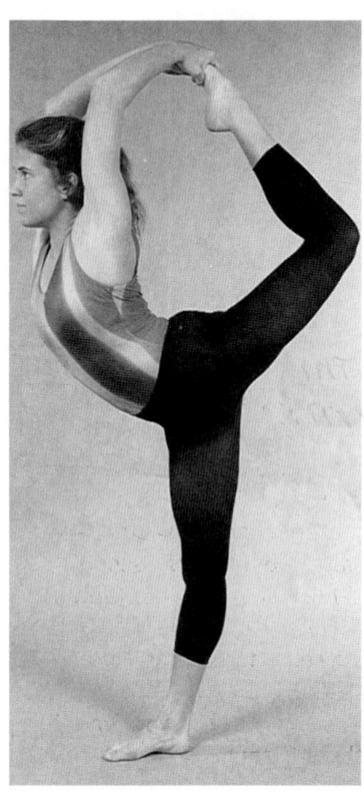

Figure 4-4

Good flexibility is essential to successful performance in many sport activities.

The elasticity of skin contractures caused by scarring, ligaments, joint capsules, and musculotendinous units can be improved to varying degrees over time through stretching. With the exception of bony structure, age, and gender, all the other factors that limit flexibility also may be altered to increase range of joint motion.

Active and Passive Range of Motion

Active range of motion, also called *dynamic flexibility*, refers to the degree to which a joint can be moved by a muscle contraction, usually through the midrange of movement. Dynamic flexibility is not necessarily a good indicator of the stiffness or looseness of a joint because it applies to the ability to move a joint efficiently, with little resistance to motion.[59]

Passive range of motion, sometimes called *static flexibility*, refers to the degree to which a joint may be passively moved to the endpoints in the range of motion. No muscle contraction is involved to move a joint through a passive range.

When a muscle actively contracts, it produces a joint movement through a specific range of motion. However, if passive pressure is applied to an extremity, it is capable of moving farther in the range of motion. It is essential in sport activities that an extremity be capable of moving through a nonrestricted range of motion. For example, a hurdler who cannot fully extend the knee joint in a normal stride is at considerable disadvantage because stride length and thus speed will be reduced significantly (Figure 4-4).

Passive range of motion is important for injury prevention. In many sports situations, a muscle is forced to stretch beyond its normal active limits. If the muscle does not have enough elasticity to compensate for this additional stretch, the musculotendinous unit will likely be injured.

Stretching Techniques

The maintenance of a full, nonrestricted range of motion has long been recognized as critical to injury prevention and as an essential component of a conditioning program.[6] See *Focus Box:* "Guidelines and precautions for stretching." The goal of any effective flexibility program should be to improve the range of motion at a given articulation by altering the extensibility of the musculotendinous units that produce movement at that joint.[31] Exercises that stretch these musculotendinous units over a period of time increase the range of movement possible at a given joint.[64]

Stretching techniques for improving flexibility have evolved over the years. The oldest technique for stretching is called ballistic stretching, which makes use of repetitive bouncing motions. A second technique, known as static stretching, involves stretching a muscle to the point of discomfort and then holding it at the point for an extended time. This technique has been used for many years. A third technique involves a group of stretching techniques known collectively as proprioceptive neuromuscular facilitation (PNF) and uses alternating contractions and stretches.[60] Researchers have had considerable discussion about which of these techniques is most effective for improving range of motion.

Agonist versus antagonist muscles Prior to a discussion of the three different stretching techniques, it is essential to define the terms *agonist* and *antagonist.* Most joints in the body are capable of more than one movement. The knee joint, for example, is capable of flexion and extension. Contraction of the quadriceps group of muscles on the front of the thigh causes knee extension, whereas contraction of the hamstring muscles on the back of the thigh produces knee flexion.

To achieve knee extension, the quadriceps group contracts while the hamstring muscles relax and stretch. The muscle that contracts to produce a movement, in this case the quadriceps, is referred to as the agonist muscle. The muscle being stretched in response to contraction of the agonist muscle is called the antagonist muscle. In knee extension, the antagonist muscle would be the hamstring group. Some degree of balance in strength between agonist and antagonist muscle groups is necessary to produce

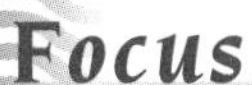

Focus

Guidelines and precautions for stretching

The following guidelines and precautions should be incorporated into a sound stretching program:

- Warm up using a slow jog or fast walk before stretching vigorously.
- To increase flexibility, the muscle must be overloaded or stretched beyond its normal range but not to the point of pain.
- Stretch only to the point where you feel tightness or resistance to stretch or perhaps some discomfort. Stretching should not be painful.
- Increases in range of motion will be specific to whatever joint is being stretched.
- Exercise caution when stretching muscles that surround painful joints. Pain is an indication that something is wrong and should not be ignored.
- Avoid overstretching the ligaments and capsules that surround joints.
- Exercise caution when stretching the lower back and neck. Exercises that compress the vertebrae and their disks may cause damage.
- Stretching from a seated position rather than a standing position takes stress off the low back and decreases the chances of back injury.
- Stretch those muscles that are tight and inflexible.
- Strengthen those muscles that are weak and loose.
- Always stretch slowly and with control.
- Be sure to continue normal breathing during a stretch. Do not hold your breath.
- Static and PNF techniques are most often recommended for individuals who want to improve their range of motion.
- Ballistic stretching should be done only by those who are already flexible or are accustomed to stretching and should be done only after static stretching.
- Stretching should be done at least three times per week to see minimal improvement. It is recommended that you stretch five or six times per week to see maximum results.

4-3

Critical Thinking Exercise

A freshman collegiate football player has had a history of multiple hamstring strains throughout his high school career. He is very concerned that because of the intensity of preseason workouts, he is likely to reinjure his hamstring. He asks the athletic trainer if there is anything that he should be doing to minimize the chances of reinjury.

? What recommendations should the athletic trainer make?

normal smooth, coordinated movement and to reduce the likelihood of muscle strain caused by muscular imbalance.[59]

Dynamic (Ballistic) Stretching

Ballistic stretching involves a bouncing movement in which repetitive contractions of the agonist muscle are used to produce quick stretches of the antagonist muscle. The ballistic stretching technique, although apparently effective in improving range of motion, has been criticized in the past because increased range of motion is achieved through a series of jerks or pulls on the resistant muscle tissue. The concern was that if the forces generated by the jerks are greater than the tissues' extensibility, muscle injury may result.

ballistic stretching Older stretching technique that uses repetitive bouncing motions.

Certainly successive forceful contractions of the agonist muscle that result in stretching of the antagonist muscle may cause muscle soreness. For example, forcefully kicking a soccer ball fifty times may result in muscular soreness of the hamstrings (antagonist muscle) as a result of eccentric contraction of the hamstrings to control the dynamic movement of the quadriceps (agonist muscle). Ballistic stretching that is controlled usually does not cause muscle soreness.[65] In fact, in the athletic population, ballistic stretching is now referred to as *dynamic stretching* and has seen a resurgence in popularity. The argument has been that dynamic stretching exercises are more closely related to the types of activities that athletes engage in and should be considered more functional.[50] So dynamic stretching exercises are routinely recommended for athletes prior to beginning an activity (Figure 4-5A).

Dynamic stretching exercises are recommended prior to beginning an activity.

Ballistic doesn't cause soreness

Figure 4-5

Stretching techniques.
A, Dynamic (ballistic) stretch for hip flexors. **B,** Static stretch for knee extensors. **C,** Slow-reversal-hold-relax PNF techniques for hamstrings. **D,** Slump-stretch for sciatic nerve. **E,** Myofascial stretching for piriformis.

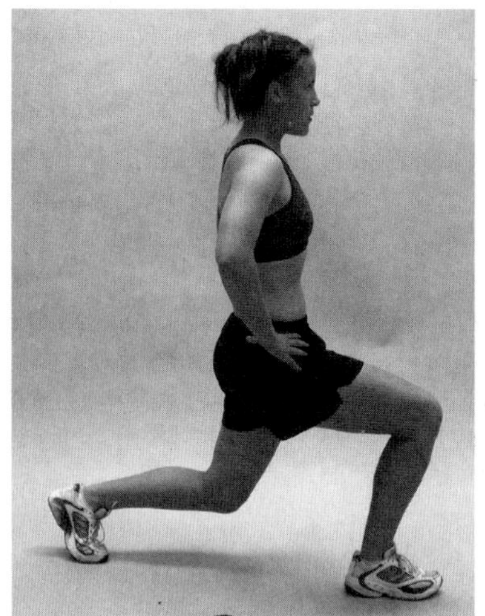
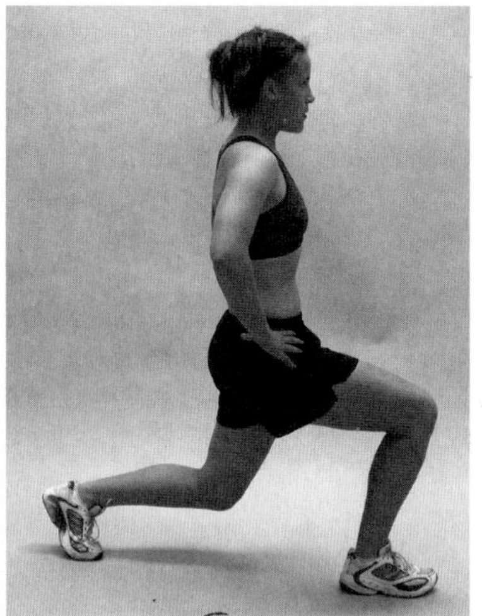

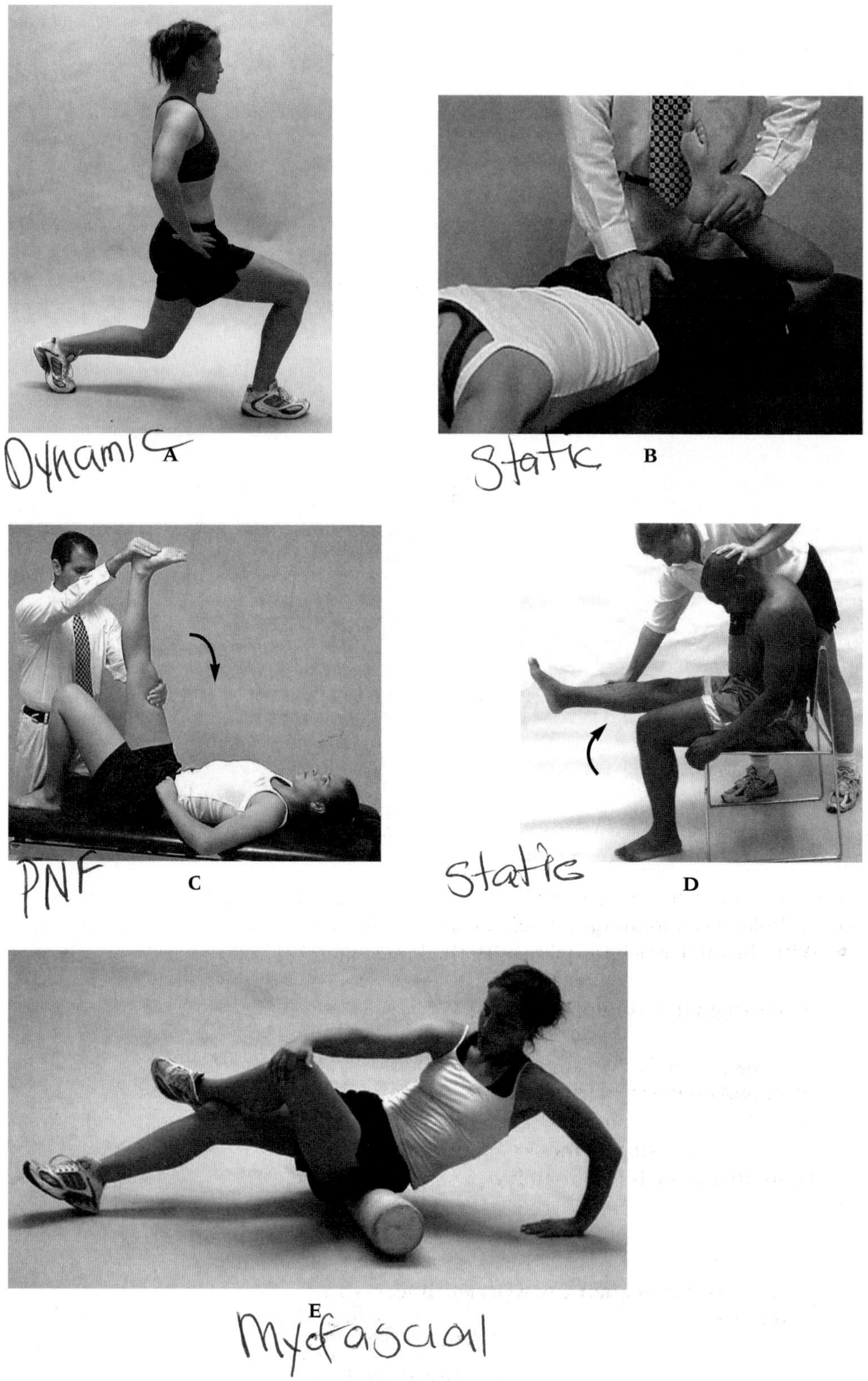

A

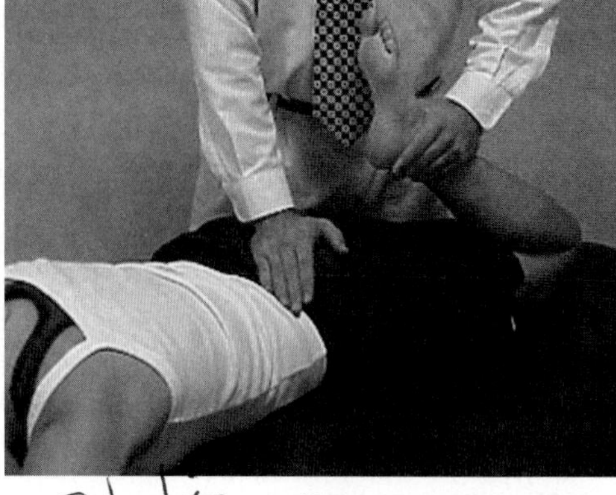

B

C

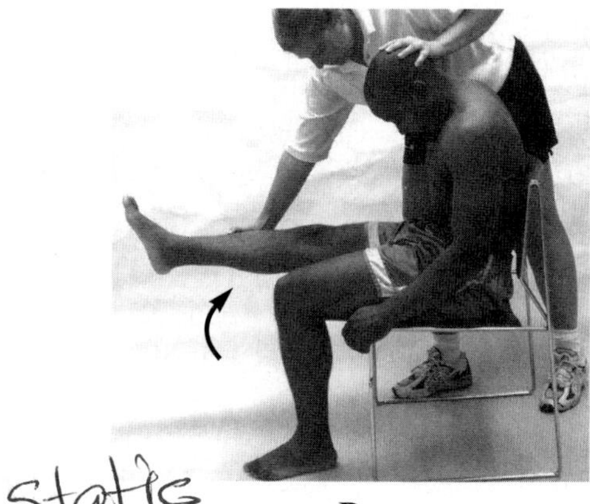

D

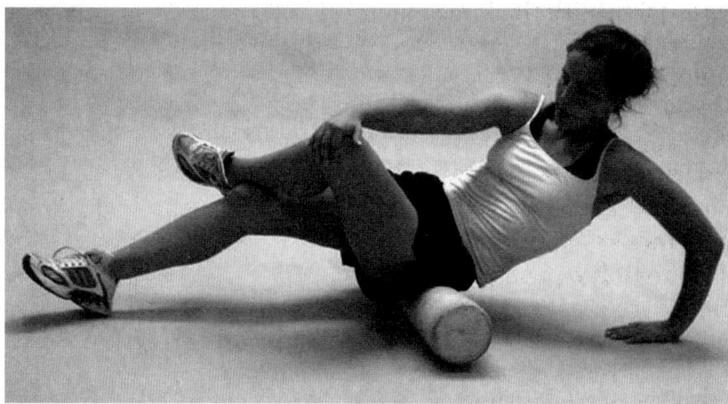

E

Static Stretching

The **static stretching** technique is a widely used and effective technique of stretching. This technique involves passively stretching a given antagonist muscle by placing it in a maximal position of stretch and holding it there for an extended time (Figure 4-5B). Recommendations for the optimal time for holding this stretched position vary from as short as three seconds to as long as sixty seconds.[36] Recent data indicate that thirty seconds may be an optimal time to hold the stretch. The static stretch of each muscle should be repeated three or four times.[8]

static stretching Passively stretching an antagonist muscle by placing it in a maximal stretch and holding it there.

Much research has been done comparing ballistic and static stretching techniques for the improvement of flexibility. It has been shown that both static and ballistic stretching are effective in increasing flexibility and that there is no significant difference between the two. However, static stretching offers less danger of exceeding the extensibility limits of the involved joints because the stretch is more controlled. Ballistic stretching is apt to cause muscular soreness, whereas static stretching generally does not and is commonly used in injury rehabilitation of sore or strained muscles.[59]

Static stretching is certainly a much safer stretching technique, especially for sedentary or untrained individuals. However, many physical activities involve dynamic movement. Thus, stretching as a warm-up for these types of activities should begin with static stretching followed by ballistic stretching, which more closely resembles the dynamic activity.

PNF Stretching Techniques

Proprioceptive neuromuscular facilitation (PNF techniques) were first used by physical therapists for treating patients who had various types of neuromuscular paralysis.[60] More recently PNF exercises have been used as a stretching technique for increasing flexibility.

proprioceptive neuromuscular facilitation (PNF) Stretching techniques that involve combinations of alternating contractions and stretches.

A number of different PNF techniques are currently being used for stretching, including slow-reversal-hold-relax, contract-relax, and hold-relax techniques. All involve some combination of alternating contraction and relaxation of both agonist and antagonist muscles. All three techniques use a ten-second push phase followed by a ten-second relax phase.

Using a hamstring stretching technique as an example (Figure 4-5C), the slow-reversal-hold-relax technique would be done as follows:[60]

- With the athlete lying supine with the knee extended and the ankle flexed to 90 degrees, the athletic trainer passively flexes the hip joint to the point at which there is slight discomfort in the muscle.
- At this point the athlete begins pushing against the athletic trainer's resistance by contracting the hamstring muscle.
- After pushing for ten seconds, the hamstring muscles are relaxed and the agonist quadriceps muscle is contracted while the athletic trainer applies passive pressure to further stretch the antagonist hamstrings. This action should move the leg so that there is increased hip joint flexion.
- The relaxing phase lasts for ten seconds, after which the athlete again pushes against the athletic trainer's resistance, beginning at this new position of increased hip/joint flexion.
- This push-relax sequence is repeated at least three times.

The contract-relax and hold-relax techniques are variations on the slow-reversal-hold-relax method. In the contract-relax method, the hamstrings are isotonically contracted so that the leg actually moves toward the floor during the push phase. The hold-relax method involves an isometric hamstring contraction against immovable resistance during the push phase. During the relax phase, both techniques involve the relaxation of hamstrings and quadriceps while the hamstrings are passively stretched. This same basic PNF technique can be used to stretch any muscle in the body. The PNF stretching techniques are perhaps best performed with a partner, although they may also be done using a wall as resistance (see Chapter 16).[60]

Figure 4-6

Stretch reflex. The muscle spindle produces a reflex resistance to stretch, and the Golgi tendon organ causes a reflex relaxation of the muscle in response to stretch.

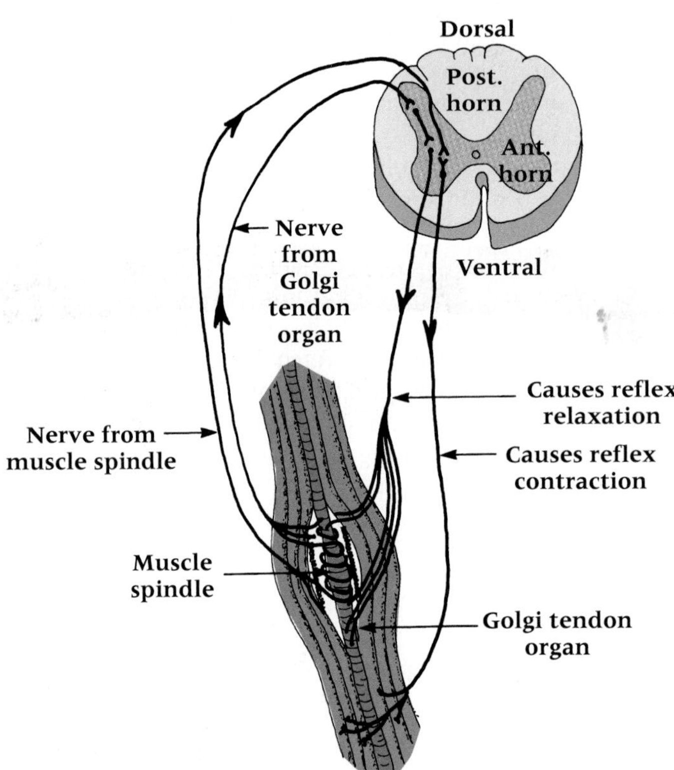

Stretching Neural Structures

The athletic trainer should be able to differentiate between tightness in the musculotendinous unit and abnormal neural tension. When the athlete performs both active and passive multiplanar movements, tension is created in the neural structures that exacerbates pain, limits range of motion, and increases neural symptoms including numbness and tingling. For example, the slump stretch position is used to detect an increase in nerve/root tension in the sciatic nerve and stretching should be done to assist in relieving tension (Figure 4-5D).

Stretching Fascia

Tight fascia can significantly limit motion. If there is damage to the fascia due to injury, disease, or inflammation, it will create pain and motion restriction. Thus it may be necessary to release tightness in the area of injury. Stretching of tight fascia can either be done manually or using a firm foam roller (Figure 4-5E). Myofascial release as a treatment technique is discussed in detail in Chapter 16.

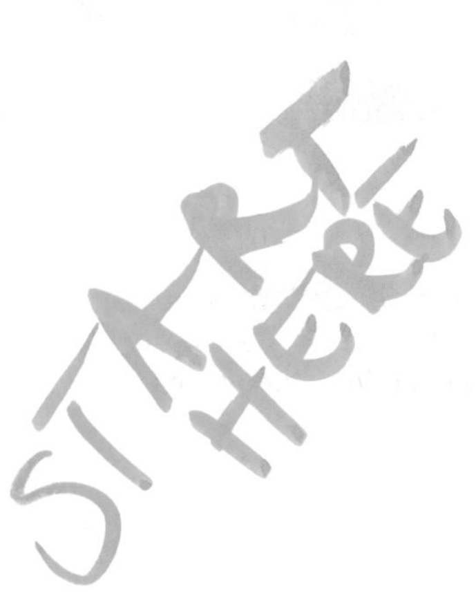

Neurophysiologic Basis of Stretching

All three stretching techniques are based on a neurophysiologic phenomenon involving the *stretch reflex* (Figure 4-6).[60] Every muscle in the body contains mechanoreceptors that, when stimulated, inform the central nervous system of what is happening with that muscle. Two of these receptors are important in the stretch reflex: the *muscle spindles* and the *Golgi tendon organs.* Both types of receptors are sensitive to changes in muscle length. The Golgi tendon organs are also affected by changes in muscle tension.

When a muscle is stretched, the muscle spindles are also stretched, sending a volley of sensory impulses to the spinal cord that informs the central nervous system that the muscle is being stretched. Impulses return to the muscle from the spinal cord, which causes the muscle to reflexively contract, thus resisting the stretch.[48] If the stretch of

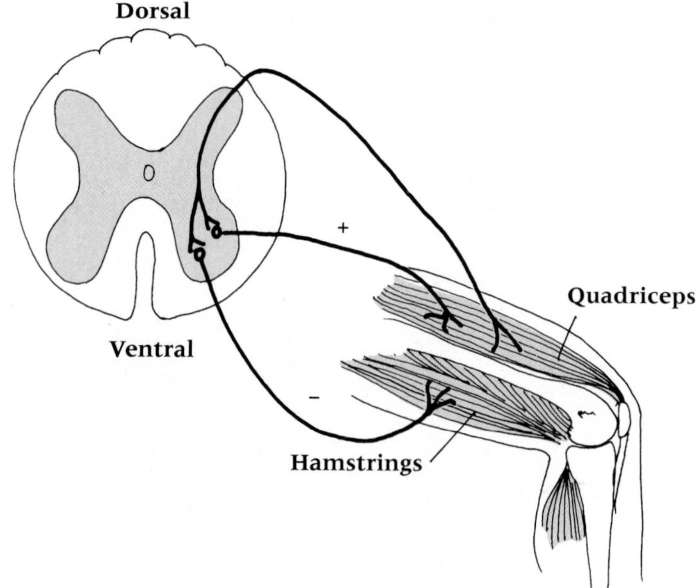

Figure 4-7

A contraction of the agonist will produce relaxation in the antagonist. Reciprocal inhibition.

the muscle continues for an extended period of time (at least six seconds), the Golgi tendon organs respond to the change in length and the increase in tension by firing off sensory impulses of their own to the spinal cord. The impulses from the Golgi tendon organs, unlike the signals from the muscle spindle, cause a reflex relaxation of the antagonist muscle. This reflex relaxation serves as a protective mechanism that will allow the muscle to stretch through relaxation before the extensibility limits are exceeded, causing damage to the muscle fibers.[60]

With the jerking, bouncing motion of ballistic stretching, the muscle spindles are being repetitively stretched; thus there is continuous resistance by the muscle to further stretch. The ballistic stretch is not continued long enough to allow the Golgi tendon organs to have any relaxing effect.

The static stretch involves a continuous sustained stretch lasting anywhere from six to sixty seconds, which is sufficient time for the Golgi tendon organs to begin responding to the increase in tension. The impulses from the Golgi tendon organs have the ability to override the impulses coming from the muscle spindles, allowing the muscle to reflexively relax after the initial reflex resistance to the change in length. Thus lengthening the muscle and allowing it to remain in a stretched position for an extended period of time is unlikely to produce any injury to the muscle.

The effectiveness of the PNF techniques may be attributed in part to these same neurophysiologic principles. The slow-reversal-hold-relax technique discussed previously takes advantage of two additional neurophysiologic phenomena.[60] The maximal isometric contraction of the muscle that will be stretched during the ten-second push phase again causes an increase in tension, which stimulates the Golgi tendon organs to effect a reflex relaxation of the antagonist muscle even before the muscle is placed in a position of stretch. This relaxation of the antagonist muscle during contractions is referred to as **autogenic inhibition**.

autogenic inhibition
The relaxation of the antagonist muscle during contractions.

During the relaxing phase the antagonist is relaxed and passively stretched while a maximal isotonic contraction of the agonist muscle pulls the extremity further into the agonist pattern. In any synergistic muscle group, a contraction of the agonist muscle causes a reflex relaxation in the antagonist muscle, allowing it to stretch and protecting it from injury. This phenomenon is referred to as *reciprocal inhibition* (Figure 4-7). Thus with the PNF techniques the additive effects of autogenic inhibition and reciprocal inhibition should theoretically allow the muscle to be stretched to a greater degree than is possible with static stretching or the ballistic technique.[60]

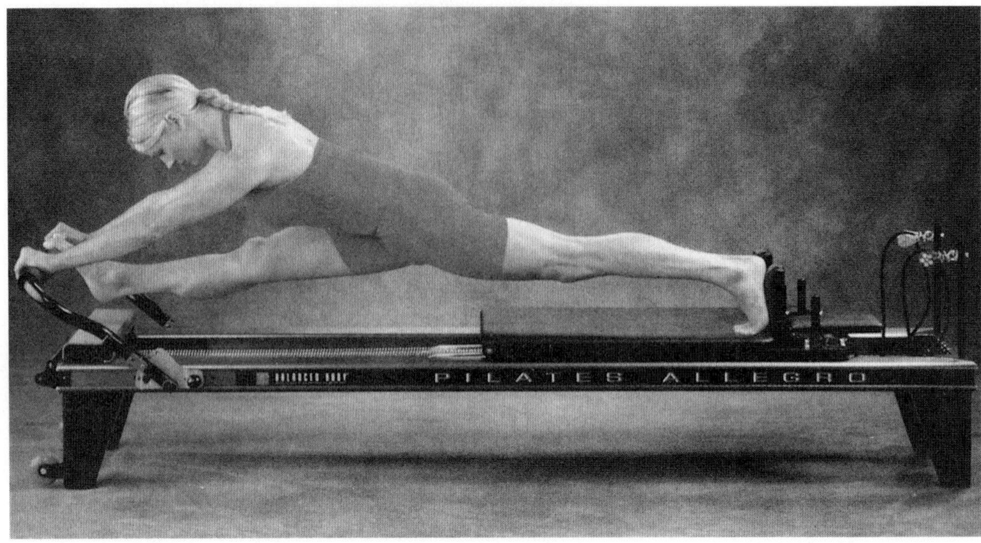

Figure 4-8

Pilates exercises are designed to improve muscle control, flexibility, coordination, and strength. (Photo courtesy Balanced Body, Inc., Sacramento, CA)

Practical Application Although all three stretching techniques have been demonstrated to effectively improve flexibility, there is still considerable debate as to which technique produces the greatest increases in range of movement. In the past, the dynamic technique has not been recommended because of the potential for causing muscle soreness. However, most sport activities are ballistic in nature (e.g., kicking, running), and those activities use the stretch reflex to enhance performance. In highly trained individuals, it is unlikely that dynamic stretching will result in muscle soreness. Static stretching is perhaps the most widely used technique. It is a simple technique and does not require a partner. A fully nonrestricted range of motion can be attained through static stretching over time.[24,67]

The PNF stretching techniques can produce dramatic increases in range of motion during one stretching session. Studies comparing static and PNF stretching suggest that PNF stretching can produce greater improvement in flexibility over an extended training period.[60,66] The major disadvantage of PNF stretching is that it requires a partner for stretching, although stretching with a partner may have some motivational advantages. An increasing number of athletic teams are adopting the PNF technique as the method of choice for improving flexibility.

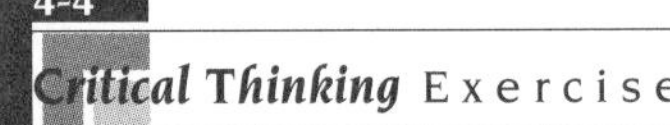
4-4 *Critical Thinking* Exercise

A college swimmer has been engaged in an off-season weight-training program to increase her muscular strength and endurance. Although she has seen some improvement in her strength, she is concerned that she also seems to be losing flexibility in her shoulders, which she feels is critical to her performance as a swimmer. She has also noticed that her muscles are hypertrophying to some degree and is worried that this may be causing her to lose flexibility. She has just about decided to abandon her weight-training program altogether.

? What can the athletic trainer recommend to her that will allow her to continue to improve her muscular strength and endurance while simultaneously maintaining or perhaps even improving her flexibility?

The Pilates Method

The Pilates method is a somewhat different approach to stretching for improving flexibility. This method has become extremely popular and widely used among personal fitness trainers and physical therapists. Pilates is an exercise technique devised by German-born Joseph Pilates, who established the first Pilates studio in the United States before World War II. The Pilates method is a conditioning program that improves muscle control, flexibility, coordination, strength, and tone. The basic principles of Pilates exercise are to make people more aware of their bodies as single integrated units, to improve body alignment and breathing, and to increase efficiency of movement. Unlike other exercise programs, the Pilates method does not require the repetition of exercises but instead consists of a sequence of carefully performed movements, some of which are carried out on specially designed equipment (Figure 4-8). Each exercise is designed to stretch and strengthen the muscles involved. There is a specific breathing pattern for each exercise to help direct energy to the areas being worked, while relaxing the rest of the body. The Pilates method works many of the deeper muscles together, improving

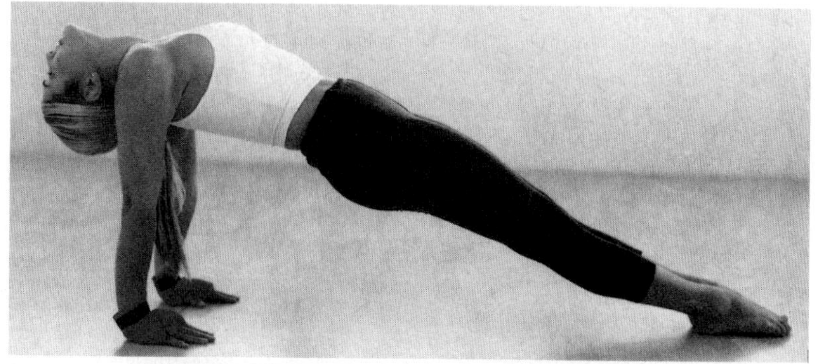

Figure 4-9

Yoga uses a variety of positions to increase flexibility in the body. (Photo courtesy International Dance Exercise Association, San Diego, CA)

coordination and balance, to achieve efficient and graceful movement. Instead of seeking an ideal or perfect body, the goal is for the practitioner to develop a healthy self-image through the attainment of better posture, proper coordination, and improved flexibility. This method concentrates on body alignment, lengthening all of the muscles of the body into a balanced whole, and building endurance and strength without putting undue stress on the lungs and heart. Pilates instructors believe that problems such as soft-tissue injuries can cause bad posture, which can lead to pain and discomfort. Pilates exercises aim to correct this.

Normally a beginner sees a Pilates instructor on a one-to-one basis for the first session. The instructor assesses the client's physical condition and asks the client about any problems and about the client's lifestyle. The client is then shown a series of exercises that work joints and muscles through a range of movement appropriate for the client's needs. A class in a studio might involve working on specially designed equipment that primarily uses resistance against tensioned springs to isolate and develop specific muscle groups. Mat work classes involve a repertoire of exercises on a floor mat only. This type of class has become very popular in health clubs and gyms and is often compared to other forms of body conditioning. In fact, the Pilates mat exercises are generally less strenuous that mat exercises in most other conditioning classes.

Yoga

Yoga originated in India approximately 6,000 years ago. Its basic philosophy is that most illness is related to poor mental attitudes, posture, and diet. Practitioners of yoga maintain that stress can be reduced through combined mental and physical approaches. Yoga can help an individual cope with stress-induced behaviors like overeating, hypertension, and smoking. Yoga's meditative aspects are believed to help alleviate psychosomatic illnesses. Yoga aims to unite the body and mind to reduce stress. For example, Dr. Chandra Patel, a yoga expert, has found that persons who practice yoga can reduce their blood pressure indefinitely as long as they continue to practice yoga. Yoga involves various body postures and breathing exercises. Hatha yoga uses a number of positions through which the practitioner may progress, beginning with the simplest and moving to the more complex (Figure 4-9). The various positions are intended to increase mobility and flexibility. However, practitioners must use caution when performing yoga positions. Some positions can be dangerous, particularly for someone who is inexperienced in yoga technique.

Slow, deep, diaphragmatic breathing is an important part of yoga. Many people take shallow breaths, however, breathing deeply, fully expanding the chest when inhaling helps lower blood pressure and heart rate. Deep breathing has a calming effect on the body. It also increases production of endorphins.

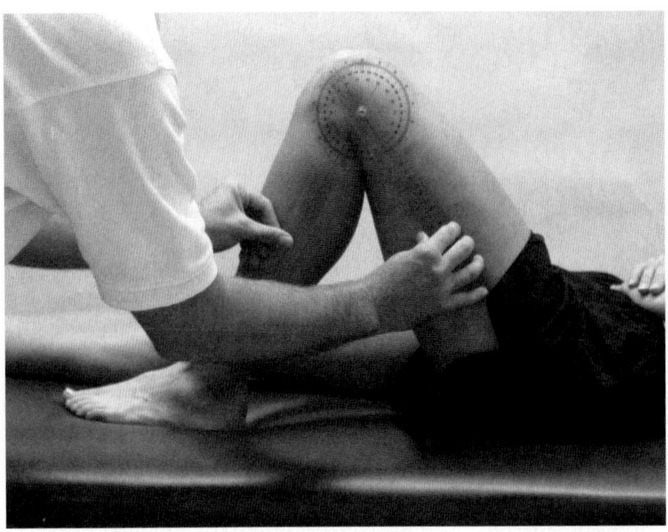

Figure 4-10

A goniometer can be used to measure joint angles and range of motion.

The Relationship between Strength and Flexibility

It is often said that strength training has a negative effect on flexibility.[64] For example, we tend to think of athletes who have highly developed muscles as having lost much of their ability to move freely through a full range of motion. Occasionally an athlete develops so much bulk that the physical size of the muscle prevents a normal range of motion. It is certainly true that strength training that is not properly done can impair movement; however, weight training, if done properly through a full range of motion, will not impair flexibility. Proper strength training probably improves dynamic flexibility and, if combined with a rigorous stretching program, can greatly enhance powerful and coordinated movements that are essential for success in many athletic activities. In all cases a heavy weight-training program should be accompanied by a strong flexibility program.

Measuring Range of Motion

Accurate measurement of the range of joint motion is difficult. Various devices have been designed to accommodate variations in the size of the joints and the complexity of movements in articulations that involve more than one joint. Of these devices, the simplest and most widely used is the goniometer (Figure 4-10). A goniometer is a large protractor with measurements in degrees. By aligning the two arms parallel to the longitudinal axis of the two segments involved in motion about a specific joint, it is possible to obtain relatively accurate measures of range of movement. The goniometer has its place in a rehabilitation setting, where it is essential to assess improvement in joint flexibility for the purpose of modifying injury rehabilitation programs.[30,57]

THE IMPORTANCE OF MUSCULAR STRENGTH, ENDURANCE, AND POWER

muscular strength
The maximum force that can be applied by a muscle during a single maximum contraction.

The development of **muscular strength** is an essential component of a training program for every athlete. By definition, strength is the ability of a muscle to generate force against some resistance. Most movements in sports are explosive and must include elements of both strength and speed if they are to be effective. If a large amount of force is generated quickly, the movement can be referred to as a *power* movement. Without the ability to generate power, an athlete will be limited in his or her performance capabilities.[59]

muscular endurance
The ability to perform repetitive muscular contractions against some resistance.

Muscular strength is closely associated with muscular endurance. **Muscular endurance** is the ability to perform repetitive muscular contractions against some resistance for an extended period of time. As muscular strength increases, there tends to be a corresponding increase in endurance.[44,69] For example, an athlete can lift a weight twenty-five times. If muscular strength is increased by 10 percent through weight training, it is likely that the maximum number of repetitions would be increased because it is easier for the athlete to lift the weight.

Skeletal Muscle Contractions

Skeletal muscle is capable of three different types of contraction: *isometric contraction, concentric contraction,* and *eccentric contraction.*[63] An isometric contraction occurs when the muscle contracts to increase tension but there is no change in the length of the muscle. Considerable force can be generated against some immovable resistance even though no movement occurs. In concentric contraction, the muscle shortens in length as a contraction is developed to overcome or move some resistance. In eccentric contraction the resistance is greater than the muscular force being produced, and the muscle lengthens while continuing to contract. Concentric and eccentric contractions are both considered to be dynamic movements.[63]

It is critical to understand that functional movements involve acceleration, deceleration, and stabilization in all three planes of motion simultaneously. Functional movements are controlled by neuromuscular mechanoreceptors located within the muscle.[20]

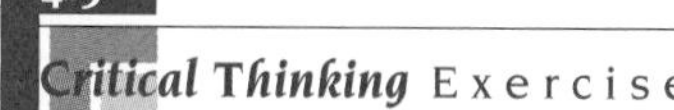

4-5

Critical Thinking Exercise

A college freshman on the varsity basketball team lacks motivation to improve her strength and conditioning over the summer and during the off-season. The coaches are frustrated with her attitude and come to the athletic trainer for advice.

? How can the athletic trainer convince the athlete of the importance of strength and conditioning?

Skeletal muscle is capable of three types of contractions:
- Isometric
- Concentric
- Eccentric

Fast-Twitch versus Slow-Twitch Fibers

All fibers in a particular motor unit are either *slow-twitch* or *fast-twitch* fibers, each of which has distinctive metabolic and contractile capabilities. Slow-twitch fibers are also referred to as type I fibers. They are more resistant to fatigue than are fast-twitch fibers; however, the time required to generate force is much greater in slow-twitch fibers.[43] Because they are relatively fatigue resistant, slow-twitch fibers are associated primarily with long-duration, aerobic-type activities.[34]

Fast-twitch fibers (also referred to as type II fibers) are capable of producing quick, forceful contractions but have a tendency to fatigue more rapidly than do slow-twitch fibers. Fast-twitch fibers are useful in short-term, high-intensity activities, which mainly involve the anaerobic system. Fast-twitch fibers are capable of producing powerful contractions, whereas slow-twitch fibers produce a long-endurance type of force. There are two subdivisions of fast-twitch fibers. Although both types of fast-twitch fibers are capable of rapid contraction, type IIa fibers are moderately resistant to fatigue, whereas type IIb fibers fatigue rapidly and are considered the "true" fast-twitch fibers.[34]

There are three basic types of muscle fibers:
- Slow-twitch type I
- Fast-twitch type IIa
- Fast-twitch type IIb

Any given muscle contains both types of fibers, and the ratio in an individual muscle varies with each person.[43] Those muscles whose primary function is to maintain posture against gravity require more endurance and have a higher percentage of slow-twitch fibers. Muscles that produce powerful, rapid, explosive strength movements tend to have a much greater percentage of fast-twitch fibers. Because this ratio is genetically determined, it may play a large role in determining ability for a given sport activity. Sprinters and weight lifters, for example, have a large percentage of fast-twitch fibers in relation to slow-twitch fibers.[15] Conversely, marathon runners generally have a higher percentage of slow-twitch fibers.

The metabolic capabilities of both fast-twitch and slow-twitch fibers may be improved through specific strength and endurance training. It now appears that there can be an almost complete change from slow-twitch to fast-twitch and from fast-twitch to slow-twitch fiber types in response to training.[51]

Physiological and Biomechanical Factors That Determine Levels of Muscular Strength

Muscular strength is proportional to the cross-sectional diameter of the muscle fibers. The greater the cross-sectional diameter or the bigger a particular muscle, the stronger it is, and thus the more force it is capable of generating. The size of a muscle tends to increase in cross-sectional diameter with weight training. This increase in muscle size is referred to as **hypertrophy**.[42] Conversely, a decrease in the size of a muscle is referred to as **atrophy**.

hypertrophy
Enlargement of a muscle caused by an increase in the size of its cells in response to training.

atrophy
Decrease of a muscle caused by a decrease in the size of its cells because of inactivity.

Size of the Muscle

Strength is a function of the number and diameter of muscle fibers composing a given muscle. The number of fibers is an inherited characteristic; thus an athlete with a large number of muscle fibers to begin with has the potential to hypertrophy to a much greater degree than does someone with relatively fewer fibers.[25]

Explanations for Muscle Hypertrophy

A number of theories have been proposed to explain why a muscle hypertrophies in response to strength training.[38] Some evidence exists that the number of muscle fibers increase because fibers split in response to training.[58] However, this research has been conducted in animals and should not be generalized to humans. It is generally accepted that the number of fibers is genetically determined and does not seem to increase with training.

Another hypothesis is that because the muscle is working harder in weight training, more blood is required to supply that muscle with oxygen and other nutrients. Thus the number of capillaries is increased. This hypothesis is only partially correct; few new capillaries are formed during strength training, but a number of dormant capillaries may become filled with blood to meet the increased demand for blood supply.

A third theory to explain this increase in muscle size seems the most credible. Muscle fibers are composed primarily of small protein filaments, called myofilaments, which are the contractile elements in muscle. These myofilaments increase in both size and number as a result of strength training, causing the individual muscle fibers themselves to increase in cross-sectional diameter.[51] This increase is particularly true in men, although women also see some increase in muscle size.[1] More research is needed to further clarify and determine the specific causes of muscle hypertrophy.

Improved Neuromuscular Efficiency

Typically with weight training, an athlete sees some remarkable gains in strength initially, even though muscle bulk does not necessarily increase. This gain in strength must be attributed to something other than muscle hypertrophy. For a muscle to contract, an impulse must be transmitted from the nervous system to the muscle. Each muscle fiber is innervated by a specific motor unit. By overloading a particular muscle, as in weight training, the muscle is forced to work efficiently. Efficiency is achieved by getting more motor units to fire, causing a stronger contraction of the muscle.[71] Consequently, it is not uncommon to see extremely rapid gains in strength when a weight-training program is first begun due to an improvement in neuromuscular function.[52]

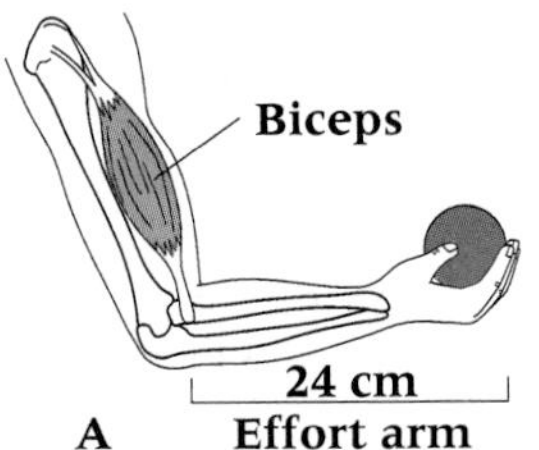

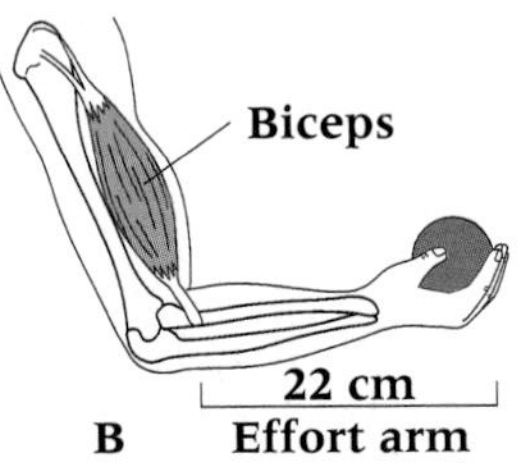

Figure 4-11

The position of attachment of the muscle tendon on the arm can affect the ability of that muscle to generate force. Person B should be able to generate greater force than person A because the tendon attachment is closer to the resistance.

Other Physiological Adaptations to Resistance Exercise

In addition to muscle hypertrophy there are a number of other physiological adaptations to resistance training.[9] The strength of noncontractile structures, including tendons and ligaments, is increased. The mineral content of bone is increased, making the bone stronger and more resistant to fracture. Maximal oxygen uptake is improved when resistance training is of sufficient intensity to elicit heart rates at or above training levels. Several enzymes important in aerobic and anaerobic metabolism also increase.[15,51]

Biomechanical Factors

Strength in a given muscle is determined not only by the physical properties of the muscle itself but also by biomechanical factors that dictate how much force can be generated through a system of levers to an external object. If we think of the elbow joint as one of these lever systems, we would have the biceps muscle producing flexion of this joint (Figure 4-11). The position of attachment of the biceps muscle on the lever arm, in this case the forearm, will largely determine how much force this muscle is capable of generating.[29] If there are two persons, A and B, and person B has a biceps attachment that is farther from the center of the joint than is person A's, then person B should be able to lift heavier weights because the muscle force acts through a longer lever (moment) arm and thus can produce greater torque around the joint.

The length of a muscle determines the tension that can be generated.[32] By varying the length of a muscle, different tensions may be produced. This length-tension relationship is illustrated in Figure 4-12. At position B in the curve, the interaction of the crossbridges between the actin and myosin myofilaments within the sarcomere is at a maximum. Setting a muscle at this length will produce the greatest amount of tension. At position A the muscle is shortened, and at position C the muscle is lengthened. In either case the interaction between the actin and myosin myofilaments through the crossbridges is greatly reduced, and the muscle is not capable of generating significant tension.

Overtraining

Overtraining can have a negative effect on the development of muscular strength. The statement "if you abuse it you will lose it" is applicable. Overtraining can result in psychological breakdown (staleness) or physiological breakdown, which may involve musculoskeletal injury, fatigue, or sickness. Engaging in proper and efficient resistance training, eating a proper diet, and getting appropriate rest can minimize the potential negative effects of overtraining.

Reversibility

If strength training is discontinued or interrupted, the muscle will atrophy, decreasing in both strength and mass. Adaptations in skeletal muscle that occur in response to resistance training may begin to reverse in as little as forty-eight hours. It does appear that consistent exercise of a muscle is essential to prevent reversal of the hypertrophy that occurs due to strength training.

Techniques of Resistance Training

There are a number of different techniques of resistance training for strength improvement, including isometric exercise, progressive resistance exercise, isokinetic exercise, circuit training, and plyometric exercise. Regardless of which of these techniques is used, one basic principle of training is extremely important. For a muscle to improve in strength, it must be forced to work at a higher level than it is accustomed to working at. In other words, the muscle must be *overloaded.* Without overload the muscle will be able to maintain strength as long as training is continued against a resistance the muscle is accustomed to. To most effectively build muscular strength, weight training requires a consistent, increasing effort against progressively increasing resistance.[23] Progressive resistance exercise is based primarily on the principles of overload and progression. If this principle of overload is applied, all five training techniques will produce improvement of muscular strength over a period of time.

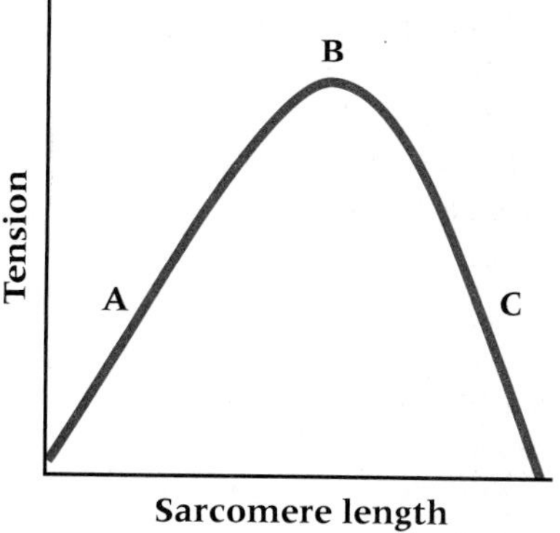

Figure 4-12

Because of the length-tension relation in muscle, the greatest tension is developed at point B, with less tension developed at points A and C.

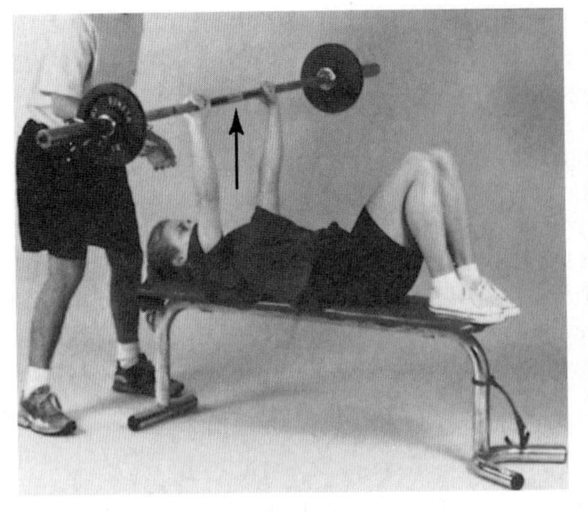

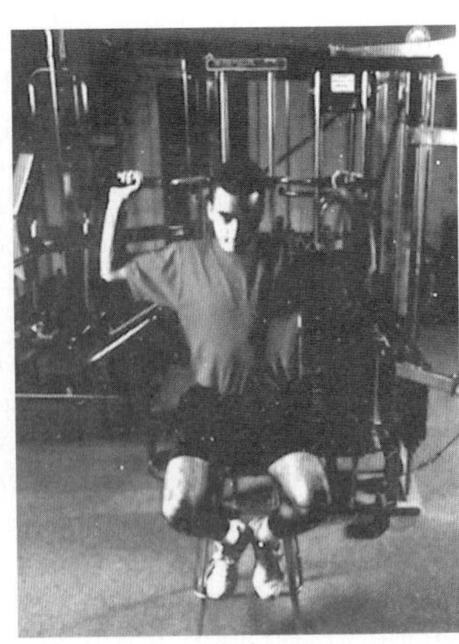

Figure 4-13

A, Barbells and dumbbells are free weights that assist the athlete in developing isotonic strength. **B,** Many machine exercise systems provide a variety of exercise possibilities for the athlete.

Isometric Exercise

isometric exercise
Contracts the muscle statically without changing its length.

An **isometric exercise** involves a muscle contraction in which the length of the muscle remains constant while tension develops toward a maximal force against an immovable resistance.[7] The muscle should generate a maximal force for ten seconds at a time, and this contraction should be repeated five to ten times per day. Isometric exercises are capable of increasing muscular strength; unfortunately, strength gains are specific to the joint angle at which training is performed. At other angles, the strength curve drops off dramatically because of a lack of motor activity at that angle.

Another major disadvantage of isometric exercises is that they tend to produce a spike in systolic blood pressure that can result in potentially life-threatening cardiovascular accidents.[59] This sharp increase in blood pressure results from an individual holding his or her breath and increasing intrathoracic pressure. Consequently, the blood pressure experienced by the heart is increased significantly. This phenomenon has been referred to as the Valsalva effect. To avoid or minimize this increase in pressure, it is recommended that breathing be continued during the maximal contraction.

Isometric exercises are useful in the rehabilitation of certain injuries; this use is discussed in the rehabilitation sections in Chapters 18 through 26.

Progressive Resistance Exercise

A second technique of resistance training is perhaps the most commonly used and the most popular technique for improving muscular strength. *Progressive resistance exercise* training uses exercises that strengthen muscles through a contraction that overcomes some fixed resistance produced by equipment such as dumbbells, barbells, or various weight machines (Figure 4-13). Progressive resistance exercise uses isotonic contractions which generate force while the muscle is changing in length.[23]

concentric (positive) contraction
The muscle shortens while contracting against resistance.

eccentric (negative) contraction
The muscle lengthens while contracting against resistance.

Isotonic contractions Isotonic contractions may be either concentric or eccentric. An athlete who is performing a biceps curl offers a good example of an isotonic contraction. To lift the weight from the starting position, the biceps muscle must contract and shorten in length. This shortening contraction is referred to as a **concentric**, or **positive, contraction**. If the biceps muscle does not remain contracted when the weight is being lowered, gravity will cause the weight to simply fall back to the starting position. Thus, to control the weight as it is being lowered, the biceps muscle must continue to contract while at the same time gradually lengthening. A contraction in which the muscle is lengthening while still applying force is called an **eccentric**, or **negative, contraction**.[39]

Eccentric contractions versus concentric contractions It is possible to generate greater amounts of force against resistance with an eccentric contraction than with a concentric contraction. This greater force occurs because eccentric contractions require a much lower level of motor unit activity to achieve a certain force than do concentric contractions. Because fewer motor units are firing to produce a specific force, additional motor units may be recruited to generate increased force. In addition, oxygen utilization is much lower during eccentric exercise than during comparable concentric exercise. Thus eccentric contractions are more resistant to fatigue than are concentric contractions. The mechanical efficiency of eccentric exercise may be several times higher than that of concentric exercise.[63]

Concentric contractions accelerate movement, whereas eccentric contractions decelerate motion. For example, the hamstrings must contract eccentrically to decelerate the angular velocity of the lower leg during running. Likewise, the external rotators in the rotator cuff muscles surrounding the shoulder contract eccentrically to decelerate the internally rotating humerus during throwing. Because of the excessive forces involved with these eccentric contractions, injury to the muscles is quite common. Thus, eccentric exercise must be routinely incorporated into the strength training program to prevent injury to those muscles that act to decelerate movement.

Free weights versus machine weights Various types of exercise equipment can be used with progressive resistance exercise, including free weights (barbells and dumbbells) or exercise machines such as those made by Universal, Nautilus, Cybex, Eagle, and Body Master. Dumbbells and barbells require the use of iron plates of varying weights that can be changed easily by adding or subtracting equal amounts of weight to both sides of the bar. The exercise machines have a stack of weights that are lifted through a series of levers or pulleys. The stack of weights slides up and down on a pair of bars that restrict the movement to only one plane. Weight can be increased or decreased simply by changing the position of a weight key.

There are advantages and disadvantages to both free weights and exercise machines. The exercise machines are relatively safe to use compared to free weights. It is also a simple process to increase or decrease the weight on exercise machines by moving a single weight key, although changes can generally be made only in increments of ten or fifteen pounds. The iron plates used with free weights must be added or removed from each side of the barbell or dumbbell.

Figure 4-14 shows examples of different isotonic strengthening exercises.

Spotting for free weight exercises When training with free weights, it is essential that the lifter have a partner who can assist in performing a particular exercise. This assistance is particularly critical when the weights to be lifted are extremely heavy. A *spotter* has three functions: to protect the lifter from injury, to make recommendations on proper lifting technique, and to help motivate the lifter. *Focus Box:* "Proper spotting techniques" provides some guidelines for correct spotting techniques.

Focus

Proper spotting techniques

- Make sure the lifter uses the proper grip.
- Check to see that the lifter is in a safe, stable position.
- Make sure the lifter moves through a complete range of motion at the appropriate speed.
- Make sure the lifter inhales and exhales during the lift.
- When spotting dumbbell exercises, spot as close to the dumbbells as possible above the elbow joint.
- Make sure the lifter understands how to get out of the way of missed attempts, particularly with overhead techniques.
- Stand behind the lifter.
- If heavy weights exceed the limits of your ability to control the weight, use a second spotter.
- Communicate with the lifter to know how many reps are to be done, whether a liftoff is needed, and how much help the lifter wants in completing a rep.
- Always be in a position to protect both the lifter and yourself from injury.

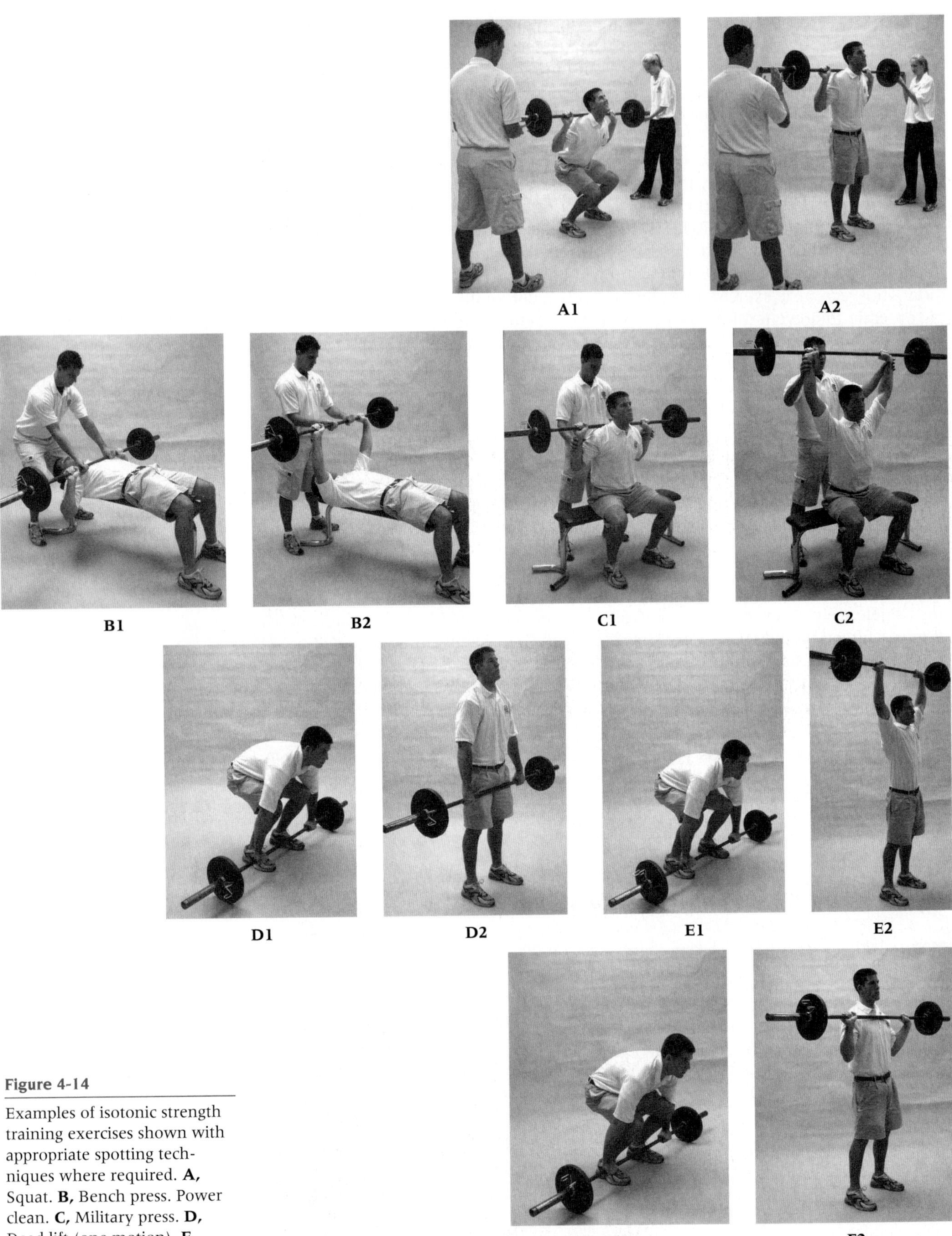

Figure 4-14

Examples of isotonic strength training exercises shown with appropriate spotting techniques where required. **A,** Squat. **B,** Bench press. Power clean. **C,** Military press. **D,** Dead lift (one motion). **E,** Snatch (one motion). **F,** Power clean (one motion).

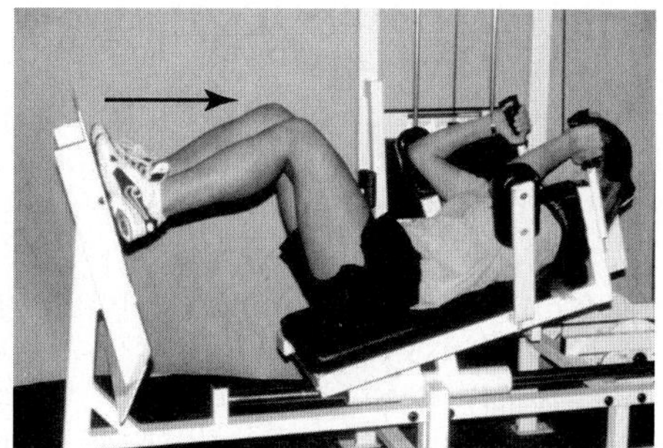

Figure 4-14—continued

G, Leg press.

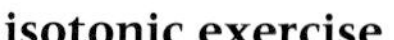

Isotonic training Regardless of which type of equipment is used, the same principles of **isotonic exercise** may be applied. In progressive resistance exercise, it is essential to incorporate both concentric and eccentric contractions. Research has clearly demonstrated that the muscle should be overloaded and fatigued both concentrically and eccentrically for the greatest strength improvement to occur.[43,51]

isotonic exercise Shortens and lengthens the muscle through a complete range of motion.

When an athlete is training specifically to develop muscular strength, the concentric, or positive, portion of the exercise should require one to two seconds and the eccentric, or negative, portion of the lift should require two to four seconds. The ratio of negative to positive should be approximately one to two. Physiologically, the muscle will fatigue much more rapidly concentrically than eccentrically.

Athletes who have trained with both free weights and machines realize the difference in the amount of weight that can be lifted. Unlike the machines, free weights have no restricted motion and can thus move in many different directions, depending on the forces applied. With free weights, an element of muscular control on the part of the lifter to prevent the weight from moving in any direction other than vertical will usually decrease the amount of weight that can be lifted.[35]

One problem often mentioned in relation to isotonic training is that the amount of force necessary to move a weight through a range of motion changes according to the angle of pull of the contracting muscle. The amount of force is greatest when the angle of pull is approximately 90 degrees. In addition, once the inertia of the weight has been overcome and momentum has been established, the force required to move the resistance varies according to the force that the muscle can produce through the range of motion. Thus, it has been argued that a disadvantage of any type of isotonic exercise is that the force required to move the resistance is constantly changing throughout the range of movement.

Certain exercise machines are designed to minimize this change in resistance by using a cam system (Figure 4-15). The cam has been individually designed for each piece of equipment so that the resistance is variable throughout the movement. The cam system attempts to alter resistance so that the muscle can handle a greater load—at

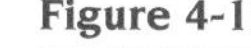

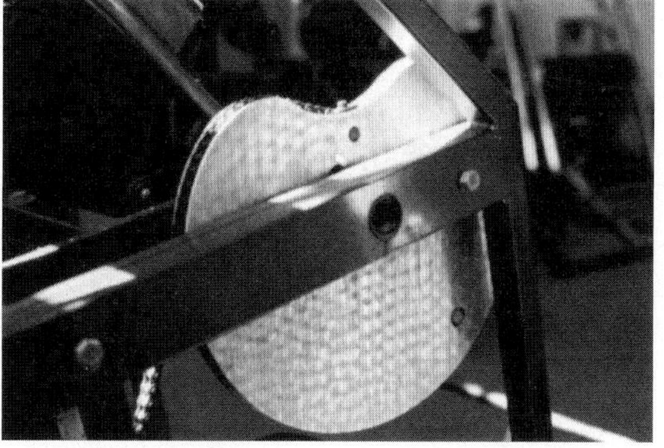

Figure 4-15

The cam system on the Nautilus equipment is designed to equalize the resistance throughout the full range of motion.

the points at which the joint angle or muscle length is at a mechanical disadvantage, the cam reduces the resistance to muscle movement. Whether this design does what it claims is debatable. This change in resistance at different points in the range is called accommodating resistance, or variable resistance.

Progressive resistance exercise techniques Perhaps the single most confusing aspect of progressive resistance exercise is the terminology used to describe specific programs. The following list of terms and their operational definitions may help clarify the confusion:

- Repetitions—The number of times a specific movement is repeated.
- Repetitions maximum (RM)—The maximum number of repetitions at a given weight.
- One repetition maximum (1RM)—The maximum amount of weight that can be lifted one time.
- Set—A particular number of repetitions.
- Intensity—The amount of weight or resistance lifted.
- Recovery period—The rest interval between sets.
- Frequency—The number of times an exercise is done in one week.

A considerable amount of research has been done in the area of resistance training to determine optimal techniques in terms of the intensity or the amount of weight to be used, the number of repetitions, the number of sets, the recovery period, and the frequency of training. It is important to realize that there are many different effective techniques and training regimens. Regardless of specific techniques used, it is certain that to improve strength the muscle must be overloaded in a progressive manner.[57] This overload is the basis of progressive resistance exercise. The amount of weight used and the number of repetitions must be enough to make the muscle work at a higher intensity than it is used to working at. This overload is the single most critical factor in any strength-training program. The strength-training program must also be designed to meet the specific needs of the athlete.

There is no such thing as an optimal strength-training program. Achieving total agreement on a program of resistance training—with specific recommendations about repetitions, sets, intensity, recovery time, and frequency—among researchers or other experts in resistance training is impossible. However, the following general recommendations will provide an effective resistance-training program.

For any given exercise, the amount of weight selected should be sufficient to allow six to eight repetitions maximum (RM) in each of three sets with a recovery period of sixty to ninety seconds between sets. Initial selection of a starting weight may require some trial and error to achieve this 6 to 8 RM range. If at least three sets of six repetitions cannot be completed, the weight is too heavy and should be reduced. If it is possible to do more than three sets of eight repetitions, the weight is too light and should be increased.[10] Progression to heavier weights is determined by the ability to perform at least 8 RM in each of three sets. An increase of about 10 percent of the current weight being lifted should still allow at least 6 RM in each of three sets.

Occasionally, athletes may be tested at 1RM to determine the greatest amount of weight that can be lifted one time. Extreme caution should be exercised when trying to determine 1RM. Attention should be directed toward making sure the athlete has had ample opportunity to warm up and that the lifting technique is correct before attempting a maximum lift. Determining 1RM should be done very gradually to minimize the chances of injuring the muscle.

A particular muscle or muscle group should be exercised consistently every other day. Thus the frequency of weight training should be at least three times per week but no more than four times per week. It is common for serious weight trainers to lift every day; however, they exercise different muscle groups on successive days. For example, Monday, Wednesday, and Friday may be used for upper body muscles, whereas Tuesday, Thursday, and Saturday are used for lower body muscles.

Training for muscular strength versus endurance Muscular endurance is the ability to perform repeated muscle contractions against resistance for an extended period

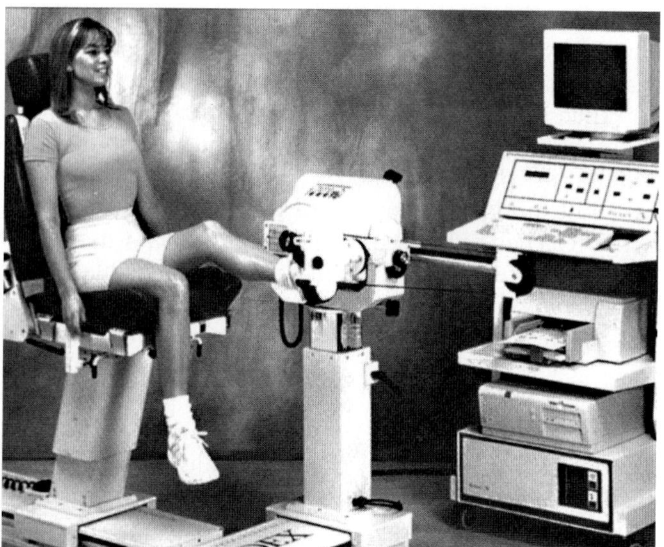

Figure 4-16

During isokinetic exercise the speed of movement is constant regardless of the force applied by the athlete.

of time. Most weight-training experts believe that muscular strength and muscular endurance are closely related.[59] As one improves, the other tends to improve also.

When weight training for strength, use heavier weights with a lower number of repetitions. Conversely, endurance training uses relatively lighter weights with a greater number of repetitions.

Endurance training should consist of three sets of ten to fifteen repetitions using the same criteria for weight selection, progression, and frequency as recommended for progressive resistance exercise.[7] Thus, suggested training regimens for muscular strength and endurance are similar in terms of sets and numbers of repetitions. Persons who possess great levels of strength also tend to exhibit greater muscular endurance when asked to perform repeated contractions against resistance.

Isokinetic Exercise

An **isokinetic exercise** involves a muscle contraction in which the length of the muscle is changing while the contraction is performed at a constant velocity.[58] In theory, maximal resistance is provided throughout the range of motion by the machine. The resistance provided by the machine will move only at some preset speed regardless of the force applied to it by the individual. Thus the key to isokinetic exercise is not the resistance but the speed at which the resistance can be moved.[16]

isokinetic exercise
Resistance is given at a fixed velocity of movement with accommodating resistance.

Currently, only one isokinetic device is available commercially—Biodex (Figure 4-16). Isokinetic devices rely on hydraulic, pneumatic, or mechanical pressure systems to produce constant velocity of motion. Isokinetic devices are capable of resisting both concentric and eccentric contractions at a fixed speed to exercise a muscle.

A major disadvantage of an isokinetic unit is its cost. The unit comes with a computer and printing device and is used primarily as a diagnostic and rehabilitative tool in the treatment of various injuries.

Isokinetic devices are designed so that regardless of the amount of force applied, the resistance can be moved only at a certain speed. That speed will be the same whether maximal force or only half the maximal force is applied. Consequently, when training isokinetically, it is absolutely necessary to exert as much force against the resistance as possible (maximal effort) for maximal strength gains to occur. This need for maximal effort is one of the major problems with an isokinetic strength-training program.

Anyone who has been involved in a weight-training program knows that on some days it is difficult to find the motivation to work out. Because isokinetic training does not require a maximal effort, it is easy to "cheat" and not go through the workout at a high level of intensity. In a progressive resistance exercise program, the individual knows how much weight has to be lifted with how many repetitions. Thus, isokinetic training is often more effective if a partner system is used as a means of motivation toward a maximal effort.

When isokinetic training is done properly with a maximal effort, it is theoretically possible that maximal strength gains are best achieved through the isokinetic training method in which the velocity and force of the resistance are equal throughout the range of motion. However, there is no conclusive research to support this theory. Whether changing force capability is in fact a deterrent to improving the ability to generate force against some resistance is debatable.

In the athletic training setting, isokinetics are perhaps best used as a rehabilitative and diagnostic tool rather than as a training device.[58]

Circuit Training

circuit training
Exercise stations that consist of various combinations of weight training, flexibility, calisthenics, and aerobic exercises.

Circuit training employs a series of exercise stations that consist of various combinations of weight training, flexibility, calisthenics, and brief aerobic exercises. Circuits may be designed to accomplish many different training goals. With circuit training the individual moves rapidly from one station to the next and performs whatever exercise is to be done at that station within a specified time period. A typical circuit would consist of eight to twelve stations, and the entire circuit would be repeated three times.

Circuit training is most definitely an effective technique for improving strength and flexibility. Certainly, if the pace or the time interval between stations is rapid and if workload is maintained at a high level of intensity with heart rate at or above target training levels, the cardiorespiratory system may benefit from this circuit. However, little research evidence exists to show that circuit training is effective in improving cardiorespiratory endurance. It should be, and is most often, used as a technique for developing and improving muscular strength and endurance.

Calisthenic Strengthening Exercises

Calisthenics, or free exercise, is one of the more easily available means of developing strength. Isotonic movement exercises can be graded according to intensity by using gravity as an aid, by ruling gravity out, by moving against gravity, or by using the body or body part as a resistance against gravity. Most calisthenics require the athlete to support the body or move the total body against the force of gravity. Push-ups are a good example of a vigorous antigravity free exercise. To be considered maximally effective, the isotonic calisthenic exercise, like all types of exercise, must be performed in an exacting manner and in full range of motion. In most cases, ten or more repetitions are performed for each exercise and are repeated in sets of two or three.

Some free exercises use an isometric, or holding, phase instead of a full range of motion. Examples of these exercises are back extensions and sit-ups. When the exercise produces maximum muscle tension, it is held between six and ten seconds and then repeated one to three times.

Plyometric Exercise

plyometric exercise
This type of exercise maximizes the myotatic, or stretch, reflex.

Plyometric exercise is a technique that includes specific exercises that encompass a rapid stretch of a muscle eccentrically, followed immediately by a rapid concentric contraction of that muscle for the purpose of facilitating and developing a forceful explosive movement over a short period of time.[2,19] The greater the stretch put on the muscle from its resting length immediately before the concentric contraction, the greater the resistance the muscle can overcome. Plyometric exercises emphasize the speed of the eccentric phase.[18] The rate of the stretch is more critical than the magnitude of the stretch. An advantage to plyometric exercises is that they can help develop eccentric control in dynamic movements.[61]

Plyometric exercises involve hops, bounds, and depth jumping for the lower extremity and use medicine balls and other types of weighted equipment for the upper extremity. Depth jumping is an example of a plyometric exercise in which an individual jumps to the ground from a specified height and then quickly jumps again as soon as ground contact is made.[19]

Plyometrics place a great deal of stress on the musculoskeletal system. The learning and perfection of specific jumping skills and other plyometric exercises must be technically correct and specific to the athlete's age, activity, physical development, and skill development.[56]

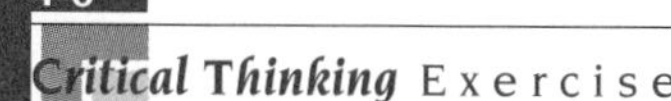

4-6 Critical Thinking Exercise

A high school shot-putter has been working intensely on weight training to improve his muscular power. In particular he has been concentrating on lifting extremely heavy free weights using a low number of repetitions (three sets of six to eight repetitions). Although his strength has improved significantly over the last several months, he is not seeing the same degree of improvement in his throws, even though his coach says that his technique is very good.

? The athlete is frustrated with his performance and wants to know if there is anything else he can do in his training program that might enhance his performance.

Strength Training for the Female Athlete

Strength training is critical for the female athlete. Significant muscle hypertrophy in the female athlete is dependent on the presence of the hormone testosterone. Testosterone is considered a male hormone, although all females possess some testosterone in their systems. Females with higher testosterone levels tend to have more masculine characteristics, such as increased facial and body hair, a deeper voice, and the potential to develop a little more muscle bulk.[49]

Both males and females experience initial rapid gains in strength due to an increase in neuromuscular efficiency as discussed previously.[71] However, in the female, these rapid initial strength gains tend to plateau after three to four weeks. Minimal improvement in muscular strength will be realized during a continuing strength-training program because the muscle will not continue to hypertrophy to any significant degree.

Perhaps the most critical difference between males and females regarding physical performance is the ratio of strength to body weight. The reduced *strength-to-body-weight ratio* in females is the result of their higher percentage of body fat. The strength-to-body-weight ratio may be significantly improved through weight training by decreasing the percentage of body fat while increasing lean weight.

Strength Training in Adolescents

The principles of resistance training discussed previously may be applied to the young athlete. There are certainly a number of sociological questions regarding the advantages and disadvantages of younger, in particular prepubescent, athletes engaging in rigorous strength-training programs, From a physiological perspective, experts have for years debated the value of strength training in young athletes. Recently, a number of studies have indicated that if properly supervised, young athletes can improve strength, power, endurance, balance, and proprioception; develop a positive body image; improve sport performance; and prevent injuries. A prepubescent child can experience gains in levels of muscle strength without significant muscle hypertrophy.[27]

An athletic trainer supervising a conditioning program for a young athlete should certainly incorporate resistive exercise into the program. However, close supervision, proper instruction, and appropriate modification of progression and intensity based on the extent of physical maturation of the individual is critical to the effectiveness of the resistive exercises.[55] A strengthening program that uses calisthenic strengthening exercises with body weight as resistance should be encouraged.

CARDIORESPIRATORY ENDURANCE

By definition, **cardiorespiratory endurance** is the ability to perform whole-body, large muscle activities for extended periods of time. The cardiorespiratory system provides a means by which oxygen is supplied to the various tissues of the body.[33] Athletes find cardiorespiratory endurance critical both for performance and for preventing undue fatigue that may predispose them to injury.

cardiorespiratory endurance
Ability to perform activities for extended periods of time.

Transport and Utilization of Oxygen

Basically, transport of oxygen throughout the body involves the coordinated function of four components: the heart, the lungs, the blood vessels, and the blood. The improvement of cardiorespiratory endurance through training occurs because of the increased capability of each of these four elements to provide necessary oxygen to the

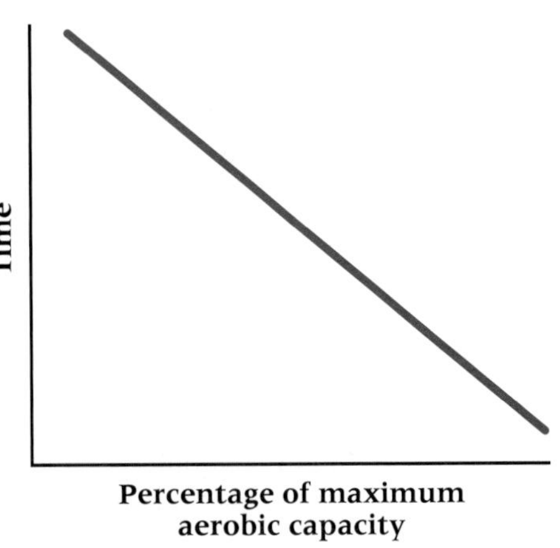

Figure 4-17

The greater the percentage of maximum aerobic capacity required during an activity, the less time the activity may be performed.

working tissues. The greatest rate at which oxygen can be taken in and used during exercise is referred to as *maximum aerobic capacity* ($\dot{V}O_2max$).[47] The performance of any activity requires a certain rate of oxygen consumption that is about the same for all persons, depending on the level of fitness. Generally, the greater the rate or intensity of the performance of an activity, the greater the oxygen consumption. Each person has his or her own maximal rate of oxygen consumption. That person's ability to perform an activity (or to fatigue) is closely related to the amount of oxygen required by that activity and is limited by the person's maximal rate of oxygen consumption. Apparently, the greater the percentage of maximum oxygen consumption required during an activity, the less time the activity may be sustained (Figure 4-17).

The maximal rate at which oxygen can be used is a genetically determined characteristic; a person inherits a certain range of maximum aerobic capacity, and the more active that person is, the higher the existing maximum aerobic capacity will be in that range.[33] A training program allows an athlete to increase maximum aerobic capacity to its highest limit within that athlete's range. Maximum aerobic capacity is most often presented in terms of the volume of oxygen used relative to body weight per unit of time (ml/kg/min). A normal maximum aerobic capacity for most college-age athletes would fall somewhere in the range of 45 to 60 ml/kg/min.[14] A world-class male marathon runner may have a maximum aerobic capacity in the 70 to 80 ml/kg/min range.

Three factors determine the maximal rate at which oxygen can be used: external respiration involving the ventilatory process or pulmonary function; gas transport, which is accomplished by the cardiovascular system (i.e., the heart, blood vessels, and blood); and internal respiration, which involves the use of oxygen by the cells to produce energy. Of these three factors the most limiting is generally the ability to transport oxygen through the system; thus the cardiovascular system limits the overall rate of oxygen consumption. A high maximum aerobic capacity within an athlete's inherited range indicates that all three systems are working well.

Effects on the Heart

The heart is the main pumping mechanism, circulating oxygenated blood throughout the body to the working tissues. As the body begins to exercise, the muscles use oxygen at a much higher rate, and the heart must pump more oxygenated blood to meet this increased demand. The heart is capable of adapting to this increased demand through several mechanisms. Heart rate shows a gradual adaptation to an increased workload by increasing proportionally to the intensity of the exercise and will plateau at a given level after about two to three minutes (Figure 4-18).

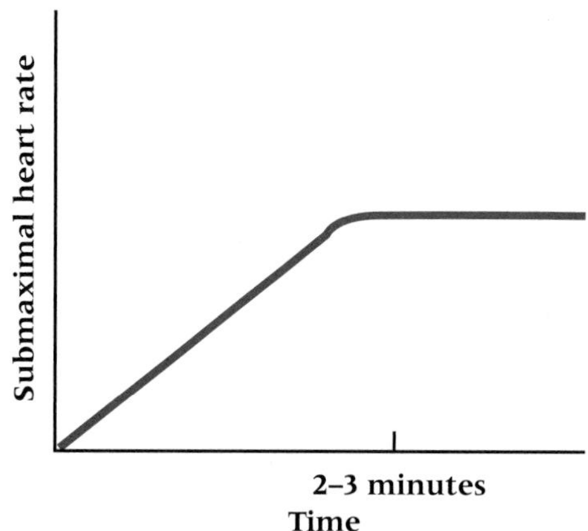

Figure 4-18

Two to three minutes are required for heart rate to plateau at a given workload.

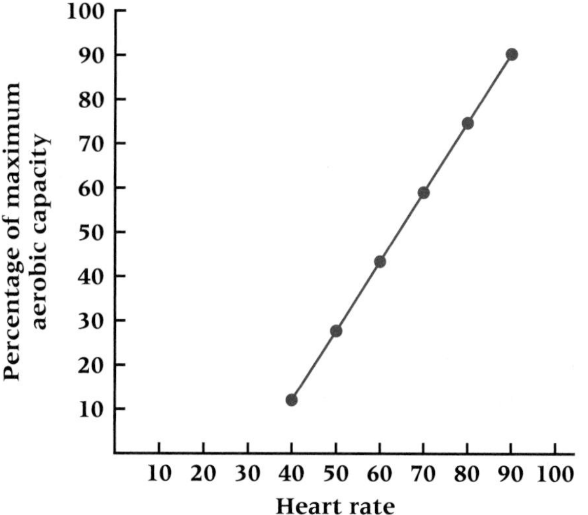

Figure 4-19

Maximal heart rate is achieved at about the same time as maximum aerobic capacity.

Monitoring heart rate is an indirect method of estimating oxygen consumption. In general, heart rate and oxygen consumption have a linear relationship, although at very low intensities and at high intensities this linear relationship breaks down (Figure 4-19).[11] During higher-intensity activities, maximal heart rate may be achieved before maximal oxygen consumption, which will continue to rise.[43] The greater the intensity of the exercise, the higher the heart rate. Because of these existing relationships it should become apparent that the rate of oxygen consumption can be estimated by taking heart rate.[15]

A second mechanism by which the heart is able to adapt to increased demands during exercise is to increase the stroke volume—the volume of blood being pumped out with each beat.[14] The heart pumps out approximately 70 ml of blood per beat. Stroke volume can continue to increase only to the point at which there is simply not enough time between beats for the heart to fill up. This point occurs at about 40 percent of maximal heart rate, and above this level increases in the volume of blood being pumped out per unit of time must be caused entirely by increases in heart rate (Figure 4-20).[51]

Stroke volume and heart rate together determine the volume of blood being pumped through the heart in a given unit of time. Approximately 5 L of blood are pumped through the heart during each minute at rest. This figure is referred to as the

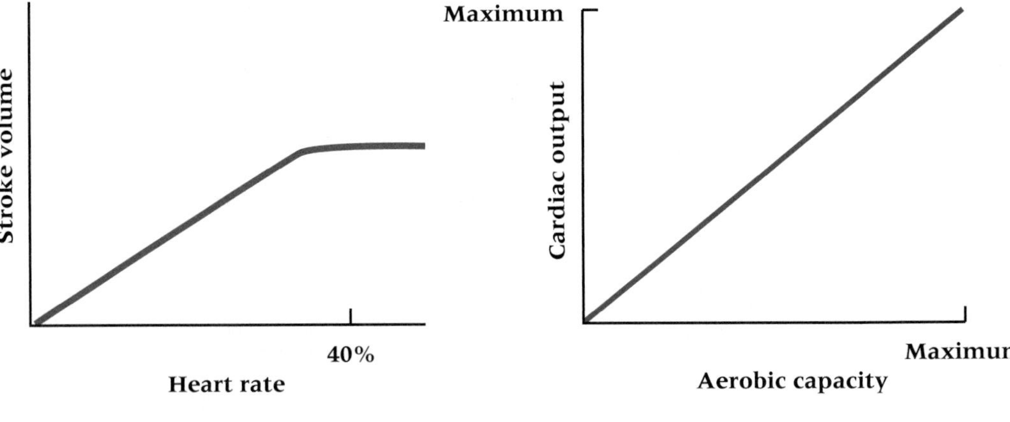

Figure 4-20 (left)

Stroke volume plateaus at 40 percent of maximal heart rate.

Figure 4-21 (right)

Cardiac output limits maximum aerobic capacity.

cardiac output, which indicates how much blood the heart is capable of pumping in exactly one minute. Thus, cardiac output is the primary determinant of the maximal rate of oxygen consumption possible (Figure 4-21). During exercise, cardiac output increases to approximately four times that experienced during rest in the normal individual and may increase as much as six times in the elite endurance athlete.

training effect
Stroke volume increases while heart rate is reduced at a given exercise load.

A **training effect** that occurs with regard to cardiac output of the heart is that the stroke volume increases while exercise heart rate is reduced at a given standard exercise load. The heart becomes more efficient because it is capable of pumping more blood with each stroke. Because the heart is a muscle, it will hypertrophy to some extent, but this hypertrophy is in no way a negative effect of training.

Training Effect

$$\text{Cardiac output} = \text{Increased stroke volume} \times \text{Decreased heart rate}$$

Effects on Work Ability

Cardiorespiratory endurance plays a critical role in the athlete's ability to resist fatigue. Fatigue is closely related to the percentage of maximum aerobic capacity that a particular workload demands.[59] For example, Figure 4-22 presents two athletes, A and B. Athlete A has a maximum aerobic capacity of 50 ml/kg/min, whereas athlete B has a maximum aerobic capacity of only 40 ml/kg/min. If athletes A and B are both exercising at the same intensity, athlete A will be working at a much lower percentage of maximum aerobic capacity than athlete B is. Consequently, athlete A should be able to sustain his or her activity over a much longer period of time. Athletic performance may be impaired if the ability to use oxygen efficiently is impaired. Thus, improvement of cardiorespiratory endurance should be an essential component of any training program.

The Energy Systems

Various sports activities involve specific demands for energy. For example, sprinting and jumping are high-energy activities, requiring a relatively large production of energy for a short time. Long-distance running and swimming, on the other hand, are mostly low-energy activities per unit of time, requiring energy production for a prolonged time. Other physical activities demand a blend of both high- and low-energy output. These various energy demands can be met by the different processes in which energy can be supplied to the skeletal muscles.

ATP: The Immediate Energy Source

Energy is produced from the breakdown of nutrient foodstuffs.[51] This energy is used to produce adenosine triphosphate (ATP), which is the ultimate usable form of energy for muscular activity. ATP is produced in the muscle tissue from blood glucose

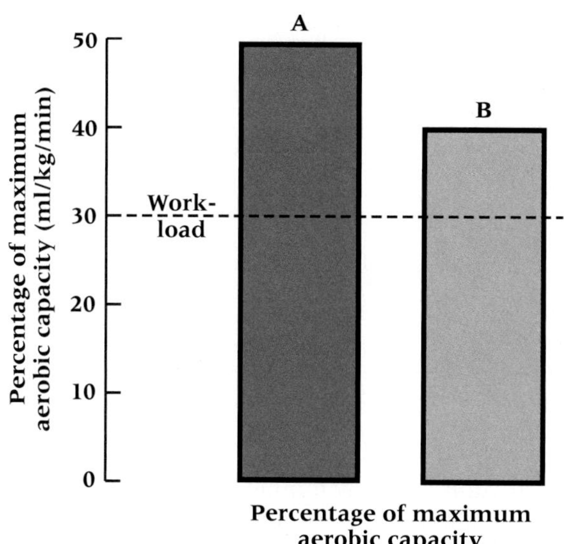

Figure 4-22

Athlete A should be able to work longer than Athlete B as a result of lower utilization of maximum aerobic capacity.

or glycogen. Glucose is derived from the breakdown of dietary carbohydrates. Glucose not needed immediately is stored as glycogen in the resting muscle and liver. Stored glycogen in the liver can later be converted back to glucose and transferred to the blood to meet the body's energy needs. Fats and proteins can also be metabolized to generate ATP.

Once much of the muscle and liver glycogen is depleted, the body relies more heavily on fats stored in adipose tissue to meet its energy needs. The longer the duration of an activity, the greater the amount of fat that is used, especially during the later stages of endurance events. During rest and submaximal exertion, both fat and carbohydrates are used as energy substrate in approximately a 60 percent to 40 percent ratio.[51]

Regardless of the nutrient source that produces ATP, it is always available in the cell as an immediate energy source. When all available sources of ATP are depleted, more must be regenerated for muscular contraction to continue.

Aerobic versus Anaerobic Metabolism

Two major energy systems function in muscle tissue: anaerobic and aerobic metabolism. Each of these systems generates ATP. During sudden outbursts of activity in intensive, short-term exercise, ATP can be rapidly metabolized to meet energy needs. After a few seconds of intensive exercise, however, the small stores of ATP are used up. The body then turns to glycogen as an energy source. Glycogen can be metabolized within the muscle cells to generate ATP for muscle contractions.[51]

Both ATP and muscle glycogen can be metabolized without the need for oxygen. Thus this energy system involves anaerobic metabolism (occurring in the absence of oxygen). As exercise continues, the body has to rely on the metabolism of carbohydrates (more specifically, glucose) and fats to generate ATP. This second energy system requires oxygen and is therefore referred to as aerobic metabolism (occurring in the presence of oxygen).[51]

In most activities both aerobic and anaerobic systems function simultaneously. The degree to which the two major energy systems are involved is determined by the intensity and duration of the activity. If the intensity of the activity is such that sufficient oxygen can be supplied to meet the demands of working tissues, the activity is considered to be *aerobic.* Conversely, if the activity is of high enough intensity or the duration is such that there is insufficient oxygen available to meet energy demands, the activity becomes *anaerobic.* Consequently, an oxygen debt is incurred that must be paid back during the recovery period. For example, short bursts of muscle contraction,

TABLE 4-1 Comparison of Aerobic versus Anaerobic Activities

	Mode	Relative Intensity	Performance	Frequency	Duration	Miscellaneous
Aerobic activities	Continuous, long-duration, sustained activities	Less intense	60% to 90% of maximum range	At least three but not more than six times per week	20 to 60 min	Less risk to sedentary or older individuals
Anaerobic activities	Explosive, short-duration, burst-type activities	More intense	90% to 100% of maximum range	Three to four times per week	10 sec to 2 min	Used in sport and team activities

as in running or swimming sprints, use predominantly the anaerobic system. However, endurance events depend a great deal on the aerobic system. Most sports use a combination of both anaerobic and aerobic metabolism (Table 4-1).

Training Techniques for Improving Cardiorespiratory Endurance

Cardiorespiratory endurance may be improved through a number of different methods. Largely, the amount of improvement possible will be determined by an individual's initial levels of cardiorespiratory endurance.

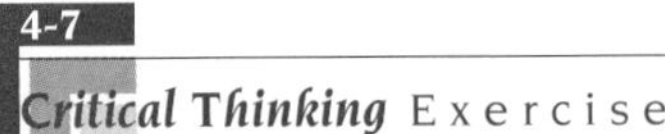

4-7 *Critical Thinking* Exercise

A female soccer player has a grade 1 ankle sprain that is likely to keep her out of practice for about a week. She has worked extremely hard on her fitness levels and is concerned that not being able to run for an entire week will hurt her cardiorespiratory fitness.

? What types of activity should the athletic trainer recommend during her rehabilitation period that can help her maintain her existing level of cardiorespiratory endurance?

Continuous Training

Continuous training involves four considerations:

- *Mode* or type of activity
- *Frequency* of the activity
- *Duration* of the activity
- *Intensity* of the activity

Mode The type of activity used in continuous training must be aerobic.[15] Aerobic activities are those that elevate the heart rate and maintain it at that level for an extended time. Aerobic activities generally involve repetitive, whole-body, large-muscle movements performed over an extended time. Examples of aerobic activities are running, jogging, walking, cycling, swimming, rope skipping, stair climbing, and cross-country skiing. The advantage of these aerobic activities as opposed to more intermittent activities such as racquetball, squash, basketball, or tennis is that aerobic activities are easy to regulate by either speeding up or slowing down the pace. Because the given intensity of the workload elicits a given heart rate, these aerobic activities allow athletes to maintain heart rate at a specified or target level. Intermittent activities involve variable speeds and intensities that cause the heart rate to fluctuate considerably. Although these intermittent activities improve cardiorespiratory endurance, their intensity is much more difficult to monitor.

Frequency To see at least minimal improvement in cardiorespiratory endurance, it is necessary for the average person to engage in no fewer than three sessions per week.[5] If possible, an individual should aim for four or five sessions per week. A competitive athlete should be prepared to train as often as six times per week. Everyone should take at least one day per week off to allow for both psychological and physiological rest.

Duration For minimal improvement to occur, an individual must participate in at least twenty minutes of continuous activity with the heart rate elevated to its working level.[5] Recent evidence suggests that even shorter exercise bouts of as little as twelve minutes may be sufficient to show improvement. Generally, the greater the duration of the workout, the greater the improvement in cardiorespiratory endurance. The competitive athlete should train for at least forty-five minutes with the heart rate elevated to training levels.

Intensity Of the four factors being considered, the most critical factor is the intensity of training, even though recommendations regarding training intensities vary. Intensity is particularly critical in the early stages of training, when the body is forced to make a lot of adjustments to increase workload demands.

Because heart rate is linearly related to the intensity of the exercise and to the rate of oxygen consumption, it becomes a relatively simple process to identify a specific workload (pace) that will make the heart rate plateau at the desired level. By monitoring heart rate, we know whether the pace is too fast or too slow to get the heart rate into a target range.[5]

Several formulas identify a target training heart rate.[5] Exact determination of maximal heart rate involves exercising an individual at a maximal level and monitoring the heart rate using an electrocardiogram. This process is difficult outside a laboratory. However, an approximate estimate of maximal heart rate for both males and females is 220 beats per minute. Maximal heart rate is related to age. As age increases, maximal heart rate decreases. Thus, a relatively simple estimation of maximal heart rate (HR) would be Maximal HR = 220 − Age. If an athlete is working at 70 percent of maximal rate, the target heart rate can be calculated by multiplying 0.7 × (220 − Age).

Another commonly used formula that takes into account the current level of fitness is the Karvonen equation.[40]

$$\text{Target training HR} = \text{Resting HR} + (0.6 \times [\text{Maximal HR} - \text{Resting HR}])$$

Regardless of the formula used, to see minimal improvement in cardiorespiratory endurance, the heart rate should be elevated to at least 70 percent of its maximal rate.[15] A trained individual ought to be able to sustain a heart rate at the 85 percent level.

Interval Training

Unlike continuous training, interval training involves more intermittent activities. **Interval training** consists of alternating periods of relatively intense work and active recovery. It allows for performance of much more work at a more intense workload over a longer period of time than does working continuously.[49]

interval training Alternating periods of work with active recovery.

It is most desirable in continuous training to work at an intensity of about 60 percent to 80 percent of maximal heart rate. Obviously, sustaining activity at a relatively high intensity over a twenty-minute period would be extremely difficult. The advantage of interval training is that it allows work at this 80 percent or higher level for a short period of time followed by an active period of recovery during which an individual may be working at only 30 percent to 45 percent of maximum heart rate.[12] Thus, the intensity of the workout and its duration can be greater than with continuous training.

Most sports are anaerobic, involving short bursts of intense activity followed by some type of active recovery period (for example, football, basketball, soccer, or tennis). Training with the interval technique allows the athlete to be more sport-specific during the workout. With interval training the overload principle is applied by making the training period much more intense.

There are several important considerations in interval training. The training period is the amount of time that continuous activity is actually being performed, and the recovery period is the time between training periods. A set is a group of combined training and recovery periods, and repetitions are the number of training and recovery periods per set. Training time or distance refers to the rate or distance of the training period. The training-recovery ratio indicates a time ratio for training versus recovery.

An example of interval training would be a soccer player running sprints. An interval workout would involve running ten 120-yard sprints with a 45-second walking recovery period between sprints. During this training session the soccer player's heart rate would probably increase to 85 percent to 90 percent of maximal level during the dash and should probably fall to the 30 percent to 45 percent level during the recovery period.

Fartlek Training

Fartlek, a training technique that is a type of cross-country running, originated in Sweden. *Fartlek* literally means "speed play." It is similar to interval training in that the athlete must run for a specified period of time; however, specific pace and speed are not identified. The course for a fartlek workout should be some type of varied terrain with some level running, some uphill and downhill running, and some running through obstacles such as trees or rocks. The object is to put surges into a running workout, varying the length of the surges according to individual purposes. One advantage of fartlek training is that because the terrain is always changing, the course may prevent boredom and may actually be relaxing.

To improve cardiorespiratory endurance, fartlek training must elevate the heart rate to at least minimal training levels. Fartlek may be utilized best as an off-season conditioning activity or as a change-of-pace activity to counteract the boredom of training using the same activity day after day.

Equipment for Improving Cardiorespiratory Endurance

The extent and variety of fitness and exercise equipment available to the consumer is at times mind boggling (Figure 4-23). Prices of equipment can range from $2 for a jump rope to $60,000 for certain computer-driven isokinetic devices. It is certainly not necessary to purchase expensive exercise equipment to see good results. Many of the same physiological benefits can be achieved from using a $2 jump rope as from running on a $10,000 treadmill. *Focus Box:* "Guidelines for choosing aerobic exercise equipment" identifies and discusses some of the more widely used pieces of exercise equipment.

FITNESS ASSESSMENT

Fitness testing provides the coach, athletic trainer, or strength and conditioning coach with information about the effectiveness of the conditioning program for an individual athlete. Testing may be done in a pretest/posttest format to determine significant improvement from some baseline measure. Tests may be used to assess flexibility, muscular strength, endurance, power, cardiorespiratory endurance, speed, balance, or agility, depending on the stated goals of the training and conditioning program. A variety of established tests can be used to assess these parameters. *Focus Box:* "Fitness testing" lists various tests that can be administered along with recommended references to consult for specific testing procedures and for in-depth testing directions.

PERIODIZATION IN TRAINING AND CONDITIONING

Sports conditioning often falls into three seasons: off-season, preseason, and in-season.

Serious athletes no longer engage only in preseason conditioning and in-season competition. Sports conditioning is a year-round endeavor. *Periodization* is an approach to conditioning that brings about peak performance while reducing injuries and overtraining in the athlete through a training and conditioning program that is followed throughout the various seasons.[13] Periodization takes into account that athletes have different training and conditioning needs during different seasons and modifies the program according to individual needs (Table 4-2, page 124).[21]

Macrocycle

Periodization organizes a training and conditioning program into cycles. The complete training period, which could be a year in the case of seasonal sports or perhaps four years for an Olympic athlete, is referred to as a *macrocycle.* With seasonal sports the

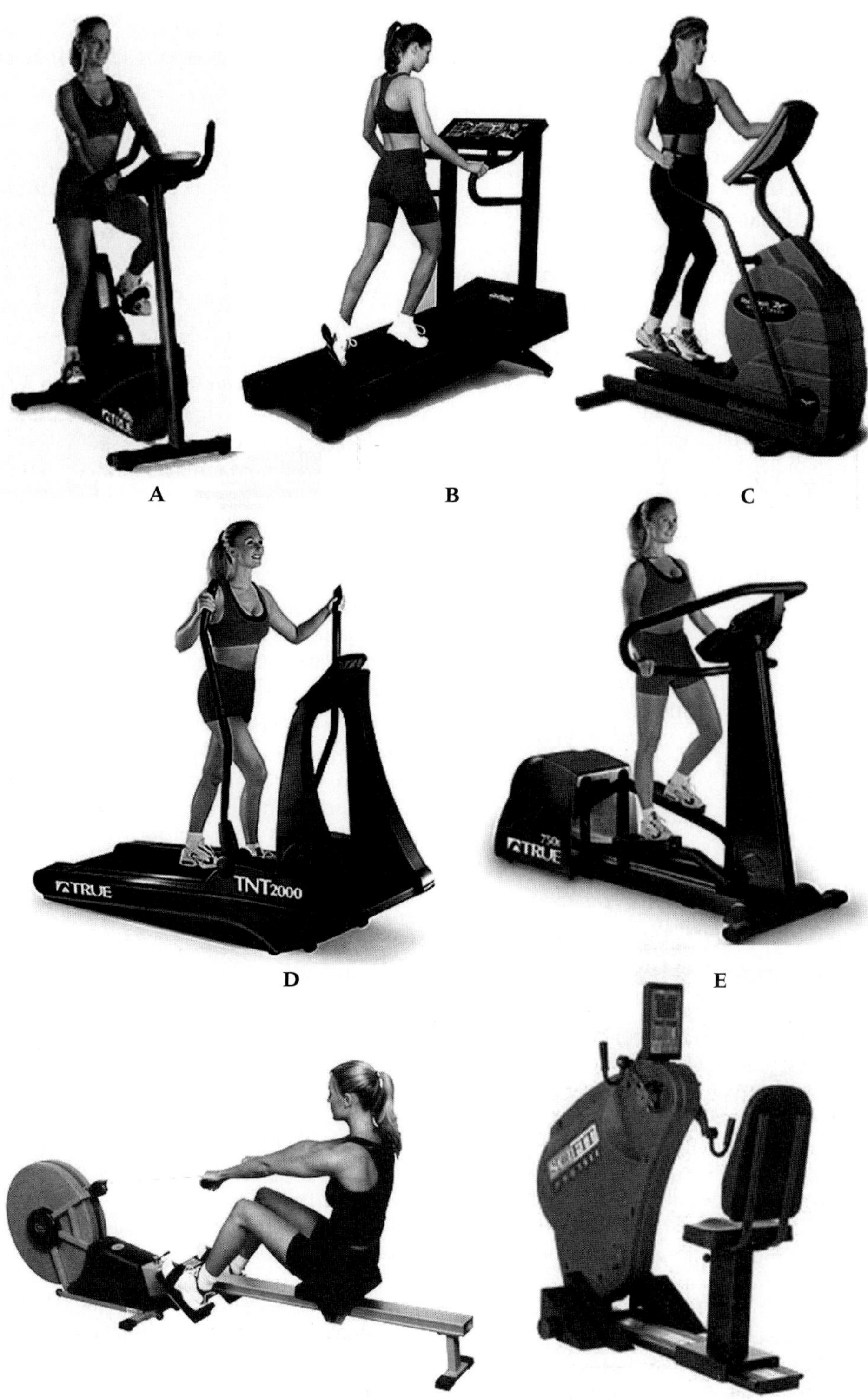

Figure 4-23

Types of fitness equipment for improving cardiorespiratory endurance. **A,** Exercise bicycle. **B,** Treadmill. **C,** Stair climber. **D,** Cross-country ski machine. **E,** Elliptical trainer. **F,** Rowing machine. **G,** Upper body ergometer.

macrocycle can be divided into a preseason, an in-season, and an off-season. Throughout the course of the macrocycle, intensity, volume, and specificity of training are altered so that an athlete can achieve peak levels of fitness for competition. As competition approaches, training sessions change gradually and progressively from high-volume, low-intensity, non–sport-specific activity to low-volume, high-intensity, sport-specific training.[70]

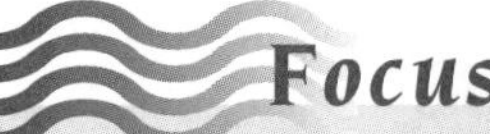

Guidelines for choosing aerobic exercise equipment

Exercise bicycle (Figure 4-23A)

Most models work only the lower body, but some have pumping handlebars for arms and shoulders. Some can be programmed for various workouts, such as climbing hills. Some models let you pedal backward, which enhances the work on your hamstring muscles. Look for

- smooth pedaling motion
- a comfortable seat
- handlebars that adjust to your height
- pedal straps to keep your feet from slipping and to make your legs work on the upstroke, too
- easy-to-adjust workload
- solid construction

Treadmill (Figure 4-23B)

Some machines have adjustable inclines to simulate hills and make workouts more strenuous. Some can be programmed for various preset workouts. Look for

- easily adjustable speed and incline
- a running surface that is wide and long enough for your stride and that absorbs shock well
- a strong motor that can handle high speeds and a heavy load

Stair climber (Figure 4-23C)

Some larger models simulate real stair climbing. But most home models have pedals that work against your weight as you pump your legs; this feature puts less strain on your knees since you don't take real steps. Some people prefer pedals that remain parallel to the floor; others like pivoting pedals. Models with independent pedals provide a more natural stepping motion. Look for

- smooth stepping action
- large, comfortable pedals with no wobble
- easily adjustable resistance
- comfortable handlebars or rails for balance

Cross-country ski machine (Figure 4-23D)

These machines work most muscle groups. They simulate the outdoor sport: your feet slide in the tracks, and your hands pull on cords or poles, either independently or in synchronized movements. Machines with cords rather than poles may provide an especially strenuous upper-body workout. Look for

- a base that is long enough to accommodate your stride
- adjustable leg and arm resistance
- smooth action

Elliptical trainer (Figure 4-23E)

An elliptical exercise machine allows for a no-impact cardiovascular workout that mimics a combination of walking, stair climbing and cross-country skiing using an elliptical-shaped stride while standing upright using a forward or reverse motion. Look for

- an electronically adjustable ramp that allows the incline to be raised or lowered
- resistance that can be adjusted

Rowing machine (Figure 4-23F)

A rowing machine provides a fuller workout than does running or cycling because it tones muscles in the upper body. Most machines have hydraulic pistons to provide variable resistance; many larger models use a flywheel. Piston models have hydraulic arms and are cheaper and more compact than are flywheel models, which have a smoother action that is usually more like real rowing. One new model actually has a flywheel in a water tank to mimic real rowing. Look for

- seats and oars that move smoothly
- footrests that pivot

Upper body ergometer (UBE) (Figure 4-23G)

An upper body ergometer is essentially a stationary bicycle that you pedal with the arms rather than the legs. These machines are most often used to help maintain cardiorespiratory endurance in rehabilitation programs for individuals with injuries to the lower extremities who, for whatever reason, cannot use weight bearing activities. A UBE may also be used as a training and conditioning tool to help increase muscular endurance for the upper extremities. Look for

- easily adjustable speed and resistance
- a comfortable seat that provides some support and stabilization for the lower back
- smooth, quiet action

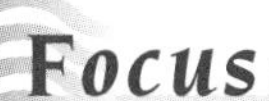

Focus

Fitness testing

Muscle strength, power, endurance

One repetition maximum tests
Timed push-ups
Timed sit-ups
Chin-ups
Bar dips
Flexed arm hang
Vertical jump

Flexibility

Sit-and-reach test
Trunk extension test
Shoulder lift test

Cardiorespiratory endurance

Cooper's 12-minute walk/run
1.5 mile run
Harvard step test

Speed

6-second dash
10- to 60-yard dash

Agility

T-test
Edgren side step
SEMO agility test

Balance

Stork test

Fitness testing references

Baumgartner T, Jackson A: *Measurement for evaluation in physical education and exercise science,* Dubuque, Iowa, 1999, WCB/McGraw-Hill.

Prentice W: *Fitness and wellness for life,* ed 6, Dubuque, Iowa, 1999, WCB/McGraw-Hill.

Semenick D: Testing procedures and protocols. In Baechle T, editor: *Essentials of strength training and conditioning,* Champaign, Ill, 1994, Human Kinetics.

Mesocycles

Within the macrocycle are a series of *mesocycles,* each of which may last for several weeks or even months. A mesocycle is further divided into *transition, preparatory,* and *competition* periods.[70]

Transition period The transition period begins after the last competition and comprises the early part of the off-season. The transition period is generally unstructured, and the athlete is encouraged to participate in sport activities on a recreational basis. The idea is to allow the athlete to escape both physically and psychologically from the rigor of a highly organized training regimen.

Preparatory period The preparatory period occurs primarily during the off-season when there are no upcoming competitions. The preparatory period has three phases: the hypertrophy/endurance phase, the strength phase, and the power phase.

TABLE 4-2 Periodization Training

Season	Period/Phase	Type of Training Activity
Off-season	Transition period	Unstructured Recreational
	Preparatory period Hypertrophy/endurance phase	Cross-training Low intensity High volume Non–sport-specific
	Strength phase	Moderate intensity Moderate volume More sport-specific
Preseason	Power phase	High intensity Decreased volume Sport-specific
In-season	Competition period	High intensity Low volume Skill-training Strategy Maintenance of strength and power gained during the off-season

4-8

Critical Thinking Exercise

Following the end of the competitive season, a college football player took the months of December and January off from intense training. He played only basketball and occasionally rode an exercise bike, thus completing the transitional period of the macrocycle. It is now time for him to begin the preparatory phase of training.

? What activities should he begin with, and how should these activities progress over the next several months?

During the hypertrophy/endurance phase, which occurs in the early part of the off-season, training is at a low intensity with a high volume of repetitions, using activities that may or may not be directly related to a specific sport. The goal is to develop a base of endurance on which more intense training can occur. This phase may last from several weeks to two months.

During the strength phase, which also occurs during the off-season, the intensity and volume progress to moderate levels. Weight-training activities should become more specific to the sport or event.

The third phase, or power phase, occurs in the preseason. The athlete trains at a high intensity at or near the level of competition. The volume of training is decreased so that full recovery is allowed between sessions.

Competition period In certain cases the competition period may last for only a week or less. With seasonal sports, however, the competition period may last for several months. In general this period involves high-intensity training at a low volume. As training volume decreases, an increased amount of time is spent on skill training or strategy sessions. During the competition period, it may be necessary to establish microcycles, which are periods lasting from one to seven days. During a weekly microcycle, training should be intense early in the week and should progress to moderate and finally to light training the day before a competition. The goal is to make sure that the athlete will be at peak levels of fitness and performance on days of competition.[14]

Cross Training

The concept of cross training is an approach to training and conditioning for a specific sport that involves substituting alternative activities that have some carryover value to that sport. For example, a swimmer could engage in jogging, running, or aerobic exercise to maintain levels of cardiorespiratory conditioning. Cross training is particularly useful in both the transition and early preparatory periods. It adds variety to the training regimen, thus keeping training during the off-season more interesting and exciting. However, while cross training can be effective in maintaining levels of cardiorespiratory endurance, it is not sport-specific and thus should not be used during the preseason.

SUMMARY

- Proper physical conditioning for sports participation should prepare the athlete for a high-level performance while helping to prevent injuries inherent to that sport.
- Year-round conditioning is essential in most sports to assist in preventing injuries. Periodization is an approach to conditioning that attempts to bring about peak performance while reducing injuries and overtraining in the athlete by developing a training and conditioning program to be followed throughout the various seasons.
- Physical conditioning must follow the SAID principle, which is an acronym for specific adaptation to imposed demands. Conditioning must work toward making the body as lean as possible, commensurate with the athlete's sport.
- A proper warm-up should precede conditioning, and a proper cooldown should follow. It takes at least fifteen to thirty minutes of gradual warm-up to bring the body to a state of readiness for vigorous sports training and participation. Warming up consists of a general, unrelated activity followed by a specific, related activity.
- Optimum flexibility is necessary for success in most sports. Too much flexibility can allow joint trauma to occur, and too little flexibility can result in muscle tears or strains. Ballistic stretching exercises should be avoided. The safest means of increasing flexibility are static stretching and the proprioceptive neuromuscular facilitation (PNF) technique, consisting of slow-reversal-hold-relax, contract-relax, and hold-relax methods.
- Strength is the capacity to exert a force or the ability to perform work against a resistance. There are many ways to develop strength, including isometric, isotonic, and isokinetic muscle contraction. Isometric exercise generates heat energy by forcefully contracting the muscle in a stable position that produces no change in the length of the muscle. Isotonic exercise involves shortening and lengthening a muscle through a complete range of motion. Isokinetic exercise allows resisted movement through a full range at a specific velocity. Circuit training uses a series of exercise stations to improve strength and flexibility. Plyometric training uses a quick, eccentric contraction to facilitate a more explosive concentric contraction.
- Cardiorespiratory endurance is the ability to perform whole-body, large-muscle activities repeatedly for long periods of time. Maximal oxygen consumption is the greatest determinant of the level of cardiorespiratory endurance. Most sport activities involve some combination of both aerobic and anaerobic metabolism. Improvement of cardiorespiratory endurance may be accomplished through continuous, interval, or fartlek training.

Websites

Health and Fitness Worldguide Forum: http://www.worldguide.com/main/hf.html

Includes coverage of anatomy, strength, cardiovascular exercise, eating well, and sports medicine.

Stretching and Flexibility: Everything you ever wanted to know: http://www.cmcrossroads.com/bradapp/docs/rec/ stretching/

Prepared by Brad Appleton, website presents detailed information on stretching and stretching techniques, including normal ranges of motion, flexibility, how to stretch, the physiology of stretching, and types of stretching (including PNF).

National Strength and Conditioning Association (NSCA): http://www.nsca-lift.org

Website for an organization that focuses on strength and conditioning to support and disseminate research-based knowledge and its practical application and to improve athletic performance and fitness.

Fitness World: http://www.fitnessworld.com

Presents information about fitness in general and includes access to Fitness Management magazine.

Kaiser Permanente Health Reference: http://www.kaisersantaclara.org

Click on Cardiovascular Exercise and find several topics including how to start, target heart rate, and injuries.

Solutions to Critical Thinking EXERCISES

4-1 Although athletes should make every effort to maintain existing levels of fitness during the rehabilitation period, to improve their fitness to competitive levels, athletes in any sport must practice or engage in that specific activity. The football player must begin a heavy strength-training program for the upper body immediately in the postseason and must continue to progressively return to heavy lifting with the lower extremities as soon as the healing process will allow. It is essential for this player to progressively increase the intensity and variety of conditioning drills that specifically relate to performance at his particular position.

4-2 The warm-up should begin with a five- to seven-minute slow jog during which the athlete should break into a light sweat. At that point, she should engage in stretching (using either static or PNF techniques), concentrating on quadriceps, hamstrings, groin, and hip abductor muscles. Each specific stretch should be repeated four times, and the stretch should be held for fifteen to twenty seconds. Once the workout begins, the athlete should gradually and moderately increase the intensity of her activity. She may also find it effective to stretch during the cooldown period after the workout.

4-3 The athletic trainer should recommend that the athlete engage in a regular, consistent flexibility program using either static or PNF stretching techniques. Stretching should be done several times a day if possible. The athlete should also be instructed to engage in full range of motion strength training for the hamstrings. The athletic trainer should also explain that when the athlete feels tightness or discomfort during a training session, he should stop the activity immediately to avoid making a hamstring strain more severe.

4-4 Weight training will not have a negative effect on flexibility as long as the lifting technique is done properly. Lifting the weight through a full range of motion will serve to improve strength and simultaneously maintain range of motion. A female swimmer is not likely to bulk up to the point that muscle size will affect range of motion. It is also important to recommend that this athlete continue to incorporate active stretching into her training regimen.

4-5 The athletic trainer can discuss the rationale for strength and conditioning with the athlete. Helping the athlete understand why it is important to increase strength and endurance can increase her motivation. In addition to improving performance and efficiency, muscular endurance and strength is also critical in preventing athletic injuries. The athletic trainer should work with the coaches to provide a periodization program that will keep the athlete's interest and prevent atrophy from occurring.

4-6 The shot put, like many other dynamic movements in sports, requires not only great strength but also the ability to generate that strength rapidly. To develop muscular power, this athlete must engage in dynamic, explosive training techniques that will help him develop his ability. Power lifting techniques should be helpful. Plyometric exercises using weights for added resistance will help him improve his speed of muscular contraction against some resistive force.

4-7 Because this athlete suffers from a lower extremity injury in which weight bearing is limited, alternative activities such as swimming or riding a stationary exercise bike should be incorporated into her rehabilitation program immediately. If the pressure on her ankle when riding an exercise bike is too painful, she may find it helpful initially to use a bike that incorporates upper extremity exercise. The athletic trainer should recommend that this soccer player engage in a minimum of thirty minutes of continuous training as well as some higher-intensity interval training to maintain both aerobic and anaerobic fitness.

4-8 During the early part of the preparatory period, training should be at a low intensity with a high volume of repetitions, using activities that may or may not be directly related to football. This phase may last from several weeks to two months. The intensity and volume of these activities should progress to moderate levels. Weight-training activities should eventually become more specific to football. Just before the preseason, the athlete should train at a high intensity, and the volume of training should decrease to allow full recovery between sessions.

REVIEW QUESTIONS AND CLASS ACTIVITIES

1. Why is year-round conditioning so important for injury prevention?
2. In terms of injury prevention, list as many advantages as you can for conditioning.
3. How does the SAID principle relate to sports conditioning and injury prevention?
4. What is the value of proper warm-up and cooldown to sports injury prevention?
5. Critically observe how a variety of sports use warm-up and cooldown procedures.
6. Compare ways to increase flexibility and how they may decrease or increase the athlete's susceptibility to injury.
7. How may increasing strength decrease susceptibility to injury?
8. Compare different techniques of increasing strength. How may each technique be an advantage or a disadvantage to the athlete in terms of injury prevention?
9. Discuss the relationships among maximal oxygen consumption, heart rate, stroke volume, and cardiac output.
10. Differentiate between aerobic and anaerobic training methods.
11. How is continuous training different from interval training?

REFERENCES

1. Akima H, Takahashi H, Kuno SY: Early phase adaptations of muscle use and strength to isokinetic training, *Med Sci Sports Exer* 31(4): 588, 1999.
2. Allerheiligen W: Speed development and plyometric training. In Baechle T, editor: *Essentials of strength training and conditioning,* Champaign, Ill, 2000, Human Kinetics.
3. Allerheiligen W: Stretching and warm-up. In Baechle T, editor: *Essentials of strength training and conditioning,* Champaign, Ill, 2000, Human Kinetics.
4. Alter M: *The science of flexibility,* Champaign, Ill, 2004, Human Kinetics.
5. American College of Sports Medicine: *Guidelines for exercise testing and prescription,* Philadelphia, 2000, William and Wilkens.
6. Armiger P: Preventing musculotendinous injuries: a focus on flexibility, *Athletic Therapy Today* 5(4):20, 2000.
7. Baker D, Wilson G, Carlyon B: Generality vs. specificity: a comparison of dynamic and isometric measures of strength and speed-strength, *Eur J Appl Physiol* 68:350,1994.
8. Bandy WD, Irion JM, Briggler M: The effect of static stretch and dynamic range of motion training on the flexibility of the hamstring muscles, *J Orthop Sports Phys Ther* 27(4):295, 1998.
9. Bassett DR, Howley ET: Limiting factors for maximum oxygen uptake and determinants of endurance performance, *Med Sci Sports Exer* 32(1):70, 2000.
10. Berger R: *Conditioning for men,* Boston, 1973, Allyn & Bacon.

11. Bergh U, Ekblom B, Astrand PO: Maximal oxygen uptake "classical" versus "contemporary" viewpoints, *Med Sci Sports Exer* 32(1): 85, 2000.
12. Billat LV: Interval training for performance: a scientific and empirical practice. Special Recommendations for middle- and long distance running. Part I: aerobic interval training. *Sports Med* 31(1):13, 2001.
13. Blanke D: Flexibility. In Mellion M, editor: *Sports medicine secrets,* Philadelphia, 1999, Hanley & Belfus.
14. Bompa TO: *Periodization training for sports,* Champaign, Ill, 1999, Human Kinetics.
15. Brooks G, Fahey T, White T: *Exercise physiology: human bioenergetics and its applications,* Mountain View, Calif, 2000, Mayfield.
16. Brown LE: *Isokinetics in human performance,* Champaign, Ill, 2000, Human Kinetics.
17. Burke DG, Culligan CJ, Holt LE: The theoretical basis of proprioceptive neuromuscular facilitation, *Strength Cond Res* 14(4):496, 2000.
18. Chimera N, Swanik K, Swanik C: Effects of plyometric training on muscle activation strategies and performance in female athletes, *J Ath Train* 39(1):24, 2004.
19. Chu DA: Plyometics in sports injury rehabilitation and training, *Athletic Therapy Today* 4(3):7, 1999.
20. Clark M: *Integrated training for the new millennium,* Calabasas, Calif, 2001, National Academy of Sports Medicine.
21. Conroy M: The use of periodization in the high school setting, *Strength Cond J* 21(1):52, 1999.
22. Cross KM, Worrell TW: Effects of a static stretching program on the incidence of lower extremity musculotendinous strains, *J Ath Train* 34(1):11, 1999.
23. DeLorme TL, Watkins AL: *Progressive resistance exercise,* New York, 1951, Appleton-Century-Crofts.
24. DePino GM, Webright WG, Arnold BL: Duration of maintained hamstring flexibility after cessation of an acute static stretching protocol, *J Ath Train* 35(1):56, 2000.
25. Faulkner J, Green H, White T. Response and adaptation of skeletal muscle to changes in physical activity. In Bouchard C, Shepard R, Stephens J, editors: *Physical activity, fitness, and health,* Champaign, Ill, 1994, Human Kinetics.
26. Fleck S, Kraemer W: *Designing resistance training programs,* Champaign, Ill, 1997, Human Kinetics.
27. Gardner PJ: Youth strength training. *Athletic Therapy Today* 8(1):42, 2003.
28. Gravelle BL, Blessing DL: Physiological adaptation in women concurrently training for strength and endurance, *J Strength Cond* 14(1): 5, 2000.
29. Goldberg L: *Strength ball training,* Champaign, Ill, 2002, Human Kinetics.
30. Green W: *The clinical measurement of joint motion,* Rosemont, Ill, 1994, American Academy of Orthopedic Surgeons.
31. Gribble P, Prentice W: Effects of static and hold-relax stretching on hamstring range of motion using the FlexAbility LE1000, *J Sport Rehabil* 8(3):195, 1999.
32. Harman E: The biomechanics of resistance exercise. In Baechle T, editor: *Essentials of strength training and conditioning,* Champaign, Ill, 2000, Human Kinetics.
33. Hawley J, Myburgh K, Noakes T: Maximal oxygen consumption: a contemporary perspective. In Fahey T, editor: *Encyclopedia of sports medicine and exercise physiology,* New York, 1995, Mayfield.
34. Hickson R, Hidaka C, Foster C: Skeletal muscle fiber type, resistance training, and strength-related performance, *Med Sci Sports Exerc* 26:593, 1994.
35. Hilbert S, Plisk SS: Free weights versus machines, *Strength Cond J* 21(6):66, 1999.
36. Holcomb WR: Improved stretching with proprioceptive neuromuscular facilitation, *Strength Cond J* 22(1):59, 2000.
37. Holt LE, Pelham TW, Burke DG: Modifications to the standard sit-and-reach flexibility protocol, *J Ath Train* 34(1):43, 1999.
38. Jones M, Trowbridge C: Four ways to a safe, effective strength training program, *Athletic Therapy Today* 3(2):4, 1998.
39. Kaminski TW, Wabbersen CV, Murphy RM: Concentric versus enhanced eccentric hamstring strength training: clinical implications, *J Ath Train* 33(3):216, 1998.
40. Karvonen MJ, Kentala E, Mustala O: The effects of training on heart rate: a longitudinal study, *Ann Med Exp Biol* 35:305, 1957.
41. Knight K, Ingersoll C, Bartholomew J: Isotonic Contractions Might Be More Effective Than Isokinetic Contractions in Developing Muscle Strength, *J Sport Rehab* 10(2):124, 2001.
42. Kraemer W: General adaptation to resistance and endurance training programs. In Baechle T, editor: *Essentials of strength training and conditioning,* Champaign, Ill, 2000, Human Kinetics.
43. Kraemer W, Fleck S: *Strength training for young athletes,* Champaign, Ill, 2004, Human Kinetics.
44. Kraemer W, Hakkinen K, Kraemer W: *Strength training for sport.* Cambridge, Mass, Blackwell Science, 2001.
45. Kraemer W, Patton J, Gordon S: Compatibility of high-intensity strength and endurance training on hormonal and skeletal muscle adaptations, *J App Physiol* 78:976, 1995.
46. Kubukeli ZN, Noakes TD, Dennis SC: Training techniques to improve endurance exercise performances. *Sports Med* 32(8):489, 2002.
47. Laursen PB, Jenkins DG: The scientific basis for high-intensity interval training: optimizing training programmes and maximising performance in highly trained endurance athletes. *Sports Med* 32(1): 53, 2002.
48. Logan GA, Wallis EL: Recent findings in learning and performance. Paper presented at the Southern Section Meeting, California Association for Health, Physical Education, and Recreation, Pasadena, Calif, 1960.
49. MacDougall D, Sale D: Continuous vs. interval training: a review for the athlete and coach, *Can J Appl Sport Sci* 6:93, 1981.
50. Mann D, Whedon C: Functional stretching: implementing a dynamic stretching program. *Athletic Therapy Today* 6(3):10, 2001.
51. McArdle W, Katch F, Katch V: *Exercise physiology, energy, nutrition, and human performance,* Philadelphia, 2001, Lea & Febiger.
52. McComas A: Human neuromuscular adaptations that accompany changes in activity, *Med Sci Sports Exerc* 26(12):1498, 1994.
53. Merce J, Dufek J, Bates B: Analysis of peak oxygen consumption and heart rate during elliptical and treadmill exercise, *J Sport Rehab* 10(1):48, 2001.
54. Middlesworth M: More than ergonomics: warm-up and stretching key to injury prevention. *Athletic Therapy Today* 7(2):32, 2002.
55. Moreno, A: The practicalities of adolescent resistance training. *Athletic Therapy Today* 8(3):26, 2003.
56. Moss RI: Physics, plyometrics, and injury prevention. *Athletic Therapy Today* 7(2):44, 2002.
57. Norkin C, White D: *Measurement of joint motion: a guide to goniometry,* Philadelphia, 1995, F. A. Davis.
58. Perrin DH: *Isokinetic exercise and assessment,* Champaign, Ill, 1993, Human Kinetics.
59. Prentice W: *Fitness and wellness for life,* ed 7, Dubuque, Iowa, 1999, WCB/McGraw-Hill.
60. Prentice W: Proprioceptive neuromuscular facilitation techniques. In Prentice W: *Rehabilitation techniques in sports medicine,* and athletic training, St. Louis, 2004, McGraw-Hill.
61. Radcliffe JC, Farentinos RC: *High-powered plyometrics,* Champaign, Ill, 1999, Human Kinetics.
62. Rubley M, Brucker J, Knight K: Flexibility retention 3 weeks after a 5-day training regime, *J Sport Rehab* 10(2):105, 2001.
63. Sanders M: Weight training and conditioning. In Sanders B: *Sports physical therapy,* Norwalk, Conn, 1997, Appleton & Lange.

64. Schilling BK, Stone MH: Stretching: acute effects on strength and power performance, *Strength Cond J* 22(1):44, 2000.
65. Sharkey J: Is ballistic stretching back? *Ultra Fit Australia* 22:22,1995.
66. Spernoga S, Uhl T, Arnold B: Duration of maintained hamstring flexibility after a 1-time modified hold-relax stretching protocol, *J Ath Train* 36(1): 44, 2001.
67. Surburg P: Flexibility/range of motion. In Winnick JP, editor, *The Brockport physical fitness training guide*, Champaign, Ill, 1999, Human Kinetics.
68. Thomas M: The functional warm-up, *Strength Cond* 22(2): 51, 2000.
69. Walker M, Sussman D, Tamburello M: Relationship between maximum strength and relative endurance for the empty-can exercise, *J Sport Rehab* 12(1):31, 2003.
70. Wathen D: Periodization: concepts and applications. In Baechle T, editor: *Essentials of strength training and conditioning*, Champaign, Ill, 2000, Human Kinetics.
71. Wilkerson G, Colson M, Short N: Neuromuscular changes in female collegiate athletes resulting from a plyometric jump-training program, *J Ath Train* 39(1):17, 2004.
72. Zentz C: Warm up to perform up, *Athletic Therapy Today* 5(2): 59, 2000.

ANNOTATED BIBLIOGRAPHY

Alter M: *The science of flexibility*, Champaign, Ill, 2004, Human Kinetics.

This text explains the principles and techniques of stretching and details the anatomy and physiology of muscle and connective tissue. It includes guidelines for developing a flexibility program, illustrated stretching exercises, and warm-up drills.

Anderson B: *Stretching*, Bolinas, Calif, 2000, Shelter.

An extremely comprehensive best-selling text on stretching exercises for the entire body.

Baechle T, editor: *Essentials of strength training and conditioning*, Champaign, Ill, 2000, Human Kinetics.

A book from the National Strength Coaches Association that explains the science, theory, and practical application of various aspects of conditioning in a very concise, easily understood text.

Brooks G, Fahey T, White T: *Exercise physiology: human bioenergetics and its applications*, Mountain View, Calif, 2000, Mayfield.

An up-to-date, advanced text in exercise physiology that contains a comprehensive listing of the most current journal articles relative to exercise physiology.

Chu D: *Jumping into plyometrics*, Champaign, Ill, 1998, Human Kinetics.

This text helps the athlete develop a safe plyometric training program with exercises designed to improve quickness, speed, upper body strength, jumping ability, balance, and coordination. It is well illustrated.

Foss M, Keteyian S: *Fox's physiological basis for exercise and sport*, Dubuque, Iowa, 1998, McGraw-Hill.

A complete text that discusses the rationale and physiological principles underlying various aspects of an exercise program. Cardiorespiratory endurance is among several facets of fitness emphasized in this text.

Moran G, McGlynn G: *Dynamics of strength training*, St. Louis, 2000, McGraw-Hill

Provides a comprehensive resource using an individualized approach to strength training, including conditioning and cardiorespiratory fitness. Emphasizes the physiological basis of muscle strength and endurance. Illustrates the most efficient and effective training techniques.

Prentice W: *Fitness and wellness for life*, ed 7, Dubuque, Iowa, 1999, WCB/ McGraw-Hill.

A comprehensive fitness text that covers all aspects of a training and conditioning program.

Wiksten D, Peters C: *The athletic trainer's guide to strength and endurance training*, Thoroghfare, NJ, 2000, Slack.

Layout offers ease of reference, sport-specific programs, information on nutritional supplements, and illustrations on weight training and supplemental routines.

Nutritional Considerations

Chapter 5

When you finish this chapter you should be able to

- Distinguish the six classes of nutrients and describe their major functions.
- Explain the importance of good nutrition in enhancing performance and preventing injuries.
- Assess the advantages or disadvantages of supplementing nutrients in the athlete's diet.
- Discuss the advantages and disadvantages of consuming a preevent meal.
- Differentiate between body weight and body composition.
- Explain the principle of caloric balance and how to assess it.
- Assess body composition using skinfold calipers.
- Evaluate methods for losing and gaining weight.
- Recognize the signs of bulimia nervosa and anorexia nervosa.

The relation of nutrition, diet, and weight control to overall health and fitness is an issue of critical importance to an athlete. Athletes who practice sound nutritional habits reduce the likelihood of injury by maintaining a higher standard of healthful living.[53] We know that eating a well-balanced diet can positively contribute to the development of strength, flexibility, and cardiorespiratory endurance.[65] Unfortunately, misconceptions, fads, and in many cases, superstitions regarding nutrition affect dietary habits, particularly in the athletic population.[42]

Many athletes associate successful performance with the consumption of special foods or supplements.[38] An athlete who is performing well may be reluctant to change dietary habits regardless of whether the diet is physiologically beneficial to overall health.[69] There is no question that the psychological aspect of allowing the athlete to eat whatever he or she is most comfortable with can greatly affect performance. The problem is that these eating habits tend to become accepted as beneficial and may become traditional when in fact they may be physiologically detrimental to athletic performance. Thus, many nutrition "experts" tend to disseminate nutritional information based on traditional rather than experimental information.[69] The athletic trainer must possess a strong knowledge of nutrition so that he or she may serve as an informational resource for the athlete.[25,43]

NUTRITION BASICS

Nutrition is the science of the substances that are found in food that are essential to life. A substance is essential if it must be supplied by the diet.[69] There are six classes of nutrients: carbohydrates (CHO), fats, proteins, vitamins, minerals, and water. Nutrients are necessary for three major roles: growth, repair, and maintenance of all tissues; the regulation of body processes; and the production of energy.[67]

The six classes of nutrients are carbohydrates, fats, proteins, vitamins, minerals, and water.

Nutrient density describes foods that supply adequate amounts of vitamins and minerals in relation to their caloric value. The so-called junk foods provide excessive amounts of calories from fat and sugar in relation to vitamins and minerals and therefore are not nutrient dense. However, many people live on junk foods that displace more nutrient-dense foods from their diet.[58] This behavior is not healthful in the long run.[67]

Nutrient-dense foods supply adequate amounts of vitamins and minerals in relation to caloric value.

ENERGY SOURCES

Carbohydrates

Athletes have increased energy needs. Carbohydrates are the body's most efficient source of energy and should be relied on to fill that need.[55] For the athlete, carbohydrate intake should account for 55 percent to 70 percent of total caloric intake. The following sections describe different forms of carbohydrates and their role in the production of energy and the maintenance of health.[67]

Sugars

Carbohydrates are sugar, starches, or fiber.

Carbohydrates are classified as simple (sugars) or complex (starch and most forms of fiber). Sugars are further divided into monosaccharides and disaccharides. Monosaccharides, or single sugars, are found mostly in fruits, syrups, and honey. Glucose (blood sugar) is a monosaccharide. Milk sugar (lactose) and table sugar (sucrose) are combinations of two monosaccharides and are called disaccharides. Because sugar contributes little in the way of other nutrients, the amount of sugar eaten should account for less than 15 percent of the total caloric intake.

Starches

Starches are complex carbohydrates. A starch is made up of long chains of glucose units. During the digestion process, the starch chain is broken down and the glucose units are free to be absorbed. Food sources of starch, such as rice, potatoes, and breads, often provide vitamins and minerals in addition to serving as the body's principal source of glucose. Many people believe that starchy foods contribute to obesity. However, most of these foods are eaten with fats from butter, margarine, sauces, and gravies that make the food more enjoyable but contribute an excess of calories.

Glycolysis is the process that breaks down glucose to produce energy.

The body cannot use starches and many sugars directly from food for energy. It must obtain the simple sugar glucose (blood sugar). During digestion and metabolism, starches and disaccharide sugars are broken down and converted to glucose. The glucose that is not needed for immediate energy is stored as glycogen in the liver and muscle cells. Glucose can be released from glycogen later if needed. The body, however, can store only a limited amount of glucose as glycogen. Any extra amount of glucose is converted to body fat. When the body experiences an inadequate intake of dietary carbohydrate, it uses protein to make glucose, but the protein is then diverted from its own important functions. Therefore, a supply of glucose must be kept available to prevent the use of protein for energy. This is called the protein-sparing action of glucose.

Fiber

In recent years, researchers have given considerable attention to the importance of fiber in the diet. Fiber forms the structural parts of plants and is not digested by humans. Fiber is not found in animal sources of food. There are two kinds of dietary fiber: soluble and insoluble. Soluble fiber includes gums and pectins; cellulose is the primary insoluble form. Sources of soluble fiber are oatmeal, legumes, and some fruits. Food sources of insoluble fiber include whole grain breads and bran cereals.

Because it is not digested, fiber passes through the intestinal tract and adds bulk. Fiber aids normal elimination by reducing the amount of time required for wastes to move through the digestive tract, which is believed to reduce the risk of colon cancer. Also, increased fiber intake is thought to reduce the risk of coronary artery disease. Soluble forms of fiber bind to cholesterol passing through the digestive tract and prevent its absorption, which can reduce blood cholesterol levels. Foods rich in saturated fats (meats, in particular) often take the place of fiber-rich foods in the diet, thus increasing cholesterol absorption and formation. Consumption of adequate amounts of fiber has been associated with lowered incidences of obesity, constipation, colitis, appendicitis, and diabetes.

The recommended amount of fiber in the diet is approximately twenty-five grams per day.[61] Unfortunately, the average person consumes only ten to fifteen grams per day. Fiber intake should be increased by increasing the amount of whole grain cereal products and fruits and vegetables in the diet rather than by using fiber supplements. Excessive consumption of fiber may cause intestinal discomfort as well as increased losses of calcium and iron.

5-1

Critical Thinking Exercise

A female softball player has been told by her coach that she is slightly overweight and needs to lose a few pounds. The athlete has been watching television and reading about how important it is to limit the dietary intake of fat for losing weight. She has decided to go on a diet that is essentially fat free and is totally convinced that this will help her lose weight.

? What should the athletic trainer tell her about avoiding the excessive intake of fat as a means of losing weight?

Fats

Fats are another essential component of the diet. They are the most concentrated source of energy, providing more than twice the calories per gram when compared with carbohydrates or proteins. Fat is used as a primary source of energy. Some dietary fat is needed to make food more flavorful and for sources of the fat-soluble vitamins. Also, a minimal amount of fat is essential for normal growth and development.

Dietary fat represents approximately 40 percent to 50 percent of the total caloric intake. A substantial amount of the fat is from saturated fatty acids. This intake is believed to be too high and may contribute to the prevalence of obesity, certain cancers, and coronary artery disease. The recommended intake should be limited to less than 30 percent of total calories, with saturated fat reduced to less than 10 percent of total calories.[61]

Saturated versus Unsaturated Fat

Fats may be saturated or unsaturated.

Both plant and animal foods provide sources of dietary fat. About 95 percent of the fat consumed is in the form of triglycerides. Depending on their chemical nature, fatty acids may be saturated or unsaturated. The unsaturated fatty acids can be subdivided into monounsaturates or polyunsaturates. Therefore the terms *saturated, monounsaturated,* and *polyunsaturated* are used to describe the chemical nature of the fat in foods. The triglycerides that make up food fats are usually mixtures of saturated and unsaturated fatty acids but are classified according to the type that predominates. In general, fats containing more unsaturated fatty acids are from plants and are liquid at room temperature. Saturated fatty acids are derived mainly from animal sources.

Trans fatty acids have physical properties generally resembling saturated fatty acids, and their presence tends to harden oils. Often found in cookies, crackers, dairy products, meats, and fast foods, trans fatty acids increase the risk of heart disease by boosting levels of bad cholesterol. Because they are not essential and provide no known health benefit, there is no safe level of trans fatty acids and people should eat as little of them as possible while consuming a nutritionally adequate diet.

Other Fats

Phospholipids and sterols represent the remaining 5 percent of fats. Phospholipids include lecithin; cholesterol is the best known sterol. Cholesterol is consumed in the diet from animal foods; it is not supplied by plant sources of food. Generally, it is wise to avoid eating foods high in cholesterol. Although cholesterol is essential to many body functions, the body can manufacture cholesterol from CHO, proteins, and especially saturated fat. Thus there is little if any need to consume additional amounts of cholesterol in the diet. The American Heart Association recommends consuming less than 300 mg per day.

One type of unsaturated fatty acid seems to serve as a protective mechanism against certain disease processes. The omega-3 fatty acids apparently have the capability of reducing the likelihood of diseases such as heart disease, stroke, and hypertension. These fatty acids are found in cold-water fish. However, experts do not recommend the use of fish oil supplements as a source of omega-3 fatty acids.

Fat Substitutes

Fat-free products containing artificial fat substitutes, such as Simplese and Olean, are now available to the consumer. These products contain no cholesterol and 80 percent fewer calories than similar products made with fat. Despite FDA approval of these fat substitutes, some individuals have reported abdominal cramping and diarrhea when using them.[10]

Proteins

Dietary recommendations: CHO, 60 percent; fats, 25 percent; proteins, 15 percent.

Proteins make up the major structural components of the body. They are needed for growth, maintenance, and repair of all body tissues. In addition, proteins are needed to make enzymes, many hormones, and antibodies that help fight infection. In general, the body prefers not to use much protein for energy; instead it relies on fats and carbohydrates. Protein intake should be around 12 percent to 15 percent of total calories.

Amino Acids

Proteins are made up of amino acids.

The basic units that make up proteins are smaller compounds called amino acids. Most of the body's proteins are made up of about twenty amino acids. Amino acids can be linked together in a wide variety of combinations, which is why there are so many different forms and uses of proteins. Most of the amino acids can be produced as needed in the body. The others cannot be made to any significant degree and therefore must be supplied by the diet. The amino acids obtained through food are referred to as the essential amino acids. The amount of protein as well as the levels of the individual essential amino acids is important for determining the quality of diet. A diet that contains large amounts of protein will not support growth, repair, and maintenance of tissues if the essential amino acids are not available in the proper proportions.[37]

Most of the proteins from animal foods contain all the essential amino acids that humans require and are called complete, or high-quality, proteins. Incomplete proteins, that is, those sources of protein that do not contain all the essential amino acids, usually are from plant sources of food.

Protein Sources and Need

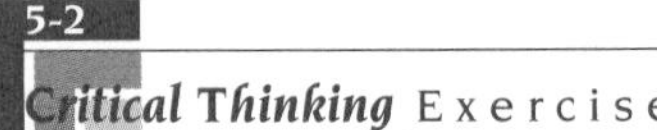

A volleyball player complains that she constantly feels tired and lethargic even though she thinks that she is eating well and getting a sufficient amount of sleep. A teammate has suggested that the player begin taking vitamin supplements, which the teammate claims gives her more energy and makes her more resistant to fatigue. The athlete comes to the athletic trainer to ask advice about what kind of vitamins she needs to take.

? What facts should the athletic trainer explain to the athlete about vitamin supplementation, and what recommendations should he or she make?

Most athletes do not have difficulty meeting protein needs because the typical diet is rich in protein, and many athletes consume more than twice the recommended levels of protein. There is no advantage to consuming more protein, particularly in the form of protein supplements. If more protein is supplied than needed, the body must convert the excess to fat for storage. This conversion can create a situation in which excess water is removed from cells, leading to dehydration and possible damage to the kidneys or liver. Protein supplements may also create imbalances of the chemicals that make up proteins, the amino acids, which is not desirable. A condition of the bones, osteoporosis, has been linked to a diet that contains too much protein.[7]

Increased physical activity increases a person's need for energy, not necessarily for protein.[37] The increases in muscle mass that result from conditioning and training are associated with only a small increase in protein requirements that can easily be met with the usual diet. Therefore an athlete does not need protein supplements.

REGULATOR NUTRIENTS

Vitamins

Although vitamins are required in extremely small amounts when compared with water, proteins, carbohydrates, and fats, they perform essential functions, primarily as regulators of body processes.[7] Thirteen vitamins have specific roles in the body, many of which are still being explored. In the past, letters were assigned as names for vitamins. Today, most are known by their scientific names. Vitamins are classified into two groups: fat-soluble vitamins, which are dissolved in fats and stored in the body, and water-soluble vitamins, which are dissolved in watery solutions and are not stored. Table 5-1 lists the vitamins and indicates their primary functions.

TABLE 5-1 Vitamins

Vitamin	Major Function	Most Reliable Sources	Deficiency	Excess (Toxicity)
A	Maintains skin and other cells that line the inside of the body; bone and tooth development; growth; vision in dim light	Liver, milk, egg yolk, deep green and yellow fruits and vegetables	Night blindness; dry skin; growth failure	Headaches, nausea, loss of hair, dry skin, diarrhea
D	Normal bone growth and development	Exposure to sunlight; fortified dairy products; eggs and fish liver oils	Rickets in children—defective bone formation leading to deformed bones	Appetite loss, weight loss, failure to grow
E	Prevents destruction of polyunsaturated fats caused by exposure to oxidizing agents; protects cell membranes from destruction	Vegetable oils, some in fruits and vegetables, whole grains	Breakage of red blood cells leading to anemia	Nausea and diarrhea; interferes with vitamin K absorption if vitamin D is also deficient; not as toxic as other fat-soluble vitamins
K	Production of blood-clotting substances	Green leafy vegetables; normal bacteria that live in intestines produce K that is absorbed	Increased bleeding time	
Thiamin	Needed for release of energy from carbohydrates, fats, and proteins	Cereal products, pork, peas, and dried beans	Lack of energy, nerve problems	
Riboflavin	Energy from carbohydrates, fats, and proteins	Milk, liver, fruits and vegetables, enriched breads and cereals	Dry skin, cracked lips	
Niacin	Energy from carbohydrates, fats, and proteins	Liver, meat, poultry, peanut butter, legumes, enriched breads and cereals	Skin problems, diarrhea, mental depression, and eventually death (rarely occurs in U.S.)	Skin flushing, intestinal upset, nervousness, intestinal ulcers
B_6	Metabolism of protein; production of hemoglobin	White meats, whole grains, liver, egg yolk, bananas	Poor growth, anemia	Severe loss of coordination from nerve damage
B_{12}	Production of genetic material; maintains central nervous system	Foods of animal origin	Neurological problems, anemia	
Folate (Folic acid)	Production of genetic material	Wheat germ, liver, yeast, mushrooms, green leafy vegetables, fruits	Anemia	
C (Ascorbic acid)	Formation and maintenance of connective tissue; tooth and bone formation; immune function	Fruits and vegetables	Scurvy (rare); swollen joints, bleeding gums, fatigue, bruising	Kidney stones, diarrhea
Pantothenic acid	Energy from carbohydrates, fats, proteins	Widely found in foods	Not observed in humans under normal conditions	
Biotin	Use of fats	Widely found in foods	Rare under normal conditions	

Fat-Soluble Vitamins

Fat-soluble vitamins: A, D, E, and K.

Vitamins A, D, E, and K are fat soluble. They are found in the fatty portions of foods and in oils. Because they are stored in the body's fat, it is possible to consume excess amounts and show the effects of vitamin poisoning.

Water-Soluble Vitamins

Water-soluble vitamins: C, thiamin, riboflavin, niacin, B_6, B_{12}, folate, biotin, and panothenic acid.

The water-soluble vitamins consist of vitamin C, known as ascorbic acid, and the B-complex vitamins, most now referred to by their scientific names. B-complex vitamins include thiamin, riboflavin, niacin, B_6, folate, B_{12}, biotin, and pantothenic acid. Although vitamins are not metabolized for energy, thiamin, riboflavin, niacin, biotin, and pantothenic acid are used to regulate the metabolism of CHO, proteins, and fats to obtain energy. Vitamin B_6 regulates the body's use of amino acids. Folate and vitamin B_{12} are important in normal blood formation. Vitamin C is used for building bones and teeth, maintaining connective tissues, and strengthening the immune system. Unlike fat-soluble vitamins, water-soluble vitamins cannot be stored to any significant extent in the body and should be supplied in the diet each day.[7]

Antioxidants

Antioxidants: vitamin C, vitamin E, and beta-carotene.

Certain nutrients, called antioxidants, may prevent premature aging, certain cancers, heart disease, and other health problems.[30] An antioxidant protects vital cell components from the destructive effects of certain agents, including oxygen. Vitamin C, vitamin E, and beta-carotene are antioxidants. Beta-carotene is a plant pigment that is found in dark green, deep yellow, or orange fruits and vegetables. The body can convert beta-carotene to vitamin A. In the early 1980s, researchers reported that smokers who ate large quantities of fruits and vegetables rich in beta-carotene were less likely to develop lung cancer than were other smokers.[45] Since that time, more evidence is accumulating about the benefits of a diet rich in the antioxidant nutrients.[45]

Some experts believe that athletes should increase their intake of antioxidants, even if it means taking supplements. Others are more cautious.[45] Excess beta-carotene pigments circulate throughout the body and may turn the skin yellow. However, the pigment is not believed to be toxic like its nutrient cousin, vitamin A is. On the other hand, increasing intake of vitamins C and E is not without some risk. Excess vitamin C is not well absorbed; the excess is irritating to the intestines and creates diarrhea. Although less toxic than vitamins A or D, too much vitamin E causes health problems.

Vitamin Deficiencies

The illness that results from a lack of any nutrient, especially those nutrients, such as vitamins, that are needed only in small amounts, is referred to as a deficiency disease.[46] Vitamin deficiency diseases are rare. Adequate amounts of the different vitamins, as with other nutrients, can be obtained if a wide variety of foods is eaten. For most people, vitamin supplements are a waste of money and can cause toxic effects if too many are taken. Many individuals think that vitamins are "foods" and are safe. However, in large doses, vitamins have druglike effects on the body. Table 5-1 describes some of vitamins' toxicity problems.

Minerals

More than twenty mineral elements have an essential role in the body and therefore must be supplied in the diet. These essential minerals are listed in Table 5-2. Most minerals are stored in the body, especially in the liver and bones. Magnesium is needed in energy-supplying reactions; sodium and potassium are important for the transmission of nerve impulses. Iron plays a role in energy metabolism but is also combined with a protein to form hemoglobin, the compound that transports oxygen in red blood cells. Calcium has many important functions: it is necessary for proper bone and teeth formation, blood clotting, and muscle contraction. In general, minerals have roles that are

TABLE 5-2 Minerals

Mineral	Major Role	Most Reliable Sources	Deficiency	Excess
Calcium	Bone and tooth formation; blood clotting; muscle contraction; nerve function	Dairy products	May lead to osteoporosis	Calcium deposits in soft tissues
Phosphorus	Skeletal development; tooth formation	Meats, dairy products, and other protein-rich foods	Rarely seen	
Sodium	Maintenance of fluid balance	Salt (sodium chloride) added to foods and sodium-containing preservatives		May contribute to the development of hypertension
Iron	Formation of hemoglobin; energy from carbohydrates, fats, and proteins	Liver and red meats, enriched breads and cereals	Iron-deficiency anemia	Can cause death in children from supplement overdose
Copper	Formation of hemoglobin	Liver, nuts, shellfish, cherries, mushrooms, whole grain breads and cereals	Anemia	Nausea and vomiting
Zinc	Normal growth and development	Seafood and meats	Skin problems, delayed development, growth problems	Interferes with copper use; may decrease high-density lipoprotein levels
Iodine	Production of the hormone thyroxin	Iodized salt, seafood	Mental and growth retardation; lack of energy	
Fluorine	Strengthens bones and teeth	Fluoridated water	Teeth are less resistant to decay	Damage to tooth enamel

too numerous to detail within the scope of this book. Eating a wide variety of foods is the best way to obtain the minerals needed in the proper concentrations.[7]

Water

Water is the most essential of all the nutrients and should be the nutrient of greatest concern to the athlete.[67] It is the most abundant nutrient in the body, accounting for approximately 60 percent of the body weight, although this varies considerably (+/−10%) among different individuals due to age and percent of body fat. Water is essential for all the chemical processes that occur in the body, and an adequate supply of water is necessary for energy production and normal digestion of other nutrients. Although water does not supply any energy (calories), an adequate supply of water is needed for energy production in all cells. Water also takes part in digestion and maintaining the proper environment inside and outside of cells. Water is also necessary for temperature control and for the elimination of waste products of nutrient and body metabolism. Too little water leads to dehydration, and severe dehydration frequently leads to death. The average adult requires a minimum of 2.5 liters or about 10 glasses of water per day.

The body has a number of mechanisms designed specifically to maintain body water at near-normal level. Too little water leads to accumulation of solutes in the blood. These solutes signal the brain that the body is thirsty while signaling the kidney to conserve water. Excessive water dilutes these solutes, which signals the brain to stop drinking and the kidneys to get rid of the excess water.

Replacing fluid after heavy sweating is far more important than replacing electrolytes.

Water is the only nutrient that is of greater importance to the athlete than to those people who are more sedentary, especially when the athlete is engaging in prolonged exercise carried out in a hot, humid environment. Such a situation may cause excessive sweating and subsequent losses of large amounts of water. When the body burns carbohydrate and fat for energy, it produces a great deal of heat. During exercise, that heat is lost from the body primarily by sweating. Sweating is how the body uses water to keep itself from overheating. Restriction of water during this time will result in dehydration. Symptoms of dehydration include fatigue, vomiting, nausea, exhaustion, fainting, and possibly death.

Electrolyte Requirements

Electrolytes: sodium, chloride, potassium, magnesium, and calcium.

Electrolytes, including sodium, chloride, potassium, magnesium, and calcium, are electrically charged ions dissolved in body water. Among many other roles, electrolytes maintain the balance of water inside and outside the cell. In other words, electrolytes especially sodium, are essential in helping the body rehydrate quickly.[3,12] Electrolyte replenishment may be needed when a person is not fit, suffers from extreme water loss, participates in a marathon, or has just completed an exercise period and is expected to perform at near-maximum effort within the next few hours. In most cases, electrolytes can be sufficiently replaced with a balanced diet, which can, if necessary, be salted slightly more than usual. Free access to water and sports drinks (ad libitum) before, during, and after activity should be the rule (see Chapter 6). In some people, electrolyte losses can produce muscle cramping and intolerance to heat. Sweating results not only in body water loss but in some electrolyte loss as well.[56]

During cold weather, water is not as critical as it is in hot weather. Therefore a stronger electrolyte solution that allows a slower, more steady release of fluid from the stomach should be used. In hot weather or in cold weather, thirst is not an indicator of hydration.

NUTRIENT REQUIREMENTS AND RECOMMENDATIONS

A nutrient requirement is that amount of the nutrient that is needed to prevent the nutrient's deficiency disease. Nutrient needs vary among individuals within a population. A recommendation for a nutrient is different from the requirement for a nutrient. Scientists establish recommendations for nutrients and calories based on extensive scientific research and assessment of present dietary intakes.[20]

In the past, the *U.S. Recommended Dietary Allowances (US RDA)* have served as the benchmarks of nutritional adequacy in the United States. Over the past several years new information has emerged about nutrient requirements that necessitated updating of the RDAs.[22] RDAs have been changed to *Dietary Reference Intakes (DRIs)*, which are established using an expanded concept that includes indicators of good health and the prevention of chronic disease, as well as possible adverse effects of overconsumption.[20] The DRIs include not only recommended intakes (RDA) intended to help individuals meet their daily nutritional requirements, but also tolerable upper intake levels (ULs), which help individuals avoid harm from consuming too much of a nutrient; estimated average requirements (EAR), which are the average daily nutrient intake level estimated to meet the requirement of half the healthy individuals in a particular age group; and Adequate Intake (AI), which is the recommended average daily intake level based on experimentally developed estimates of nutrient intake that are used when the RDA cannot be determined.[20] Table 5-3 shows the latest DRIs. (Appendix B shows nutrient recommendations for Canadians.)

Food Labels

Food labels on packages help consumers to make more informed food selections (Figure 5-1). Concern over the amount of fat, cholesterol, sodium, and fiber in the typical American diet led the drive for a more health-conscious label. For more than a decade, the US RDA appeared on nutrient labels. In the early 1990s, the old food

ability, prevent graying hair, or cure muscular dystroph amounts of vitamin E by consuming whole-grain prod

The B-complex vitamins that are involved in obtain proteins are often abused by athletes who believe tha increased need for these nutrients is easily fulfilled wh tious foods while training.[63] If athletes do not increas will lose weight because of their high level of caloric e

If an athlete is not eating a well balanced diet, takir day would be helpful and in fact is recommended by n that minimum DRIs are met.

Mineral Supplementation

Obtaining adequate levels of certain minerals can be Calcium and iron intakes may be low for those ath products, red meats, or enriched breads and cereals i their money and overdosing, however, athletes mu whether they need extra minerals. The following sect can be low in the diet and some suggestions for imp that supplements may not be necessary.

Calcium Deficiency

Calcium is the most abundant mineral in the body. It as well as for muscle contraction and the conduction importance of obtaining adequate calcium supplies th recognized. If calcium intake is too low to meet need from the bones. Over time, the bones become weake films. These bones are brittle and often break sponta **osteoporosis** and is estimated to be eight times mor men. It becomes a serious problem for women after r

The AI for young adults is 1,000 mg (an eight-ou 300 mg of calcium). Unfortunately about 25 percent c consume less than 300 mg of calcium per day, well b ets and alcohol consumption also increase calcium e causes calcium to be retained in bones, so physical younger females who exercise to extremes so that th upset are prone to develop premature osteoporos preferably as calcium carbonate or citrate rather than females who have a family history of osteoporosis.

Milk products are the most reliable sources of calci milk and other dairy products upset their stomach. lactase that is needed to digest milk sugar lactose. Th tose intolerance, or **lactase deficiency**.[67] The undig testine, where the bacteria that normally reside the produce large quantities of intestinal gas, which caus lactose-intolerant people also suffer from diarrhea. duced the missing enzyme, lactase. Lactase is availal that can be added to foods before eating or taken alc

Iron Deficiency

Iron deficiency is also a common problem, especiall can result in iron-deficiency **anemia** (see Chapter form hemoglobin. With anemia, the oxygen-carryi reduced so that muscles cannot obtain enough oxy leaves a person feeling tired and weak. Obviously, a level while suffering from an iron deficiency.

labels we centages

The Foc

The Basi designed America food gro amples c group) fc etary Gu percenta cording t sic Four each wit apex of t provide suggeste

TABLE 5-3 Dietary Reference Intakes: Recommended Levels for Individual Intake from the Food and Nutrition Board, Institute of Medicine–National Academy of Sciences[20]

Life-Stage Group		Vitamin D (μg/d)[a,b]	Thiamin (mg/d)	Riboflavin B_1 (mg/d)	Niacin (mg/d)[b]	B_6 (μg/d)	Folate (μg/d)[d]	B_{12} (mg/d)	Pantothenic Acid (mg/d)	Biotin (μg/d)	Choline[e] (mg/d)	Vitamin A (μg/d)	Vitamin C (mg/d)	Vitamin E (mg/d)	Vitamin K (μg/d)
Males	14–18 yr	5*	1.2	1.3	16	1.3	400	2.4	5*	25*	550*	900	75	15	75*
	19–30 yr	5*	1.2	1.3	16	1.3	400	2.4	5*	25*	550*	900	90	15	120*
	31–50 yr	5*	1.2	1.3	16	1.3	400	2.4	5*	30*	550*	900	90	15	120*
	51–70 yr	10*	1.2	1.3	16	1.7	400	2.4	5*	30*	550*	900	90	15	120*
	>70 yr	15*	1.2	1.3	16	1.7	400	2.4[f]	5*	30*	550*	900	90	15	120*
Females	14–18 yr	5*	1.0	1.0	14	1.2	400[g]	2.4[f]	5*	25*	400*	700	65	15	75*
	19–30 yr	5*	1.1	1.1	14	1.3	400[g]	2.4	5*	30*	425*	700	75	15	90*
	31–50 yr	5*	1.1	1.1	14	1.3	400[g]	2.4	5*	30*	425*	700	75	15	90*
	51–70 yr	10*	1.1	1.1	14	1.5	400[g]	2.4[f]	5*	30*	425*	700	75	15	90*
	<70 yr	15*	1.1	1.1	14	1.5	400	2.4[f]	5*	30*	425*	700	75	15	90*
Pregnancy	>18 yr	5*	1.4	1.4	18	1.9	600[h]	2.6	6*	30*	450*	750	80	15	75*
	19–30 yr	5*	1.4	1.4	18	1.9	600[h]	2.6	6*	30*	450*	770	85	15	90*
	31–50 yr	5*	1.4	1.4	18	1.9	600[h]	2.6	6*	30*	450*	770	85	15	90*
Lactation	≤18 yr	5*	1.5	1.6	17	2.0	500	2.8	7*	35*	550*	1,200	115	19	75*
	19–30 yr	5*	1.5	1.6	17	2.0	500	2.8	7*	35*	550*	1,300	120	19	90*
	31–50 yr	5*	1.5	1.6	17	2.0	500	2.8	7*	35*	550*	1,300	120	19	90*

Continued

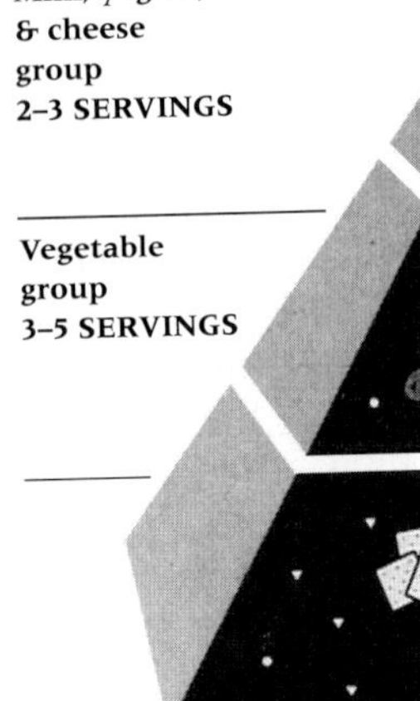

Figure 5-2 The food pyramid offers examples of appropriate food selections important to an athlete's diet.

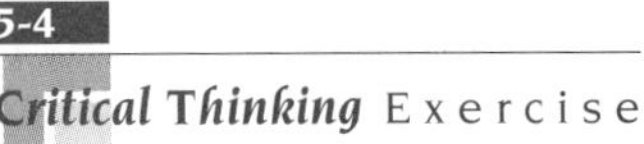

5-4 Critical Thinking Exercise

A high-school football player has become interested in body building. He is most interested in seeing an increase in muscle mass. He is religious about his weight training but has heard that increasing protein intake will cause the muscles to hypertrophy more quickly.

? What advice can the athletic trainer give him about taking commercially produced protein supplements?

Protein Supplementation

Athletes often believe that more protein is needed to build bigger muscles.[39] It is true that a relatively small amount of extra protein is needed by athletes who are developing muscles in a training program. Many athletes, particularly those who are training with heavy weights or who are bodybuilders, routinely take protein supplements that are commercially produced and marketed.[37,39] To build muscle, athletes should consume 1 to 1.5 grams of extra protein per kilogram (0.5 to 0.7 grams per pound) of body weight every day. This range goes from slightly above to about double the protein RDA (0.8 grams per kilogram of desirable body weight). Anyone eating a variety of foods, but especially protein-rich foods, can easily meet the higher amounts. Thus, athletes do not need protein supplements, because their diets typically exceed even the most generous protein recommendations. An active adult will most likely require 0.6 grams per pound, or 66 percent more than the RDA.[20]

Creatine Supplementation

Creatine is a naturally occurring organic compound synthesized by the kidneys, liver, and pancreas. Creatine also can be obtained from ingesting meat and fish that contain approximately five grams per kilogram. Creatine has an integral role in energy metabolism.[5]

There are two main types of creatine: free creatine and phosphocreatine. Phosphocreatine is stored in skeletal muscle and is used during anaerobic activity to produce ATP with the assistance of the enzyme creatine kinase. With creatine supplementation, phosphocreatine depletion is delayed and performance is enhanced through the maintenance of the normal metabolic pathways.[41]

The positive physiological effects of creatine include increasing the resynthesis of ATP, thus allowing for increased intensity in a workout; functioning as a lactic acid buffer, thus prolonging maximal effort and improving exercise recovery time during maximal intensity activities; stimulating protein synthesis; decreasing total cholesterol while improving the HDL-to-LDL ratio; decreasing total triglycerides; and increasing fat-free mass.[5] It has been suggested that creatine supplementation may reduce the incidence of muscle cramps.[27] Side effects of creatine supplementation include weight gain, due primarily to an increase in total body water;[48] gastrointestinal disturbances, and renal dysfunction. These are apparently no other known long-term side effects.

It has been suggested that an initial loading phase should consist of twenty grams of creatine and 120 ounces of water each day for six days. The recommended amount for improving performance after the loading phase is five to ten grams per day for four weeks.[5,68] Oral supplementation with creatine may enhance muscular performance during high-intensity resistance exercise.[41,66]

In August 2000 the NCAA Committee on Competitive Safeguards and Medical Aspects of Sports banned the distribution to student athletes of all muscle-building substances, including creatine, by NCAA member institutions. The use of creatine itself is not banned.

Sugar and Performance

Ingesting large quantities of glucose in the form of honey, candy bars, or pure sugar immediately before physical activity may have a significant impact on performance.[50] As carbohydrates are digested, large quantities of glucose enter the blood. This increase in blood sugar (glucose) levels stimulates the release of the hormone insulin. Insulin allows the cells to use the circulating glucose so that blood glucose levels soon return to normal.[55] It was hypothesized that a decline in blood sugar levels was detrimental to performance and endurance. However, recent evidence indicates that the effect of eating large quantities of carbohydrates is beneficial rather than negative.

Nevertheless, some athletes are sensitive to high-carbohydrate feedings and experience problems with increased levels of insulin. Also, some athletes cannot tolerate large amounts of the simple sugar fructose. For these individuals, too much fructose leads to intestinal upset and diarrhea. Athletes should test themselves with various high-carbohydrate foods to see if they are affected (but not before a competitive event).[42]

Caffeine and Performance

Caffeine is a central nervous system stimulant. Most people who consume caffeine in coffee, tea, or carbonated beverages are aware of its effect of increasing alertness and decreasing fatigue. Chocolate contains compounds that are related to caffeine and have the same stimulating effects. However, large amounts of caffeine cause nervousness, irritability, increased heart rate, and headaches.[22] Also, headaches are a withdrawal symptom experienced when a person tries to stop consuming caffeinated products.[46]

Although small amounts of caffeine do not appear to harm physical performance, cases of nausea and light-headedness have been reported. Caffeine enhances the use of fat during endurance exercise, thus delaying the depletion of glycogen stores.[18] This delay would help endurance performance. Caffeine also helps make calcium more available to the muscle during contraction, allowing the muscle to work more efficiently. However, Olympic officials rightfully consider caffeine to be a drug. It should not be present in an Olympic competitor's blood in levels greater than that resulting from drinking five or six cups of coffee.

Alcohol and Performance

Alcohol provides energy for the body; each gram of pure alcohol (ethanol) supplies seven calories. However, sources of alcohol provide little other nutritional value with regard to vitamins, minerals, and proteins. The depressant effects of alcohol on the central nervous system include decreased physical coordination, slowed reaction times, and decreased mental alertness. Also, this drug increases the production of urine, resulting in body water losses (diuretic effect). Therefore, the use of alcoholic beverages by the athlete is not recommended before, during, or after physical activity.[32]

Eating Organic, Natural, or Health Foods

Many athletes are concerned about the quality of the foods they eat—not just the nutritional value of the food but also its safety. Organic foods are grown without the use of synthetic fertilizers and pesticides. Those who advocate the use of organic farming methods claim that these foods are nutritionally superior and safer than the same products grown using chemicals such as pesticides and synthetic fertilizers.[16]

Technically, the description of organic food is meaningless. All foods (except water) are organic; that is, they contain the element carbon. Organically produced foods are often more expensive than the same foods that have been produced by conventional means. There is no advantage to consuming organic food products. They are not more nutritious than foods produced by conventional methods. Nevertheless, for some athletes, the psychological benefit of believing that they are doing something good for their bodies justifies the extra cost.

Natural foods have been subjected to little processing and contain no additives such as preservatives or artificial flavors.[64] Processing can protect nutritional value. Preservatives save food that would otherwise spoil and have to be destroyed. Furthermore, many foods in their natural form are poisonous. The green layer often found under the skin of potatoes is poisonous if eaten in large amounts. Poisonous mushrooms and molds in peanuts cause liver cancer.

Both organic and natural foods could be described as health foods. However, there is no benefit derived from eating a diet consisting of health foods, even for the athlete.

Using Herbal Supplements

The use of herbs as natural alternatives to drugs and medicines has clearly become a trend among American consumers. Most herbs, as edible plants, are safe to ingest as foods; as natural medicines, they are claimed to have few side effects, although occasionally a mild, allergic reaction may occur.[21,46]

Herbs can offer the body nutrients that are reported to nourish the brain, glands, and hormones. Unlike vitamins, which work best when taken with food, herbs do not need to be taken with other foods, since they provide their own digestive enzymes.[23]

Herbs in their whole form are not drugs. As medicine, herbs are essentially body balancers that work with the body's functions so that it can heal and regulate itself. Herbal formulas can be general for overall strength and nutrient support or specific to a particular ailment or condition.

Hundreds of herbs are widely available today at all quality levels. They are readily available at health food stores. However, unlike both food and medicine, no federal or governmental controls regulate the sale of herbs to ensure the quality of the products being sold.[23] The consumer of herbal products must exercise extreme caution.

The *Focus Box:* "Most widely used herbs and purposes for use" lists the most popular and widely used herbal products sold in health food stores. Some additional potent and complex herbs, such as capsicum, lobelia, sassafras, mandrake tansy, canada snake root, wormwood, woodruff, poke root, and rue may be useful in small amounts and as catalysts, but should not be used alone.

Focus

Most widely used herbs and purposes for use

cayenne—used for weight loss
cascara—used as a laxative, can cause dehydration
dong quai—to treat menstrual symptoms
echinacea—to promote wound healing and strengthen the immune system
fever few—to prevent and relieve migraine headaches, arthritis, and PMS
garlic—used as an antibiotic, antibacterial, antifungal agent to prevent and relieve coronary artery disease by reducing total blood cholesterol and triglyceride levels and raising HDL levels
garcina cambagia—used to promote loss of fat
ginkgo biloba—used to improve blood circulation, especially in the brain
ginseng—used to reduce impotence, weakness, lethargy, and fatigue
**guarana*—used as a stimulant, contains large amounts of caffeine, often in weight loss products
kava—used to reduce anxiety, relax muscle tension, produce analgesic effects, act as a local anesthetic, provide antibacterial benefit
**ma huang (ephedrine)*—derived from the ephedra plant, it has been used in China for medicinal purposes including increased energy, appetite suppression, increased fat burning, and preservation of muscle tissue from breaking down. It is a central nervous system stimulant drug which was used in many diet pills. In 1995, the FDA revealed adverse reactions to ephedrine such as heart attacks, strokes, paranoid psychosis, vomiting, fever, palpitations, convulsions, and comas. In 2003, it was banned by the FDA.
mate—CNS stimulant
saw palmetto—used to treat inflamed prostate; also used as a diuretic and as a sexual enhancement agent
senna—used as a laxative, can cause water and electrolyte loss
St. John's wort—used as an antidepressant; also used to treat nervous disorders, depression, neuralgia, kidney problems, wounds, and burns
valerian—used to treat insomnia, anxiety, stress
yohimbe—used to increase libido and blood flow to sexual organs in the male

*Banned by some athletic organizations and/or the FDA

Ephedrine

Ephedrine is a stimulant that has been used as an ingredient in diet pills, illegal recreational drugs, and legitimate over-the-counter medications to treat congestion and asthma.[49] Ephedrine is similar to an amphetamine. In December 2003, the FDA banned the use of ephedrine as a dietary supplement. For several years the FDA has warned consumers about the potential dangers of using ephedrine.[33] In recent years both the NCAA and minor league baseball have banned the use of ephedrine by their athletes. However some companies continue to sell dietary products that contain ephedrine or other stimulants despite the fact that these supplements have caused numerous problems. Ephedrine is know to produce the following adverse reactions: heart attack, stroke, tachycardia, paranoid psychosis, depressions, convulsions, fever, coma, vomiting, palpitations, hypertension, and respiratory depression.[49,71]

Practicing Vegetarianism

Vegetarians: total vegetarians, lactovegetarians, ovolactovegetarians, and semivegetarians.

Vegetarianism has emerged as an alternative to the usual American diet. All vegetarians use plant foods to form the foundation of their diet; animal foods are either totally excluded or included in a variety of eating patterns.[15] Athletes who choose to become vegetarians do so for economic, philosophical, religious, cultural, or health reasons. Vegetarianism is no longer considered to be a fad if it is practiced intelligently. However, the vegetarian diet may create deficiencies if nutrient needs are not carefully considered. Athletes who follow this eating pattern must plan their diet carefully so that their calorie needs are met.[15] Types of vegetarian dietary patterns are categorized as follows:

- *Total vegetarians, or vegans:* People who consume plant but no animal foods; meat, fish, poultry, eggs, and dairy products are excluded from their diet. This diet is adequate for most adults if they give careful consideration to obtaining enough calories, vitamin B12, and the minerals calcium, zinc, and iron.
- *Lactovegetarians:* Individuals who consume milk products along with plant foods; meat, fish, poultry, and eggs are excluded from their diet. Iron and zinc levels can be low in this form of vegetarianism.
- *Ovolactovegetarians:* People who consume dairy products and eggs in their diet along with plant foods; meat, fish, and poultry are excluded. Again, obtaining sufficient iron could be a problem.
- *Semivegetarians:* People who consume animal products but exclude red meats. Plant products still form an important part of the diet. This diet is usually adequate.

PREEVENT NUTRITION

The importance and content of the preevent meal has been heatedly debated among coaches, athletic trainers, and athletes.[29] The trend has been to ignore logical thinking about what should be eaten before competition and to upholding the tradition of "rewarding" the athlete for hard work by serving foods that may hamper performance. For example, the traditional steak-and-eggs meal before football games is great for coaches and athletic trainers; however, the athlete gains nothing from this meal. The important point is that too often people are concerned primarily with the preevent meal and fail to realize that those nutrients consumed over several days before competition are much more important than what is eaten three hours before an event. The purpose of the preevent meal should be to provide the competitor with sufficient nutrient energy and fluids for competition while taking into consideration the digestibility of the food and, most important, the eating preferences of the individual athlete. (See *Focus Box:* "The pregame meal.") Figure 5-3 gives examples of preevent meals.

Athletes should be encouraged to become conscious of their diets. However, no experimental evidence exists to indicate that performance may be enhanced by altering a diet that is basically sound. There are a number of ways that a nutritious diet may be achieved, and the diet that is optimal for one athlete may not be the best for another. In many instances, the individual will be the best judge of what he or she should or

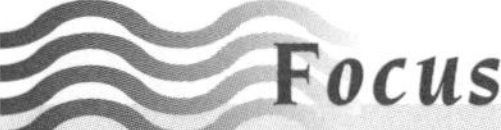

The pregame meal

- Try to achieve the largest possible storage of carbohydrates (glycogen) in both resting muscle and the liver. This storage is particularly important for endurance activities but may also be beneficial for intense, short-duration exercise.
- A stomach that is full of food during contact sports is subject to injury. Therefore, the type of food eaten should allow the stomach to empty quickly. Carbohydrates are easier to digest than are fats or proteins. A meal that contains plenty of carbohydrates will leave the stomach and be digested faster than a fatty meal. It would be wise to replace the traditional steak-and-eggs preevent meal with a low-fat one containing a small amount of pasta, tomato sauce, and bread.
- Foods should not cause irritation or upset to the gastrointestinal tract. Foods high in cellulose and other forms of fiber, such as whole grain products, fruits, and vegetables, increase the need for defecation. Highly spiced foods or gas-forming foods (such as onions, baked beans, or peppers) must also be avoided because any type of disturbance in the gastrointestinal tract may be detrimental to performance. Carbonated beverages and chewing gum also contribute to the formation of gas.
- Liquids consumed should be easily absorbed and low in fat content and should not act as a laxative. Whole milk, coffee, and tea should be avoided. Water intake should be increased, particularly if the temperature is high.
- A meal should be eaten approximately three to four hours before the event or before exercising. This timing allows for adequate stomach emptying, but the individual will not feel hungry during activity.
- The athlete should not eat any food that he or she dislikes. Most important, the individual must feel psychologically satisfied by any preevent meal. If not, performance may be impaired more by psychological factors than by physiological factors.
- Prolonged fasting and diet programs that severely restrict caloric intake are scientifically undesirable and can be medically dangerous.
- Fasting and diet programs that severely restrict caloric intake result in the loss of large amounts of water, electrolytes, minerals, glycogen stores, and other fat-free tissue (including proteins within fat-free tissues), with minimal amounts of fat loss.
- Mild calorie restriction (500 to 1,000 calories less than the usual daily intake) results in a smaller loss of water, electrolytes, minerals, and other fat-free tissue and is less likely to cause malnutrition.
- Dynamic exercise of large muscles helps maintain fat-free tissue, including muscle mass and bone density, and results in losses of body weight. Weight loss resulting from an increase in energy expenditure is primarily in the form of fat weight.
- A nutritionally sound diet resulting in mild calorie restriction coupled with an endurance exercise program, along with behavioral modification of existing eating habits, is recommended for weight reduction. The rate of sustained weight loss should not exceed 1 kg (2 lb) per week.
- To maintain proper weight control and optimal body fat levels, a lifetime commitment to proper eating habits and regular physical activity is required.

should not eat in the preevent meal or before exercising. It seems that a person's best guide is to eat whatever he or she is most comfortable with.

Liquid Food Supplements

Recently, liquid food supplements (Gatorade Nutrition Shake, Exceed) have been recommended as extremely effective preevent meals and are being used by high school, college, university, and professional teams with some indications of success.[51] These supplements supply from 225 to 400 calories per average serving. Athletes who have used these supplements report elimination of the usual pregame symptoms of dry mouth, abdominal cramps, leg cramps, nervous defecation, and nausea.

MEAL 1	
3/4 c Orange juice	3/4 c Orange juice
1/2 c Cereal with 1 tsp sugar	1–2 Pancakes with:
1 Slice whole wheat toast with:	1 tsp Margarine
1 tsp Margarine	2 tbsp Syrup
1 tsp Honey or jelly	8 oz Skim or lowfat milk
8 oz Skim or lowfat milk	Water
Water	(Approximately 450–500 kcal)
(Approximately 450–500 kcal)	
MEAL 2	
1 c Vegetable soup	1 c Spaghetti with tomato sauce and cheese
1 Turkey sandwich with:	1/2 c Sliced pears (canned) on 1/4 c cottage cheese
2 Slices bread	1–2 Slices (Italian) bread with 1–2 tsp margarine (avoid garlic)
2 oz Turkey (white or dark)	1/2 c Sherbet
1 oz Cheese slice	1–2 Sugar cookies
2 tsp Mayonnaise	4 oz Skim or lowfat milk
8 oz Skim or lowfat milk	Water
Water	(Approximately 700 kcal)
(Approximately 550–600 kcal)	

Figure 5-3

Sample preevent meals.

Under ordinary conditions, it usually takes approximately four hours for a full meal to pass through the stomach and the small intestine. Pregame emotional tension often delays the emptying of the stomach; therefore the undigested food mass remains in the stomach and upper bowel for a prolonged time, even up to or through the actual period of competition, and frequently results in nausea, vomiting, and cramps. This unabsorbed food mass is of no value to the athlete. Team physicians who have experimented with the liquid food supplements say that a major advantage to the supplements is that they clear both the stomach and the upper bowel before game time, thus making available the caloric energy that would otherwise still be in an unassimilated state. There is merit in the use of such food supplements for pregame meals.[51]

Eating Fast Foods

Eating fast food is a way of life in American society.[57] Athletes, especially young athletes, have for the most part grown up as fast-food junkies. Furthermore, travel budgets and tight schedules dictate that fast food is a frequent choice for coaches on road trips.[57] Aside from occasional problems with food flavor, the biggest concern in consuming fast foods, as can be seen in Table 5-4, is that 40 percent to 50 percent of the calories consumed are from fats. To compound this problem, these already sizable meals are now being "supersized" at a more affordable price for those who want maximum fat, salt, and calories in a single sitting.[46]

On the positive side, fast-food restaurants have broadened their menus to include whole wheat breads and rolls, salad bars, and low-fat milk products. Many of the larger fast-food restaurants provide nutritional information for consumers upon request or from well-stocked racks.[46] *Focus Box:* "Tips for selecting fast foods" provides suggestions for eating more healthfully at fast-food restaurants.

Glycogen Supercompensation

For endurance events, maximizing the amount of glycogen that can be stored, especially in muscles, may make the difference between finishing first or at the end of the pack. Athletes can increase glycogen supplies in muscle and liver by reducing the training program a few days before competing and by significantly increasing carbohydrate intake during the week before the event.[50] By reducing training for at least forty-eight hours before the competition, the athlete can eliminate any metabolic waste products that may hinder performance. The high-carbohydrate diet restores glycogen levels in

5-5

Critical Thinking **Exercise**

A recreational runner has been training to run his first marathon. He feels good about his level of conditioning but wants to make certain that he does everything that he can do to maximize his performance. He is concerned about eating the right type of foods both before and during the marathon to help ensure that he does not become excessively fatigued.

? What recommendations should the athletic trainer make regarding glycogen supercompensation, the preevent meal, and food consumption during the event?

TABLE 5-4 Fast-Food Choices and Nutritional Value

Food	Calories	Protein (g)	CHO (g)	Fat (g)	Calories from Fat (%)	Cholesterol (mg)	Sodium (mg)
Hamburgers							
McDonald's hamburger	263	12.4	28.3	11	38.6	29.1	506
Dairy Queen single hamburger w/cheese	410	24	33	20	43.9	50	790
Hardee's 1/4 pound cheeseburger	506	28	41	26	46.2	61	1,950
Wendy's double hamburger, white bun	560	4.1	24	34	54.6	125	575
McDonald's Big Mac	570	24.6	39.2	35	55.2	83	45
Burger King Whopper sandwich	640	27	42	41	57.6	94	842
Jack in the Box Jumbo Jack	485	26	38	26	48.2	64	905
Chicken							
Arby's chicken breast sandwich	592	28	56	27	41.0	57	1,340
Burger King chicken sandwich	688	26	56	40	52.3	82	1,423
Dairy Queen chicken sandwich	670	29	46	41	55.0	75	870
Church's Crispy Nuggets (one; regular)	55	3	4	3	49.0	—	125
Kentucky Fried Chicken Nuggets (one)	46	2.82	2.2	2.9	56.7	11.9	140
Fish							
Church's Southern fried catfish	67	4	4	4	53.7	—	151
Long John Silver's Fish & More	978	34	82	58	53.3	88	2,124
McDonald's Filet-O-Fish	435	14.7	35.9	25.7	53.1	45.2	799
Others							
Hardee's hot dog	346	11	26	22	57.2	42	744
Jack in the Box taco	191	8	1.6	11	51.8	21	406
Arby's roast beef sandwich (regular)	350	22	32	15	38.5	39	590
Hardee's roast beef sandwich	377	21	36	17	40.5	57	1,030
French fries							
Arby's french fries	211	2	33	8	34.1	6	30
McDonald's french fries (regular)	220	3	26.1	11.5	47.0	8.6	109
Wendy's french fries (regular)	280	40	35	14	45.0	15	95
Shakes							
Dairy Queen	710	14	120	19	24.0	50	260
McDonald's							
Vanilla	352	9.3	59.6	8.4	21.4	30.6	201
Chocolate	383	9.9	65.5	9	21.1	29.7	300
Strawberry	362	9	62.1	8.7	22.3	32.2	207
Soft drinks							
Coca-Cola	154	—	40	—	—	—	6
Diet Coke	0.9	—	0.3	—	—	—	16
Sprite	142	—	36	—	—	—	45
Tab	1	—	1	—	—	—	30
Diet Sprite	3	—	0	—	—	—	9

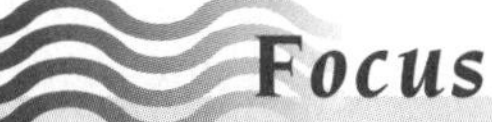

Tips for selecting fast foods

- Limit deep-fried foods such as fish and chicken sandwiches and chicken nuggets, which are often higher in fat than plain burgers are. If you are having fried chicken, remove some of the breading before eating.
- Order roast beef, turkey, or grilled chicken, where available, for a lower fat alternative to most burgers.
- Choose a small order of fries with your meal rather than a large one, and request no salt. Add a small amount of salt yourself if desired. If you are ordering a deep-fat-fried sandwich or one that is made with cheese and sauce, skip the fries altogether and try a plain baked potato (add butter and salt sparingly) or a dinner roll instead of a biscuit; or, try a side salad to accompany your meal instead.
- Choose regular sandwiches instead of "double," "jumbo," "deluxe," or "ultimate" sandwiches. And order plain types rather than those with the works, such as cheese, bacon, mayonnaise, and special sauce. Pickles, mustard, ketchup, and other condiments are high in sodium. Choose lettuce, tomatoes, and onions.
- At the salad bar, load up on fresh greens, fruits, and vegetables. Be careful of salad dressings, added toppings, and creamy salads (potato salad, macaroni salad, coleslaw). These can quickly push calories and fat to the level of other menu items or higher.
- Many fast-food items contain large amounts of sodium from salt and other ingredients. Try to balance the rest of your day's sodium choices after a fast-food meal.
- Alternate water, low-fat milk, or skim milk with a soda or a shake.
- For dessert, or a sweet-on-the-run, choose low-fat frozen yogurt where available.
- Remember to balance your fast-food choices with your food selections for the whole day.

muscle and the liver. This practice is called **glycogen supercompensation**. The basis for the practice is that the quantity of glycogen stored in muscle directly affects the endurance of that muscle.[50]

glycogen supercompensation High-carbohydrate diet.

Glycogen supercompensation is accomplished over a six-day period divided into three phases. In phase 1 (days 1 and 2), training should be hard and dietary intake of carbohydrates restricted. During phase 2 (days 3 through 5), training is cut back and the individual eats plenty of carbohydrates. Studies have indicated that glycogen stores may be increased from 50 percent to 100 percent, theoretically enhancing endurance during a long-term event. Phase 3 (day 6) is the day of the event, during which a normal diet must be consumed.

The effect of glycogen supercompensation in improving performance during endurance activities has not as yet been clearly demonstrated. It has been recommended that glycogen supercompensation not be done more than two to three times during the course of a year. Glycogen supercompensation is only of value in long-duration events that produce glycogen depletion, such as a marathon.[46]

Recommendations for Restoring Muscle Glycogen After Exercise

When the time period between exercise sessions is relatively short (less than 8 hours), the athlete should begin consuming carbohydrates to restore supplies of muscle glycogen as soon as possible after the workout to maximize recovery between sessions.[16] Given that complete muscle glycogen restoration takes at least 20 to 24 hours, athletes should not waste time. They should ingest approximately 0.45 to 0.55 grams of carbohydrate per pound of body weight for each of the first four hours after exercise or until they eat their next large meal. During this period nutrient-rich carbohydrate foods like fruits and vegetables or a high carbohydrate drink are recommended.[36] Over a 24-hour period, carbohydrate intake should range from 2.3 grams to as much as 5.5 grams per pound of body weight, depending on the intensity of the activity.[6] Pasta, potatoes, oatmeal, or a sports drink are recommended.[36]

Fat Loading

Some endurance athletes tried fat loading in place of carbohydrate loading. Their intent was to have a better source of energy at their disposal. The deleterious effects of this procedure outweigh any benefits that may be derived. Associated with fat loading is cardiac protein and potassium depletion, causing arrhythmias and increased levels of serum cholesterol as a result of the ingestion of butter, cheese, cream, and marbled beef.

5-6

Critical Thinking Exercise

A female softball player has a problem controlling her weight. Her body fat percentage has been measured at 25 percent and she asks the athletic trainer what she needs to do to be able to lose some weight quickly and then to maintain her body weight thereafter.

? How should the athletic trainer respond?

WEIGHT CONTROL AND BODY COMPOSITION

Gain or loss of weight in an athlete often poses a problem because the individual's ingrained eating habits are difficult to change.[26] The athletic trainer's inability to adequately supervise the athlete's meal program in terms of balance and quantity further complicates the problem. An intelligent and conscientious approach to weight control requires that the athletic trainer, the coach, and the athlete have some knowledge of what is involved.[60] Such understanding allows athletes to better discipline themselves as to the quantity and kinds of foods they should eat.[28]

Body Composition

Ideal body weight is most often determined by consulting age-related height and weight charts such as those published by life insurance companies. Unfortunately, these charts are inaccurate because they involve broad ranges and often fail to take individual body types into account. Health and performance, rather than body weight, may best be related to body composition.[31]

Body composition refers to both the fat and nonfat components of the body. That portion of total body weight that is composed of fat tissue is referred to as the percentage of body fat. The total body weight that is composed of nonfat or lean tissue, which includes muscles, tendons, bones, and connective tissue, is referred to as lean body weight. Body composition measurements provide an accurate determination of precisely how much weight an athlete may gain or lose.[14]

The average college-age female has between 20 percent and 25 percent of her total body weight made up of fat. The average college-age male has between 12 percent and 15 percent body fat. Male endurance athletes may get their fat percentage as low as 8 percent to 12 percent, and female endurance athletes may reach 10 percent to 18 percent. Body fat percentage should not go below 3 percent in males and 12 percent in females, because below these percentages the internal organs tend to lose their protective padding of essential fat, potentially subjecting them to injury.[11]

Being overweight and being obese are different conditions. Being overweight implies having excess body weight relative to physical size and stature. Being overweight may not be a problem unless a person is also overfat, which means that the percentage of total body weight that is made up of fat is excessive. **Obesity** implies an extreme amount of excessive fat, much greater than what would be considered normal. Females with body fat above 30 percent and males with body fat above 20 percent are considered to be obese.[11]

obesity
Excessive amount of body fat.

Two factors determine the amount of fat in the body: the number of fat, or adipose, cells and the size of the adipose cell. Proliferation, or hyperplagia, of adipose cells begins at birth and continues to puberty. It is thought that after early adulthood the number of fat cells remains fixed, although some evidence suggests that the number of cells is not necessarily fixed.[17] Adipose cell size also increases gradually, or hypertrophies, to early adulthood and can increase or decrease as a function of caloric balance. In adults, weight loss or gain is primarily a function of the change in cell size, not cell number. Obese adults tend to exhibit a great deal of adipose cell hypertrophy.

The **adipose cell** stores triglyceride (a form of liquid fat). This liquid fat moves in and out of the cell according to the energy needs of the body, which are determined to some extent by activity type. The greatest amount of fat is used in activities of moderate intensity and long duration. The greater the amount of triglyceride contained in the adipose cell, the greater the amount of total body weight composed of fat. One pound of body fat is made up of approximately 3,500 calories stored as triglyceride within the adipose cell.

adipose cell Stores triglyceride.

Assessing Body Composition

Among the several methods of assessing **body composition** are measurement of skinfold thickness;[2] hydrostatic, or underwater, weighing; and measurement of electrical impedance.

body composition Percent body fat plus lean body weight.

Skinfold Measurements

The method of measuring the thickness of skinfolds is based on the fact that about 50 percent of the fat in the body is contained in the subcutaneous fat layers and is closely related to total fat. The remainder of the fat in the body is found around organs and vessels and serves a shock-absorptive function. The skinfold technique measures the thickness of the subcutaneous fat layer with a skinfold caliper (Figure 5-4). Its accuracy is relatively low; however, expertise in measurement is easily developed and the time required for this technique is considerably less than for the others. It has been estimated that error in skinfold measurement is plus or minus 3 percent to 5 percent.[17]

Researchers have offered several different techniques for measuring body composition via skinfolds. A technique proposed by Jackson and Pollack,[31] which measures the thigh, triceps, suprailiac, abdomen, and chest skinfolds is widely used.[44]

Hydrostatic weighing Hydrostatic (underwater) weighing involves placing a subject in a specially designed underwater tank to determine body density.[17] Fat tissue is less dense than lean tissue. Therefore the more body fat present, the more the body floats (buoyancy) and the less it weighs in water. Body composition is calculated by comparing the weight of the submerged individual with the weight before entering the tank. If done properly, this technique is very accurate. Unfortunately, the tank and equipment are expensive and generally not available to most coaches and physical educators. In addition, there are other drawbacks with this technique. It is time consuming (especially for large groups), and subjects must exhale completely and hold their breath while underwater. Many students have real problems and fears with this aspect of the technique.

Bioelectrical impedance The second technique involves the measurement of resistance to the flow of electrical current through the body between selected points.[2] This technique is based on the principle that electricity will choose to flow through the tissue that offers the least resistance or impedance. Fat is generally a poor conductor of electrical energy, whereas lean tissue is a fairly good conductor. Thus the higher the percentage of body fat, the greater the resistance to the passage of electrical energy. Very simply, this method predicts the percentage body fat by measuring bioelectrical impedance.[2] It should be mentioned that bioelectrical impedance measures can be affected by levels of hydration. If the body is dehydrated, the measurement will tend to overestimate percentage of body fat relative to measurements taken when there is normal hydration. The equipment available for taking these measurements is, again, fairly expensive and generally includes the use of computer software.

Determining Body Mass Index

A relatively easy way to determine the extent of overweight or obesity is to use a person's body weight and height measurements to calculate body mass index (BMI). BMI is a ratio of body weight to height. This technique represents a method for measuring

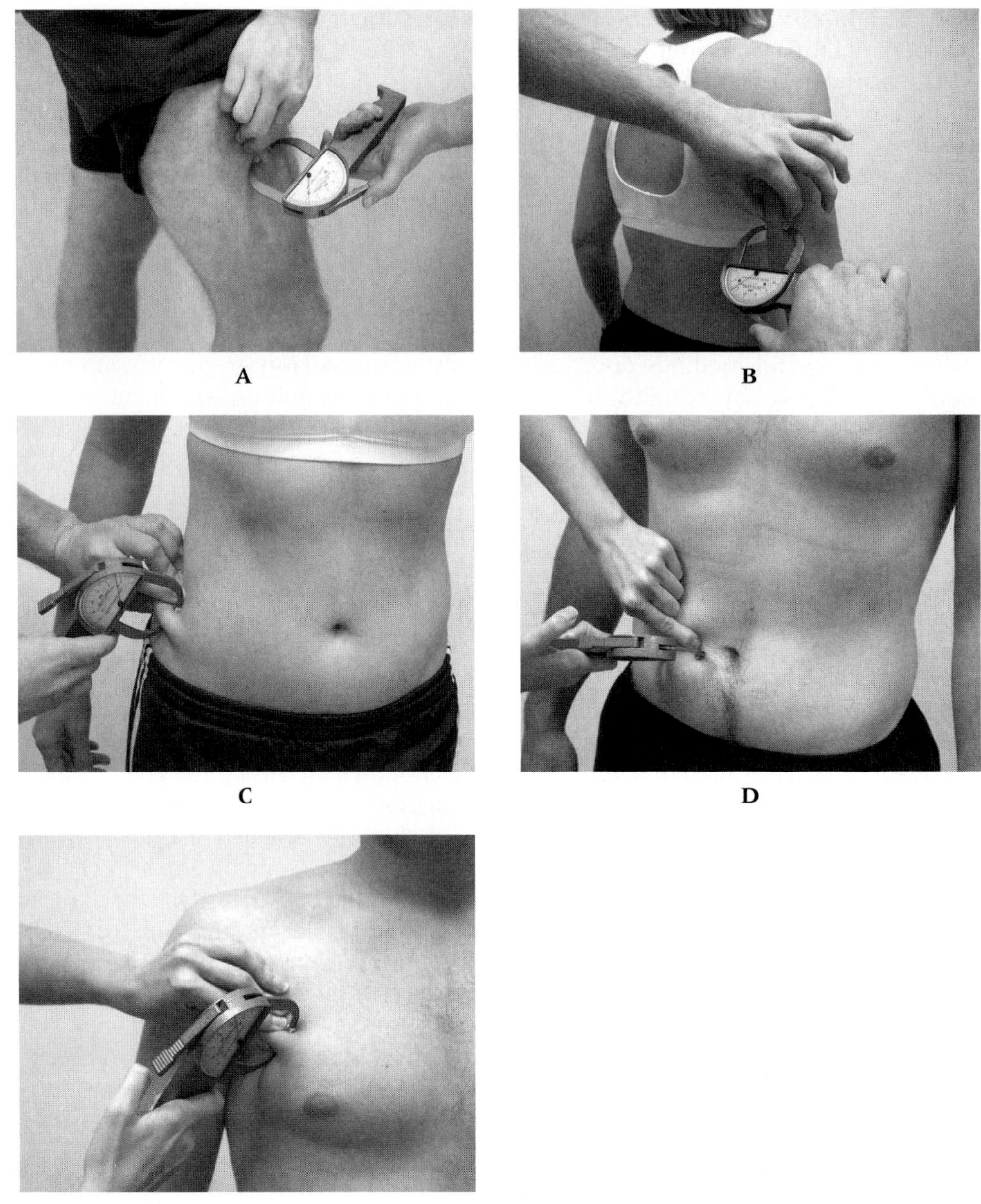

Figure 5-4

Measuring body composition. **A,** Thigh. **B,** Triceps. **C,** Suprailiac. **D,** Abdomen, **E,** Chest.

health risks from obesity using height/weight measurements. Health problems associated with excess body fat tend to be associated with a BMI of more than 25. A BMI of 25 to 30 indicates that a person is overweight. A BMI of 30 or more indicates a state of obesity.[46] *Focus Box:* "Determining body mass index (BMI)" will help you calculate BMI.

Assessing Caloric Balance

Changes in body weight are almost entirely the result of changes in caloric balance.[40]

Caloric balance = Number of calories consumed − Number of calories expended

If more calories are consumed than expended, this positive caloric balance results in weight gain. Conversely, weight loss results from a negative caloric balance in which more calories are expended than are consumed. Caloric balance may be calculated by maintaining accurate records of both the number of calories consumed in the

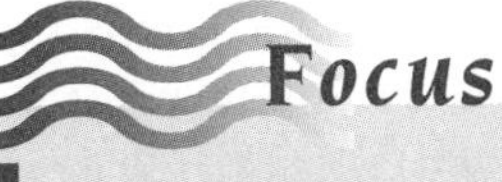

Determining body mass index (BMI) as a means of examining overweight and obesity

1. Weigh yourself to determine body weight in pounds.
2. Divide your weight in pounds by 2.2 to determine kilograms.
3. Measure your height in inches.
4. Multiply your height in inches by 2.54 and divide by 100 to convert your height to meters.
5. Multiply your height in meters by your height in meters to get your height in meters squared.
6. Divide your weight in kilograms by your height in meters squared to determine your BMI.

1. ________ Divided by 2.2 = ________
   Weight (lbs) Weight (kg)
2. ________ Times 2.54 divided by 100 = ________
   Height (in) Height (m)
3. ________ Times ________ = ________
   Height (m) Height (m) Height (m^2)
4. ________ Divided by ________ = ________
   Weight (kg) Height (m^2) Body Mass Index

diet and the number of calories expended for metabolic needs and in activities performed during the course of a day.

Caloric Consumption or Intake

Positive caloric balance leads to weight gain; negative caloric balance leads to weight loss.

Caloric balance is determined by the number of calories consumed regardless of whether the calories are contained in fat, carbohydrate, or protein. There are differences in the caloric content of these foodstuffs:

Carbohydrate = 4 calories per gram
Protein = 4 calories per gram
Fat = 9 calories per gram
Alcohol = 7 calories per gram

Estimations of caloric intake for college athletes range between 2,000 and 5,000 calories per day. Estimations of caloric expenditure range between 2,200 and 4,400 calories on average. Energy demands will be considerably higher in endurance-type athletes, who may require as many as 7,000 calories per day.[43]

Low carbohydrate diets and weight loss For many years it was recommended that fat intake be limited as a means of controlling weight. Recently the recommendation has been to severely limit the intake of carbohydrate in the diet. There are many different versions of a low-carbohydrate diet, all of which recommend a strict reduction in the consumption of carbohydrates. Most low-carb diets replace carbohydrates with a high-fat and moderate protein diet. The low-calorie and low-fat diets that have been recommended for years have failed to realize that dietary fat is not necessarily converted into body fat. However carbohydrates are readily converted into fat. When eating a high-carbohydrate meal, the increased blood glucose stimulates insulin production by the pancreas. Insulin allows blood glucose to be used by the cells, but it also causes fat to be deposited, and it stimulates the brain to produce hunger signals. So there is a tendency to eat more carbohydrates, and the cycle repeats. It has been shown that most overweight people became overweight due to a condition called *hyperinsulinemia*—elevated insulin levels in the blood. Restricting carbohydrate intake halts this cycle by decreasing insulin levels. Carbohydrate restriction also increases the levels of glucagon which is a hormone that causes body fat to be burned and aids in removing cholesterol deposits in the arteries. Severely restricting carbohydrate intake puts the body into a state of ketosis in which blood glucose levels stabilize, insulin level drops, and because the body is burning fat, fairly rapid weight loss occurs.

Caloric Expenditure

Calories may be expended by three different processes: basal metabolism, work (work is defined as any activity that requires more energy than sleeping), and excretion. When estimating caloric expenditure, it is first necessary to determine the amount of calories (energy) needed to support basal metabolism. This is the minimal amount of energy required to sustain the body's vital functions such as respiration, heartbeat, circulation, and maintenance of body temperature during a twenty-four-hour period. The basal metabolic rate (BMR) is the rate at which calories are spent for these maintenance activities. BMR is most accurately determined in a laboratory through a measurement process known as indirect calorimetry, which measures a person's oxygen uptake to predict BMR. Measurement of BMR using this procedure is generally done as soon as the subject awakes, in a quiet, warm environment, and after a twelve-hour fast.

Once BMR has been determined, it is necessary to calculate the energy requirements of all physical activities done in a twenty-four-hour period. This is the second component of energy needs, referred to as work. There is a wide variation in energy output for work. It is determined by the type, intensity, and duration of a physical activity. Body size is also a factor; heavier people expend more energy in an activity than do lighter people. Specific energy expenditures may be determined by consulting charts that predict energy used in an activity based on (1) the time spent in each activity in minutes and (2) the metabolic costs of each activity in kilocalories per minute per pound (kcal/min/lb) of body weight.

Methods of Weight Loss

An individual has several ways to go about losing weight: dieting, increasing the amount of physical exercise, or a combination of diet and exercise.

Weight loss through dieting alone is difficult, and in most cases dieting alone is an ineffective means of weight control. Long-term weight control through dieting alone is successful only 2 percent of the time.[67] About 35 percent to 45 percent of weight decrease due to dieting results from a loss of lean tissue. The minimum caloric intake should not go below 1,000 to 1,200 calories per day for a female and not below 1,200 to 1,400 calories per day for a male.[54]

Weight loss through exercise involves an 80 percent to 90 percent loss of fat tissue with almost no loss of lean tissue. Weight loss through exercise alone is almost as difficult as losing weight through dieting. However, exercise will not only result in weight reduction but may also enhance cardiorespiratory endurance, improve strength, and increase flexibility.[11] For these reasons, exercise has some distinct advantages over dieting in any weight-loss program.

The most efficient method of decreasing the percentage of body weight that is fat is through some combination of diet and exercise. A moderate caloric restriction combined with a moderate increase in caloric expenditure will result in a negative caloric balance. This method is relatively fast and easy compared with either of the other methods because habits are being moderately changed.

In any weight-loss program, the goal should be to lose 1.5 to 2 pounds per week. Weight loss of more than 4 to 5 pounds per week may be attributed to dehydration as opposed to a loss of body fat.[11] A weight-loss program must emphasize the long-haul approach. It generally takes a long time to put on extra weight, and there is no reason to expect that true loss of excess body fat can be accomplished in a relatively short time. The American College of Sports Medicine has made specific recommendations for weight loss.[4]

Methods of Weight Gain

The aim of a weight-gaining program should be to increase lean body mass, that is, muscle as opposed to body fat. Muscle mass should be increased only by muscle work combined with an appropriate increase in dietary intake. Muscle mass cannot be increased by the intake of any special food or vitamin.

The recommended rate of weight gain is approximately one to two pounds per week. Each pound of lean body mass gained represents a positive caloric balance. This positive balance is an intake in excess of an expenditure of approximately 2,500 calories. One pound of fat represents the equivalent of 3,500 calories; lean body tissue contains less fat, more protein, and more water and represents approximately 2,500 calories. To gain one pound of muscle, an excess of approximately 2,500 calories is needed; to lose one pound of fat, approximately 3,500 calories in excess of intake must be expended in activities. Adding 500 to 1,000 calories daily to the usual diet will provide the energy needs of gaining one to two pounds per week and fuel the increased energy expenditure of the weight-training program. Weight training must be part of the weight-gaining program. Otherwise, the excess intake of energy will be converted to fat.[15]

5-7

Critical Thinking Exercise

An ice hockey attackman has an excellent level of fitness and has superb skating ability and stick work. He is convinced that the only thing keeping him from moving to the next level is his low body weight. In recent years he has engaged more in weight-training activities to improve his muscular endurance and, to a lesser extent, to increase his strength.

? What recommendations should the athletic trainer make for him to be successful in his weight-gaining efforts?

Disordered Eating

Disordered eating can be defined as a spectrum of abnormal eating behaviors, ranging from mild food restriction and occasional binging and purging, to severe conditions of bulimia nervosa and anorexia nervosa. Disordered eating is a multifactorial disorder that includes social, familial, physiological, and psychological components. In the athletic population, the incidence of disordered eating behaviors and pathologic eating disorders is significantly higher than in the general population.[72] This relatively high incidence in athletes has been attributed to the athlete's attempt to control body weight or body composition in an effort to improve his or her performance. In addition to the emotional stress and social pressures characteristic of eating disorders, there are also serious physiological effects that can compound one another and ultimately affect the athlete's overall health and performance. Recently a brief (four measurements and a fourteen-item questionnaire) physiologic screening test has been developed to detect eating disorders in collegiate female athletes.[9] Athletic trainers working with young athletes, particularly active females, should be educated about these disorders and work within their resources to develop strategies for prevention and management.[62]

Bulimia Nervosa

The bulimic person is commonly female, ranging in age from adolescence to middle age. It is estimated that 1 out of every 200 American girls, ages twelve to eighteen years (1 percent to 2 percent of the population), will develop patterns of bulimia nervosa, anorexia nervosa, or both.[52] The bulimic individual typically gorges herself with thousands of calories after a period of starvation and then purges herself through induced vomiting and further fasting or through the use of laxatives or diuretics. This secretive binge-eating–purging cycle may go on for years.

Typically the bulimic athlete is white and belongs to a middle-class or upper-middle-class family. She is perfectionistic, obedient, overcompliant, highly motivated, successful academically, well liked by her peers, and a good athlete.[60] She most commonly participates in gymnastics, track, and dance. Male wrestlers and gymnasts may also develop bulimia nervosa. (See *Focus Box:* "Identifying the athlete with an eating disorder.")

Binge-purge patterns of eating can cause stomach rupture, disruption of heart rhythm, and liver damage. Stomach acids brought up by vomiting cause tooth decay and chronically inflame the mucous lining of the mouth and throat.

5-8

Critical Thinking Exercise

A tennis coach observes that one of her players has lost a significant amount of weight. Along with this loss of weight, this athlete's level of play has begun to decrease. The coach becomes seriously concerned when another player tells the coach that she thinks her roommate was purposely throwing up after a team meal on a recent road trip. After briefly questioning the athlete about her eating habits, the coach asks the athletic trainer to become involved in dealing with this situation.

? How should the athletic trainer respond to this request?

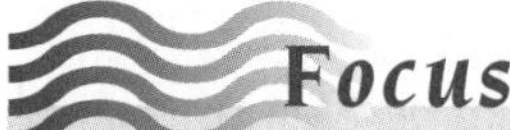

Identifying the athlete with an eating disorder

The athlete with an eating disorder may display the following signs:

- Social isolation and withdrawal from friends and family
- A lack of confidence in athletic abilities
- Ritualistic eating behavior (e.g., organizing food on plate)
- An obsession with counting calories
- An obsession with constantly exercising, especially just before a meal
- An obsession with weighing self
- A constant overestimation of body size
- Patterns of leaving the table directly after eating to go into the restroom
- Problems related to eating disorders (e.g., malnutrition, menstrual irregularities, or chronic fatigue)
- Family history of eating disorders

Anorexia Nervosa

It has been estimated that 30 percent to 50 percent of all individuals diagnosed as having anorexia nervosa also develop some symptoms of bulimia nervosa. Anorexia nervosa is characterized by a distorted body image and a major concern about weight gain. As with bulimia nervosa, anorexia nervosa affects mostly females. It usually begins in adolescence and can be mild without major consequences or can become life threatening. As many as 15 percent to 21 percent of individuals diagnosed as anorexic ultimately die from this disorder. Despite being extremely thin, the athlete sees herself as too fat. These individuals deny hunger and are hyperactive, engaging in abnormal amounts of exercise such as aerobics or distance running.[59] In general, the anorexic individual is highly secretive, and the coach and athletic trainer must be sensitive to eating problems. Early intervention is essential. Any athlete with signs of bulimia nervosa or anorexia nervosa must be confronted in a kind, empathetic manner by the coach or athletic trainer. When detected, individuals with eating disorders must be referred for psychological or psychiatric treatment. Unfortunately, simply referring an anorexic person to a health education clinic is not usually effective. The key to the treatment of anorexia nervosa seems to be getting the patient to realize that a problem exists and that he or she could benefit from professional help. The individual must voluntarily accept such help if treatment is to be successful.[46]

Anorexia Athletica

Anorexia athletica is a condition specific to athletes that is characterized by several of the features common to anorexia nervosa, but without the self-starvation practices. Athletes with anorexia athletica may exhibit a variety of signs including disturbance of body image, a weight loss greater than 5 percent of body weight, gastrointestinal complaints, primary amenorrhea, menstrual dysfunction, absence of medical illness explaining the weight reduction, excessive fear of becoming obese, binging or purging, compulsive eating, and/or restriction of caloric intake.

Female Athlete Triad Syndrome

Female athlete triad syndrome is a potentially fatal problem that involves a combination of an eating disorder (either bulimia or anorexia), amenorrhea, and osteoporosis (diminished bone density). The incidence of this syndrome is uncertain; however, some studies have suggested that eating disorders in female athletes may be as high as 62 percent in certain sports, with amenorrhea being common in at least 60 percent of female athletes. However, the major risk of this syndrome is that the bone lost in osteoporosis may not be regained.[44]

SUMMARY

- The classes of nutrients are carbohydrates, fats, proteins, vitamins, minerals, and water. Carbohydrates, fats, and proteins provide the energy required for muscular work during activity and also play a role in the function and maintenance of body tissues. Vitamins are substances found in food that have no caloric value but are necessary to regulate body processes. Vitamins may be either fat soluble (vitamins A, D, E, and K) or water soluble (B-complex vitamins and vitamin C). Minerals are necessary in most physiological functions of the body. Water is the most essential of all the nutrients and should be of great concern to anyone involved in physical activity.
- A nutritious diet consists of eating a variety of foods in amounts recommended in the food pyramid. A diet that meets those recommended amounts does not need nutrient supplementation.
- Protein supplementation during weight training is not necessary if a nutritious diet is maintained. Many males and especially females may require calcium supplementation to prevent osteoporosis. It may be necessary to supplement the diet with extra iron to prevent iron-deficiency anemia.
- Organic or natural foods have no beneficial effect on performance. Vegetarian diets can provide all the essential nutrients if care is taken and the diet is well thought out and properly prepared.
- The preevent meal should be higher in carbohydrates, easily digested, eaten three to four hours before an event, and psychologically pleasing.
- Glycogen supercompensation involves maximizing resting stores of glucose in the muscles, blood, and liver before a competitive event.
- Body composition indicates the percentage of total body weight composed of fat tissue versus the percentage composed of lean tissue. The size and number of adipose cells determine percentage of body fat. Percentage of body fat can be assessed by measuring the thickness of the subcutaneous fat at specific areas of the body with a skinfold caliper.
- Changes in body weight are caused almost entirely by a change in caloric balance, which is a function of the number of calories taken in and the number of calories expended. Weight can be lost either by increasing caloric expenditure through exercise or by decreasing caloric intake through dieting. Diets generally do not work. The recommended technique for losing weight involves a combination of moderate calorie restriction and a moderate increase in physical exercise during the course of each day. Weight gain should be accomplished by increasing caloric intake and engaging in a weight-training program. It is possible to gain weight and lose fat, thus changing body composition. Equal volumes of muscle weigh more than fat.
- Anorexia is a disease in which a person suffers a pathological weight loss because of a psychological aversion to food and eating. Bulimia is an eating disorder that involves binging and subsequent purging.

Websites

Gatorade Sports Science Institute: http://www.gssiweb.com/

This website provides information for coaches, athletic trainers, physicians, nutritionists, and others in the field of sports medicine, sports nutrition, and exercise science.

Healthy Biz 2000: http://www.healthybiz2000.com/

This site provides information about sports nutrition and nutritional supplements for fitness and weight loss.

Food and Nutrition Information Center: http://www.nalusda.gov/fnic

This site is part of the information centers at the National Agricultural Library and offers access to information on healthy eating habits, food composition, and many additional resources.

Yahoo Health and Nutrition Information: http://www.yahoo.com/Health/Nutrition

This site includes diet analysis information, nutritional facts, and links to many other informative sites.

Eating Disorders: http://www.eating_disorder.com/

Eating disorder information can be found here, including information about anorexia, bulimia, and overeating as well as information about how to access support groups.

Athletes and Eating Disorders: http://www.uq.net.au/eda/documents/start/html

This site is part of the Eating Disorders Resources website; it gives some statistics from a recent NCAA study and has a section on the coaches' responsibility. The site also includes information about warning signs and the female athlete triad.

The American Dietetic Association: http://www.eatright.org

This site includes access to the journal published by the American Dietetic Association and provides informative nutritional tips as well as gateways to nutrition and related sites.

Solutions to Critical Thinking EXERCISES

5-1 The important consideration for weight control is the total number of calories that are consumed relative to the total number of calories expended. It makes no difference whether the calories consumed are CHO, fat, or protein. Fat contains more than twice the number of calories that either CHO or protein contains, so an athlete can eat significantly more food and still have about the same caloric intake if the diet is high in CHO. This athlete should be told that it is also essential to consume at least some fat, which is necessary for the production of several enzymes and hormones.

5-2 For an athlete who is truly consuming anything close to a well-balanced diet, vitamin supplementation is generally not necessary. However, if taking a one-a-day type of vitamin supplement makes the athlete feel better, there is no harm. Her tiredness could be related to a number of medical conditions (e.g., mononucleosis). An iron-deficiency anemia may be detected through a laboratory blood test. The athletic trainer should refer the athlete to a physician for blood work.

5-3 This athlete should be referred to the team physician and nutritionist. From her history, the athletic trainer can assume she is not consuming enough iron by not eating meats or other nutritious foods. Iron is essential for hemoglobin formation and energy formation. In addition, since she is not eating vegetables, she is not receiving an adequate amount of Vitamin K. Vitamin K is important in blood coagulation. By not eating a well balanced diet, she lacks Vitamin K, which is found in green leafy vegetables.

5-4 A small amount of protein (slightly above to about double the protein RDA) is needed for developing muscles in a training program. However, an athlete can easily meet these necessary higher amounts by eating a variety of foods, especially protein-rich foods. Thus, athletes do not need protein supplements, because their diets typically exceed protein recommendations.

5-5 The amount of glycogen that can be stored in the muscle and liver can be increased by reducing the training program a few days before competing and by significantly increasing carbohydrate intake during the week before the event. Nutrients consumed over several days before competition are much more important than what is eaten three hours before an event. The purpose of the preevent meal should be to provide the competitor with sufficient nutrient energy and fluids for competition while taking into consideration the digestibility of the food. Glucose-rich drinks taken at regular intervals are beneficial for highly intense and prolonged events that severely deplete glycogen stores.

5-6 The athletic trainer should recommend that this athlete set a goal of 18 to 20 percent body fat. If the softball player needs to lose weight, she must consume fewer calories than she is burning off, and this is not something that can be achieved in a short period of time. It also must be explained that weight control is simply a matter of achieving caloric balance and making lifestyle changes in terms of eating and exercise habits to achieve caloric balance.

5-7 This athlete must understand the importance of adding lean tissue muscle mass rather than increasing his percentage of body fat. His caloric intake must be increased so that he is in a positive caloric balance of about 500 calories per day. Additional calorie intake should consist primarily of CHO. Additional supplementation with protein is not necessary. It is absolutely essential that this athlete incorporate a weight-training program using heavy weights that will overload the muscle, forcing it to hypertrophy over a period of time.

5-8 Treating eating disorders is difficult even for health care professionals specifically trained to counsel these individuals. The athletic trainer should approach the athlete, not with accusation, but with support, showing concern about her weight loss and expressing a desire to help her secure appropriate counseling. Remember that the athlete must first be willing to admit that she has an eating disorder before treatment and counseling will be effective. Eliciting the support of close friends and family can help with treatment.

REVIEW QUESTIONS AND CLASS ACTIVITIES

1. What is the value of good nutrition in terms of an athlete's performance and injury prevention?
2. Ask coaches of different sports about the type of diet they recommend for their athletes and their rationale behind the diet.
3. Have a nutritionist talk to the class about food myths and fallacies.
4. Have each member of the class prepare a week's food diary; then compare it with other class members' diaries.
5. What are the daily dietary requirements according to the food pyramid? Should the requirements of the typical athlete's diet differ from those requirements? If so, in what ways?
6. Have the class debate the value of vitamin and mineral supplements.
7. Describe the advantages and disadvantages of supplementing iron and calcium.
8. Is there some advantage to preevent nutrition?
9. Are there advantages or disadvantages in a vegetarian diet for the athlete?
10. What is the current thinking on the value of creatine as a nutritional supplement?
11. What is the primary concern of using herbs?
12. Discuss the importance of athletes monitoring their body composition.
13. Explain the most effective technique for losing weight.
14. Contrast the signs and symptoms of bulimia nervosa and anorexia nervosa. If an athletic trainer is aware of an athlete who may have an eating disorder, what should he or she do?

REFERENCES

1. Allred J: Too much of a good thing? An overemphasis on eating low-fat foods may be contributing to the alarming increase in overweight among U.S. adults, *J Am Diet Assoc* 95:417, 1995.

2. Amato H, Wenos D: Bioelectrical impedance of hydration effects on muscular strength and endurance in college wrestlers, *J Ath Train* 28(2):170, 1993.
3. American College of Sports Medicine: Position stand on exercise and fluid replacement, *Med Sci Sports Exerc* 28:1, 1996.
4. American College of Sports Medicine: Proper and improper weight loss programs, *Med Sci Sports Exerc* 15:ix, 1983.
5. American College of Sports Medicine: The physiological and health effects of oral creatine supplementation, *Med Sci Sports Exerc* 32(3):706, 2000.
6. American Dietetic Association and Canadian Dietetic Association: Position of the American Dietetic Association and Canadian Dietetic Association: nutrition for physical fitness and athletic performance of adults, *J Am Diet Assoc* 93:691, 1993.
7. Anderson J, Stender M, Rodando P: Nutrition and bone in physical activity and sport. In Wolinsky I, Hickson J: *Nutrition in exercise and sport,* Boca Raton, 1998, CRC Press.
8. Antonio J: *Sports supplements,* Philadelphia, 2001, Lippincott, Williams and Wilkins.
9. Black D, Larkin L, Coster D: Physiologic screening test for eating disorders/disordered eating among female collegiate athletes, *J Ath Train* 38(4):286, 2003.
10. Blackburn H: Olestra and the FDA, *N Engl J Med* 334(15):984, 1996.
11. Brownell K, Fairbum C: *Eating disorders and obesity: a comprehensive handbook,* New York, 2002, Guilford Press.
12. Casa D, Armstrong L, Hillman S: National Athletic Trainers Association position statement: fluid replacement for athletes, *J Ath Train* 35(2):212, 2000.
13. Clarkson P et al: Methods and strategies for weight loss in athletics, roundtable, *Sports Science Exchange* 9(1):1998.
14. Clarkson PM: Nutritional supplements for weight gain, *Sports Science Exchange* 11(1):1, 1998.
15. Coleman E: Nutritional concerns of vegetarian athletes, *Sports Med Digest* 17(2):1, 1995.
16. Coyle E: Highs and lows of carbohydrate diets, *Sports Science Exchange* 17(2):1, 2004.
17. DeLorenzo A et al: Comparison of different techniques to measure body composition in moderately active adolescents, *British Journal of Sports Medicine* 32(3):215, 1998.
18. Dodd S, Herb R, Powers S: Caffeine and exercise performance: an update, *Sports Med* 15:14, 1993.
19. Food and Drug Administration: Food labeling: reference daily intakes, *Federal Register* 59(2):427, 1994.
20. Food and Nutrition Board, National Academy of Sciences—National Research Council: Recommended dietary allowances, ed 12, Washington, DC, 1998, U.S. Government Printing Office.
21. Foster S: *101 medicinal herbs.* Loveland, Colo, 1998, Interweave Press.
22. Friedman-Kester K: Do food triggers give you a headache? *Athletic Therapy Today* 6(6):42, 2001.
23. Friedman-Kester K: Herbal remedies are drugs, too! *Athletic Therapy Today* 7(4):40, 2002.
24. Friedman-Kester K: RDAs, RDIs—R U confused? *Athletic Therapy Today* 6(3):56, 2001.
25. Friedman-Kester K: The function of functional foods. *Athletic Therapy Today* 7(3):46, 2002.
26. Gorinski R: In pursuit of the perfect body composition: do dietary strategies make a difference? *Athletic Therapy Today* 6(6):54, 2001.
27. Greenwood M, Kreider R, Greenwood L: Cramping and injury incidence in collegiate football players are reduced by creatine supplementation, *J Ath Train* 38(3), 2003.
28. Gutgesell M, Moreau K, Thompson D: Weight concerns, problem eating behaviors, and problem drinking behaviors in female college athletes, *J Ath Train* 38(1):62, 2003.
29. Hale CW: The precompetition meal. *Athletic Therapy Today* 6(3):21, 2001.
30. Hoffman R, Garewal H: Antioxidants and the prevention of coronary heart disease, *Arch Int Med* 155:241, 1995.
31. Jackson AS, Pollack M: Generalized equations for predicting body density of women, *Med Sci Sports Exer* 12:175, 1980.
32. Jackson C: *Nutrition for recreational athletes,* Boca Raton, 1995, CRC Press.
33. Johnson, KD: Ephedra and ma huang consumption: do the benefits outweigh the risks? *Strength Cond* 23(5):32, 2001.
34. Kirshner E, Lewis R, O'Connor P: Bone mineral density and dietary intake of college gymnasts, *Med Sci Sports Exerc* 24(4):543, 1995.
35. Kleiner S: Fluids for performance, *Athletic Therapy Today* 5(1):51, 2000.
36. Kleiner SM: Postexercise-recovery nutrition. *Athletic Therapy Today* 6(2):40, 2001.
37. Kleiner SM: Protein power. *Athletic Therapy Today* 7(1):24, 2002.
38. Kleiner SM: *Power eating,* Champaign, Ill, 2001, Human Kinetics.
39. Kleiner SM: The scoop on protein supplements. *Athletic Therapy Today* 6(1):52, 2001.
40. Kleiner SM: Top-ten rules for healthy weight control. *Athletic Therapy* 7(2):38,
41. Krieder R, Ferreira M, Wilson M: Effects of creatine supplementation on body composition, strength, and sprint performance, *Med Sci Sports Exerc* 30(1):73, 1998.
42. Larson-Duyff R: *The American Dietetic Association's complete food and nutrition guide,* New York, 1998, Wiley.
43. Massad S, Headley S: Nutrition assessment: considerations for athletes, *Athletic Therapy Today* 4(6):6, 1999.
44. Merrick MA: Osteoporosis and the female athlete. *Athletic Therapy Today* 6(3):42, 2001.
45. Papas A, Quillen J: *Antioxidant status: diet, nutrition, and health,* Boca Raton, 1998, CRC Press.
46. Payne W, Hahn D: *Focus on health,* ed 8, St. Louis, 2004, McGraw-Hill.
47. Peterson D: Athletes and iron deficiency: is it true anemia or "sport anemia"? *Physician Sports Med* 26(2):24, 1998.
48. Powers M, Arnold B, Weltman A: Creatine supplementation increases total body water without altering fluid distribution, *J Ath Train* 38(1):44, 2003.
49. Powers M: Ephedra and its application to sport performance: another concern for the athletic trainer?, *J Ath Train* 36(4):420, 2001.
50. Rauch L, Rodger I, Wilson J: The effects of carbohydrate loading on muscle glycogen content and cycling performance, *Int J Sports Med* 5(l):25, 1995.
51. Reimers K: The role of liquid supplements in weight gain, *Strength Cond* 17(l):64, 1995.
52. Rhea DJ, Jambor EA, Wiginton K: Preventing eating disorders in female athletes. *JOHPER* 67(4):66, 1996.
53. Rodriguez N: The role of nutrition in injury prevention and healing, *Athletic Therapy Today* 4(6):27, 1999.
54. Sanborn CF, Horea M, Siemers BJ, Dieringer KI: Disordered eating and the female athlete triad. *Clin Sports Med* 19(2):199, 2000.
55. Schlabach G: Carbohydrate strategies for injury prevention, *J Ath Train* 29(3):244, 1994.
56. Shi X, Gisolfi CV: Fluid and carbohydrate replacement during intermittent exercise, *Sports Med* 25(3):157, 1998.
57. Skolnik H: Sport nutrition in a fast-food society: eating on the road, *Athletic Therapy Today* 4(6):22, 1999.
58. Steen S: Sports nutrition for children, *Athletic Therapy Today* 4(6):48, 1999.
59. Sundgot-Borgen J: Eating disorders in athletes. In Sundgot-Borgen J, editor: *Nutrition in sport,* Oxford, 2000, Blackwell.
60. Turk JC, Prentice WE: Collegiate coaches' knowledge of eating disorders, *J Ath Train* 34(1):19, 1999.
61. U.S. Department of Agriculture and U.S. Department of Health and Human Services: *Nutrition and your health: dietary guidelines for Americans,* ed 5, Washington, DC, 2000.

62. Vaughn J, King K, Cottrell R: Collegiate athletic trainers confidence in helping female athletes with eating disorders, *J Ath Train* 39(1): 71, 2004.
63. Vinci D: Negotiating the maze of nutritional ergogenic aids. *Athletic Therapy Today* 8(2):28, 2003.
64. Vinci DM: What's for lunch? *Athletic Therapy Today* 8(1):50, 2003.
65. Vinci, DM: The training room: developing a sports-nutrition game plan. *Athletic Therapy Today* 7(5):52, 2002.
66. Volek J, et al: Creatine supplementation enhances muscular performance during high-intensity resistance exercise, *J Am Diet Assoc* 97:765, 1997.
67. Wardlaw GM, Insel PM: *Perspectives in nutrition,* ed 6, St Louis, 2003, Mosby.
68. Wilder N, Deivert R, Hagerman F: The effects of low-dose creatine supplementation versus creatine loading in collegiate football players, *J Ath Train* 36(2):124, 2001.
69. Williams M: *Nutrition for fitness and sports,* Boston, 2004, McGraw-Hill.
70. Williams M: The use of nutritional ergogenic aids in sports: is it an ethical issue? *Int J Sport Nutr* 4:120, 1994.
71. Winterstein A, Storrs C: Herbal Supplements: Considerations for the athletic trainer, *J Ath Train* 36(4):425, 2001.
72. Zawila L, Steib C, Hoogenboom B: The female, collegiate, cross-country runner: nutritional knowledge and attitudes, *J Ath Train* 38(1):67, 2003.

ANNOTATED BIBLIOGRAPHY

American Dietetic Association, Dyrugff R: *Complete food and nutrition guide,* Minnetonka, Minn, 2002, Chronimed Publishing.

This extensive text is packed with information concerning every aspect of eating and food safety. This book is highly recommended for individuals who aspire to the highest understanding of healthful eating.

Clark N: *Sport nutrition guidebook: eating to fuel your active lifestyle,* Champaign, Ill, 2003, Human Kinetics.

Provides real-life case studies of nutritional advice given to athletes; the book also provides recommendations for pregame meals.

Sheldan M: *Wellness encyclopedia for food and nutrition.* New York, 2000, Rebus.

The encyclopedia covers every type of whole, fresh food found in supermarkets, specialty shops, and health-food stores. It also presents the latest information on what makes up a healthy diet and on the connection between diet and disease protection.

Wardlaw GM, Insel PM: *Perspectives in nutrition,* ed 6, St Louis, 2003, McGraw-Hill.

This comprehensive text deals with all aspects of nutrition.

Weil A: *Eating well for optimum health: the essential guide to food, diet, and nutrition,* New York, 2000, Knopf.

This text offers a thorough rundown of nutritional basics and a primer on micronutrients such as vitamins, minerals, and fiber.

Williams M: *Nutrition for fitness and sport,* Boston, 2004, McGraw-Hill.

This textbook provides thorough coverage of the role nutrition plays in enhancing health, fitness, and sport performance. Current research and practical activities are incorporated throughout.

Hendler S, Rorvik, D: *PDR for nutritional supplements,* Montvale, NJ, 2001, Medical Economics Company.

From the Publishers of the Physicians' Desk Reference, this new resource gathers solid clinical evidence about the use of dietary supplements from the available medical literature and presents it in a unique and authoritative manner.

Environmental Considerations

Chapter 6

When you finish this chapter you should be able to

- Describe the physiology of hyperthermia.
- Recognize the clinical signs of heat stress and how they can be prevented.
- Identify the causes of hypothermia and the major cold disorders and how they can be prevented.
- Examine the problems that high altitude might present to the athlete and explain how they can be managed.
- Review how an athlete should be protected from exposure to the sun.
- Describe precautions that should be taken in a lightning storm.
- List the problems that air pollution presents to the athlete and how they can be avoided.
- Discuss what effect circadian dysrhythmia can have on athletes and the best procedures for handling this problem.
- Compare the effect of synthetic versus natural turf on the incidence of injury.

Environmental stress can adversely affect an athlete's performance and in some instances can pose a serious health threat. The environmental categories that are of major concern to athletic trainers, particularly those involved in outdoor sports, include hyperthermia, hypothermia, altitude, exposure to the sun, lightning storms, air pollution, and circadian dysrhythmia (jet lag).

HYPERTHERMIA

A major concern in sports is the problem of **hyperthermia**. Over the years, hyperthermia has caused a number of athlete deaths in high school, college, and at the professional level.[66]

hyperthermia Elevated body temperature.

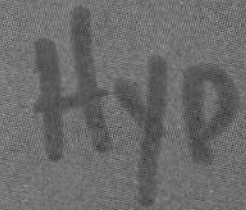

It is vitally important that the athletic trainer and the coaching staff have knowledge about temperature and humidity factors to assist them in planning practice. The athletic trainer must clearly understand when environmental heat and humidity are at a dangerous level and must make recommendations to the coaches accordingly. In addition, the athletic trainer must recognize and properly manage the clinical symptoms and signs of heat stress.

Heat Stress

Regardless of the level of physical conditioning, athletes must take extreme caution when exercising in hot, humid weather. Prolonged exposure to extreme heat can result in heat illness.[52] Heat stress is preventable, but each year many athletes suffer illness and even death from some heat-related cause.[9] Athletes who exercise in hot, humid environments are particularly vulnerable to heat stress.[16]

Heat can be gained or lost through:
- Metabolic heat production
- Conductive heat exchange
- Convective heat exchange
- Radiant heat exchange
- Evaporative heat loss

The physiological processes in the body will continue to function only as long as body temperature is maintained within a normal range.[44] The maintenance of normal temperature in a hot environment depends on the body's ability to dissipate heat. Body temperature can be affected by five factors, described in the following sections.

Metabolic Heat Production

Normal metabolic function in the body results in the production and radiation of heat. Consequently, metabolism will always cause an increase in body heat that depends on the intensity of the physical activity. The higher the metabolic rate, the more heat produced.

Conductive Heat Exchange

Physical contact with other objects can result in either a heat loss or a heat gain. A football player competing on artificial turf on a sunny August afternoon will experience an increase in body temperature simply by standing on synthetic turf.

Convective Heat Exchange

Body heat can be either lost or gained, depending on the temperature of the circulating medium. A cool breeze will always tend to cool the body by removing heat from the body surface. Conversely, if the temperature of the circulating air is higher than the temperature of the skin, body heat increases.

Radiant Heat Exchange

Radiant heat from sunshine causes an increase in body temperature. Obviously, the effects of this radiation are much greater in the sunshine than in the shade.[24] On a cloudy day, the body also emits radiant heat energy; thus, radiation may result in either heat loss or heat gain. During exercise the body attempts to dissipate heat produced by metabolism by dilating superficial arterial and venous vessels, thus channeling blood to the superficial capillaries in the skin.

Evaporative Heat Loss

Sweat glands in the skin allow water to be transported to the surface, where it evaporates, taking large quantities of heat with it. When the temperature and radiant heat of the environment become higher than body temperature, the loss of body heat becomes highly dependent on the process of sweat evaporation.

The rate of sweating is critical for an athlete to dissipate heat. A normal person can sweat off about one quart of water per hour for about two hours. However, certain individuals can lose as much as 2 quarts of water (4 pounds) per hour.[55] *Focus Box:* "Variations in Sweat Rates" identifies factors that influence sweat rates. Sweating does not cause heat loss. The sweat must evaporate for heat to be dissipated. But the air must be relatively free of water for evaporation to occur. Heat loss through evaporation is severely impaired when the relative humidity reaches 65 percent and virtually stops when the humidity reaches 75 percent.

Focus

Variations in sweat rates

Sweat rates can vary considerably from one athlete to another and are determined by a number of factors:

- Athlete's height and weight (heavier athletes sweat more)
- Degree of acclimatization (well acclimated athletes sweat earlier and more)
- Fitness level (fit athletes sweat more)
- Hydration status
- Environmental conditions
- Clothing
- Intensity and duration of activity
- Heredity

It should be obvious that heat-related problems have the greatest chance of occurring on days when the sun is bright and the temperature and relative humidity are high. However, cramps, heat exhaustion, and heatstroke can occur whenever the body's ability to dissipate heat is impaired.

Monitoring the Heat Index

The athletic trainer must exercise common sense when overseeing the health care of athletes who are training or competing in the heat. Obviously, when the combination of heat, humidity, and bright sunshine is present, extra caution is warranted. The universal wet bulb globe temperature (WBGT) index provides the athletic trainer with an objective means for determining necessary precautions for practice and competition in hot weather.[51] The index incorporates readings from several different thermometers. The dry bulb temperature (DBT) is recorded from a standard mercury thermometer. The wet bulb temperature (WBT) uses a wet wick or piece of gauze wrapped around the end of a thermometer that is swung around in the air. Globe temperature (GT) measures the sun's radiation and has a black metal casing around the end of the thermometer. Once the three readings have been taken, the following formula is used to calculate the WBGT index:

$$\text{WBGT} = 0.1 \times \text{DBT} + 0.7 \times \text{WBT} + \text{GT} \times 0.2$$

If only a web bulb and dry bulb temperature is taken the WBGT index is calculated using the following modified formula:

$$\text{WBGT} = 0.3 \times \text{DBT} + 0.7 \times \text{WBT}$$

Using this formula yields a universally accepted WBGT index (Table 6-1) on which recommendations relative to outdoor activity are based. Table 6-2 is a modification of the WBGT index that indicates activity restrictions for outdoor physical conditioning in hot weather.

The DBT and WBT can be measured easily using a *psychrometer.* It consists of two identical thermometers—the wet bulb thermometer, so called because its bulb is covered with a jacket of tight-fitting muslin cloth that can be saturated with distilled water, and the dry bulb thermometer. When the cloth is soaked and the thermometers are properly ventilated, the wet bulb temperature will be lower than the dry bulb temperature (actual air temperature) because of cooling due to the evaporation of water from the cloth. The drier the air is, the greater the evaporation, and thus the more wet bulb temperature is depressed. In some units such as the Physio-Dyne, ventilation is provided by a suction fan (aspiration psychrometer) (Figure 6-1A) or by whirling the thermometers at the end of a chain (sling psychrometer) (Figure 6-1B). Newer psychrometers use special digital sensors (Figure 6-1C). Recording the temperature requires about ninety seconds. Either instrument is relatively inexpensive and easy to use, although it appears that the old sling psychrometer may have the greatest accuracy.[17]

TABLE 6-1 Universal WBGT Index

		Easy Work		Moderate Work		Hard Work	
Heat Category	**WBGT °F**	**Work/Rest***	**Water per Hour**	**Work/Rest***	**Water per Hour**	**Work/Rest***	**Water per Hour**
1	78–81.9	No limit	1/2 qt	No limit	3/4 qt	40/20 min	3/4 qt
2	82–84.9	No limit	1/2 qt	50/10 min	3/4 qt	30/30 min	1 qt
3	85–87.9	No limit	3/4 qt	40/20 min	3/4 qt	30/30 min	1 qt
4	88–89.9	No limit	3/4 qt	30/30 min	3/4 qt	20/40 min	1 qt
5	>90	50/10 min	1 qt	20/40 min	1 qt	10/50 min	1 qt

*Rest means minimal physical activity (sitting or standing) and should be accomplished in the shade if possible.

TABLE 6-2 Activity Restrictions for Outdoor Physical Conditioning in Hot Weather

WBGT[a] (°F)	Flag Color[c]	**Guidance[b] for nonacclimatized personnel in boldface** *Guidance for fully acclimatized personnel in italics*
<78.0°F	**No flag**	**Extreme exertion may precipitate heat illness.** *Normal activity*
78.0°F–82.0°F	Green	**Use discretion in planning intense exercise.** *Normal activity* Pay special attention to at-risk individuals in both cases.
82.1°F–86.0°F	Yellow	**Limit intense exercise to 1 hour; limit total outdoor exercise to 2.5 hours.** *Use discretion in planning intense physical activity.* Pay special attention to at-risk individuals in both cases. Be on high alert; watch for early signs and symptoms in both cases.
86.1°F–89.9°F	Red	**Stop outdoor practice sessions and outdoor physical conditioning.** *Limit intense exercise to 1 hour; limit total outdoor exercise to 4 hours.* Be on high alert; watch for early signs and symptoms throughout.
≥90°F	**Black**	**Cancel all outdoor exercise requiring physical exertion.** *Cancel all outdoor exercise involving physical exertion.*

[a]WGBT is wet bulb globe temperature.
Calculation of WBGT: $0.7\ T_{wb} + 0.2\ T_{bg} + 0.1\ T_{db}$, where T_{wb} is wet bulb temperature; T_{bg} is black globe temperature; T_{db} is dry bulb temperature
[b]Guidelines assume that athletes are wearing summer-weight clothing and that all activities are constantly supervised by an athletic trainer to assure early detection of problems. When equipment must be worn, as in football, please use guidelines one step below. For example, if WBGT is 86°F (yellow) then use the guidelines for red.
[c]Flag color indicates a warning flag, which is placed in a location visible from a practice field, that is used to notify everyone using that facility what the conditions are and the restrictions that should be applied.
Modified from Nunnelly SA, Reardon MJ: Prevention of heat illness. In *Medical aspects of harsh environments: Volume I.*. Pandolf KB, Burr RE, editors: Washington, DC, 2002, TMM Publications.

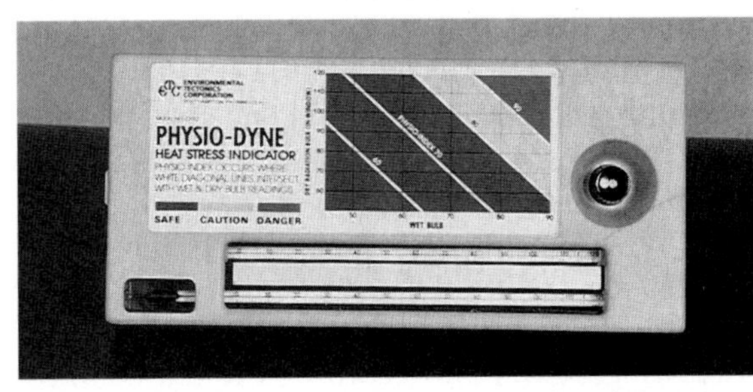

A

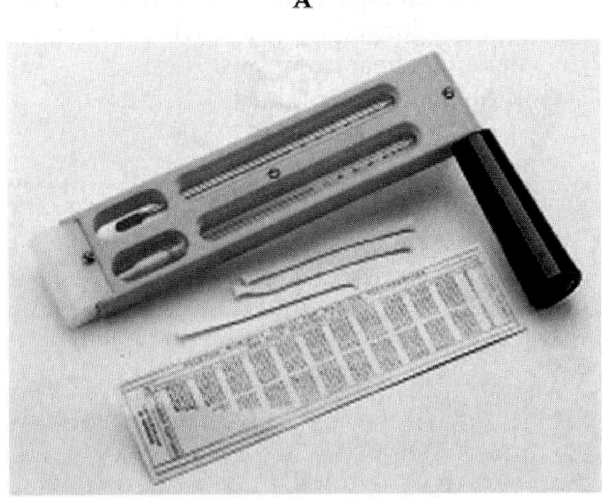

B

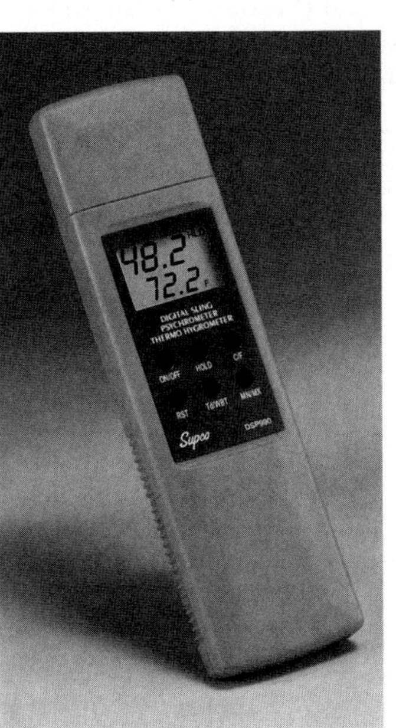

C

Figure 6-1

A, A Physio-Dyne, **B,** a sling psychrometer, or **C,** a digital psychrometer may be used to determine the WBGT heat index.

Exertional Heat Illnesses

In 2003, a consensus statement on exertional heat illnesses was prepared by an interassociation task force that included input from experts representing eighteen professional sports medicine organizations.[39] Exercising in a hot, humid environment can cause various forms of heat illness, including heat rash, heat syncope, heat cramps, heat exhaustion, exertional heatstroke, and exertional hyponatremia.[43] A position statement from NATA on exertional heat illness can be found in Appendix C.

Heat Rash

Heat rash, also called prickly heat, is a benign condition associated with a red, raised rash accompanied by sensations of prickling and tingling during sweating. It usually occurs when the skin is continuously wet with unevaporated sweat. The rash is generally localized to areas of the body that are covered with clothing. Continually toweling the body can help prevent the rash from developing.[61]

Heat Syncope

Heat syncope, or heat collapse, is associated with rapid physical fatigue during overexposure to heat. It is usually caused by standing in heat for long periods or by not being accustomed to exercising in the heat. It is caused by peripheral vasodilation of superficial vessels, hypotension, or a pooling of blood in the extremities, which results in dizziness, fainting, and nausea. Heat syncope is quickly relieved by laying the athlete down in a cool environment and replacing fluids.[61]

Heat Cramps

Heat cramps occur because of some imbalance between water and electrolytes.

Heat cramps are extremely painful muscle spasms that occur most commonly in the calf and abdomen, although any muscle can be involved (Table 6-3). The occurrence of heat cramps is related to excessive loss of water and several electrolytes or ions (sodium, chloride, potassium, magnesium, and calcium), but especially sodium, that are each essential elements in muscle contraction.

Profuse sweating involves losses of large amounts of water and small quantities of sodium, potassium, magnesium, and calcium, thus destroying the balance in the concentration of these elements within the body. This imbalance will ultimately result in painful muscle contractions and cramps. The person most likely to get heat cramps is one who is in fairly good condition but who is not acclimatized to the heat.

Heat cramps may be prevented by adequate replacement of sodium, chloride, potassium, magnesium, calcium, and most important, fluids.[8] Ingestion of salt tablets may help prevent cramps. Simply salting food a bit more heavily can replace sodium; bananas are particularly high in potassium; and calcium is present in milk, cheese, and dairy products. The immediate treatment for heat cramps is ingestion of large quantities of fluids, preferably a sports drink, and mild prolonged stretching with ice massage of the muscle in spasm. An athlete who experiences heat cramps will generally not be able to return to practice or competition for the remainder of the day, because cramping is likely to reoccur.

Exertional Heat Exhaustion

Exertional heat exhaustion results from dehydration.

Exertional heat exhaustion is a more moderate form of heat illness that occurs from environmental heat stress and strenuous physical exercise. In exertional heat exhaustion an athlete becomes dehydrated to the point that he or she is unable to sustain adequate cardiac output and thus cannot continue intense exercise. Mild hyperthermia is characteristic of heat exhaustion, with a rectal temperature of less than 104 degrees and no evidence of central nervous system (CNS) dysfunction. Obtaining an accurate rectal temperature measurement is essential for the athletic trainer to differentiate between heat exhaustion and heat stroke. See *Focus Box:* "Measuring rectal temperature" for a description of the procedure. An athlete who is experiencing heat exhaustion

Measuring rectal temperature is critical to differentiate heat stroke and heat exhaustion.

TABLE 6-3 **Heat Disorders: Treatment and Prevention**

Disorder	Cause	Clinical Features and Diagnosis	Treatment	Prevention
Heat syncope	Rapid physical fatigue during overexposure to heat	Pooling of blood in extremities leading to dizziness, fainting, and nausea	Lay athlete down in a cool environment and replenish fluids	Gradually acclimatize to exercising in a hot humid environment
Exertional heat cramps	Hard work in heat; sweating heavily; imbalance between water and electrolytes (sodium)	Muscle twitching and cramps, usually after midday; spasms in arms, legs, abdomen	Ingesting large amounts of fluid, mild stretching, and ice massage of affected muscle	Acclimatize athlete properly; provide large quantities of fluids; increase intake of calcium, sodium, and potassium slightly
Exertional heat exhaustion	Prolonged sweating leading to dehydration and an inability to sustain adequate cardiac output	Excessive thirst, dry tongue and mouth; weight loss; fatigue; weakness; incoordination; mental dullness; low urine volume; slightly elevated body temperature; high serum protein and sodium; reduced swelling	Bed rest in cool room, IV fluids if drinking is impaired; increase fluid intake to 6 to 8 L/day; sponge with cool water; keep records of body weight and fluid balance; provide semiliquid food until salination is normal	Supply adequate fluids Provide adequate rest and opportunity for cooling
Exertional heatstroke	Thermoregulatory failure of sudden onset	Abrupt onset, CNS abnormalities including headache, vertigo, and fatigue; flushed skin; relatively less sweating than seen with heat exhaustion; rapidly increasing pulse rate that may reach 160 to 180; increased respiration; blood pressure seldom rises; rapid rise in temperature to 104°F (40°C); athlete feels as if he or she is burning up; diarrhea, vomiting; could lead to permanent brain damage; circulatory collapse may produce death	Take immediate emergency measures to reduce temperature (e.g., immersion in ice water bath or sponge cool water and air fan over body, massage limbs); remove to hospital as soon as possible	Ensure proper acclimatization, proper hydration Educate those supervising activities conducted in the heat Adapt activities to the environment Screen participants with past history of heat illness for malignant hyperthermia
Exertional hyponatremia	Fluid/electrolyte disorder resulting in low concentration of sodium in the blood	Progressively worsening headache, nausea and vomiting, swelling in hands and feet, lethargy or apathy, low blood sodium, compromised CNS	Do not try to rehydrate; transport to medical facility; sodium levels must be increased and fluid levels decreased	Hydrate with sports drinks; increase sodium intake; make sure fluid intake equals fluid loss

Focus

Measuring rectal temperature

Monitoring temperature with a thermometer inserted into the rectum is the most exact way of determining core temperature. Normal rectal temperature is 99.6°F (37.5°C).

- Shake the thermometer down to below the 97°F mark (36.1°C).
- Cover the tip of the thermometer with lubricating or petroleum jelly.
- Place the athlete on his or her stomach.
- Spread the buttocks and gently insert the thermometer about an inch into the rectum. Never force it. Hold the buttocks together to keep the thermometer from falling out.
- Do not release your grip on the thermometer.
- Leave the thermometer in place for three minutes.
- To read the temperature, slowly turn the thermometer until you can see the line of mercury.
- Wash the thermometer carefully in soap and warm water after each use. Store in a safe place.

will show signs and symptoms of dehydration and/or electrolyte depletion that include pale skin; profuse sweating; stomach cramps with nausea, vomiting, or diarrhea; headache; persistent muscle cramps; and dizziness with loss of coordination.

An athlete who has exertional heat exhaustion must be immediately removed from play and taken to a shaded or air-conditioned area. Excess clothing or equipment should be removed and the athlete should lie down with his or her legs elevated. Cooling efforts should continue until rectal temperature has lowered to 101 degrees. Rehydration should begin immediately with water or a sports drink as long as the athlete is not nauseated or vomiting. If the athlete cannot take fluids orally, intravenous fluid replacement should be initiated by a physician. The athletic trainer should continually monitor heart rate, blood pressure, and core temperature. If rapid improvement is not observed the athlete must be transported to an emergency facility. Before returning to play, the athlete must be completely rehydrated and should be cleared by a physician.

Exertional Heatstroke

Unlike heat cramps and exertional heat exhaustion, exertional heatstroke is a serious, life-threatening emergency (Table 6-3). It is the most severe form of heat illness and is induced by strenuous physical exercise and increased environmental heat stress. It is characterized by CNS abnormalities and potential tissue damage resulting from a significantly elevated body temperature. As body temperature rises, extreme circulatory and metabolic stresses can produce damage and severe physiological dysfunction that can ultimately result in death.

Heatstroke can occur suddenly and without warning.[27] The specific cause of heatstroke is unknown. It is clinically characterized by sudden collapse with CNS dysfunction, such as altered consciousness, seizures, confusion, emotional instability, irrational behavior, or decreased mental acuity. Measured rectal temperature is at 104°F or higher. Additionally the victim will be flushed and will have hot skin with sweating about 75 percent of the time, although about 25 percent of the cases will have less sweating than would be seen with heat exhaustion. Other symptoms include shallow, fast breathing; a rapid, strong pulse; nausea, vomiting, or diarrhea; headache, dizziness, or weakness; decreased blood pressure; and dehydration. The heatstroke victim experiences a breakdown of the thermoregulatory mechanism due to excessively high body temperature, and the body loses the ability to dissipate heat through sweating.[54]

6-1

Critical Thinking Exercise

A wrestler collapses during a match and exhibits signs of profuse sweating, pale skin, mildly elevated temperature (102°F), dizziness, hyperventilation, and rapid pulse. When questioned by the athletic trainer, the wrestler indicates that earlier in the day he took diuretic medication to facilitate water loss in an effort to help him make weight.

? What type of heat illness is the athlete experiencing, and what does the athletic trainer need to do to manage this situation appropriately?

6-2

Critical Thinking Exercise

A high school football team is doing conditioning outside. The temperature is 80 degrees with 85 percent humidity. The players have their helmets on and are running 100-yard sprints. One player looks like he is becoming fatigued and slightly disoriented. Thirty yards into the sprint, the athlete collapses.

? What is the immediate course of action to treat this athlete? What is wrong with the athlete?

Heatstroke is a life-threatening emergency.

The possibility of death from heatstroke can be significantly reduced if the victim's body temperature is lowered to normal as soon as possible. The longer that the body temperature is elevated to 104°F or higher, the higher the mortality rate. Thus the key to managing this condition is aggressive and immediate whole-body cooling.[63] Get the athlete into a cool environment, strip off all clothing, and immerse the athlete in a cold water bath (35° to 58°F).[18] If it is not possible to immerse the athlete in cold water, sponge him or her down with cool water and fan with a towel. Try to lower rectal temperature to 101°F. Call the rescue squad. It is imperative that the victim be transported to a hospital as quickly as possible, however it is recommended that the victim be cooled down first and transported second if onsite rapid cooling and adequate medical supervision are available. If rescue squad transport is delayed, it may be necessary to transport the victim in whatever vehicle happens to be available. Following an exertional heat stroke the athlete should avoid exercise for a minimum of one week and gradually return to full practice after being completely asymptomatic and cleared by a physician.

Malignant hyperthermia Malignant hyperthermia is a rare, genetically inherited muscle disorder that causes hypersensitivity to anesthesia and extreme exercise in hot environments. It is characterized by muscle breakdown.[45] This disorder causes muscle temperatures to increase faster than core temperatures, and its symptoms are similar to those of heatstroke. The athlete complains of muscle pain after exercise, and rectal temperature remains elevated for ten to fifteen minutes after exercise. During this period, muscle tissue is destroyed and breakdown products of muscle may damage the kidneys and cause acute renal failure.[25] The condition may be fatal if not treated immediately. Muscle biopsy is necessary for diagnosis. Athletes with malignant hyperthermia should be disqualified from competing in hot, humid environments.[28]

Acute exertional rhabdomyolysis Acute exertional rhabdomyolysis is a syndrome that is characterized by sudden catabolic destruction and degeneration of skeletal muscle accompanied by leakage of myoglobin (muscle protein) and muscle enzymes into the vascular system.[5] It can occur in healthy individuals during intense exercise in extremely hot and humid environmental conditions. It can result in either the gradual onset of muscle weakness, swelling, and pain; the presence of darkened urine and renal dysfunction; or, in severe cases, sudden collapse, renal failure, and death. Rhabdomyolysis has been associated with individuals with sickle-cell trait. If rhabdomyolysis is suspected, the athlete should be referred to a physician immediately.

Exertional Hyponatremia

Hyponatremia is a condition involving a fluid/electrolyte disorder that results in an abnormally low concentration of sodium in the blood.[10] It is most often caused by ingesting so much fluid before, during, and after exercise that the concentration of sodium is decreased. It also can occur due to too little sodium in the diet or in ingested fluids over a period of prolonged exercise. An individual with a high rate of sweating and a significant loss of sodium, who continues to ingest large quantities of fluid over a several hour period of exercise (as in a marathon or triathlon), is particularly vulnerable to developing hyponatremia. Hyponatremia can be avoided completely by making certain that fluid intake during exercise does not exceed fluid loss and that sodium intake is adequate.

The signs and symptoms of exertional hyponatremia may include a progressively worsening headache; nausea and vomiting; swelling of the hands and feet; lethargy, apathy, or agitation; and low blood sodium (<130 mmol/L). Ultimately, a very low concentration of sodium can compromise the central nervous system creating a life-threatening situation.[39]

If the athletic trainer suspects exertional hyponatremia and blood sodium levels cannot be determined onsite, measures to rehydrate the athlete should be delayed and the athlete should be transported immediately to a medical facility.[39] At the medical facility the delivery of sodium, certain diuretics, or intravenous solutions may be necessary. A physician should clear the athlete before he or she is allowed to return to play.

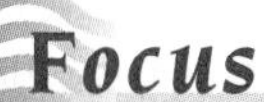

NATA recommendations for preventing heat illness[10]

- Ensure that appropriate medical care is available.
- Conduct a thorough physician-supervised preparticipation exam to identify susceptible individuals.
- Acclimatize athletes over ten to fourteen days.
- Educate athletes and coaches regarding prevention, recognition, and treatment of heat illnesses.
- Educate athletes to balance fluid intake with sweat and urine losses to maintain adequate hydration.
- Encourage athletes to sleep six to eight hours per night in a cool environment.
- Monitor environmental conditions and develop guidelines for altering practice sessions based on those conditions.
- Provide an adequate supply of water or sports drinks to maintain hydration.
- Weigh high-risk athletes before and after practice to make certain they are not dehydrated.
- Minimize the amount of equipment and clothing worn in hot humid conditions.
- Minimize warm-up time in hot humid conditions.
- Allow athletes to practice in shaded areas and use cooling fans when possible.
- Have appropriate emergency equipment available (e.g., fluids, ice, immersion tank, rectal thermometer, telephone or radio).

Preventing Heat Illness

The athletic trainer should understand that heat illness is preventable if he or she exercises some common sense and caution. An athlete can only perform at an optimal level when dehydration and hyperthermia are minimized by the ingestion of ample volumes of fluid during exercise and when commonsense precautions are used to keep cool.[56] *Focus Box:* "NATA recommendations for preventing heat illness" summarizes NATA-recommended guidelines for preventing heat illness.[59] The following factors should be considered when planning a training or competitive program that is likely to take place during hot weather.

The prevention of hyperthermia involves:
- Gradual acclimatization
- Identification of susceptible individuals
- Lightweight uniforms
- Routine weight record keeping
- Unrestricted fluid replacement
- Well-balanced diet
- Routine temperature and humidity readings

Dehydration

An athlete who does not replenish fluids is likely to become dehydrated. Whenever an individual is exercising, some dehydration will occur, since it is difficult to balance fluid loss through sweating with fluid intake. An individual is said to have mild dehydration when fluids lost are less than 2 percent of normal body weight.[39] Even mild dehydration can impair cardiovascular and thermoregulatory response and can reduce the capacity for exercise and have a negative effect on performance.[42,56] Individuals who are becoming dehydrated may exhibit any or all of the following symptoms and signs: thirst, dry mouth, headache, dizziness, irritability, lethargy, excessive fatigue, and possibly cramps. Obviously, an athlete who is dehydrated needs to replace fluids and should be moved to a cool environment. The athlete should rehydrate with a sports drink that contains carbohydrates and electrolytes (particularly sodium and potassium) and should not return to full activity until he or she is symptom free and has returned to normal body weight. It is important to note that fluid replacement should not exceed fluid loss.

Mild dehydration is the loss of less than 2% of body weight.

Fluid intake should equal fluid loss.

Fluid and Electrolyte Replacement

During hot weather it is essential that athletes continually replace fluids lost through evaporation by drinking large quantities of water or other beverages.[21]

The average adult doing minimal physical activity requires a minimum of 2.5 liters of water or about ten glasses of water a day. A normal sweat-loss rate for a person during an hour of exercise ranges between 0.8 and 3 liters with an average of 1.5 liters per hour. Because water is so vital, the healthy body carefully manages its internal water levels. When body weight drops by 1 to 2 percent (1.5 to 3 pounds in a 150-pound individual), he or she begins to feel thirsty. Drinking water and other beverages eventually returns the internal water levels to normal. However, if thirst signals are ignored and body water continues to decrease, dehydration results. People who are dehydrated cannot generate enough energy, and they feel weak. Dehydration is more likely to occur when an individual is outdoors and is sweating heavily while engaging in some strenuous activity. To prevent dehydration, an athlete should make sure to replace the lost water by drinking plenty of fluids and not relying on thirst as a signal that it's time to have a drink. By the time thirst develops, the body is already slightly dehydrated. Many people ignore their thirst, or if they do heed it, they don't drink enough, especially during physical activity. Most people replace only about 50 percent of the water they lose through sweating. For this reason, athletes should consume fluids before, during, and after practice and competition.

Athletes must have unlimited access to water. There is no acceptable reason for allowing or causing an athlete to become hypohydrated.[59] Failure to permit ad libitum access to fluids will not only undermine an athlete's performance, but may also predispose the athlete to unnecessary heat-related illnesses (Figure 6-2).

A number of adverse physiological and potentially pathological effects can be caused by hypohydration, including reduced muscular strength and endurance, decreased blood and plasma volume, altered cardiac function, impaired thermoregulation, decreased kidney function, reduced glycogen stores, and loss of electrolytes.[59]

Sports drinks are more effective than water for fluid replacement.

Using sports drinks During physical activity, it is essential to replace fluids lost through sweating.[56] It has been shown that replacing lost fluids with a sports drink is more effective than using water alone.[50] Research has shown that because of the flavor, an athlete is likely to drink more sports drinks than plain water. In addition, sports drinks replace both fluids and electrolytes that are lost in sweat, and they also provide energy to the working muscles. Water is a good thirst quencher, but it is not a good rehydrator because it actually "turns off" thirst before the body is completely rehydrated. Water also "turns on" the kidneys prematurely, so an individual loses fluid in the form of urine more quickly than when he or she is drinking a sports drink. The small amount of sodium in sports drinks allows the body to hold onto the fluid consumed rather than losing it through urine.[57]

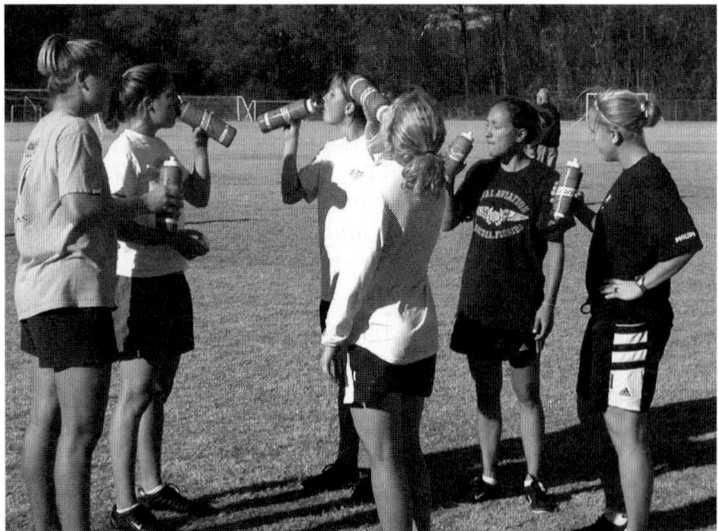

Figure 6-2

Athletes must have unlimited access to fluids, especially in hot weather.

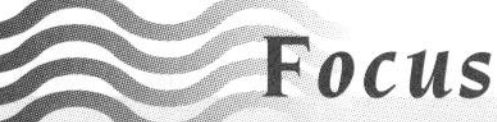

Recommendations for fluid replacement*

- Athletes should begin all exercise sessions well hydrated.
- Establish a hydration protocol for fluid replacement.
- To ensure proper hydration, the athlete should consume seventeen to twenty ounces of water or a sports drink two to three hours before exercise and then seven to ten ounces twenty minutes before exercise.
- Fluid replacement beverages should be easily accessible during activity and should be consumed at a minimal rate of seven to ten ounces every ten to twenty minutes.
- During activity, the athlete should consume the maximal amount of fluid that can be tolerated, but it is important that fluid intake does not exceed fluid loss.
- A cool, flavored beverage at refrigerator temperature is recommended.
- The addition of proper amounts of carbohydrates and electrolytes to a fluid replacement solution is recommended for exercise events that last longer than forty-five to fifty minutes or are intense.
- For vigorous exercise lasting less than one hour, the addition of carbohydrates and electrolytes does enhance physical performance.
- A 6 percent carbohydrate solution appears to be optimal (fourteen grams of carbohydrate per eight-ounce serving). A concentration greater than 8 percent slows gastric emptying.
- Adding a modest amount of sodium (0.3 to 0.7 grams per liter) is acceptable to stimulate thirst and increase fluid intake.

*Based on recommendations from the National Athletic Trainers' Association,[15] American College of Sports Medicine,[2] and Gatorade Sport Science Institute.[56]

Not all sports drinks are the same. How a sports drink is formulated dictates how well it works to provide rapid rehydration and energy. The optimal level of carbohydrate is 14 grams per 8 ounces of water for the quickest fluid absorption. Thus, sports drinks should be used without diluting. Sports drinks with too much carbohydrate are absorbed more slowly. Most sports drinks contain no carbonation or artificial preservatives, so they are satisfying during exercise and cause no stomach bloating. Also, most sports drinks contain a minimal number of calories. It has been shown that sports drinks are effective not only for endurance exercise but also for improving performance during both endurance activities and short-term, high-intensity activities such as soccer, basketball, and tennis that last from thirty minutes to an hour.[39] (See *Focus Box:* "Recommendations for fluid replacement.") A position statement from NATA on fluid replacement for athletes can be found in Appendix D.

Gradual Acclimatization

Gradual acclimatization is a critical consideration in avoiding heat stress. Acclimatization should involve not only becoming accustomed to heat but also becoming acclimatized to exercising in hot temperatures.[52] A good preseason conditioning program, started well before the advent of the competitive season and carefully graded as to intensity, is recommended.[59] Progressive exposure should occur over a seven- to ten-day period.[59] During the first five or six days, an 80 percent acclimatization can be achieved on the basis of a two-hour practice period in the morning and a two-hour practice period in the afternoon. Each practice period should be broken down into twenty minutes of work alternated with twenty minutes of rest in the shade.

Identifying Susceptible Individuals

Athletes with a large muscle mass are particularly prone to heat illness.[17] Body build must be considered when determining individual susceptibility to heat stress. Overweight individuals may have as much as 18 percent greater heat production than underweight individuals, because metabolic heat is produced proportionately to surface area. It has been found that heat illness victims tend to be overweight. Death from heatstroke increases at a ratio of approximately four to one as body weight increases.[17]

Women are apparently more physiologically efficient in body temperature regulation than men are. Although women possess as many heat-activated sweat glands as men do, they sweat less and manifest a higher heart rate when working in heat.[50] Although slight differences exist, the same precautionary measures apply to both genders.

Other individuals who are susceptible to heat stress include those with relatively poor fitness levels, those with a history of heat illness, and anyone with a febrile condition.[59]

Selecting Appropriate Uniforms

Uniforms should be selected on the basis of temperature and humidity. Initial practices should be conducted in short-sleeved T-shirts, shorts, and socks, and athletes should be moved gradually into short-sleeved net jerseys, lightweight pants, and socks as acclimatization proceeds. All early-season practices and games should be conducted in lightweight uniforms with short-sleeved net jerseys and socks. Rubberized suits should never be used.[59]

Maintaining Weight Records

Careful weight records of all players must be kept. Weights should be measured both before and after practice for at least the first two weeks of practice. If a sudden increase in temperature or humidity occurs during the season, weight should be recorded again for a period of time. A loss of 3 percent to 5 percent of body weight will reduce blood volume and could lead to a health threat.[67]

6-3
Critical Thinking Exercise

A high school football coach in southern Louisiana is concerned about the likelihood that several of his players will suffer heat-related illness during preseason football practice in the first two weeks of August. The school has recently hired an athletic trainer, and the coach has come to the athletic trainer to ask what can be done to minimize the risk of heat-related illnesses.

? What recommendations or intervention strategies can the athletic trainer implement to help the athletes avoid heat-related illnesses?

Monitoring Temperature and Humidity Readings

Dry bulb and wet bulb temperature readings should be taken on the field before practice to monitor the heat index.[51] Modifications to the practice schedule should be made according to the severity of existing environmental conditions. The purchase of a physiodyne or sling psychrometer for this purpose is recommended (see Figure 6-1).

Clinical Indications and Treatment

Focus Box: "Environmental conduct of sports, particularly football" and Table 6-3 (page 166) list the clinical symptoms of the various hyperthermia conditions and the indications for treatment. Although the Focus Box calls particular attention to some of the procedures for football, the precautions in general apply to all sports. Because of the specialized equipment worn by the players, football requires special consideration. Many football uniforms are heat traps and serve to compound the environmental heat problem, which is not true of lighter uniforms.

Guidelines for Athletes Who Intentionally Lose Weight

Wrestlers or other athletes who purposely dehydrate themselves as a means of making weight are predisposing themselves to heat-related illness and may in fact be creating a potentially life-threatening situation. Weight loss to make some predetermined weight limit should absolutely not be accomplished through dehydration. The process must be gradual over a period of several weeks, or even months, and should result from a reduction in the percentage of body fat relative to lean body mass. The NCAA and many state high school federations have recently established guidelines for weight loss and set policies for how and when a wrestler can weigh in officially.

HYPOTHERMIA

Many sports played in cold weather do not require heavy protective clothing; thus, weather becomes a factor in injury susceptibility.

Cold weather is a frequent adjunct to many outdoor sports in which the sport itself does not require heavy protective clothing; consequently, the weather becomes a pertinent factor in injury susceptibility.[69] In most instances, the activity itself enables the athlete to increase the metabolic rate sufficiently to function physically in a normal

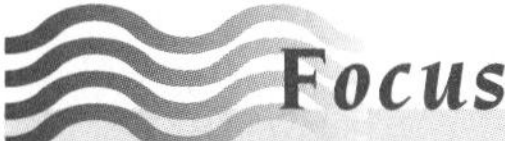

Focus

Environmental conduct of sports, particularly football

I. General warning
   A. Most adverse reactions to environmental heat and humidity occur during the first few days of training.
   B. It is necessary to become thoroughly acclimatized to heat to successfully compete in hot or humid environments.
   C. Occurrence of a heat injury indicates poor supervision of the sports program.

II. Athletes who are most susceptible to heat injury
   A. Individuals unaccustomed to working in the heat.
   B. Overweight individuals, particularly large linemen.
   C. Eager athletes who constantly compete at capacity.
   D. Ill athletes who have an infection, fever, or gastrointestinal disturbance.
   E. Athletes who receive immunization injections and subsequently develop temperature elevations.

III. Prevention of heat injury
   A. Take complete medical history and provide physical examination.
      1. Include history of previous heat illnesses or fainting in the heat.
      2. Include inquiry about sweating and peripheral vascular defects.
   B. Evaluate general physical condition and type and duration of training activities for previous month.
      1. Extent of work in the heat.
      2. General training activities.
   C. Measure temperature and humidity on the practice or playing fields. (WBGT index)
      1. Make measurements before and during training or competitive sessions.
      2. Adjust activity level to environmental conditions.
         a. Decrease activity if hot or humid.
         b. Eliminate unnecessary clothing when hot or humid.
   D. Acclimatize athletes to heat gradually.
      1. Acclimatization to heat requires work in the heat.
         a. Use recommended type and variety of warm weather workouts for preseason training.
         b. Provide graduated training program for first seven to ten days and on other abnormally hot or humid days.
      2. Adequate rest intervals and fluid replacement should be provided during the acclimatization period.
   E. Monitor body weight loss during activity in the heat.
      1. Body fluid should be replaced as it is lost.
         a. Allow additional fluid as desired by players.
         b. Provide salt on training tables (no salt tablets should be taken).
         c. Weigh athletes each day before and after training or competition.
            (1) Treat athlete who loses excessive weight each day.
            (2) Treat well-conditioned athlete who continues to lose weight for several days.
   F. Monitor clothing and uniforms.
      1. Provide lightweight clothing that is loose fitting at the neck, waist, and sleeves; use shorts and T-shirt at beginning of training.
      2. Avoid excessive padding and taping.
      3. Avoid the use of long stockings, long sleeves, double jerseys, and other excess clothing.
      4. Avoid the use of rubberized clothing or sweatsuits.
      5. Provide clean clothing daily—all items.
   G. Provide rest periods to dissipate accumulated body heat.
      1. Rest athletes in cool, shaded area with some air movement.
      2. Avoid hot brick walls or hot benches.
      3. Instruct athletes to loosen or remove jerseys or other garments.
      4. Provide fluids during the rest period.

IV. Trouble signs: stop activity!

Headache	Visual disturbance	Unsteadiness	Diarrhea	Weak, rapid pulse	Faintness
Nausea	Fatigue	Collapse	Cramps	Pallor	Chill
Mental slowness	Weakness	Unconsciousness	Seizures	Flush	Cyanotic appearance
Incoherence		Vomiting	Rigidity		

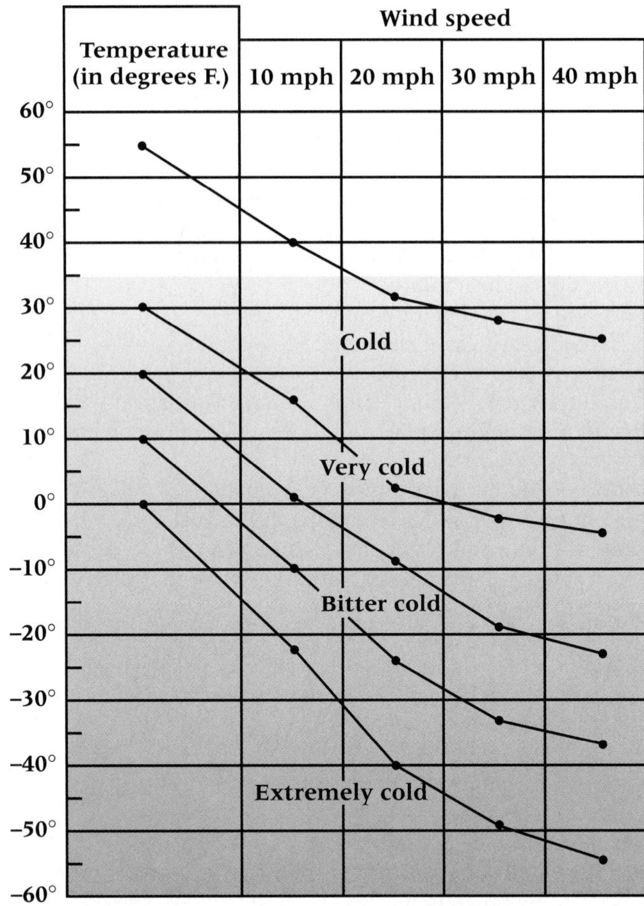

Figure 6-3

Low temperatures can pose serious problems for the athlete, but wind chill could be a critical factor.

manner and dissipate the resulting heat and perspiration through the usual physiological mechanisms.[13] An athlete may fail to warm up sufficiently or may become chilled because of relative inactivity for varying periods of time demanded by the particular sport, either during competition or training; consequently, the athlete is exceedingly prone to injury. Low temperatures alone can pose some problems, but when such temperatures are further accentuated by wind, the chill factor becomes critical (Figure 6-3).[11] For example, a runner proceeding at a pace of 10 mph directly into a wind of 5 mph creates a chill factor equivalent to a 15-mph headwind.

Low temperatures accentuated by wind and dampness can pose major problems for athletes.

A third factor, dampness or wetness, further increases the risk of hypothermia. Air at a temperature of 50°F is relatively comfortable, but water at the same temperature is intolerable. The combination of cold, wind, and dampness creates an environment that easily predisposes the athlete to hypothermia.

Sixty-five percent of the heat produced by the body is lost through radiation. This loss occurs most often from the warm, vascular areas of the head and neck, which may account for as much as 50 percent of total heat loss.[59] Twenty percent of heat loss is through evaporation, of which two-thirds is through the skin and one-third is through the respiratory tract.[68]

As an athlete's muscular fatigue builds up during strenuous physical activity in cold weather, the rate of exercise begins to drop and may reach a level where the body heat loss to the environment exceeds the metabolic heat protection, resulting in definite impairment of neuromuscular responses and exhaustion.[13] A relatively small drop in body core temperature can induce shivering sufficient to materially affect an athlete's neuromuscular coordination. Shivering ceases below a body temperature of 85° to 90°F (29.4° to 32.2°C). Death is imminent if the core temperature rises to 107°F (41.6°C) or drops to between 77° and 85°F (25° and 29°C).

Prevention

Apparel for competitors must be geared to the weather.[30] The function of such apparel is to provide a semitropical microclimate for the body and to prevent chilling. Several fabrics available on the market are waterproof and windproof but permit the passage of heat and allow sweat to evaporate. The clothing should not restrict movement, should be as lightweight as possible, and should consist of material that will permit the free passage of sweat and body heat that would otherwise accumulate on the skin or the clothing and provide a chilling factor when activity ceases. The athlete should routinely dress in thin layers of clothing that can easily be added or removed as the temperature decreases or increases. Continuous adjustment of these layers will reduce sweating and the likelihood that clothing will become damp or wet. Again, wetness or dampness plays a critical role in the development of hypothermia. To prevent chilling, athletes should wear warm-up suits before exercising, during activity breaks or rest periods, and at the termination of exercise. Activity in cold, wet, and windy weather poses some problems because such weather reduces the insulating value of clothing; consequently, the individual may be unable to achieve energy levels equal to the subsequent body heat losses. Runners who wish to continue outdoor work in cold weather should use lightweight insulating clothing and, if breathing cold air seems distressful, should use ski goggles and a ski face mask or should cover the mouth and nose with a free-hanging cloth.[3]

Dress in thin layers of clothing that can be added and removed.

Inadequate clothing, improper warm-up, and a high chill factor form a triad that can lead to musculoskeletal injury, chilblains, frostbite, or the minor respiratory disorders associated with lower tissue temperatures. For work or sports in temperatures below 32°F (0°C), it is advisable to add a layer of protective clothing for every 5 mph of wind.

As is true in a hot environment, athletes exercising in a cold environment need to replace fluids. Dehydration causes reduced blood volume, which means less fluid is available for warming the tissues.[58,59] Athletes performing in a cold environment should be weighed before and after practice, especially in the first two weeks of the season.[43] Severe overexposure to a cold climate occurs less often than hyperthermia does in a warm climate; however, it is still a major risk of winter sports, long-distance running in cold weather, and swimming in cold water.[30]

Common Cold Injuries

Local cooling of the body can result in tissue damage ranging from superficial to deep. Exposure to a damp, freezing cold can cause frost nip. In contrast, exposure to dry temperatures well below freezing more commonly produces a deep, freezing type of frostbite.

Cold injuries in sports include:
- Frost nip
- Frostbite

Below-freezing temperatures may cause ice crystals to form between or within the cells and may eventually destroy the cell. Local capillaries can be injured, blood clots may form, and blood may be shunted away from the injury site to ensure the survival of the nonaffected tissue.

Frost Nip

Frost nip involves ears, nose, cheeks, chin, fingers, and toes. It commonly occurs when there is a high wind, severe cold, or both. The skin initially appears very firm, with cold, painless areas that may peel or blister in twenty-four to seventy-two hours. Affected areas can be treated early by firm, sustained pressure of the hand (without rubbing), by blowing hot breath on the spot, or if the injury is to the fingertips, by placing them in the armpits.

Frostbite

Chilblains result from prolonged and constant exposure to cold for many hours. In time, there is skin redness, swelling, tingling, and pain in the toes and fingers. This adverse response is caused by problems of peripheral circulation and can be avoided by preventing further cold exposure.

Superficial frostbite involves only the skin and subcutaneous tissue. The skin appears pale, hard, cold, and waxy. Palpating the injured area will reveal a sense of hardness but with yielding of the underlying deeper tissue structures. When rewarming, the superficial frostbite will at first feel numb, then will sting and burn. Later the area may produce blisters and be painful for a number of weeks.[41]

Deep frostbite is a serious injury indicating tissues that are frozen. This medical emergency requires immediate hospitalization. As with frost nip and superficial frostbite, the tissue is initially cold, hard, pale or white, and numb. Rapid rewarming is required, including hot drinks, heating pads, or hot water bottles that are 100° to 110°F (38° to 43°C). During rewarming, the tissue will become blotchy red, swollen, and extremely painful. Later the injury may become gangrenous, causing a loss of tissue.

ALTITUDE

Most athletic events are not conducted at high altitudes.

Most athletic events are not conducted at extreme altitudes. For example, Mexico City's elevation, which is 7,600 feet high, is considered moderate, yet at this height there is a 7 percent to 8 percent decrease in maximum oxygen uptake.[65] This loss in maximum oxygen uptake represents a 4 percent to 8 percent deterioration in an athlete's performance in endurance events, depending on the duration of effort and lack of wind resistance.[37] Often, the athlete's body compensates for this decrease in maximum oxygen uptake with corresponding tachycardia.[65] When the body is suddenly without its usual oxygen supply, hyperventilation can occur. Many of these responses result from the athlete having fewer red blood cells than necessary to adequately capture the available oxygen in the air.[20,37]

Adaptation to Altitude

A major factor in altitude adaptation is the problem of oxygen deficiency. With a reduction in barometric pressure, the partial pressure of oxygen in inspired air is also low. Under these circumstances, the existing circulating red blood cells become less saturated, depriving tissue of needed oxygen.[48]

An individual's adaptation to high altitude depends on whether he or she is a native, resident, or visitor to the area. Natives of areas with high altitudes (e.g., the Andes and Nepal) have a larger chest capacity, more alveoli, more capillaries that transport blood to tissue, and a higher red blood cell level.[20] In contrast, the resident or the individual who stays at a high altitude for months or years makes a partial adaptation. His or her later adaptation includes the conservation of glucose, an increased number of mitochondria (the sources of energy in a cell), and increased formation of hemoglobin. In the visitor or the person who is in an early stage of adaptation to high altitude, a number of responses represent a physiological struggle. The responses include increased breathing, increased heart action, increased hemoglobin in circulating blood, increased blood alkalinity, and increased myoglobin as well as changes in the distribution of blood flow and cell enzyme activity. Dehydration has also been linked to altitude sickness.[1]

There are many uncertainties about when to have an athlete go to an area of high altitude to train and compete.[12] Experts believe that having the athlete arrive two to three weeks before competition provides the best adjustment period, whereas others believe that, for psychological as well as physiological reasons, bringing in the athlete three days before competition is enough time.[65] This shorter adjustment period allows for the recovery of the acid-base balance in the blood but does not provide enough time for the athlete to achieve a significant adjustment in blood volume and maximum cardiac output.[65]

6-4

***Critical Thinking* Exercise**

A track athlete from Florida is traveling to Colorado to compete in a week-long track meet. She is concerned because she will be competing at a much higher altitude than she has been training at in Florida. She wants to make certain that she has a chance to adapt to the higher altitude.

? What should the athletic trainer recommend to maximize her ability to compete at the higher altitude?

practice at track meet

Altitude Illnesses

Coaches and athletic trainers must understand that some of their athletes may become ill when suddenly subjected to high altitudes.[74] These illnesses include acute mountain sickness, pulmonary edema, and when present in some athletes, an adverse reaction to the sickle cell trait.

Acute Mountain Sickness

One out of three individuals who go from a low to a moderate altitude of 7,000 to 8,000 feet will experience mild to moderate symptoms of acute mountain sickness.[6] Symptoms include headache, nausea, vomiting, sleep disturbance, and dyspnea, which may last up to three days.[65] These symptoms have been attributed to a tissue disruption in the brain that affects the sodium and potassium balance. This imbalance can cause excess fluid retention within the cells and the subsequent occurrence of abnormal pressure.[65]

Pulmonary Edema

At an altitude of 9,000 to 10,000 feet, high-altitude pulmonary edema may occur. Characteristically, lungs at this altitude will accumulate a small amount of fluid within the alveolar walls.[65] In most individuals this fluid is absorbed in a few days, but in some it continues to collect and forms pulmonary edema. Symptoms of high-altitude pulmonary edema are dyspnea, cough, headache, weakness, and in some cases, unconsciousness.[65] The treatment of choice is to move the athlete to a lower altitude as soon as possible and give oxygen. The condition rapidly resolves once the athlete is at a lower altitude.[64]

Sickle-Cell Trait Reaction

Approximately 8 percent to 10 percent of African Americans (approximately 2 million persons) have the sickle cell trait. In most, the trait is benign. The sickle cell trait relates to an abnormality of the structure of the red blood cell and its hemoglobin content.[26] When the abnormal hemoglobin molecules become deoxygenated as a result of exercise at a high altitude, the cells tend to clump together. This process causes an abnormal sickle shape to the red blood cell, which can be destroyed easily. This condition can cause an enlarged spleen, which in some cases has been known to rupture at high altitudes (see Chapter 29).[65]

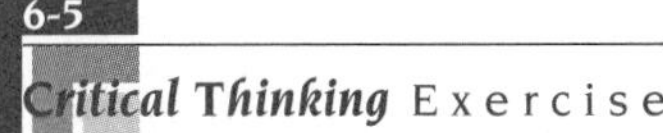

A track athlete is competing in a day-long outdoor track meet. She is extremely concerned about getting sunburned and has liberally applied sunscreen with an SPF of 30 during the early morning. It is a hot, sunny day, and she is sweating heavily. She is worried that her sunscreen has worn off and asks the athletic trainer for more sunscreen. The athletic trainer hands her sunscreen with an SPF of 15 and she complains that it is not strong enough to protect her.

? What can the athletic trainer tell the athlete to assure her that she will be well protected by the sunscreen she has been given?

OVEREXPOSURE TO SUN

Athletes, along with coaches, athletic trainers, and other support staff, frequently spend a great deal of time outdoors in direct sunlight. Precautions to protect these individuals from overexposure to ultraviolet light by applying sunscreens are often totally ignored.

Long-Term Effects on Skin

The most serious effects of long-term exposure to ultraviolet light are premature aging of the skin and skin cancer.[24] Lightly pigmented individuals are more susceptible to these maladies. Premature aging of the skin is characterized by dryness, cracking, and a decrease in the elasticity of the skin. Skin cancer is the most common malignant tumor found in humans and has been epidemiologically and clinically associated with exposure to ultraviolet radiation. Damage to DNA is suspected as the cause of skin cancer, but the exact cause is unknown. The major types of skin cancer are basal cell carcinoma, squamous cell carcinoma, and malignant melanoma. Fortunately, the rate of cure exceeds 95 percent with early detection and treatment.[24]

Using Sunscreens

Sunscreens applied to the skin can help prevent many of the damaging effects of ultraviolet radiation. A sunscreen's effectiveness in absorbing the sunburn-inducing radiation is expressed as the sun protection factor **(SPF).** An SPF of 6 indicates that an athlete can be exposed to ultraviolet light six times longer than without a sunscreen before the skin will begin to turn red. Higher numbers provide greater protection. However, athletes who have a family or personal history of skin cancer may experience

SPF
Sun protection factor.

significant damage to the skin even when wearing an SPF-15 sunscreen. Therefore, these individuals should wear an SPF-30 sunscreen.

Sunscreen should be worn regularly by athletes, coaches, and athletic trainers who spend time outside, particularly if the individual has a fair complexion, light hair, blue eyes, or skin that burns easily.[22] People with dark complexions should also wear sunscreens to prevent sun damage.[24]

Sun exposure causes a premature aging of skin (wrinkling, freckling, prominent blood vessels, coarsening of skin texture), induces the formation of precancerous growths, and increases the risk of developing basal and squamous cell skin cancers. Because 60 percent to 80 percent of our lifetime sun exposure is often obtained by age twenty, everyone over six months of age should use sunscreens.

Sunscreens are needed most between the months of March and November but should be used year-round. They are needed most between the hours of 10 A.M. and 4 P.M. and should be applied fifteen to thirty minutes before sun exposure. Although clothing and hats provide some protection from the sun, they are not a substitute for sunscreens (a typical white cotton T-shirt provides an SPF of only 5). Reflected sunlight from water, sand, and snow may effectively increase sun exposure and the risk of burning.

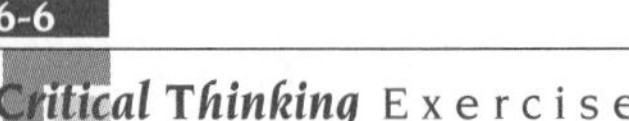

6-6 **Critical Thinking** Exercise

A lacrosse team is practicing on a remote field with no indoor facility in close proximity. The weather is rapidly worsening with the sky becoming dark and the wind blowing harder. Twenty minutes are left in the practice session, and the coach is hoping to finish practice before it begins to rain. Suddenly, there is a bolt of lightning and an immediate burst of thunder.

? How should the athletic trainer manage this extremely dangerous situation?

LIGHTNING SAFETY

Research indicates that lightning is the number two cause of death by weather phenomena, accounting for 110 deaths per year.[49,72] As a result of the inherent danger associated with electrical storms to athletes and staff who practice and compete outdoors, the NATA has established a position statement with specific guidelines for athletic trainers.[70] Each institution should develop a specific emergency action plan to be implemented in case of a lightning storm that includes establishing a chain of command to determine who should monitor both the weather forecast and changing weather of a threatening nature, and to determine who makes the decision both to remove from, and ultimately to return a team to, the practice field based on specific preestablished criteria.[71] If you hear thunder or see lightning, you are in immediate danger and should seek a protective shelter in an indoor facility at once. An indoor facility is recommended as the safest protective shelter. However, if an indoor facility is not available, an automobile is a relatively safe alternative. If neither of these is available, the following guidelines are recommended. Avoid standing near large trees, flagpoles, or light poles. Choose an area that is not on a hill. As a last alternative, find a ditch, ravine, or valley. At times, the only natural forewarning that might precede a strike is feeling your hair stand on end and your skin tingle. At this point, you are in imminent danger of being struck by lightning and should drop to the ground, assuming a crouched position immediately. Do not lie flat. Should a ground strike occur near you, lying flat increases the body's surface area that is exposed to the current traveling through the ground.[72] Avoid standing water (pools), showers, telephones, and metal objects at all times (metal bleachers, umbrellas, etc.).[7]

The most dangerous storms give little or no warning.

The most dangerous storms give little or no warning; thunder and lightning are not heard or seen. Lightning is always accompanied by thunder, although 20 percent to 40 percent of thunder cannot be heard because of atmospheric disturbances. The **flash-to-bang** method provides an estimation of how far away lightning is occurring.[7] From the time lightning is sighted, count the number of seconds until the bang occurs and divide by 5 to calculate the number of miles away the lightning is occurring.[60] When the flash-to-bang count is at 30 there is inherent danger, and conditions should be closely monitored. When the count is 15, everyone should leave the field immediately and seek safe shelter.[60]

flash-to-bang
Number of seconds from lightning flash until the sound of thunder divided by five.

Both the NATA and the National Severe Storms Service recommend that 30 minutes should pass after the last sound of thunder is heard or lightning strike is seen before resuming play.[60] This is enough time to allow the storm to pass and move out of lightning strike range. The perilous misconception that it is possible to see lightning coming and

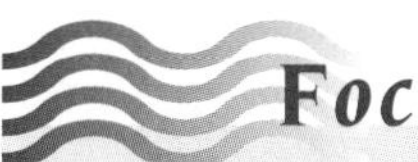

Lightning safety[70]

The following checklist includes basic guidelines that should be followed during an electrical storm.

- In situations in which thunder or lightning may be present and you feel your hair stand on end and skin tingle, immediately assume a crouched position—drop to your knees, place your hands and arms on your legs, and lower your head. Do not lie flat.
- If thunder and/or lightning can be heard or seen, stop activity and seek protective shelter immediately. An indoor facility is recommended as the safest protective shelter. However, if an indoor facility is not available, an automobile is a relatively safe alternative. If neither of these options is available, you should avoid standing under large trees and telephone poles. If the only alternative is a tree, choose a small tree in a wooded area that is not on a hill. As a last alternative, find a ravine or valley. In all instances outdoors, assume the aforementioned crouched position.
- Avoid standing water and metal objects at all times (e.g., metal bleachers, metal cleats, umbrellas, etc.).
- Allow 30 minutes to pass after the last sound of thunder or lightning strike before resuming play.

have time to act before it strikes could prove to be fatal. In reality, the lightning that we see flashing is actually the return stroke flashing upward from the ground to the cloud, not downward. When you see the lightning strike, it already has hit.[72]

Focus Box: "Lightning safety" identifies guidelines that should be followed during an electrical storm. The NATA position statement dealing with lightning safety for athletics and recreation appears in Appendix E.

Lightning Detectors

A lightning detector is a hand-held instrument with an electronic system to detect the presence and the distance of lightning/thunderstorm activity occurring within a 40 mile distance (Figure 6-4). It allows you to know the level of activity of the storm, and it determines whether the storm is moving towards, away, or parallel to your position. When the lightning detector detects a lightning stroke, it emits an audible warning tone and lights the range indicator allowing you to see the distance to the last, closest, detected lightning strike. Lightning detectors are under $200 and are thus an inexpensive alternative to contracting with a weather service to provide information on potentially dangerous weather conditions over a pager system.

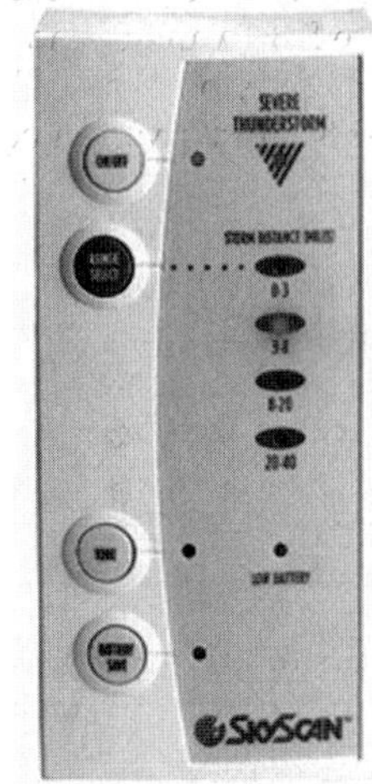

Figure 6-4

Portable hand-held lightning detector. (Courtesy Novalynx Corp., Grass Valley, CA)

AIR POLLUTION

Air pollution is a major problem in urban areas with large industries and heavy automobile traffic. Because athletes are outside for long periods of time during training or competition, they may be more susceptible to the effects of air pollution than is a sedentary individual who remains indoors.[4] There are two types of pollution: photochemical haze and smog. Photochemical haze consists of nitrogen dioxide and stagnant air that are acted on by sunlight to produce ozone.[4] Smog is produced by the combination of carbon monoxide and sulphur dioxide, which emanates from the combustion of a fossil fuel such as coal.

Air pollution is a major problem in urban areas with large industries and heavy automobile traffic.

Ozone

Ozone is a form of oxygen in which three atoms of the element combine to form the molecule O_3. It is produced by a reaction of oxygen (O_2), nitrogen oxides, and hydrocarbon plus sunlight.[31]

When individuals are engaged in physical tasks requiring minimum effort, an increase in ozone in the air does not usually reduce functional capacity in normal work output. However, when individuals increase their work output (e.g., during exercise), their work capacity is decreased. The athlete may experience shortness of breath, coughing, chest tightness, pain during deep breathing, nausea, eye irritation, fatigue, lung irritation, and a lowered resistance to lung infections. Over a period of time, individuals may to some degree become desensitized to ozone. Asthmatics are at greater risk when ozone levels increase.

Sulfur Dioxide

Sulfur dioxide (SO_2) is a colorless gas that is a component of burning coal or petroleum. As an air contaminant it causes an increased resistance to air movement in and out of the lungs, a decreased ability of the lungs to rid themselves of foreign matter, shortness of breath, coughing, fatigue, and increased susceptibility to lung diseases. Sulfur dioxide causes an adverse effect mostly on asthmatics and other sensitive individuals. Nose breathing lessens the effects of sulfur dioxide because the nasal mucosa acts as a sulfur dioxide scrubber.[31]

Carbon Monoxide

Carbon monoxide (CO) reduces hemoglobin's ability to transport and release oxygen in the body.

Carbon monoxide (CO) is a colorless, odorless gas. In general, it reduces hemoglobin's ability to transport oxygen and restricts the release of oxygen to the tissue. Besides interfering in performance during exercise, carbon monoxide exposure interferes with various psychomotor, behavioral, and attention-related activities.[31]

Prevention

To avoid problems created by air pollution, the athlete must stop or significantly decrease physical activity during periods of high pollution. If activity is conducted, it should be performed when commuter traffic has lessened and when ambient temperature has lowered. Ozone levels rise during dawn, peak at midday, and are much reduced after the late-afternoon rush hour. Running should be avoided on roads containing a concentration of auto emissions and carbon monoxide.[31]

CIRCADIAN DYSRHYTHMIA (JET LAG)

Jet power has made it possible to travel thousands of miles in just a few hours. Athletes and athletic teams are now quickly transported from one end of the country to the other and to foreign lands. For some athletes, such travel induces a particular physiological stress, resulting in a syndrome that is identified as *circadian dysrhythmia* and that reflects a desynchronization of the athlete's biological and biophysical time clock.[29]

6-7

***Critical Thinking* Exercise**

A college tennis team from the West Coast must travel to the East Coast to play a scheduled match. The coach has done a lot of traveling and knows that traveling from west to east seems to be more difficult than traveling east to west. This match is important, and the tennis coach asks the athletic trainer for advice to help the athletes minimize the effects of jet lag.

? What can the athletic trainer recommend to help the athletes adjust to the new time zone in as short a time as possible?

The term *circadian* (from the Latin *circa dies,* "about a day") implies a period of time of approximately twenty-four hours. The body maintains many cyclical mechanisms (circadian rhythms) that follow a pattern (e.g., the daily rise and fall of body temperature or the tidal ebb and flow of the cortical steroid secretion, which produces other effects on the metabolic system that are in themselves cyclical in nature). Body mechanisms adapt at varying rates to time changes. Some adjust immediately (e.g., protein metabolism), whereas others take time (e.g., the rise and fall of body temperature, which takes approximately eight days to adjust). Other body mechanisms, such as the adrenal hormones, which regulate metabolism and other body functions, may take as long as three weeks to adjust. Even intellectual proficiency, or the ability to think, clearly is cyclical.

The term *jet lag* refers to the physical and mental effects caused by traveling rapidly across several time zones.[62] It results from the disruption of both circadian rhythms and the sleep-wake cycle. As the length of travel increases over several time zones, the effects of jet lag become more profound.

Disruption of circadian rhythms has been shown to cause fatigue, headache, problems with the digestive system, and changes in blood pressure, heart rate, hormonal

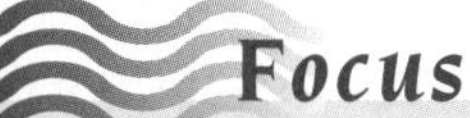

Minimizing the effects of jet lag

- Depart for a trip well rested.
- Preadjust circadian rhythms by getting up and going to bed one hour later for each time zone crossed when traveling west and one hour earlier for each time zone crossed when traveling east.
- When traveling west, eat light meals early and heavy meals late in the day. When traveling east, eat a heavy meal earlier in the day.
- Drink plenty of fluids to avoid dehydration, which occurs because of dry, high-altitude, low-humidity cabin air.
- Consume caffeine in coffee, tea, or soda when traveling west. Caffeine should be avoided when traveling east.
- Exercise or training should be done later in the day if traveling west and earlier in the day if traveling east.
- Reset watches according to the new time zone after boarding the plane.
- If traveling west, get as much sunlight as possible on arrival.
- On arrival, immediately adopt the local time schedule for training, eating, and sleeping. Forget about what time it is where you came from.
- Avoid using alcohol before, during, and after travel.

release, endocrine secretions, and bowel habits.[73] Any of these changes may have a negative effect on athletic performance and may predispose the athlete to injury.[23,77]

Younger individuals adjust more rapidly to time zone changes than do older people, although the differences are not great. The stress induced in jet travel occurs only when flying either east or west at high speed. There is 30 percent to 50 percent faster adaptation in individuals flying westward than in individuals flying eastward.[36] In fact, flying from the west to the east has been demonstrated to decrease performance.[75] Travel north or south has no effect on the body unless several time zones are crossed in an east or west progression. The changes in time zones, illumination, and environment prove somewhat disruptive to the human physiological mechanisms, particularly when a person flies through five or more time zones, as occurs in some international travel.[36] Some people are more susceptible to the syndrome than are others, but the symptoms can be sufficiently disruptive to interfere with an athlete's ability to perform maximally in a competitive event.[40] In some cases, an athlete will become ill for a short period of time with anorexia, severe headache, blurred vision, dizziness, insomnia, or extreme fatigue. The negative effects of jet lag can be reduced by paying attention to the guidelines in *Focus Box:* "Minimizing the effects of jet lag."

SYNTHETIC TURF

Synthetic turf was first used in the Houston Astrodome in 1966 and was first marketed under the trade name AstroTurf. The artificial surface was said to be more durable, offer greater consistency, require less maintenance, be more "playable" during inclement weather, and offer greater performance characteristics such as increased speed and resiliency. Since the late 1960s, a number of companies have manufactured synthetic surfaces that are variations of AstroTurf. Today synthetic surfaces have a relatively new option in "resilient infill turf," which claims to be more similar to natural grass and is considerably less expensive than other types of synthetic turf.[13] It is made of polyethylene and polypropylene yarns that sit on a base of either sand or crumbled rubber pellets or a combination of both. The consumer can choose from a number of artificial turf products, including AstroTurf, Nexturf, FirstTurf, FieldTurf, AstroPlay, Sof-Step 200, HomeField, SpinTurf, and Avery SportsTurf.[1]

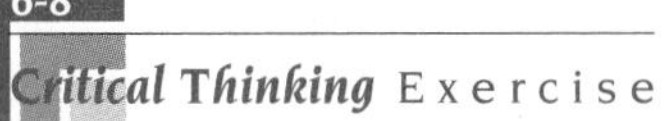

A collegiate athletic director says that he is trying to make a decision about replacing a natural grass playing field with a new synthetic playing surface. He asks the athletic trainer to provide him with recommendations relative to the incidence of injury on natural grass versus synthetic turf.

? What can the athletic trainer tell him?

There has been an ongoing debate over the advantages and disadvantages of synthetic surfaces compared to natural surfaces.[46] From an injury perspective, there is not enough conclusive evidence in the literature to indicate that a synthetic surface is more likely to cause injury than a natural surface.[19,47,48,60] Empirically, it seems that most athletes, coaches, and athletic trainers agree that injuries are more likely to occur on synthetic surfaces than on natural grass, and most of these individuals would rather practice and play on natural grass. In recent years the trend in many colleges, universities, and professional arenas has been to move away from synthetic surfaces, replacing them with natural grass. New hybrid grasses are now available that are more durable.

It has been argued that synthetic surfaces lose their inherent shock absorption capability as they age.[46] It has been demonstrated that training injuries are more likely to occur if training always occurs on artificial turf.[23] Higher speeds are said to be possible on artificial surfaces; thus, injuries involving collision can potentially be more severe because of increased force on impact.[8] A shoe that does not "stick" to the artificial surface but still provides solid footing will significantly reduce the likelihood of injury.[35]

Two injuries that seem to occur more frequently in athletes competing on an artificial surface are abrasions and turf toe (a hyperextension of the great toe). The incidence of abrasions can be greatly reduced by wearing pads on the elbows and knees. Turf toe is less likely to occur if the shoe has a stiff, firm sole.

SUMMARY

- Environmental stress can adversely affect an athlete's performance and pose a serious health problem.
- Hyperthermia is one of sport's major concerns. In times of high temperatures and humidity, athletes should always exercise caution. The key to preventing heat-related illness is rehydration, acclimatization, and common sense. Losing 2 percent or more of body weight due to fluid loss could pose a potential health problem.
- Cold weather requires athletes to wear the correct apparel and to warm up properly before engaging in sports activities. The wind chill factor must always be considered when performing. As is true in a hot environment, athletes in cold conditions must ingest adequate fluids. Extreme cold exposure can cause conditions such as frost nip, chilblains, and frostbite.
- An athlete going from a low to a high altitude in a short time may encounter problems with performance and may perhaps experience some health problems. Researchers are unsure about how much time it takes for adaptation to occur and about when to bring the athlete to the higher altitude, especially for an endurance event. Many athletic trainers believe that three days at the higher altitude will provide enough time for adaptation to occur. Others believe that a much longer time period is needed. An athlete who experiences a serious illness because of his or her presence at a particular altitude must be returned to a lower altitude as soon as possible.
- Air pollution can produce a major decrement to performance and, in some cases, can cause illness. Increased ozone levels can cause respiratory distress, nausea, eye irritation, and fatigue. Sulfur dioxide, a colorless gas, can also cause physical reactions in some athletes and can be a serious problem for asthmatics. Carbon monoxide, a colorless and odorless gas, reduces hemoglobin's ability to use oxygen and, as a result, adversely affects performance.
- Travel through different time zones can place a serious physiological stress on the athlete. This stress is called circadian dysrhythmia, or jet lag. This disruption of biological rhythm can adversely affect performance and may even produce health problems. The athletic trainer must pay careful attention to helping the athlete acclimatize to time-zone shifting.
- There is inconclusive evidence that the incidence of injury on artificial surfaces is higher than on natural surfaces, although most coaches, athletes, and athletic trainers seem to prefer practicing and playing on natural grass. Two frequently seen injuries that occur on artificial turf are turf toe and abrasions.

Websites

National Lightning Safety Institute (NLSI): http://www.lightningsafety.com/

The National Lightning Safety Institute provides consulting, education, training, and expert witnesses relating to lightning hazard mitigation.

FEMA: Extreme Heat Fact Sheet: http://www.fema.gov/library/hazards/extremeheat/heatf.shtm

Doing too much on a hot day, spending too much time in the sun, or staying too long in an overheated place can cause heat-related illnesses.

OnHealth: Heat Illness (Heat Exhaustion, Heatstroke, Heat Cramps): http://my.webmd.com/medical_information/condition_centers/default.htm

Prolonged or intense exposure to hot temperatures can cause heat-related illnesses, such as heat exhaustion, heat cramps, and heatstroke (also known as sunstroke).

A Hypothermia Treatment Technology Website: http://www.hypothermia-ca.com/

OA Guide to Hypothermia & Cold Weather Injuries: http://www.princeton.edu/~oa/safety/hypocold.shtml

National Athletic Trainers Association: http://www.nata.org

This site contains detailed position papers on heat illness, fluid replacement, and lightning safety.

Sports Turf Managers Association: www.sportsturfmanager.com

Gatorade Sport Science Institute: http://www.gssiweb.com

This site provides the most up-to-date recommendations for fluid replacement and preventing heat illnesses.

Solutions to Critical Thinking EXERCISES

6-1 The wrestler is experiencing heat exhaustion, which results from inadequate fluid replacement or dehydration. If conscious, the athlete should be forced to drink large quantities of water. By far the most rapid method of fluid replacement is for a physician to use an IV (fluids administered intravenously). It is desirable but not necessary to move the athlete to a cooler environment. The athlete should be counseled about the dangers of using diuretic medication.

6-2 The athletic trainer may suspect that the athlete is experiencing a heat stroke. The course of action includes checking the athlete's vitals (airway, breathing, circulation) and activating the emergency action plan. Remove his helmet and as much excess clothing as is appropriate. The first priority is to cool the individual down as quickly as possible by immersing him in a cold water tub. Continuously monitor his vital signs until the rescue squad arrives. The athlete's core temperature should be around 100°F before he is removed from the cold tub. If a cold tub is not available, use cold packs or cold water spray. Move the athlete into the shade or to a cooler environment, if possible.

6-3 The athletic trainer should explain to the coach that heat-related illnesses are, for the most part, preventable. The athletes should come into preseason practice at least partially acclimatized to working in a hot, humid environment and during the first week of practice should become fully acclimatized. Temperature and humidity readings should be monitored, and practice should be modified according to conditions. Practice uniforms should maximize evaporation and minimize heat absorption to the greatest extent possible. Weight records should be maintained to identify individuals who are becoming dehydrated. Most important, the athletes must keep themselves hydrated by constantly drinking large quantities of water both during and between practice sessions.

6-4 The safest recommendation would be for the athlete to travel to Colorado two to three weeks before the event. If this arrival time is not practical, she should be in Colorado for at least three days before her first event.

6-5 The sun protection factor (SPF) indicates the sunscreen's effectiveness in absorbing the sunburn-inducing radiation. An SPF of 15 indicates that an athlete can be exposed to ultraviolet light 15 times longer than without a sunscreen before the skin will begin to turn red. Therefore the athlete needs to understand that a higher SPF does not indicate a greater degree of protection. She must simply apply the sunscreen with an SPF of 15 twice as often as would be necessary with a sunscreen with an SPF of 30.

6-6 As soon as lightning is observed, the athletic trainer should immediately end practice and get the athletes under cover. If an indoor facility is not available, automobiles are a relatively safe alternative. The athletes should avoid standing under large trees or telephone poles. As a last alternative, athletes should assume a crouched position in a ditch or ravine. If possible, athletes should avoid any standing water or metal objects around the fields.

6-7 Most important, the athletes should leave for the trip well rested. The day before leaving, the athletes should go to bed and get up three hours earlier than normal. Athletes should reset their watches according to the new time zone once they board the plane. During the trip they should drink plenty of fluids to prevent dehydration, but they should avoid caffeine. Their largest meal should be eaten earlier in the day. On arrival, athletes should immediately adopt the local time schedule for training, eating, and sleeping, and they should get as much sunlight as possible. Training sessions should be done earlier in the day.

6-8 The athletic trainer should inform the athletic director that the trend seems to be moving toward natural grass fields. The research data collected over the years has not clearly indicated that there is a difference in injury rates between natural grass and synthetic turf. However, it does seem that most athletes, coaches, and athletic trainers would prefer natural turf. It should also be stressed that the newer synthetic surfaces are more like natural grass and may perhaps warrant additional investigation.

REVIEW QUESTIONS AND CLASS ACTIVITIES

1. How do temperature and humidity cause heat disorders?
2. What steps should be taken to avoid heat disorders?
3. Describe the symptoms and signs of the most common heat disorders.
4. How is heat lost from the body to produce hypothermia?
5. What should an athlete do to prevent heat loss?
6. Identify the physiological basis for the body's susceptibility to a cold disorder.

7. Describe the symptoms and signs of the major cold disorders affecting athletes.
8. How should athletes protect themselves from the effects of ultraviolet radiation from the sun?
9. What precautions can be taken to minimize the possibility of injury during an electrical storm?
10. What concerns should an athletic trainer have when athletes are to perform an endurance sport at high altitudes?
11. What altitude illnesses might be expected among some athletes, and how should those illnesses be managed?
12. What adverse effects could high air concentrations of ozone, sulfur dioxide, and carbon monoxide have on the athlete? How should they be dealt with?
13. How can the adverse effects of circadian dysrhythmia be avoided or lessened?
14. What are two common injuries in athletes who compete on artificial turf?

REFERENCES

1. A dehydration link to altitude sickness?; *Physician Sportsmed* 30(10):13, 2002.
2. American College of Sports Medicine: position stand on exercise and fluid replacement, *Med and Sci Sports Exerc* 28(17), 1996.
3. Armstrong LE, Epstein Y, Greenleaf JE: Heat and cold illnesses during distance running, *Med Sci Sports Exerc* 28(12), 1996.
4. Atkinson G: Air pollution and exercise, *Sports Exercise and Injury* 3(1):2, 1997.
5. Baxter R, Moore J: Diagnosis and Treatment of Acute Exertional Rhabdomyolysis, *J Ortho Sports Phys Ther* 33(3):124, 2003.
6. Bellis F: Acute mountain sickness: an unexpected management problem, *British Journal of Sports Medicine* 36(2):147, 2002.
7. Bennett B: A model lightning safety policy for athletics, *J Ath Train* 32(3):251, 1997.
8. Bergeron MF: Averting heat cramps, *Physician Sportsmed* 30(11):14, 2002.
9. Bernard TE: Risk management for preventing heat illness in athletes, *Athletic Therapy Today* 1(4):19, 1996.
10. Binkley H, Beckett J, Casa D: National Athletic Trainers' Association position statement: exertional heat illnesses, *J Ath Train* 37(3):329, 2002.
11. Bodine KL: Avoiding hypothermia: caution, forethought and preparation, *Sports Medicine Alert* 6(1):6, 2000.
12. Bovard R, Schoene RB, Wappes JR: Don't let altitude sickness bring you down, *Physician Sportsmed* 23(2):87, 1995.
13. Brukner P: Exercise in the cold. In Brukner P, editor: *Clinical sports medicine*, ed 2, Sydney, McGraw-Hill, 2002.
14. Brzozowski-Gardner C: New options under foot. *Athletic Management* 13(3):47, 2001.
15. Casa DJ, Armstrong LE, Hillman S: National Athletic Trainers' Association position statement: fluid replacement for athletes, *J Ath Train* 35(2):212, 2000.
16. Casa DJ: Exercise in the heat. I. Fundamentals of thermal physiology, performance implications, and dehydration, *J Ath Train* 34(3):246, 1999.
17. Casa DJ: Exercise in the heat. II. Critical concepts in rehydration, exertional heat illnesses, and maximizing athletic performance, *J Ath Train* 34(3):253, 1999.
18. Clements J, Casa DJ, Knight C: Ice-water immersion and cold-water immersion provide similar cooling rates in runners with exercise-induced hyperthermia, *J Ath Train* 37(2):146, 2002.
19. Conklin AR: Grass gets greener: Division 1-A football programs are gradually switching from synthetic turf to grass—and the reasons behind the shift may surprise you, *Sports Med Update* 15(1):11, 2000.
20. Coote JH: Medicine and mechanisms in altitude sickness: recommendations, *Sports Med* 20(3):148, 1995.
21. Coyle E: Fluid and carbohydrate replacement during exercise: how much and why? *Sports Science Exchange* 7(50):1, 1994.
22. Davis JL: Sun and active patients: preventing cumulative skin damage, *Physician Sportsmed* 28(7):79, 2000.
23. Davis JO et al: *Jet lag and athletic performance*, Colorado Springs, 1986, United States Olympic Committee Sports Medicine Council.
24. Davis M: Ultraviolet therapy. In Prentice W, editor: *Therapeutic modalities in sports medicine*, St. Louis, 2003, McGraw-Hill.
25. Ehlers G, Ball T, Liston L: Creatine kinase levels are elevated during 2-a-day practices in collegiate football players, *J Ath Train* 37(2):151, 2002.
26. Eichner ER: Sickle cell trait, exercise, and altitude, *Physician Sportsmed* 14(11):144, 1986.
27. Epstein Y, Moran D, Shapiro Y: Exertional heat stroke: a case series, *Med Sci Sports Exerc* 31(2):224, 1999.
28. Folinsbee LJ: Air pollution and exercise. In Welsh RP, Shephard RJ, editors: *Current therapy in sports medicine 1985–1986*, Philadelphia, 1985, Decker.
29. French J: Circadian rhythms, jet lag, and the athlete. In Torg J, Shephard R, editors: *Current therapy in sports medicine*, St Louis, 1995, Mosby.
30. Fritz R, Perrin D: Cold exposure injuries: prevention and treatment. In Ray R, editor: *Clinics in sports medicine*, Philadelphia, 1989, Saunders.
31. Gong H: How pollution and airborne allergens affect exercise, *Physician Sportsmed* 23(7):35, 1995.
32. Grose K, Mickey C, Bierhals A: Conditioning injuries associated with artificial turf in two preseason football training programs, *J Ath Train* 32(4):304, 1997.
33. Gutierrez G: Solar injury and heat illness, *Physician Sportsmed* 23(7):43, 1995.
34. Harrelson GL, Fincher L, Robinson J: Acute exertional rhabdomyolysis and its relationship to sickle cell trait, *J Ath Train* 30(4):309, 1995.
35. Heidt RS, Dormer SG, Crawley PW: Differences in friction and torsional resistance in athletic shoe–turf surface interfaces, *Am J Sports Med* 24(6):834, 1996.
36. Herbert DL: Does "jet lag" for teams traveling west-to-east adversely affect performance? *Sports Med Stand Malpract Report* 8(3):43, 1996.
37. Hoffman J: Exercise at altitude. In Hoffman J, editor: *Physiological aspects of sport training and performance*, Champaign, Ill., Human Kinetics, 2002.
38. Hunter SL et al: Malignant hyperthermia in a college football player, *Physician Sportsmed* 15(12):77, 1987.
39. Inter-Association Task Force on Exertional Heat Illnesses Consensus Statement, *NATA News* 6:24, 2003.
40. Johnson R, Tulin B: *Travel fitness*, Champaign, Ill, 1995, Human Kinetics.
41. Kanzanbach TL, Dexter WW: Cold injuries: protecting your patients from the dangers of hypothermia and frostbite, *Post Graduate Medicine* 105(1):72, 1999.
42. Kay D, Marino FE: Fluid ingestion and exercise hyperthermia: implications for performance, thermoregulation, metabolism, and development of fatigue, *Journal of Sports Sciences* 18(2):71, 2000.
43. Kleiner, DM: A new exertional heat illness scale. *Athletic Therapy Today* 7(6):65, 2002.
44. Knochel JP: Management of heat conditions, *Athletic Therapy Today* 1(4):30, 1996.
45. Kozack JK, MacIntyre DL: Malignant hyperthermia, *Phys Ther* 81:945, 2001.
46. Kraeger DR: Playing surfaces in sports. In Baker CL et al, editors: *The Hughston Clinic sports medicine book*, Baltimore, 1995, Williams & Wilkins.
47. Lemack L: The artificial turf debate. *Sports Med Update* 15(1):14, 2000.
48. Levine B, Stray-Gundersen J: Exercise at high altitudes. In Torg J, Shephard R, editors: *Current therapy in sports medicine*, St Louis, 1995, Mosby.

49. Lightning casualties on the rise in recreational and sports settings, *Athletic therapy* 6(5):33, 2001.
50. McArdle WD, Katch FI, Katch VL: *Exercise physiology,* Philadelphia, 2001, Lea & Febiger.
51. McCann DJ, Adams WC: Wet bulb globe temperature index and performance in competitive distance runners, *Med Sci Sports Exerc* 29(7):955, 1997.
52. Mellion MB, Shelton GL: Thermoregulation, heat illness, and safe exercise in the heat. In Mellion MB, editor: *Office sports medicine,* ed 2, Philadelphia, 1996, Hanley & Belfus.
53. Montain SJ, Maughan RJ, Sawka MN: Fluid replacement strategies for exercise in hot weather, *Athletic Therapy Today* 1(4):24, 1996.
54. Moss RI: Another look at sudden death and exertional hyperthermia. *Athletic Therapy Today* 7(3):44, 2002.
55. Murray B: Fluid replacement: the American College of Sports Medicine position stand. *Sports Science Exchange* 9(4):1, 1996.
56. Murray R: Dehydration, hyperthermia, and athletes: science and practice, *J Ath Train* 31(3):248, 1996.
57. Murray R: Guidelines for fluid replacement during exercise. *Australian Journal of Nutrition and Dietetics* 53(4 suppl):S17, 1996.
58. Murray R: Practical advice for exercising in cold weather. In Murray R: *Endurance training for performance,* Barrington, Ill, 1995, Gatorade Sports Science Institute.
59. *NCAA sports medicine handbook, 2004–2005,* Indianapolis, 2004, National Collegiate Athletic Association.
60. Noncontact knee injuries in the NFL: the role of field surface and footwear. *Sports Med Digest* 19(4):37, 1997.
61. Pandolf K: Avoiding heat illness during exercise. In Torg J, Shephard R, editors: *Current therapy in sports medicine,* St Louis, 1995, Mosby.
62. Reilly T, Atkinson G, Waterhouse J: Travel fatigue and jet lag, *Journal of Sports Sciences* 15(3):365, 1997.
63. Sandor RP: Heat illness: on-site diagnosis and cooling. *Physician Sportsmed* 25(6):35, 1997.
64. Schoene RB, Bracker MD: High-altitude pulmonary edema: the disguised killer, *Physician Sportsmed* 16(8):103, 1988.
65. Shephard RJ: Adjustment to high altitude. In Welsh RP, Shephard RJ, editors: *Current therapy in sports medicine 1985–1986,* Philadelphia, 1985, Decker.
66. Sparling PB, Milford-Stafford M: Keeping sports participants safe in hot weather, *Physician Sportsmed* 27(7):27, 1999.
67. Thein L: Environmental conditions affecting the athlete, *J Orthop Sports Phys Ther* 21(3):158, 1995.
68. Thompson RL, Hayward JS: Wet-cold exposure and hypothermia: thermal and metabolic responses to prolonged exercise in rain, *J App Physiol* 81(3):1128, 1996.
69. Vellerand A: Exercise in the cold. In Torg J, Shephard R, editors: *Current therapy in sports medicine,* St Louis, 1995, Mosby.
70. Walsh K, Bennett B, Cooper M: National Athletic Trainers' Association position statement: lightning safety for athletics and recreation, *J Ath Train* 35(4):471, 2000.
71. Walsh K, Hanley M, Graner S: A survey of lightning policy in selected division I colleges, *J Ath Train* 32(3):206, 1997.
72. Walters F: Position stand on lightning and thunder: the Athletic Health Care Services of the District of Columbia Public Schools, *J Ath Train* 28(3):201, 1993.
73. Waterhouse J: Identifying some determinants of "jet lag" and its symptoms: a study of athletes and other travellers. *British Journal of Sports Medicine* 36(1):54, 2002.
74. White-Clergerie AM: Mountaineering without oxygen: courting death? *Physician Sportsmed* 15(3):38, 1987.
75. Worthen JB, Wasde CE: Direction of travel and visiting team athletic performance: support for a circadian dysrhythmia hypothesis, *Journal of Sport Behavior* 22(2):279, 1999.
76. www.lycos.com
77. Youngstedt SD, O'Connor PJ: The influence of air travel on athletic performance, *Sports Med* 28(3):197, 1999.

ANNOTATED BIBLIOGRAPHY

Haymes EM, Wells CL: *Environment and human performance,* Champaign, Ill, 1986, Human Kinetics.

This text examines sports performance during a variety of environmental conditions. Two hundred and fifty references are reported.

Strauss RH, editor: *Sports medicine,* Philadelphia, 1996, Saunders.

This book provides four pertinent chapters on the subject of environmental disorders that could affect the athlete.

Johnson R, Tulin B: *Travel fitness.* Champaign, Ill, 1995, Human Kinetics.

Chapters include health and fitness in transit; coping with jet lag; getting to sleep; taking your workout on the road; avoiding excess baggage; how to eat right on your next trip; managing your travel stress; and coming home strong.

NCAA sports medicine handbook, 2004–2005, Indianapolis, 2005. National Collegiate Athletic Association.

This handbook contains guidelines and recommendations for preventing heat illness and hypohydration, for cold, for stress, and for lightning safety.

Maughan R, Murray R: *Sports drinks: basic science and practical aspects,* Boca Raton, Fla, 2001, CRC Press.

Provides a review of current knowledge on issues relating to the formulation of sports drinks and the physiological responses to their ingestion during physical activity.

Graver D, Armstrong, L: *Exertional heat illness,* Champaign, Ill, 2003, Human Kinetics.

This text focuses on all aspects of heat illness and is a good resource for the athletic trainer.

Chapter 7

Protective Gear and Sports Equipment

When you finish this chapter you should be able to

- Fit selected protective equipment properly (e.g., football helmets, shoulder pads, and running shoes).
- Differentiate between good and bad features of selected protective devices.
- Contrast the advantages and disadvantages of customized versus off-the-shelf foot and ankle protective devices.
- Rate the protective value of various materials used in sports to make pads and orthotic devices.
- List the steps in making a customized foam pad with a thermomoldable shell.

Because of the nature of sports activity, injuries often occur. One of the main responsibilities of the athletic trainer is to try to minimize the likelihood of injury. A number of factors either singly or collectively can contribute to the incidence of injury. Certainly the selection, fitting, and maintenance of protective equipment are critical in injury prevention. Thus it is essential that the athletic trainer have some knowledge about the types of protective equipment available for a particular sport and how that equipment should best be fitted and maintained to reduce the possibility of athletic injury.[44]

This protection is particularly important in direct contact and collision sports such as football, hockey, and lacrosse, but it can also be important in indirect contact sports such as basketball and soccer. When protective sports equipment is selected and purchased, a major commitment is made to safeguard athletes' health and welfare.

SAFETY STANDARDS FOR SPORTS EQUIPMENT AND FACILITIES

There is serious concern about the standards for protective sports equipment, particularly material durability standards. These concerns include who should set the standards, the mass production of equipment, equipment testing methods, and requirements for wearing protective equipment. Standards are also needed for protective equipment maintenance, repair, and replacement. Too often, old, worn-out, and ill-fitting equipment is passed down from the varsity players to the younger and often less-experienced players, compounding their risk of injury.[47] It is critical for those responsible for purchasing athletic equipment to be less concerned with the color, look, and style of a piece of equipment and more concerned with its ability to prevent injury.[51] Many national organizations are addressing these issues. Engineering, chemistry, biomechanics, anatomy, physiology, physics, computer science, and other related disciplines are applied to solve problems inherent in safety standardization of sports equipment and facilities. *Focus Box:* "Equipment regulatory agencies" lists agencies that regulate protective sports equipment.

Old, worn-out, poorly-fitted equipment should never be passed down to younger, less-experienced players because it compounds their chances for injury.

LEGAL CONCERNS IN USING PROTECTIVE EQUIPMENT

As with other aspects of sports participation, there is increasing litigation related to the use of protective equipment. Both manufacturers and those who purchase sports

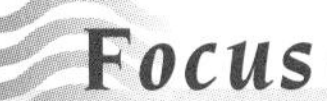

Equipment regulatory agencies

American National Standards Institute
1819 L Street NW
Washington, DC 20036
(202) 293-8020
http://www.ansi.org

American Society for Testing Materials
100 Barr Harbor Drive
West Conshohocken, PA 19428-2959
(610) 832-9585
http://www.astm.org

Athletic Equipment Manufacturers Association
Dorothy Cutting
Cornell University Athletic Department
P.O. Box 729
Ithaca, NY 14851
(607) 255-4115
http://www.wisc.edu/ath/aema/

Hockey Equipment Certification Council
18103 Trans Canada Highway
Kirkland, QC H9J324
Canada
(514) 697-9900
http://www.hecc.net

National Athletic Trainers' Association
2952 Stemmons Freeway
Dallas, TX 75247-6196
(214) 637-6282
http://www.nata.org

National Collegiate Athletic Association
700 W. Washington Street
P.O. Box 6222
Indianapolis, IN 46206-6222
http://www.ncaa.org

National Association of Intercollegiate Athletics
6120 S. Yale Avenue
Suite 1450
Tulsa, OK 74136
(918) 494-8828
http://www.naia.org

National Federation of State High School Athletic Associations
P.O. Box 690
Indianapolis, IN 46200
(317) 972-6900
http://www.nfhs.org

National Operating Committee on Standards for Athletic Equipment
P.O. Box 12290
Overland, KS 66282-2290
http://www.nocsae.org

Sporting Goods Manufacturers Association
200 Castlewood Drive
North Palm Beach, FL 33418
(561) 842-4100
http://sgma@ix.netcom.com

U.S. Consumer Product Safety Commission
4330 East-West Highway
Bethesda, MD 20814-4408
(301) 504-0990
http://www.cpsc.gov

equipment must foresee all possible uses and misuses of the equipment and must warn the user of any potential risks inherent in using or misusing that equipment.

If an injury occurs as the result of an athlete using a piece of equipment that is determined to be defective or inadequate for its intended purpose, the manufacturer is considered liable. If a piece of protective equipment is modified in any way by an athlete, coach, or athletic trainer (e.g., removing some pads from inside a football helmet), the liability on the part of the manufacturer is voided, and the individual who modified the equipment becomes liable. *The best way for an athletic trainer to avoid litigation is to follow exactly the manufacturer's instructions for using and maintaining protective equipment.*

If an athletic trainer modifies a piece of equipment and an athlete wearing that equipment is injured, it is likely that any lawsuit would involve both the athletic trainer individually and the employing institution. This becomes a case of tort (described in Chapter 3) in which the injured athlete must show that the athletic trainer

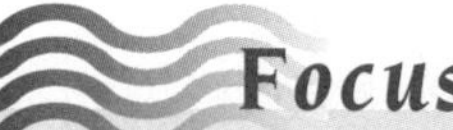

Guidelines for selecting, purchasing, and fitting protective gear and sports equipment to help minimize liability

- Buy sports equipment from reputable manufacturers.
- Buy the safest equipment that resources will permit.
- Make sure that all equipment is assembled correctly.
- Ensure that the person who assembles equipment is competent to do so and follows the manufacturer's instructions to the letter.
- Maintain all equipment properly, according to the manufacturer's guidelines.
- Use equipment only for the purpose for which it was designed.
- If an athlete is wearing some type of immobilization device (i.e., cast, brace), make certain that this does not violate the rules of that sport.[15]
- Warn athletes who use the equipment about all possible risks that using the equipment could entail.
- Use great caution in constructing or customizing of any piece of equipment.
- Do not use defective equipment.
- Routinely inspect all equipment for defects and render all defective equipment unusable.

was negligent in his or her decision to alter a piece of equipment and that the negligence resulted in injury. The athletic trainer would then be legally liable for that action. (See *Focus Box:* "Guidelines for selecting, purchasing, and fitting protective gear and sports equipment to help minimize liability.")

EQUIPMENT RECONDITIONING AND RECERTIFICATION

The National Operating Committee on Standards for Athletic Equipment (NOCSAE) is an organization that has established voluntary test standards to reduce head injuries by establishing minimum safety requirements for football helmets/face masks, baseball/softball batting helmets, baseballs and softballs, and lacrosse helmets/face masks. These standards are adopted by various regulatory bodies for sports, including the NCAA and the National Federation of State High School Associations (NFSHSA). Factors such as the type of helmet and the amount and intensity of usage will determine the condition of each helmet over a period of time. The NOCSAE helmet standard is not a warranty, but simply a statement that a particular helmet model met the requirements of performance tests when it was manufactured or reconditioned. NOCSAE does recommend that the consumer adhere to a program of periodically having used helmets reconditioned and recertified. Because of the difference in the amount and intensity of usage on each helmet, the consumer should use discretion regarding the frequency with which certain helmets are to be reconditioned and recertified. Helmets which regularly undergo the reconditioning and recertification process can meet standard performance requirements for many seasons, depending on the model and usage. *Focus Box:* "Purchasing and reconditioning helmets" provides some guidelines.

7-1

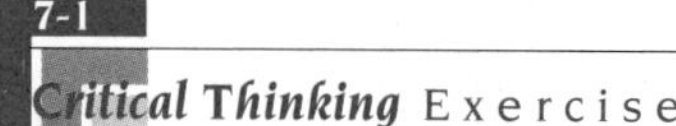

Critical Thinking Exercise

An athletic training student must acquire a basic understanding of protective sports equipment.

? What competencies in protective sports equipment must student athletic trainers have?

USING OFF-THE-SHELF VERSUS CUSTOM PROTECTIVE EQUIPMENT

"Off-the-shelf" equipment is premade and packaged by the manufacturer and when taken out of the package may be used immediately without modification. Examples of off-the-shelf equipment would be neoprene sleeves, sorbethane shoe inserts, and protective ankle braces. Customized equipment is constructed according to the individual characteristics of the athlete. Using off-the-shelf items may cause problems with sizing and exact fit. In contrast, a custom-made piece of equipment can be specifically sized and made to fit the protective and support needs of the individual.

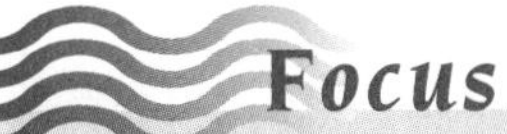

Guidelines for purchasing and reconditioning helmets

- Purchase only NOCSAE-approved helmets.
- Purchase helmets for the appropriate skill level. For example, do not purchase youth helmets for high school football.
- Assign a code number to each helmet purchased and record the date of purchase.
- Fit helmets according to manufacturer's recommendations.
- Recheck helmets for proper fit during the season.
- Review written warranty information and comply with manufacturer's requirement(s) for cleaning/reconditioning/recertification.
- Replace or repair broken or damaged helmets before returning to service.
- Develop a written accounting of player use, inspections, reconditioning, recertification and disposal of each helmet.
- Clean helmets according to manufacturer's recommendations on a regular schedule during the season and at the end of the season prior to off-season storage.
- Recertify/recondition each football helmet according to manufacturer's warranty.
- Recertify/recondition helmets every two years using a certified NOCSAE-approved vendor if no warranty exists or after the warranty expires.

HEAD PROTECTION

Direct collision sports such as football and hockey require special protective equipment, especially for the head. Football provides more frequent opportunities for body contact than does hockey, but hockey players generally move faster and therefore create greater impact forces. Besides direct head contact, hockey has the added injury elements of swinging sticks and fast-moving pucks. Other sports using fast-moving projectiles are baseball, with its pitched ball and swinging bat, lacrosse, and track and field, with the javelin, discus, and shot, which can also produce serious head injuries.[12]

Football Helmets

NOCSAE has developed standards for football helmet certification. An approved helmet must protect against concussive forces that may injure the brain. Collisions that cause concussions are usually with another player or the turf.[35]

Football helmets must withstand repeated blows that are of high mass and low velocity.

Schools must provide the athlete with quality equipment, especially football helmets. All helmets must have NOCSAE certification. However, a helmet that is certified is not necessarily completely fail-safe. Athletes as well as their parents must be apprised of the dangers that are inherent in any sport, particularly football.[35]

To make this danger especially clear, NOCSAE has adopted the following recommended warning to be placed on all football helmets:

> WARNING: Do not strike an opponent with any part of this helmet or face mask. This is a violation of football rules and may cause you to suffer severe brain or neck injury, including paralysis or death. Severe brain or neck injury may also occur accidentally while playing football. NO HELMET CAN PREVENT ALL SUCH INJURIES. USE THIS HELMET AT YOUR OWN RISK.

Each player's helmet must have this visible, exterior warning label or a similar one ensuring that players have been made aware of the risks involved in the game of American football. The warning label must be attached to each helmet by both the manufacturer and the reconditioner.[25] It is important to have each player read this warning, after which it is read aloud by the equipment manager. The athlete then should sign a statement agreeing that he or she understands this warning.

There are a variety of different football helmets available on the market (Figure 7-1), although the number of companies producing these helmets has decreased significantly

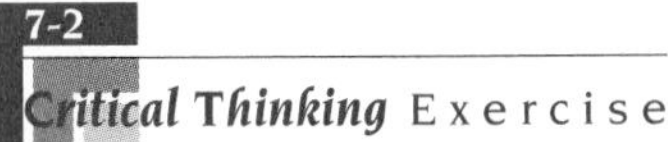

Freshman or junior varsity high school football players are issued their equipment. These athletes and their parents know very little about the equipment's potential for preventing injury. The athletic trainer is given the responsibility to reduce legal liability by educating the players and their parents about the equipment safety limits.

? What steps should the athletic trainer take?

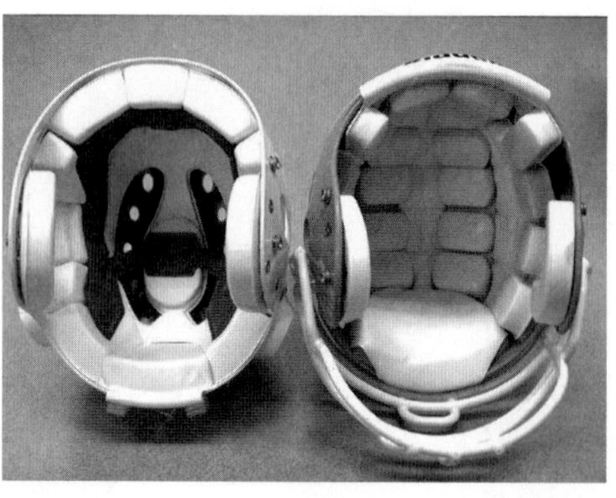

A

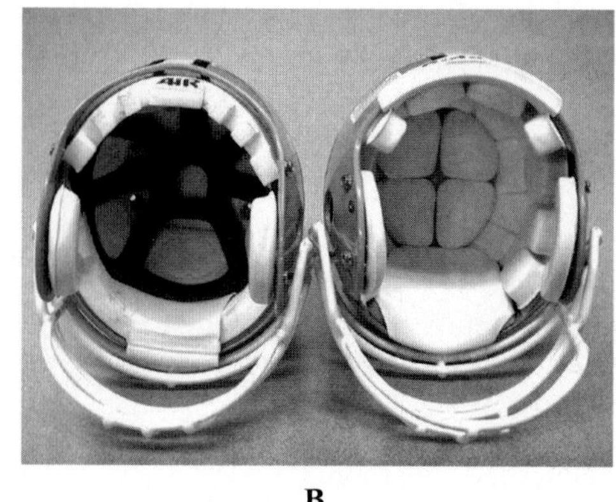

B

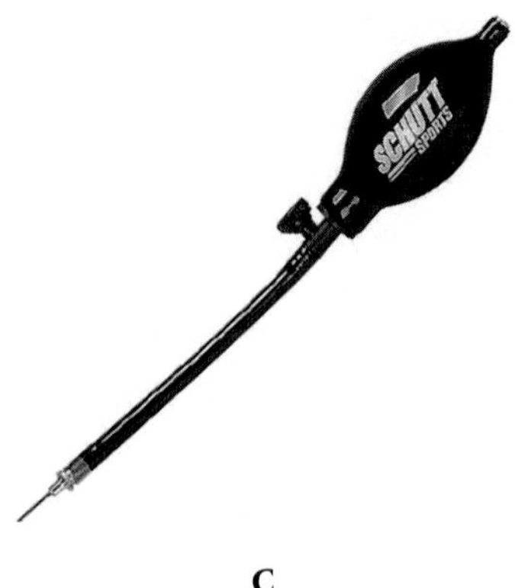

C

Figure 7-1

A, B, The air- and fluid-filled padded football helmets.
C, Helmet air pump.

over the years. This decrease in the number of helmet manufacturers can be attributed primarily to the number of lawsuits and liability cases that have forced many companies out of business.

The lightweight Revolution helmet from Riddell marks the first significant structural change in football helmet design in nearly 25 years (Figure 7-2).[40] The protective shell has been computer designed and extends to the jaw area to provide protection to the side of the head and the jaw as well as improved front-to-back fit and stability. The distance between the helmet shell and the head has been increased. The padding inflates to provide a custom fit to every player's head shape. The face guard system is designed to isolate the attachment points of the face guard from the shell, thus reducing jarring to the player from low-level impacts to the face guard.

Fitting a Football Helmet

When fitting a football helmet, always wet the player's hair to simulate playing conditions; this makes the initial fitting easier. Closely follow the manufacturer's directions for a proper fit. (See *Focus Box:* "Properly fitting the helmet.") The football helmet must be routinely checked for proper fit, especially in the first few days that it is worn. A check for snugness should be made by inserting a credit card between the head and the liner. Fit is proper when the credit card is resisted firmly when moved back and forth. If air bladder helmets are used by a team that travels to a different altitude and air pressure, the helmet fit must be routinely rechecked.

Chin straps are also important in maintaining the proper head and helmet relationship. Three basic types of chin straps are in use today: a two-snap, a four-snap, and a six-snap strap. Many coaches prefer the four-snap chin strap because it keeps

Figure 7-2

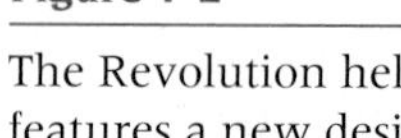

The Revolution helmet features a new design and different shape for football helmets. (Courtesy Riddell Inc.)

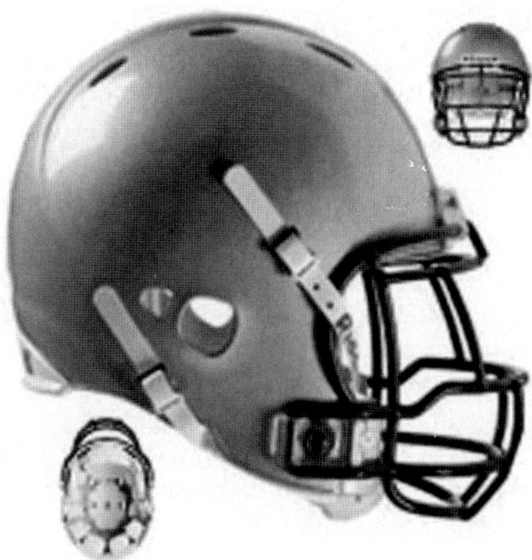

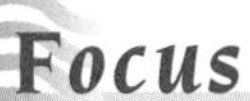

Properly fitting the helmet

In general, the helmet should adhere to the following fit standards:

- The helmet should fit snugly around all parts of the player's head (front, sides, and crown), and there should be no gaps between the pads and the head or face.
- It should cover the base of the skull. The pads placed at the back of the neck should be snug but not to the extent of discomfort.
- It should not come down over the eyes. It should set (front edge) ¾ inch (1.91 cm) above the player's eyebrows (approximately two finger widths).
- The ear holes should match.
- It should not shift when manual pressure is applied.
- It should not recoil on impact.
- The chin strap should be an equal distance from the center of the helmet. Straps must keep the helmet from moving up and down or side to side.
- The cheek pads should fit snugly against the sides of the face.
- The face mask should be attached securely to the helmet, allowing a complete field of vision, and should be positioned three finger widths from the nose.

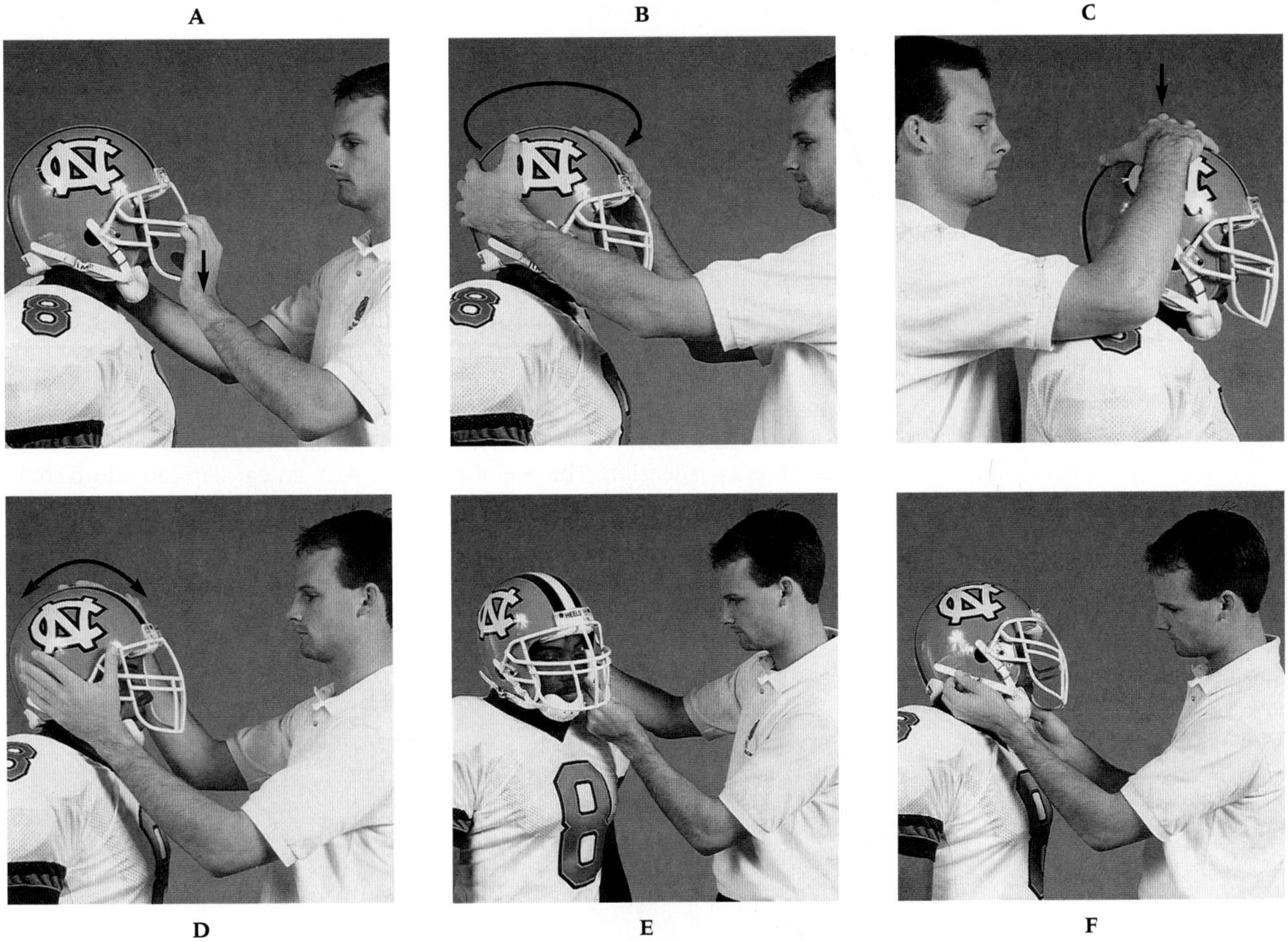

A B C

D E F

Figure 7-3

Fitting a football helmet. **A,** Pull down on face mask; helmet must not move. **B,** Turn helmet to position on the athlete's head. **C,** Push down on helmet; there must be no movement. **D,** Try to rock helmet back and forth; there must be no movement. **E,** Check for a snug jaw pad fit. **F,** Proper adjustment of the chin strap is necessary to ensure proper helmet fit.

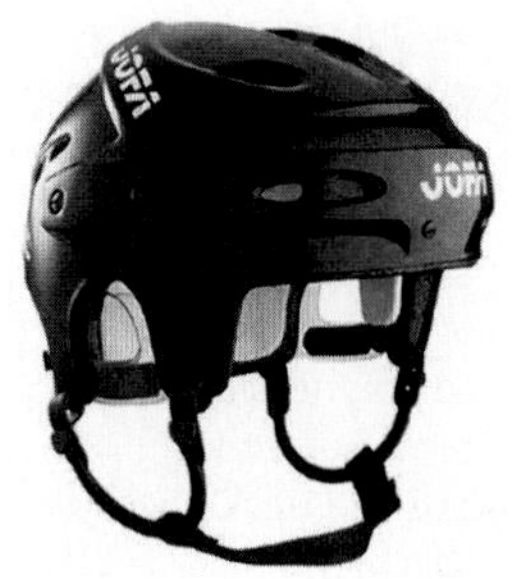

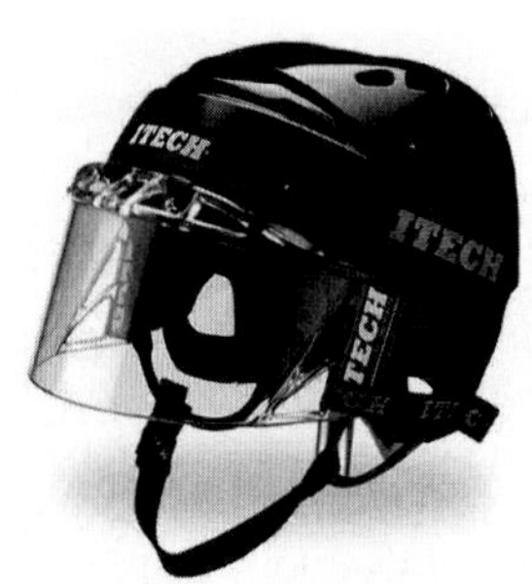

Figure 7-4

Ice hockey helmets.

7-3 Critical Thinking Exercise

The athletic trainer explains the helmet's limitations to a football team.

? Why does the football helmet have a warning label?

the helmet from tilting forward and backward. The chin strap should always be locked so that it cannot be released by a hard external force to the helmet (Figure 7-3).

Jaw pads are also essential to keep the helmet from rocking laterally. They should fit snugly against the player's cheekbones. Certification of a helmet's ability to withstand the forces of the game is of no avail if the helmet is not properly fitted or maintained.

Even high-quality helmets are of no use if not properly fitted or maintained.

Ice Hockey Helmets

Like football helmets, ice hockey helmets have been upgraded and standardized.[35] Blows to the head in ice hockey, in contrast to football, are usually singular rather than multiple. An ice hockey helmet must withstand not only high-velocity impacts (e.g., being hit with a stick or a puck, which produces low mass and high velocity) but also the high-mass–low-velocity forces produced by running into the boards or falling on the ice. In each instance, the hockey helmet, like the football helmet, must be able to disperse the impact over a large surface area through a firm exterior shell and, at the same time, be able to decelerate forces that act on the head through a proper energy-absorbing liner. It is essential for all hockey players to wear protective helmets that carry the stamp (Figure 7-4) of approval from the Canadian Standards Association (CSA).

Ice hockey helmets must withstand the high-velocity impact of a stick or puck and the low-velocity forces from falling or hitting a board.

Baseball/Softball Batting Helmets

Like ice hockey helmets, the baseball/softball batting helmet must withstand high-velocity impacts.[35] Unlike football and ice hockey, baseball and softball have not produced a great deal of data on batting helmets. It has been suggested, however, that baseball and softball helmets do little to adequately dissipate the energy of the ball during impact (Figure 7-5). A possible solution is to add external padding or to improve the helmet's suspension. The use of a helmet with an ear flap can afford some additional protection to the batter. Each runner and on-deck batter is required to wear a baseball or softball helmet that carries the NOCSAE stamp, which is similar to the warning on football helmets.

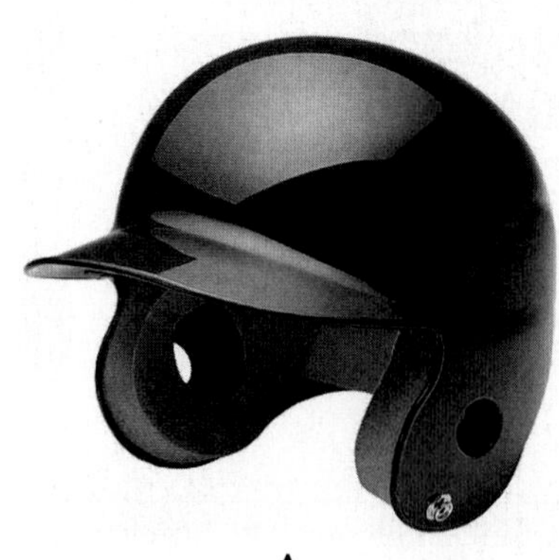

A

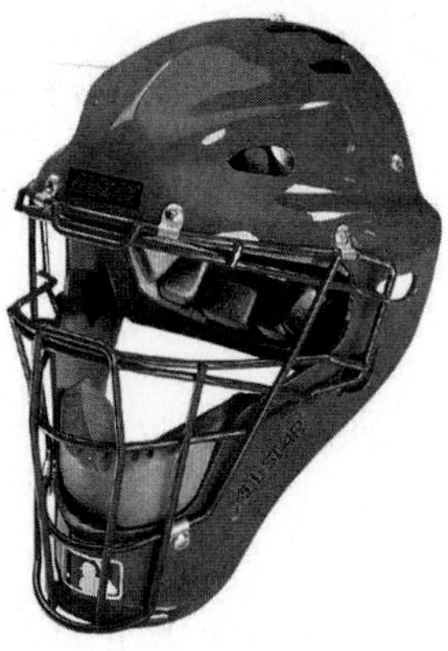

B

Figure 7-5

There is some question about how well baseball batting helmets protect against high-velocity impacts. **A,** Batters helmet. **B,** Catcher's helmet and mask.

Cycling Helmets

Unlike other helmets discussed, cycling helmets are designed to protect the head during one single impact. Football, hockey, and baseball helmets are more durable and can survive repeated impacts. Many states require the use of cycling helmets, especially by adolescents (Figure 7-6).

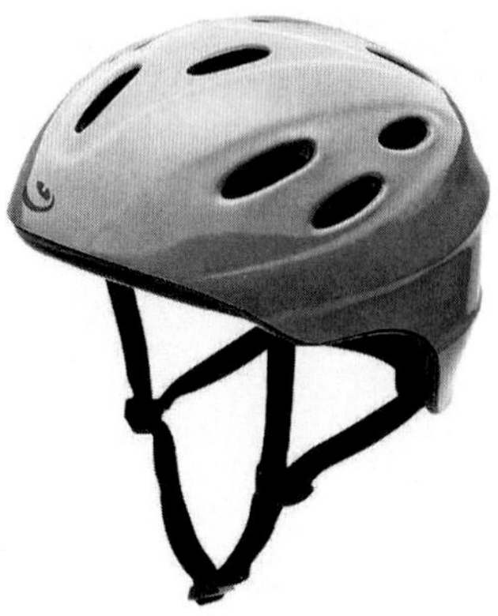

Figure 7-6

Cycling helmet.

Soccer Headgear

Recently several companies have been actively marketing headgear to be worn by soccer players for the purpose of reducing concussions and other head injuries that occur from heading a soccer ball.[9] The headgear is essentially a headband with a piece of foam in the front that is about 1½ to 2 inches wide. To date there are no studies that demonstrate that this headgear is effective in reducing the incidence of concussions or other head injuries. It is far more likely that a soccer player will get a concussion from hitting his or her head on another player, the goalpost, or the ground rather than from heading a soccer ball.

FACE PROTECTION

Devices that provide face protection fall into five categories: full face guards, throat protection, mouth guards, ear guards, and eye protection devices.

Face Guards

Face guards are used in a variety of sports to protect against flying or carried objects during a collision with another player (Figure 7-7). Since the adoption of face guards and mouth guards for use in football, the incidence of facial injuries (i.e. lacerations, nose fractures, eye injuries, etc.) has dramatically decreased. However, the number of concussions and, to some extent, neck injuries has increased, because the head is more often used to make initial contact. The catcher in baseball, the goalie in hockey, and the lacrosse player should all be adequately protected against facial injuries, particularly lacerations and fractures (Figure 7-8).

A variety of face masks and bars is available to the player, depending on the position played and the degree of protection needed.[20] In football, no face guard should have less than two bars. Proper mounting of the face mask and bars is imperative for maximum safety. All mountings should be made in such a way that the bar attachments are flush with the helmet. A 3-inch (7.62 cm) space should exist between the top of the face guard and the lower edge of the helmet. No helmet should be drilled more than one time on each side, and this drilling must be done by a factory-authorized

In sports, the face may be protected by:

- Face guards
- Mouth guards
- Ear guards
- Eye protection devices
- Throat protection devices

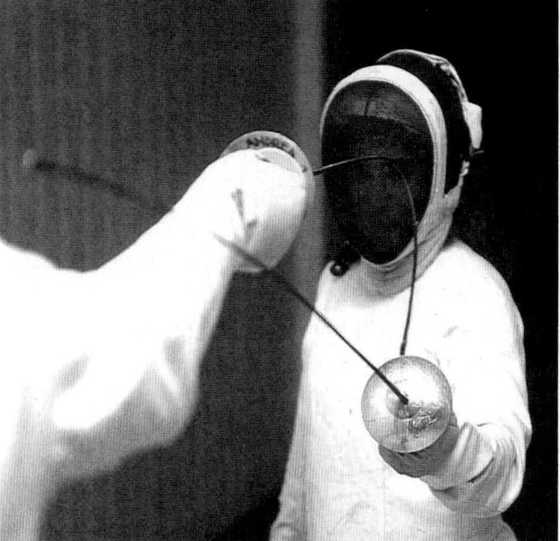

Figure 7-7

Sports such as fencing require complete face protection.

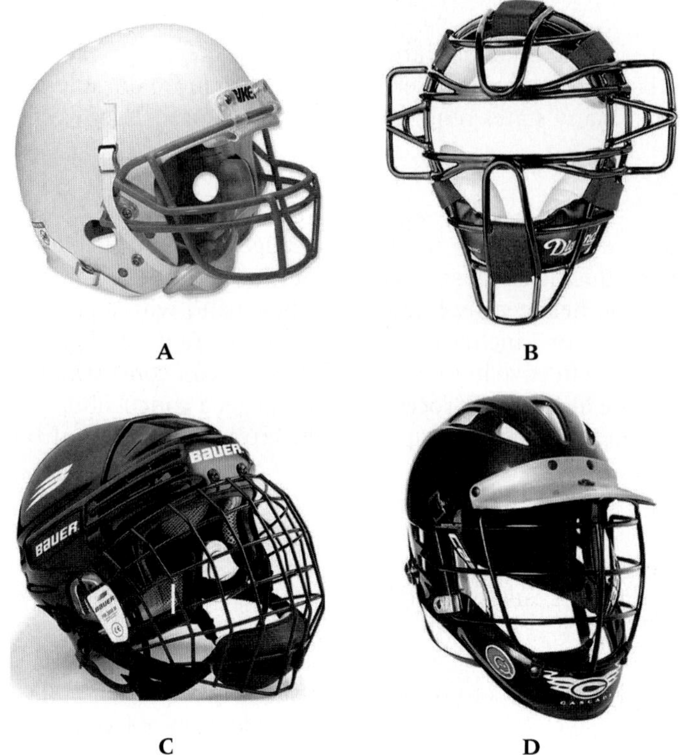

Figure 7-8

A, Football face mask.
B, Baseball catcher's face mask.
C, Ice hockey face mask.
D, Lacrosse face mask.

reconditioner. Attachment of a bar or face mask not specifically designed for the helmet can invalidate the manufacturer's warranty.

Ice hockey face masks have been shown to reduce the incidence of facial injuries. In high school, face masks are required not just for the goalie but for all players. Helmets should be equipped with commercial plastic-coated wire mask guards, which must meet standards set by the Hockey Equipment Certification Council (HECC) and the American Society for Testing Materials (ASTM).[25] The openings in the guard must be small enough to prevent a hockey stick from entering. Plastic guards such as polycarbonate face shields have been approved by the HECC, ASTM, and the CSA Committee on Hockey Protective Equipment. The rule also requires that goalkeepers wear commercial throat protectors in addition to face protectors. The National Federation of High School Associations (NFHSA) rule is similar to the NCAA rule that requires players to wear face guards.

Throat (Laryngotracheal) Protection

A laryngotracheal injury, though relatively uncommon, can be fatal.[35] Baseball catchers, lacrosse goalies, and ice hockey goalies are most at risk. Throat protection should be mandatory for these sports (Figure 7-9).

Mouth Guards

A properly fitted mouth guard protects the teeth, absorbs blows to the chin, and can prevent concussion.

The majority of dental traumas can be prevented if the athlete wears a correctly fitted, customized, intraoral mouth guard (Figure 7-10).[31,36] In addition to protecting the teeth, the intraoral mouth guard absorbs the shock of chin blows and helps prevent a possible cerebral concussion.[2] Mouth guards also serve to minimize lacerations to lips and cheeks and fractures to the mandible. The mouth protector should give the athlete proper and tight fit, comfort, unrestricted breathing, and unimpeded speech during competition. A loose mouthpiece will soon be ejected onto the ground or left unused in the locker room.[2] The athlete's air passages should not be obstructed in any way by the mouthpiece. It is best when the mouthpiece is retained on the upper jaw and projects backward only as far as the last molar, thus permitting speech. Maximum

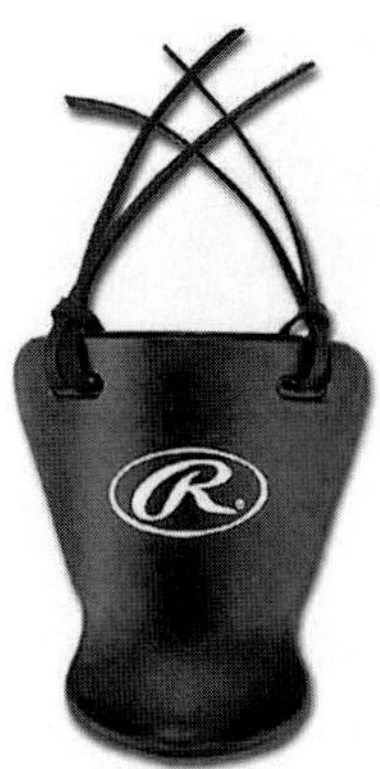

Figure 7-9

A throat protector can be attached to the face mask in baseball, softball, lacrosse, and ice hockey.

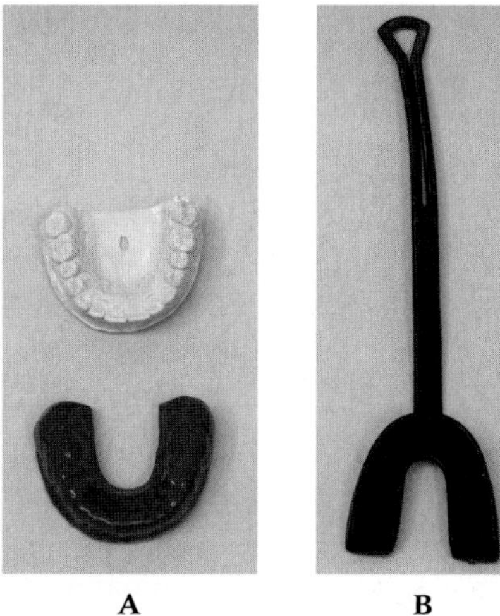

Figure 7-10

Mouthpieces. **A,** Custom fit from a mold and **B,** heat moldable.

protection is afforded when the mouth guard is composed of a flexible, resilient material and is formed to fit to the teeth and upper jaw.[30]

Cutting down mouth guards to cover only the front teeth should never be permitted. This invalidates the manufacturer's warranty against dental injuries, and a cut-down mouth guard can potentially become dislodged and lead to an obstructed airway.

The three types of mouth guards generally used in sports are the stock variety, the commercial mouth guard formed after submersion in boiling water, and the custom fabricated type, which is formed over a mold made from an impression of the athlete's maxillary arch.[35]

Many high schools and colleges now require that mouth guards be worn at all times during participation. For example, the NCAA football rules mandate that all players wear a properly manufactured mouth guard. A time-out is charged to a team if a player fails to wear the mouth guard.[23] To assist enforcement, official mouth guards are increasingly made in a highly visible color.

7-4

***Critical Thinking* Exercise**

The ice hockey team has traditionally been responsible for obtaining their own mouth guards. Lately, however, several players have complained about their mouth guards and do not want to wear them. The athletic trainer would like to purchase the supplies necessary to make custom fabricated mouth guards.

? How can the athletic trainer justify this request to the athletic department?

Ear Guards

With the exception of wrestling, water polo, and boxing, most contact sports do not make a special practice of protecting the ears. All these sports can cause irritation of the ears to the point that permanent deformity can ensue. To avoid this problem, special ear guards should be worn routinely (Figure 7-11).

Eye Protection Devices

The National Society to Prevent Blindness estimates that the highest percentage of eye injuries are sports or play related. Most injuries are from blunt trauma. Protective devices must be sport-specific.

Glasses

For the athlete who must wear corrective lenses, glasses can be both a blessing and a nuisance. They may slip on sweat, get bent when hit, fog from perspiration, detract from peripheral vision, and be difficult to wear with protective headgear. Even with all these disadvantages, properly fitted and designed glasses can provide adequate protection and withstand the rigors of the sport. Athletes should wear polycarbonate lenses, which are virtually unbreakable.[55] These are the newest type of lenses available, and they are certainly the safest. If the athlete has glass lenses, they must be

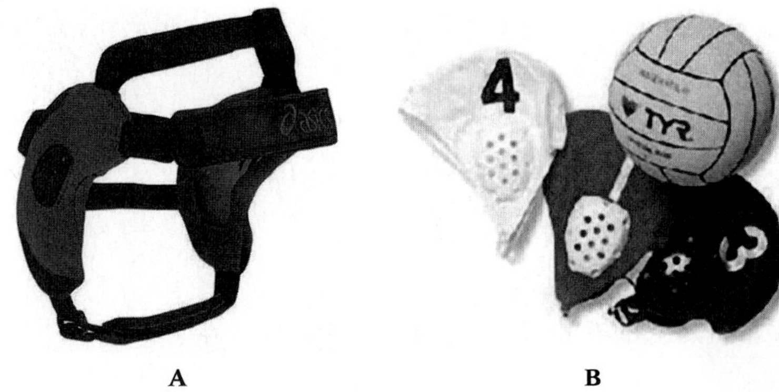

Figure 7-11

Ear protection. **A,** Wrestler's ear guard. **B,** Water polo player's ear protection.

case-hardened to prevent them from splintering on impact. When a case-hardened lens breaks, it crumbles, eliminating the sharp edges that may penetrate the eye. The cost of this process is relatively low. The only disadvantages are that the glasses are heavier than average and may be scratched more easily than regular glasses.[26]

Another possible sports advantage of glass-lensed glasses is that they can be created so the lenses will become color tinted when exposed to ultraviolet rays from the sun and then return to a clear state when removed from the sun's rays. These lenses are known as photochromic lenses. Plastic lenses for glasses are popular with athletes. They are much lighter weight than glass lenses and they can be made scratch resistant with a special coating.

Contact Lenses

The athlete who can wear contact lenses without discomfort can avoid many of the inconveniences of glasses. The greatest advantage to contact lenses is probably the fact that they "become a part of the eye" and move with it.

Contact lenses come mainly in two types: the corneal type, which covers just the iris of the eye, and the scleral type, which covers the entire front of the eye, including the white. Peripheral vision as well as astigmatism and corneal waviness is improved through the use of contact lenses. Unlike regular glasses, contact lenses do not normally cloud during temperature changes. They also can be tinted to reduce glare. For example, yellow lenses can be used against ice glare and blue ones against glare from snow. One of the main difficulties with contact lenses is their high cost compared with regular glasses. Some other serious disadvantages of wearing contact lenses are the possibility of corneal irritation caused by dust getting under the lens and the possibility of a lens becoming dislodged during body contact. In addition, only certain individuals can wear contacts with comfort, and some individuals are unable to ever wear them because of certain eye idiosyncrasies. Athletes currently prefer the soft, hydrophilic lenses to the hard type. Adjustment time for the soft lenses is shorter than for the hard, they can be more easily replaced, and they are more adaptable to the sports environment. There are also disposable lenses and lenses that can be worn for an extended period. In the last few years, the cost of contact lenses has dropped significantly.

The advent of two eye surgery procedures, radial kerotectomy (RK) and laser in-situ keratomileusis (LASIK), has potentially reduced the need for individuals to wear vision-correcting glasses or contact lenses. Although relatively expensive, the LASIK procedure has proven to be a safe and effective technique for correcting faulty vision.

Eye and Glasses Guards

Eye protection must be worn by all athletes who play sports that use fast-moving projectiles.

It is essential that athletes take special precautions to protect their eyes, especially in sports that use fast-moving projectiles and implements, such as handball or racquetball (Figure 7-12).[26] Besides the more obvious sports of ice hockey, lacrosse, and baseball, the racquet sports can also cause serious eye injury. Athletes not wearing glasses should wear closed eye guards to protect the orbital cavity. Athletes who normally

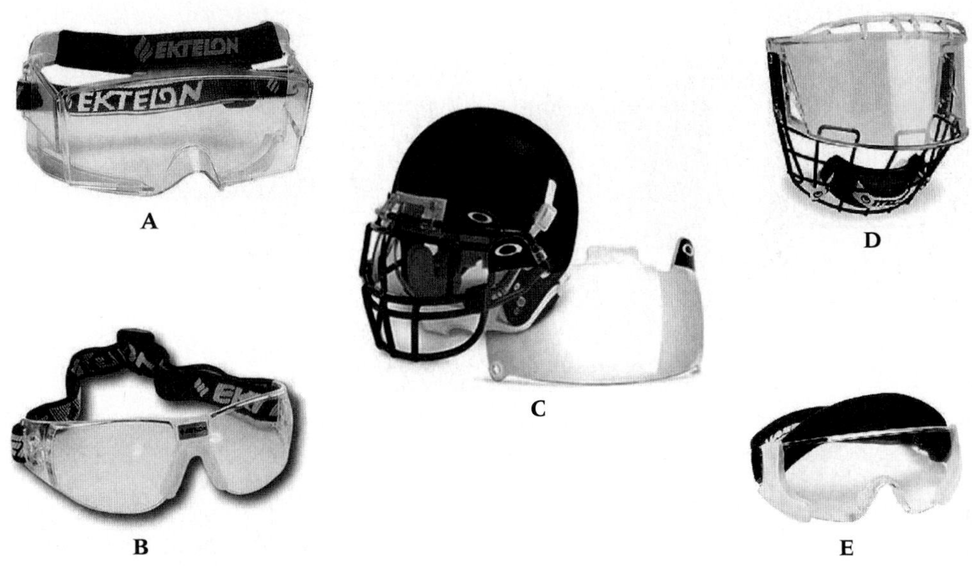

Figure 7-12

A & B, Athletes playing sports that involve small, fast projectiles should wear closed eye guards. **C,** Polycarbonate shield for a football helmet. **D,** Shield for an ice hockey face mask. **E,** Lacrosse/field hockey goggle.

wear glasses with plastic or case-hardened lenses are to some degree already protected against eye injury from an implement or projectile; however, greater safety is afforded by the polycarbonate frame that surrounds and fits over the athlete's glasses. The protection that the guard affords is excellent, but it hinders vision in some planes. Polycarbonate eye shields can be attached to football face masks, hockey helmets, and baseball and softball helmets.

Neck Protection

Experts in cervical injuries consider the major value of commercial and customized cervical collars to be mostly a reminder to the athlete to be cautious rather than to provide a definitive restriction (see Figure 7-16B on page 200).

TRUNK AND THORAX PROTECTION

Trunk and thorax protection is essential in many contact and collision sports. Sports such as football, ice hockey, baseball, and lacrosse use extensive body protection. Areas that are most exposed to impact forces must be properly covered with some material that offers protection against soft-tissue compression. Of particular concern are the external genitalia and the exposed bony protuberances of the body that have insufficient soft tissue for protection, such as shoulders, ribs, and spine (Figure 7-13).

As discussed earlier, the problem that arises in wearing protective equipment is that, although it is armor against injury to the athlete wearing it, it can also serve as a weapon against all opponents. Standards must become more stringent in determining

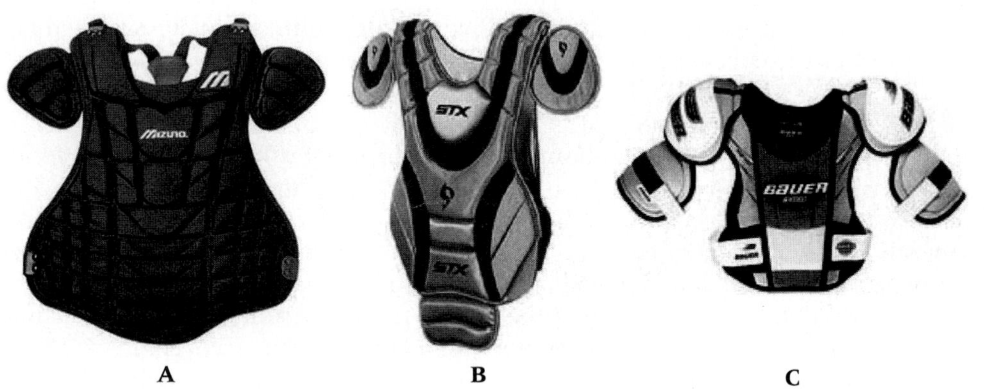

Figure 7-13

Chest and thorax protectors. **A,** Baseball catcher's chest protector. **B,** Lacrosse goalie chest protector. **C,** Ice hockey thorax protector and shoulder pads.

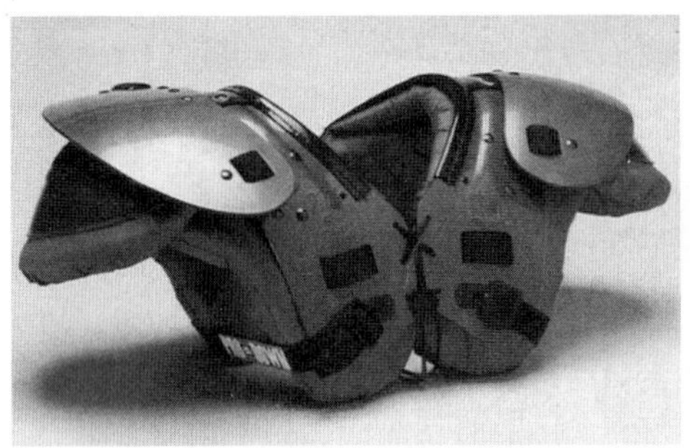

A

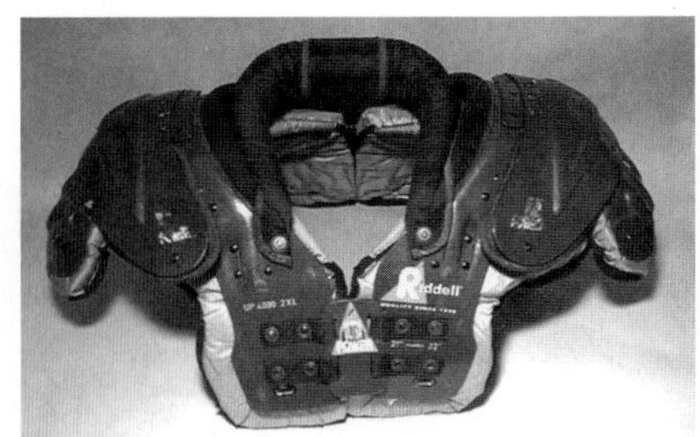

B

Figure 7-14

Shoulder pads protect both the shoulder and thorax. **A,** Non-cantilever. **B,** Cantilever pads.

what equipment is absolutely necessary for body protection and at the same time is not itself a source of trauma. Proper fit and proper maintenance of equipment are essential.

Football Shoulder Pads

There are two general types of shoulder pads: cantilevered and noncantilevered (Figure 7-14). The player who uses the shoulder a great deal in blocking and tackling requires the bulkier cantilevered type, whereas the quarterback or a receiver might prefer to use the noncantilever pads that don't restrict shoulder motion as much as the cantilevered pads. Over the years, the shoulder pad's front and rear panels have been extended along with the cantilever. The following are rules for fitting the football shoulder pad (Figure 7-15):

- The width of the shoulder is measured to determine the proper size of pad.
- The inside shoulder pad should cover the tip of the shoulder in a direct line with the lateral aspect of the shoulder.
- The epaulets and cups should cover the deltoid muscle and allow movements required by the athlete's specific position.
- The neck opening must allow the athlete to raise the arm overhead but not allow the pad to slide back and forth.
- If a split-clavicle shoulder pad is used, the channel for the top of the shoulder must be in the proper position.
- Straps underneath the arm must hold the pads firmly in place, but not so they constrict soft tissue. A collar and drop-down pads may be added to provide more protection.

Some athletic trainers use a combination of football and ice hockey shoulder pads to prevent injuries high on the upper arm and shoulder. A pair of supplemental shoulder pads are placed under the football pads (Figure 7-16 on page 200). The deltoid cap of the hockey pad is connected to the main body of the hockey pad by an adjustable lace. The distal end of the deltoid cap is held in place by a Velcro strap. The chest pad is adjustable to ensure proper fit for any size athlete. The football shoulder pads are placed over the hockey pads. The athletic trainer should observe for a proper fit. Larger football pads may be needed. A neck collar can be attached to the shoulder pads and has been shown to be effective in minimizing neck movement (Figure 7-16B).[19]

Sports Bras

To be effective, a bra should hold the breasts tightly to the chest.

Manufacturers have made significant efforts to develop athletic support bras for women who participate in all types of physical activity. In the past, the primary concern was for breast protection against external forces that could cause bruising. Most sports bras are now designed to minimize excessive vertical and horizontal movements of the breasts that occurs with running and jumping.[42]

To be effective, a bra should hold the breasts to the chest and prevent stretching of the Cooper's ligament, which causes premature sagging (see Figure 7-17 on page 200). Metal parts (snaps, fasteners, underwire support) rub and abrade the skin.

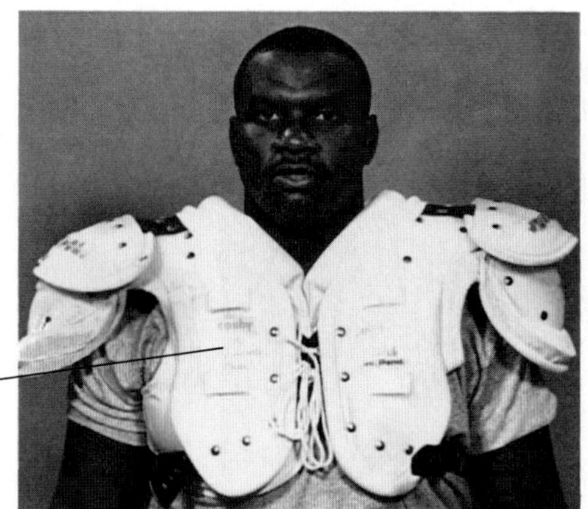

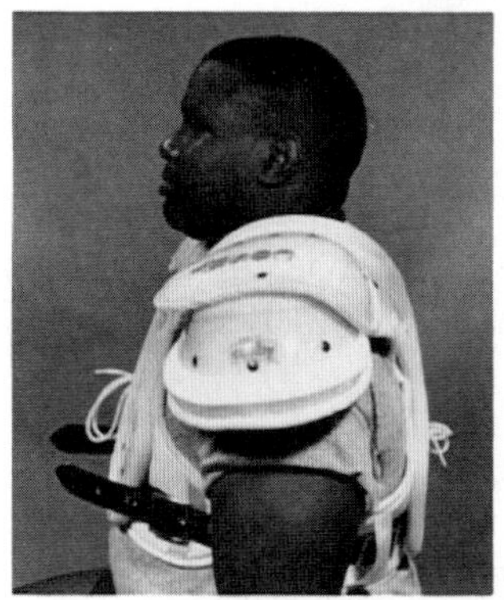

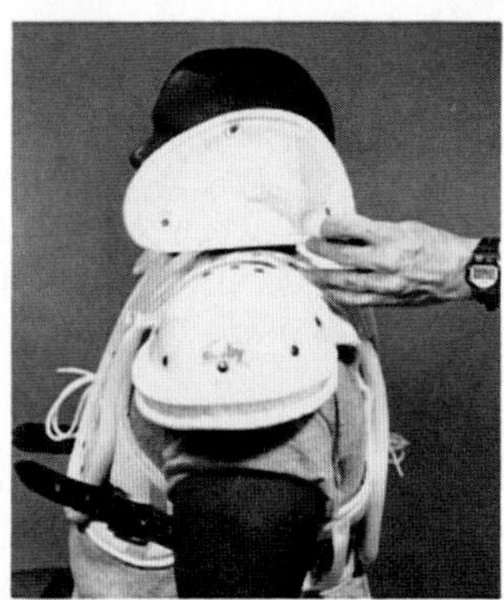

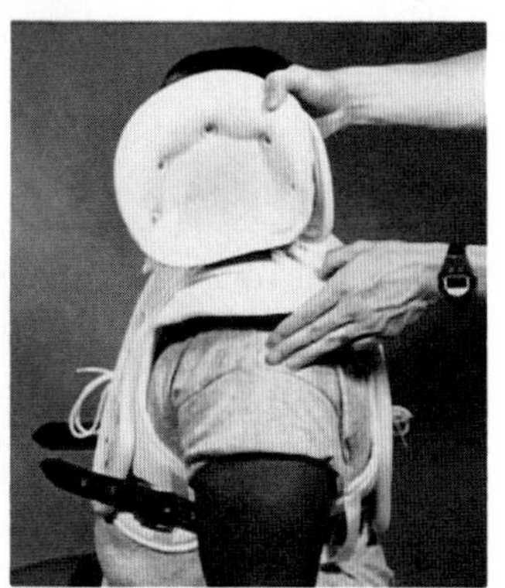

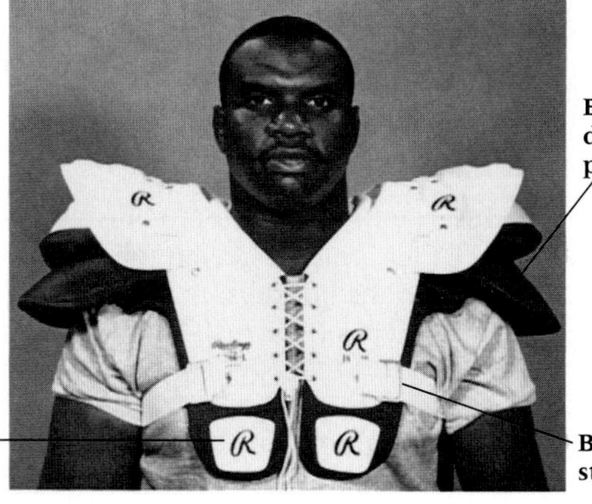

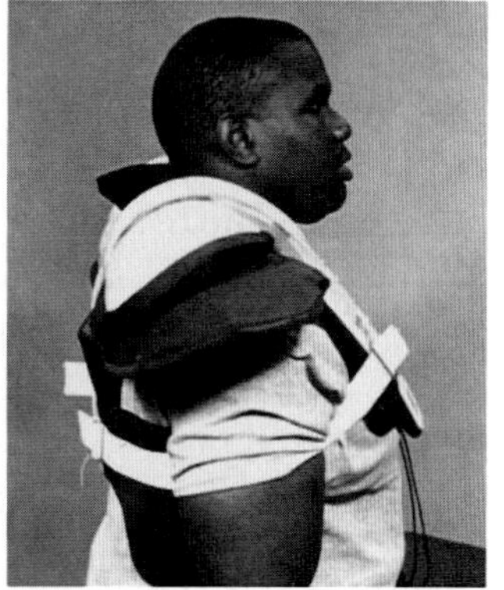

Figure 7-15

Football shoulder pads should be made to protect the player against direct force to the entire shoulder complex.

Nonsupport bras lack sufficient padding, and seams over nipples compound the rubbing of the bra on the nipple, which can lead to irritation.[8]

Several styles of sports bras are now available:

1. For women with smaller breasts it is not as critical to provide compression or support and thus a less elastic, lightweight bra is sufficient (Figure 7-18A on page 201).
2. A compressive pullover bra is perhaps the most common and is recommended for women with medium-size breasts. Compressive bras function like wide elastic bandages, binding the breasts to the chest wall (Figure 7-18B on page 201).
3. Support bras are a bit more heavy duty and provide good upward support with elastic material and an underwire. They tend to have wide bands under the breasts with elastic shoulder straps in the back. They are designed for women with larger breasts (Figure 7-18C on page 201).

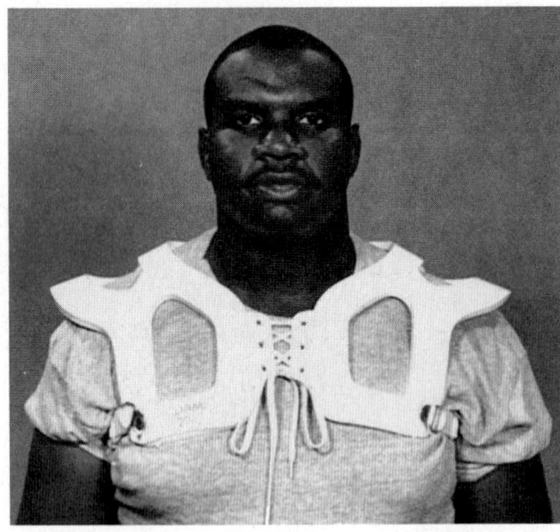
A

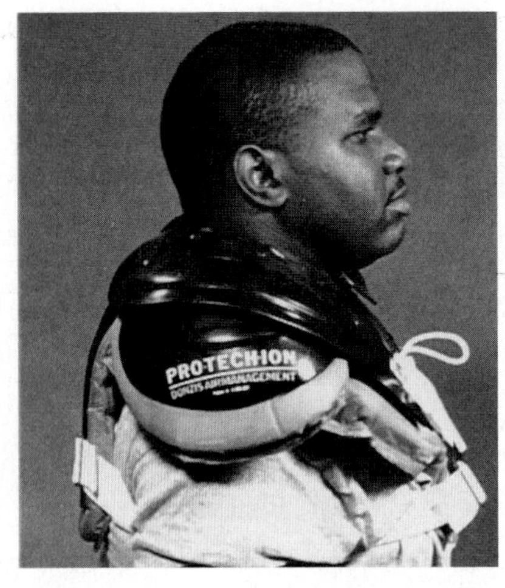

B

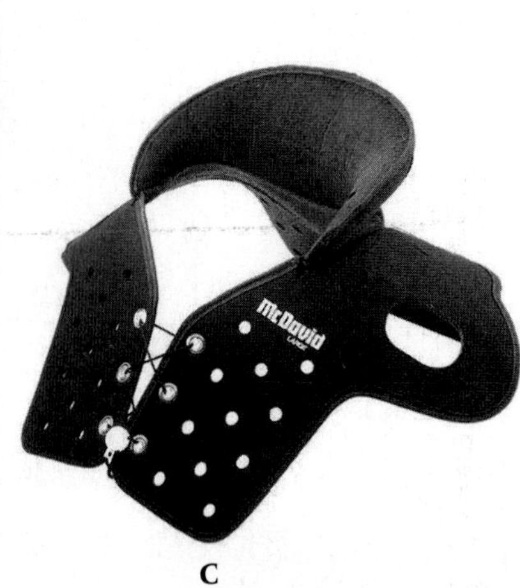

C

Figure 7-16

A, B, Customized foam is placed on the underside of the shoulder pad to provide additional protection.
C, A cowboy collar can be attached to the shoulder pad.

In contact sports, additional padding may be placed inside the cup if needed. Women competing in ice hockey, for example, wear protective plastic chest pieces that attach to their shoulder pads to protect the breast tissue from contusions (Figure 7-18D).

Thorax and Rib Protection

Several manufacturers provide equipment for thorax protection. Many of the thorax protectors and rib belts can be modified by replacing stock pads with customized thermomoldable plastic protective devices.[35] Recently, many lightweight pads have been developed to protect the athlete against external forces. A jacket for the protection of a rib injury incorporates a pad composed of air-inflated, interconnected cylinders that protect against severe external forces (Figure 7-19). This same principle has been used in the development of other protective pads.

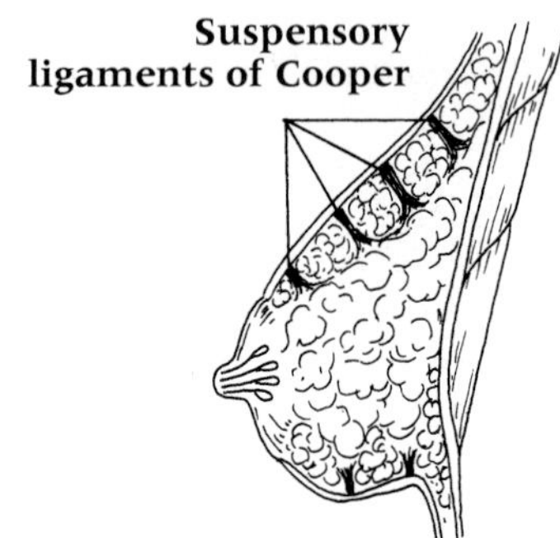

Figure 7-17

Stretching of Cooper's ligament causes premature sagging.

Hips and Buttocks

Pads in the region of the hips and buttocks are often needed in collision and high-velocity sports such as hockey and football. Other athletes needing protection in this region are amateur boxers, snow skiers, equestrians, jockeys, and water skiers. Two popular commercial pads are the girdle and belt types (Figure 7-20).

Groin and Genitalia

Sports involving high-velocity projectiles (e.g., hockey, lacrosse, and baseball) require cup protection for male participants. It comes as an off-the-shelf item that fits into place in a jockstrap, or athletic supporter (Figure 7-21 on page 202).

LOWER EXTREMITY PROTECTIVE EQUIPMENT

Footwear

It is essential that the athletic trainer and equipment personnel make every effort to fit their athletes with proper shoes and socks.

Socks

All athletic socks should be clean and dry and without holes. Socks of the wrong size can irritate the skin.

Poorly fitted socks can cause abnormal stresses on the foot. For example, socks that are too short crowd the toes, especially the fourth and fifth ones. Socks that are too long can wrinkle and cause skin irritation. All athletic socks should be clean, dry, and without holes to avoid irritations. Manufacturers are now providing different types of socks for various sports. The composition of the sock's material also should be noted. Cotton socks can be too bulky, whereas a combination of materials such as cotton and polyester is less bulky and dries faster.

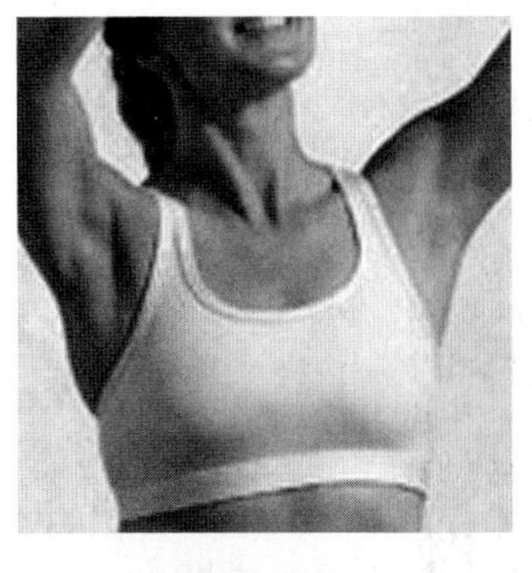
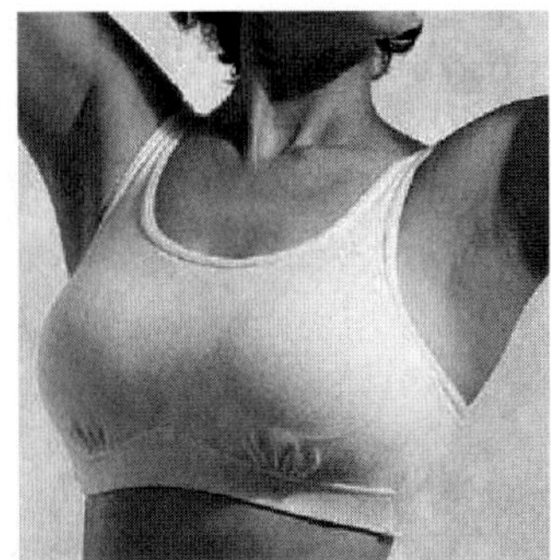
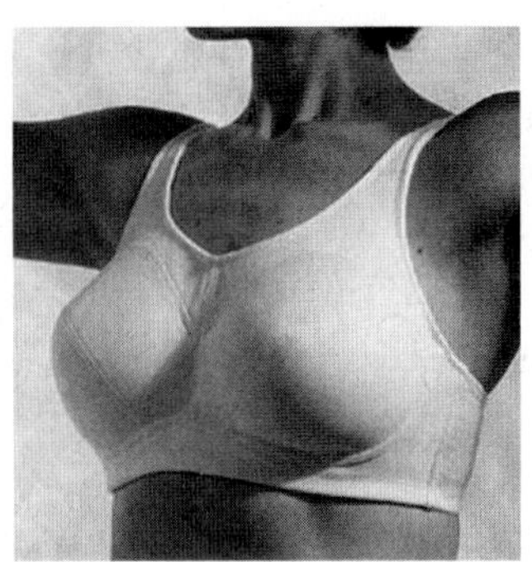
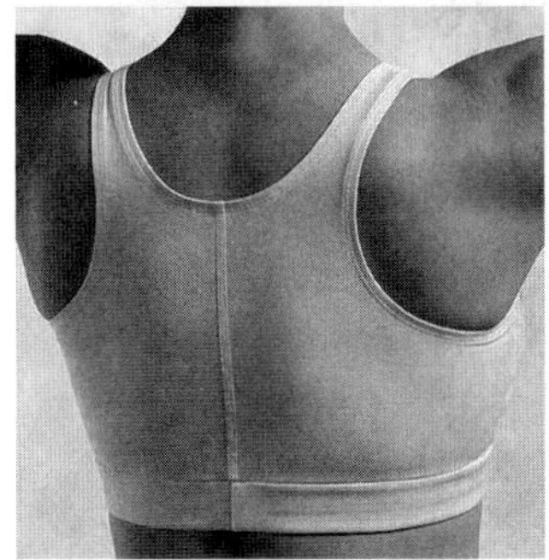
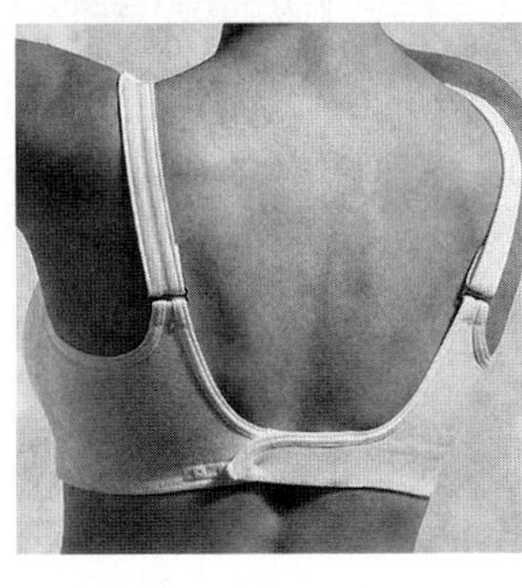
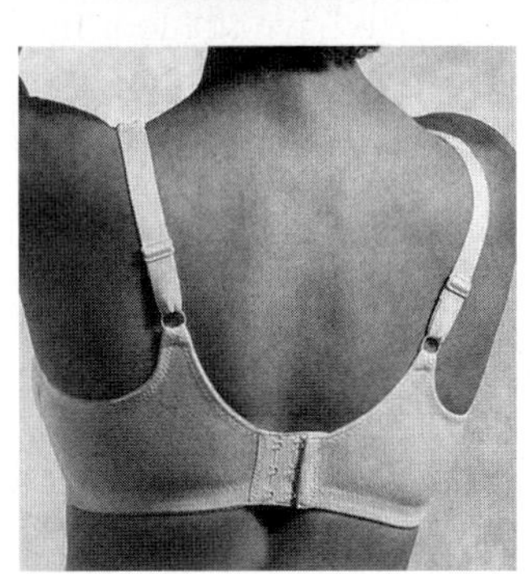
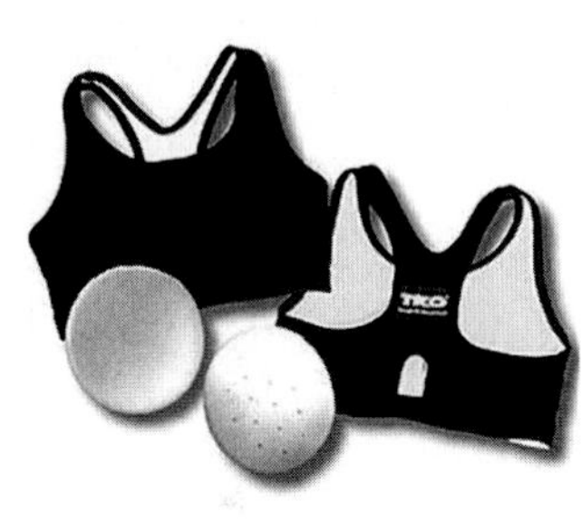

A B C D

Figure 7-18

Sports bras. **A,** Lightweight pullover bra. **B,** Compressive bra. **C,** Support bra with underwire. **D,** Protective sports bra with cup inserts.

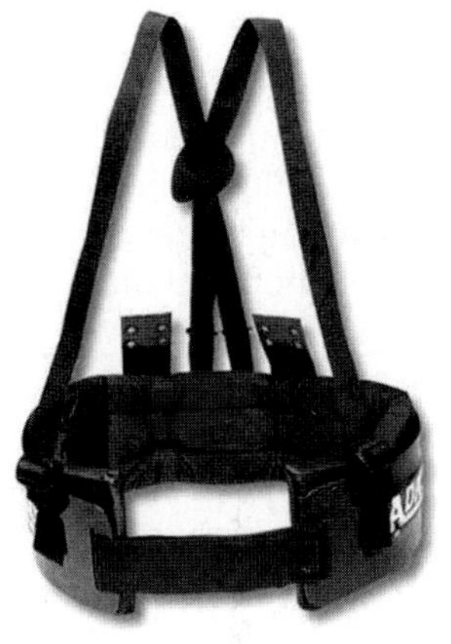
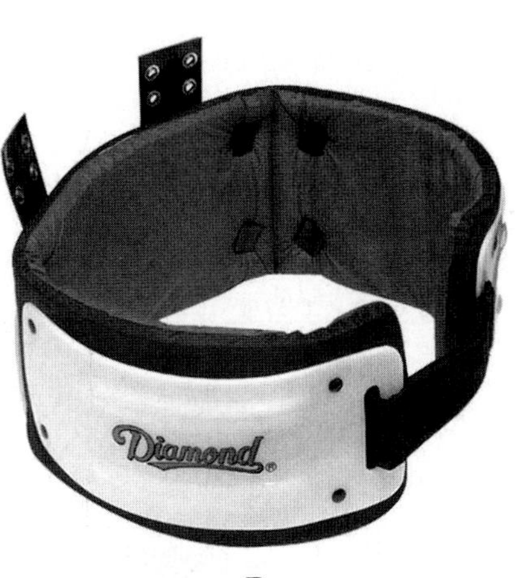

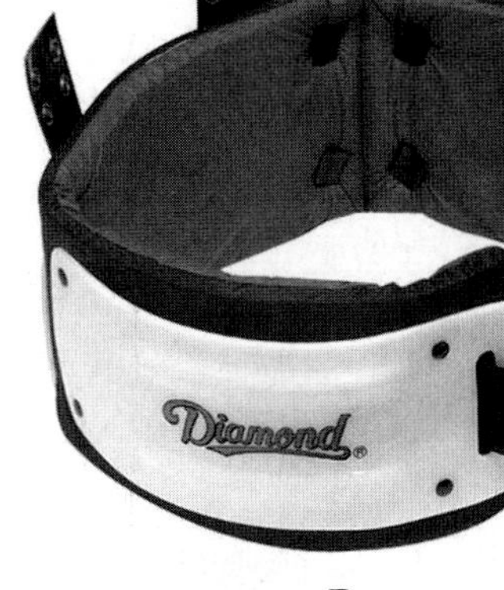

A B

Figure 7-19

Protective rib belts.

A B

Figure 7-20

Girdle-style hip and coccygeal pads.

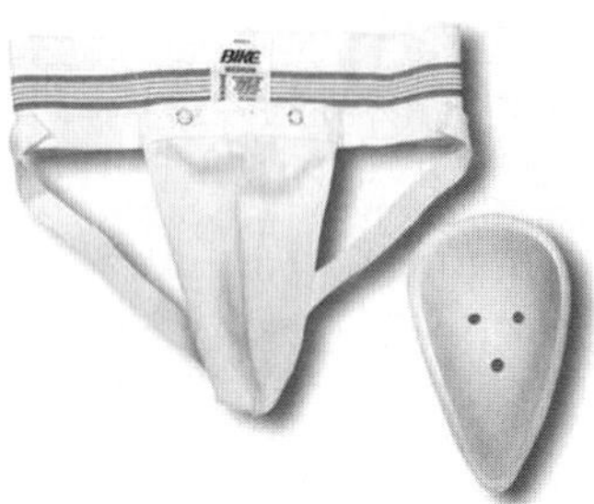

Figure 7-21

A cup, held in place by an athletic supporter, used for protecting the genitals against high-velocity projectiles.

Shoe Selection

The athletic and fitness shoe manufacturing industry has become extremely sophisticated and offers a number of options when it comes to purchasing shoes for different activities.[46] Figure 7-22 shows the major parts of a shoe. The following guidelines can help in selecting the most appropriate shoe:[13]

- *Toe Box.* There should be plenty of room for the toes in the fitness shoe. Most experts recommend a ½- to ¾-inch distance between the longest toe and the front of the shoe. A few fitness shoes are made in varying widths. If an athlete has a very wide or narrow foot, most shoe salespersons can recommend a specific shoe for that foot. The best way to make sure there is adequate room in the toe box is to have the foot measured and then try on the shoe.
- *Sole.* The sole should possess two qualities. First, it must provide a shock absorptive function; second, it must be durable. Most shoes have three layers on the sole: a thick, spongy layer, which absorbs the force of the foot strike under the heel; a midsole, which cushions the midfoot and toes; and a hard rubber layer, which comes in contact with the ground. The average runner's feet strike the ground between 1,500 and 1,700 times per mile. Thus it is essential that the force of the heel strike be absorbed by the spongy layer to prevent overuse injuries from occurring in the ankles and knees. Heel wedges are sometimes inserted either on the inside or outside surface of the sole underneath the heel counter to accommodate and correct for various structural deformities of the foot that may alter normal biomechanics of the running gait. A flared heel may be appropriate for running shoes but is not recommended in aerobic or court shoes. The sole must provide good traction and must be made of tough material that is resistant to wear. Most of the better-known brands of shoes have well-designed, long-lasting soles.
- *Heel counters.* The heel counter is the portion of the shoe that prevents the foot from rolling from side to side at heel strike. The heel counter should be firm but well fitted to minimize movement of the heel up and down or side to side. A good heel counter may prevent ankle sprains and painful blisters.
- *Shoe uppers.* The upper part of the shoe is made of some combination of nylon and leather. The uppers should be lightweight, quick drying, and well ventilated. The uppers should have some type of extra support in the saddle area, and there should be some extra padding in the area of the Achilles tendon just above the heel counter.

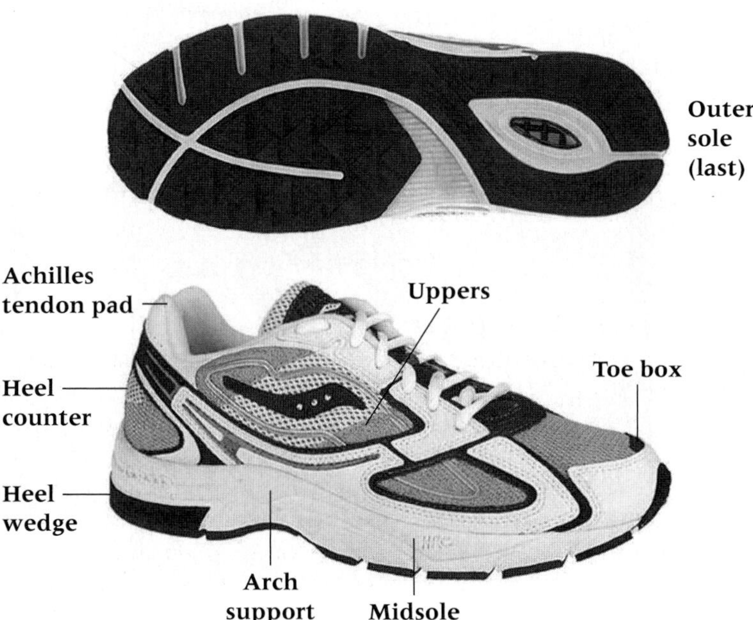

Figure 7-22

Parts of a well-designed sport shoe.

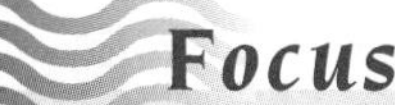

Focus

Proper running shoe design and construction

To avoid injury to the athlete, the running shoe should meet the following requirements:[21]

- Have a strong heel counter that fits well around the foot and locks the shoe around the foot.
- Always have good flexibility in the forefoot where toes bend.
- Preferably have a fairly high heel for the athlete with a tight Achilles tendon.
- Have a midsole that is moderately soft but does not flatten easily.
- Have a heel counter that is high enough to surround the foot but still allows room for an orthotic insert, if needed.
- Have a counter that is attached to the sole to avoid the possibility of it coming loose from its attachment.
- Always be of quality construction. A properly fitted shoe will bend where the foot bends.

- *Arch support.* The arch support should be made of some durable yet soft supportive material and should smoothly join with the insole. The support should not have any rough seams or ridges inside the shoe, which may cause blisters.
- *Price.* Unfortunately, in many instances price is the primary consideration in buying athletic shoes. When buying athletic shoes, remember that in many activities shoes are important for performance and prevention of injury. Thus it is worth a little extra investment to buy a quality pair of shoes.

Shoe fitting Fitting athletic shoes can be difficult.[6] Frequently the athlete's left foot varies in size and shape from the right foot. Therefore measuring both feet is imperative. To fit the sports shoe properly, the athlete should approximate the conditions under which he or she will perform, such as wearing athletic socks, jumping up and down, or running. It is also desirable to fit the athlete's shoes at the end of the day to accommodate the gradual increase in foot volume that occurs during weight-bearing. The athlete must carefully consider this shoe choice because he or she will be spending countless hours in those shoes (see *Focus Box:* "Proper running shoe design and construction" for suggestions about shoe fitting).[16]

7-5

Critical Thinking Exercise

A high school basketball player asks the athletic trainer for advice on purchasing a pair of basketball shoes.

? What fitting factors must be taken into consideration when purchasing basketball shoes?

During performance conditions the new shoe should feel snug but not too tight. The sports shoe should be long enough that all toes can be fully extended without being cramped. Its width should permit full movement of the toes, including flexion, extension, and some spreading. A good point to remember is that the wide part of the shoe should match the wide part of the foot to allow the shoe to crease evenly when the athlete is on the balls of the feet. The shoe should bend (or "break") at its widest part; when the break of the shoe and the ball joint coincide, the fit is correct. However, if the break of the shoe is in back of or in front of the normal bend of the foot (metatarsophalangeal joint), the shoe and the foot will oppose one another, causing abnormal skin and structural stresses to occur. Two measurements must be considered when fitting shoes: (1) the distance from the heel to the metatarsophalangeal joint and (2) the distance from the heel to the end of the longest toe. An individual's feet may be equal in length from the heels to the balls of the feet but different between the heels and the toes. One type of shoe is not appropriate for all athletes in a particular sport. Shoes therefore should be selected for the longer of the two measurements. Other factors to consider when buying the sports shoe are the stiffness of the sole and the width of the shank, or narrowest part of the sole. A shoe with a sole that is too rigid and nonyielding places a great deal of extra strain on the foot tendons. A shoe with a shank that is too narrow also causes extra strain because it fails to adequately support the athlete's inner, longitudinal arches.[46] Lacing techniques can help adjust the width of the shoe to the foot. *Focus Box:* "Shoe lacing techniques" provides some

A properly fitted shoe will bend where the foot bends

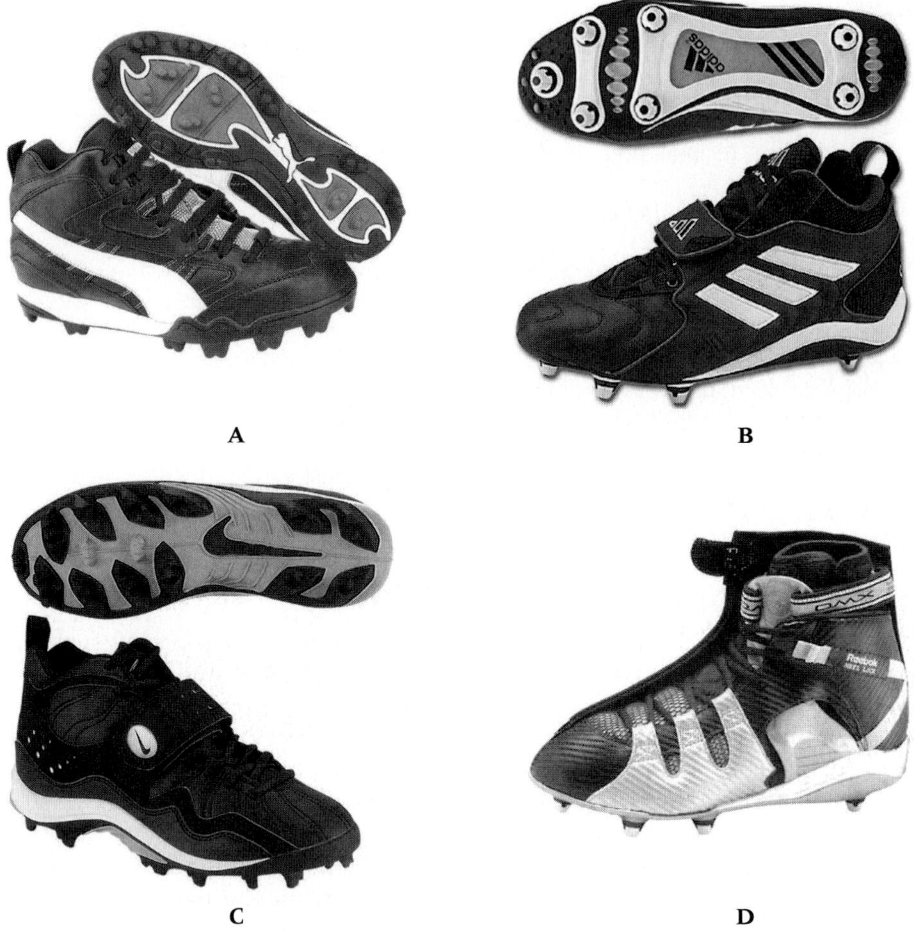

Figure 7-23

Variations in cleated shoes: the longer the cleat, the higher the incidence of injury.

suggestions for alternative lacing techniques. Two other shoe features to consider are insoles to reduce friction and arch supports.

The cleated shoe The cleated shoe presents some additional fitting problems. For example, American football uses the multi–short-cleated, soccer-type polyurethane sole with cleats no longer than ½ inch (1.27 cm) (Figure 7-23). Specially soled shoes are also worn when playing on a synthetic surface. Whenever cleated shoes are used, the cleats must be properly positioned under the two major weight-bearing joints and must not be felt through the soles of the shoes (see Table 7-1 for shoe comparisons).[46]

TABLE 7-1 Shoe Comparisons

	Tennis	Aerobic	Running
Flexibility	Firm sole, more rigid than running shoe	Sole between running and tennis shoe	Flexible ball of foot
Uppers	Leather or leather with nylon	Leather or leather with nylon	Nylon or nylon mesh
Heel flare	None	Very little	Flared for stability
Cushioning	Less than a running shoe	Between running and tennis shoe	Heel and sole well padded
Soles	Polyurethane	Rubber or polyurethane	Carbon-based material for greater durability
Tread	Flattened	Flat or pivot dot	Deep grooves for grip

Foot Orthotics

An orthotic is a device for correcting biomechanical problems that exist in the foot that can potentially cause an injury.[19,53] The orthotic is a plastic, thermoplastic, rubber, sorbethane, or leather support that is placed in the shoe as a replacement for the existing insole.[41] Ready-made orthotics can be purchased in sporting goods or shoe stores. Some athletes need orthotics that are custom made by a physician, podiatrist, athletic trainer, or physical therapist. These are more expensive but can be well worth the expense if the athlete's feet cause pain and discomfort, especially when exercising (Figure 7-24).

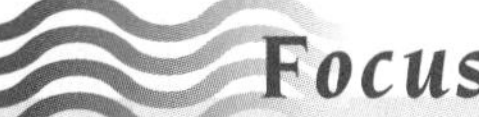

Shoe lacing techniques

A shoe that doesn't fit just right may be adjusted to provide a more secure, comfortable, and supportive fit by using specific lacing techniques to accommodate a narrow heel, a high/low arch, or a wider foot. Athletic shoes with a large number of eyelets make it easier to adjust the laces for a custom fit.

Narrow foot or heel (Technique A)

If the shoe has two rows of eyelets that appear to zig-zag use the row furthest from the tongue tightening from the outer eyelets and pulling the body of the shoe towards the center. If there is only one row of eyelets, follow a normal lacing pattern up to the last pair of holes. At the last hole, tighten the laces and thread into the last hole leaving a loop on each side. Cross the laces and thread them each through the loop on the other side before tightening and tying.

Wide Foot (Technique B)

If the shoe has two rows of eyelets that appear to zig-zag use the row closest to the tongue. If there is only a single row, thread laces through the first set of eyelets and then straight up each side without criss-crossing at all. Continue this way for two or three holes until the laces are above the forefoot and can tighten without squeezing. Then begin criss-crossing and finish lacing as normal.

Low Arch (pes planus) (Technique C)

Beginning at the bottom, criss-cross lace shoes as normal halfway up the eyelets. Use the loop lacing technique used for a narrow heel the rest of the way.

High arches (pes cavus) (Technique D)

Begin lacing as normal, criss-crossing and stopping after the first set of holes. Thread laces straight up each side, criss-crossing only before threading the last hole.

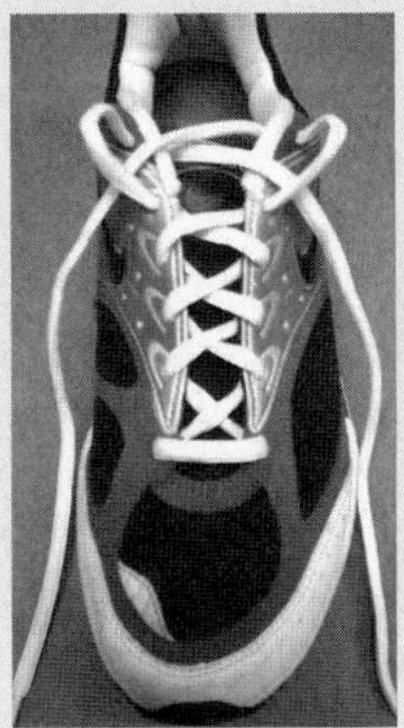

A

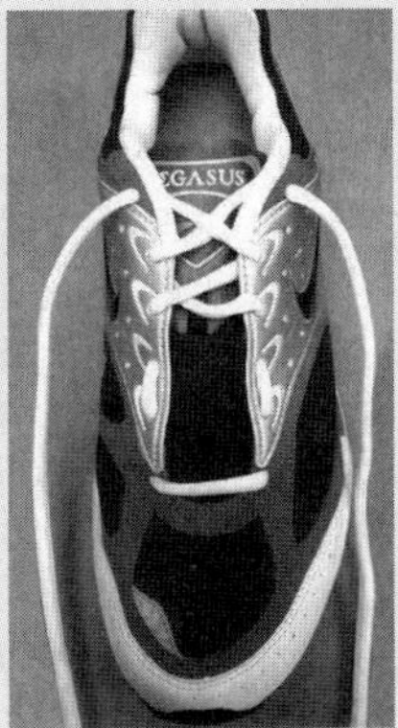

B

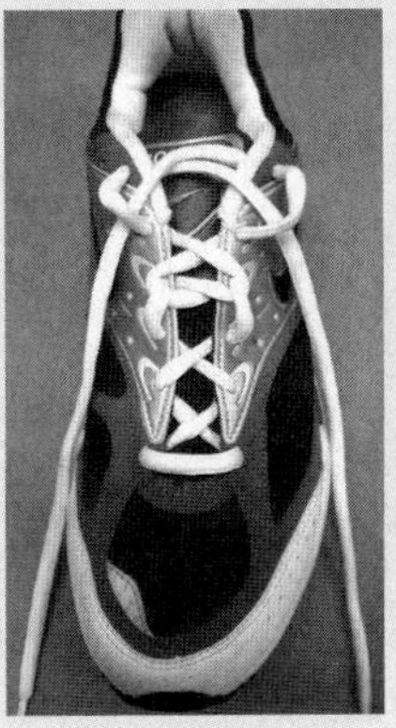

C

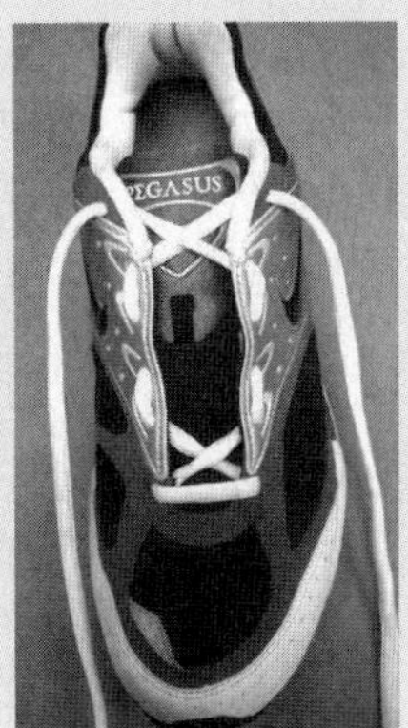

D

Figure 7-24

Commercially manufactured orthotic devices.

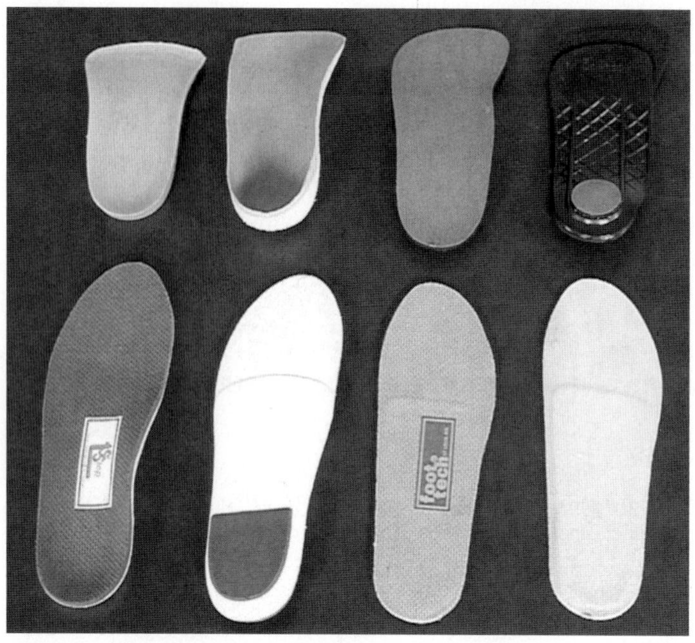

Figure 7-25

Heel cups and pads, including lifts of orthotic felt.

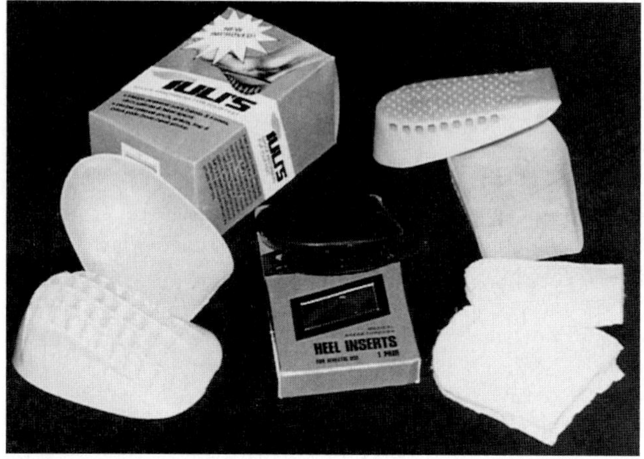

Heel Cups

Heel cups should be used for a variety of conditions including plantar fasciitis, a heel spur, Achilles tendonitis, and heel bursitis (Figure 7-25). Heel cups may be either hard plastic or spongy rubber. The heel cup helps to compress the fat pad under the heel, providing more heel cushioning during weight-bearing activities.

Off-the-Shelf Foot Pads

Indiscriminate use of commercial foot orthotics may give the athlete a false sense of security.

Off-the-shelf foot pads are intended for use by the general public and are not usually designed to withstand the rigors of sports activities. Off-the-shelf pads that are suited for sports are generally not durable enough for hard, extended use. If money is no object, the ready-made off-the-shelf pad, which is replaced more often, has the advantage of saving time. Off-the-shelf pads are manufactured for almost every type of common structural foot condition, ranging from corns and bunions to fallen arches and pronated feet. Off-the-shelf foot pads are commonly used before more customized orthotic devices are made. These products offer a compromise to the custom-made foot orthotics by providing some biomechanical control.[16] Indiscriminate use of these

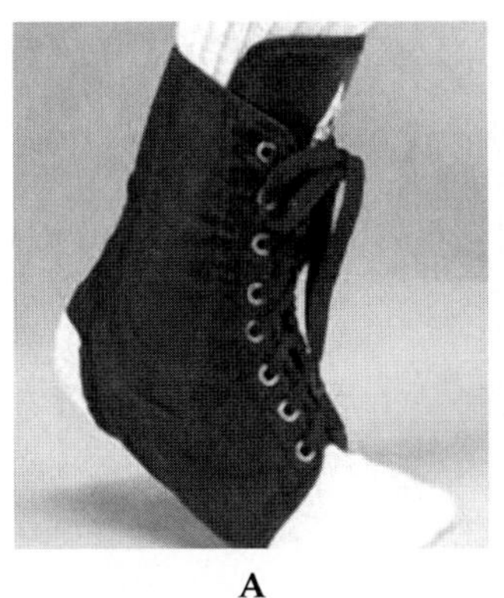
A

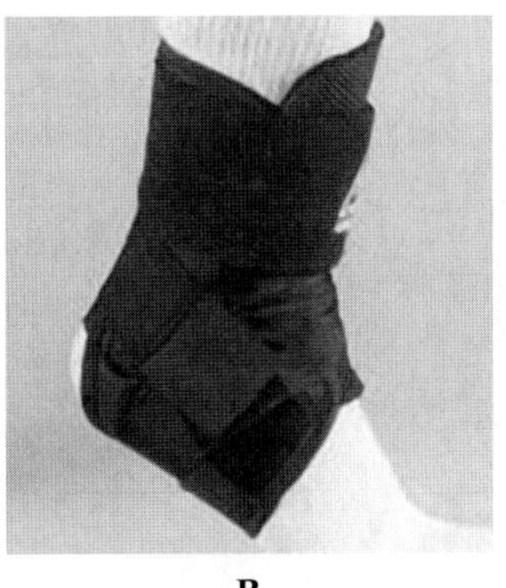
B

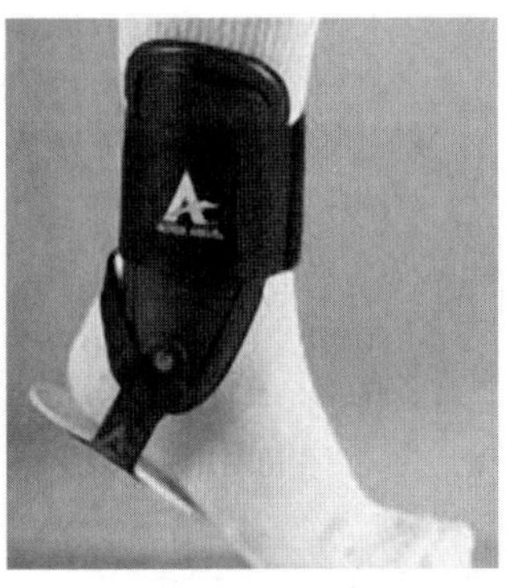
C

Figure 7-26

Commercial ankle supports for an injured ankle. **A,** Lace up brace. **B,** Lace up with straps brace. **C,** Rigid support brace.

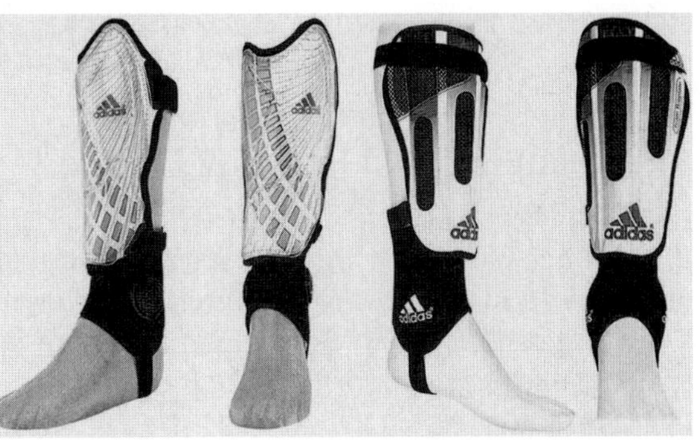

Figure 7-27

Soccer shin guards.

aids, however, may intensify the pathological condition or cause the athlete to delay seeing the team physician or team podiatrist for evaluation.[24]

For the most part, foot devices are fabricated and customized from a variety of materials such as foam, felt, plaster, aluminum, and spring steel (see the section titled "Construction of Protective and Supportive Devices," later in this chapter).

Ankle Supports

Ankle stabilizers, either alone or in combination with ankle taping, are becoming increasingly popular in sports (Figure 7-26).[14,58] There has been significant debate regarding the efficacy of ankle supports in the prevention of ankle sprains.[15,27] Most studies indicate that bracing is effective in reducing ankle injury,[33,43,50] while other studies have shown no effects[7,21] or even negative effects.[34,37] Bracing probably has little or no effect on performance; any change in performance is due to the athlete's perception of support and comfort.[3] When compared with ankle taping, these devices do not loosen significantly during exercise.[14,54] Recent studies have focused on the proprioceptive effects and how ankle braces influence balance, postural sway, and joint position sense.[22,29,56]

7-6

***Critical Thinking* Exercise**

A basketball player with a history of ankle sprains needs support during practice.

? Which type of ankle support is cost-efficient and most reliable: tape or commercial supports?

Shin and Lower Leg

The shin is an area of the body that is commonly neglected in contact and collision sports. Commercially marketed hard-shelled, molded shin guards are used in field hockey and soccer (Figure 7-27).

Thigh and Upper Leg

Thigh and upper leg protection is necessary in collision sports such as hockey, football, and soccer. Generally, pads slip into ready-made pockets in the uniform (Figure 7-28A). In some instances, customized pads should be constructed and held in place with tape or an elastic wrap. Neoprene sleeves can be used for support following strain to the hamstring, groin, or quadriceps muscles (Figure 7-28B).

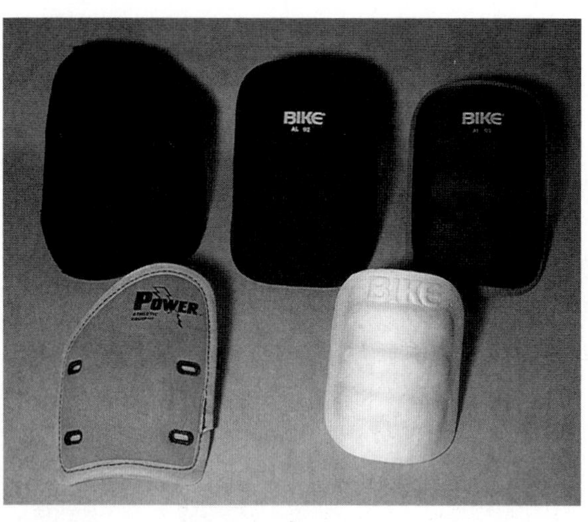

A

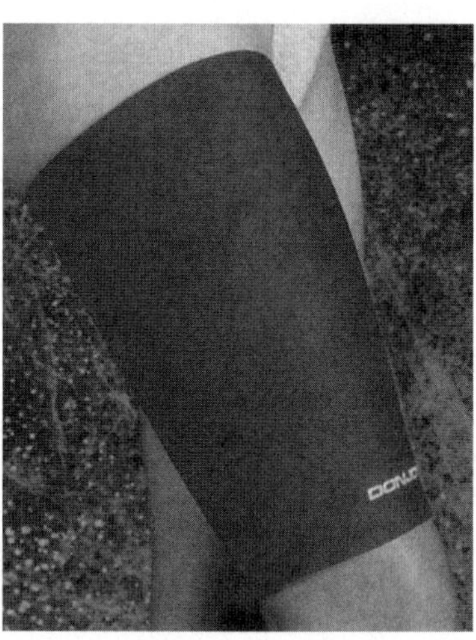

B

Figure 7-28

A, Protective thigh pads.
B, Neoprene thigh sleeve.

Knee Supports and Protective Devices

Knee Pads

Elastic knee pads or guards are extremely valuable in sports in which the athlete falls or receives a direct blow to the anterior aspect of the knee. An elastic sleeve containing a resilient pad may help dissipate an anterior striking force but fails to protect the knee against lateral, medial, or twisting forces.

Knee Braces

Because of the high incidence of injury to the knee joint, manufacturers have designed a host of different knee braces for a variety of purposes.[49] *Protective knee braces* are used prophylactically to prevent injuries to the medial collateral ligament in contact sports such as football (Figure 7-29A).[39,48] Although these protective braces have been widely used in the past, the American Orthopedic Society for Sports Medicine has expressed concern about their efficacy in reducing injuries to the collateral ligaments. Several studies have actually shown an increase in the incidence of injuries to the medial collateral ligament in athletes wearing these braces.[48] Others have shown a positive influence on joint position sense[28] but little or no effect on performance.[21]

Rehabilitative braces are widely used following surgical repair or reconstruction of the knee joint to allow for controlled progressive immobilization (Figure 7-29B).[4] These braces have hinges that can be easily adjusted to allow range of motion to be progressively increased over time.

Functional knee braces may be worn both during and following the rehabilitative period to provide support during functional activities (Figure 7-29C).[1,11] Functional braces can be purchased ready made or can be custom made.[52] Some physicians strongly recommend that their patients consistently[38] wear these braces during physical activity, whereas others do not feel that they are necessary.[10,57]

Neoprene braces with medial and lateral supports may be used by individuals who have sustained injury to the collateral ligaments and feel that they need extra support medially and laterally (Figure 7-29D).

A variety of *neoprene sleeves* may also be used to provide some support for patellofemoral conditions (Figure 7-29E).[5]

ELBOW, WRIST, AND HAND PROTECTION

As with the lower extremity, the upper extremity requires protection from injury and prevention of further injury after trauma. Although the elbow joint is less commonly injured than the ankle, knee, or shoulder, it is still vulnerable to instability, contusion, and muscle strain. A variety of off-the-shelf protective neoprene sleeves and pads and hinged adjustable rehabilitative braces can offer protection to the elbow (Figure 7-30).[45]

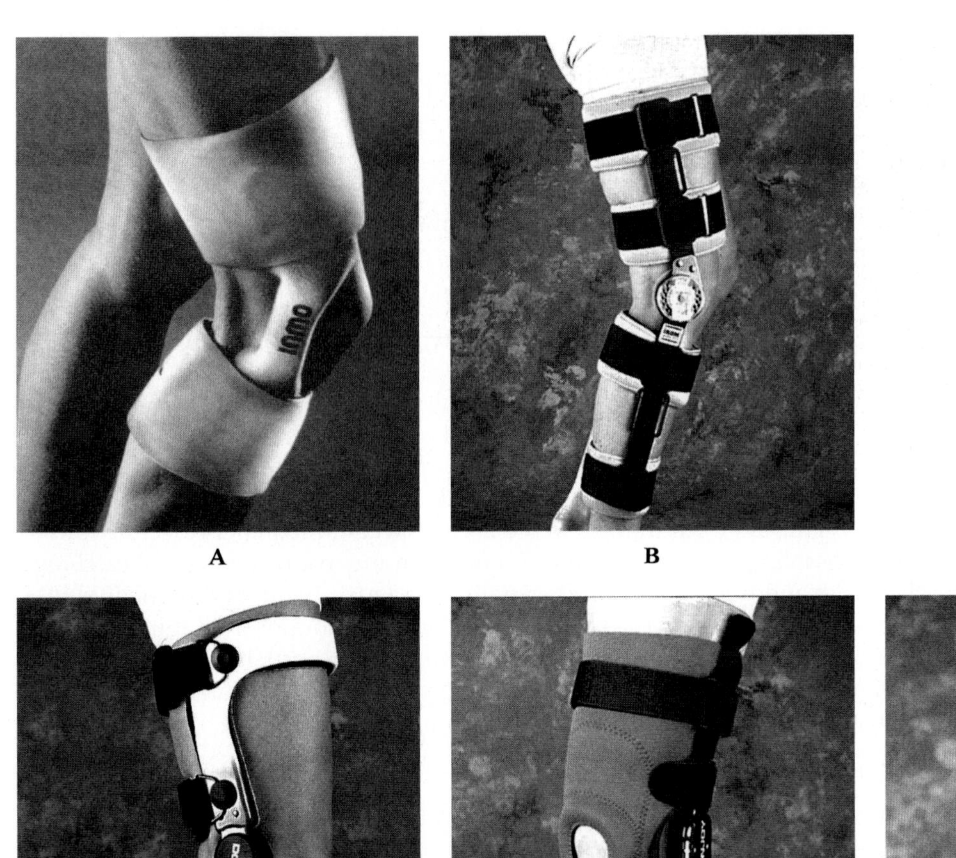

A B C D E

Figure 7-29

Knee braces. **A,** Prophylactic knee brace. **B,** Rehabilitative brace. **C,** Functional brace. **D,** Neoprene with medial support-brace. **E,** Neoprene brace.

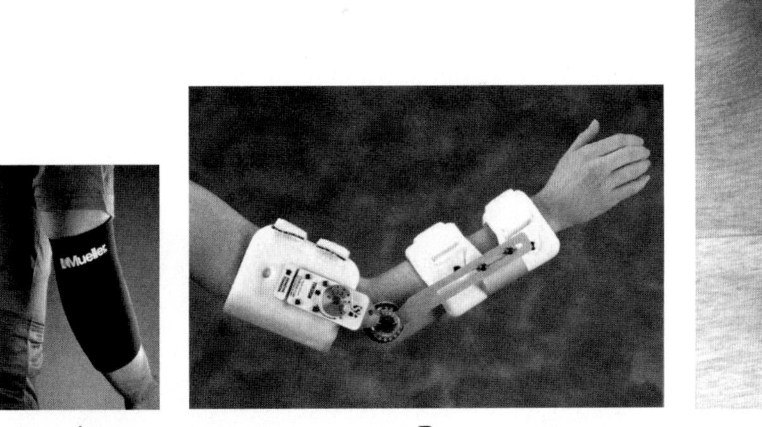

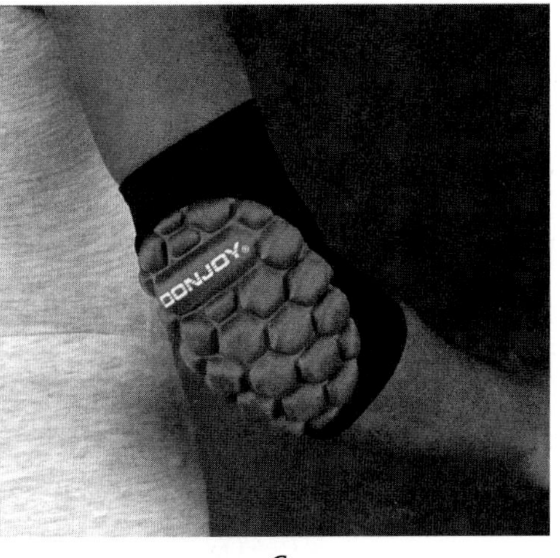

A B C

Figure 7-30

A, Neoprene elbow sleeve. **B,** Hinged rehabilitative elbow brace. **C,** Elbow pad.

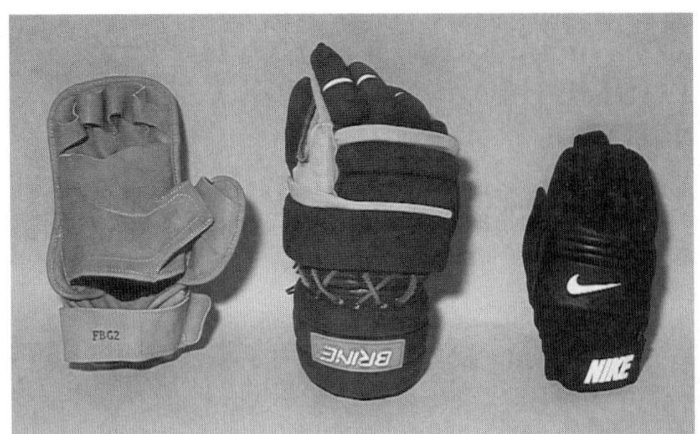

Figure 7-31

The hand is an often neglected area of the body in sports.

In sports medicine, injuries to the wrist, hand, and fingers are often trivialized and considered insignificant. But injuries to the distal aspect of the upper extremity can be functionally disabling, especially in those sports that involve throwing and catching.[1] In both contact and noncontact sport activities the wrist, hand, and particularly the fingers are susceptible to fracture, dislocation, ligament sprains, and muscle strains. Protective gloves are essential in preventing injuries in sports like lacrosse and ice hockey (Figure 7-31). It is also common to use both off-the-shelf and custom-molded splints both for support and to immobilize an injury.

CONSTRUCTION OF PROTECTIVE AND SUPPORTIVE DEVICES

The athletic trainer should be able to design and construct protective and supportive devices when necessary. Certainly the athletic trainer must understand the theoretical basis for constructing protective pads and supports. However, the ability to construct an effective and appropriate protective device is more of an art than a science.

Custom Pad and Orthotic Materials

Many different materials are available to the athletic trainer attempting to protect or support an injured area. In general, these materials can be divided into soft and hard materials (Figure 7-32).

Soft Materials

The primary soft-material media found in athletic training rooms are cotton, gauze pads, adhesive felt or adhesive foam rubber felt, and an assortment of foam rubber.

Gauze padding is less versatile than other pad materials. It is assembled in varying thicknesses and can be used as an absorbent or protective pad.

Cotton is probably the cheapest and most widely used material in sports. It has the ability to absorb, to hold emollients, and to offer a mild padding effect.

Adhesive felt (moleskin) or *sponge rubber* material contains an adhesive mass on one side, thus combining a cushioning effect with the ability to be held in a specific spot by the adhesive mass. It is a versatile material that is useful on all body parts.

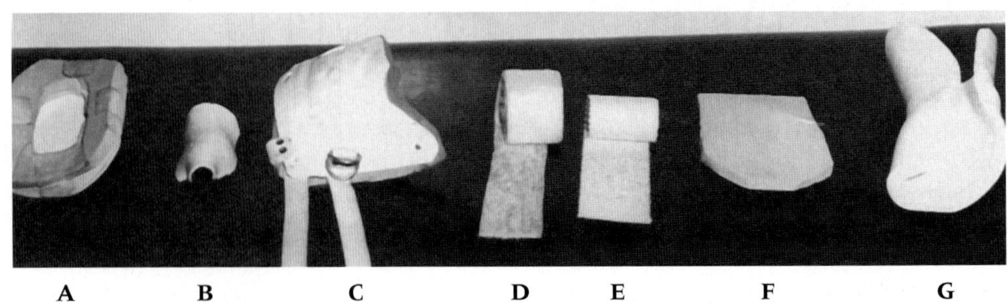

Figure 7-32

Types of sports orthoses. **A,** Orthoplast with a foam rubber doughnut. **B,** Orthoplast splint. **C,** Orthoplast rib protector with a foam rubber pad. **D,** Fiberglass material for splint construction. **E,** Plaster of paris material for cast construction. **F,** Foam rubber pad. **G,** Aloplast foam moldable material for protective pad construction.

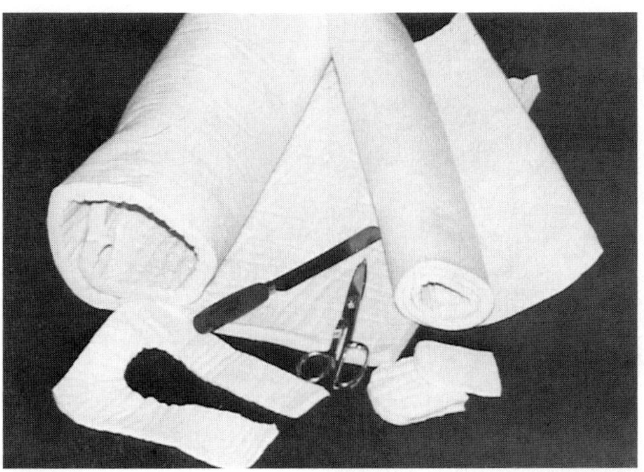

Figure 7-33

Orthopedic felt, both ½- and ¼-inch wide, with broad-blade knife and large scissors for contouring.

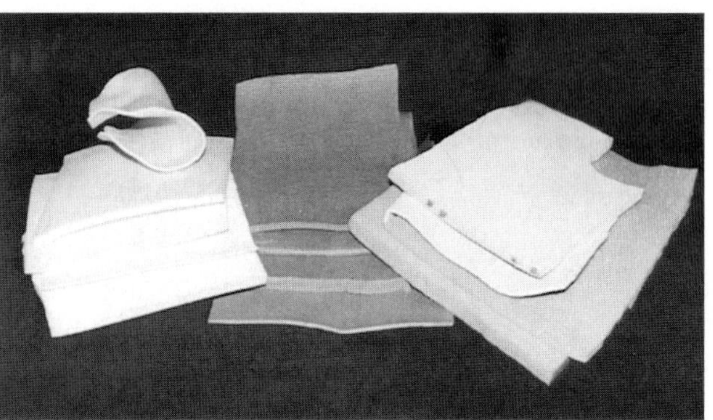

Figure 7-34

Foam assortment: *left,* thermomoldable; *center,* closed celled; *right,* open celled.

Felt is a material composed of matted wool fibers pressed into varying thicknesses that range from ¼ to 1 inch (0.6 to 2.5 cm). Its benefit lies in its comfortable, semiresilient surface, which gives a firmer pressure than most sponge rubbers. Because felt absorbs perspiration, it clings to the skin, and it has less tendency to move than sponge rubber does (Figure 7-33). Because of its absorbent qualities, felt should be replaced daily. Currently, it is most often used as support and protection for a variety of foot conditions.

Foams are currently the materials most often used for providing injury protection in sports. They come in many different thicknesses and densities (Figure 7-34). They are usually resilient, nonabsorbent, and able to protect the body against compressive forces. Some foams are open celled, whereas others are closed. The closed-cell type is preferable in sports because it rebounds and returns to its original shape quickly. Foams can be easily worked through cutting, shaping, and faceting. Some foams are thermomoldable and, when heated, become highly pliant and easy to shape. When cooled, they retain the shape in which they were formed. A new class of foams are composed of viscoelastic polymers. Sorbothane is one example. This foam has a high energy-absorbing quality, but it also has a high density, making it heavy. Used in inner soles in sports shoes, foam helps prevent blisters and also effectively absorbs anterior/posterior and medial/lateral ground reaction forces. Foams generally range from ⅛ to ½ inch (0.3 to 1.25 cm) in thickness.

Nonyielding Materials

A number of hard, nonyielding materials are used in athletic training for making protective shells and splints.

Thermomoldable plastics Plastic materials are widely used in sports medicine for customized orthotics. They can brace, splint, and shield a body area. They can provide casting for a fracture; support for a foot defect; or a firm, nonyielding surface to protect a severe contusion.

Plastics used for these purposes differ in their chemical composition and reaction to heat. The three major categories are heat-forming plastics, heat-setting plastics, and heat-plastic foams.

Heat-forming plastics are of the low-temperature variety and are the most popular in athletic training. When heated to 140° to 180°F (60° to 82.2°C), depending on the material, the plastic can be accurately molded to a body part. Aquaplast (polyester sheets) and Orthoplast (synthetic rubber thermoplast) are popular types.

Heat-forming plastics of the low-temperature variety are the most popular in athletic training.

Heat-setting plastics require relatively higher temperatures for shaping. They are rigid and difficult to form, usually requiring a mold rather than being formed directly

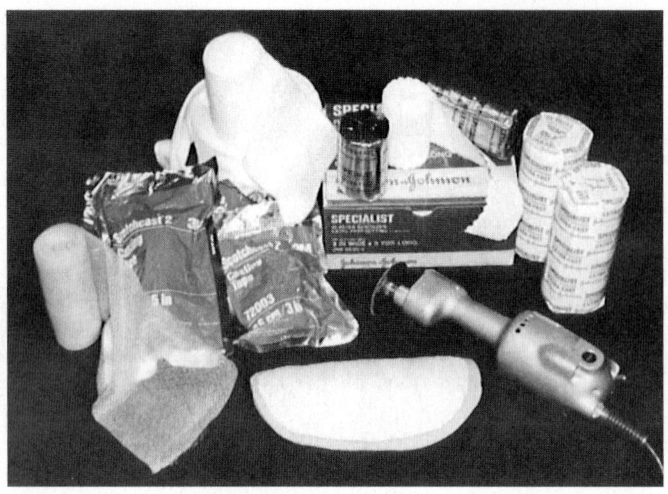

Figure 7-35

Casting material: *left*, fiberglass; *right*, plaster including cast saw used to trim pictured shin guard.

to the body part. High-impact vinyl (polyvinyl chloride), Kydex (polyvinyl chloride acrylic), and Nyloplex (heat-plastic acrylic) are examples of the more commonly used thermoforming plastics.

Heat-plastic foams are plastics that have differences in density as a result of the addition of liquids, gas, or crystals. They are commonly used as shoe inserts and other body padding. Aloplast and Plastazote (polyethylene foams) are two commonly used products.

Usually the plastic is heated until soft and malleable. It is then molded into the desired shape and allowed to cool, thereby retaining its shape. Various pads and other materials can also be fastened in place. The rules and regulations of various sport activities may place limitations on the use of rigid thermomoldable plastics.

Casting materials Applying casts to injured body areas has long been a practice in sports medicine. The material of choice is fiberglass, which uses resin and a catalytic converter, plus water, to produce hardening. Besides casts, this material makes effective shells for splints and protective pads. Once hardened, the fiberglass is trimmed to shape with a cast saw (Figure 7-35).

Tools Used for Customizing

Many different tools are needed to work with the various materials used to customize protective equipment. These tools include adhesives, adhesive tapes, heat sources, and shaping tools.

Adhesives A number of adhesives are used in constructing custom protective equipment. Many cements and glues join plastic to plastic or join other combinations of materials.

Adhesive tape Adhesive tape is a major tool in holding various materials in place. Linen and elastic tape can hold pads to a rigid backing or to adhesive felt (moleskin) and can be used to protect against sharp edges (see Chapter 8).

Heat sources To form thermomoldable plastics, a heat source must be available. Three sources are commonly found in training rooms: the commercial moist heat unit, a hot air gun or hair dryer, and a convection oven with a temperature control. The usual desired temperature is 160° F (71° C) or higher.

Shaping tools Commonly, the tools required to shape custom devices are heavy-duty scissors, sharp-blade knives, and cast saws.

Fastening material Once formed, customized protective equipment often must be secured in place. Fastening this equipment requires the availability of a great variety of different materials. For example, if something is to be held securely, Velcro can be used when a device must be continually put on and removed. Leather can be cut and riveted in place to form hinge straps with buckles attached. Various types of laces can

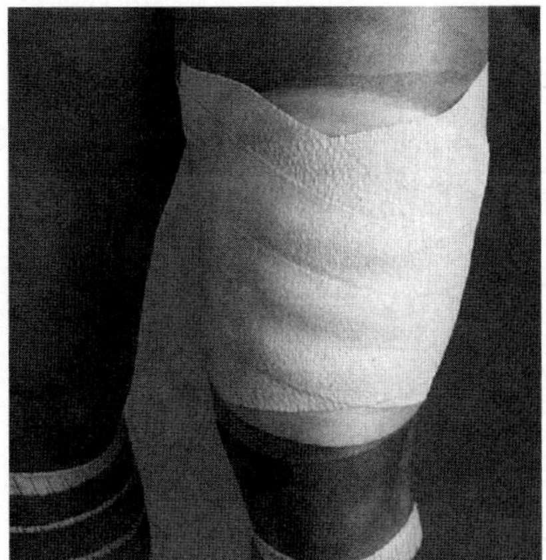

Figure 7-36

Hard shell pad wrapped on the thigh.

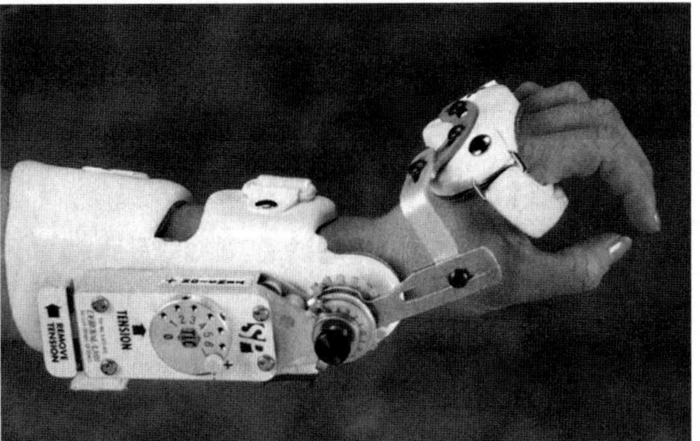

Figure 7-37

A dynamic splint for the hand and fingers.

be laced through eyelets to hold something in place. Tools that allow for this type of construction include a portable drill, a hole punch, and an ice pick.

Customized Hard-Shell Pads

A hard-shell pad is often required for an athlete who has acquired an injury, such as a painful contusion (bruise), that must be completely protected from further injury. *Focus Box:* "How to construct a hard-shell pad" provides the procedures needed to customize such a pad (Figure 7-36).

Dynamic Splints

Occasionally it is necessary to fabricate and apply a dynamic splint in treating injuries to the hand and fingers (Figure 7-37). Most often, an occupational therapist would make a dynamic splint; however, the athletic trainer is certainly capable of designing such a splint. A dynamic splint is used to provide long-duration tension on a healing structure (usually a tendon) so that it can return to normal function. Dynamic splints use a combination of thermoplastic material, Velcro, and pieces of rubber band or elastic to provide dynamic assistance.

7-7

***Critical Thinking* Exercise**

A soccer player has incurred a number of contusions to the right quadriceps muscle.

? How does the athletic trainer customize a hard-shell protective thigh pad for the soccer player?

Focus

How to construct a hard-shell pad

1. Select proper material and tools, which might include
   a. Thermomoldable plastic sheet (Orthoplast, Hexalite)
   b. Scissors
   c. Felt material
2. Palpate and mark the margins of the tender area that needs protection.
3. Cut a felt piece to fit in the area of tenderness.
4. Heat plastic until malleable.
5. Place heated plastic over felt and wrap in place with an elastic wrap.
6. When cooled, remove elastic wrap and felt pad.
7. Trim shell to desired shape; a protective shell has now been made to provide a "bubble" relief.
8. If needed, add a softer inner layer of foam to distribute and lessen force further.
   a. Cut a doughnut-type hole in softer foam material the same size as the injury site.
   b. Cut foam the same shape as the hard shell.
   c. Use tape or an adhesive to affix the foam to the shell.

SUMMARY

- The proper selection and proper fitting of sports equipment are essential in the prevention of many sports injuries. Because of the number of current litigations, sports equipment standards regarding the durability of the material and the fit and wear requirements of the equipment are of serious concern. Manufacturers must foresee all possible uses and misuses of their equipment and warn the user of any potential risks.
- Sports professionals must be concerned about head protection in many collision and contact sports. The football helmet must be used only for its intended purpose and not as a weapon. To avoid unwarranted litigation, a warning label must be placed on the outside of the helmet indicating that the helmet is not fail-safe and must be used as intended. Properly fitting the helmet is of critical importance.
- Face protection is of major importance in sports that have fast-moving projectiles, use implements that are in close proximity to other athletes, and facilitate body collisions. Protecting teeth and eyes is of particular significance. The customized mouth guard, fitted to individual requirements, provides the best protection for the teeth and also protects against concussions. Eyes must be protected against projectiles and sports implements. The safest eye guard for the athlete wearing contact lenses or glasses is the closed type that completely protects the orbital cavity.
- Many sports require protection of various parts of the athlete's body. American football players, ice hockey players, and baseball catchers are examples of players who require body protection. Commonly, the protection is for the shoulders, chest, thighs, ribs, hips, buttocks, groin, genitalia (male athletes), and breasts (female athletes).
- Footwear is essential to prevent injuries. Socks must be clean, without holes, and made of appropriate materials. Shoes must be suited to the sport and must be properly fitted. The wide part of the foot must match the wide part of the shoe. If the shoe has cleats, they must be positioned at the metatarsophalangeal joints.
- Currently, there are many off-the-shelf pieces of specialized, protective equipment on the market. They may be designed to support ankles, knees, or other body parts. In addition to stock equipment, athletic trainers often construct customized equipment out of a variety of materials to pad injuries or support feet. Professionals such as orthopedists and podiatrists may devise orthopedic footwear and orthotic devices to improve the biomechanics of the athlete's foot.

Websites

Riddell: http://riddell.com/

Riddell is an equipment manufacturing company, and this site gives information about the safety of the products they sell and the necessary standards for safety equipment.

Healthyway Sporting Protective Eyewear: http://www.hb.sympatico.ca/contentshealth/HEALTHYWAY/archive/feature_vis3c.html

This site emphasizes the importance of protective eyewear for young athletes and provides links to related informative sites.

National Operating Committee on Standards for Athletic Equipment: http://www.nocsae.org

National Institute for Sports Science and Safety (NISSS): http://www.nisss.org/

Provides information on research, design, and testing of sports equipment and sports protective equipment.

The Training Room: http://www.thetrainingroom.com

Provides information on sports orthopedic braces, orthotics, protective sports equipment, and athletic injury treatment.

Athletic Protective Equipment: http://www.rapidwear.com/

Provides information on a variety of protective equipment.

Douglas Protective Equipment: http://www.douglaspads.com/

Manufacturer and distributor of football, hockey, and baseball protective padding. Custom fitting players at all levels for over twelve years.

The Sports Authority: http://www.thesportsauthority.com

Provides a wide selection of protective equipment for virtually all sports.

Solutions to Critical Thinking EXERCISES

7-1 The athletic training student must acquire the following protective equipment competencies:

- Identify good-quality and poor-quality commercial protective equipment
- Properly fit commercial protective equipment
- Construct protective and supportive devices

7-2 The athletic trainer should initiate the following steps:

1. Call a team meeting in which he or she fully explains the risks entailed in the use and fitting of the equipment.
2. Report and repair any defective pieces of equipment are immediately.
3. Send out a letter to each parent or guardian explaining equipment limitations. This letter must be signed and returned to the athletic trainer.
4. Call a meeting of parents, team members, and coaches in which he or she further explains equipment limitations.

7-3 The athletic trainer explains that the helmet cannot prevent serious neck injuries. Striking an opponent with any part of the helmet or face mask can place abnormal stress on cervical structures. Most severe neck injuries occur from striking an opponent with the top of the helmet; this action is known as axial loading.

7-4 Mouth guards serve several important purposes in preventing injury in athletics, especially contact sports such as ice hockey. Mouth guards help to prevent or minimize lacerations, fractures, and possibly reduce the incidence of cerebral concussions. For a mouth guard to work effectively, proper fit is essential and needs to not interfere with breathing or speech. A custom fabricated mouth guard is produced from a mold of each individual athlete causing the fit to be more precise. If the fit is improved, athletes are more likely to wear their mouth guards.

7-5 The athletic trainer provides the following advice:

- Shoes should be purchased to fit the larger foot.
- Athlete should wear athletic socks when fitting shoes.
- Shoes should be purchased at the end of the day.
- Shoes should feel snug but comfortable when the athlete jumps up and down and performs cutting motions.
- Shoe length and width should allow full toe function.
- Wide part of foot should match wide part of shoe.
- Shoe should bend at its widest part.
- Each foot should be measured from the heel to the end of the largest toe.

7-6 A verified commercial ankle support provides more consistent support for a longer period of time and is more cost-efficient.

7-7 To construct a hard-shell protective thigh pad, the athletic trainer follows these steps:

1. Mark the area on the athlete to be protected.
2. Cut a foam piece to temporarily cover the injury.
3. Heat thermomoldable plastic and place over the foam piece to form a bubble.
4. Cut a plastic sheet to form to the athlete's thigh.
5. Create a doughnut-shaped foam lining to surround the injury.
6. Secure the foam doughnut to the plastic piece.
7. Secure the pad in place with elastic wrap.

REVIEW QUESTIONS AND CLASS ACTIVITIES

1. What are the legal responsibilities of the equipment manager, athletic trainer, and coach in terms of protective equipment?
2. Invite an attorney to class to discuss product liability and its impact on the athletic trainer.
3. What are the various sports with high risk factors that require protective equipment?
4. How can the athletic trainer select and use safety equipment to decrease the possibility of sports injuries and litigation?
5. Why is continual inspection and/or replacement of used equipment important?
6. What are the standards for fitting football helmets? Are there standards for any other helmets?
7. Invite your school equipment manager to class to demonstrate all the protective equipment and how to fit it to the athlete.
8. Why are mouth guards important, and what are the advantages of custom-made mouth guards over the stock type?
9. What are the advantages and disadvantages of glasses and contact lenses in athletic competition?
10. How do you fit shoulder pads for the different-sized players and their positions?
11. Why is breast protection necessary? Which types of sports bras are available and what should the athlete look for when purchasing one?
12. How do you properly fit shoes? What type of shoes should you use for the various sports and the different floor and field surfaces?

REFERENCES

1. Alexy C, De Carlo M: Rehabilitation and use of protective devices in hand and wrist injuries. In Rettig AC, editor: *Hand and wrist injuries. Clinic in sports medicine,* vol 17, no 3, July 1998.
2. Amis T, Di Somma E, Bacha F, Wheatley J: Influence of intra-oral maxillary sports mouthguards on the airflow dynamics of oral breathing, *Med Sci Sports Exerc* 32(2):284, 2000.
3. Beriau M, Cox W, Manning J: Effects of ankle braces upon agility course performance in high school athletes, *J Ath Train* 29(3):224, 1994.
4. Beynnon B, Good L, Risberg M: The effect of bracing on proprioception of knees with anterior cruciate ligament injury, *J Ortho Sports Phys Ther* 32(1):32, 2002.
5. Birmingham TB, Inglis JT, Kramer JF: Effect of a neoprene sleeve on knee joint kinesthesis: influence of different testing procedures, *Med Sci Sports Exerc* 32(2):304, 2000.
6. Bone S: If the shoe fits ..., *Athletic Therapy Today* 6(6):52, 200l.
7. Bot SDM, van Mechelen W: The effect of ankle bracing on athletic performance, *Sports Med* 27(3):171, 1999.
8. *Breast support for female athletes, Sport research review/Nike sport research review* 1:1, 2002.
9. Broglio S, Yan-Ying J, Broglio M: The efficacy of soccer headgear, *J Ath Train* 38(3), 2003.
10. Brownstein B. Migration and design characteristics of functional knee braces, *J Sport Rehabil* 7(1):33, 1998.
11. Carlson L: Use of functional knee braces after ACL reconstruction, *Athletic Therapy Today* 7(3):48, 2002.
12. Caswell S, Deivert R: Lacrosse helmet designs and the effects of impact forces, *J Ath Train* 37(2):164, 2002.
13. Cuddy S: The right running shoe: the first step in avoiding running injuries. *Sports Med Update* 13(3):8, 1998.
14. Davis PF, Trevino SG: Ankle injuries. In Baxter DE, editor: *The foot and ankle in sport,* St Louis, 1995, Mosby.
15. Fiolkowski P: Considerations in the use of ankle braces, *Athletic Therapy Today* 3(4):38, 1998.
16. Frey C: The shoe in sports. In Baxter DE, editor: *The foot and ankle in sport,* St Louis, 1995, Mosby.
17. Garth W, Flowers K: Efficacy of knee sleeves in the management of patellofemoral dysfunction, *Athletic Therapy Today* 3(4):23, 1998.
18. Gorden J, Straub S, Swanik C: Effects of football collars on cervical hyperextension and lateral flexion, *J Ath Train* 38(3), 2003.

19. Gross MT: The impact of custom semirigid foot orthotics on pain and disability for individuals with plantar fasciitis, *Journal of Ortho Sports Phys Ther* 32(4):149, 2002.
20. Halstead PD: Performance testing updates in head, face, and eye protection, *J Ath Train* 36(3):322, 2001.
21. Hartsell H: Effects of bracing on isokinetic torque for the chronically unstable ankle, *J Sport Rehabil* 8(2):83, 1999.
22. Hartsell H: The effects of external bracing on joint position sense awareness for the chronically unstable ankle, *J Sport Rehabil* 9(4):279, 2000.
23. Hawn K, Visser M, Sexton P: Enforcement of mouthguard use and athlete compliance in National Collegiate Athletic Association men's collegiate ice hockey competition, *J Ath Train* 37(2):204, 2002.
24. Hermann TJ: Taping and padding of the foot and ankle. In Sammarco GI, editor: *Rehabilitation of the foot and ankle,* St Louis, 1995, Mosby.
25. Hodgson VR, Thomas LM: *Biomechanical study of football head impacts using a head model—condensed version.* Final report prepared for National Operating Committee on Standards for Athletic Equipment (NOCSAE), 1975.
26. International Federation of Medicine: Position statement: eye injuries and eye protection in sports, *Athletic Therapy Today* 4(5):6, 1999.
27. Kaminski T: The history and current use of ankle brace technology, *Athletic Therapy Today* 3(4):32, 1998.
28. Kaminski TW, Perrin D: Effect of prophylactic knee bracing on balance and joint position sense, *J Ath Train* 31(2):131, 1996.
29. Kinzey SJ, Ingersoll CD, Knight KL: The effects of selected ankle appliances on postural control, *J Ath Train* 32(4):300, 1997.
30. Labella CR, Smith RW, Sigurdsson A: Effect of mouth guards on dental injuries and concussions in college basketball, *Med Sci Sports Exerc* 34(1)41, 2002.
31. Lahti H: Dental injuries in ice hockey games and training, *Med Sci Sports Exerc* 34(3):400, 2002.
32. Liggett C, Tandy R, Young J: The effects of prophylactic knee bracing on running gait, *J Ath Train* 30(2):159, 1995.
33. Lindley T: Taping and semirigid bracing may not affect ankle functional range of motion, *J Ath Train* 30(2):109, 1995.
34. Locke A et al: Long-term use of a soft-shell prophylactic ankle stabilizer on speed, agility, and vertical jump performance, *J Sport Rehabil* 6(3):235, 1997.
35. Lord JL: Protective equipment in high-risk sports. In Birrer RB, editor: *Sports medicine for the primary care physician,* ed 3, Boca Raton, Fla, 2004, CRC Press.
36. McCrory P: Do mouthguards prevent concussion?, *British Journal of Sports Medicine* 35(2):81, 2001.
37. Metcalfe RC, Schlabach GA, Looney MA et al: A comparison of moleskin tape, linen tape, and lace-up brace on joint restriction and movement performance, *J Ath Train* 32(2):136, 1997.
38. Miller J et al: Dynamic analysis of custom-fitted functional knee braces: EMG and brace migration during physical activity, *J Sport Rehabil* 8(2):109, 1999.
39. Montgomery DL: Prophylactic knee braces. In Torg JS, Shephard RJ, editors: *Current therapy in sports medicine,* St Louis, 1995, Mosby.
40. New Revolution helmet being put to the test for improved safety on the field, *Sports Medicine Alert* 8(7):55, 2002.
41. Nigg BM, Nurse MA, Stefanyshyn DJ: Shoe inserts and orthotics for sport and physical activities, *Med Sci Sports Exerc* 31(7 Suppl.): S421,1999.
42. Page KA, Steele JR: Breast motion and sports brassiere design: implications for future research, *Sports Med* 27(4):205, 1999.
43. Paris D, Vardaxis V, Kokkaliaris J: Ankle ranges of motion during extended activity periods while taped and braced, *J Ath Train* 30(3):223, 1995.
44. Peterson L, Renstrom P: Sports and protective equipment. In Peterson, L, editor: *Sports injuries: their prevention and treatment,* ed 3, Champaign, Ill, 2001, Human Kinetics.
45. Pincivero D, Rijke A, Heinrichs K et al: The effects of a functional elbow brace on medial joint stability: a case study, *J Ath Train* 29(3):232, 1994.
46. Prentice W: *Fitness and wellness for life,* ed 7, Winston-Salem, NC, 2004, Kendall-Hunt.
47. Rules and equipment. In *Coaching youth football,* ed 3, Champaign, Ill, 2001, Human Kinetics, 63–90.
48. Sauers E, Harter R: Efficacy of prophylactic knee braces: current research perspectives, *Athletic Therapy Today* 3(4):14, 1998.
49. Scriber K: The history and current use of knee brace technology, *Athletic Therapy Today* 3(4):7, 1998.
50. Sharpe SR, Knapik J, Jones B: Ankle braces effectively reduce recurrence of ankle sprains in female soccer players, *J Ath Train* 32(1):21, 1997.
51. Steinbach P. Armor for all. With player safety paramount, the purchasing of football equipment must ensure adequate supply and proper fit of helmets, shoes and everything in between, *Athletic Business* 26(8):96, 2002.
52. Styf J: The effects of functional knee bracing on muscle function and performance, *Sports Med* 28(2):77, 1999.
53. Swanik CB: Orthotics in sports medicine, *Athletic Therapy Today* 5(1):5, 2000.
54. Vaes P et al: Influence of ankle strapping, taping, and nine braces on talar tilt: a stress roentgenologic comparison, *J Sport Rehabil* 7(3):157, 1998.
55. Vinger PF: A practical guide for sports eye protection. *Physician Sportsmed* 28(6):49, 2000.
56. Wilkerson GB: Biomechanical and neuromuscular effects of ankle taping and bracing, *J Ath Train* 37(4):436, 2002.
57. Wojtys EM, Huston LJ: Functional knee braces—the 25-year controversy. In Chan KM, editor: *Controversies in orthopedic sports medicine.* Champaign, Ill, 2002, Human Kinetics.
58. Yaggie J, Kinzey S: A comparative analysis of selected ankle orthoses during functional tasks, *Journal Sport Rehabil* 10(3):174, 2001.

ANNOTATED BIBLIOGRAPHY

Hunter S, Dolan M, Davis M: *Foot orthotics in therapy and sport,* Champaign, Ill, 1995, Human Kinetics.

This text takes a detailed look at the fabrication of orthotic devices.

Nicholas JA, Hirshman EB, editors: *The upper extremity in sports medicine,* St Louis, 1995, Mosby.

This book includes a special chapter on protective equipment for the shoulder, elbow, wrist, and hand.

Street S, Runkle D: *Athletic protective equipment: care, selection and fitting,* Boston, 2000, McGraw-Hill.

This reference book provides an overview of available athletic equipment and its usage. The text is a resource for athletic trainers, coaches, and physical education teachers.

Bandaging and Taping

Chapter 8

When you finish this chapter you should be able to

- Explain the need for and demonstrate the application of a cloth ankle wrap.
- Explain the need for and demonstrate the application of triangular and cravat bandages.
- Demonstrate site preparation for taping.
- Demonstrate basic skill in the use of taping in sports.
- Demonstrate the skillful application of tape for a variety of musculoskeletal problems.

Bandaging and taping techniques are used routinely by athletic trainers. They may be used to accomplish a variety of specific objectives, including:

- providing compression to minimize swelling in the initial management of injury.
- reducing the chances of injury by applying tape prophylactically before an injury occurs.
- providing additional support to an injured structure.

Correctly and effectively applying a bandage or a "tape job" to a specific body part is a skill usually left to the athletic trainer. It is true that athletic trainers have been instructed in and generally become highly proficient in applying a variety of bandaging and taping techniques to accomplish the objectives listed. Certainly bandaging and taping skills are not difficult. They can be mastered by anyone willing to spend time practicing and learning what works best in a given situation. Of course certain taping and bandaging techniques are more advanced and should be used only by those with some advanced experience. However, there are some very basic techniques that can be easily applied with only a little training.

BANDAGING

A **bandage**, when properly applied, may contribute to recovery from sports injuries. Bandages carelessly or improperly applied may cause discomfort, allow wound contamination, and/or hamper repair and healing. In all cases bandages must be firmly applied—neither so tightly that circulation is impaired nor so loosely that the **dressing** is allowed to slip.

bandage
Strip of cloth or other material used to cover a wound or hold a dressing in place.

dressing
Covering, protective or supportive, that is applied to an injury or wound.

Bandages used on sports injuries consist of gauze, cotton cloth, and elastic wrapping.

Gauze comes in three forms: (1) a roller bandage for holding dressings and compresses in place, (2) padding in the prevention of blisters on a taped ankle, and (3) sterile pads for wounds.

Cotton cloth is used primarily for cloth ankle wraps and for triangular and cravat bandages.

Elastic Bandages

The *elastic bandage* is extremely popular with athletic trainers because of its extensibility, which allows it to conform to most parts of the body. Elastic wraps are active bandages; they let the athlete move without restriction. They act as controlled compression bandages where hemorrhage or swelling must be prevented, and they can also help support soft tissue.

A *cohesive elastic bandage* exerts constant, even pressure. It is lightweight and contours easily to the body part. The bandage is composed of two layers of nonwoven rayon, which are separated by strands of spandex material. The cohesive elastic bandage is coated with a substance that makes the material adhere to itself, eliminating the need for metal clips or adhesive tape to hold it in place.

Elastic bandages are commonly used in the athletic training room. The width and length vary according to the body part to be bandaged. The sizes most frequently used are the 2-inch (5 cm) width by 6-yard (5.5 m) length for hand, finger, toe, and head bandages; the 3-inch (7.5 cm) width by 10-yard (9 m) length for the extremities; and the 4-inch (10 cm) or 6-inch (15 cm) width by 10-yard (9 m) length for thigh, groin, and trunk. For ease and convenience in the application of the elastic bandage, the strips of material are first rolled into a cylinder. When a bandage is selected, it should be a single piece that is free from wrinkles, seams, and any other imperfections that may cause skin irritation.[15]

Wrinkles or seams in roller bandages may irritate skin.

Application

To apply a roller bandage, hold it in the preferred hand with the loose end extending from the bottom of the roll.

Application of the elastic bandage must be executed in a specific manner to maximize its effectiveness. When an elastic bandage is about to be placed on a body part, the roll should be held in the preferred hand with the loose end extending from the bottom of the roll. The back surface of the loose end is placed on the injured area and held in position by the other hand. The bandage cylinder is then unrolled and passed around the injured area. As the hand pulls the material from the roll, it also standardizes the bandage pressure and guides the bandage in the proper direction. To anchor and stabilize the bandage, a number of turns, one on top of the other, are made. Circling a body part requires the athletic trainer to alternate the bandage roll from one hand to the other and back again.

8-1

***Critical Thinking* Exercise**

A freshman football player has a chronically weak ankle that he has sprained several times before. He wants to have the ankle taped before games and practices but has never had it taped before.

? What can the athletic trainer do to minimize the occurrence of blisters and ensure that the tape provides support?

To provide maximum benefit, an elastic bandage should be applied uniformly and firmly but not too tightly (Figure 8-1). Excessive or unequal pressure can hinder the normal blood flow within the part. The following points should be considered when using the elastic bandage:

1. A body part should be wrapped in the position of maximum muscle contraction to ensure unhampered movement or circulation.
2. It is better to use a large number of turns with moderate tension than a limited number of turns applied too tightly.
3. Each turn of the bandage should be overlapped by at least one half of the overlying wrap to prevent the separation of the material while the athlete is engaged in activity. Separation of the bandage turns tends to pinch and irritate the skin and also leaves a space where swelling/edema can collect.

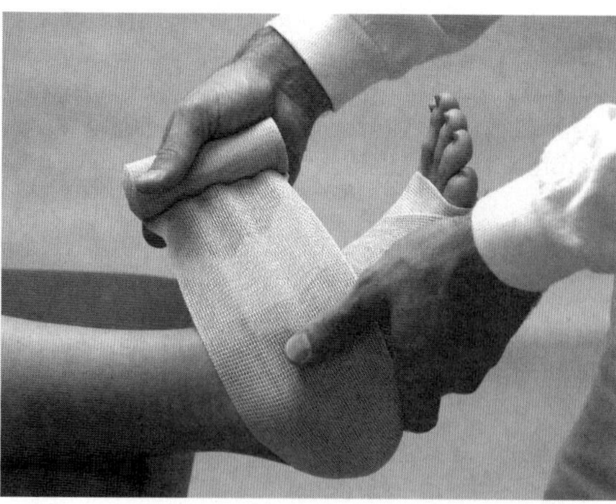

Figure 8-1

Elastic bandages should be applied with firm, even pressure.

4. When limbs are wrapped, fingers and toes should be checked often for signs of circulation impairment. Abnormally cold or cyanotic phalanges are signs of excessive bandage pressure.

The usual anchoring of elastic bandages consists of several circular wraps directly overlying each other. Whenever possible, anchoring is commenced at the smallest circumference of a limb and is then moved upward. Wrists and ankles are the usual sites for anchoring bandages of the limbs. Bandages are applied to these areas in the following manner:

Begin anchoring bandages at the smallest part of the limb.

1. The loose end of the elastic bandage is laid obliquely on the anterior aspects of the wrist or ankle and held in this position. The roll is then carried posteriorly under and completely around the limb and back to the starting point.
2. The triangular portion of the uncovered oblique end is folded over the second turn.
3. The folded triangle is covered by a third turn, which finishes a secure anchor.

After an elastic bandage has been applied, it is held in place by a locking technique. The method most often used to finish a wrap is to firmly tie or pin the bandage or place adhesive tape over several overlying turns.

Once a bandage has been put on and has served its purpose, it can be removed either by unwrapping or by carefully cutting with bandage scissors. Whatever method of bandage removal is used, the athletic trainer must take extreme caution to avoid additional injury.

Elastic Bandage Techniques

Any time an athletic trainer applies an elastic bandage to the athlete, the trainer must always check for decreased circulation and blueness of the extremity as well as for a blood capillary refill.

Check circulation after applying an elastic wrap.

Ankle and foot spica The ankle and foot **spica** bandage (Figure 8-2) is primarily used in sports for the compression of new injuries and for holding wound dressings in place.

spica
A figure-eight bandage with one of the two loops larger than the other.

Materials needed Depending on the size of the ankle and foot, a 2-inch (5 cm) or 3-inch (7.5 cm) wrap is used.

Position of the athlete The athlete sits with his or her ankle and foot extended over the edge of a table.

Procedure

1. Place an anchor around the foot near the metatarsal arch.
2. Bring the elastic bandage across the instep and around the heel, and return to the starting point.
3. Repeat the procedure several times, with each succeeding revolution progressing upward on the foot and the ankle.
4. Overlap each spica over the preceding layer by approximately three fourths.

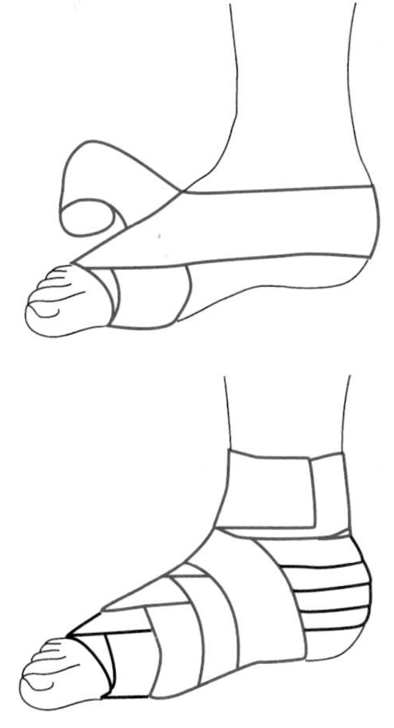

Figure 8-2

Ankle and foot spica.

Spiral bandage

The spiral bandage (Figure 8-3) is widely used in sports for covering a large area of a cylindrical part.

Materials needed Depending on the size of the area, a 3-inch (7.5 cm) or 4-inch (10 cm) wrap is required.

Position of the athlete If the wrap is for the lower limb, the athlete bears weight on the opposite leg.

Procedure

1. Anchor the elastic spiral bandage at the smallest circumference of the limb and wrap upward in a spiral against gravity.
2. To prevent the bandage from slipping down on a moving extremity, fold two pieces of tape lengthwise and place them on the bandage at either side of the limb, or spray tape adherent on the injured area.
3. After the bandage is anchored, carry it upward in consecutive spiral turns, each overlapping the other by at least ½ inch.

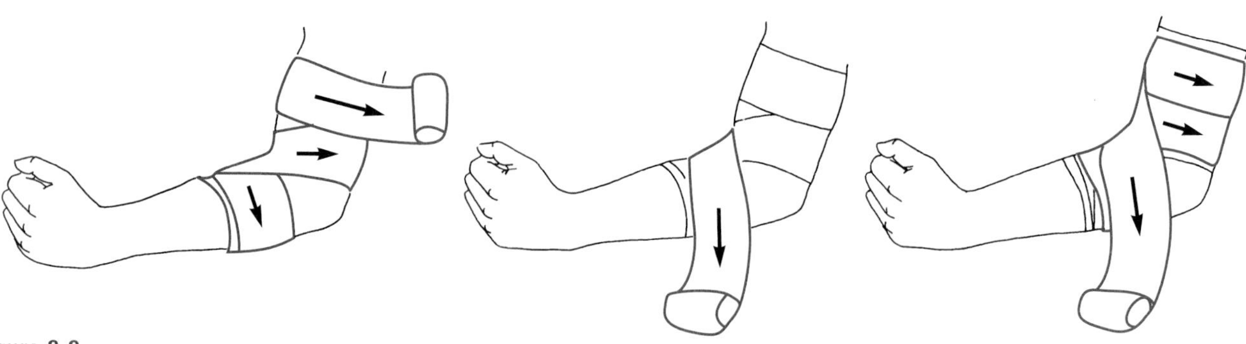

Figure 8-8

Elastic elbow figure-eight bandage.

3. After anchoring the bandage around the arm on the injured side, carry the wrap around the back under the unaffected arm and across the chest to the injured shoulder.
4. Encircle the affected arm again by the bandage, which continues around the back. Every figure-eight pattern moves progressively upward with an overlap of at least half of the previous underlying wrap.

Elbow figure-eight bandage The elbow figure-eight bandage (Figure 8-8) can be used to secure a dressing in the antecubital fossa or to restrain full extension in hyperextension injuries. When it is reversed, it can be used on the posterior aspect of the elbow.

8-3 *Critical Thinking* Exercise

A wrestler sustains a left shoulder point injury. The athletic trainer cuts a sponge rubber doughnut to protect the shoulder point from further injury.

? How is the doughnut held in place?

Materials needed One 3-inch (7.5 cm) elastic roll and 1½-inch (3.8 cm) adhesive tape.

Position of the athlete The athlete flexes his or her elbow between 45 degrees and 90 degrees, depending on the restriction of movement required.

Procedure

1. Anchor the bandage by encircling the lower arm.
2. Bring the roll obliquely upward over the posterior aspect of the elbow.
3. Carry the roll obliquely upward, crossing the antecubital fossa; then pass once again completely around the upper arm and return to the beginning position by again crossing the antecubital fossa.
4. Continue the procedure as described, but for every new sequence move upward toward the elbow one half the width of the underlying wrap.

Gauze hand and wrist figure eight A figure-eight bandage (Figure 8-9) can be used for mild wrist and hand support and for holding dressings in place.

Figure 8-9

Hand and wrist figure-eight bandage.

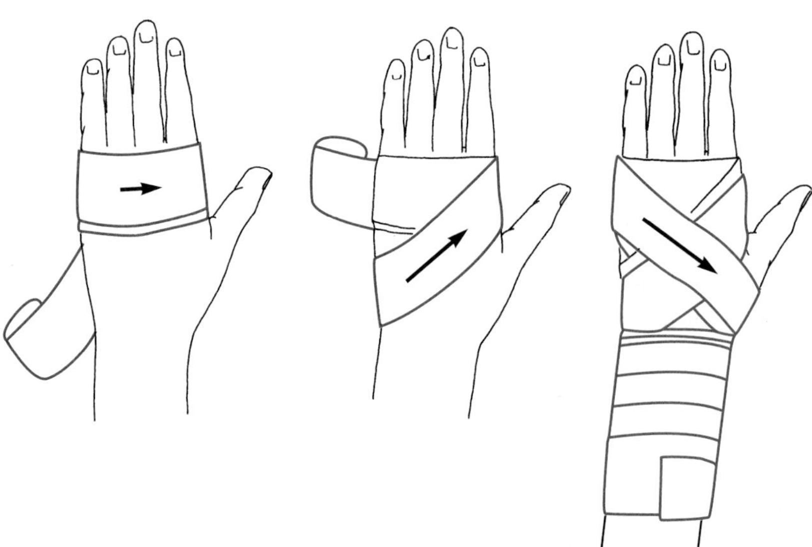

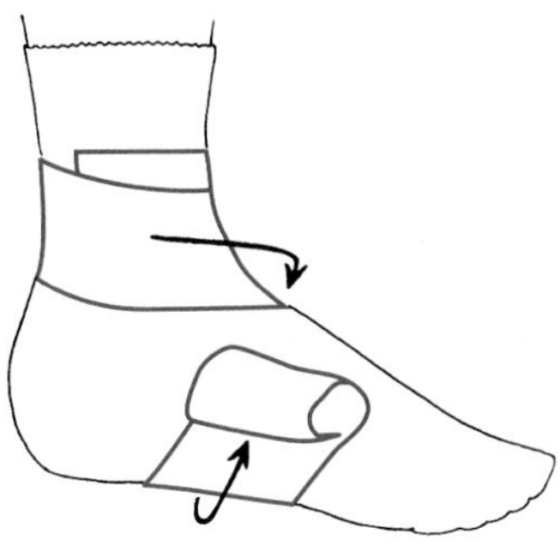

Materials needed One roll of ½-inch (1.25 cm) gauze, ½-inch (1.25 cm) tape, and scissors.

Position of the athlete The athlete positions his or her elbow at a 45-degree angle.

Procedure

1. The anchor is executed with one or two turns of the bandage around the palm of the hand.
2. The roll is then carried obliquely across the anterior or posterior portion of the hand, depending on the position of the wound, to the wrist, which it circles once; then it is returned to the primary anchor.
3. As many figure eights as needed are applied.

Cloth Ankle Wrap

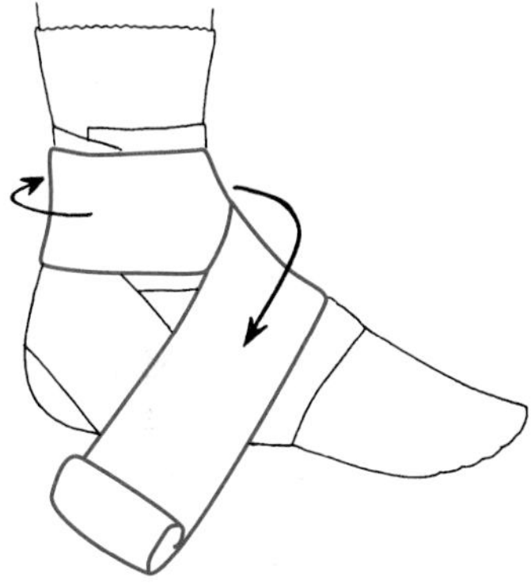

Figure 8-10

Ankle wrap.

Because tape is so expensive, the ankle wrap is an inexpensive and expedient means of mildly protecting ankles (Figure 8-10). Due to an increase in the use of ankle braces and supports, the cloth ankle wrap is used infrequently in an athletic training setting.

Materials needed Each wrap should be 1½ to 2 inches (3.8 to 5 cm) wide and 72 to 96 inches (180 to 240 cm) long to ensure complete coverage and protection. The purpose of this wrap is to give mild support against lateral and medial motion of the ankle. It is applied over a sock.

Position of the athlete The athlete sits on a table, extending the leg and positioning the foot at a 90-degree angle. To avoid any distortion, it is important that the ankle be neither overflexed nor overextended.

Procedure

1. Start the wrap above the instep around the ankle, circle the ankle, and move it at an acute angle to the inside of the foot.
2. From the inside of the foot, move the wrap under the arch, coming up on the outside and crossing at the beginning point, and continue around the ankle, hooking the heel.
3. Move the wrap up, inside, over the instep, and around the ankle, hooking the opposite side of the heel. This completes one series of the ankle wrap.
4. Complete a second series with the remaining material.
5. For additional support, apply two heel locks with adhesive tape over the ankle wrap.

Triangular and Cravat Bandages

Triangular and cravat bandages can be applied easily and quickly.

Triangular and cravat bandages, usually made of cotton cloth, may be used if roller types are not applicable or available. The triangular and cravat bandages are primarily used as first aid devices.[15] They are valuable in emergency bandaging because they are easy and quick to apply. In sports the more diversified roller bandages are usually available and lend themselves more to the needs of the athlete. The principal use of the triangular bandage in athletic training is for arm slings. There are two basic kinds of slings, the cervical arm sling and the shoulder arm sling, and each has a specific purpose.

Cervical arm sling The cervical arm sling (Figure 8-11) is designed to support the forearm, wrist, and hand. A triangular bandage is placed around the neck and under the bent arm that is to be supported.

Materials needed One triangular bandage.

Position of the athlete The athlete stands with the affected arm bent at approximately a 70-degree angle.

Procedure

1. Position the triangular bandage under the injured arm with the apex facing the elbow.
2. Carry the end of the triangle nearest the body over the shoulder of the uninjured arm. Allow the other end to hang down loosely.
3. Pull the loose end over the shoulder of the injured side.

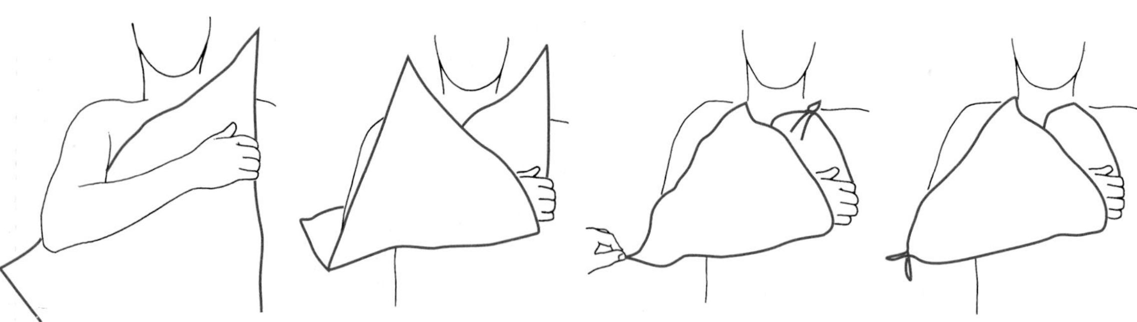

Figure 8-11

Cervical arm sling.

4. Tie the two ends of the bandage in a square knot behind the neck. For the sake of comfort, the knot should be on either side of the neck, not directly in the middle.
5. Bring the apex of the triangle around to the front of the elbow and fasten by twisting the end, then tying in a knot.

If greater arm stabilization is required than that afforded by a sling, an additional bandage can be swathed about the upper arm and body.

Shoulder arm sling The shoulder arm sling (Figure 8-12) is suggested for forearm support when there is an injury to the shoulder girdle or when the cervical arm sling is irritating to the athlete.

Materials needed One triangular bandage and one safety pin.

Position of the athlete The athlete stands with his or her injured arm bent at approximately a 70-degree angle.

Procedure

1. Place the upper end of the shoulder sling over the uninjured shoulder side.
2. Bring the lower end of the triangle over the forearm and draw it between the upper arm and the body, swinging it around the athlete's back and then upward to meet the other end, where a square knot is tied.
3. Bring the apex end of the triangle around to the front of the elbow and fasten with a safety pin.

Sling and swathe The sling and swathe combination is designed to stabilize the arm securely in cases of shoulder dislocation or fracture (Figure 8-13).

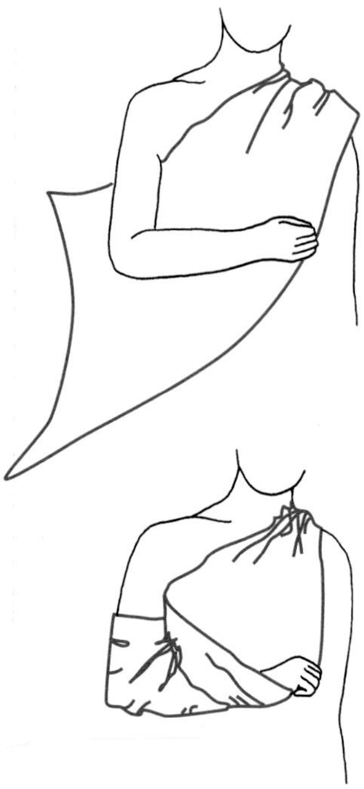

Figure 8-12

Shoulder arm sling.

NONELASTIC AND ELASTIC ADHESIVE TAPING

Historically, taping has been an important part of athletic training. In recent years athletic taping has become decreasingly important as an adjunct to sports medicine because current research questions long-held ideas about the effectiveness of taping.[17,22,28] The psychological effect of taping on the athlete is currently unknown.

Tape Usage

Injury Care

When used for sports injuries, adhesive tape offers a number of possibilities:

- Retention of wound dressings.[16]
- Stabilization of compression bandages that control external and internal hemorrhaging.[16]
- Support of recent injuries to prevent additional insult that might result from the activities of the athlete.[5]
- Stabilization of an injury while the athlete is undergoing an exercise rehabilitation procedure.[5]

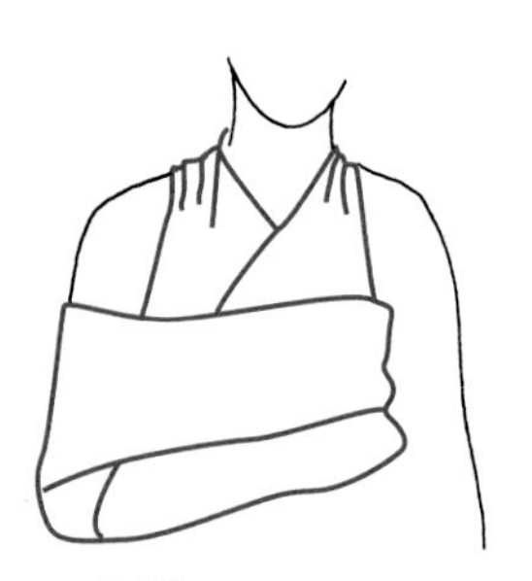

Figure 8-13

Sling and swathe.

Injury Protection

Protecting against acute injuries is another major use of tape support. This protection can be achieved by limiting the motion of a body part or by securing some special device.

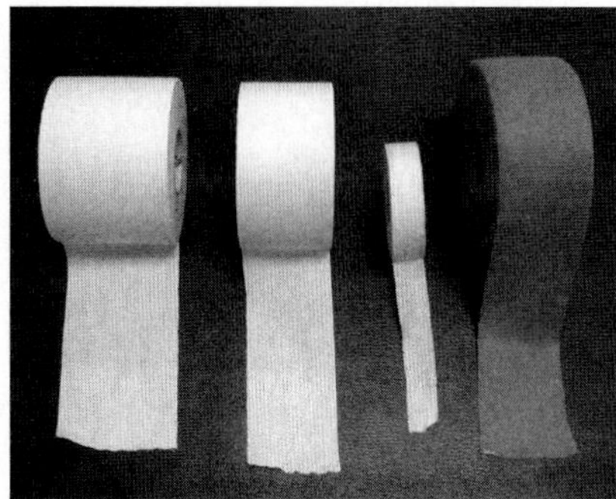

Figure 8-14

Nonelastic adhesive tape 2″, 1½″, ½″, and Leukotape.

Nonelastic Adhesive Tape

Nonelastic adhesive tape has great adaptability for use in sports because of its uniform adhesive mass, adhering qualities, and lightness and because of the relative strength of the backing materials.[21] All these qualities are of value in holding wound dressings in place and in supporting and protecting injured areas. This tape comes in a variety of sizes; widths of ½, 1, 1½, and 2 inches (1.25, 2.5, 3.75, and 5 cm) are commonly used in sports medicine (Figure 8-14). When linen tape is purchased, factors such as cost, grade of backing, quality of adhesive mass, and properties of unwinding should be considered.

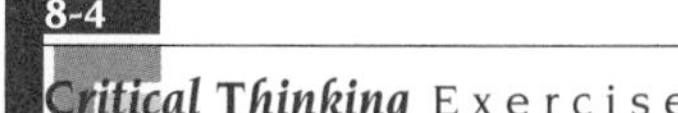

8-4 **Critical Thinking** Exercise

An athlete falls and sustains a dislocated right shoulder.

? How should the athlete be transported safely to the hospital?

Tape Grade

White adhesive tape is most often graded according to the number of longitudinal and vertical fibers per inch of backing material.[4] The heavier and more costly backing contains 85 or more longitudinal fibers and 65 vertical fibers per square inch. The lighter, less expensive grade has 65 or fewer longitudinal fibers and 45 vertical fibers.

When purchasing linen tape, consider:
- Grade of backing
- Quality of adhesive mass
- Winding tension

Adhesive Mass

As a result of improvements in adhesive mass, certain essentials should be expected from tape. It should adhere readily when applied and should maintain this adherence in the presence of profuse perspiration and activity. Besides sticking well, the mass must contain as few skin irritants as possible and must be able to be removed easily without leaving a mass residue or pulling away the superficial skin.

Winding Tension

The winding tension of a tape roll is important to the athletic trainer. The demands of sport activity place a unique demand on the unwinding quality of tape; if tape is to be applied for protection and support, there must be even and constant unwinding tension. In most cases, a proper wind needs little additional tension to provide sufficient tightness.

Increasingly, tape with varying elasticity is being used in sports medicine.

Elastic Adhesive Tape

Elastic adhesive tape is commonly used in sports medicine, often in combination with nonelastic adhesive tape. Because of its conforming qualities, elastic tape is used for small, angular body parts, such as the feet, wrist, hands, and fingers. As with nonelastic adhesive tape, elastic tape comes in a variety of widths (1, 2, 3, and 4 inch) (Figure 8-15).

Tape Storage

When storing tape, take the following steps:

1. Store in a cool place such as in a low cupboard.
2. Stack so that the tape rests on its flat top or bottom to avoid distortion.

Store tape in a cool place, and stack it flat.

Figure 8-15

Elastic adhesive tape.
A, 2″ and 1″ light wrap tape.
B, 3″, 2″, and 1″ elastic tape.

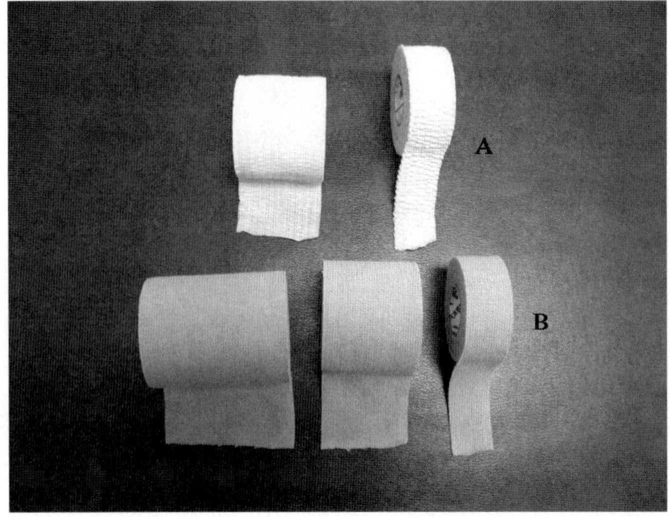

Using Adhesive Tape in Sports

Preparation for Taping

Skin should be cleansed and hair should be shaved before tape is applied.

The athletic trainer must pay special attention when applying tape directly to the skin.[23] A list of supplies needed for proper taping appears later in this chapter. Perspiration, oil, and dirt prevent tape from adhering to the skin. Whenever tape is used, the skin surface should be cleaned with soap and water to remove all dirt and oil. Also, hair should be shaved to prevent additional irritation when the tape is removed (Figure 8-16A). A quick-drying tape adherent spray can be used to help the tape adhere to the skin, although it is not absolutely necessary (Figure 8-16B). Also, at certain points such as over bony prominences, the tape can produce friction blisters. Extra foam or gauze pads (heel and lace pads) with a small amount of lubricant can help to minimize the occurrence of blisters (Figure 8-16C). Taping directly on skin provides maximum sup-

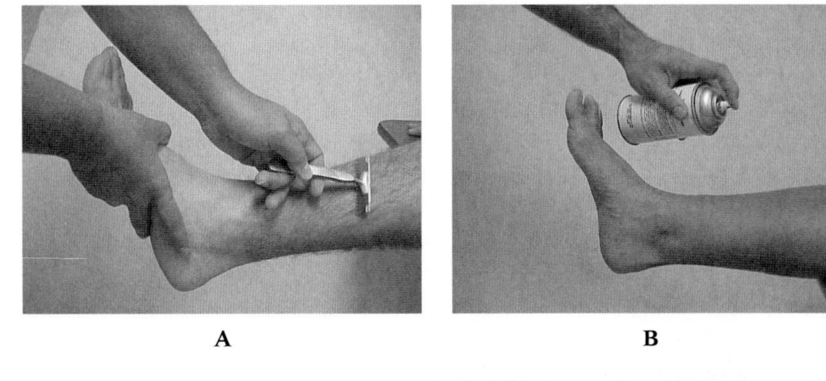

A B

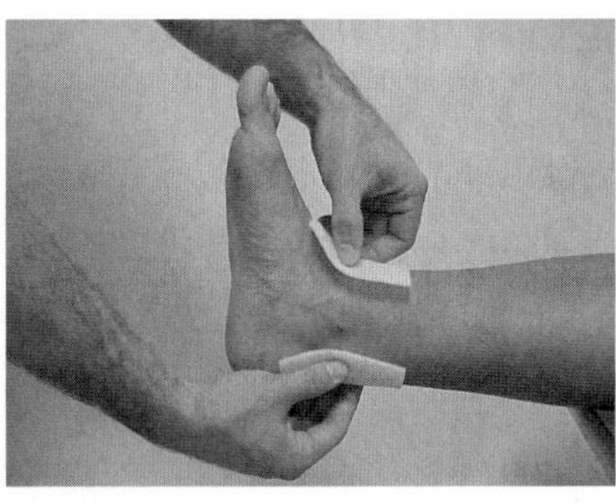

C

D

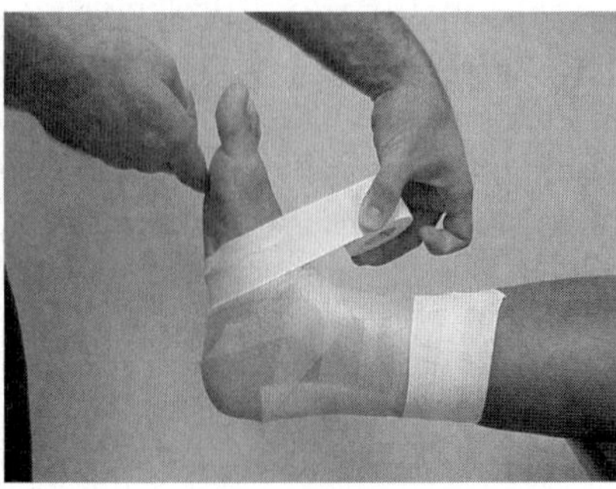

E

Figure 8-16

Taping preparation. **A,** Shaving. **B,** Applying tape adherent. **C,** Placing heel and lace pads. **D,** Applying one layer of under wrap. **E,** Applying anchor strips.

port. However, applying tape day after day can lead to skin irritation. A roll of foam that is thin, porous, extremely lightweight, and resilient, called underwrap or prewrap, easily conforms to the contours of the part to be taped and protects the skin to some degree. Underwrap material should be applied only one layer thick (Figure 8-16D). The underwrap should be anchored both proximally and distally (Figure 8-16E).

Proper Taping Technique

The correct tape width depends on the area to be covered. The more acute the angles, the narrower the tape must be to fit the many contours. For example, the fingers and toes usually require ½- or 1-inch (1.25 or 2.5 cm) tape; the ankles require 1½-inch (3.75 cm) tape; and the larger skin areas such as thighs and back can accommodate 2- to 3-inch (5 to 7.5 cm) tape with ease.

NOTE: Supportive tape improperly applied can aggravate an existing injury or can disrupt the mechanics of a body part, causing an initial injury to occur.

Tearing Tape

Athletic trainers use various techniques to tear tape (Figure 8-17). The tearing method should permit the operator to keep the tape roll in hand most of the time.[30] The following is a suggested procedure:

1. Hold the tape roll in the preferred hand with the middle finger hooked through the center of the tape roll and the thumb pressing its outer edge.
2. With the other hand, grasp the loose end between the thumb and index finger.
3. With both hands in place, pull both ends of the tape so that it is tight. Next, make a quick, scissorslike move to tear the tape. In tearing tape, one hand moves away from the body and the other hand moves toward the body. Remember, do not try to bend or twist the tape to tear it.

To tear tape, move hands quickly in opposite directions.

When tearing is properly executed, the torn edges of the nonelastic adhesive tape are relatively straight, without curves, twists, or loose threads sticking out. Once the first thread is torn, the rest of the tape tears easily. Learning to tear tape effectively from many different positions is essential for speed and efficiency. Many tapes other than the linen-backed type cannot be torn manually but require a knife, scissors, or razor blade.

Rules for Tape Application

The following are a few of the important rules to be observed in the use of adhesive tape. In practice the athletic trainer will identify others.

1. *If the part to be taped is a joint, place it in the position in which it is to be stabilized.* If the part is musculature, make the necessary allowance for contraction and expansion.
2. *Overlap the tape at least half the width of the tape below.* Unless tape is overlapped sufficiently, the active athlete will separate it, exposing the underlying skin to irritation and allowing a space in which swelling/edema can occur.

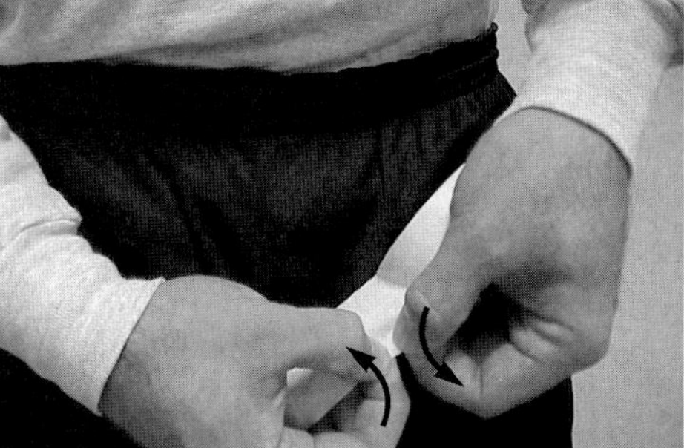

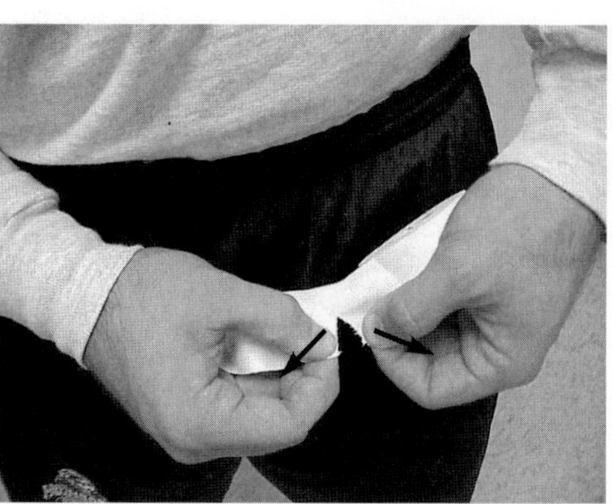

Figure 8-17

Technique for tearing adhesive tape.

3. *Avoid continuous taping.* Tape continuously wrapped around a part may cause constriction. Make one turn at a time and tear each encirclement to overlap the starting end by approximately 1 inch. This rule is particularly true of the nonyielding linen-backed tape.
4. *Keep the tape roll in the hand whenever possible.* By learning to keep the tape roll in the hand, seldom putting it down, and by learning to tear the tape, an athletic trainer can develop taping speed and accuracy.
5. *Smooth and mold the tape as it is laid on the skin.* To save additional time, smooth and mold tape strips to the body part as they are put in place; this is done by stroking the top with the fingers, palms, and heels of both hands.
6. *Allow tape to fit the natural contour of the skin.* Each strip of tape must be placed with a particular purpose in mind. Linen-backed tape is not sufficiently elastic to bend around acute angles but must be allowed to fall as it may, fitting naturally to the body contours. Failing to allow this fit creates wrinkles and gaps that can result in skin irritations.
7. *Start taping with an anchor piece and finish by applying a lock strip.* Commence taping, if possible, by sticking the tape to an anchor piece that encircles the part. This placement affords a good medium for the stabilization of succeeding tape strips so that they will not be affected by the movement of the part.
8. *Where maximum support is desired, tape directly over skin.* In cases of sensitive skin, prewrap may be used as tape bases. With prewrap, some movement can be expected between the skin and the base.[3]
9. *Do not apply tape if skin is hot or cold from a therapeutic treatment.*

Removing Adhesive Tape

Tape usually can be removed from the skin by hand, by tape scissors or tape cutters, or by chemical solvents.[30]

Peel the skin from the tape, not the tape from the skin.

Manual removal When pulling tape from the body, be careful not to tear or irritate the skin. Tape must not be wrenched in an outward direction from the skin but should be pulled in a direct line with the body (Figure 8-18). Remember to remove the skin carefully from the tape and not to peel the tape from the skin. Use one hand to gently pull the tape in one direction, and the opposite hand to gently press the skin away from the tape.

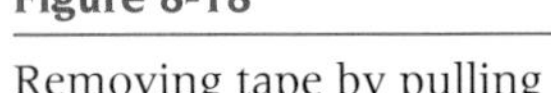

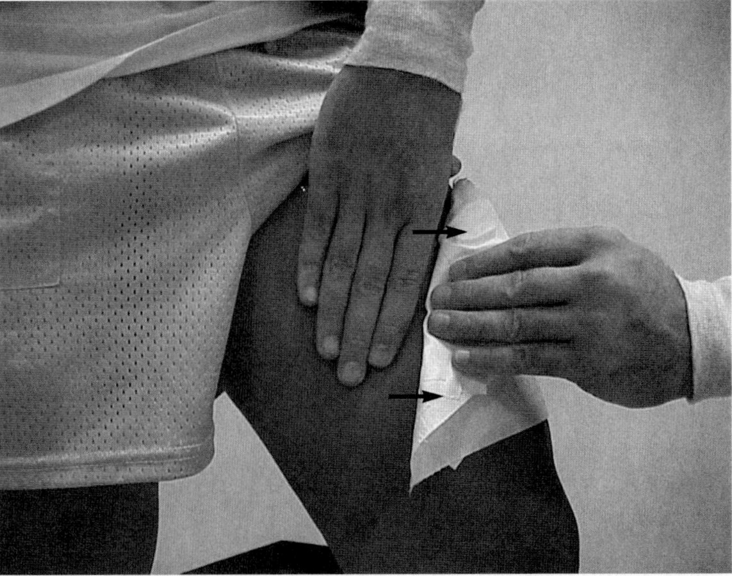

Figure 8-18

Removing tape by pulling in a direct line with the body.

Use of tape scissors or cutters The characteristic tape scissors have a blunt nose that slips underneath the tape smoothly without gouging the skin. Take care to avoid cutting the tape too near the site of the injury, so the scissors do not aggravate the condition. Cut on the uninjured side.

Taping Supplies

Effective taping requires the availability of numerous supplies:

1. Razor—hair removal
2. Soap—cleaning skin
3. Alcohol—oil removal from skin
4. Adhesive spray—tape adherent
5. Prewrap material—skin protection
6. Heel and lace pads
7. White nonelastic adhesive tape (½ inch, 1 inch, 1½-inch, and 2 inch [1.25 cm, 2.5 cm, 3.8 cm, and 5 cm])
8. Elastic adhesive tape (1 inch, 2 inch, and 3 inch [2.5 cm, 5 cm, and 7.5 cm])
9. Felt and foam padding material
10. Tape scissors
11. Tape cutters
12. Elastic bandages (2 inch, 3 inch, 4 inch, and 6 inch [5 cm, 7.5 cm, 10 cm, and 15 cm])

Common Taping Procedures

The Arch

Arch technique no. 1: with pad support Arch taping with pad support strengthens weakened arches (Figure 8-19). NOTE: The longitudinal arch should be lifted. CAUTION: When applying tape around the forefoot, be aware that the metatarsals must have room to spread when bearing weight.

Materials needed One roll of 1½-inch (3.8 cm) tape, tape adherent, and a ⅛- or ¼-inch (0.3 or 0.6 cm) adhesive foam rubber pad or wool felt pad, cut to fit the longitudinal arch.

Site preparation Clean foot of dirt and oil; if hairy, shave dorsum of foot. Spray area with tape adherent.

Position of the athlete The athlete lies face down on the table with the foot that is to be taped extending approximately 6 inches (15 cm) over the edge of the table. To ensure proper position, allow the foot to hang in a relaxed position.

Procedure

1. Place a series of strips of tape directly around the arch or, if added support is required, around an arch pad and the arch. The first strip should go just above the metatarsal arch (1).
2. Each successive strip overlaps the preceding piece about half the width of the tape (2 through 4).

CAUTION: Avoid putting on so many strips of tape that the action of the ankle is hampered.

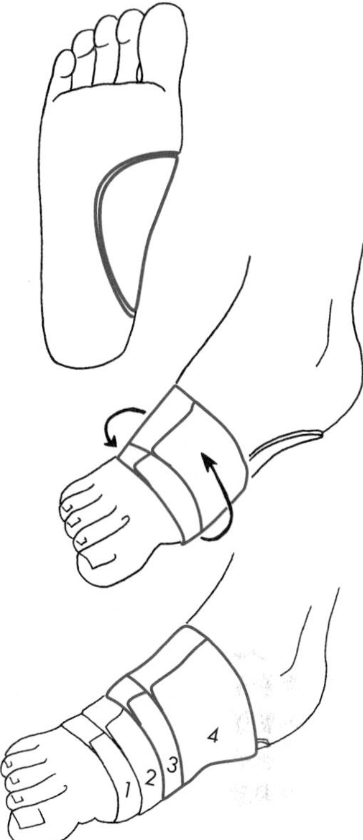

Figure 8-19

Arch taping technique no. 1, including an arch pad and circular tape strips.

Arch technique no. 2: the X for the longitudinal arch Use the figure-eight method for taping the longitudinal arch (Figure 8-20).

Materials needed One roll of 1-inch (2.5 cm) tape and tape adherent.

Site preparation Same as for arch technique no. 1.

Position of the athlete The athlete lies face down on the table with the affected foot extending approximately 6 inches (15 cm) over the edge of the table. To ensure proper position, allow the foot to hang in a relaxed position.

Procedure

1. Lightly place an anchor strip around the ball of the foot, making certain not to constrict the action of the toes (1).

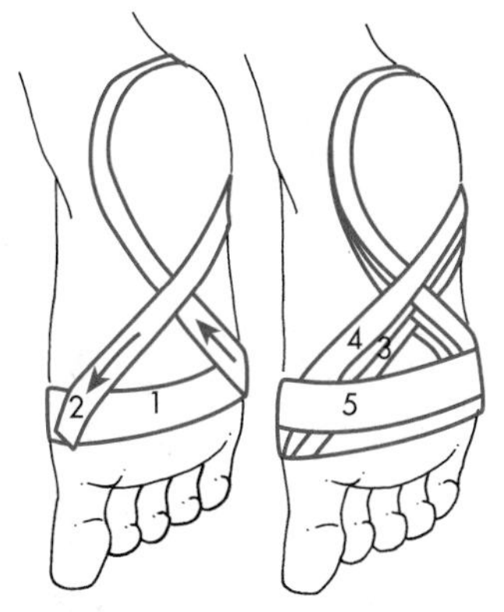

Figure 8-20

Arch taping technique no. 2 (X taping).

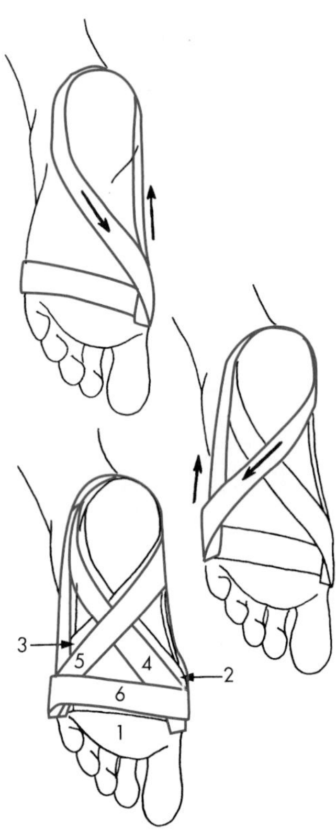

Figure 8-21

Teardrop arch taping technique no. 3 with double X and forefoot support.

2. Start tape strip 2 from the lateral edge of the anchor. Move it upward at an acute angle, cross the center of the longitudinal arch, encircle the heel, and descend. Then cross the arch again and end at the medial aspect of the anchor (2). Repeat three or four times (3 and 4).
3. Lock the taped Xs with a single piece of tape placed around the ball of foot (5).

After all the X strips are applied, cover the entire arch with 1½-inch (3.8 cm) circular tape strips.

Arch technique no. 3: the X teardrop arch and forefoot support As its name implies, this taping both supports the longitudinal arch and stabilizes the forefoot into good alignment (Figure 8-21).

Materials needed One roll of 1-inch (2.5 cm) tape and tape adherent.

Position of the athlete The athlete lies face down on the table with the foot to be taped extending approximately 6 inches (15 cm) over the edge of the table.

Procedure

1. Place an anchor strip around the ball of the foot (1).
2. Start tape strip 2 on the side of the foot, beginning at the base of the great toe. Take the tape around the heel, crossing the arch and returning to the starting point (2).
3. The pattern of the third strip of tape is the same as the second strip except that it is started on the little toe side of the foot (3). Repeat two or three times (4 and 5).
4. Lock each series of strips by placing tape around the ball joint (6). A completed procedure usually consists of a series of three strips.

Arch technique no. 4: fan arch support The fan arch technique supports the entire plantar aspect of the foot (Figure 8-22).

Materials needed One roll of 1-inch (2.5 cm) tape, one roll of 1½-inch (3.8 cm) tape, and tape adherent.

Position of athlete The athlete lies face down on the table with the foot to be taped extending approximately 6 inches (15 cm) over the edge of the table.

Procedure

1. Using the 1-inch (2.5 cm) tape, place an anchor strip around the ball of the foot (1).
2. Starting at the third metatarsal head, take the tape around the heel from the lateral side and meet the strip where it began (2 and 3).
3. Start the next strip near the second metatarsal head and finish it on the fourth metatarsal head (4).

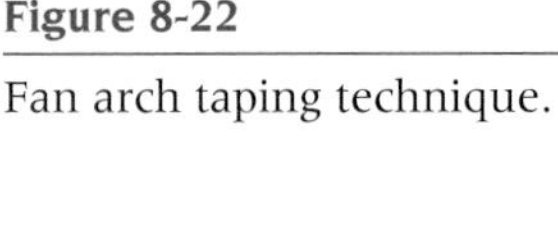

Figure 8-22

Fan arch taping technique.

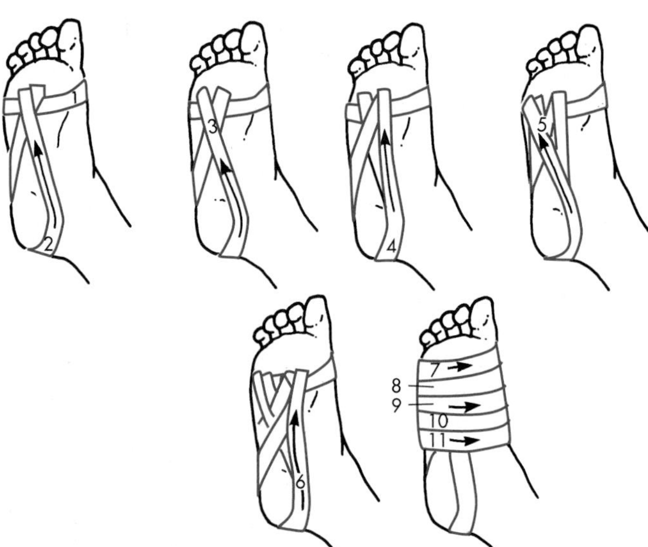

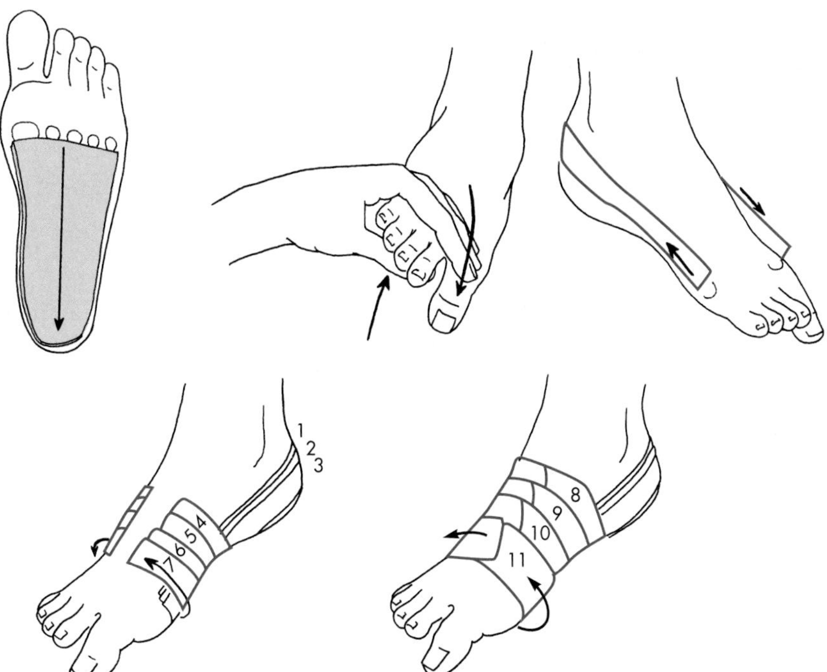

Figure 8-23

LowDye taping technique.

4. Begin the last strip on the fourth metatarsal head and finish it on the fifth metatarsal head (5). The technique, when completed, forms a fan-shaped pattern covering the metatarsal region (6).
5. Lock strips using 1½-inch (3.8 cm) tape and encircling the complete arch (7 through 11).

LowDye technique The LowDye technique is an excellent method for managing the fallen medial longitudinal arch, foot pronation, arch strains, and plantar fasciitis.[13,27] Moleskin is cut in 3-inch (7.5 cm) strips to the shape of the sole of the foot. It should cover the head of the metatarsal bones and the calcaneus bone (Figure 8-23).

Materials needed One roll of 1-inch (2.5 cm) tape, one roll of 2-inch (5 cm) tape, and moleskin.

Position of the athlete The athlete sits with the foot in a neutral position with the great toe and medial aspect of the foot in plantar flexion.

Procedure

1. Apply the moleskin to the sole of the foot, pulling it slightly downward before attaching it to the calcaneus.
2. Grasp the forefoot with the thumb under the distal 2 to 5 metatarsal heads, pushing slightly upward, with the tips of the second and third fingers pushing downward on the first metatarsal head. Apply two or three 1-inch (2.5 cm) tape strips laterally, starting from the distal head of the first metatarsal bone (1 through 3). Keep these lateral strips below the outer malleolus.
3. Secure the moleskin and lateral tape strip by circling the forefoot with four 2-inch (5 cm) strips (4 through 7). Start at the lateral dorsum of the foot, circle under the plantar aspect, and finish at the medial dorsum of the foot. Apply four strips of 2-inch stretch tape that encircle the arch (8 through 11).

A variation of this method is to use two 2-inch (5 cm) moleskin strips, one at the ball of the foot and the other at the base of the fifth metatarsal. Cross the strips and extend them along the plantar surface of the foot. For anchors, apply 2-inch (5 cm) elastic tape around the forefoot, lateral to medial, giving additional support.[13,27]

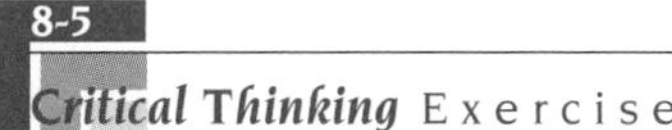

A football lineman has a severe right foot pronation with a fallen medial longitudinal arch. He is subject to arch strains.

? What taping technique is designed for this situation?

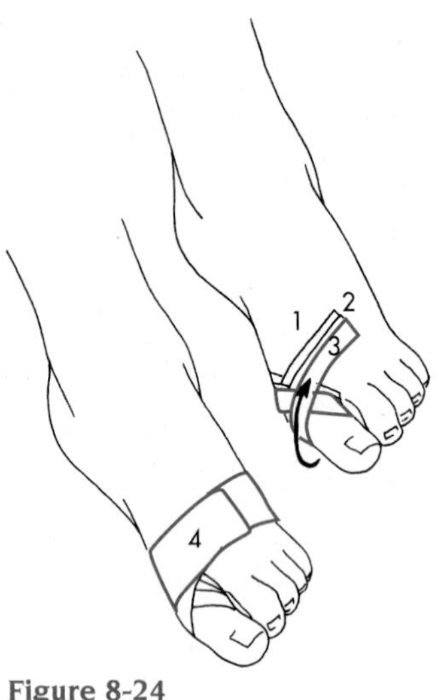

Figure 8-24

Taping for a sprained great toe.

The Toes

The sprained great toe This procedure is used for taping a sprained great toe (Figure 8-24).

Materials needed One roll of 1-inch (2.5 cm) tape and tape adherent and one roll of 1½-inch (3.8 cm) tape.

Site preparation Clean foot of dirt and oil, shave hair from toes, and spray area with tape adherent.

Position of the athlete The athlete assumes a sitting position.

Procedure

1. The greatest support is given to the joint by a half-figure-eight taping (1 through 3). Start the series at an acute angle on the top of the foot and swing down between the great and first toes, first encircling the great toe and then coming up, over, and across the starting point. Repeat this process, starting each series separately.
2. After the required number of half-figure-eight strips are in position, place 1½-inch lock piece around the ball of the foot (4).

Bunions

Materials needed One roll of 1-inch (2.5 cm) tape, tape adherent, and ¼-inch (0.6 cm) sponge rubber or felt (Figure 8-25).

Position of the athlete The athlete assumes a sitting position.

Procedure

1. Cut the ¼-inch sponge rubber to form a wedge between the great and second toes.
2. Place anchor strips to encircle the midfoot and distal aspect of the great toe (1 and 2).
3. Place two or three strips on the medial aspect of the great toe to hold the toe in proper alignment (3 through 5).
4. Lock the ends of the strips with tape (6 and 7).

Turf toe Turf toe taping is designed to prevent excessive hyperextension of the metatarsophalangeal joint (Figure 8-26).

Materials needed One roll of 1½-inch (3.8 cm) adhesive tape, one roll of 1-inch (2.5 cm) adhesive tape, and tape adherent.

Site preparation Shave hair off the top of the forefoot and great toe. Spray the area with tape adherent.

Position of the athlete The great toe is in a neutral position.

Procedure

1. Apply a one 1-inch (2.5 cm) tape strip around the great toe. Using 1½-inch (3.8 cm) tape, apply two arch anchors to the midarch area.
2. On the middle of the great toe, attach three 1-inch (2.5 cm) tape strips to create a checkrein.
3. Attach the checkrein to the arch anchor tapes, strip-crossing the metatarsophalangeal joint line.
4. Lock both ends of the checkrein in place.

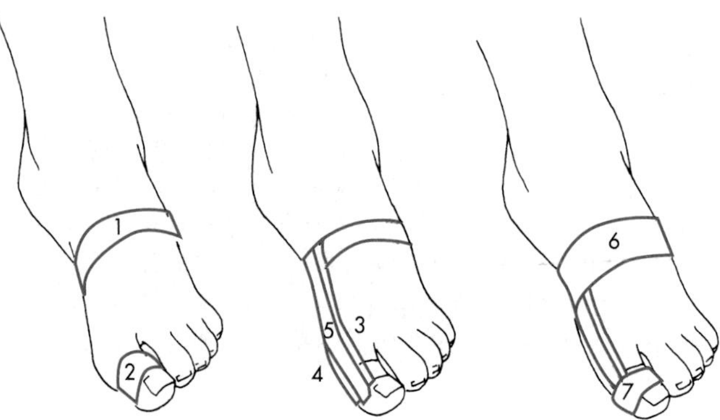

Figure 8-25

Bunion taping.

Hammer, or clawed, toes This technique is designed to reduce the pressure of the bent toes against the shoe (Figure 8-27).[26]

Materials needed One roll of ½- or 1-inch (1.25 or 2.5 cm) adhesive tape and tape adherent.

Position of the athlete The athlete sits on the table with the affected leg extended over the edge.

Procedure

1. Tape one affected toe; then lace under the adjacent toe and over the next toe.
2. Tape can be attached to the next toe or can be continued and attached to the fifth toe.

Fractured toes This technique splints the fractured toe with a nonfractured one (Figure 8-28).

Materials needed One roll of ½- or 1-inch (1.25 or 2.5 cm) tape, ⅛-inch (0.3 cm) sponge rubber, and tape adherent.

Position of the athlete The athlete assumes a sitting position.

Procedure

1. Cut a ⅛-inch (0.3 cm) sponge rubber wedge and place it between the affected toe and a healthy one.
2. Wrap two or three strips of tape around both toes.

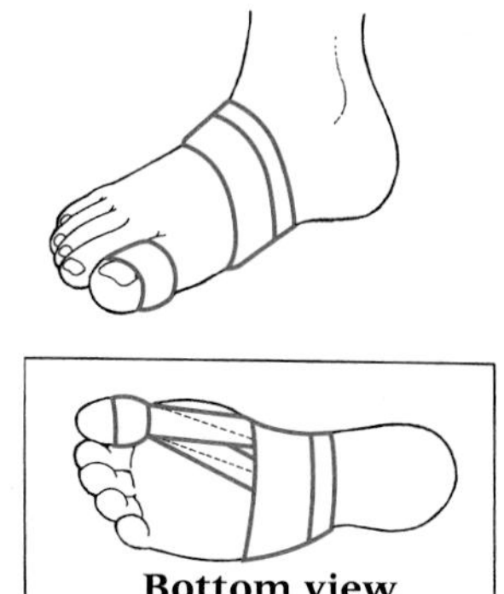

Figure 8-26

Turf toe taping.

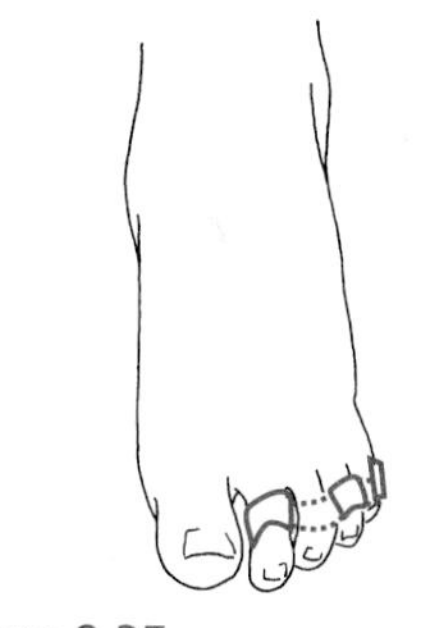

Figure 8-27

Hammer, or clawed, toe taping.

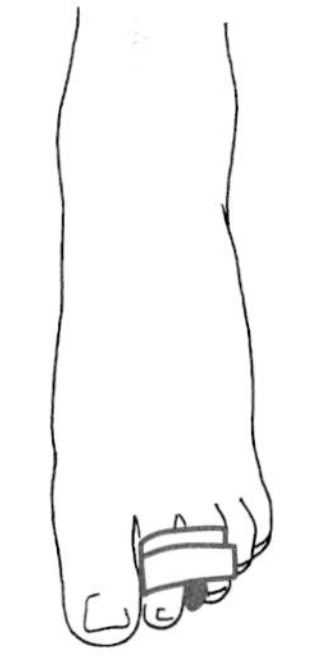

Figure 8-28

Fractured toe taping.

The Ankle Joint

The combination of foam prewrap plus tape provides significantly better ankle support during exercise than does taping directly on the skin. Both procedures diminish over time, but prewrap appears to decline more slowly. It is most effective immediately after initial application because it provides some minor resistance to ankle inversion movements.[10,18,32]

Ankle joint taping is most appropriate for sports with short bursts of at-risk activity, such as high jumping, and for endurance sports, such as soccer or basketball. Whether ankle braces are as effective as ankle taping has been debated and remains controversial.[1,6,12,20,24,25]

Routine prophylactic (preventative) taping

Materials needed One roll of 1½-inch (3.8 cm) tape, tape adherent, and underwrap (Figure 8-29).

Site preparation Ankle taping applied directly to the athlete's skin affords the greatest support; however, when it is applied and removed daily, skin irritation will occur. To avoid this problem, apply an underwrap material. Before taping, follow these procedures:

1. Clean foot and ankle thoroughly.
2. Shave all the hair off the foot and ankle.
3. Apply a coating of tape adherent to protect the skin and offer an adhering base.
4. Apply a gauze pad coated with friction-reducing material such as grease over the instep and to the back of the heel.
5. If underwrap is used, apply a single layer. The tape anchors extend beyond the underwrap and adhere directly to the skin.
6. Do not apply tape if skin is cold or hot from a therapeutic treatment.

Position of the athlete The athlete sits on the table with the leg extended and the foot held at a 90-degree angle.

Procedure

1. Place an anchor around the ankle approximately 5 or 6 inches (12.5 or 15 cm) above the malleolus.
2. Apply two strips in consecutive order, starting behind the outer malleolus, taking care that the second strip overlaps the first by half the width of the tape (2 and 3).
3. After applying the strips, wrap seven or eight circular strips around the ankle, from the point of the anchor downward, until the malleolus is completely covered (4 through 12).

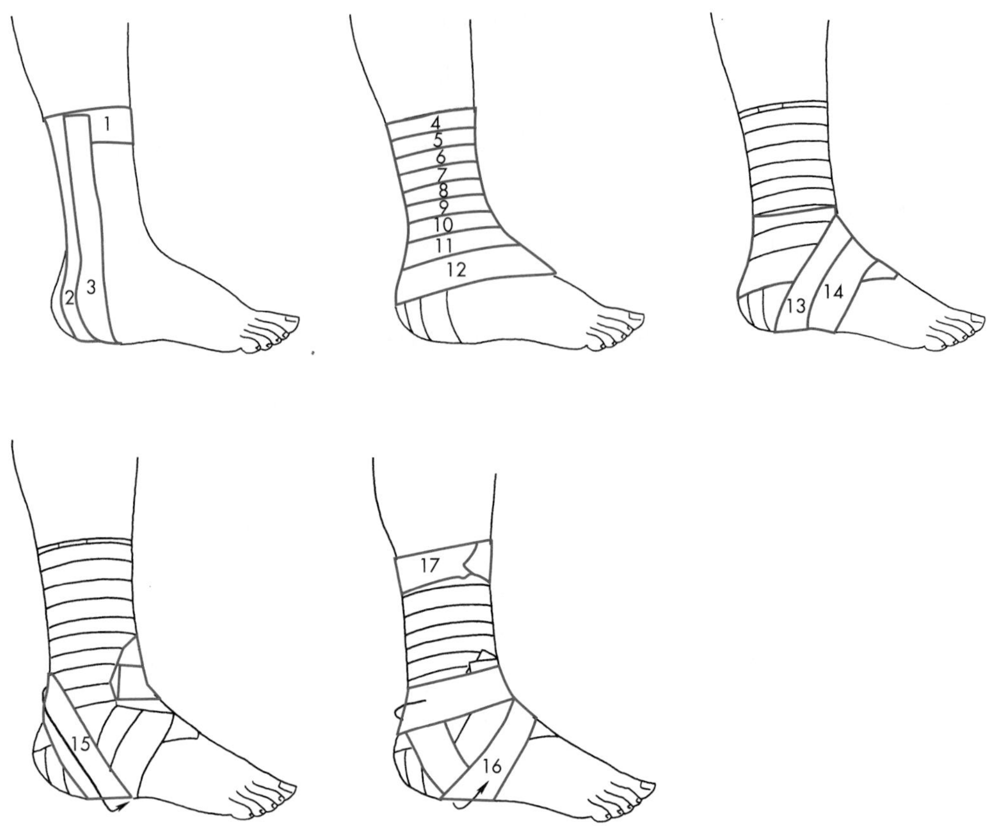

Figure 8-29

Routine noninjury ankle taping.

4. Apply two or three arch strips from lateral to medial, giving additional support to the arch (13 and 14).
5. Additional support is given by a heel lock. Starting high on the instep, bring the tape along the ankle at a slight angle, hooking the heel, leading under the arch, then coming up on the opposite side, and finishing at the starting point. Tear the tape to complete half of the heel lock (15). Repeat on the opposite side of the ankle (16). Finish with a band of tape around the ankle (17).

Closed basket weave (Gibney) technique The closed basket weave, or Gibney, technique offers strong tape support and is primarily used in athletic training for newly sprained or chronically weak ankles (Figure 8-30). A U-shaped felt pad can be used with this taping technique to provide focal compression and thus assist in controlling swelling. The technique for controlling swelling initially following injury is discussed in detail in Chapter 12.

Materials needed One roll of 1½-inch (3.8 cm) tape, underwrap, and tape adherent.

Position of the athlete The athlete sits on the table with the leg extended and the foot at a 90-degree angle.

Procedure

1. Place one anchor piece around the ankle approximately 5 or 6 inches (12.5 or 15 cm) above the malleolus just below the belly of the gastrocnemius muscle. Place a second anchor around the instep directly over the styloid process of the fifth metatarsal (1 and 2).
2. Apply the first strip posteriorly to the malleolus and attach it to the ankle anchor (3). NOTE: When applying strips, pull the foot into eversion for an inversion strain and into a neutral position for an eversion strain.
3. Start the first Gibney directly under the malleolus and attach it to the foot anchor (4).
4. In an alternating series, place three strips and three Gibneys on the ankle with each piece of tape overlapping at least half of the preceding strip (5 through 8).

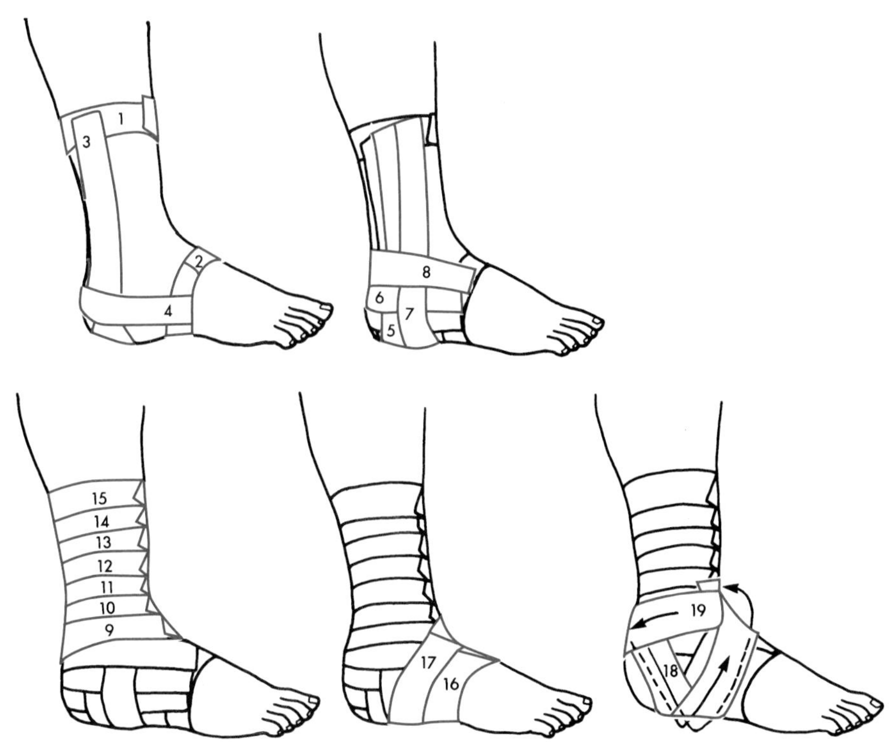

Figure 8-30

Closed basket weave ankle taping.

5. After applying the basket weave series, continue the Gibney strips up the ankle, thus giving circular support (9 through 15).
6. For arch support, apply two or three circular strips laterally to medially (16 and 17).
7. After completing the conventional basket weave, apply two or three heel locks to ensure maximum stability (18 and 19).

Open basket weave This modification of the closed basket weave, or Gibney, technique is designed to give freedom of movement in dorsiflexion and plantar flexion while providing lateral and medial support and allowing swelling room. Taping in this pattern may be used immediately after an acute sprain in conjunction with a pressure bandage and cold applications because it allows for swelling (Figure 8-31).

Materials needed One roll of 1½-inch (3.8 cm) tape and tape adherent.

Position of the athlete The athlete sits on the table with the leg extended and the foot held at a 90-degree angle.

Procedure

1. The procedures are the same as for the closed basket weave (Figure 8-30) with the exception of incomplete closures of the Gibney strips (11 through 17).
2. Lock the gap between the Gibney ends with two pieces of tape running on either side of the instep (18 through 21). NOTE: Application of a 1½-inch (3.8 cm) elastic bandage over the open basket weave affords added control of swelling; however, the athlete should remove it before going to bed. Apply the elastic bandage distal to proximal to prevent swelling from moving into the toes.

Of the many ankle taping techniques in use today, those using combinations of strips, basket weaves, and heel locks offer the best support.

Continuous-stretch tape technique This technique provides a fast alternative to other taping methods for the ankle (Figure 8-32).[23]

Materials needed One roll of 1½-inch (3.8 cm) linen tape, one roll of 2-inch (5 cm) stretch tape, tape adherent, and underwrap.

Position of the athlete The athlete sits on the table with the leg extended and the foot at a 90-degree angle.

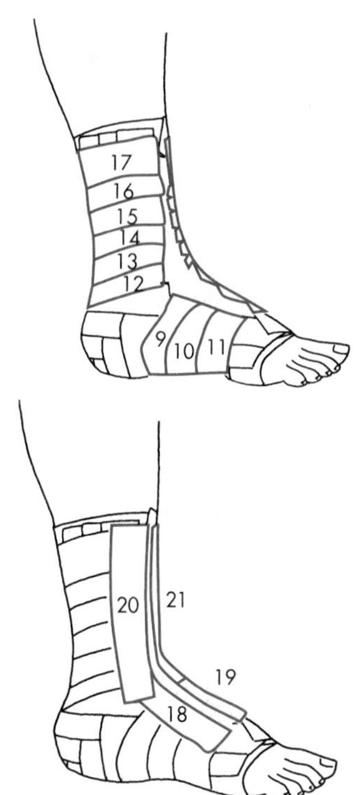

Figure 8-31

Open basket weave ankle taping.

Chapter 9 Mechanisms and Characteristics of Sports Trauma

When you finish this chapter you should be able to

- Analyze the biomechanical factors in sports injuries.
- Distinguish the major biomechanical forces occurring in sports injuries.
- Categorize the most common exposed skin injuries.
- Review the normal structures of soft tissue and identify the specific mechanical forces that cause skin, internal soft-tissue, synovial joint, and bone injuries.
- Define the terminology that describes injuries incurred during sports participation.
- Describe the various types of bone fractures and explain how they occur.
- Explain how a nerve is injured.

trauma
A physical injury or wound sustained in sport and produced by an external or internal force is called trauma.

Many factors produce mechanical injuries or trauma in sports. **Trauma** is defined as a physical injury or wound sustained in sport and produced by an external or internal force (Figure 9-1).[6] This chapter provides a foundation for the identification, understanding, and management of sports injuries. It examines mechanical forces and tissue characteristics of sports injuries and the classification of these injuries.[16]

9-1 Critical Thinking Exercise

To effectively present and manage sports injuries, the athletic trainer must understand tissue susceptibility to sports trauma.

? What should the athletic trainer know about tissue properties?

MECHANICAL INJURY

"Force or mechanical energy is that which changes the state of rest or uniform motion of matter. When a force applied to any part of the body results in a harmful disturbance in function and or structure, a mechanical injury is said to have been sustained."[22] Injuries related to sports participation can be caused by external forces directed on the body or can occur internally within the body.[23] Understanding sports injuries requires a knowledge of tissue susceptibility to trauma and the mechanical forces involved.

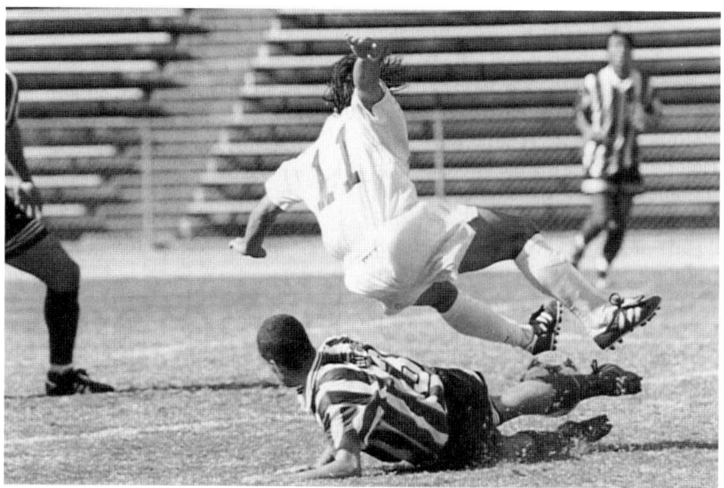

Figure 9-1

A sports injury can be sustained from an external or internal force.

Tissue Properties

Tissues have relative abilities to resist a particular load. The stronger the tissue, the greater the magnitude of load it can withstand. Strength pressure, or power, is often used to imply a force. A force can be defined as a push or pull.[25] Tissue properties are described according to engineering terminology.[18] A **load** can be a singular force or a group of outside or internal forces acting on the body. The resistance to a load is called a mechanical **stress**, and the internal response is a deformation, or change in dimensions. Deformation is also defined as a mechanical **strain**. All human tissue is **viscoelastic;** it has both viscous and elastic properties, allowing for deformation. Tissue such as bone is brittle and has fewer viscoelastic properties than soft tissue. Tissue also is anisotropic, responding with greater or lesser strength depending on the direction of the load that is being applied. When tissue is deformed to the extent that its elasticity is almost fully exceeded, a **yield point** has been reached. When the yield point has been exceeded, **mechanical failure** occurs, resulting in tissue damage.[2]

load
Outside force or forces acting on tissue.

stress
The internal reaction or resistance to an external load.

strain
Extent of deformation of tissue under loading.

viscoelastic
Any material whose mechanical properties vary depending on rate of load.

Human tissue is viscoelastic—it has both viscous and elastic properties.

yield point
Elastic limit of tissue.

mechanical failure
Elastic limit of tissue is exceeded, causing tissue to break.

Tissue Stresses

There are five primary tissue stresses leading to sports injuries: tension, stretching, compression, shearing, and bending.[18]

Tension is that force which pulls or stretches tissue. Muscle strains and ligament sprains both occur due to increased tension.

Stretching beyond the yield point leads to rupturing of soft tissue or fracturing of a bone. Examples of stretching injuries are sprains, strains, and avulsion fractures.

Compression is a force that, with enough energy, crushes tissue. When the force can no longer be absorbed, injury occurs. Constant submaximum compression over a period of time can cause the contacted tissue to develop abnormal wear. Compression occurs when a muscle or bone is stretched directly or when cartilage bone is directly loaded. Arthritic changes, fractures, and contusions are commonly caused by compression force.

Tissue stresses
- Tension
- Stretching
- Compression
- Shearing
- Bending

Shearing is a force that moves across the parallel organization of the tissue. Injury occurs once shearing has exceeded the inherent strength of a tissue. Shearing stress can result in skin injuries such as blisters, rips of the hands, abrasions, or vertebral disk injuries (Figure 9-2).

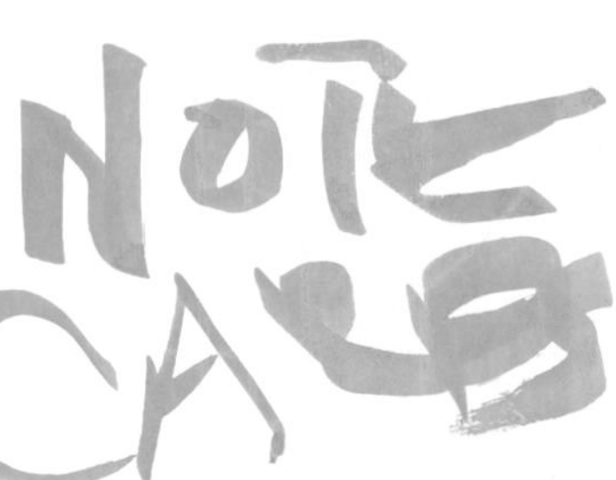

Bending is a force on a horizontal beam or bone that places stresses within the structure, causing it to bend or strain.[25] This force is known as three-point bending (Figure 9-3). Compression occurs parallel to the beam's length if the force is on the concave side, and tension occurs if the force is on the convex side. Shear stress is also caused in two directions within the bending beam.[25] Bending strain can also occur perpendicular to or along the length of a beam, with compression, tension, and shearing occurring. Injuries to the hip and femur are examples of this type of bending strain. A torsion, or twisting, load causes compression and tension in a spiral pattern,

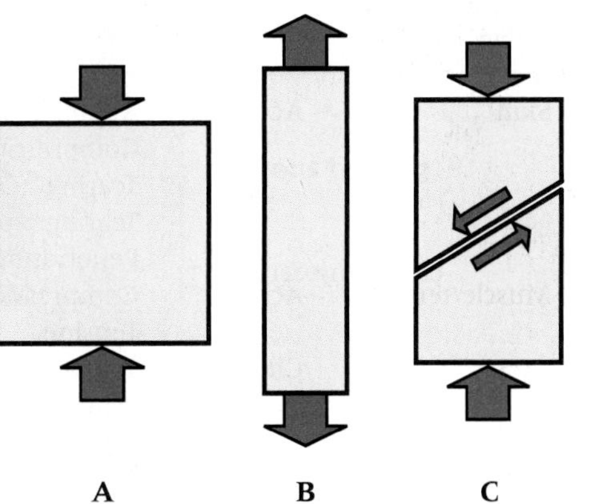

Figure 9-2
Mechanical forces that can cause injury. **A,** Compression. **B,** Tension. **C,** Shear.

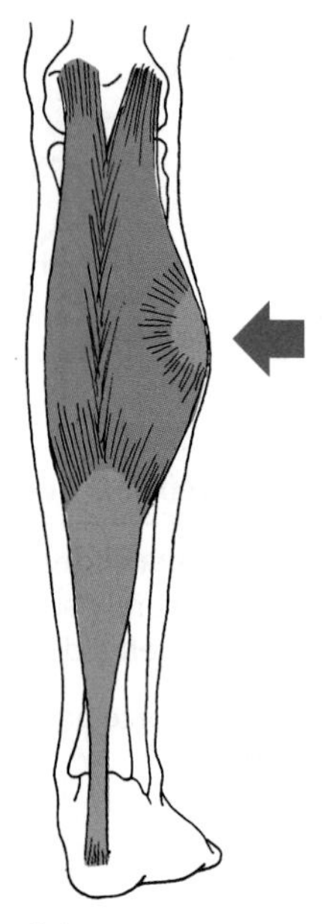

Figure 9-6

A contusion is caused by a compression force.

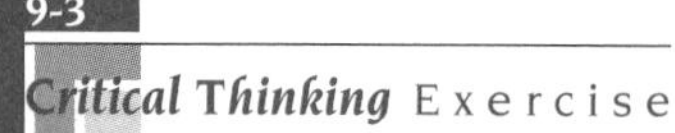

9-3 Critical Thinking Exercise

A shortstop is hit in the shin by a batted ball that took a bad hop.

? What is the force and type of injury sustained by this athlete?

the fibrous tendon. The fibrous wrapping of a muscle may become a flat sheet of connective tissue (aponeurosis) that attaches to other muscles. Tendons and aponeuroses are extremely resilient to injuries. They will pull away from a bone, a bone will break, or a muscle will tear before tendons and aponeuroses are injured. Skeletal muscles are generally well supplied with blood vessels that permeate throughout their structure. Arteries, veins, lymph vessels, and bundles of nerve fibers spread into the perimysium. A complex capillary network goes throughout the endomysium, coming into direct contact with the muscle fibers.[35]

Acute Muscle Injuries

Contusions

A bruise, or contusion, occurs from a sudden traumatic blow to the body. The intensity of a contusion can range from superficial to deep tissue compression and hemorrhage (Figure 9-6).

Interrupting the continuity of the circulatory system results in a flow of blood and lymph into the surrounding tissues. A hematoma (blood tumor) is formed by the localization of the extravasated blood into a clot, which becomes encapsulated by a connective tissue membrane. The speed of healing of a contusion, as with all soft-tissue injuries, depends on the extent of tissue damage and internal bleeding.

A contusion can penetrate to the skeletal structures, causing a bone bruise. The extent to which an athlete may be hampered by this condition depends on the location of the bruise and the force of the blow. Typical in cases of severe contusion are the following:

1. The athlete reports being struck by a hard impact.
2. The impact causes pain and a transitory paralysis caused by pressure on and shock to the motor and sensory nerves.
3. Palpation often reveals a hardened area, indurated because of internal hemorrhage.
4. Ecchymosis, or tissue discoloration, may take place.

Muscle contusions are usually rated by the extent to which the muscle is able to produce range of motion in a part (see Chapter 10). A blow to a muscle can be so great that the related fascia is ruptured, allowing muscle tissue to protrude through it.

Strains

A strain is a stretch, tear, or rip in the muscle or adjacent tissue such as the fascia or muscle tendons (Figure 9-7). The cause of muscle strain is often obscure. Most often a strain is produced by an abnormal muscular contraction. The cause of this abnormality has been attributed to many factors. One popular theory suggests that a fault in the reciprocal coordination of the agonist and antagonist muscles takes place. The cause of this fault or incoordination is a mystery. However, possible explanations are that it may be related to an electrolyte imbalance caused by profuse sweating, or to a strength imbalance between agonist and antagonist muscles.

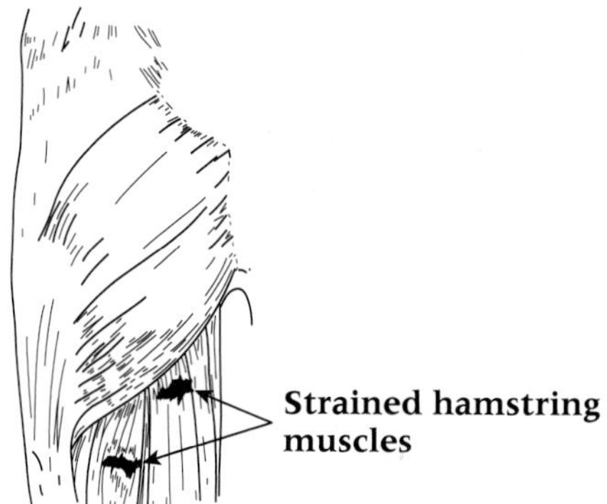

Figure 9-7

A muscle strain results in tearing or separation of fibers.

A strain may range from a minute separation of connective tissue and muscle fibers to a complete tendinous avulsion or muscle rupture (grade 1, 2, or 3).[12] The resulting pathology is similar to that of the contusion or sprain, with capillary or blood vessel hemorrhage.

- *Grade 1 strain.* Some muscle fibers have been stretched or actually torn. There is some tenderness and pain on active motion. Movement is painful, but full range of motion is usually possible.
- *Grade 2 strain.* A number of muscle fibers have been torn, and active contraction of the muscle is extremely painful. Usually a depression or divot can be felt somewhere in the muscle belly at the place at which the muscle fibers have been torn. Some swelling may occur because of capillary bleeding; therefore, some discoloration is possible.
- *Grade 3 strain.* A complete rupture of a muscle has occurred in the area of the muscle belly at the point at which muscle becomes tendon or at the tendinous attachment to the bone. There is significant impairment to or perhaps total loss of movement. Initially, pain is intense but quickly diminishes because of complete nerve fiber separation.

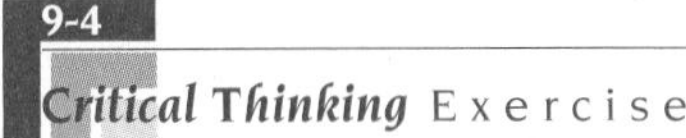

While performing an arm tackle, a football player severely injures his upper arm.

? What injury mechanism has occurred, and what is the subsequent injury produced?

Tendon Injuries

The tendon contains wavy parallel collagenous fibers that are organized in bundles surrounded by a gelatinous material that decreases friction. A tendon attaches a muscle to a bone and concentrates a pulling force in a limited area. Tendons can produce and maintain a pull from 8,700 to 18,000 pounds per square inch. When a tendon is loaded by tension, the wavy collagenous fibers straighten in the direction of the load; when the tension is released, the collagen returns to its original shape. In tendons, collagen fibers will break if their physiological limits have been reached. A breaking point occurs after a 6 percent to 8 percent increase in length (Figure 9-8). Because a tendon is usually double the strength of the muscle it serves, tears commonly occur at the muscle belly, musculotendinous junction, or bony attachment.[8] Clinically, however, a constant abnormal tension on tendons increases elongation by the infiltration of fibroblasts, which will cause more collagenous tissue to be produced. Repeated microtraumas can evolve into chronic muscle strain that resorbs collagen fibers and eventually weakens the tendon.[30] Collagen resorption occurs in the early period of sports conditioning and during the immobilization of a part. During resorption, collagenous tissues are weakened and susceptible to injury; therefore a gradually paced conditioning program and early mobilization in the rehabilitation process are necessary.

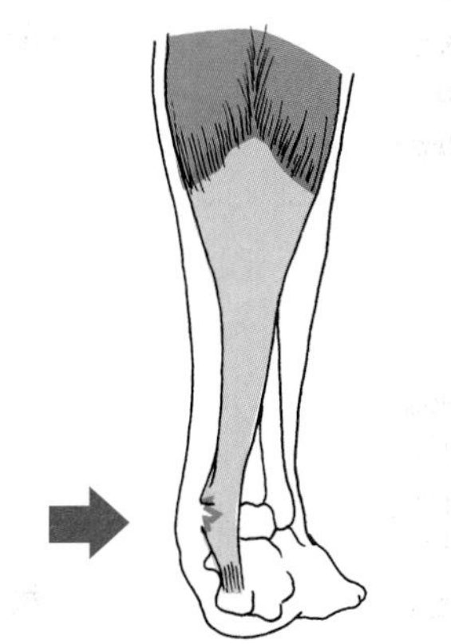

Figure 9-8

Tendon injuries occur due to excessive tension in the musculotendinous unit.

Muscle Spasms

A spasm is a reflex reaction caused by trauma of the musculoskeletal system. The two types of spasms are the **clonic** type, with alternating involuntary muscular contraction and relaxation in quick succession, and the **tonic** type, with rigid muscle contraction that lasts a period of time. Muscle spasms may lead to a muscle strain.

clonic
Involuntary muscle contraction characterized by alternate contraction and relaxation in rapid succession.

tonic
Muscle contraction characterized by constant contraction that lasts for a period of time.

Overexertional Muscle Problems

One constant problem in conditioning and fitness training is overexertion. Even though the gradual pattern of overloading the body is the best way for ultimate success, many athletes and even coaches believe that "if there is no pain, there is no gain."

Exercise overload is reflected in muscle soreness, decreased joint flexibility, and general fatigue that occurs twenty-four hours after activity. Four specific indicators of possible overexertion are acute muscle soreness, delayed muscle soreness, muscle stiffness, and muscle cramping.

Muscle soreness Overexertion in strenuous muscular exercise often results in muscular pain. Most people, at one time or another, have experienced muscle soreness, usually resulting from some physical activity to which they are unaccustomed. The older a person gets, the more easily muscle soreness seems to develop.

The two major types of muscle soreness associated with severe exercise are acute and delayed-onset muscle soreness (DOMS).

There are two types of muscle soreness. The first type is *acute-onset muscle soreness,* which accompanies fatigue. This muscle pain is transient and occurs during and immediately after exercise. The second type of soreness involves delayed muscle pain that appears approximately twelve hours after injury. This *delayed-onset muscle soreness* (DOMS) becomes most intense after twenty-four to forty-eight hours and then gradually subsides so that the muscle becomes symptom-free after three or four days. This second type of pain is described as a syndrome of delayed muscle pain leading to increased muscle tension, swelling, stiffness, and resistance to stretching.[9]

Delayed-onset muscle soreness is thought to result from several possible causes. It may occur from very small tears in the muscle tissue, which seems to be more likely with eccentric or isometric contractions. It may also occur because of disruption of the connective tissue that holds muscle tendon fibers together.[10]

Muscle soreness may be prevented by beginning an exercise at a moderate level and gradually increasing the intensity of the exercise over time. Treatment of muscle soreness usually involves static or PNF stretching activities. Like other conditions discussed in this chapter, muscle soreness can be treated with ice applied within the first forty-eight to seventy-two hours.[9]

Muscle stiffness Muscle stiffness does not produce pain. It occurs when a group of muscles have been worked hard for a long period of time. The fluids that collect in the muscles during and after exercise are absorbed into the bloodstream at a slow rate. As a result, the muscle becomes swollen, shorter, and thicker and therefore resists stretching. Light exercise, massage, and passive mobilization assist in reducing stiffness.

Muscle cramps Cramps are painful involuntary skeletal muscle contractions.[14] Muscle cramps are different than heat cramps (discussed in Chapter 6) which occur in individuals who are performing hard muscular work in a hot environment and are sweating profusely. Muscle cramps are most likely to occur in well-developed individuals and develop when a muscle, already in a shortened position, involuntarily contracts. This most often occurs at rest, usually at night, asymetrically in either the gastrocnemius or small foot muscles.[37]

Muscle Guarding

Following injury, the muscles that surround the injured area contract to, in effect, splint that area, thus minimizing pain by limiting movement. Quite often this splinting is incorrectly referred to as a muscle spasm. The terms *spasm* and *spasticity* are more correctly associated with increased tone or contractions of muscle that occur because of some upper motor neuron lesion in the brain. Thus, *muscle guarding* is a more appropriate term for the involuntary muscle contractions that occur in response to pain following musculoskeletal injury.[7]

Myofascial Trigger Points

A *myofascial trigger point* is a discreet, hypersensitive nodule found within a taut band of skeletal muscle and/or fascia.[11] Palpation of this nodule reveals an area of harder-than-normal consistency. Trigger points are classified as being latent or active, depending on their clinical characteristics. A *latent trigger point* does not cause spontaneous pain, but may restrict movement or cause muscle weakness. The individual presenting with muscle restrictions or weakness may become aware of pain originating from a latent trigger point only when pressure is applied directly over the point. An *active trigger point* causes pain at rest. Firm pressure applied over the point usually elicits a "jump sign," with the patient crying out, wincing, or withdrawing from the stimulus. It is tender to palpation with a referred pain pattern that is similar to the patient's pain complaint. This referred pain is not felt at the site of the trigger-point origin but rather at a remote point. The pain is often described as spreading or radiating. Referred pain is an important characteristic of a trigger point. It differentiates a trigger point from a tender point, which is associated with pain at the site of palpation only. They are palpable within

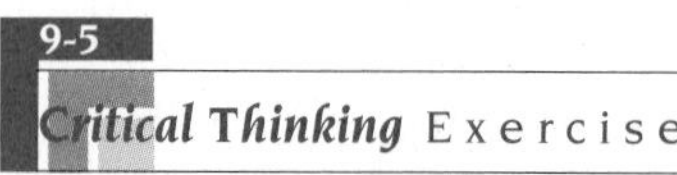

A tennis player with a pronounced topspin style of hitting a backhand stroke sustains a painful elbow.

? What are the forces and type of elbow injury sustained by the tennis player, and what are ways to prevent this problem?

muscles as cordlike bands within a sharply circumscribed area of extreme tenderness. Trigger points are found most commonly in muscles involved in postural support.[7] Acute trauma or repetitive microtrauma may lead to the development of stress on muscle fibers and the formation of trigger points.

Chronic Musculotendinous Injuries

Chronic injuries usually progress slowly over a long period of time. Often, repeated acute injuries can lead to a chronic condition. A constant irritation caused by poor performance techniques or a constant stress beyond physiological limits can eventually result in a chronic condition. These injuries are often attributed to overuse microtraumas.[31]

Chronic muscle injuries are representative of a low-grade inflammatory process with a proliferation of fibroblasts and scarring. The acute injury that is improperly managed or that allows an athlete to return to activity before healing has completely occurred can cause chronic injury. The athletic trainer should be especially knowledgeable about five chronic muscle conditions: myositis, tendinitis, tenosynovitis, ectopic calcification, and muscle atrophy and contracture.

Myositis/fasciitis In general, the term *myositis* means inflammation of muscle tissue. More specifically, it can be considered a fibrositis, or connective tissue inflammation. Fascia that supports and separates muscle can also become chronically inflamed after injury. A typical example of this condition is plantar fasciitis.

Tendinitis Tendinitis has a gradual onset, diffuse tenderness because of repeated microtraumas, and degenerative changes. Obvious signs of tendinitis are swelling and pain.

Tenosynovitis Tenosynovitis is inflammation of the synovial sheath surrounding a tendon. In its acute state there is rapid onset, articular crepitus, and diffuse swelling. In chronic tenosynovitis the tendons become locally thickened, with pain and articular crepitus present during movement (Figure 9-9).

Ectopic calcification Striated muscles can become chronically inflamed, resulting in myositis. An **ectopic** calcification known as *myositis ossificans* can occur in a muscle that directly overlies a bone. Two common sites for this condition are the quadriceps region of the thigh and the brachial muscle of the arm. In myositis ossificans, osteoid material that resembles bone rapidly accumulates. If there is no repeated injury, the growth may subside completely in nine to twelve months, or it may mature into a calcified area, at which time surgical removal can be accomplished with little fear of recurrence. Occasionally, tendinitis leads to deposits of minerals, primarily lime, and is known as *calcific tendinitis*.

ectopic
Located in a place different from normal.

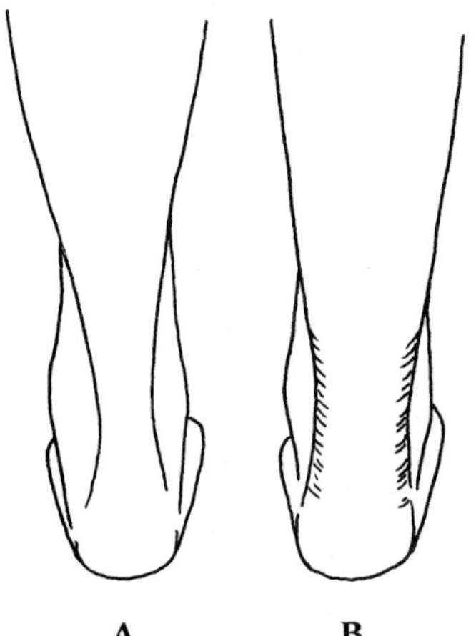

Figure 9-9
Tenosynovitis is an inflammation of the sheath covering a tendon. **A,** Normal. **B,** Inflamed.

9-6

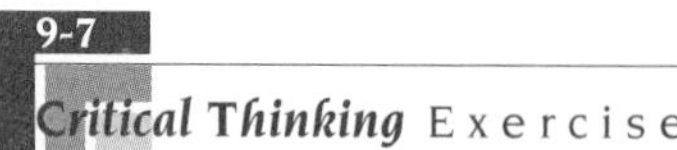

Critical Thinking Exercise

A football player sustains repeated contusions to the left quadriceps muscle.

? What should he be most concerned about?

9-7

Critical Thinking Exercise

A football player who plays wide receiver sustains repeated blows to his left quadriceps muscle.

? What type of injury could be sustained from repeated compressive forces to the quadriceps muscle?

Atrophy and contracture Two complications of muscle and tendon conditions are atrophy and contracture. Muscle atrophy is the wasting away of muscle tissue. Its main cause in athletes is immobilization of a body part, inactivity, or loss of nerve stimulation. A second complication in sport injuries is muscle contracture, an abnormal shortening of muscle tissue in which there is a great deal of resistance to passive stretch. A contracture is associated with a joint that, because of muscle injury, has developed unyielding and resisting scar tissue.

SYNOVIAL JOINTS

A joint in the human body is defined as the point at which two bones join together. A joint must also transmit forces between articulating bones.[22]

Anatomical Characteristics

The joint consists of cartilage and fibrous connective tissue. Joints are classified as immovable (synarthrotic), slightly movable (amphiarthrotic), and freely movable (diarthrotic). Diarthrotic joints are also called synovial articulations. Anatomical characteristics of synovial articulations consist of four features: they have a capsule or ligaments, the capsule is lined with a synovial membrane, the opposing bone surfaces contain hyaline or articular cartilage, and there is a joint space (joint cavity) containing a small amount of fluid (synovial fluid) (Figure 9-10). In addition, nerves and blood are supplied to the synovial articulation, and muscles cross the joint or are intrinsic to it.[35]

Joint Capsule

Bones of the diarthrotic joint are held together by a cuff of fibrous tissue known as the capsule, or capsular ligament. It consists of bundles of collagen and functions primarily to maintain a relative joint position. It is extremely strong and can withstand cross-sectional forces of 500 kg/cm^2. Parts of the capsule become slack or taut, depending on the joint movements.

Ligaments

Ligaments are sheets or bundles of collagen fibers that form a connection between two bones. Ligaments fall into two categories: ones that are considered intrinsic and ones that are extrinsic to the joint. Intrinsic ligaments occur where the articular capsule has become thickened in some places. Extrinsic ligaments are separate from the capsular thickening.[35]

Ligaments and capsules, found in synovial joints, are similar in composition to tendons; however, ligaments and capsules contain elastic fibers and collagen fibers that

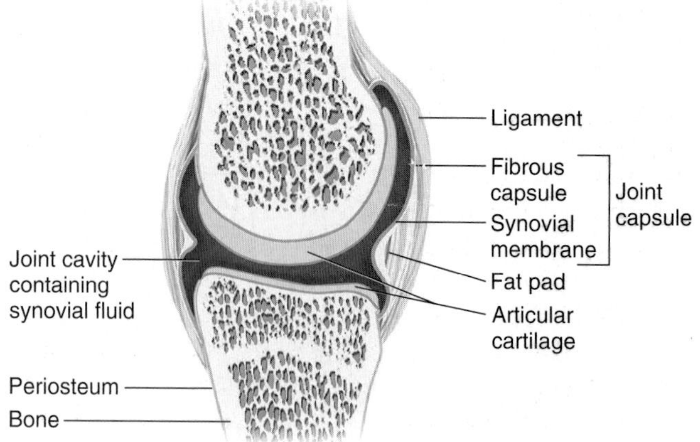

Figure 9-10

General anatomy of a synovial joint.

have a wavy, irregular, spiral configuration. Ligaments are strongest in their middle and weakest at their ends. When an intact ligament is traumatically stretched, the injury often produces an avulsion-type fracture or tear at the ends rather than in the middle. Tears in the middle of the ligament are referred to as *midsubstance tears.* Avulsion fractures are more common when bone tissue is comparatively weaker than ligamentous tissue—for instance, in older individuals or postmenopausal women in whom significant osteoporosis has occurred or in children in whom the epiphyseal plates are relatively wide and soft.[35]

Constant compression or tension will cause ligaments to deteriorate; intermittent compression and tension will increase strength and growth.

A primary factor in ligamentous injury is the viscoelastic tissue properties of ligaments and capsules. Viscoelasticity refers to extensibility when loaded that is time dependent. Constant compression or tension causes ligaments to deteriorate, whereas intermittent compression and tension increases strength, especially at the bony attachment. Chronic inflammation of ligamentous, capsular, and fascial tissue causes a shrinkage of collagen fibers; therefore, repeated microtraumas over time make capsules and ligaments highly susceptible to major acute injuries.

Ligaments act as protective backups for the joint. Primary protection occurs from the dynamic aspect of muscles and their tendons.[1] In a fast-loading situation, ligament failure ultimately will occur; however, the capsule and ligament provide maximum protection during rapid movements. Nevertheless, capsular and ligamentous tissues are highly sensitive to movement deprivation stress through joint immobilization.[1] Capsular and ligamentous tissue respond to Roux's law of functional adaptation: An organ will adapt itself structurally to an alteration, quantitative or qualitative, of function.[22]

Synovial Membrane and Synovial Fluid

Lining the synovial articular capsule is a synovial membrane made of connective tissue with flattened cells and villi (small projections) on its inner aspect. Fluid is secreted and absorbed by the synovial membrane. Synovial fluid has the consistency of egg white and acts as a joint lubricant. It has the ability to vary its viscosity. During slow movement, the fluid thickens; during fast movement it thins. This variation in viscosity is produced by the presence of hyaluronic acid.[35]

Articular Cartilage

Cartilage, a connective tissue, provides firm and flexible support. It occurs throughout the body and consists of three types: hyaline (articular), fibrous, and elastic. Cartilage is a semifirm connective tissue with a predominance of ground substance in the extracellular matrix. Within the ground substance are varying amounts of collagenous and elastic fibers. Cartilage has a bluish white or gray color and is semiopaque. It has no direct blood or nerve supply. Hyaline cartilage composes part of the nasal septum, the larynx, the trachea, the bronchi, and the articular ends of bones of the synovial joints. Fibrocartilage makes up the vertebral disks, symphysis pubis, and menisci of the knee joint. Elastic cartilage is found in the external ear and the eustachian tube.

As mentioned previously, the ends of the bones in a diarthrotic joint are covered by hyaline cartilage, which cushions the bone ends. Its general appearance is smooth and pearly. Hyaline cartilage acts like a sponge in relation to synovial fluid. As movement occurs, the articular cartilage helps provide both static and dynamic stability; it also absorbs and squeezes out the fluid as pressures vary between the joint surfaces. Because of its great strength, cartilage can be deformed without damage and can still return to its original shape. However, cartilaginous degeneration, producing microtrauma, may occur during the abnormal compressional forces that take place over time. Hyaline cartilage has no direct blood supply; it receives its nourishment from the synovial fluid, or more specifically, from the synovial membrane located at its edges. Deeper aspects of the cartilage are fed by spaces (lacunae) in the adjacent bone. The articular cartilage provides three major functions: motion control, stability, and load transmission.[24]

Motion Control

The shape of the articular cartilage determines what motion will occur. An enarthrodial joint, or a ball-and-socket joint such as the hip, is considered a universal joint, allowing movement in all planes. In contrast, a hinge joint such as the interphalangeal joint allows movement in only one plane.

Stability

Bones that form a joint have articulating surfaces that are at least somewhat congruent with one another and that produce varying degrees of stability, depending on their particular shape. The less congruent the articulating surfaces, the greater the instability.

Load Transmission

The articular cartilage assists in transmitting a joint load smoothly and uniformly across the articulating surface.

Additional Synovial Joint Structures

Fat

In some joints, such as the knee and elbow, pads of fat lie between the synovial membrane and the capsule. These pads of fat tend to fill in the spaces between the bones that form joints. As movement occurs, they move in and out of these spaces.

Articular (Fibrocartilage) Disks

Some diarthrotic joints have an additional fibrocartilaginous disk. These disks vary in shape and are connected to the capsule. They are found in joints in which two planes of movement exist, and they may act to disperse the synovial fluid between the joint surfaces. In some joints, a fibrocartilaginous disk is referred to as a meniscus.

Nerve Supply

The articular capsule, ligaments, outer aspects of the synovial membrane, and fat pads of the synovial joint are well supplied with nerves. The inner aspect of the synovial membrane, cartilage, and articular disks, if present, have nerves as well. Mechanoreceptors (encapsulated nerve endings) provide information about the relative position of the joint and are found in the fibrous capsule and ligaments. Mechanoreceptors are myelinated, whereas nonmyelinated fibers are pain receptors or blood vessel suppliers.[32]

Types of Synovial Joints

Synovial joints are subdivided into six types: ball-and-socket, hinge, pivot, ellipsoidal, saddle, and gliding.[35] Ball-and-socket joints allow all possible movement (e.g., shoulder and hip joints). Hinge joints allow only flexion and extension (e.g., elbow joint). Pivot joints permit rotation around an axis (e.g., cervical atlas and axis, proximal ends of radius and ulna). Ellipsoidal joints have an elliptical convex head in an elliptical concave socket (e.g., wrist joint). Saddle-shaped joints are reciprocally concavo-convex (e.g., carpometacarpal joint of the thumb). Gliding joints allow a small amount of gliding back and forth or sideways (e.g., joints between the carpal and tarsal bones and all the joints between the articular processes of the vertebrae).[39]

Functional Synovial Joint Characteristics

Synovial joints differ in their ability to withstand trauma, depending on their skeletal, ligamentous, and muscular organization. Table 9-2 provides a general guide to the relative strength of selected articulations in terms of sports participation.

Synovial Joint Stabilization

Muscle tension is important in limiting synovial joint movement. Limitation may be the result of contacting another anatomic structure. When the joint capsule is overstretched, a reflex contraction of muscles in the area occurs to prevent overstretching.

TABLE 9-2 **General Relative Strength Grades in Selected Articulations**

Articulation	Skeleton	Ligaments	Muscles
Ankle	Strong	Moderate	Weak
Knee	Weak	Moderate	Strong
Hip	Strong	Strong	Strong
Lumbosacral	Weak	Strong	Moderate
Lumbar vertebrae	Strong	Strong	Moderate
Thoracic vertebrae	Strong	Strong	Moderate
Cervical vertebrae	Weak	Moderate	Strong
Sternoclavicular	Weak	Weak	Weak
Acromioclavicular	Weak	Moderate	Weak
Glenohumeral	Weak	Moderate	Moderate
Elbow	Moderate	Strong	Strong
Wrist	Weak	Moderate	Moderate
Phalanges (toes and fingers)	Weak	Moderate	Moderate

This reaction demonstrates Hilton's law, which states that the joint capsule, the muscles moving that joint, and the skin overlying the insertion of the muscles have the same nerve supply. Ligaments, for the most part, are not extensible but can be extended as a result of the collagen fibers being arranged in bundles at right angles to one another. As the angles of the bundles are changed, ligaments can be extended without lengthening the collagen fiber.

Ligaments and capsular structures are important to joint stability. Characteristically, joints that are shallow and relatively poor fitting must depend on their capsular structures or muscles for major support. The knee is an example of an articulation that lacks bony congruence and depends mainly on muscles and ligaments for its support.

Besides moving limbs, muscles also provide joint stabilization to a greater or lesser extent and absorb the forces of load transmission. Muscles help stabilize joints in the following ways: muscles that cross joints assist in maintaining proper articular alignment, and some muscles attach directly to the articular capsule (shunt muscles) and, when stretched, also tighten the capsule. By becoming taut, the shunt muscles prevent the articulations from separating and also assist in maintaining proper alignment.

Articular Capsule and Ligaments

Capsular and ligamentous tissue helps maintain anatomical integrity and structural alignment of synovial joints. Unlike tendons, however, these tissues contain elastic fibers, and their collagenous fibers, although they have many configurations, are irregular and have a spiral arrangement. Ligaments, which attach bone to bone, are generally strongest in the middle and weakest at the ends. Compared to ligaments and capsular tissues, with their fast, protective response, muscles respond much more slowly. For example, a muscle begins to develop protective tension within just a few hundredths of a second when overly stretched, but will not fully respond until approximately one-tenth of a second has elapsed.

Synovial Joint Trauma

A major factor in joint injuries is the viscoelastic tissue properties of ligaments and capsules (Table 9-3). Constant compression or tension can cause ligaments or capsular tissue to deteriorate. In contrast, intermittent compression and tension will, over time, increase overall strength, including that of the bony attachments of the connective tissue. Like tension forces, torsional or twisting forces that exceed the relative strength of collagen fibers can produce injury. Although occurring less often, a shearing action that cuts across the collagen fiber can traumatize capsular and ligamentous tissue. Tissue damage may occur when articular cartilage fails to properly transmit the

9-8

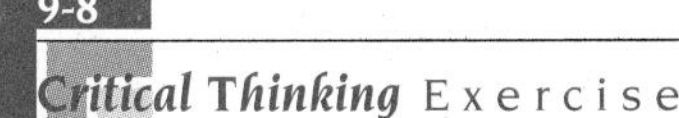

A basketball player steps on another player's foot and sustains a lateral ankle injury.

? What forces are applied, and what type of injury has been incurred?

TABLE 9-3 Synovial Joint Trauma

Primary Tissue	Type	Mechanical Forces	Condition
Capsule	Acute	Tension/compression	Sprains Dislocation/subluxation Synovial swelling
	Chronic	Tension/compression/ shearing	Capsulitis Synovitis Bursitis
Articular cartilage (hyaline)	Chronic	Compression/shearing	Osteochondrosis Traumatic arthritis

applied loads. In other words, the bones and hyaline cartilage that form a joint become out of accordance with each other's compressional forces over a period of time and predispose the joint to degenerative changes.

Synovial Joint Injury Classification

Acute Joint Injuries

The major injuries that happen to synovial joints are sprains, subluxations, and dislocations.

Joint Sprains A sprain, one of the most common and disabling injuries seen in sports, is a traumatic joint twist that results in stretching or total tearing of the stabilizing connective tissues (Figure 9-11). When a joint is forced beyond its normal anatomical limits, microscopic and gross pathologies occur. Specifically, there is injury to ligaments and to the articular capsule and synovial membrane. According to the extent of injury, sprains are graded in three degrees. A grade 1 sprain is characterized by some pain, minimum loss of function, mild point tenderness, little or no swelling, and no abnormal motion when tested. With a grade 2 sprain there is pain, moderate loss of function, swelling, and in some cases slight to moderate instability.[11] A grade 3 (or severe) sprain is extremely painful initially, with loss of function, severe instability, tenderness, and swelling. A grade 3 sprain may also represent a subluxation that has been reduced spontaneously.

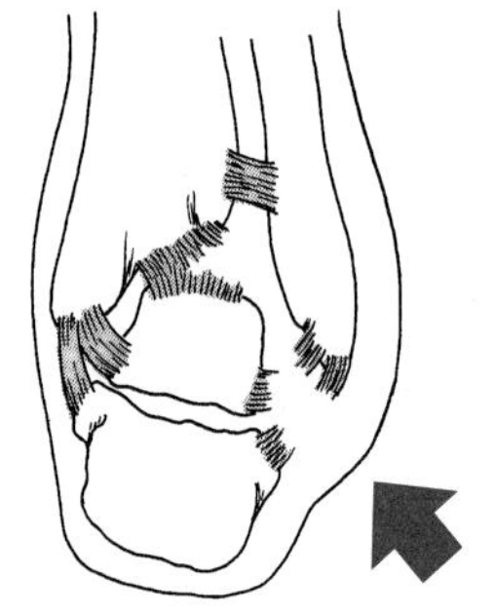

Figure 9-11

A sprain mainly involves injury to ligamentous and capsular tissue; however, muscle tendons can be secondarily strained.

Effusion of blood and synovial fluid into the joint cavity during a sprain produces joint swelling, local temperature increase, pain or point tenderness, and skin discoloration (ecchymosis). Ligaments and capsules, like tendons, can experience forces that completely rupture or produce an avulsion fracture. Ligaments and capsules heal slowly because of a relatively poor blood supply; however, their nerves are plentiful, often producing a great deal of pain when injured.[38]

The joints that are most vulnerable to sprains in sports are the ankles, knees, and shoulders. Sprains occur less often to the wrists and elbows. Because it is often difficult to distinguish between joint sprains and tendon strains, the athletic trainer should expect the worst possible condition and manage it accordingly. Repeated joint twisting can eventually result in chronic inflammation, degeneration, and arthritis.

Acute synovitis The synovial membrane of a joint can be acutely injured by a contusion or a sprain. Irritation of the membrane causes an increase in fluid production, and swelling occurs. The result is joint pain during motion, along with skin sensitivity from pressure at certain points. In a few days, with proper care, effusion and extravasated blood are absorbed, and swelling and pain diminish.

Subluxations, dislocations, and diastasis Dislocations are second to fractures in terms of disabling the athlete. The highest incidence of dislocations involves the fingers, followed by the shoulder joint (Figure 9-12). Dislocations, which result primarily from forces causing the joint to go beyond its normal anatomical limits, are divided into two classes: subluxations and luxations. Subluxations are partial dislocations in which an incomplete separation between two articulating bones occurs. Luxations are

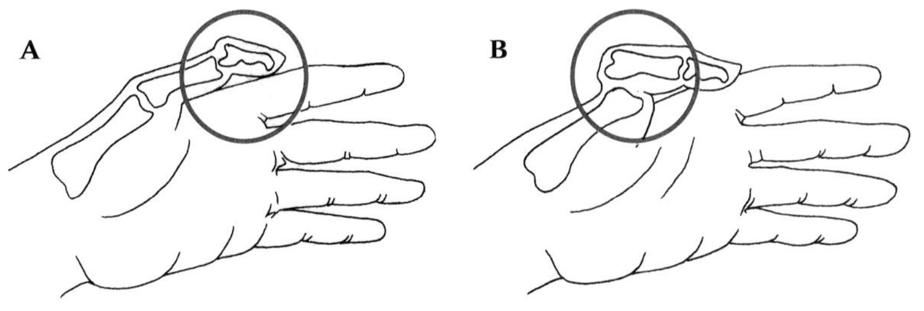

Figure 9-12

A point that is forced beyond its anatomical limits can become **A,** partially dislocated (subluxated), or **B,** completely dislocated (luxated).

complete dislocations, presenting a total disunion of bone apposition between the articulating surfaces. A diastasis is of two types: a disjointing of two bones parallel to one another, such as the radius and ulna; and the rupture of a "solid" joint, such as the symphysis pubis.[1] A diastasis commonly occurs with a fracture.

Several factors are important in recognizing and evaluating dislocations:

1. There is a loss of limb function. The athlete usually complains of having fallen or of having received a severe blow to a particular joint and then suddenly being unable to move that part.
2. Deformity is almost always apparent. Because the deformity can often be obscured by heavy musculature, it is important for the athletic trainer to palpate the injured site to determine the loss of normal body contour. Comparison of the injured side with its normal counterpart often reveals distortions.
3. Swelling and point tenderness are immediately present.

At times, X-ray examination of the dislocation, as with a fracture, is the only absolute diagnostic measure. First-time dislocations or joint separations may result in a rupture of the stabilizing ligamentous and tendinous tissues surrounding the joint and in avulsion, or pulling away from the bone. Trauma is often so violent that small chips of bone are torn away with the supporting structures, or the force may separate growth epiphyses or cause a complete fracture of the neck in long bones. These possibilities indicate the importance of administering complete and thorough medical attention to first-time dislocations. It has often been said, "Once a dislocation, always a dislocation." In most cases this statement is true because once a joint has been either subluxated or completely luxated, the connective tissues that bind and hold it in its correct alignment are stretched to such an extent that the joint will be extremely vulnerable to subsequent dislocations. Chronic, recurring dislocations may take place without severe pain because of the somewhat slack condition of the stabilizing tissues.

A first-time dislocation should always be considered a possible fracture.

A first-time dislocation should always be considered and treated as a possible fracture. Once the athletic trainer has ascertained that the injury is a dislocation, a physician should be consulted for further evaluation. However, before the patient is taken to the physician, the injury should be properly splinted and supported to prevent any further damage.

Chronic Joint Injuries

Like other chronic physical injuries or problems occurring from sports participation, chronic synovial joint injuries stem from microtraumas and overuse. The two major categories in which they fall are osteochondrosis and osteoarthritis (traumatic arthritis), or inflammation of surrounding soft tissues such as the bursal capsule and the synovium.[17] Another general expression for the chronic synovial conditions of the child or adolescent is articular epiphyseal injury. A major cause of chronic joint injury such as osteoarthritis is failure of the muscle to control or limit deceleration. Athletes can avoid such injuries by avoiding chronic fatigue and training when tired and by wearing protective gear to enhance active absorption of impact forces.[29]

9-9

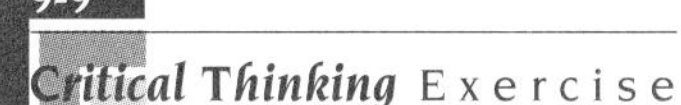
Critical Thinking Exercise

A young female gymnast has a pronounced knee malalignment. She complains of a left knee locking, pain, and swelling.

? What is the gymnast's possible condition?

Osteochondrosis Osteochondrosis is a category of conditions of which the causes are not well understood. In general, the term refers to degenerative changes in the

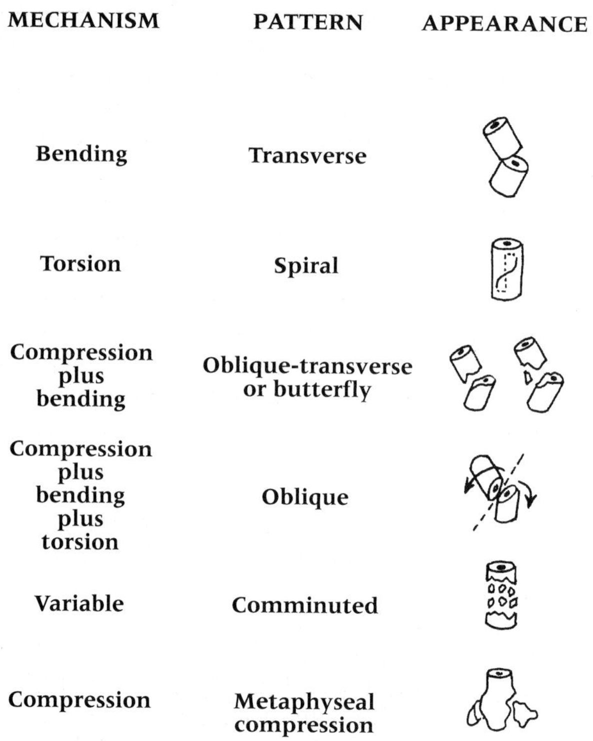

Figure 9-15

Mechanisms, patterns, and appearances of acute bone fractures.

MECHANISM	PATTERN	APPEARANCE
Bending	Transverse	
Torsion	Spiral	
Compression plus bending	Oblique-transverse or butterfly	
Compression plus bending plus torsion	Oblique	
Variable	Comminuted	
Compression	Metaphyseal compression	

trauma; in other words, the bone breaks directly at the site where a force is applied. A fracture that occurs some distance from where force is applied is called an indirect fracture. A sudden, violent muscle contraction or repetitive abnormal stress to a bone can also cause a fracture. Fractures must be considered among the most serious hazards of sports and should be routinely suspected in musculoskeletal injuries. The next sections present more detailed descriptions of acute fractures.[21]

Depressed fracture Depressed fractures occur most often in flat bones such as those found in the skull. They are caused by falling and striking the head on a hard, immovable surface or by being hit with a hard object. Such injuries also result in gross pathology of soft areas.

Greenstick fracture Greenstick fractures are incomplete breaks in bones that have not completely ossified, such as the bones of adolescents. This injury occurs most frequently in the convex bone surface, while the concave surface remains intact. The name is derived from the similarity of the fracture to the break in a green twig taken from a tree.

9-11

Critical Thinking Exercise

An alpine skier catches his right ski tip and severely twists the lower leg.

? What type of serious injury could be created by this mechanism?

Impacted fracture Impacted fractures can result from a fall from a height, which causes a long bone to receive, directly on its long axis, a force of such magnitude that the osseous tissue is compressed. This stress telescopes one part of the bone on the other. Impacted fractures require immediate splinting by the athletic trainer and traction by the physician to ensure a normal length of the injured limb.

Longitudinal fracture Longitudinal fractures are those in which the bone splits along its length. They are often the result of an athlete jumping from a height and landing in such a way as to impart force or stress to the long axis.

Spiral fracture Spiral fractures have an S-shaped separation. They are common in football and skiing, sports in which the foot is firmly planted when the body is suddenly rotated in an opposing direction.

Oblique fracture Oblique fractures are similar to spiral fractures. Oblique fractures occur when one end of the bone receives sudden torsion or twisting while the other end is fixed or stabilized.

Serrated fracture Serrated fractures, in which the two bony fragments have a sawtooth, sharp-edged fracture line, are usually caused by a direct blow. Because of the sharp and jagged bone edges, extensive internal damage, such as the severance of vital blood vessels and nerves, often occurs.

Transverse fracture Transverse fractures occur in a straight line, more or less at right angles to the bone shaft. A direct outside blow usually causes this injury.

Comminuted fracture Comminuted fractures consist of three or more fragments at the fracture site. This injury could be caused by a hard blow or a fall in an awkward position. These fractures impose a difficult healing situation because of the displacement of the bone fragments. Soft tissues are often interposed between the fragments, causing incomplete healing. Such cases may need surgical intervention.

Contrecoup fracture Contrecoup fractures occur on the side opposite to the point at which trauma was initiated. Fracture of the skull is, at times, a contrecoup fracture. An athlete may be hit on one side of the head with such force that the brain and internal structures compress against the opposite side of the skull, causing a fracture.

Blowout fracture Blowout fractures occur to the wall of the eye orbit as the result of a blow to the eye.

Avulsion fracture An avulsion fracture is the separation of a bone fragment from its cortex at an attachment of a ligament or tendon. This fracture usually occurs as a result of a sudden, powerful twist or stretch of a body part. A ligamentous avulsion can occur, for example, when a sudden eversion of the foot causes the deltoid ligament to avulse bone away from the medial malleolus. A tendinous avulsion can occur when an athlete falls forward while suddenly bending a knee, which causes a patellar fracture. The stretch of the patellar tendon pulls a portion of the inferior patellar pole apart. Figure 9-16 illustrates a tendinous avulsion of the sartorius muscle.

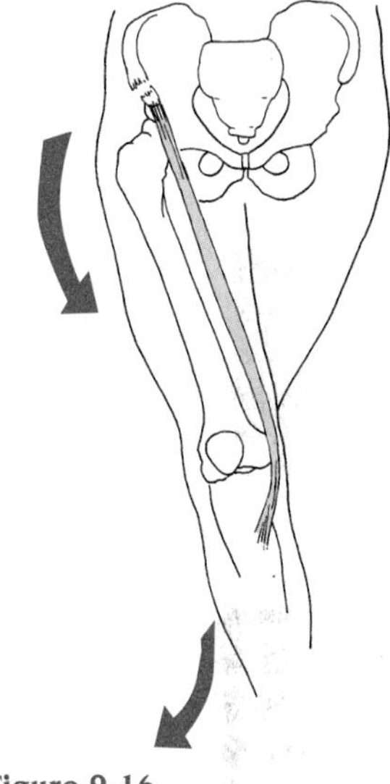

Figure 9-16

Tendinous avulsion fracture of the sartorius muscle.

Stress fractures Stress fractures have been variously called march, fatigue, and spontaneous fractures, although stress fracture is the most commonly used term. The exact cause of this fracture is not known, but there are a number of likely possibilities: an overload caused by muscle contraction, an altered stress distribution in the bone accompanying muscle fatigue, a change in the ground reaction force such as movement from a wood surface to a grass surface, or the performance of a rhythmically repetitive stress that leads up to a vibratory summation point, which appears to be the most likely cause.[22] Rhythmic muscle action performed over a period of time at a subthreshold level causes the stress-bearing capacity of the bone to be exceeded, hence, a stress fracture. A bone may become vulnerable to fracture during the first few weeks of intense physical activity or training. Weight-bearing bones undergo bone resorption and become weaker before they become stronger. The sequence of events results from increased muscular forces plus an increased rate of remodeling that leads to bone resorption, weakening of the out surface of the bone, and rarefaction, which progresses to produce increasingly more severe fractures.[33] The four progressively severe fractures are focal microfractures, periosteal or endosteal response (stress fractures), linear fractures (stress fractures), and displaced fractures.

Typical causes of stress fractures in sports are as follows:

1. Coming back into competition too soon after an injury or illness.
2. Going from one event to another without proper training in the second event.
3. Starting initial training too quickly.
4. Changing habits or the environment (e.g., running surfaces, the bank of a track, or shoes).

Susceptibility to fracture can also be increased by a variety of postural and foot conditions. Flatfeet, a short first metatarsal bone, or a hypermobile metatarsal region can predispose an athlete to stress fractures (see Chapter 18).

Early detection of the stress fracture may be difficult. Because of their frequency in a wide range of sports, stress fractures always must be suspected in susceptible body areas that fail to respond to usual management. Until there is an obvious reaction in the bone, which may take several weeks, X-ray examination may fail to reveal any change. Although nonspecific, a bone scan can provide early indications in a given area.

The signs of a stress fracture are swelling, focal tenderness, and pain. In the early stages of the fracture, the athlete complains of pain when active but not at rest. Later,

9-12

***Critical Thinking* Exercise**

A long jumper experiences a sudden sharp pain in the region of the left ischial tuberosity during a jump.

? What injuries are possible through this mechanism?

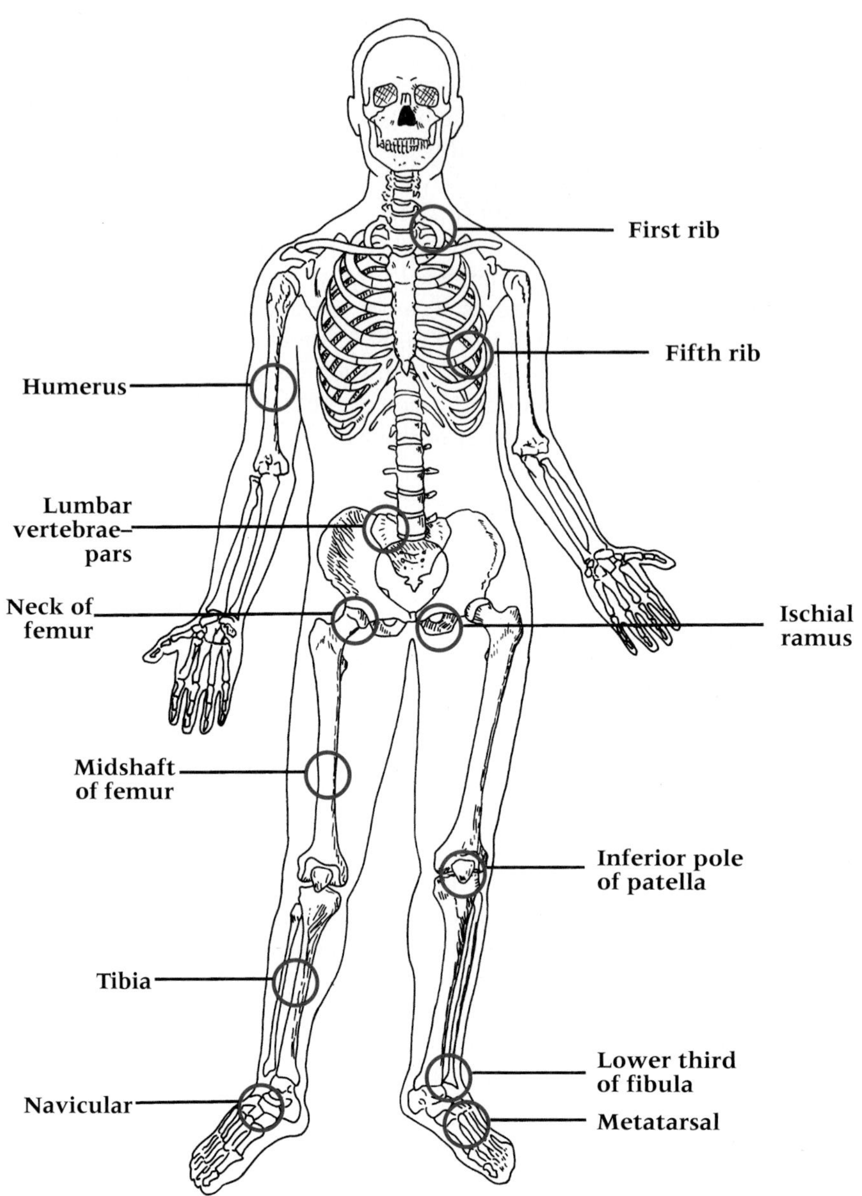

Figure 9-17

The most common stress fracture sites.

9-13

***Critical Thinking* Exercise**

A track athlete training for a marathon is complaining of pain in the lower leg. She consults with her physician, who determines that she has a stress fracture. When she returns to practice, she is confused about how a stress fracture is different from a real fracture.

? How should the athletic trainer explain the difference between the two, and what is the course of management?

the pain is constant and becomes more intense at night. Percussion, by light tapping on the bone at a site other than the suspected fracture, will produce pain at the fracture site.

The most common sites of stress fracture are the tibia, fibula, metatarsal shaft, calcaneus, femur, pars interarticularis of the lumbar vertebrae, ribs, and humerus (Figure 9-17).

The management of stress fractures varies with the individual athlete, injury site, and extent of injury. Stress fractures that occur on the compression side of bone heal more rapidly and are managed more easily compared with those on the tension side. Stress fractures on the tension side can rapidly produce a complete fracture.

Epiphyseal conditions Three types of epiphyseal growth site injuries can be sustained by children and adolescents performing sports activities. They are injury to the epiphyseal growth plate, or physis articular epiphyseal injuries, and apophyseal injuries. The most prevalent age range for these injuries is from ten to sixteen years.

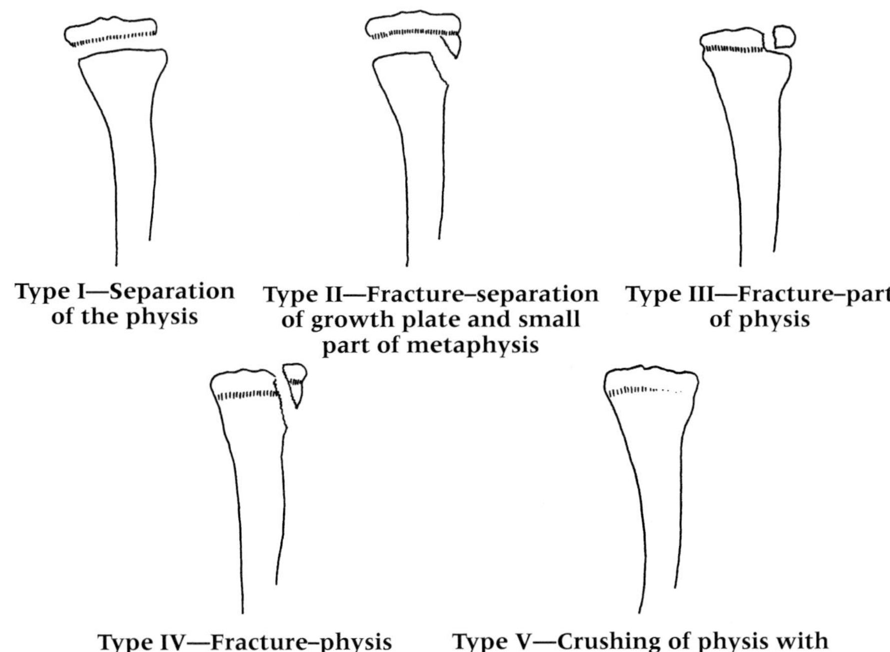

Figure 9-18

Salter-Harris classification of long bone epiphyseal injuries in children.

Epiphyseal growth plate injuries (Figure 9-18) have been classified by Salter-Harris into five types as follows:[4]

- Type I—complete separation of the physis in relation to the metaphysis without fracture to the bone.
- Type II—separation of the growth plate and a small portion of the metaphysis.
- Type III—fracture of the physis.
- Type IV—fracture of a portion of the physis and metaphysis.
- Type V—no displacement of the physis, but the crushing force can cause a growth deformity.

Apophyseal injuries The young, physically immature athlete is particularly prone to apophyseal injuries. The apophyses are traction epiphyses in contrast to the pressure epiphyses of the long bones. These apophyses serve as origins or insertions for muscles on growing bone that provide bone shape but not length. Common apophyseal avulsion conditions found in sports are Sever's disease and Osgood-Schlatter's disease (see Chapter 20).

A musculoskeletal injury to a child or adolescent should always be considered a possible epiphyseal condition.

NERVE TRAUMA

A number of abnormal nerve responses can be attributed to athletic participation or injury. The most frequent type of nerve injury is neuropraxia produced by a direct trauma. A laceration can cut nerves, causing complications in healing of the injury. Fractures and dislocation can avulse or abnormally compress nerves.

Anatomical Characteristics

Nerve tissue provides sensitivity and communication from the central nervous system (brain and spinal cord) to the muscles, sensory organs, various systems, and the periphery. The basic nerve cell is the neuron. The neuron cell body contains a large nucleus and branched extensions called dendrites, which respond to neurotransmitter substances released from other nerve cells. From each nerve cell arises a single axon, which conducts the nerve impulses. Large axons found in peripheral nerves are

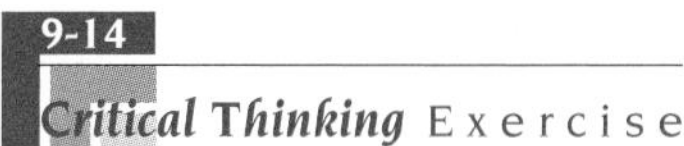

An 11-year-old soccer player fell on an outstretched hand during practice. There is obvious deformity in her right wrist.

? What is a possible complication with a fracture in this wrist?

enclosed in neurilemmal sheaths composed of Schwann cells and satellite cells, which are tightly wound around the axon. In the central nervous system, various types of neuroglial cells including astrocytes, oligodendrocytes, ependymal cells, and microglia function collectively to bind neurons together and provide a supportive framework for the nervous tissue.[35]

Nerve Injuries

The two main forces that cause major nerve injury responses are compression and tension. As with injuries to other tissues in the body, the injurious forces to nerves may be acute or chronic.

Physical trauma to nerves in general produces pain as part of the inflammatory process (see Chapter 10). Any number of traumas directly affecting nerves can also produce a variety of sensory responses, including pain. For example, a sudden nerve stretch or pinch can produce muscle weakness as well as a sharp burning pain that radiates down a limb. **Neuritis**, a chronic nerve problem, can be caused by a variety of forces that usually have been repeated or continued for a long period of time. Symptoms of neuritis can range from minor nerve problems to paralysis.

neuritis
Inflammation of a nerve.

Pain that is felt at a point of the body other than its actual origin is known as **referred pain.**[15] Another potential cause of referred pain is a trigger point, which occurs in the muscular system but refers pain to some other distant body part.

referred pain
Pain that is felt at a point of the body other than its origin.

BODY MECHANICS AND INJURY SUSCEPTIBILITY

If you carefully study the mechanical structure of the human body, it is amazing that humans can move so effectively in the upright posture. Not only must the body overcome constant gravitational force, but it also must be manipulated through space by a complex system of somewhat inefficient levers, fueled by a machinery that operates at an efficiency level of approximately 30 percent. The bony levers that move the body must overcome considerable resistance in the form of inertia and muscle viscosity and must work in most instances at an extremely unfavorable angle of pull. All these factors mitigate the effectiveness of lever action to the extent that most movement is achieved at an efficiency level of less than 25 percent.

When determining the mechanical reasons for sports injuries to the musculoskeletal system, many factors can be identified. Hereditary, congenital, or acquired defects may predispose an athlete to a specific type of injury. Anomalies in anatomical structure or in body build (somatotype) may make an athlete prone to injuries. The habitually incorrect application of skill is a common cause of overuse injuries.

Microtrauma and Overuse Syndrome

Injuries as a result of abnormal and repetitive stress and microtraumas fall into a class with certain identifiable syndromes.[36] Such stress injuries frequently result in either limitation or curtailment of sports performance. Most of these injuries in athletes are directly related to the dynamics of running, throwing, or jumping. The injuries may result from constant and repetitive stresses placed on bones, joints, or soft tissues; from forcing a joint into an extreme range of motion; or from prolonged strenuous activity. Some of the injuries falling into this category may be relatively minor; still, they can be disabling. Among injuries classified as repetitive stress and microtrauma are Achilles tendinitis; shin splints; stress fractures, particularly of the fibula and second and fifth metatarsal bones; Osgood-Schlatter's disease; runner's and jumper's knee; patellar chondromalacia; apophyseal avulsion, especially in the lower extremities of growing athletes; and intertarsal neuroma.

Postural Deviations

Postural deviations are often an underlying cause of sports injuries.[36] Postural malalignment may be the result of unilateral muscle and soft-tissue asymmetries or bony asymmetries. As a result, the athlete engages in poor mechanics of movement (pathomechanics). Many sports activities are unilateral, thus leading to asymmetries in body development. The resulting imbalance is manifested by a postural deviation as the body seeks to reestablish itself in relation to its center of gravity. Often, such deviations are a primary cause of injury. For example, a consistent pattern of knee injury may be related to asymmetries within the pelvis and the legs (short-leg syndrome). Unfortunately, not much in the form of remedial work is usually performed. As a result, an injury often becomes chronic—sometimes to the point that participation in a sport must be halted. When possible, the athletic trainer should seek to ameliorate or eliminate faulty postural conditions through therapy. A number of postural conditions offer genuine hazards to athletes by making them exceedingly prone to specific injuries. Some of the more important are discussed in the chapters on foot and leg anomalies, spinal anomalies, and various stress syndromes.

SUMMARY

- "When a force applied to any part of the body results in a harmful disturbance in function or structure, a mechanical injury is said to have been sustained."[17] Engineering terminology is used to describe tissue properties and sport injuries. Examples of this terminology are *load, stress, deformation, viscoelastic, anisotropic, yield point,* and *tissue failure.*
- The five primary stresses leading to tissue trauma are tension, stretching, compression, shearing, and bending. Bending strain can produce a torque on a bone followed by injury. A torsion, or twisting, load can produce a spiral fracture along the long axis of a bone.
- Soft tissue (nonbony tissue) is categorized as noncontractile and contractile (muscle) tissues.
- Skin trauma can occur from a variety of forces (e.g., friction, scraping, compression, tearing, cutting, and puncturing) that produce blisters, skin bruises, lacerations, skin avulsions, incisions, and puncture wounds.
- Skeletal muscle trauma from sports participation can involve any aspect of the muscle-tension unit. Forces that injure muscles are compression, tension, and shearing. Acute muscle injuries include contusions and strains. Avulsion fractures and muscle ruptures can occur from an acute episode. Chronic muscle conditions are myositis, fasciitis, tendinitis, and tenosynovitis. Chronic muscle irritation can cause ectopic calcification; muscle disuse can cause atrophy; and immobilization can cause joint contracture.
- Sports injuries to the synovial joints are common. Anatomically, synovial joints have relative strengths or weaknesses based on their ligamentous or capsular type and their muscle arrangements. Forces that can injure synovial joints are tension, compression, torsion, and shear. Sprains involve acute injury to ligaments or the joint capsule. A grade 3 sprain may cause ligament rupture or an avulsion fracture. Acute synovial joint injuries that go beyond the third degree may result in a dislocation. Two major chronic synovial joint conditions are osteochondrosis and traumatic arthritis. Other chronic conditions are bursitis, capsulitis, and synovitis.
- Because of their shape, long bones are anatomically susceptible to fractures caused by changes in direction of the force applied to them. Mechanical forces that cause injury are compression, tension, bending, torsion, and shear. Bending and torsional forces are forms of tension. Acute fractures include avulsion, blowout, comminuted, depressed, greenstick, impacted, longitudinal, oblique, serrated, spiral, transverse, and contrecoup types. Stress fractures are commonly the result of overload to a given bone area. Stress fractures are apparently caused by an altered stress distribution or by the performance of a rhythmically repetitive action that leads to a vibratory summation and thus a fracture. Three major epiphyseal injuries in sports occur to the growth plate, the articular cartilage, and the apophysis.

- Nerve trauma can be produced by overstretching or compression. Like other injuries, nerve injuries can be acute or chronic. The sudden stretch of a nerve can cause a burning sensation. A variety of traumas to nerves can produce acute pain or a chronic pain such as neuritis.
- An athlete with faulty body mechanics has an increased potential for injury.

Websites

Biomechanics World Wide: http://www.per.ualberta.ca/biomechanics

This site enables the reader to search the biomechanics journals for recent information regarding mechanism of injury.

Cramer First Aider: http://www.cramersportsmed.com/first_aider.com

American Red Cross: http://www.redcross.org

National Institute of Health: http://www.nih.gov

Wheeless' Textbook of Orthopedics: http://www.wheelessonline.com

Solutions to Critical Thinking EXERCISES

9-1 All human tissue has viscous and elastic properties. The resistance of tissue is dependent on its viscoelastic characteristics and the types of forces that are applied.

9-2 The friction force produced by sliding into home base causes a serious abrasion skin injury.

9-3 The ball created a compressive force that crushed tissue, causing a secondary contusion.

9-4 The football player has sustained a tension force to the long head of the biceps tendon that caused a rupture or severe strain.

9-5 The mechanism of this elbow injury is repeated tension to the extensor tendons attached to the lateral epicondyle, causing microtraumas. Stress to this area can be reduced by increasing the grip circumference and flattening the backhand stroke.

9-6 Repeated contusion of any muscle may lead to the development of myositis ossificans. The key to treating myositis ossificans is prevention. An initial contusion to any muscle should be immediately protected with padding to prevent reinjury.

9-7 Repeated contusions to the quadriceps could produce an ectopic calcification known as myositis ossificans.

9-8 In stepping on another player's foot, the basketball player produces an abnormal ankle torsion and lateral ankle tension, stretching and tearing ligaments.

9-9 Knee malalignment produces abnormal compression and shearing forces on the lateral menisci, which can lead to osteochondritis dissecans and osteochondritis.

9-10 The athletic trainer should suspect that the wrestler has developed bursitis from constantly kneeling on the mat. Inflammation may best be treated by rest, ice, antiinflammatory medication, and protective padding of the knee.

9-11 Catching the ski tip produces a torsional force that could cause a boot-top spiral fracture.

9-12 During the jump, a powerful stretch of the biceps femoris could cause a serious strain or an avulsion fracture in the region of the ischial tuberosity.

9-13 A stress fracture is not an actual break of the bone, it is simply an irritation of the bone. Treatment of a stress fracture requires about fourteen days of rest. However, the athletic trainer should point out that a stress fracture can become a true fracture if it is not rested; if that happens, four to six weeks of immobilization in a cast is necessary. Thus, it is critical that this athlete rest for the required amount of time.

9-14 An epiphyseal condition, such as an epiphyseal growth plate fracture, can occur in children and adolescents and needs to be considered with any musculoskeletal injury. These injuries can impair growth and further skeletal development.

REVIEW QUESTIONS AND CLASS ACTIVITIES

1. Describe the mechanics that produce inert and contractile sports injuries.
2. Describe the mechanical forces that injure skin.
3. What forces injure muscle tissue?
4. Describe all types of acute muscle injuries.
5. Describe all types of chronic muscle injuries.
6. Describe the major acute injuries occurring to joints.
7. What mechanical forces traumatize the musculotendinous unit and the synovial joint? How are the forces similar to one another, and how are they different?
8. What forces gradually weaken tendons and ligaments?
9. Contrast two chronic synovial joint injuries.
10. List the structural characteristics that make a long bone susceptible to fracture.
11. What mechanical forces cause acute fracture of a bone?
12. How do stress fractures probably occur?
13. Describe the most common epiphyseal conditions that result from sports participation.
14. What are the relationships of postural deviations to sports injuries?
15. Discuss the concept of pathomechanics as it relates to microtraumas and overuse syndromes.

REFERENCES

1. Akeson WH et al: The biology of ligaments. In Hunter LY, Funk FJ Jr, editors: *Rehabilitation of the injured knee,* St Louis, 1984, Mosby.
2. American Academy of Orthopaedic Surgeons: *Athletic training and sports medicine,* Park Ridge, Ill, 1991, American Academy of Orthopaedic Surgeons.

3. Barak T et al: Basic concepts of orthopaedic manual therapy. In Malone T, McPhail T, editors: *Orthopaedic and sports physical therapy,* ed 3, St Louis, 1996, Mosby.
4. Blavelt CT, Nelson FRT: *A manual of orthopaedic terminology,* ed 6, Philadelphia, PA, 1998, Elsevier.
5. Brinker M: *Review of orthopaedic trauma,* Philadelphia, 2001, WB Saunders.
6. Browner B: *Skeletal trauma: basic science, management, and reconstruction,* Philadelphia, 2002, WB Saunders.
7. Brukner P, Khan K: Sports injuries. In Brukner P, editor, *Clinical sports medicine,* ed 2, Sydney, 2002, McGraw-Hill.
8. Butterwick DJ: Recognition of complete muscle or tendon ruptures. *Athletic Therapy Today* 7(l):43, 2002.
9. Byrnes WB, Clarkson PM: Delayed onset muscle soreness and training. In Katch FL, Freedson PS, editors: *Clinics in sports medicine,* vol 5, Philadelphia, 1986, Saunders.
10. Cleary M, Kimura I, Sitler M: Temporal pattern of the repeated bout effect of eccentric exercise on delayed-onset muscle soreness, *J Ath Train* 37(1):32, 2002.
11. Delee J, Drez D, Miller M: *Delee & Drez's orthopaedic sports medicine: principles and practice,* Philadelphia, 2002, WB Saunders.
12. Delforge G: *Musculoskeletal trauma: implications for sports injury management,* Champaign, Ill, 2002, Human Kinetics.
13. DiFiori JP: Overuse injuries in young athletes: an overview, *Athletic Therapy Today* 7(6):25, 2002.
14. Dumke CL: Muscle cramps are not all created equal. *Athletic Therapy Today* 8(3):42, 2003.
15. Fine PG: The biology of pain. In Heil J, editor: *Psychology of sport injury,* Champaign, Ill, 1993, Human Kinetics.
16. Gallaspie J, May D: *Signs and symptoms of athletic injuries,* St. Louis, 1996, McGraw-Hill.
17. Geesink RGT et al: Stress response of articular cartilage, *Int J Sports Med* 5:100, 1984.
18. Gomez M: *Biomechanics of soft-tissue injury,* Tuscon, Ariz, 2000, Lawyers & Judges Publishing Company.
19. Gonza ER: Biomechanics of long bone injuries. In Gonza ER, Harrington IJ, editors: *Biomechanics of musculoskeletal injury,* Baltimore, 1982, Williams & Wilkins.
20. Hirsch CS, Lumwalt RE: Injuries caused by physical agents. In Kissane JM, editor: *Anderson's pathology,* ed 9, vol 1, Philadelphia, PA, 1996, Elsevier.
21. Hoppenfield S, Murthy V, Taylor K: *Treatment and rehabilitation of fractures,* Philadelphia, 2000, Lippincott Williams & Wilkins.
22. Huson A: Mechanics of joints, *Int J Sports Med* 5:83, 1984.
23. Hutson, M: Sports injuries: recognition and management, ed 3, Oxford, England, 2001, Oxford University Press.
24. James C, Uhl T: A review of articular cartilage pathology and the use of glucosamine sulfate, *J Ath Train* 36(4):413, 2001.
25. Leaveau BF: Basic biomechanics in sports and orthopaedic therapy. In Malone T, McPhail T, editors: *Orthopaedic and sports physical therapy,* ed 3, St Louis, 1996, Mosby.
26. Levine D, Prall E, Marcellin-Little D: Running and the development of osteoarthritis, Part I: Animal studies, *Athletic Therapy Today* 8(1):6, 2003.
27. Levine D: Running and the development of osteoarthritis. Part II. Human studies. *Athletic Therapy Today* 8(1):12, 2003.
28. Malone T, McPhoil T, Nitz A, editors: *Orthopaedic and sports physical therapy,* ed 2, St Louis, 1996, Mosby.
29. Markey KL: Stress fractures. In Hunter-Griffin LY, editor: *Overuse injuries. Clinics in sports medicine,* vol 6, Philadelphia, 1987, Saunders.
30. Merrick M: Secondary injury after musculoskeletal trauma: a review and update. *J Ath Train* 37(2):209, 2002.
31. Porth CM: *Pathophysiology,* ed 6, Philadelphia, 2003, Lippincott, Williams and Wilkins.
32. Riemann B, Lephart S: The sensorimotor system, Part I: The physiologic basis of functional joint stability, *J Ath Train* 37(1):71, 2002.
33. Romani W, Gieck J, Perrin D: Mechanisms and management of stress fractures in physically active persons, *J Ath Train* 37(3):306, 2002.
34. Roux W: *Die entwichlungsmechanic,* Leipzig, Germany, 1905, Englemann.
35. Saladin K: *Anatomy and physiology,* New York, 2001, McGraw-Hill.
36. Shamus E, Shamus L: *Sports injury: prevention and rehabilitation,* New York, 2001, McGraw-Hill.
37. Stone MB: Exercise-associated muscle cramps. *Athletic Therapy Today* 8(3):30, 2003.
38. Weintraub W: *Tendon and ligament healing: a new approach to sports and overuse injury,* Herndon, WV, 2003, Paradigm Publications.
39. Whiting W, Zernicke, R: *Biomechanics of musculoskeletal injury,* Champaign, Ill, 1998, Human Kinetics.
40. Wilson TC: Articular-cartilage lesions of the knee and osteoarthritis in athletes: an overview. *Athletic Therapy Today* 8 (1):20, 2003.
41. Wolff J: *Das geset der transformation der knockan,* Berlin, 1892, Hirschwald.

ANNOTATED BIBLIOGRAPHY

Blavelt CT, Nelson RRT: *A manual of orthopaedic terminology,* ed 6, Philadelphia, 1998, Elsevier.

This resource book is for all individuals who need to identify medical words or their acronyms.

Booher JM, Thibodeau GA: *Athletic injury assessment,* Boston, 2001, McGraw-Hill.

An excellent guide to the recognition, assessment, classification, and evaluation of athletic injuries.

Dandy D, Edwards D: *Essential orthopaedics and trauma,* 2003, Elsevier.

Presents essential core information for students and emphasizes common conditions and current orthopaedic practice.

Delforge G: *Musculoskeletal trauma: implications for sport injury management,* Champaign, Ill, 2003, Human Kinetics.

This text focuses on the therapeutic management of sport-related soft tissue injuries, fractures, and proprioceptive/sensorimotor impairments.

Garrick JG, Webb DR: *Sports injuries: diagnosis and management.* Philadelphia, 1999, WB Saunders.

An overview of musculoskeletal injuries that are unique to sports and exercise.

Griffith HW, Pederson M: *Complete guide to sports injuries: how to treat fractures, bruises, sprains, dislocations, and head injuries,* New York, 1997, Perigee.

Tells readers how to treat, avoid, and rehabilitate nearly 200 of the most common sports injuries, including fractures, bruises, sprains, strains, dislocations, and head injuries.

Peacinn M, Bojanic I: *Overuse injuries of musculoskeletal system,* Boca Raton, FL, 2003, CRC Press.

A comprehensive text describing overuse injuries of the tendon, tendon sheath, bursae, muscle, muscle-tendon function, cartilage, and nerve.

Williams JGP: *Color atlas of injury in sport,* Chicago, 1990, Mosby.

This excellent visual guide to the area of sports injuries covers the nature and incidence of sport injury, types of tissue damage, and regional injuries caused by a variety of sports activities.

Weintraub W: *Tendon and ligament healing: a new approach to sports and overuse injury,* Herndon, WV, 2003, Paradigm Publications.

Gives readers a clear understanding of the dynamic nature of tendons and ligaments from an excellent review of their structure, function, mechanics, injury, and healing processes.

Chapter 10 Tissue Response to Injury

When you finish this chapter you should be able to

- Contrast the three phases of the healing process.
- Classify the physiological events that must take place during each phase of healing.
- Identify those factors that may impede the healing process.
- Discuss the healing process relative to various soft tissue structures including cartilage, ligament, muscle, tendon, and nerve.
- Describe the healing process as it occurs in bone.
- Formulate a management plan for treating acute fractures.
- Define pain and discuss the various types of pain.
- Understand the neurophysiology of pain.
- Differentiate between the three mechanisms of pain control.
- Examine the various techniques for assessing pain.

10-1

***Critical Thinking* Exercise**

A volleyball player has sprained her ankle just two days prior to the beginning of the conference tournament. The athlete, her parents, and her coach are extremely concerned that she is going to miss the tournament and want to know if anything can be done to make her get well more quickly.

? What can the athletic trainer tell this athlete about the healing process?

THE HEALING PROCESS

It is essential for the athletic trainer to possess an in-depth understanding of the healing process. The healing process consists of three phases: the inflammatory response phase, the fibroblastic repair phase, and the maturation-remodeling phase. The athletic trainer should recognize both the sequence and time frames for these various phases of healing and realize that certain physiological events must occur during each of the phases. Anything that an athletic trainer does when treating a sport-related injury that interferes with this healing process will likely slow the return to full activity. The healing process must have an opportunity to accomplish what it is supposed to. At best the goal of the athletic trainer should be to try to create an environment that is conducive to the healing process. There is little that can be done to speed up the process physiologically, but there are many things that may be done during rehabilitation to impede healing. Although the phases of healing are often discussed as three separate entities, the healing process is a continuum. Phases of the healing process overlap one another and have no definitive beginning or end points (Figure 10-1).

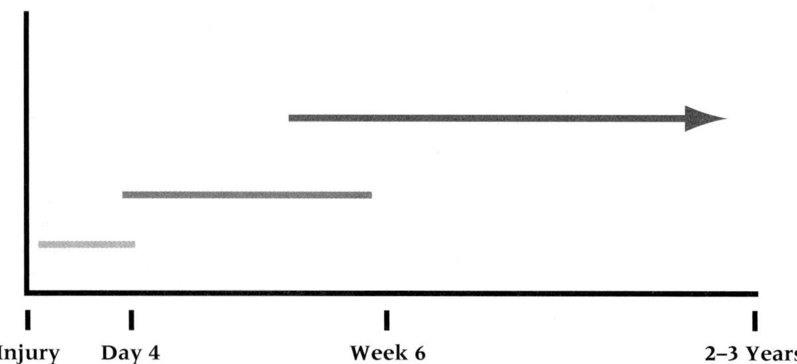

Figure 10-1

The three phases of the healing process fall along a continuum.

Inflammatory Response Phase

Once a tissue is injured, the process of healing begins immediately[2,30] (Figure 10-2A). The destruction of tissue produces direct injury to the cells of the various soft tissues.[16] Cellular injury results in altered metabolism and the liberation of materials that initiate the inflammatory response. It is characterized symptomatically by redness (*rubor*), swelling (*tumor*), tenderness and pain (*dolor*), increased temperature (*calor*), and loss of function (*functio laesa*).[25] *This initial inflammatory response is critical to the entire healing process. If this response does not accomplish what it is supposed to, or if it does not subside, normal healing cannot take place.*[15]

Figure 10-2

Healing process. **A,** Inflammatory response phase. **B,** Fibroblastic repair phase.

Continued

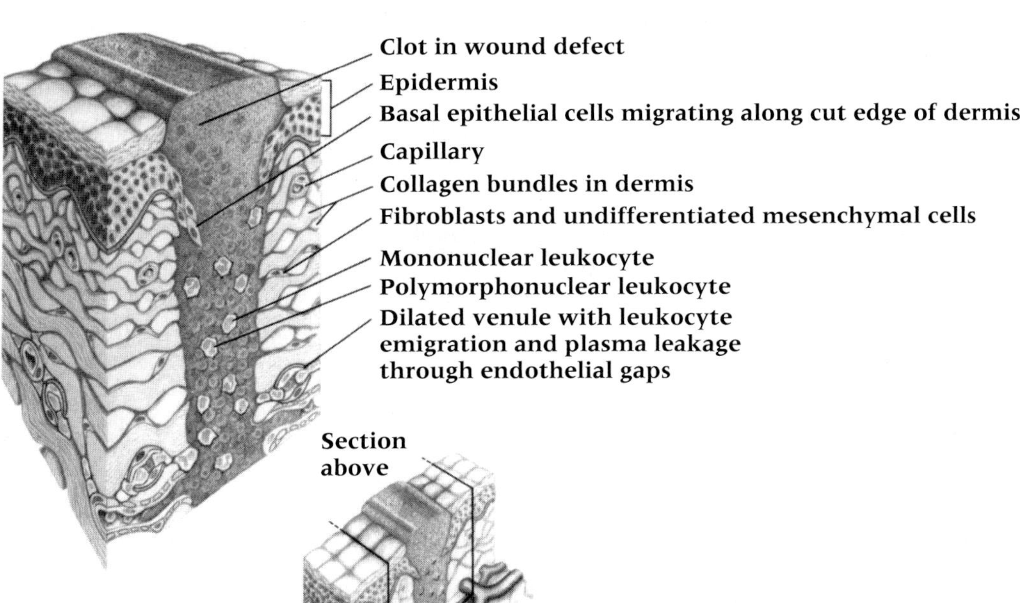

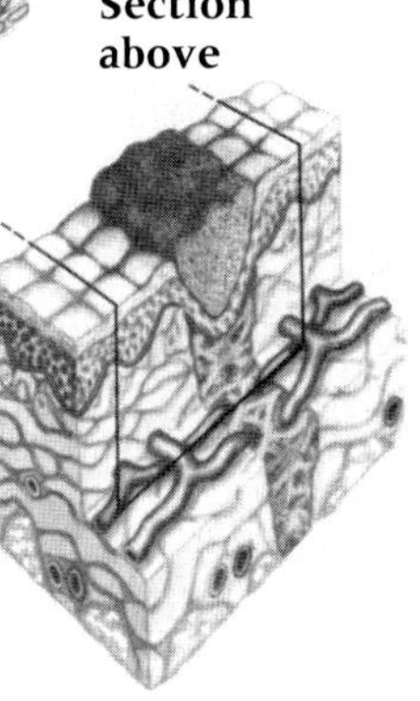

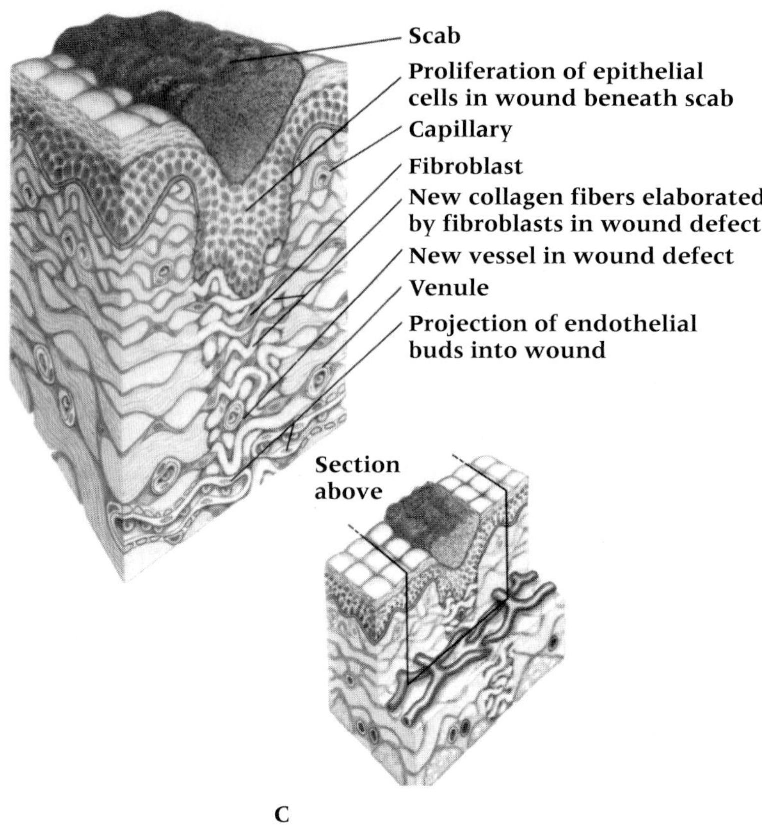

Figure 10-2—continued

Healing process **C,** Maturation-remodeling phase.

leukocytes
White blood cells.

phagocytosis
Process of ingesting microorganisms, other cells, or foreign particles, commonly performed by monocytes (white blood cells).

Signs of Inflammation
- Redness (rubor)
- Swelling (tumor)
- Tenderness (dolor)
- Increased temperature (calor)
- Loss of function (functio laesa)

vasoconstriction
Decrease in diameter of blood vessel.

chemical mediators
- Histamine
- Leukotaxin
- Necrosin

margination
Leukocytes line up along cell wall.

Inflammation is a process through which **leukocytes** and other *phagocytic cells* and exudate are delivered to the injured tissue. This cellular reaction is generally protective, tending to localize or dispose of injury by-products (for example, blood and damaged cells) through **phagocytosis** and thus setting the stage for repair, Local vascular effects, disturbances of fluid exchange, and migration of leukocytes from the blood to the tissues occur.[27]

Vascular Reaction

The vascular reaction involves vascular spasm, the formation of a platelet plug, blood coagulation, and the growth of fibrous tissue.[43] The immediate response to tissue damage is a **vasoconstriction** of the vascular walls that lasts for approximately five to ten minutes. This spasm presses the opposing endothelial linings together to produce a local anemia that is rapidly replaced by hyperemia of the area due to dilation. This increase in blood flow is transitory and gives way to slowing of the flow in the dilated vessels, which then progresses to stagnation and stasis. The initial effusion of blood and plasma lasts for twenty-four to thirty-six hours.

Chemical Mediators Three *chemical mediators, histamine, leukotaxin,* and *necrosin,* are important in limiting the amount of exudate, and thus swelling, after injury.[27] Histamine released from the injured mast cells causes vasodilation and increased cell permeability, owing to a swelling of endothelial cells and then separation between the cells. Leukotaxin is responsible for **margination,** in which leukocytes line up along the cell walls. It also increases cell permeability locally, thus affecting the passage of the fluid and white blood cells through cell walls via diapedesis to form exudate. Therefore vasodilation and active hyperemia are important in exudate (plasma) formation and in supplying leukocytes to the injured area. Necrosin is responsible for phagocytic activity. The amount of swelling that occurs is directly related to the extent of vessel damage.

Formation of a Clot

Platelets do not normally adhere to the vascular wall. However, injury to a vessel disrupts the endothelium and exposes the collagen fibers. Platelets adhere to the collagen fibers to create a sticky matrix on the vascular wall, to which additional platelets and leukocytes adhere, eventually forming a plug. These plugs obstruct local lymphatic fluid drainage and thus localize the injury response.

The initial event that precipitates clot information is the conversion of *fibrinogen* to *fibrin.* This transformation occurs because of a cascading effect beginning with the release of a protein molecule called *thromboplastin* from the damaged cell. Thromboplastin causes *prothrombin* to be changed into *thrombin,* which in turn causes the conversion of fibrinogen into a very sticky fibrin clot that shuts off blood supply to the injured area.[15] Clot formation begins around twelve hours after injury and is completed within forty-eight hours.

Blood coagulation:
Thromboplastin
↓
Prothrombin
↓
Thrombin
↓
Fibrinogen
↓
Insoluble fibrin clot

As a result of a combination of these factors, the injured area becomes walled off during the inflammatory stage of healing. The leukocytes phagocytize most of the foreign debris toward the end of the inflammatory phase, setting the stage for the fibroblastic phase. This initial inflammatory response lasts for approximately two to four days after initial injury.

Chronic Inflammation

A distinction must be made between the acute inflammatory response as previously described and chronic inflammation. *Chronic inflammation* occurs when the acute inflammatory response does not eliminate the injuring agent and restore tissue to its normal physiological state. Chronic inflammation involves the replacement of leukocytes with **macrophages, lymphocytes,** and *plasma cells.* These cells accumulate in a highly vascularized and innervated loose connective tissue matrix in the area of injury.[26]

macrophage
A phagocytic cell of the immune system.

lymphocytes
Cells that are the primary means of providing the body with immune capabilities.

The specific mechanisms that convert an acute inflammatory response to a chronic inflammatory response are unknown, but they seem to be associated with situations that involve overuse or overload with cumulative microtrauma to a particular structure.[13,26] Likewise there is no specific time frame in which the classification of acute changes to chronic inflammation. It does appear that chronic inflammation is resistant to both physical and pharmacologic treatments.[21]

Fibroblastic Repair Phase

During the fibroblastic phase of healing, proliferative and regenerative activity leading to scar formation and repair of the injured tissue follows the vascular and exudative phenomena of inflammation[19] (Figure 10-2B). The period of scar formation referred to as **fibroplasia** begins within the first few hours after injury and may last for as long as four to six weeks. During this period, many of the signs and symptoms associated with the inflammatory response subside. The patient may still indicate some tenderness to touch and will usually complain of pain when particular movements stress the injured structure. As scar formation progresses, complaints of tenderness or pain gradually disappear.[2]

fibroplasia
Period of scar formation.

During this phase, the growth of endothelial capillary buds into the wound is stimulated by a lack of oxygen, after which the wound is capable of healing aerobically. Along with increased oxygen delivery comes an increase in blood flow, which delivers nutrients essential for tissue regeneration in the area.[11]

The formation of a delicate connective tissue called *granulation tissue* occurs with the breakdown of the fibrin clot. Granulation tissue consists of *fibroblasts,* collagen, and capillaries. It appears as a reddish granular mass of connective tissue that fills in the gaps during the healing process.

granulation tissue
- fibroblasts
- collagen
- capillaries

As the capillaries continue to grow into the area, fibroblasts accumulate at the wound site, arranging themselves parallel to the capillaries. Fibroblastic cells begin to

extracellular matrix
- collagen
- elastin
- ground substance
- proteoglycans
- glycosaminoglycans

synthesize an *extracellular matrix* that contains protein fibers of *collagen* and *elastin,* a *ground substance* that consists of nonfibrous proteins called *proteoglycans, glycosaminoglycans,* and fluid. On about the sixth or seventh day, fibroblasts also begin producing collagen fibers that are deposited in a random fashion throughout the forming scar. As the collagen continues to proliferate, the tensile strength of the wound rapidly increases in proportion to the rate of collagen synthesis. As the tensile strength increases, the number of fibroblasts diminishes to signal the beginning of the maturation phase.

This normal sequence of events in the repair phase leads to the formation of minimal scar tissue. Occasionally, a persistent inflammatory response and continued release of inflammatory products can promote extended fibroplasia and excessive fibrogenesis that can lead to irreversible tissue damage.[42] Fibrosis can occur in synovial structures as with adhesive capsulitis in the shoulder, in extraarticular tissues such as tendons and ligaments, in bursae, or in muscle.

Maturation-Remodeling Phase

10-2

Critical Thinking Exercise

A football player sustains a grade 2 medial collateral ligament sprain in his left knee. The athlete expresses concern with prolonged immobilization because he does not want to lose strength.

? What methods can be used to prevent atrophy from occurring but still allow healing to take place?

The maturation-remodeling phase of healing is a long-term process (Figure 10-2C). This phase features a realignment or remodeling of the collagen fibers that make up scar tissue according to the tensile forces to which that scar is subjected. Ongoing breakdown and synthesis of collagen occur with a steady increase in the tensile strength of the scar matrix. With increased stress and strain the collagen fibers realign in a position of maximum efficiency parallel to the lines of tension. The tissue gradually assumes normal appearance and function, although a scar is rarely as strong as the normal injured tissue. Usually by the end of approximately three weeks, a firm, strong, contracted, nonvascular scar exists. The maturation phase of healing may require several years to be complete.

The Role of Progressive Controlled Mobility During the Healing Process

Wolff's law states that bone and soft tissue will respond to the physical demands placed on them, causing them to remodel or realign along lines of tensile force.[36] Therefore it is critical that injured structures be exposed to progressively increasing loads throughout the rehabilitative process.[29]

Controlled mobilization is superior to immobilization for scar formation, revascularization, muscle regeneration, and reorientation of muscle fibers and tensile properties in animal models.[33] However, a brief period of immobilization of the injured tissue during the inflammatory response phase is recommended and will likely facilitate the process of healing by controlling inflammation, thus reducing clinical symptoms. As healing progresses to the repair phase, controlled activity directed toward return to normal flexibility and strength should be combined with protective support or bracing.[23] Generally, clinical signs and symptoms disappear at the end of this phase.

10-3

Critical Thinking Exercise

A wrestler receives a sudden twist to his right shoulder, causing a grade 2 strain to the teres minor muscle.

? What hemodynamic changes occur in the first hour of this acute injury?

As the remodeling phase begins, aggressive active range-of-motion and strengthening exercises should be incorporated to facilitate tissue remodeling and realignment.[44] To a great extent, pain will dictate the rate of progression. With initial injury, pain is intense and tends to decrease and eventually subside altogether as healing progresses. Any exacerbation of pain, swelling, or other clinical symptoms during or after a particular exercise or activity indicates that the load is too great for the level of tissue repair or remodeling. The athletic trainer must be aware of the time required for the healing process and realize that being overly aggressive can interfere with that process.

Factors that Impede Healing

Extent of Injury

microtears
Overuse.

macrotears
Acute trauma.

The nature or amount of the inflammatory response is determined by the extent of the tissue injury. **Microtears** of soft tissue involve only minor damage and are most often associated with overuse. **Macrotears** involve significantly greater destruction of soft tissue and result in clinical symptoms and functional alterations. Macrotears are generally caused by acute trauma.[23]

Edema

The increased pressure caused by swelling retards the healing process, causes separation of tissues, inhibits neuromuscular control, produces reflexive neurological changes, and impedes nutrition in the injured part. Edema is best controlled and managed during the initial first-aid management period as described previously.[36]

Hemorrhage

Bleeding occurs with even the smallest amount of damage to the capillaries. Bleeding produces the same negative effects on healing as does the accumulation of edema, and its presence produces additional tissue damage and thus exacerbation of the injury.[35]

Poor Vascular Supply

Injuries to tissues with a poor vascular supply heal poorly and at a slow rate. This response is likely related to a failure in the initial delivery of phagocytic cells and fibroblasts necessary for scar formation.[35]

Separation of Tissue

Mechanical separation of tissue can significantly affect the course of healing. A wound that has smooth edges that are in good apposition will tend to heal by *primary intention* with minimal scarring. Conversely, a wound that has jagged, separated edges must heal by *secondary intention,* with granulation tissue filling the defect and excessive scarring.[34,35]

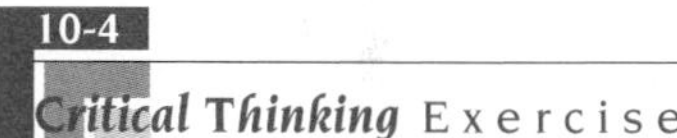

An athlete sustained a grade 2 lateral ankle sprain three weeks ago. It was given proper immediate and follow-up care.

? What repair has taken place during this time?

Muscle Spasm

Muscle spasm causes traction on the torn tissue, separates the two ends, and prevents approximation. Local and generalized ischemia may result from spasm.

Atrophy

Wasting away of muscle tissue begins immediately with injury. Strengthening and early mobilization of the injured structure retard atrophy.[34]

Corticosteroids

The use of corticosteroids in the treatment of inflammation is controversial. Steroid use in the early stages of healing has been demonstrated to inhibit fibroplasia, capillary proliferation, collagen synthesis, and increases in tensile strength of the healing scar. Their use in the later stages of healing and with chronic inflammation is debatable.[45]

Chronic inflammation can stem from repeated acute microtraumas and overuse.

Keloids and Hypertrophic Scars

Keloids occur when the rate of collagen production exceeds the rate of collagen breakdown during the maturation phase of healing. This process leads to hypertrophy of scar tissue, particularly around the periphery of the wound.

Infection

The presence of bacteria in the wound can delay healing, cause excessive granulation tissue, and frequently causes large, deformed scars.[35]

Humidity, Climate, and Oxygen Tension

Humidity significantly influences the process of epithelization. Occlusive dressings stimulate the epithelium to migrate twice as fast without crust or scab formation. The formation of a scab occurs with dehydration of the wound and traps wound drainage, which promotes infection. Keeping the wound moist allows the necrotic debris to more easily go to the surface and be shed.

10-5

Critical Thinking Exercise

A lacrosse player complains of a swollen ankle that never became completely resolved since he sustained a sprain nine months ago.

? What is the reason for this chronic swelling?

Oxygen tension relates to the neovascularization of the wound, which translates into optimal saturation and maximal tensile strength development. Circulation to the wound can be affected by ischemia, venous stasis, hematomas, and vessel trauma.

Health, Age, and Nutrition

The elastic qualities of the skin decrease with aging. Degenerative diseases, such as diabetes and arteriosclerosis, also become a concern for older patients and may affect wound healing.[41] Nutrition is important for wound healing. In particular, vitamins C (collagen synthesis and immune system), K (clotting), and A (immune system); zinc for the enzyme systems; and amino acids play critical roles in the healing process.[32]

SOFT-TISSUE HEALING

Cell Structure and Function

All organisms, from the simplest to the most complex, are composed of cells. The properties of a specific soft tissue of the body are derived from the structure and function of the cells. Individual cells contain a nucleus surrounded by cytoplasm and are enclosed by a cell membrane that selectively allows substances to enter and leave the cell. The nucleus contains chromosomes, which consist of DNA and protein. The functional and structural elements within the cell are called organelles and include mitochondria, ribosomes, endoplasmic reticulum, centrioles, and Golgi apparatus.

All tissues of the body can be defined as soft tissue except for bone. The human body has four types of soft tissue: epithelial tissue, which consists of the skin and the lining of vessels and many organs; connective tissue, which consists of tendons, ligaments, cartilage, fat, and blood vessels; muscle, which can be skeletal (striated), cardiac, or smooth; and nervous tissue, which consists of the brain, spinal cord, and nerves.[20]

Soft tissue can undergo changes and adaptations as a result of healing and of the rehabilitative process following injury. Soft-tissue adaptations include:

- metaplasia—coversion of one kind of tissue into a form that is not normal for that tissue
- dysplasia—abnormal development of tissue
- hyperplasia—excessive proliferation of normal cells in the normal tissue arrangement
- atrophy—a decrease in the size of tissue due to cell death and resorption or decreased cell proliferation
- hypertrophy—an increase in the size of a tissue without necessarily increasing the number of cells

Cartilage Healing

Cartilage has a relatively limited healing capacity.[8] When chondrocytes are destroyed and the matrix is disrupted, the course of healing is variable, depending on whether damage is to cartilage alone or also to subchondral bone. Injuries to articular cartilage alone fail to elicit clot formation or a cellular response. For the most part, the chondrocytes adjacent to the injury are the only cells that show any signs of proliferation and synthesis of matrix. Thus the defect fails to heal, although the extent of the damage tends to remain the same.[16,22]

If subchondral bone is also affected, inflammatory cells enter the damaged area and formulate granulation tissue. In this case, the healing process proceeds normally with differentiation of granulation tissue cells into chondrocytes occurring in about two weeks.[22] At approximately two months, normal collagen has been formed.[35]

Ligament Healing

The healing process in the sprained ligament follows a course of repair similar to that of other vascular tissues.[3] Immediately after injury and for approximately seventy-two hours there is a loss of blood from damaged vessels and attraction of inflammatory cells into the injured area. If a ligament is sprained outside of a joint capsule (extraarticular ligament), bleeding occurs in a subcutaneous space. If an intraarticular ligament is injured, bleeding occurs inside of the joint capsule until either clotting occurs or the pressure becomes so great that bleeding ceases.

During the next six weeks, vascular proliferation with new capillary growth begins to occur along with fibroblastic activity, resulting in the formation of a fibrin clot.[31] It is essential that the torn ends of the ligament are reconnected by bridging of this clot. A synthesis of collagen and a ground substance of proteoglycan in an intracellular matrix contributes to the proliferation of the scar that bridges the torn ends of the ligament. Initially this scar is soft and viscous, but eventually it becomes more elastic. Collagen fibers are arranged in a random woven pattern with little organization. Gradually there is a decrease in fibroblastic activity, a decrease in vascularity, and a maximum increase in the collagen density of the scar.[3] Failure to produce enough scar and failure to reconnect the ligament to the appropriate location on a bone are the two reasons why ligaments are likely to fail.

Over the next several months the scar continues to mature with the realignment of collagen occurring in response to progressive stresses and strains.[31] The maturation of the scar may require as long as twelve months to complete.[3] The exact length of time required for maturation depends on mechanical factors such as apposition of torn ends and length of immobilization.

Factors Affecting Ligament Healing

Surgically repaired extraarticular ligaments have healed with decreased scar formation and are generally stronger than unrepaired ligaments initially, although this strength advantage may not be maintained as time progresses.[39] Nonrepaired ligaments heal by fibrous scarring, effectively lengthening the ligament and producing some degree of joint instability. With intraarticular ligament tears the presence of synovial fluid dilutes the hematoma, thus preventing the formation of a fibrin clot and spontaneous healing.[39]

Several studies have shown that actively exercised ligaments are stronger than those that are immobilized. Ligaments that are immobilized for periods of several weeks after injury tend to decrease in tensile strength and also exhibit weakening of the insertion of the ligament to bone.[3] Thus it is important to minimize periods of immobilization and progressively stress the injured ligaments while exercising caution relative to biomechanical considerations for specific ligaments.[3,34]

It is not likely that the inherent stability of the joint provided by the ligament before injury will be regained. Thus to restore stability to the joint, the other structures that surround that joint, primarily muscles and their tendons, must be strengthened. The increased muscle tension provided by strength training can improve the stability of the injured joint.[20,21]

Muscle Healing

Injuries to muscle tissue involve processes of healing and repair similar to those of other tissues. Initially there will be hemorrhage and edema followed almost immediately by phagocytosis to clear debris. Within a few days there is a proliferation of ground substance, and fibroblasts begin producing a gel-type matrix that surrounds the connective tissue, leading to fibrosis and scarring. At the same time, myoblastic cells form in the area of injury, which will eventually lead to the regeneration of new myofibrils. Thus the regeneration of both connective tissue and muscle tissue has begun.[29]

Collagen fibers undergo maturation and orient themselves along lines of tensile force according to Wolff's law. Active contraction of the muscle is critical in regaining normal tensile strength.[6,29]

Regardless of the severity of the strain, the time required for rehabilitation is fairly lengthy. In many instances, rehabilitation time for a muscle strain is longer than for a ligament sprain. These incapacitating muscle strains occur most often in the large, force-producing hamstring and quadriceps muscles of the lower extremity. The treatment of hamstring strains requires a healing period of at least six to eight weeks and a considerable amount of patience. Trying to return to activity too soon often causes reinjury to the area of the musculotendinous unit that has been strained, and the healing process must begin again.

Tendon Healing

Unlike most soft tissue healing, tendon injuries pose a problem.[20] The injured tendon requires dense fibrous union of the separated ends and both extensibility and flexibility at the site of attachment.[9] Thus an abundance of collagen is required to achieve good tensile strength. Unfortunately, collagen synthesis can become excessive, resulting in fibrosis, in which adhesions form in surrounding tissues and interfere with the gliding that is essential for smooth motion.[38] Fortunately, over a period of time the scar tissue of the surrounding tissues becomes elongated in its structure because of a breakdown in the cross-links between fibrin units and thus allows the necessary gliding motion. A tendon injury that occurs where the tendon is surrounded by a synovial sheath can be potentially devastating.

A typical time frame for tendon healing would be that during the second week the healing tendon adheres to the surrounding tissue to form a single mass. During the third week, the tendon separates to varying degrees from the surrounding tissues. However, the tensile strength is not sufficient to permit a strong pull on the tendon for at least four to five weeks, the danger being that a strong contraction can pull the tendon ends apart.[28,37]

Nerve Healing

Specialized tissue, such as nerve cells, cannot regenerate once the nerve cell dies. In an injured peripheral nerve, however, the nerve fiber can regenerate significantly if the injury does not affect the cell body.[39] The proximity of the axonal injury to the cell body can significantly affect the time required for healing. The closer an injury is to the cell body, the more difficult the regenerative process. In the case of a severed nerve, surgical intervention can markedly enhance regeneration.

For regeneration to occur, an optimal environment for healing must exist.[7] When a nerve is cut, several degenerative changes occur that interfere with the neural pathways (Figure 10-3). Within the first three to five days, the portion of the axon distal to the cut begins to degenerate and breaks into irregular segments. There is also a concomitant increase in metabolism and protein production by the nerve cell body to facilitate the regenerative process. The neuron in the cell body contains the genetic material and produces chemicals necessary to maintain the axon. These substances cannot be transmitted to the distal part of the axon, and eventually there will be complete degeneration.[39]

In addition, the myelin portion of the Schwann cells around the degenerating axon also degenerates, and the myelin is phagocytized. The Schwann cells divide, forming a column of cells in place of the axon. If the cut ends of the axon contact this column of Schwann cells, the chances are good that an axon may eventually reinnervate distal structures. If the proximal end of the axon does not make contact with the column of Schwann cells, reinnervation will not occur.

The axon proximal to the cut has minimal degeneration initially and then begins the regenerative process with growth from the proximal axon. Bulbous enlargements and several axon sprouts form at the end of the proximal axon. Within about two weeks, these sprouts grow across the scar that has developed in the area of the cut and enter the column of Schwann cells. Only one of these sprouts will form the new axon, while the others will degenerate. Once the axon grows through the Schwann cell columns, remaining Schwann cells proliferate along the length of the degenerating

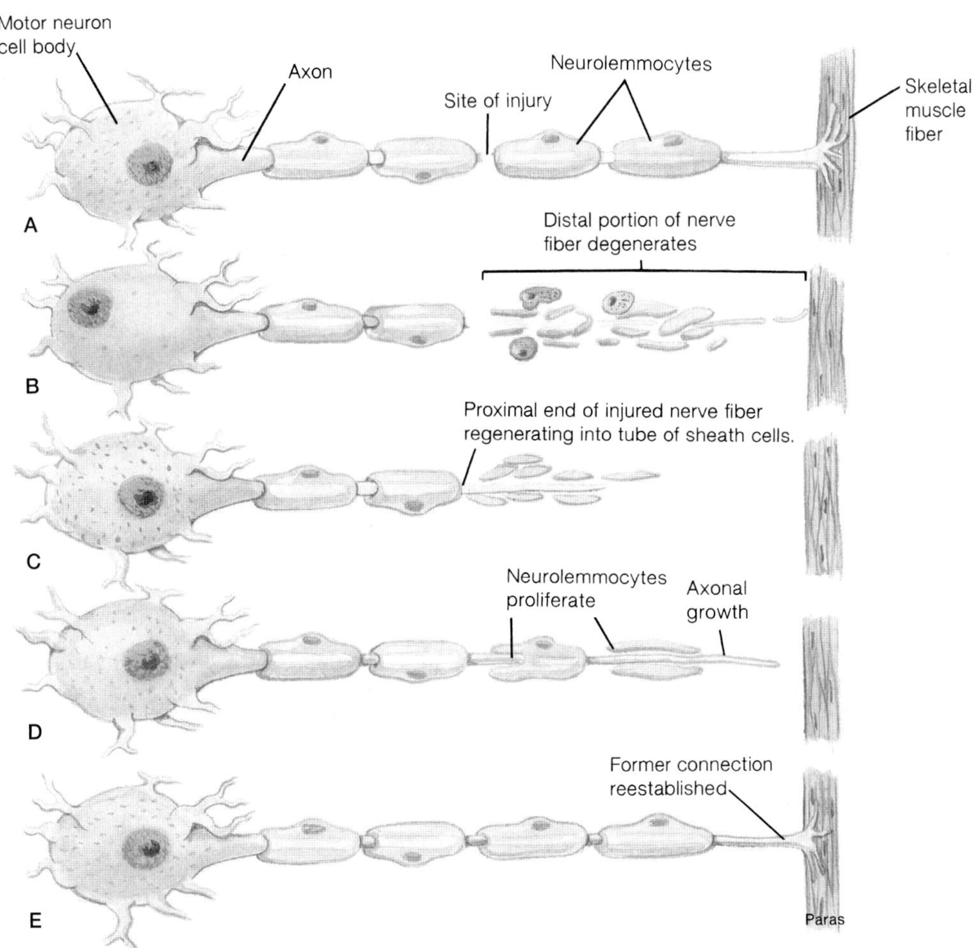

Figure 10-3

Neuron regeneration. **A,** If a neuron is severed through a myelinated axon, the proximal portion may survive but **B,** the distal portion will degenerate through phagocytosis. **C & D,** The myelin layer provides a pathway for regeneration of the axon, and **E,** innervation is restored.

fiber and form new myelin around the growing axon, which will eventually reinnervate distal structures.

Regeneration is slow, at a rate of only three to four millimeters per day. Axon regeneration can be obstructed by scar formation due to excessive fibroplasia. Damaged nerves within the central nervous system regenerate very poorly compared to nerves in the peripheral nervous system. Central nervous system axons lack connective tissue sheaths, and the myelin-producing Schwann cells fail to proliferate.[39]

Modifying Soft-Tissue Healing

The healing process is unique in each athlete. In addition, different tissues vary in their ability to regenerate. For example, cartilage regenerates to some degree from the perichondrium, striated muscle is limited in its regeneration, and peripheral nerve fibers can regenerate only if their damaged ends are opposed. Usually connective tissue will readily regenerate, but as is true of all tissue, this possibility is dependent on the availability of nutrients.

Age and general nutrition can play a role in healing. Older athletes may be more delayed in healing than younger athletes are. In an athlete with a poor nutritional status injuries may heal more slowly than normal. Athletes with certain organic disorders may heal slowly. For example, blood conditions such as anemia and diabetes often inhibit the healing process. Many of the current treatment approaches are designed to enhance the healing process. Current treatments use drugs to combat inflammation, thermal agents, therapeutic modalities, mobilization, and exercise rehabilitation.

Methods to modify soft-tissue healing include:

- Drugs to treat inflammation
- Therapeutic modalities
- Exercise and rehabilitation

The Use of Antiinflammatory Medications

It is a common practice for a physician to routinely prescribe nonsteroidal antiinflammatory drugs (NSAIDs) for patients who have sustained an injury.[7] These medications are certainly effective in minimizing pain and swelling associated with inflammation and may enhance a return to full activity. However, there are some concerns that the use of NSAIDs acutely following injury may actually interfere with inflammation, thus delaying the healing process. The use of NSAIDs will be further discussed in Chapter 17.

Therapeutic modalities

Both cold and heat are used for different conditions. In general, heat stimulates acute inflammation and cold acts as an inhibitor. Conversely, in chronic conditions, heat may serve as a depressant.[36]

A number of electrical modalities are used for the treatment of inflammation stemming from sports injuries. These procedures include penetrating heat devices such as shortwave and ultrasound therapy and electrical stimulation, including transcutaneous electrical nerve stimulation (TENS) and electrical muscle stimulation (EMS).[36]

Therapeutic exercise

A major aim of soft-tissue rehabilitation through exercise is pain-free movement, full-strength power, and full extensibility of associated muscles. The ligamentous tissue, if related to the injury, should become pain free and have full tensile strength and full range of motion. The dynamic joint stabilizers should regain full strength and power.[18]

Immobilization of a part after injury or surgery is not always good for all injuries. When a part is immobilized over an extended period of time, adverse biochemical changes occur in collagenous tissue. Early mobilization used in exercise rehabilitation that is highly controlled may enhance the healing process (see Chapter 16).[21]

BONE HEALING

Healing of injured bone tissue is similar to soft tissue healing in that all phases of the healing process may be identified, although bone regeneration capabilities are somewhat limited. However, the functional elements of healing differ significantly from those of soft tissue. The tensile strength of the scar is the single most critical factor in soft tissue healing, whereas bone has to contend with a number of additional forces including torsion, bending, and compression.[17] Trauma to bone may vary from contusions of the periosteum to closed, nondisplaced fractures to severely displaced open fractures that also involve significant soft tissue damage. When a fracture occurs, blood vessels in the bone and the periosteum are damaged, resulting in bleeding and subsequent clot formation (Figure 10-4). Hemorrhaging from the marrow is contained by the periosteum and the surrounding soft tissue in the region of the fracture. In about one week, fibroblasts have begun laying down a fibrous collagen network. The fibrin strands within the clot serve as the framework for proliferating vessels. *Chondroblast* cells begin producing fibrocartilage, creating a *callus* between the broken bones. At first, the callus is soft and firm because it is composed primarily of collagenous fibrin. The callus becomes firm and more rubbery as cartilage begins to predominate. Bone-producing cells called **osteoblasts** begin to proliferate and enter the callus, forming cancellous bone trabeculae, which eventually replace the cartilage. Finally the callus crystallizes into bone, at which point remodeling of the bone begins. The callus can be divided into two portions, the external callus located around the periosteum on the outside of the fracture and the internal callus found between the bone fragments. The size of the callus is proportional both to the damage and to the amount of irritation to the fracture site during the healing process. Also during this time, **osteoclasts** begin to appear in the area to resorb bone fragments and clean up debris.[17,39]

osteoblasts
Bone-producing cells.

osteoclasts
Cells that resorb bone.

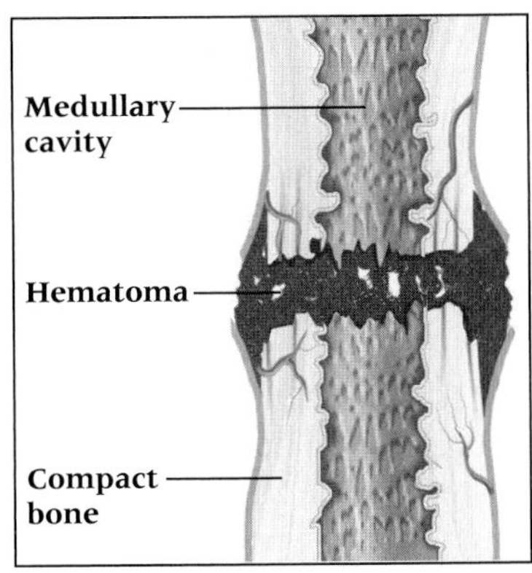

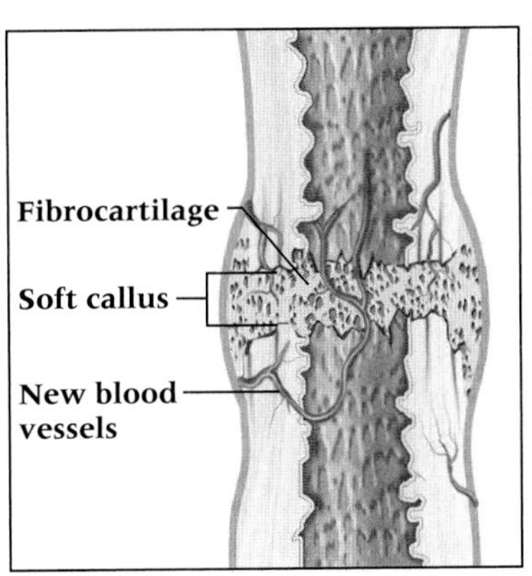

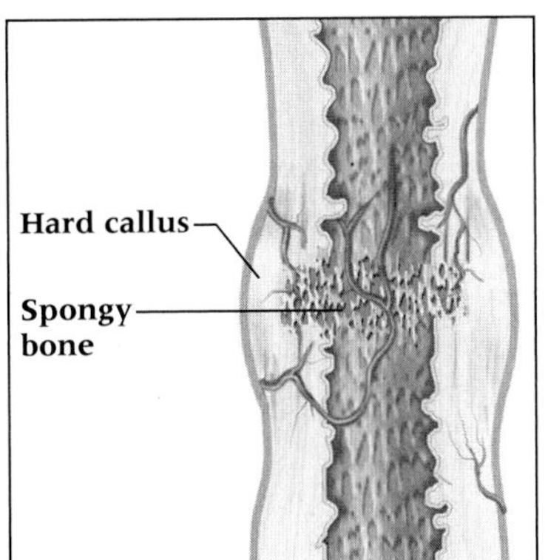

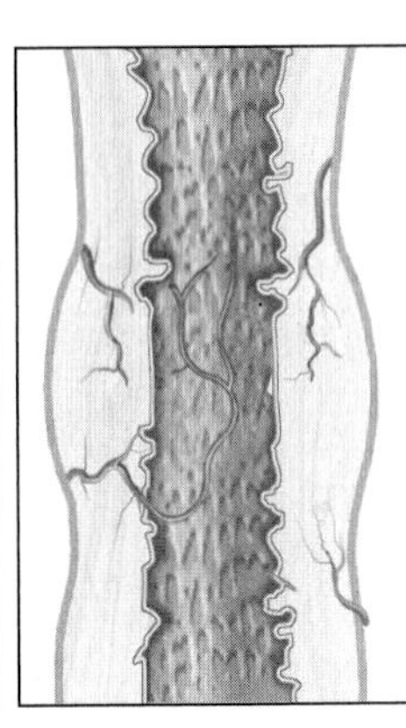

Figure 10-4

The healing of a fracture. **A,** Blood vessels are broken at the fracture line; the blood clots and forms a fracture hematoma. **B,** Blood vessels grow into the fracture and a fibrocartilage soft callus forms. **C,** The fibrocartilage becomes ossified and forms a bony callus made of spongy bone. **D,** Osteoclasts remove excess tissue from the bony callus and the bone eventually resembles its original appearance.

The remodeling process is similar to the growth process of bone in that the fibrous cartilage is gradually replaced by fibrous bone and then by more structurally efficient lamellar bone. Remodeling involves an ongoing process during which osteoblasts lay down new bone and osteoclasts remove and break down bone according to the forces placed upon the healing bone.[17] Wolff's law maintains that a bone will adapt to mechanical stresses and strains by changing size, shape, and structure. Therefore, once the cast is removed, the bone must be subjected to normal stresses and strains so that tensile strength may be regained before the healing process is complete.[5,39,46]

The time required for bone healing is variable and based on a number of factors such as severity of the fracture, site of the fracture, extensiveness of the trauma, and age of the patient. Normal periods of immobilization range from as short as three weeks for the small bones in the hands and feet to as long as eight weeks for the long bones of the upper and lower extremities. In some instances, for example, the four small toes, immobilization may not be required for healing. The healing process is certainly not complete when the splint or cast is removed. Osteoblastic and osteoclastic activity may continue for two to three years after severe fractures.

Management of Acute Fractures

In the treatment of acute fractures, the bones commonly must be immobilized completely until X-ray studies reveal that the hard callus has been formed. It is up to the physician to know the various types of fractures and the best form of immobilization for each specific fracture.[45] Fractures can keep an athlete out of participation in his or her sport for several weeks or months, depending on the nature, extent, and site of the fracture. During this period, certain conditions can seriously interfere with the healing process:

- If there is a *poor blood supply to the fractured area* and one of the parts of the fractured bone is not properly supplied by the blood, that part will die and union or healing of the fracture will not take place. This condition is known as *avascular necrosis* and often occurs in the head of the femur, the navicular bone in the wrist, the talus in the ankle, and isolated bone fragments. The condition is relatively rare among vital, healthy, young athletes except in the navicular bone of the wrist.
- *Poor immobilization of the fracture site,* resulting from poor casting by the physician and permitting motion between the bone parts, may not only prevent proper union but may also, in the event that union does transpire, cause deformity to develop.
- *Infection* can materially interfere with the normal healing process, particularly in the case of a compound fracture, which offers an ideal situation for the development of a severe streptococcal or staphylococcal infection. The increased use of modern antibiotics has considerably reduced the prevalence of these infections coincidental with or immediately after a fracture. The closed fracture is not

10-6

***Critical Thinking* Exercise**

A field hockey player falls and sustains an acute fracture of the left humerus.

? What are the healing events typical of this acute bone fracture?

Conditions that interfere with fracture healing:

- Poor blood supply
- Poor immobilization
- Infection

immune to contamination because infections within the body or poor blood supply can render it susceptible. If the fracture site should become and remain infected, the infection could interfere with the proper union of the bone.
- Soft tissues that become positioned between the severed ends of the bone—such as muscle, connective tissue, or other soft tissue immediately adjacent to the fracture—can prevent proper bone union, often necessitating surgical intervention.

Healing of Stress Fractures

10-7 Critical Thinking Exercise

A female cross-country runner sustains a stress fracture of her left tibia. Her left leg is ¾ inch shorter than the right leg.

? What is a possible cause of this injury?

As discussed in Chapter 9, stress fractures may be created by cyclic forces that adversely load a bone at a susceptible site. Fractures may be the result of axial compression or tension created by the pull of muscles. Stress on ligamentous and bony tissue can be positive and increase relative strength or can be negative and lead to tissue weakness. Bone produces an electrical potential in response to the stress of tension and compression. As a bone bends, tension is created on its convex side along with a positive electrical charge; conversely, on the concave or compressional side, a negative electrical charge is created. Torsional forces produce tension circumferentially. Constant tension caused by axial compression or stress by muscular activity can result in an increase in bone resorption and, subsequently, a microfracture. In other words, if the osteoclastic activity is greater than the osteoblastic activity, the bone becomes increasingly susceptible to stress fractures.

Like the healing of acute fractures, healing of stress fractures involves restoring a balance of osteoclastic and osteoblastic activity. Achieving this balance requires recognition of the situation as early as possible. Stress fractures that go unhealed will eventually develop into complete cortical fractures that may, over a period of time, become displaced. A decrease in activity and elimination of other factors in training that cause stress will allow the bone to remodel and to develop the ability to withstand stress.

PAIN

Pain can be defined as "an unpleasant sensory and emotional experience associated with actual or potential tissue damage, or described in terms of such damage."[1] Pain is a subjective sensation with more than one dimension and an abundance of descriptors of its qualities and characteristics. Pain is composed of a variety of human discomforts, rather than being a single entity. The perception of pain can be subjectively modified by past experiences and expectations. Much of what is done to treat athletes' pain is to change their perceptions of pain. Certainly, reducing pain is an essential part of treatment. The athletic trainer's goal is to control acute pain by encouraging the body to heal through exercise designed to progressively increase functional capacity and to return the patient to full activity as swiftly and safely as possible.

Types of Pain

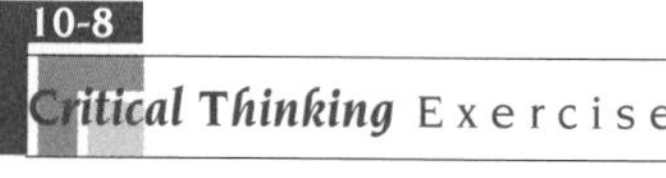

A butterfly swimmer has been experiencing low back pain for more than six months. The pain is described as aching and throbbing.

? What type of pain is this athlete experiencing?

Pain can be described according to a number of different categories, such as pain sources, acute versus chronic, and projected (referred) pain.[12]

Pain Sources

Pain sources are cutaneous, deep somatic, visceral, and psychogenic. Cutaneous pain is usually sharp, bright, and burning and can have a fast or slow onset. Deep somatic pain stems from structures such as tendons, muscles, joints, periosteum, and blood vessels. Visceral pain originates from internal organs. Visceral pain is diffused at first and later may be localized, as in appendicitis. In psychogenic pain, the individual feels pain but the cause is emotional rather than physical.[12]

Acute versus Chronic Pain

Acute pain is pain that is less than six months in duration. Tissue damage occurs and serves as a warning to the athlete. Chronic pain, on the other hand, has a duration longer than six months. The International Association for the Study of Pain describes chronic pain as that which continues beyond the usual normal healing time.[18]

Referred Pain

Referred pain occurs away from the actual site of irritation. This pain has been called an error in perception. Each referred pain site must also be considered unique to each individual. Symptoms and signs vary according to the nerve fibers affected. Response may be motor, sensory, or both. Three types of referred pain common to athletes are myofascial, sclerotomic, and dermatomic pain.

Myofascial pain As discussed in Chapter 9, **trigger points** are small hyperirritable areas within a muscle in which nerve impulses bombard the central nervous system and are expressed as a referred pain.[36] Acute and chronic musculoskeletal pain can be caused by myofascial trigger points. Such pain sites have variously been described as fibrositis, myositis, myalgia, myofasciitis, and muscular strain.

trigger points Small hyperirritable areas within a muscle.

An active trigger point is hyperirritable and causes an obvious complaint. Pain radiating from an active trigger point does not follow a usual area of distribution such as sclerotomes, dermatomes, or peripheral nerves. The trigger point pain area is called the reference zone, which could be close to the point of irritation or a considerable distance from it.[36]

Sclerotomic and dermatomic pain Deep pain may originate from sclerotomic, myotomic, or dermatomic nerve irritation or injury. A sclerotome is an area of bone or fascia that is supplied by a single nerve root. Myotomes are muscles supplied by a single nerve root. Dermatomes also are in an area of skin supplied by a single nerve root.

Sclerotomic pain is deep, aching, and poorly localized pain. Sclerotomic pain impulses can be projected to regions in the brain such as the hypothalamus, limbic system, and reticular formation and can cause depression, anxiety, fear, or anger. Autonomic changes, such as changes in vasomotor tone, blood pressure, and sweating, may also occur.

Dermatomic pain, in contrast to sclerotomic pain, is sharp and well localized. Unlike sclerotomic pain, dermatomic pain projects mainly to the thalamus and is relayed directly to the cortex, skipping autonomic and affective responses.

Nociceptors and Neural Transmission

Pain receptors known as *nociceptors,* or free nerve endings, are sensitive to mechanical, thermal, and chemical energy.[12] They are commonly found in skin, periosteum surrounding bone, teeth, meninges, and some organs.

Afferent nerve fibers transmit impulses from the nociceptors toward the brain, while *efferent* nerve fibers such as motor neurons transmit impulses from the brain toward the periphery. First-order or primary afferents transmit impulses from a nociceptor to the dorsal horn of the spinal cord. There are four different types of first-order neurons: $A\alpha$, $A\beta$, $A\delta$, and C. $A\alpha$ and $A\beta$ fibers are characterized as large-diameter afferents and $A\delta$ and C fibers as small-diameter afferents. $A\delta$ and C fibers transmit sensations of pain and temperature. $A\delta$ neurons originate from nociceptors located in skin and transmit "fast pain," while C neurons originate from both superficial tissue (skin) and deeper tissue (ligaments and muscle) and transmit "slow pain."[12]

Second-order afferent fibers carry sensory messages from the dorsal horn to the brain and are categorized as nociceptive specific. Second-order afferents receive input from $A\beta$, $A\delta$, and C fibers. Second-order afferents serve relatively large, overlapping receptor fields. Nociceptive-specific, second-order afferents respond exclusively to noxious stimulation and receive input only from $A\delta$ and C fibers. All of these neurons synapse with third-order neurons, which carry information to various brain centers where the input is integrated, interpreted, and acted upon.[12]

Facilitators and Inhibitors of Synaptic Transmission

For information to pass between neurons, a transmitter substance must be released from one neuron terminal, enter the synaptic cleft, and attach to a receptor site on the next neuron. This occurs primarily due to chemicals called *neurotransmitters.* However, it has been shown that several compounds that are not true neurotransmitters can facilitate or inhibit synaptic activity. These include *serotonin,* which is active in descending pathways; *norepinephrine,* which inhibits pain transmission between first- and second-order neurons; *substance P,* which is active in small-diameter primary afferent neurons; *enkephalins,* found in descending pathways; and β-*endorphin,* found in the central nervous system.[14]

Mechanisms of Pain Control

The neurophysiologic mechanisms of pain control have not been fully explained. To date three different models of pain control have been proposed: the gate control theory, central biasing, and the release of β-endorphin. It is likely that some as-yet-unexplained combination of these three models is responsible for pain modulation.[4]

Gate Control Theory

Sensory information coming from cutaneous receptors in the skin enters the ascending Aβ afferents and is carried to the dorsal horn of the spinal cord (Figure 10-5). Likewise, pain messages from the nociceptors are carried along Aδ and C afferent fibers and also enter the dorsal horn of the spinal cord. The substantia gelatinosa at the dorsal horn of the spinal cord inhibits or "closes the gate" to synaptic transmission coming from Aδ and C fiber afferent pathways. Sensory information coming from Aβ fibers is transmitted to higher centers in the brain. Thus the "pain message" carried along Aδ and C fibers is not transmitted to second-order neurons and never reaches sensory centers. The gate control theory of pain control occurs at the spinal cord level.[12]

Central Biasing

Stimulation of descending pathways in the spinal cord may also inhibit pain impulses carried along the Aδ and C afferent fibers (Figure 10-6). It is theorized that previous experiences, emotional influences, sensory perception, and other factors could influence the transmission of the pain messages and thus the perception of pain. This has

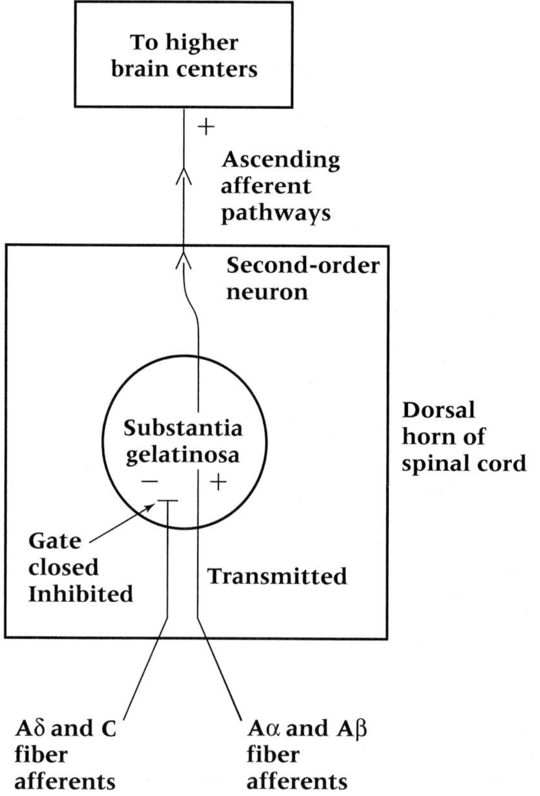

Figure 10-5

Gate control theory of pain control.

been referred to as *central biasing*. This information coming from higher centers in the brain along efferent descending pathways in the spinal cord causes a release of two neurotransmitter-like substances, enkephalin and norepinephrine, into the dorsal horn, which together act to block or inhibit the synaptic transmission of impulses from the Aδ and C afferent fibers to second-order afferent neurons.[12]

Release of β-Endorphin

It has been shown that noxious (painful) stimulation of nociceptors resulting in the transmission of pain information along Aδ and C afferents can stimulate the release of an opiate-like chemical called β-*endorphin* from the hypothalamus (Figure 10-7). β-endorphin is endogenous to the central nervous system and is known to have strong analgesic effects. The exact mechanisms by which β-endorphin produces these potent analgesic effects are unclear. Acupuncture, acupressure, and point stimulation using electrical currents are all techniques that may stimulate the release of β-endorphin.[12]

Pain Assessment

Pain is a complex phenomenon that is difficult to evaluate and quantify because it is subjective. Thus, obtaining an accurate and standardized assessment of pain is problematic. A number of validated assessment tools are available that allow the athletic trainer to develop a pain profile by identifying the type of pain an athlete is experiencing, quantifying intensity of pain, evaluating the effect of the pain experience on an athlete's level of functioning, and assessing the psychosocial impact of pain.

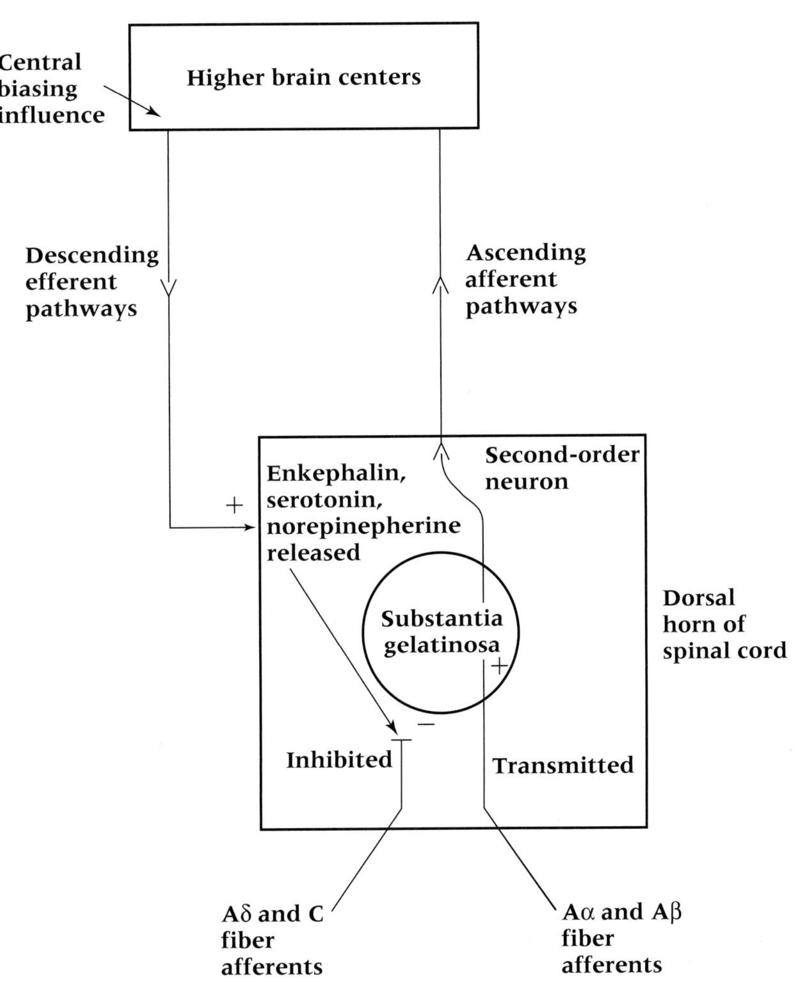

Figure 10-6

Central biasing model of pain control.

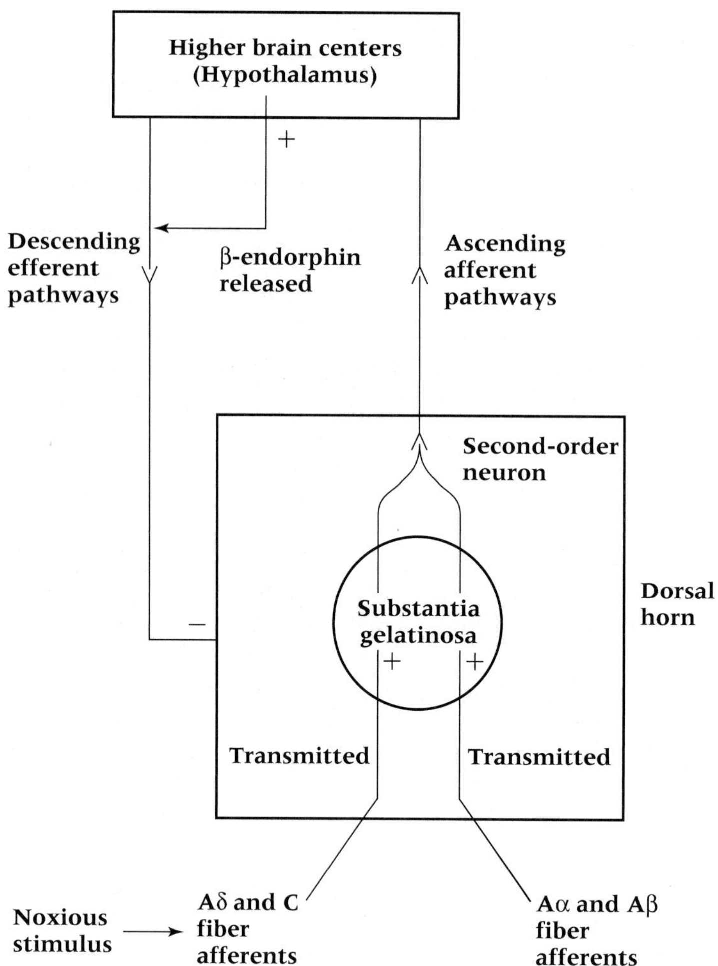

Figure 10-7

β-endorphin model of pain control.

Pain measurement tools include simple *unidimensional scales* or *multidimensional questionnaires.* Pain measurement should include both the time frame and the clinical context of the pain. With unidimensional scales, individuals with acute pain are usually asked to describe their pain "right now" and may be asked about the average intensity over a fixed period to provide information on the course of the pain. Examples of commonly used unidimensional scales include verbal rating scales, the numeric rating scale, and the visual analog scale. Multidimensional pain assessment tools are more comprehensive pain assessments that require the determination of the quality of the pain and its effect on mood and function. They are used mainly to quantify these aspects of pain, and they take longer to administer than the unidimensional scales. The McGill Pain Questionnaire is an example of a multidimensional pain assessment tool.

Visual Analogue Scales

Visual analogue scales are quick and simple tests that consist of a line, usually 10 cm in length, the extremes of which are taken to represent the limits of the pain experience. The athlete simply places a mark on that line based on the perceived level of pain. Scales can be completed daily or more often (Figure 10-8).

Pain Charts

Pain charts are used to establish spatial properties of pain. They involve a two-dimensional graphic chart on which the athlete assesses the location of pain and a number of subjective components. The athlete colors the chart in areas that correspond to pain (Figure 10-9).

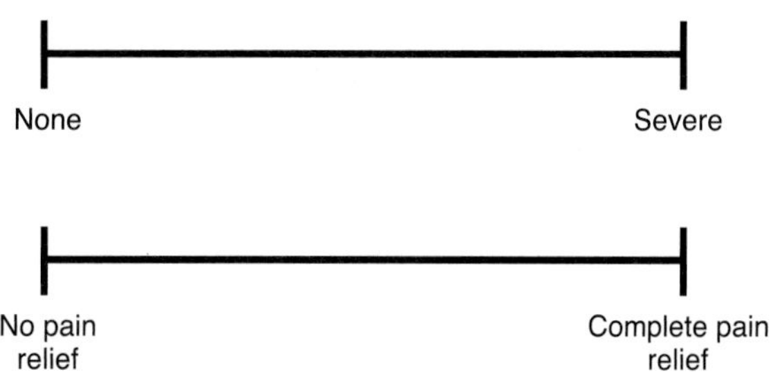

Figure 10-8

Visual analogue scale.

McGill Pain Questionnaire

The McGill Pain Questionnaire lists seventy-eight words that describe pain, which are grouped into twenty sets and divided into four categories representing dimensions of the pain experience. It may take up to twenty minutes to complete, and the questionnaire is administered every two to four weeks (Figure 10-10).

Activity Pain Indicators Profile

The Activity Pain Indicators Profile is a sixty-four question, self-report tool used to assess functional impairment associated with pain. It measures the frequency of certain behaviors, such as housework, recreation, and social activities, that produce pain.

Numeric Rating Scale

The Numeric Rating Scale is the most common acute pain profile used in sports medicine. The athlete is asked to rate pain on a scale from 1 to 10 with 10 representing the worst pain they have experienced or could imagine. Usually the scale is administered before and after treatment. When treatments provide pain relief, questions are asked about the extent and duration of the relief.

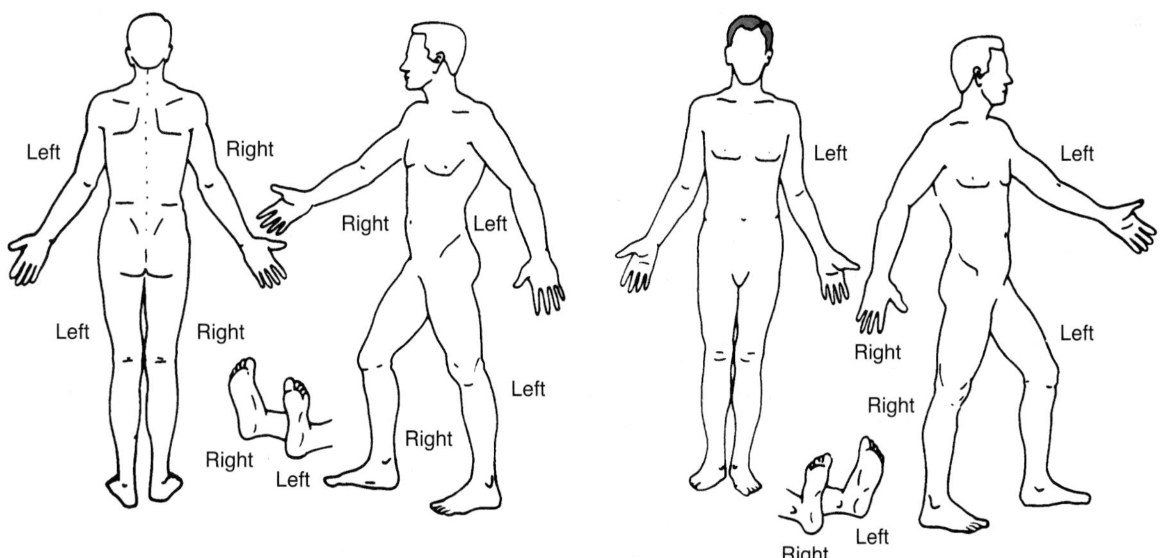

Figure 10-9

The pain chart. Use the following instructions: "Please use all of the figures to show me exactly where all your pains are, and where they radiate to. Shade or draw with *blue marker.* Only the athlete is to fill out this sheet. Please be as precise and detailed as possible. Use *yellow marker* for numbness and tingling. Use *red marker* for burning or hot areas, and *green marker* for cramping. Please remember: blue = pain, yellow = numbness and tingling, red = burning or hot areas, green = cramping." Used with permission from Melzack, R: *Pain measurement and assessment,* New York, 1983, Raven Press.

McGill Pain Questionnaire

Patient's Name ______ Date ______ Time ______ am/pm

PRI S ______ A ______ E ______ M ______ PRI (T) ______ PPI ______

(1–10) (11–15) (16) (17–20) (1–20)

1 Flickering Quivering Pulsing Throbbing Beating Pounding	11 Tiring Exhausting	
2 Jumping Flashing Shooting	12 Sickening Suffocating	
3 Pricking Boring Drilling Stabbing Lancinating	13 Fearful Frightful Terrifying	
4 Sharp Cutting Lacerating	14 Punishing Gruelling Cruel Vicious Killing	
5 Pinching Pressing Gnawing Cramping Crushing	15 Wretched Blinding	
6 Tugging Pulling Wrenching	16 Annoying Troublesome Miserable Intense Unbearable	
7 Hot Burning Scalding Searing	17 Spreading Radiating Penetrating Piercing	
8 Tingling Itchy Smarting Stinging	18 Tight Numb Drawing Squeezing Tearing	
9 Dull Sore Hurting Aching Heavy	19 Cool Cold Freezing	
10 Tender Taut Rasping Splitting	20 Nagging Nauseating Agonizing Dreadful Torturing	
	PPI 0 No pain 1 Mild 2 Discomforting 3 Distressing 4 Horrible 5 Excruciating	

Brief Momentary Transient	Rhythmic Periodic Intermittent	Continuous Steady Constant

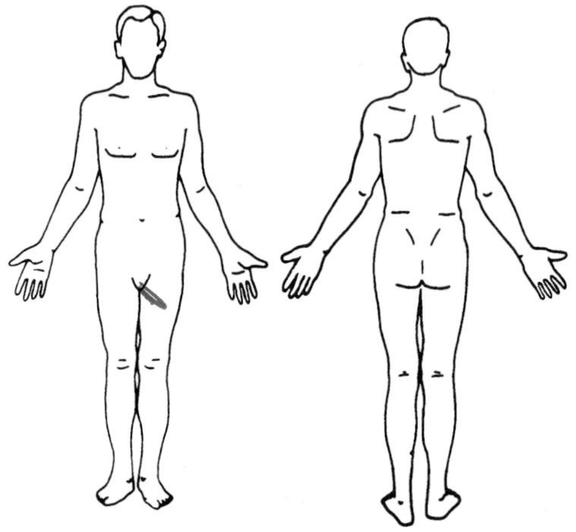

E = External
I = Internal

COMMENTS

Figure 10-10

McGill Pain Questionnaire. The descriptors fall into four groups: Sensory, 1 to 10; affective, 11 to 15; evaluative, 16; and miscellaneous, 17 to 20. The rank value for each descriptor is based on its position in the word set. The sum of the rank values is the pain rating index (PRI). The present pain intensity (PPI) is based on a scale of 0 to 5. Used with permission from Melzack, R: *Pain measurement and assessment,* New York, 1983, Raven Press.

Treating Pain

An athletic trainer can approach pain management using a variety of treatment options, including the use of therapeutic modalities as well as the use of pain medications.

Therapeutic Modalities

Many therapeutic modalities can provide pain relief. There is not one best therapeutic agent for pain control. The athletic trainer must select the therapeutic agent that is most appropriate for each athlete, based on the knowledge of the modalities and professional judgment (see Chapter 15). In no situation should the athletic trainer apply a therapeutic agent without first developing a clear rationale for the treatment. The therapeutic modalities used to control pain do little to promote tissue healing. They should be used to relieve acute pain following injury or surgery or to control pain and other symptoms, such as swelling, to promote progressive exercise. The athletic trainer should not lose sight of the effects of the modalities or the importance of progressive exercise in restoring the athlete's functional ability.

The athletic trainer can make use of the gate control mechanism of pain control by using superficial heat or cold, electrical stimulating currents, massage, and counterirritants to stimulate the large-diameter $A\alpha$ and $A\beta$ efferent nerve fibers. Noxious stimulation of acupuncture and trigger points using either electrical stimulating currents or deep acupressure massage techniques can mediate the release of β-endorphin.[12]

Medications

A physician may choose to prescribe oral or injectable medications in the treatment of the athlete. The most commonly used medications are classified as analgesics, antiinflammatory agents, or both.[10] The athletic trainer should become familiar with these drugs and note if the athlete is taking any medications (see Chapter 17). It is also important to work with the referring physician to make sure that the athlete takes the medications appropriately.

10-9

Critical Thinking Exercise

A gymnast is receiving electrical stimulation for chronic low back pain.

? What is the purpose of administering electrical stimulation for the chronic pain?

Psychological Aspect of Pain

Pain, especially chronic pain, is a subjective, psychological phenomenon. When painful injuries are treated, the total athlete must be considered, not just the pain or condition. Even in the most well-adjusted person, pain will create emotional changes. Constant pain will often cause self-centeredness and an increased sense of dependency. Chapter 11 will discuss in great detail the psychosocial aspects of dealing with injury and managing pain.

Athletes, like nonathletes, vary in their pain thresholds (Figure 10-11). Some can tolerate enormous pain, whereas others find mild pain almost unbearable. Pain is perceived as being worse at night because persons are alone, more aware of themselves, and devoid of external diversions. Personality differences can also cause differences in pain toleration. For example, athletes who are anxious, dependent, and immature have less tolerance for pain than those who are relaxed and emotionally in control.

A number of theories about how pain is produced and perceived by the brain have been advanced. Only in the last few decades has science demonstrated that pain is both a psychological and physiological phenomenon and is therefore unique to each individual. Sports activities demonstrate this fact clearly. Through conditioning, an athlete learns to endure the pain of rigorous activity and to block the sensations of a

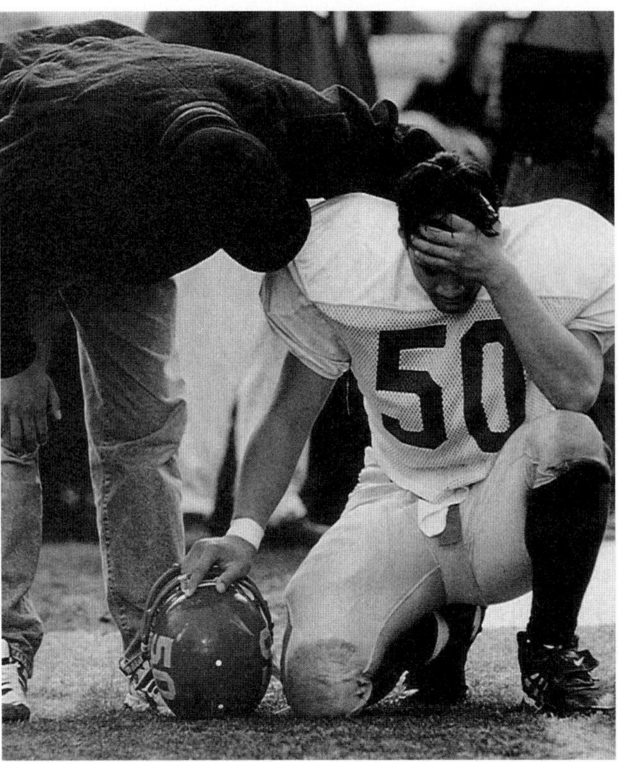

Figure 10-11

Coping with pain in sports is as much psychological as it is physical.

minor injury. It is perhaps most critical for the athletic trainer to recognize that all pain is very real to the athlete.

SUMMARY

- The three phases of the healing process are the inflammatory response phase, the fibroblastic repair phase, and the maturation-remodeling phase, which occur in sequence but overlap one another in a continuum.
- During the inflammatory response phase, debris is phagocytized (cleaned up). The fibroblastic repair phase involves the deposition of collagen fibers to form a firm scar. During the maturation-remodeling phase, collagen is realigned along lines of tensile force and the tissue gradually assumes normal appearance and function.
- Factors that may impede the healing process include edema, hemorrhage, lack of vascular supply, separation of tissue, muscle spasm, atrophy, corticosteroids, hypertrophic scars, infection, climate and humidity, age, health, and nutrition.
- The healing of soft tissues including cartilage, ligament, muscle, and nerve follows a similar course. Unlike the other tissues, nerve has the capability of regenerating.
- Bone healing following fracture involves increased activity of osteoblastic cells and osteoclastic cells.
- Pain is a response to a noxious stimulus that is subjectively modified by past experiences and expectations.
- Pain is classified as either acute or chronic and can exhibit many different patterns.
- Three models of pain control include the gate control theory, central biasing affecting the descending pathways, and the release of β-endorphin from higher centers of the brain.
- Pain perception may be influenced by a variety of cognitive processes mediated by the higher brain centers.

Websites

American Academy of Pain Management: http://www.aapainmanage.org

American Pain Society http://www.ampainsoc.org

World Union of Wound Healing Societies http://www.wuwhs.org

Solutions to Critical Thinking EXERCISES

10-1 Little can be done to speed up the healing process physiologically. This athlete must realize that certain physiological events must occur during each phase of the healing process. Any interference with this healing process during a rehabilitation program will likely slow return to full activity. The healing process must have an opportunity to accomplish what it is supposed to.

10-2 Immobilization during the inflammatory process may be beneficial, however, controlled mobilization will help the tissue to decrease atrophy and enhance the healing process. Controlled mobilization will allow the athlete to perform progressive strengthening exercises in a timely manner.

10-3 Initially, a transitory vasoconstriction with the start of blood coagulation of the broken blood vessels occurs. Dilation of the vessels in the region of injury follow, along with activation of chemical mediators via key cells.

10-4 A grade 2 lateral ankle sprain implies that the joint capsule and ligaments are partially torn. At three weeks the injury has been cleaned of debris and is undergoing the process of secondary healing. Granulation tissue fills the torn areas, and fibroblasts are beginning to form scar tissue.

10-5 In its acute phase the athlete's injury was not allowed to heal properly. As a result, the injury became chronic, with a proliferation of scar tissue, lymphocytes, plasma cells, and macrophages.

10-6 Uncomplicated acute bone healing goes through five stages: hematoma formation, cellular proliferation, callus formation, ossification, and remodeling.

10-7 Because it is shorter, the left leg has the greater stress during running. This stress creates increased tension on the tibia's concave side, causing an increase in osteoclastic activity.

10-8 The pain is considered to be chronic, deep somatic pain stemming from the low back muscles. It is conducted primarily by the C-type nerve fibers.

10-9 The purpose is to stimulate the large, rapidly conducting nerve fibers to inhibit the smaller and slower nerves that carry pain impulses.

REVIEW QUESTIONS AND CLASS ACTIVITIES

1. What are the three phases of healing and what are the approximate time frames for each of these three phases?
2. What are the physiological events associated with the inflammatory response phase of the healing process?
3. How can you differentiate between acute and chronic inflammation?
4. How is collagen laid down in the area of injury during the fibroblastic repair phase of healing?
5. Explain Wolff's law and the importance of controlled mobility during the maturation-remodeling phase of healing.
6. What are some of the factors that can have a negative impact on the healing process?
7. Compare and contrast the course of healing in cartilage, ligaments, muscle, and nerve.
8. What is a basic definition of pain?
9. What are the different types of pain?
10. What are the characteristics of the various sensory receptors?
11. How does the nervous system relay information about painful stimuli?
12. Describe how the gate control mechanism of pain modulation may be used to modulate pain.
13. How does central biasing and the descending pain control mechanism function to modulate pain?
14. What are the opiatelike substances and how do they act to modulate pain?
15. What are the different assessment scales available to help the athletic trainer determine the extent of pain perception?
16. How can pain perception be modified by cognitive factors?

REFERENCES

1. Acute Pain Management Guideline Panel: Acute pain management: operative or medical procedures and trauma, AHCPR Pub. No. 92-0032, Rockville, Md, 1992, Agency for Health Care Policy and Research, Public Health Service, U.S. Department of Health and Human Services.
2. Anonymous: The healing process, *Nursing Times* 90(16):95, 1994.
3. Arnoczky SP: Physiologic principles of ligament injuries and healing. In Scott WN, editor: *Ligament and extensor mechanism injuries of the knee,* St Louis, 1991, Mosby.
4. Aronson PA: Pain theories: a review for application in athletic training and therapy. *Athletic Therapy Today* 7(4):8, 2002.
5. Bailon-Plaza A: Beneficial effects of moderate, early loading and adverse effects of delayed or excessive loading on bone healing. *Journal of Biomechanics* 36(8):1069, 2003.
6. Bandy W, Dunleavy K: Adaptability of skeletal muscle: response to increased and decreased use. In Zachazewski J, Magee D, Quillen W: *Athletic injuries and rehabilitation,* Philadelphia, 1996, WB Saunders.
7. Black KP: Perepheral afferent nerve regeneration. In Lephart S, Fu F, editors: Proprioception and neuromuscular control in joint stability, Champaign, Ill, 2000, Human Kinetics.
8. Buckwalter JA: Articular cartilage: injuries and potential for healing, *J Orthop Sports Phys Ther* 28(4):192, 1998.
9. Clancy W: Tendon trauma and overuse injuries. In Leadbetter W, Buckwalter J, Gordon S, editors: *Sports-induced inflammation,* Park Ridge, Ill, 1990, American Academy of Orthopedic Surgeons.
10. Clark WG: *Goth's medical pharmacology,* ed 13, St Louis, 1992, Mosby.
11. Cox D: Growth factors in wound healing, *J Wound Care* 2(6):339, 1993.
12. Denegar CR, Donley PB: Managing pain with therapeutic modalities. In Prentice WE, editor: *Therapeutic modalities in sports medicine and athletic training,* ed 5, St Louis, 2003, McGraw-Hill.
13. Fantone J: Basic concepts in inflammation. In Leadbetter W, Buckwalter J, Gordon S, editors: *Sports-induced inflammation,* Park Ridge Ill, 1990, American Academy of Orthopaedic Surgeons.
14. Fine PG: The biology of pain. In Heil J, editor: *Psychology of sport injury,* Champaign, Ill, 1993, Human Kinetics.
15. Gallin J, Snyderman R, Haynes B: *Inflammation: basic principles and clinical correlates,* Baltimore, 1999, Lippincott Williams & Wilkins Publishers.

16. Gelberman R, Goldberg V, An KN, et al. *Soft tissue healing*. In Woo SLY, Buckwalter J, editors: *Injury and repair of musculoskeletal soft tissues*, Park Ridge, Ill, 1988, American Academy of Orthopaedic Surgeons.
17. Gradisar IA: Fracture stabilization and healing. In Gould JA, Davies GJ, editors: *Orthopaedic and sports physical medicine*, St Louis, 1990, Mosby.
18. Grichnick K, Ferrante FM: The difference between acute and chronic pain, *Mt Sinai J Med* 58:217, 1991.
19. Hettinga DL: Inflammatory response of synovial joint structures. In Malone T, McPhoil T, editors: *Orthopaedic and sports physical therapy*, St Louis, 1990, Mosby.
20. Houglum P: Soft tissue healing and its impact on rehabilitation, *J Sport Rehabil* 1(1):19, 1992.
21. Hubbel S, Buschbacher R: Tissue injury and healing: using medications, modalities, and exercise to maximize recovery. In Bushbacher R, Branddom R: *Sports medicine and rehabilitation: a sport specific approach*, Philadelphia, 2002, Elsevier Health Services.
22. Irrgang JJ, Pezzullo D: Rehabilitation following surgical procedures to address articular cartilage lesions in the knee, *J Orthop Sports Phys Ther* 28(4):232, 1998.
23. Kibler WB: Concepts in exercise rehabilitation of athletic injury. In Leadbetter W, Buckwalter J, Gordon S, editors: *Sports-induced inflammation*, Park Ridge, Ill, 1990, American Academy of Orthopaedic Surgeons.
24. Kocher MS: Ligament healing and augmentation. In *Proceedings, National Athletic Trainers' Association, 10th annual meeting and clinical symposia*, Champaign, Ill, 1999, Human Kinetics.
25. Leadbetter W, Buckwalter J, Gordon S, editors: *Sports-induced inflammation*, Park Ridge, Ill, 1990, American Academy of Orthopaedic Surgeons.
26. Leadbetter W: Introduction to sports-induced soft-tissue inflammation. In Leadbetter W, Buckwalter J, Gordon S, editors: *Sports-induced inflammation*, Park Ridge, Ill, 1990, American Academy of Orthopaedic Surgeons.
27. Ley K: *Physiology of inflammation* (Methods in Physiology Series), Bethesda, Md, 2001, American Physiological Society.
28. Maffulli N: Basic science of tendons. *Sports Med Arthroscopy Review* 8(1)1, 2000.
29. Malone T, Garrett W, Zachewski J: Muscle: deformation, injury and repair. In Zachazewski J, Magee D, Quillen W: *Athletic injuries and rehabilitation*, Philadelphia, 1996, WB Saunders.
30. Martinez-Hernandez A, Amenta P: Basic concepts in wound healing. In Leadbetter W, Buckwalter J, Gordon S, editors: *Sports-induced inflammation*, Park Ridge, Ill, 1990, American Academy of Orthopaedic Surgeons.
31. Molloy T: The roles of growth factors in tendon and ligament healing. *Sports Med* 33(5):381, 2003.
32. Murdoch S: Managing the inflammatory response through nutritional supplements. *Athletic Therapy Today* 6(5):46, 2001.
33. Murrell GAC, Jang D, Lily E, Best T: The effects of immobilization and exercise on tendon healing, *Journal of Science and Medicine in Sport* 2(1 Supplement):40, 1999.
34. Musacchia XJ: Disuse atrophy of skeletal muscle: animal models. In Pandolf KB, editor: *Exercise and sport sciences review*, New York, 1988, Macmillan Publishing.
35. Norris S, Provo B, Stotts N: Physiology of wound healing and risk factors that impede the healing process, *AACN Clinical Issues in Critical Care Nursing* 1(3):545, 1990.
36. Prentice WE: *Therapeutic modalities in sports medicine and athletic training*, ed 5, St Louis, 2003, McGraw-Hill.
37. Sandrey M: Acute and chronic tendon injuries: factors affecting the healing response and treatment, *Journal Sport Rehabil* 12(1):70, 2003.
38. Sandrey MA: Effects of acute and chronic pathomechanics on the normal histology and biomechanics of tendons: a review. *J Sport Rehabil* 9(4):339, 2000.
39. Seeley R, Stephens T, Tate P: *Anatomy and physiology*, St Louis, 2003, McGraw-Hill.
40. Taylor M: Treating chronic tendon injuries, *Athletic Therapy Today* 5(6):50, 2000.
41. Thompson L: Skeletal muscle adaptations with age, inactivity, and therapeutic exercise. *J Orthop Sports Phys Ther* 32(2), 2002.
42. Wahl S, Renstrom P: Fibrosis in soft-tissue injuries. In Leadbetter W, Buckwalter J, Gordon S, editors: *Sports-induced inflammation*, Park Ridge, Ill, 1990, American Academy of Orthopaedic Surgeons.
43. Walker JM: Pathomechanics and classification of cartilage lesions, facilitation of repair, *J Orthop Sport Phys Ther* 28(4):216, 1998.
44. Warren G, Ingalls C, Lowe D: What mechanisms contribute to the strength loss that occurs during and in the recovery from skeletal muscle injury?, *J Orthop Sports Phys Ther* 32(2), 2002.
45. Whiteside JA, Fleagle SB, Kalenck A: Fractures and refractures in intercollegiate athletes: An eleven-year experience, *Am J Sports Med* 9(6):369, 1981.
46. Woo SLY, Buckwalter J, editors: *Injury and repair of musculoskeletal soft tissues*, Park Ridge, Ill, 1988, American Academy of Orthopaedic Surgeons.

ANNOTATED BIBLIOGRAPHY

Damjanov I, editor: *Anderson's pathology*, ed 10, Philadelphia, 1996, Elsevier Science.

This major pathology text discusses inflammation and healing in depth.

Kloth LE, McCulloch JM: *Wound healing: alternatives in management*, Philadelphia, 2001, Davis.

This book offers an excellent discussion of factors influencing wound healing, evaluation, and methods of treatment.

Melzack R, Wall P: *Handbook of pain*, Philadelphia, 2003, Elsevier.

This book provides a summary of current knowledge of pain states and their management for all health care professionals involved in the diagnosis and treatment of patients with a wide variety of acute and chronic pain problems.

Porth CM: *Pathophysiology*, ed 4, Philadelphia, 2003, Lippincott, Williams, and Wilkins.

This in-depth text on the physiology of altered health contains an excellent discussion on inflammation, healing, and pain.

Psychosocial Intervention for Sports Injuries and Illnesses

Chapter 11

When you finish this chapter you should be able to

- Analyze the athlete's psychological response to injury.
- Recognize the importance of social support for the injured athlete.
- Explain the relationship of stress and overtraining to the risk of injury.
- Describe the role of the athletic trainer as a counselor to the injured athlete.
- Identify the psychological factors important to rehabilitating the injured athlete.
- Compare and contrast the mental training techniques that are used to manage the psychological aspects of injury.
- Recognize the different mental disorders and the appropriate referral and treatment techniques.

Certainly, the injured or ill athlete experiences physical disability. But for many athletes, the psychological and sociological consequences of injury can be as debilitating as the physical injuries.[32] These psychological and sociological reactions combined with the physical injury itself can have an adverse impact on the athlete's successful return to competition. The sports medicine team and the coach must understand how the psyche, especially feelings and emotions, enters into an athlete's reactions to serious injury or illness and ultimately how it affects the rehabilitation process (Figure 11-1).[31]

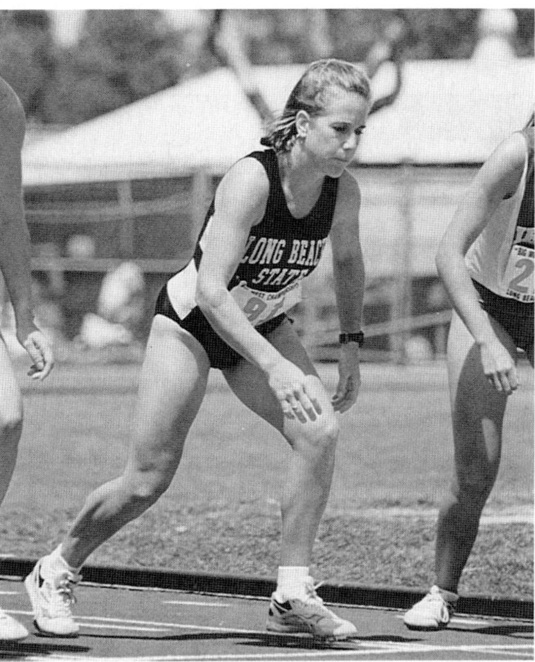

Figure 11-1

Sports participation can cause the athlete to experience either negative or positive stress.

Athletes, no matter what sport they participate in, react to serious injury and illness in a very personal way.[3] Each athlete makes unique adaptations to these challenges. Some athletes view an injury or illness as devastating; others take such a setback in stride.[14] Some athletes have problems with emotional control after sustaining a serious injury or illness. The athletic trainer must be aware that returning an athlete to full, all-out competition requires the athlete to be completely ready psychologically as well as physically. Success in sports performance requires fundamental skills such as speed, attention, concentration, stress management, and the ability to perform cognitive strategies.

Some athletes have a tendency to sustain injuries, whereas others under similar circumstances can stay injury free.[1] Countless physical and psychosocial factors can interact to predispose an athlete to injury as well as influence the effectiveness of the rehabilitation process.[1] No one personality type can be associated with accident-proneness. However, athletes who are risk takers seem to be more prone to injury. These athletes have a higher competition anxiety, demonstrate sensation-seeking behaviors, and have a high motivation for success, but they lack the appropriate coping skills to address these stressors.[1]

THE ATHLETE'S PSYCHOLOGICAL RESPONSE TO INJURY

Athletes don't all deal with injury in the same manner.[3,31] One athlete may view an injury as disastrous; another may view it as an opportunity to show courage; and a third may embrace the injury to avoid embarrassment over poor performance, to provide an escape from a losing team, or to discourage a domineering parent.[14]

Reactive phases

- Reaction to injury
- Reaction to rehabilitation
- Reaction to return

Injury might mean major changes in the way an athlete behaves socially.

Some factors are common among athletes who are adjusting to injury and rehabilitation. The severity of the injury usually determines the length of rehabilitation.[14] Generally, injuries may be classified as short-term (less than four weeks), long-term (more than four weeks), chronic (recurring), or terminating (career-ending). Regardless of the severity of the injury and the corresponding length of time required for rehabilitation, the injured athlete has to deal with a variety of emotions that may occur during three reactive phases of the injury and rehabilitation process (Figure 11-2). These reactive phases are: reaction to injury, reaction to rehabilitation, and reaction to return to competition or career termination.[14] Not all athletes have all of these reactions, nor do all reactions fall precisely into the suggested sequence. Some psychologists have applied five stages of psychological reaction to injury based on Kübler-Ross's classic model of reactions to death and dying, which includes *denial, anger, bargaining,*

Figure 11-2

Progressive reactions of athletes based on severity of injury and length of rehabilitation.

Length of rehabilitation	Reaction to injury	Reaction to rehabilitation	Reaction to return
Short (<4 weeks)	Shock Relief	Impatience Optimism	Eagerness Anticipation
Long (>4 weeks)	Fear Anger	Loss of vigor Irrational thoughts Alienation	Acknowledgment
Chronic (recurring)	Anger Frustration	Dependence or independence Apprehension	Confident or skeptical
Termination (career-ending)	Isolation Grief process	Loss of athletic identity	Closure and renewal

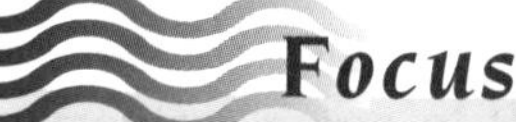

Psychological barriers to rehabilitation

- Depression or grief
- Anxiety
- Anger, agitation, or aggression
- Denial
- Sleep disturbance
- Psychosocial isolation
- Substance abuse

From NATA brochure, *Psychological hints for rehabilitation success,* Dallas, TX

depression, and *acceptance* (Figure 11-3). Other factors that can influence reactions to injury and rehabilitation are the athletes' coping skills, past history of injury, social support, and personality traits.[20]

With any type of injury, but particularly with those that require a lengthy period of rehabilitation, athletes whose whole life tends to revolve around a sport may have to make major adjustments in how they perceive themselves and may have to come to terms with how they are perceived by others.[35] Therefore, many athletes have difficulty controlling their emotions when they sustain an injury (see *Focus Box:* "Psychological barriers to rehabilitation").

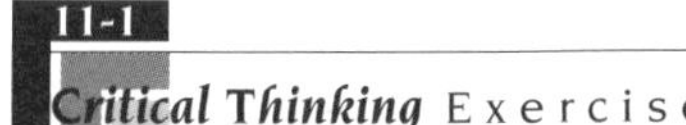

11-1 **Critical Thinking** Exercise

A world-class sprinter tears her left hamstring muscle, which eliminates her from the Olympic trials.

? What could be the psychological ramifications for this athlete?

THE ATHLETE AND THE SOCIOLOGICAL RESPONSE TO INJURY

Following injury, particularly one that requires long-term rehabilitation, athletes may have problems adjusting socially and may feel alienated from the rest of the team.[19] Athletes with an injury that requires weeks or months of rehabilitation before they can return to competition often feel that the coaches have ceased to care, that teammates have no time to spend with them, that friends are no longer around, and that their social life consists of time put into rehabilitation. Occasionally athletes feel that they have received little support from coaches and teammates.[14]

Injured athletes may understand that the coach cares but has no expertise in injury management and must be concerned with getting the team ready without them. The athletic trainer has no expertise in coaching but is primarily interested in rehabilitating injuries. Injured athletes may feel unable to maintain or regain normal relationships with teammates. The injured athlete is a reminder that injury can happen, and teammates may pull away from that constant reminder. Friendships based on athletic identification are now compromised because the athletic identification is gone; friends and team members may relate to injured athletes only in terms of what they did yesterday

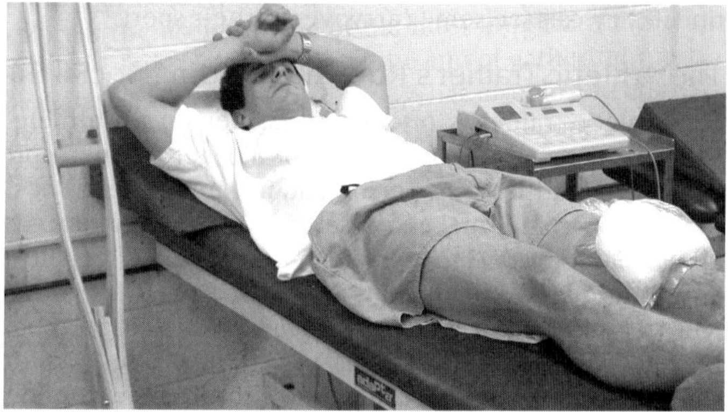

Figure 11-3

A sports injury can create in the athlete psychological reactions characteristic of a sudden loss.

Focus

Sample emergency action plan

Emergency action plan for women's ice hockey

Emergency Personnel:
Certified athletic trainer and student athletic trainer(s) on site for practice and competition; additional sports medicine staff accessible from main athletic training facility (across street from arena)

Emergency Communication:
Fixed telephone line in ice hockey satellite athletic training room (_____-_________)

Emergency Equipment:
Supplies (AED, trauma kit, splint kit, spine board) maintained in ice hockey satellite athletic training room; additional emergency equipment accessible from athletic training facility across street from arena (_____-______)

Roles of First Responders:
Immediate care of the injured or ill student athlete
Emergency equipment retrieval

Activation of emergency medical system (EMS)
911 call (provide name, address, telephone number; number of individuals injured; condition of injured; first aid treatment; specific directions; other information as requested)
Direct EMS to scene
Open appropriate doors
Designate individual to "flag down" EMS and direct to scene
Scene control: Limit scene to first aid providers and move bystanders away from area

Venue Directions:
Ice hockey arena is located on corner of ____________________ Street and ____________________ Street adjacent to ____________________. Two gates provide access to the arena: ____________________ Street: drive leads to arena as well as rear door of complex (locker room, athletic training room)

Sports Medicine Staff and Phone Numbers:

ATC in Charge	929-0000
Head ATC	929-0001
Team Physician	929-0002

From *NCAA Sports Medicine Handbook 2000–2001*.

b. Decide what emergency equipment should be available for each sport. The emergency equipment needs for football will likely be different from those of the cross-country team.

2. Establish specific procedures and policies regarding the removal of protective equipment, particularly the helmet and shoulder pads. These procedures will be discussed later in this chapter.[25,34]
3. Make sure phones are readily accessible. Cellular or digital phones are best because the athletic trainer can carry one at all times. However, a land line should also be readily available in case cell phone service is not available. If cellular phones are not available, the athletic training students, coaches, and athletes should know the location of the telephone; phones should be clearly marked. Use 911 if available, but realize that in some areas all service is not accessible by cellular phones and thus land lines should be used to access the emergency medical system.

4. The athletic trainer should be familiar with the community-based emergency health care delivery plan, including existing communication and transportation policies. It is also critical for the athletic trainer to be familiar with emergency care facility admission and treatment policies, particularly when rendering emergency care to a minor. The athletic trainer should specifically designate someone to make an emergency phone call. Most emergency medical systems can be accessed by dialing 911, which connects the caller to a dispatcher who has access to rescue squad, police, and fire personnel. The person making the emergency phone call must provide the following information:
   a. Type of emergency situation
   b. Type of suspected injury
   c. Present condition of the athlete
   d. Current assistance being given (e.g., cardiopulmonary resuscitation)
   e. Location of telephone being used
   f. Exact location of emergency (give names of streets and cross streets) and how to enter facility
5. Make sure keys to gates or padlocks are easily accessible. Both the athletic trainer and the coach should have the appropriate key.
6. Inform all coaches, athletic directors, school nurses, and maintenance personnel of the emergency plan at a meeting held annually before the beginning of the school year. Each individual must know his or her responsibilities should an emergency occur.
7. Assign someone to accompany the injured athlete to the hospital.
8. Carry contact information for all athletes, coaches, and other personnel at all times, particularly when traveling (see Figure 3-1). For minors, consent forms should also be available when traveling.
9. In certain situations at both high schools and colleges, the athletic trainer may be called upon to provide emergency services not only to athletes but also to coaches, referees, and in some cases parents and other spectators who may develop an emergent condition during the course of an athletic event. The emergency action plan should include plans for managing these situations with the help of emergency medical services and other local health care providers.

In 2002, the NATA released a position statement relative to an emergency action plan.[4] The objective was to provide guidelines for athletic trainers in the development of emergency plans and to advocate documentation of emerging planning. A summary of this position appears in Appendix F.

Cooperation between Emergency Care Providers

Emergency practice sessions for athletic trainers and EMTs should be held at least once a year.

Individuals providing emergency care to injured athletes must cooperate and act professionally. The athletic trainer should make every effort to nurture the relationship with the emergency medical technicians (EMTs) and, if possible, incorporate them into the development and implementation of the emergency action plan. Occasionally, disagreement arises between rescue squad personnel, the physician, and the athletic trainer over exactly how the injured athlete should be handled and transported. The athletic trainer is usually the first to deal with the emergency situation. The athletic trainer has generally had more training and experience in moving and transporting an injured athlete than the physician has. If an athletic trainer or physician is not available, the coach should not hesitate to call 911 to let the rescue squad handle an emergency situation. If the rescue squad is called and responds, the EMTs should have the final say on how that athlete is to be transported while the athletic trainer assumes an assistive role.

To alleviate potential conflicts, the athletic trainer should establish procedures and guidelines and should arrange practice sessions at least once a year that include everyone responsible for handling an injured athlete.[10] Rescue squad personnel may not be experienced in dealing with someone who is wearing a helmet or other protective

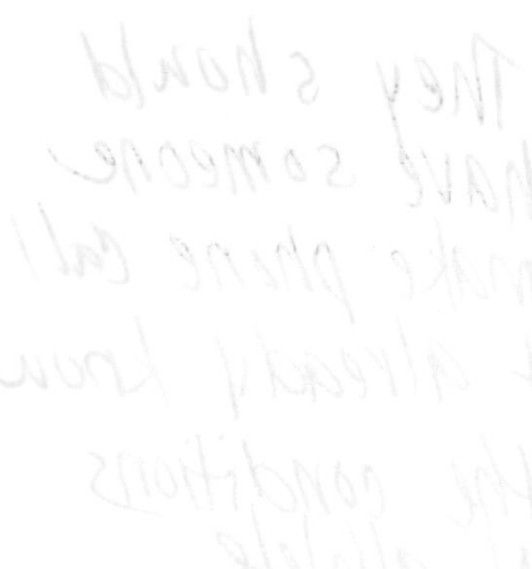

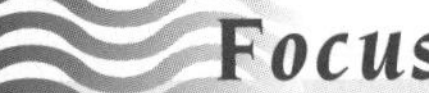

Focus

Consent form for medical treatment of a minor

By this signature, I hereby consent to allow the physician(s) and other health care provider(s) selected by myself or the school to perform a preparticipation examination on my child and to provide treatment for any injury or condition resulting from participating in athletics and activities for his or her school during the school year covered by this form. I further consent to allow said physician(s) or health care provider(s) to share appropriate information concerning my child that is relevant to participation in athletics and activities with coaches and other school personnel as deemed necessary.

________________________ __________
Parent or Guardian Date

equipment. The athletic trainer should make sure before an incident occurs that the EMTs understand the correct management of athletes wearing various types of athletic equipment.

Parent Notification

If the injured athlete is a minor, the athletic trainer should try to obtain consent from the parent to treat the athlete during an emergency.[32] *Focus Box:* "Consent form for medical treatment of a minor" provides an example of a consent form that may be signed by the parents or guardians of a minor. Consent may be given in writing either before or during an emergency. This consent is notification that the parent has been informed about what the athletic trainer thinks is wrong and what the athletic trainer intends to do, and parental permission is granted to give treatment for a specific incident. If the athlete's parents cannot be contacted, the predetermined wishes of the parent given at the beginning of a season or school year can be enacted. The athletic trainer should have these consent forms available when traveling in case the need for medical care arises. If no informed consent exists, implied consent on the part of the athlete to save the athlete's life takes precedence.

PRINCIPLES OF ON-THE-FIELD INJURY ASSESSMENT

The athletic trainer cannot deliver appropriate acute medical care to the injured athlete until some systematic assessment of the situation has been made on the playing field or court where the injury occurs.[52] This *on-the-field assessment* helps determine the nature of the injury and provides direction in the decision-making process concerning the emergency care that must be rendered (Figure 12-1).[7] The on-the-field assessment may be subdivided into a primary survey and a secondary survey.

primary survey assesses life-threatening injuries.

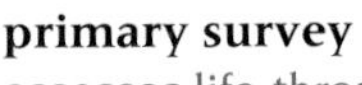

The **primary survey,** which is done initially, determines the existence of potentially life-threatening situations, including problems with airway, breathing, circulation, severe bleeding, and shock. The primary survey takes precedence over all other aspects of victim assessment and should be used to correct life-threatening situations.[36] Any athlete who has a life-threatening situation should be transported to an emergency care facility as soon as possible.

secondary survey performed after life-threatening injuries have been ruled out.

Once the primary survey has ruled out the existence of a life-threatening injury or illness, the **secondary survey** takes a closer look at the athlete's injury. The secondary survey gathers specific information about the injury from the athlete, systematically assesses vital signs and symptoms, and allows for a more detailed evaluation of the injury. The secondary survey is done to uncover problems that do not pose an immediate threat to life but that may do so if they remain uncorrected.[36]

An injured athlete who is conscious and stable will not require a primary survey. However, the unconscious athlete must be monitored for life-threatening problems throughout the assessment process.

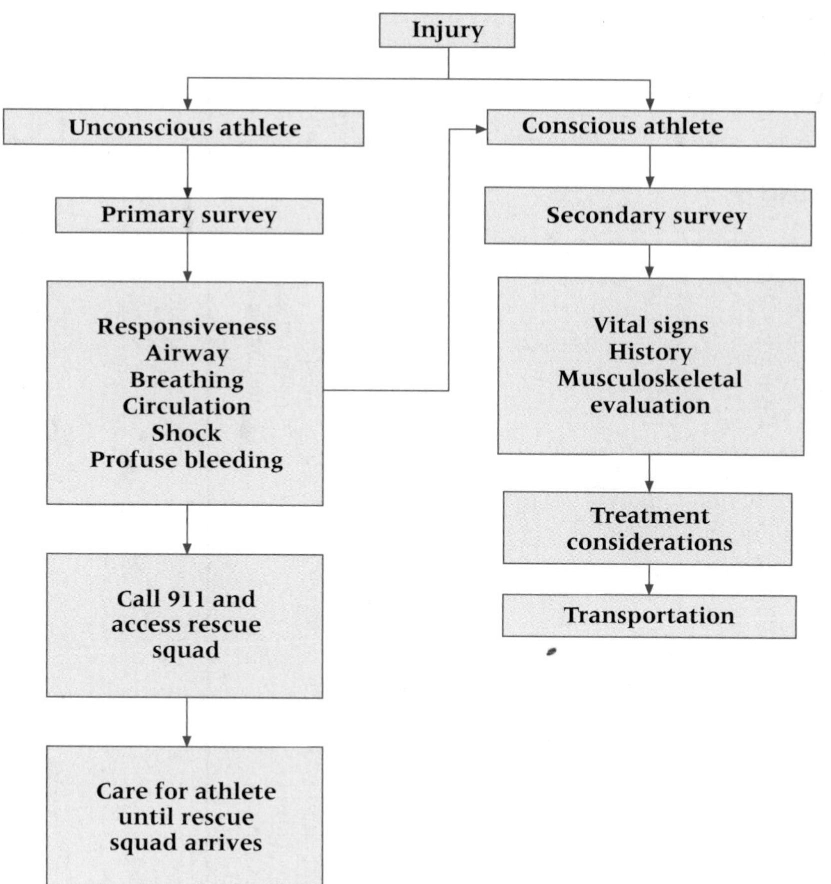

Figure 12-1

Flowchart showing the appropriate emergency procedures for the injured athlete.

THE PRIMARY SURVEY

Treatment of Life-Threatening Injuries

Life-threatening injuries take precedence over all other injuries sustained by the athlete. Situations that are considered life-threatening include those that require cardiopulmonary resuscitation (i.e., obstruction of the airway, no breathing, no circulation), profuse bleeding, and shock.

Life-threatening conditions
- Airway obstruction
- No breathing
- No circulation
- Profuse bleeding
- Shock

Dealing with the Unconscious Athlete

The state of unconsciousness provides one of the greatest dilemmas for the athletic trainer. Whether to move the athlete and allow the game to resume or to await the arrival of a physician is a decision that too often is resolved hastily and without much forethought. Unconsciousness may be defined as a state of insensibility in which the athlete exhibits a lack of conscious awareness. This condition can be brought about by a blow to either the head or the solar plexus, it may result from general shock, or it may result from fainting (syncope) due to inadequate blood flow to the brain. It is often difficult to determine the exact cause of unconsciousness (Table 12-1).

The unconscious athlete always must be considered to have a life-threatening injury, which requires an immediate primary survey. The following guidelines should be used when working with the unconscious athlete:

1. The athletic trainer should immediately note the body position and determine the level of consciousness and unresponsiveness.
2. Airway, breathing, and circulation should be established immediately.
3. Injury to the neck and spine should always be considered a possibility in the unconscious athlete.[14]

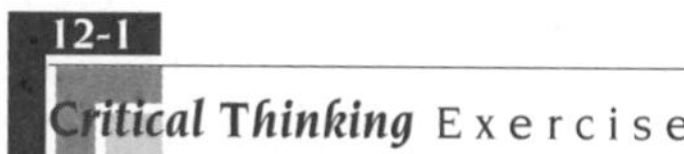

A football defensive back is making a tackle and drops his head on contact with the ball-carrier. He hits the ground and does not move. When the athletic trainer gets to him, the athlete is lying prone, is unconscious, but is breathing.

? How should the athletic trainer manage this situation?

TABLE 12-1 Evaluating the Unconscious Athlete

	Selected Conditions						
Functional Signs	**Fainting**	**Concussion**	**Grand Mal Epilepsy**	**Brain Compression and Injury**	**Heatstroke**	**Diabetic Coma**	**Shock**
Onset	Usually sudden	Usually sudden	Sudden	Usually gradual	Gradual or sudden	Gradual	Gradual
Mentality	Complete unconsciousness	Confusion or unconsciousness	Unconsciousness	Unconsciousness, gradually deepening	Delirium or unconsciousness	Drowsiness, later unconsciousness	Listlessness, later unconsciousness
Pulse	Fast and feeble	Feeble and irregular	Fast	Gradually slower	Fast and feeble	Fast and feeble	Fast and feeble
Respiration	Quick and shallow	Shallow and irregular	Noisy, later deep and slow	Slow and noisy	Difficult	Deep and sighing	Rapid and shallow, with occasional deep sigh
Skin	Pale, cold, and clammy	Pale and cold	Livid, later pale	Hot and flushed	Hot and relatively dry	Livid, later pale	Pale, cold, and clammy
Pupils	Equal and dilated	Equal	Equal and dilated	Unequal	Equal	Equal	Equal and dilated
Paralysis	None	None	None	May be present in leg, arm, or both	None	None	None
Convulsions	None	None	None	Present in some cases	Present in some cases	None	None
Breath	N/A	N/A	N/A	N/A	N/A	Acetone smell	N/A
Special features	Giddiness and sway before collapse	Signs of head injury, vomiting during recovery	Bites tongue, voids urine and feces, may injure self while falling	Signs of head injury, delayed onset of symptoms	Vomiting in some cases	In early stages, headache, restlessness, and nausea	May vomit; early stages shivering, thirst, defective vision, and ear noises

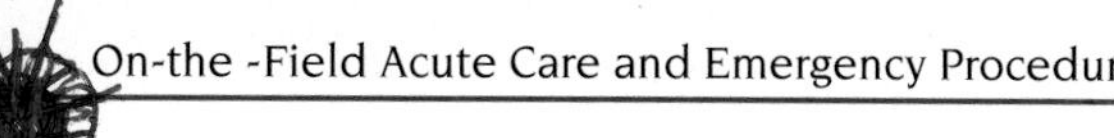

4. If the athlete is wearing a helmet, it should never be removed until neck and spine injury have been unequivocally ruled out. However, the face mask must be cut away and removed to allow for cardiopulmonary resuscitation (CPR).
5. If the athlete is supine and not breathing, airway, breathing, and circulation (ABC) should be established immediately.
6. If the athlete is supine and breathing, nothing should be done until he or she regains consciousness.
7. If the athlete is prone and not breathing, he or she should be logrolled carefully to the supine position and ABC should be established immediately.
8. If the athlete is prone and breathing, nothing should be done until he or she regains consciousness, then the athlete should be carefully logrolled onto a spine board because CPR could be necessary at any time.
9. Life support for the unconscious athlete should be monitored and maintained until emergency medical personnel arrive.
10. Once the athlete is stabilized, the athletic trainer should begin a secondary survey.

Overview of Emergency Cardiopulmonary Resuscitation

A careful evaluation of the injured person must be made to determine whether CPR should be conducted. This overview of adult CPR is not intended to be used by persons who are not certified in CPR. Because of the serious nature of CPR, individuals should routinely be recertified through the American Red Cross, the American Heart Association, or the National Safety Council.

The athletic trainer should follow the emergency action steps: *check-call-care.*[2] *Check* the scene to find out what happened and to identify other individuals who might help and then check the victim for consciousness. *Call* 911 to access the rescue squad and then initiate *care* for the victim.

Equipment Considerations

Protective equipment worn by an athlete may complicate lifesaving CPR procedures. The presence of a football, ice hockey, or lacrosse helmet as well as a face mask and various types of shoulder pads will obviously make CPR more difficult if not impossible. Over the years, significant debate has raged in the sports medicine community about removing the helmet of an athlete with suspected cervical spine injury, and a number of differing opinions have been expressed.[16,20,26,27,29,34,35,37,38,39,41,42,45,47,48,51]

It has been proposed that removing the face mask should be the first step.[42] The face mask does not hinder the evaluation of the airway, but it may hinder treatment.[12] Thus the face mask should be removed immediately when a decision is made to transport the athlete to a medical care facility, regardless of the current respiratory status. It is also recommended that the face mask be removed completely by cutting all of the loop straps rather than simply cutting the bottom two loop-straps and retracting the helmet guard. Various instruments have been recommended to remove the face mask, including wire cutters, bolt cutters, trainer's scissors, and scalpels, none of which work very well. Thus using any of these tools as a primary means of removing a face mask is not recommended. Using an electric screwdriver has been shown to be faster and produce less torque on the helmet than tools that cut through the loop straps[25] as long as the screws are not rusted. Three devices—the Anvil Pruner, the Trainer's Angel, and the FM Extractor—have been recommended for their effectiveness in quickly cutting the plastic clips (Figure 12-2).[37,53] It also has been suggested that the athletic trainer should be proficient in removing the face mask within thirty seconds.[37] Studies comparing the efficacy of using these various devices suggest that the Anvil Pruner seems to be easier to use than the Trainer's Angel.[29] Other studies have shown that the Anvil Pruner and the FM Extractor were faster in removing the face mask than the Trainer's Angel.[54] Furthermore, using a Trainer's Angel seems to cause more motion in the cervical spine than either a manual or powered screwdriver.[47]

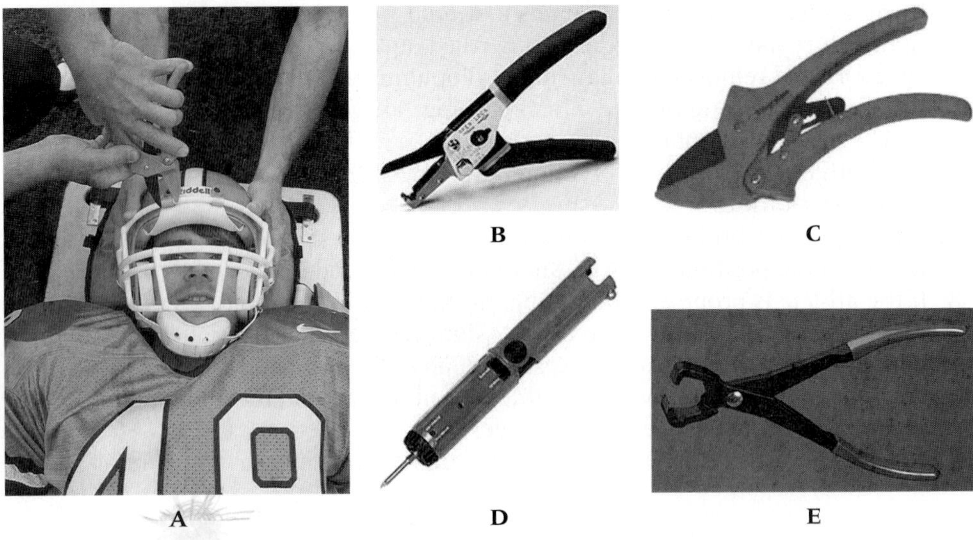

Figure 12-2

A, A number of different tools can be used to cut or remove the plastic grommets that hold the face mask. **B,** FM Extractor. **C,** Anvil Pruner. **D,** Electric cordless screwdriver. **E,** Trainers Angel.

In 1992 the Occupational Safety and Health Administration (OSHA) mandated the use of a barrier device or pocket mask to protect the athletic trainer from the transmission of bloodborne pathogens during CPR (Figure 12-7B, page 329). It is possible to slip the pocket mask under the face mask, attach the one-way mouthpiece or valve through the bars of the face mask, and begin CPR within five to ten seconds without removing the face mask.[45] Also, the use of a pocket mask appears to cause less extraneous motion in the cervical spine than does the use of either screwdrivers or the Trainer's Angel to remove the face mask.[47] It also has been shown that using a pocket mask is quicker for initiating rescue breathing than rotation of the face mask using screwdriver removal.[46]

As mentioned earlier, controversy has existed for some time as to whether the helmet and shoulder pads should be left in place or removed.[38] The current recommendation is to leave the helmet and shoulder pads in place.[34,35,56] The football helmet and chin strap should only be removed if: 1) the helmet and chin strap do not hold the head securely and immobilizing the helmet does not immobilize the head; 2) the design of the helmet and chin strap is such that, even after removal of the face mask, the airway cannot be controlled or ventilation provided; 3) the face mask cannot be removed after a reasonable period of time; or 4) the helmet prevents the athlete from being immobilized appropriately for transportation.[19] If the helmet must be removed, spinal immobilization must be maintained during removal. In most circumstances, it may be helpful to remove cheek padding and/or deflate air padding prior to removing the helmet. (See Appendix G for the NATA position statement.)

The athletic trainer must either remove both the helmet and shoulder pads or leave them both in place. Removing one or the other independently will force the cervical spine into either flexion or extension. If they are left in place, the face mask should be dealt with as recommended previously, and the jersey and shoulder pad strings or straps should be cut, spreading the shoulder pads apart so that the chest may be compressed according to CPR guidelines. Although removal of the helmet and shoulder pads has been recommended by some individuals,[13] it seems that no matter how much care is taken, removal would create unnecessary movement of the cervical spine and would delay the initiation of CPR, neither of which is best for the injured athlete.[30] If cervical neck injury is suspected, yet the athlete is conscious and breathing and does not require CPR, the athlete should be transported with the helmet, chin strap, and shoulder pads in place. The face mask should be removed in case CPR becomes necessary.

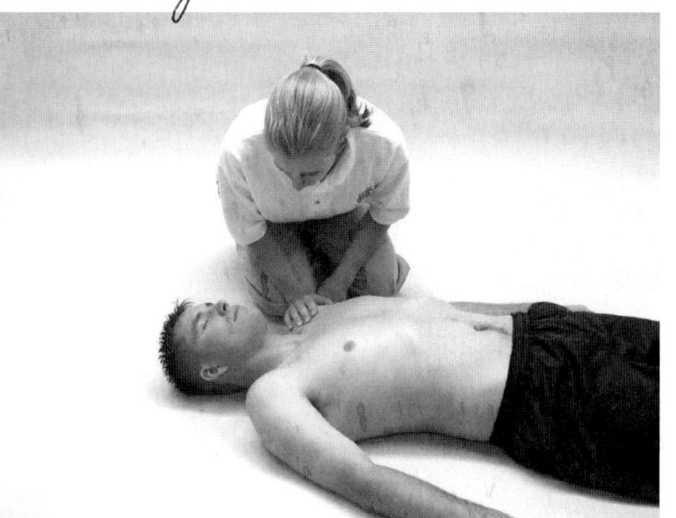

Figure 12-3

Establish unresponsiveness by gently shaking the victim and asking, "Are you okay?"

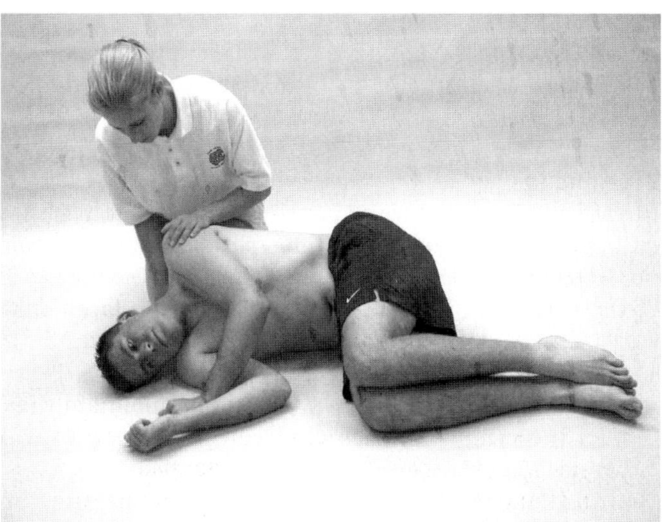

Figure 12-4

Victims who are breathing should be placed on their side in the recovery position.

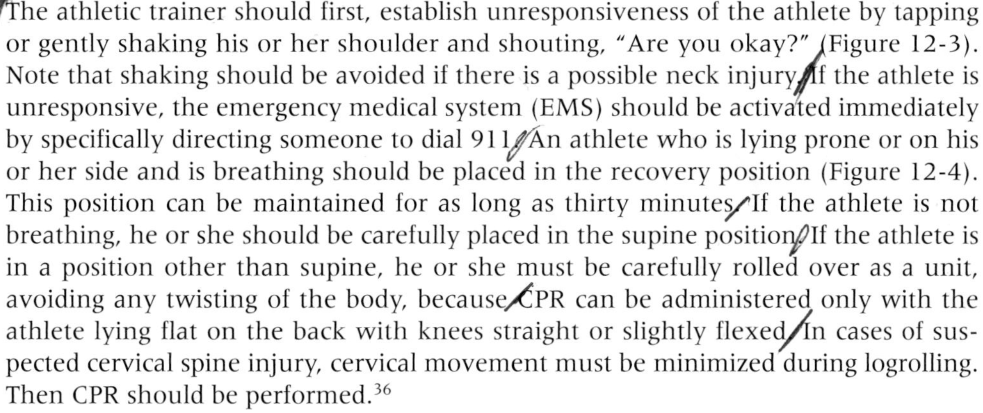

Establishing Unresponsiveness

The athletic trainer should first, establish unresponsiveness of the athlete by tapping or gently shaking his or her shoulder and shouting, "Are you okay?" (Figure 12-3). Note that shaking should be avoided if there is a possible neck injury. If the athlete is unresponsive, the emergency medical system (EMS) should be activated immediately by specifically directing someone to dial 911. An athlete who is lying prone or on his or her side and is breathing should be placed in the recovery position (Figure 12-4). This position can be maintained for as long as thirty minutes. If the athlete is not breathing, he or she should be carefully placed in the supine position. If the athlete is in a position other than supine, he or she must be carefully rolled over as a unit, avoiding any twisting of the body, because CPR can be administered only with the athlete lying flat on the back with knees straight or slightly flexed. In cases of suspected cervical spine injury, cervical movement must be minimized during logrolling. Then CPR should be performed.[36]

Opening the airway

Open the airway by using the head tilt–chin lift method (Figure 12-5A).[59] Lift under the chin with one hand while pushing down on the victim's forehead with the other,

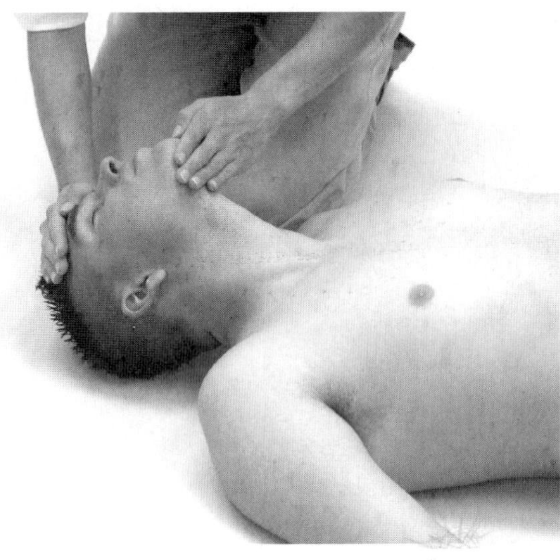

A

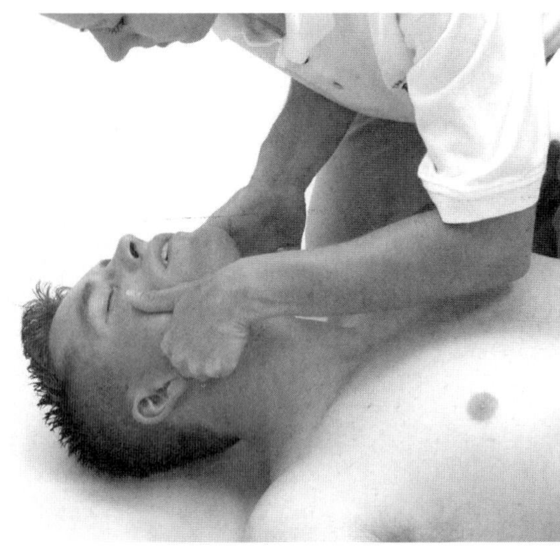

B

Figure 12-5

A, Head tilt–chin lift technique for establishing an airway.
B, Jaw thrust technique.

avoiding the use of excessive force. The tongue is the most common cause of airway obstruction; the forward lift of the jaw raises the tongue away from the back of the throat, thus clearing the airway.

NOTE: On victims with suspected head or neck injuries, perform a modified jaw thrust maneuver by grasping each side of the lower jaw at the angles, thus displacing the lower mandible forward as the head is tilted backward (Figure 12-5B).[59] In executing this maneuver, both elbows should rest on the same surface the victim is lying on. If the victim's lips close, open them by retracting the lower lip with a thumb. If the victim is not breathing, additional forward displacement of the jaw may help.

Establishing breathing

1. To determine if the victim is breathing, maintain the open airway; place your ear over the victim's mouth; observe the chest; and look, listen, and feel for breath sounds (Figure 12-6).
2. Using the hand on the athlete's forehead, pinch the nose shut, keeping the heel of the hand in place to hold the head back (if there is no neck injury). Take a deep breath, place your mouth over the athlete's mouth to provide an airtight seal, and give two slow, full breaths at a rate of 1½ to 2 seconds per inflation. Observe the chest rise and fall. Remove your mouth, and listen for the air to escape through passive exhalation. If the airway is obstructed, reposition the victim's head and try again to ventilate. If the airway is still obstructed, give fifteen chest compressions followed by a finger sweep with the index finger to clear visible objects from the mouth.[17] Be careful not to push the object further into the throat. Continue to repeat this sequence until ventilation occurs.

If available, use a bag/valve mask for artificial respiration. Although the bag/valve mask is easy to use, some instruction and practice in its use is recommended (Figure 12-7A). NOTE: OSHA has mandated the use of barrier shields by athletic trainers to minimize the risk of transmitting bloodborne pathogens (Figure 12-7B). These shields have a plastic or silicone sheet that spreads over the face and separates the athletic trainer from the athlete. Some models have a tubelike mouthpiece, which may help in situations in which the athlete is wearing a face mask.

Establishing circulation

1. To determine whether a pulse exists, locate the Adam's apple with the index and middle fingers of the hand closest to the victim's head. Then slide your fingers down into the groove on the side of the body on which you are kneeling to locate

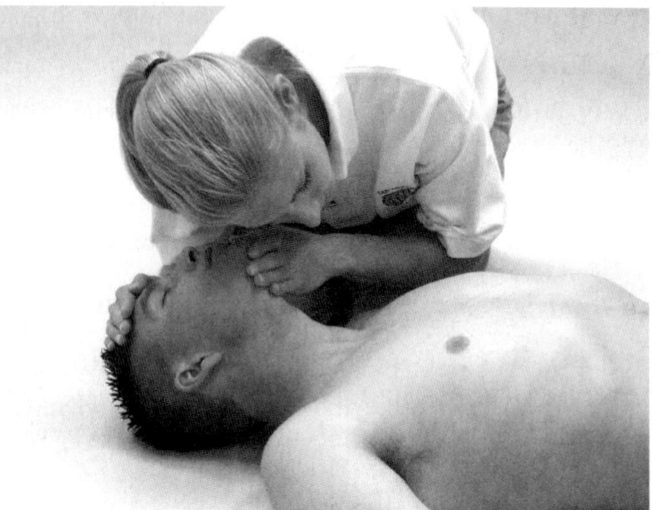
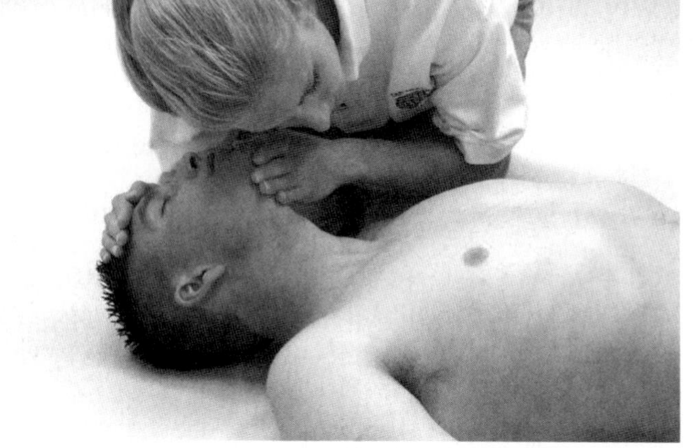

Figure 12-6

Once the airway is established look, listen, and feel for breathing.

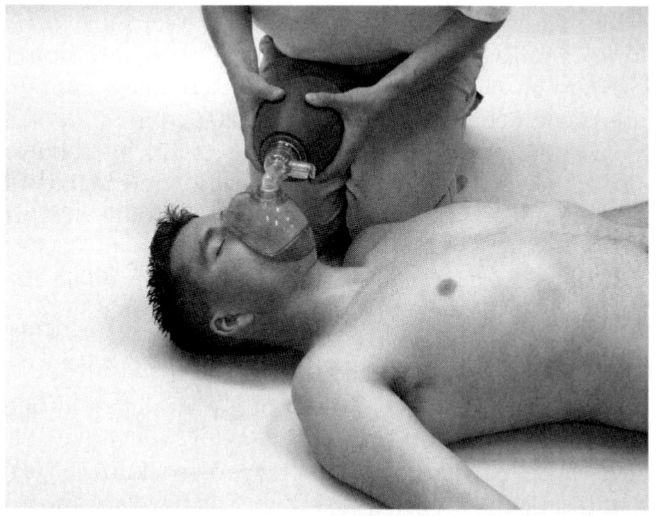

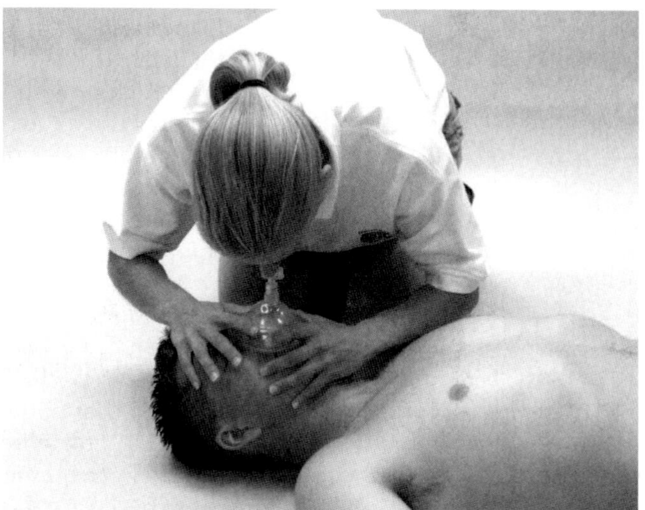

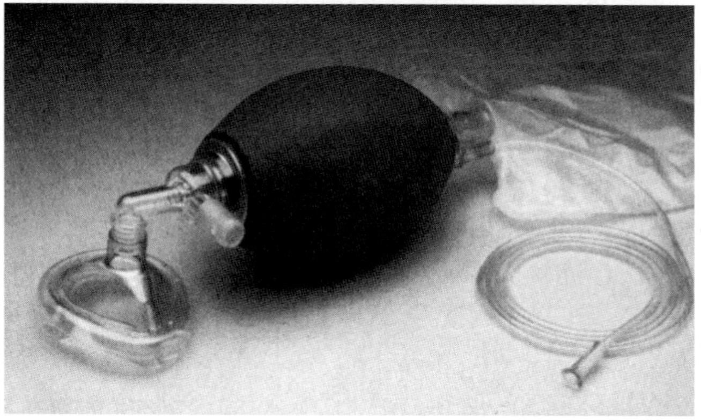

A

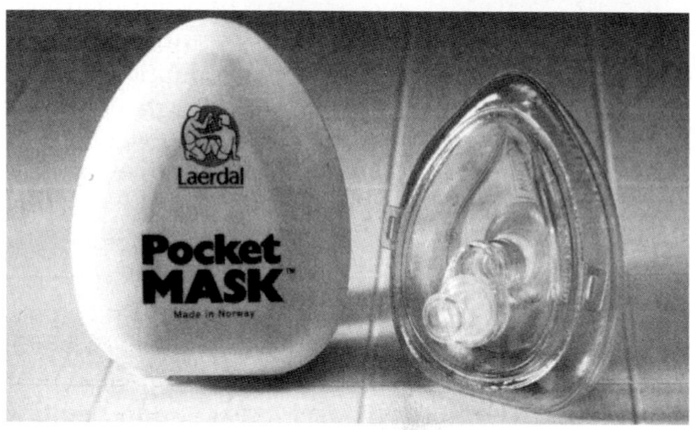

B

Figure 12-7

A, A bag/valve mask can be used for respiration. **B,** A barrier mask protects the athletic trainer from potential exposure to bloodborne pathogens.

the carotid artery. Palpate the carotid pulse with one hand for five to ten seconds while maintaining head tilt with the other hand (Figure 12-8).

2. Maintain an open airway. Position yourself close to the side of the athlete's chest. With the middle and index fingers of the hand closest to the victim's waist, locate the lower margin of his or her rib cage on the side next to you (Figure 12-9).
3. Run the fingers up along the rib cage to the xiphoid notch, where the ribs meet the sternum.
4. Place the middle finger on the notch and the index finger next to it on the lower end of the sternum.
5. Next, position the hand closest to the athlete's head on the lower half of the sternum next to the index finger of the first hand that located the notch; then place the heel of that hand on the long axis of the sternum.
6. Then remove the first hand from the notch and place it on top of the hand on the sternum so that the heels of both hands are parallel and the fingers are directed straight away from you (Figure 12-10).
7. Fingers can be extended or interlaced, but they must be kept off the chest wall.
8. Keep elbows in a locked position with arms straight and shoulders positioned over the hands, enabling the thrust to be straight down.
9. In a normal-sized adult, apply enough force to depress the sternum 1½ to 2 inches (3.8 to 5 cm). After depression, completely release the sternum to allow the heart to refill. The time of release should equal the time of compression. For one rescuer, compression must be given at the rate of 80 to 100 times per minute, maintaining a rate of fifteen chest compressions to two full breaths.
10. After four cycles of fifteen compressions and two breaths (15:2), or about one minute, recheck the pulse at the carotid artery for five seconds while maintaining the head tilt. If no pulse is found, continue the 15:2 cycle, beginning with chest compressions.

Every coach and athletic trainer should be certified in CPR and should take a refresher examination at least once a year. All assistants should be certified as well.[44]

Obstructed Airway Management

All coaches and athletic trainers must have current CPR certification.

Choking is a possibility in many sports activities; for example, an athlete may choke on a mouth guard, a broken piece of dental work, chewing gum, or even a chaw of tobacco. When such emergencies arise, early recognition and prompt, knowledgeable action are necessary to avert a tragedy. An unconscious athlete can have an obstructed airway when the tongue falls back in the throat, blocking the upper airway. Blood clots resulting from head, facial, or dental injuries may impede normal breathing, as may vomiting. When complete airway obstruction occurs, the individual is unable to speak, cough, or breathe. If the athlete is conscious, there is a tremendous effort made to breathe, the head is forced back, and the face initially is flushed and then becomes cyanotic as oxygen deprivation occurs. If partial airway obstruction is causing the choking, some air passage can be detected, but during a complete obstruction no air movement is discernible.

For the victim who is conscious and has an airway obstruction, the standing abdominal thrust technique should be performed until he or she is relieved. In cases of unconsciousness, fifteen chest compressions are applied, followed by a finger sweep with an attempt at ventilation.[2]

First, if the victim cannot cough, speak, or breathe, have someone call 911. Stand behind and to one side of the athlete. Place both arms around the waist just above the belt line, and permit the athlete's head, arms, and upper trunk to hang forward (Figure 12-11). Grasp one of your fists with the other, placing the thumb side of the grasped fists immediately below the xiphoid process of the sternum and clear of the rib cage. Then sharply and forcefully thrust the fists into the abdomen, inward, and upward, several times. This "hug" pushes up on the diaphragm, compressing the air in the lungs, creating forceful pressure against the blockage, and thus usually causing

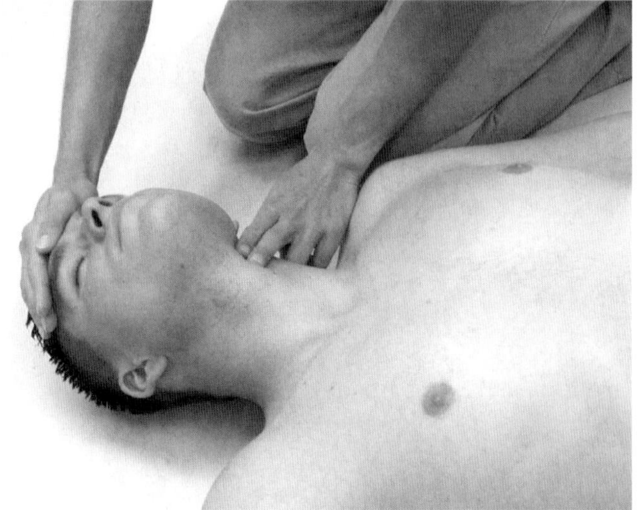

Figure 12-8

To check the carotid pulse locate the Adam's apple and then slide the index and middle fingers into the groove on the side of the body where you are kneeling.

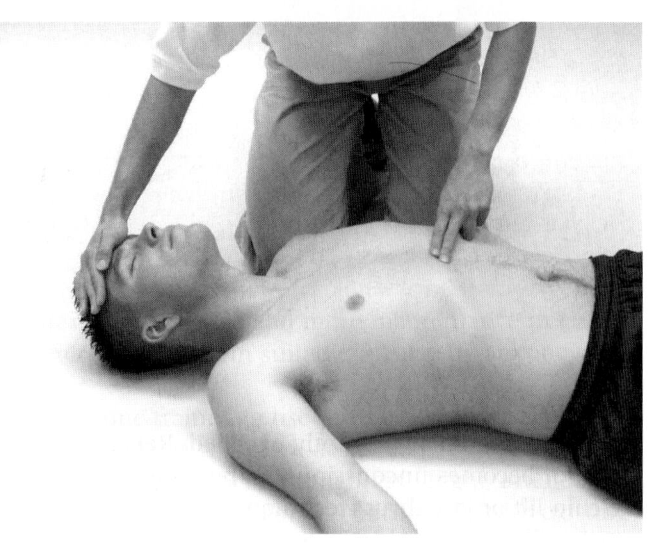

Figure 12-9

With the middle and index fingers of the hand closest to the waist, locate the lower margin of the victim's rib cage. Then run the fingers along the rib cage to the notch where the ribs meet the sternum. Place the middle finger on the notch with the index finger next to it on the lower end of the sternum.

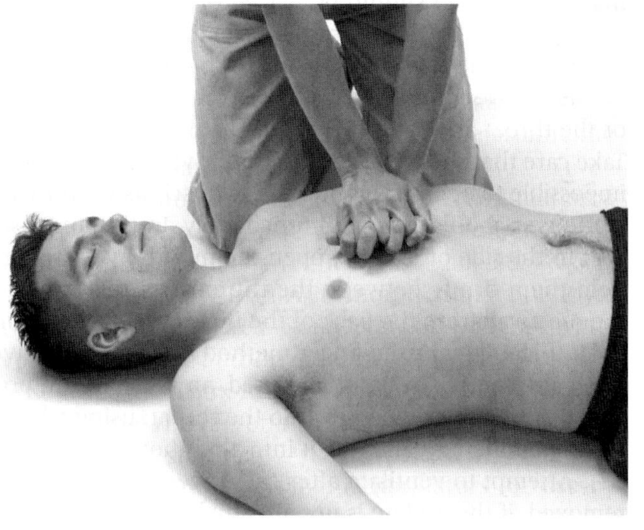

Figure 12-10

Place the heel of the hand closest to the athelete's head on the long axis of the lower half of the sternum next to the index fingers of the first hand. Remove the first hand from the notch and place it on top of the hand on the sternum with fingers extended or interlaced.

To convert Fahrenheit to centigrade (Celsius):
°C = (°F − 32) ÷ 1.8
To convert centigrade to Fahrenheit: °F = (1.8 × °C) + 32

replicating the depth and angle of insertion. Changes in body temperature can be reflected in the skin. For example, hot, dry skin might indicate disease, infection, or overexposure to environmental heat. Cool, clammy skin could reflect trauma, shock, or heat exhaustion; cool, dry skin is possibly the result of overexposure to cold.

A rise or fall of internal temperature may be caused by a variety of circumstances such as the onset of a communicable disease, cold exposure, pain, fear, or nervousness. Characteristically, a lowered body temperature is accompanied by chills with chattering teeth, blue lips, goose bumps, and pale skin.

Skin Color

For individuals who are lightly pigmented, the skin can be a good indicator of the state of health. Normal skin tone is pink. A flushed or red skin color may indicate heatstroke, sunburn, allergic reaction, high blood pressure, or elevated temperature. A pale, ashen, or white skin can mean insufficient circulation, shock, fright, hemorrhage, heat exhaustion, or insulin shock. Skin that is bluish in color (cyanotic), primarily in the lips and fingernails, usually means an airway obstruction or respiratory insufficiency. A yellowish or jaundice color may indicate liver disease or dysfunction.

Assessing skin color in a dark-skinned athlete is more difficult. These individuals normally have pink coloration of the nail beds and inside the lips, mouth, and tongue. When a dark-skinned person goes into shock, the skin around the mouth and nose will often have a grayish cast, and the tongue, the inside of the mouth, the lips, and the nail beds will have a bluish cast. Shock resulting from hemorrhage will cause the tongue and inside of the mouth to become a pale, grayish color instead of blue. Fever in these athletes can be noted by a red flush at the tips of the ears.[24]

Pupils

Some athletes normally have irregular and unequal pupils.

The pupils of the eyes are extremely sensitive to situations affecting the nervous system. Although most persons have pupils of regular outline and equal size, some individuals normally have pupils that may be irregular and unequal. This disparity requires the athletic trainer to know which athletes deviate from the norm.

A constricted pupil may indicate that the athlete is using a central nervous system depressant drug. If one or both pupils are dilated, the athlete may have sustained a head injury; may be experiencing shock, heatstroke, or hemorrhage; or may have ingested a stimulant drug (Figure 12-20). The pupils' response to light also should be noted. If one or both pupils fail to accommodate to light, there may be brain injury or alcohol or drug poisoning. When examining an athlete's pupils, the examiner should note the presence of contact lenses. Pupil response is more critical in evaluation than pupil size.

Level of Consciousness

When recognizing vital signs, the examiner must always note the athlete's level of consciousness. Normally the athlete is alert, is aware of the environment, and responds quickly to vocal stimulation. Head injury, heatstroke, and diabetic coma can alter the athlete's level of conscious awareness.

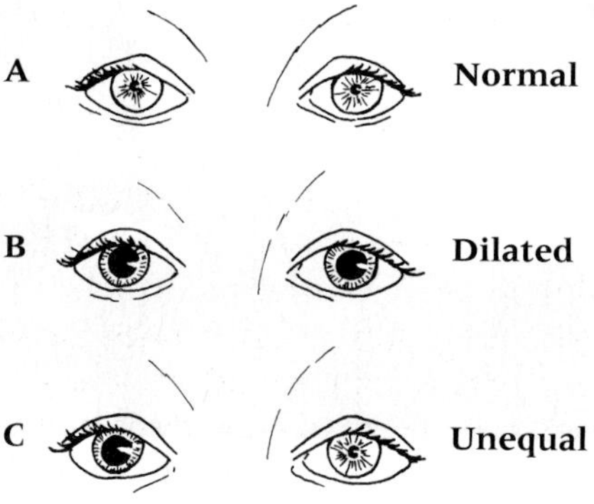

Figure 12-20

The pupils of the eyes are extremely sensitive to situations affecting the nervous system. **A,** Normal pupils. **B,** Dilated pupils. **C,** Unequal pupils.

The level of consciousness can be assessed by using several different scales: the AVPU scale, the ACDU scale, or the Glasgow Coma Scale. (See Chapter 27 for a discussion of Glasgow Coma Scale.) The AVPU scale is widely used by EMTs for assessing the neurologic status of trauma patients as originally taught in Advanced Trauma Life Support (ATLS). Both the AVPU and the ACDU scales are simpler to use than the Glasgow Coma Scale.

The AVPU scale is as follows:

- A for alert signifies that the patient is alert; awake; responsive to voice; and oriented to person, time, and place.
- V for verbal signifies that the patient responds to voice but is not fully oriented to person, time, or place.
- P for pain signifies that the patient does not respond to voice but does respond to painful stimulus such as a squeeze to the hand.
- U for unresponsive signifies that the patient does not respond to painful stimulus.

The ACDU scale is as follows:

- Alert
- Confused
- Drowsy
- Unresponsive

Movement

The inability to move a body part can indicate a serious central nervous system injury that has involved the motor system. An inability to move one side of the body (hemiplegia) could be caused by a head injury or cerebrovascular accident (stroke). Bilateral tingling and numbness or sensory or motor deficits of the upper extremity may indicate a cervical spine injury. Weakness or inability to move the lower extremities could mean an injury below the neck, and pressure on the spinal cord could lead to limited use of the limbs.[24,36]

Abnormal Nerve Response

The injured athlete's pain or other reactions to adverse stimuli can provide valuable clues to the coach or athletic trainer. Numbness or tingling in a limb with or without movement can indicate nerve or cold damage. Blocking of a main artery can produce severe pain, loss of sensation, or lack of a pulse in a limb. A complete lack of pain or of awareness of serious but obvious injury may be caused by shock, hysteria, drug usage, or a spinal cord injury. Generalized or localized pain in the injured region probably means there is no injury to the spinal cord.

Musculoskeletal Assessment

A logical process must be used to evaluate accurately the extent of a musculoskeletal injury.[52] The athletic trainer must be aware of the major signs that reveal the site, nature, and above all, severity of the injury. Detection of these signs can be facilitated by understanding the mechanism or traumatic sequence and by methodically inspecting the injury. Knowledge of the mechanism of an injury is extremely important in determining which area of the body is most affected. When the injury mechanism has been determined, the examiner proceeds to the next phase: physical inspection of the affected region. At this point, information is gathered by what is seen, heard, and felt.[31]

In an attempt to understand the mechanism of injury, a brief *history* of the complaint must be taken. The athlete is asked, if possible, about the events leading up to the injury and how it occurred and what he or she heard or felt when the injury took place. Sounds occurring at the time of injury or during manual inspection yield pertinent information about the type and extent of pathology present. Such uncommon sounds as grating or harsh rubbing may indicate fracture. Joint sounds may be detected when either arthritis or internal derangement is present. Areas of the body that have abnormal amounts of fluid may produce crepitus when palpated or moved. Such sounds as a snap, crack, or pop at the moment of injury often indicate bone fracture or injury to ligaments or tendons.

The athletic trainer should make a visual *observation* of the injured site, comparing it to the uninjured body part. The initial visual examination can disclose obvious deformity, swelling, and skin discoloration.

Finally, the region of the injury should be gently *palpated*. Feeling, or palpating, a part with trained fingers can, in conjunction with visual and audible signs, indicate the nature of the injury. Palpation is started away from the injury and gradually moves toward it. As the examiner gently feels the injury and surrounding structures with the fingertips, several factors can be revealed: the extent of point tenderness, the extent of irritation (whether it is confined to soft tissue alone or extends to the bony tissue), and deformities that may not be detected by visual examination alone.

Assessment Decisions

Decisions that can be made from the secondary survey:
- Seriousness of injury
- Type of first aid required
- Whether injury warrants physical referral
- Type of transportation needed

After a quick on-site injury inspection and evaluation, the athletic trainer should make the following decisions:

1. The seriousness of the injury.
2. The type of first aid and immobilization necessary.
3. Whether the injury warrants immediate referral to a physician for further assessment.
4. The manner of transportation from the injury site to the sidelines, training room, or hospital.

All information about the initial history, signs, and symptoms of the injury must be documented, if possible, so that they may be described in detail to the physician.

Immediate Treatment

Musculoskeletal injuries are extremely common in sports. The athletic trainer must be prepared to provide appropriate first aid immediately to control hemorrhage and associated swelling. Every first aid effort should be directed toward one primary goal—reducing the amount of swelling and inflammation resulting from the injury.[33] If swelling and inflammation can be controlled initially, the amount of time required for injury rehabilitation will be significantly reduced. Initial management of musculoskeletal injuries should include rest, ice, compression, and elevation (RICE) (see Figure 12-21).

Rest Rest after any type of injury is an extremely important component of any treatment program. Once a body part is injured, it immediately begins the healing process.[40] If the injured part is not rested and is subjected to external stresses and strains, the healing process never takes place. Consequently, the injured part does not heal, and the time required for rehabilitation is greatly increased. The number of days necessary for resting varies with the severity of the injury. Parts of the body that have experienced minor injury should rest for approximately seventy-two hours before a rehabilitation program is begun.

Figure 12-21

RICE technique: **A,** A wet compression wrap should be applied over the horseshoe pad. **B,** Ice bags should be secured in place by a dry compression wrap. **C,** The leg should be elevated during the initial treatment period.

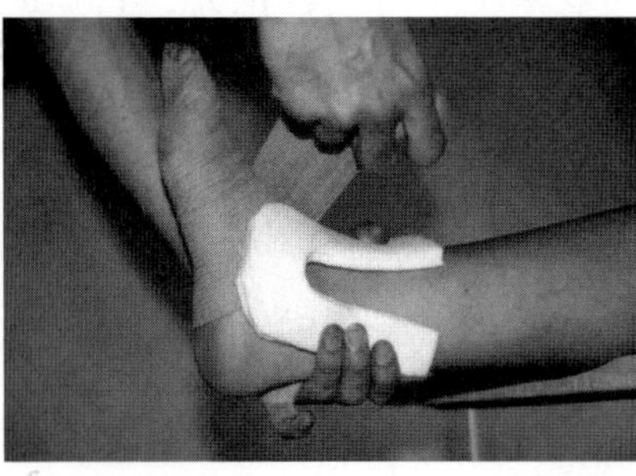

A

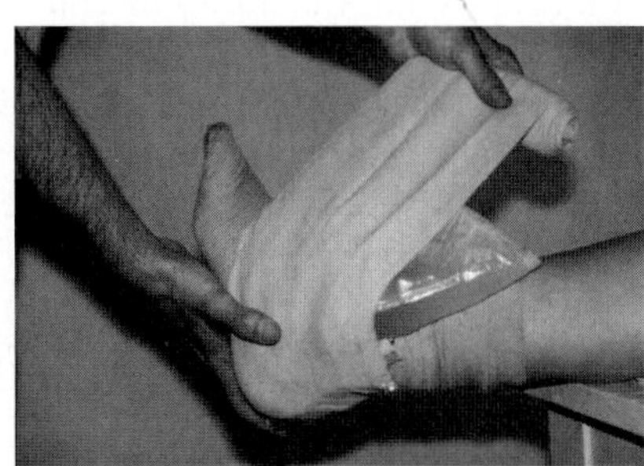

B

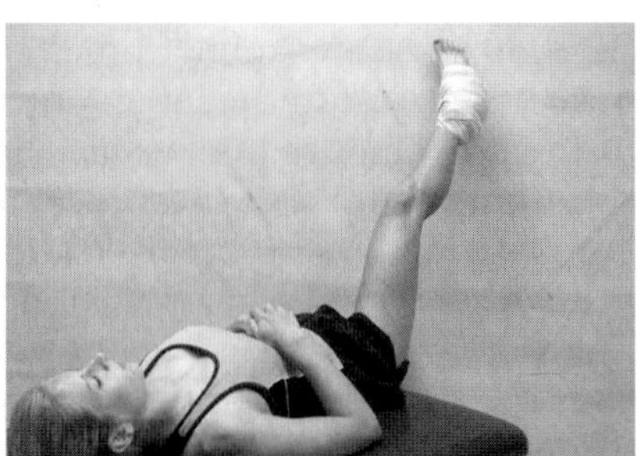

C

Ice (cold application) The initial treatment of acute injuries should use cold.[20] Therefore ice is used for most conditions involving strains, sprains, and contusions. Cold is most commonly used immediately after injury to decrease pain and promote local superficial constriction of the vessels (vasoconstriction), thus controlling hemorrhage and edema.[40] Cold applied to an acute injury will lower metabolism and tissue demands for oxygen and will reduce hypoxia.[28] This benefit extends to uninjured tissue, preventing injury-related tissue death from spreading to adjacent normal cellular structures. Cold is also used in the acute phase of inflammatory conditions such as bursitis, tenosynovitis, and tendinitis conditions in which heat may cause additional pain and swelling. Cold is also used to reduce the muscle guarding that accompanies pain. Its pain-reducing (analgesic) effect is probably one of its greatest benefits. One explanation of the analgesic effect is that cold slows the speed of nerve transmission, so the pain sensation is reduced. It is also possible that cold bombards pain receptors with so many cold impulses that pain impulses are lost. With ice treatments, the athlete usually reports an uncomfortable sensation of cold, followed by burning, then an aching sensation, and finally complete numbness.

Because the subcutaneous (under the skin) fat slowly conducts the cold temperature, applications of cold for short periods of time will be ineffective in cooling deeper tissues. For this reason, longer treatments of at least twenty minutes are recommended. However, prolonged application of cold can cause tissue damage.[28]

Cold treatments seem to be more effective in reaching deep tissues than most forms of heat are. Cold applied to the skin is capable of significantly lowering the temperature of tissues at a considerable depth. The temperature to which the deeper tissues can be lowered depends on the type of cold that is applied to the skin, the duration of its application, the thickness of the subcutaneous fat, and the region of the body to which it is applied.[28] Ice packs should be applied to the area for at least seventy-two hours after an acute injury. With many injuries, regular ice treatments may be continued for several weeks.

For best results, ice packs (crushed ice and towel) should be applied over a compression wrap. Frozen gel packs should not be used directly against the skin because they reach much lower temperatures than do ice packs. A good rule of thumb is to apply a cold pack to a recent injury for a twenty-minute period and repeat every 1 to 1½ hours throughout the waking day. Depending on the severity and site of the injury, cold may be applied intermittently for one to seventy-two hours. For example, a mild strain will probably require one day of twenty-minute periods of cold application, whereas a severe knee or ankle sprain might need three to seven days of intermittent cold. If the severity of an injury is in doubt, the best approach is to extend the time that ice is applied.

Compression In most cases immediate compression of an acute injury is considered an important adjunct to cold and elevation and in some cases may be superior to them. Placing external pressure on an injury assists in decreasing hemorrhage and hematoma formation by mechanically reducing the space available for swelling to accumulate.[36] Fluid seepage into interstitial spaces is retarded by compression, and absorption is facilitated. However, applying compression to an anterior compartment syndrome or to certain injuries involving the head and neck is contraindicated.

Many types of compression are available. An elastic wrap that has been soaked in water and frozen in a refrigerator can provide both compression and cold when applied to a recent injury. Pads can be cut from felt or foam rubber to fit difficult-to-compress body areas. For example, a horseshoe-shaped pad placed around the malleolus in combination with an elastic wrap and tape provides focal compression to reduce ankle edema.[62] Although cold is applied intermittently, compression should be maintained throughout the day and if possible throughout the night. Because of the pressure buildup in the tissues, the athlete may find it painful to leave a compression wrap in place for a long time. However, it is essential to leave the wrap in place in spite of significant pain because compression is so important in the control of swelling.

Rest, ice, compression, and elevation (RICE) are essential in the emergency care of musculoskeletal injuries.

12-5

Critical Thinking Exercise

A field hockey player trips over an opponent's stick, plantar flexing and inverting her ankle, and she falls to the turf with a grade 2 ankle sprain. She has immediate effusion and significant pain. On examination, there appears to be some laxity in the ankle joint. The athletic trainer transports the athlete to the training room so that the ankle sprain can be managed properly.

? What specifically should the athletic trainer do to most effectively control the initial swelling associated with this injury?

The compression wrap should be left in place for at least seventy-two hours after an acute injury. In many chronic overuse problems, such as tendinitis, tenosynovitis, and particularly bursitis, the compression wrap should be worn until all swelling is almost entirely gone.

Elevation Along with cold and compression, elevation reduces internal bleeding. The injured part, particularly an extremity, should be elevated to eliminate the effects of gravity on blood pooling in the extremities.[40] Elevation assists the veins, which drain blood and other fluids from the injured area, returning them to the central circulatory system. The greater the degree of elevation, the more effective the reduction in swelling. In an ankle sprain, for example, the leg should be placed so that the ankle is virtually straight up in the air. The injured part should be elevated as much as possible during the first seventy-two hours.

Emergency Splinting

A suspected fracture must be splinted before the athlete is moved.

Any suspected fracture should always be splinted before the athlete is moved.[13] Transporting a person with a fracture without proper immobilization can result in increased tissue damage, hemorrhage, and shock.[33] Conceivably, a mishandled fracture could cause death. Therefore a thorough knowledge of splinting techniques is important. Applying splints should be a simple process using commercial emergency splints.[18,33] The athletic trainer usually does not have to improvise a splint because such devices are readily available in most sports settings.

Rapid form vacuum immobilizer The rapid form vacuum immobilizer is widely used by both EMTs and athletic trainers.[43] It consists of styrofoam chips contained inside an airtight cloth sleeve that is pliable. This splint can be molded to the shape of any joint or angulated fracture through the use of Velcro straps. A handheld pump sucks the air out of the sleeve, giving it a cardboardlike rigidity. This splint is most useful for injuries that are angulated and must be splinted in the position in which they are found (Figure 12-22A).

Air splint An air splint is a clear plastic splint that is inflated with air around the affected part and can be used for extremity splinting, but its use requires some special training. This splint provides support and moderate pressure to the body part and affords a clear view of the site for X-ray examination. The inflatable splint should not be used if it will alter a fracture deformity (Figure 12-22B).

Half-ring splint For fractures of the femur, the half-ring traction splint offers the best support and immobilization but takes considerable practice to master. An open fracture must be carefully dressed to avoid additional contamination (Figure 12-22C).

Whatever the material used, the principles of good splinting remain the same. Two major concepts of splinting are to splint from one joint above the fracture to one joint below the fracture and to splint where the athlete lies. If at all possible, do not move the athlete until he or she has been splinted.

Splinting of lower-limb fractures Fractures of the ankle or leg require immobilization of the foot and knee. Any fracture involving the knee, thigh, or hip needs splinting of all the lower-limb joints and one side of the trunk.

Splinting of upper-limb fractures Fractures around the shoulder complex are immobilized by a sling and swathe bandage, with the upper limb securely bound to the body. Upper-arm and elbow fractures must be splinted, with immobilization effected in a straight-arm position to lessen bone override. Lower-arm and wrist fractures should be splinted in a position of forearm flexion and should be supported by a sling. Hand and finger dislocations and fractures should be splinted with tongue depressors, roller gauze, or aluminum splints.[49]

Splinting of the spine and pelvis Injuries involving a possible spine or pelvic fracture are best splinted and the athlete moved using a spine board. Recently, a total body rapid form vacuum immobilizer has been developed for dealing with spinal injuries (Figure 12-23). The effectiveness of this piece of equipment as an immobilization device has yet to be determined.[43]

12-6

Critical Thinking Exercise

During practice, a lacrosse player is involved in a collision on the field. When the athletic trainer reaches the athlete, the athlete's ankle is deformed and obviously fractured.

? How should the athletic trainer immobilize this injury?

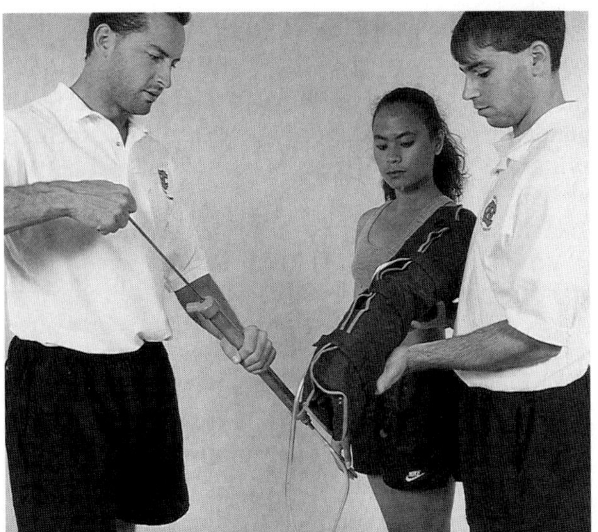

A

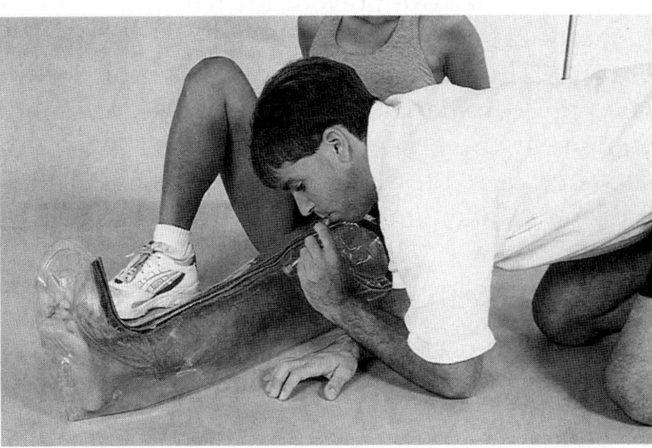

B

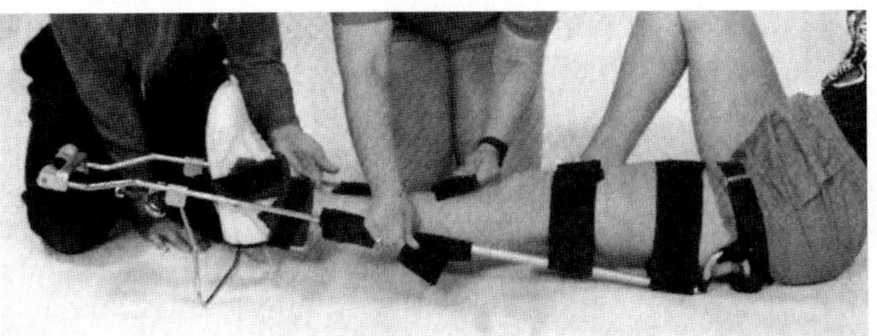

C

Figure 12-22

Examples of splints. **A,** Rapid form vacuum immobilizer. **B,** Air splint. **C,** Half-ring splint.

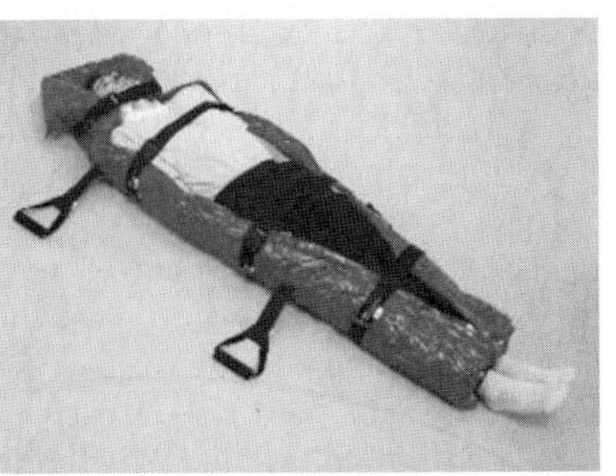

Figure 12-23

Full body mattress vacuum splint immobilizer (From MDI Immobile Inc.).

EMERGENCY EMOTIONAL CARE

Besides evaluating and responding to the emergency physical requirements of an injury, the athletic trainer must evaluate and respond appropriately to the emotions engendered by the situation. The American Psychiatric Association has set forth major principles for the emergency care of emotional reactions to trauma.[24] Those principles are as follows:

1. Accept everyone's right to personal feelings, because everyone comes from a unique background and has had different emotional experiences. Do not tell the injured person how he or she should feel. Show empathy, not pity.
2. Accept the injured person's limitations as real.
3. Accept your own limitations as a provider of first aid.

In general, the athletic trainer dealing with an injured athlete's emotions should be empathetic and calm and should make it obvious that the athlete's feelings are understood and accepted (see Chapter 11).

MOVING AND TRANSPORTING THE INJURED ATHLETE

Great caution must be taken when transporting the injured athlete.

Moving, lifting, and transporting the injured athlete must be executed with the use of techniques that will prevent further injury. Moving or transporting the athlete improperly causes more additional injuries than does any other emergency procedure.[24,36] There is no excuse for poor handling of the injured athlete. Planning should take into consideration all the possible transportation methods and the necessary equipment to execute them.[8] Capable and well-trained personnel, spine boards, stretchers, and a rescue vehicle may be needed to transport the injured athlete. Special consideration must be given to extracting the injured athlete from a pool.

Placing the Athlete on a Spine Board

In cases of suspected cervical spine injury, the athletic trainer should generally access the EMS and wait until the rescue squad arrives before attempting to move the athlete. The only exception would be if the athlete is not breathing. Then the athlete must be logrolled onto his or her back for CPR.

A suspected spinal injury requires extremely careful handling and is best left to properly trained paramedics or EMTs or to athletic trainers who are well trained and have access to the proper equipment for transport. (See the back inside cover of this text for a list of emergency equipment that should be available on the sidelines.) If such personnel are not available, the athlete should be moved under the express direction of a physician, and a spine board should be used (Figure 12-24). The most important principle in transporting an individual on a spine board is to maintain the head and neck in alignment with the long axis of the body. In such cases, it is best to have one person whose sole responsibility is to ensure and maintain proper positioning of the head and neck until the head is secured to a spine board.

Primary emergency care involves helping the athlete maintain normal breathing, treating the athlete for shock, and keeping the athlete quiet and in the position found until medical assistance arrives. Ideally, transportation should not be attempted until a physician has examined the athlete and has given permission to move him or her. Neck stabilization must be maintained throughout transportation, first to the emergency vehicle, then to the hospital, and throughout the hospital procedure.[1]

These steps should be followed when moving an athlete with a suspected neck injury:

1. The examiner must determine whether the athlete is breathing and has a pulse.
2. A spine board is retrieved for moving the athlete.
3. If the athlete is lying prone, he or she must be logrolled onto his or her back for CPR or to be secured to the spine board. An athlete with a possible cervical fracture is transported face up. An athlete with a spinal fracture in the lower trunk area may be transported face down.

a. All extremities are placed in an axial alignment (Figure 12-24A).
b. To roll the athlete over requires four or five persons, with the captain of the team protecting the athlete's head and neck. The neck must be stabilized and must not be moved from its original position, no matter how distorted it may appear.
c. The spine board is placed close to the side of the athlete (Figure 12-24B).
d. Each assistant is responsible for one of the athlete's body segments. One assistant is responsible for turning the trunk, another the hips, another the thighs, and the last the lower legs.

4. With the spine board close to the athlete's side, the captain gives the command to logroll him or her onto the board as one unit (Figure 12-24C).
5. On the board, the athlete's head and neck continue to be stabilized by the captain (Figure 12-24D).
6. If the athlete is a football player, the helmet is not removed; however, the face guard is removed or lifted away from the face for possible CPR. NOTE: To remove the face guard, the plastic fasteners holding it to the helmet should be removed.

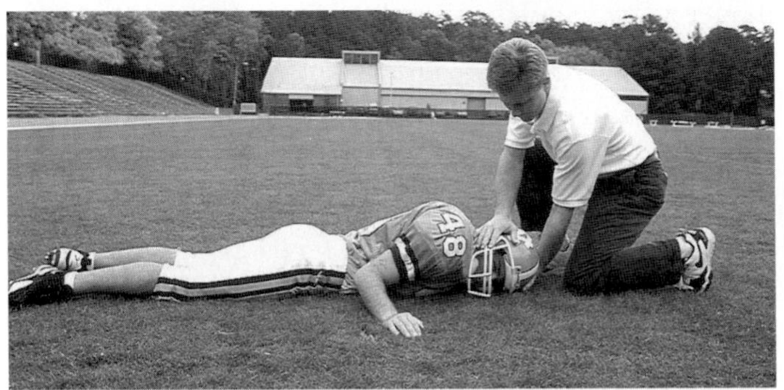

A

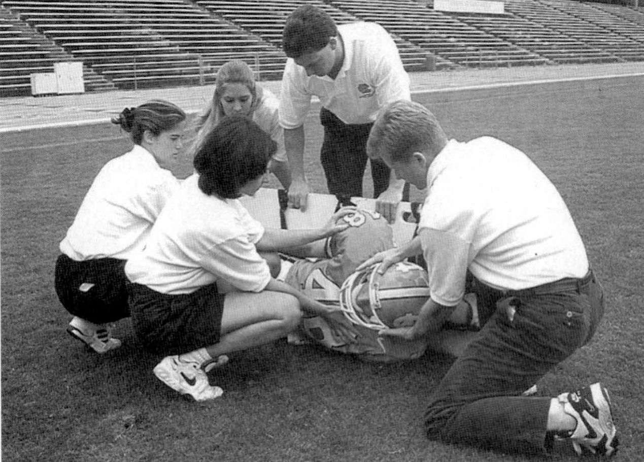

C

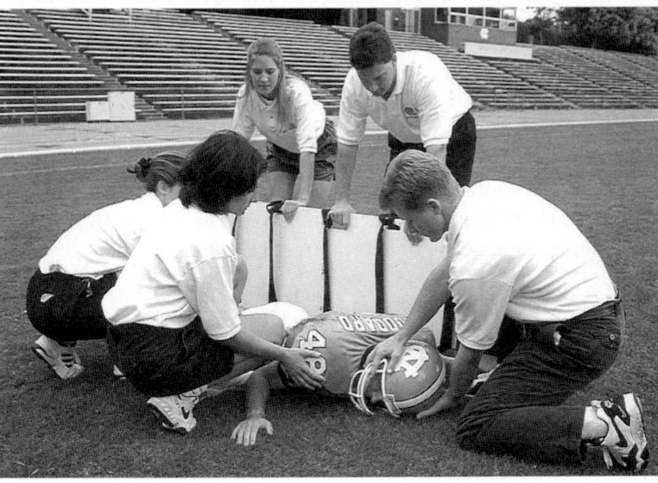

B

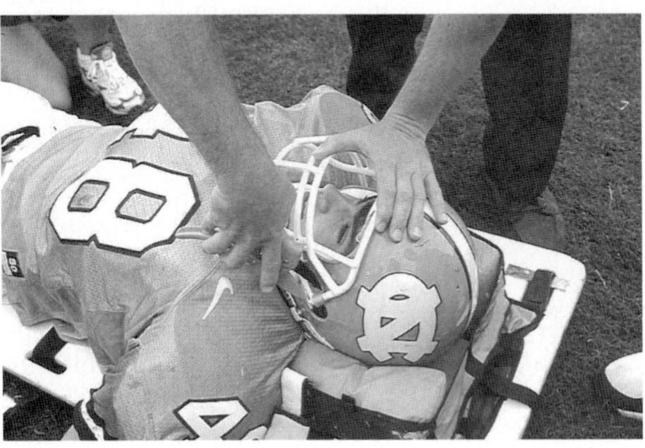

D

Figure 12-24

A, When moving an unconscious athlete, first establish whether the athlete is breathing and has a pulse. An unconscious athlete must always be treated as having a serious neck injury. If lying prone, the athlete must be turned over for CPR or be secured to a spine board for possible cervical fracture. One person (the "captain") should stabilize the athlete's neck and head. **B,** The spine board is placed as close to the athlete as possible. **C,** Each assistant is responsible for one of the athlete's segments. When the coach or athletic trainer gives the command "roll," the athlete is moved as a unit onto the spine board. **D,** The face mask is cut away while the captain continues to stabilize the athlete's neck.

Continued

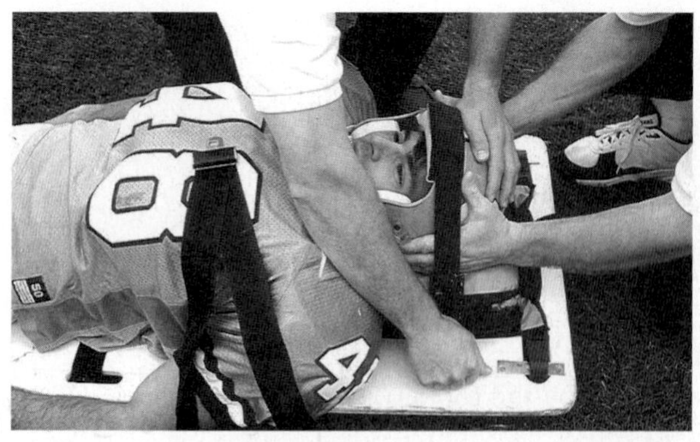

E

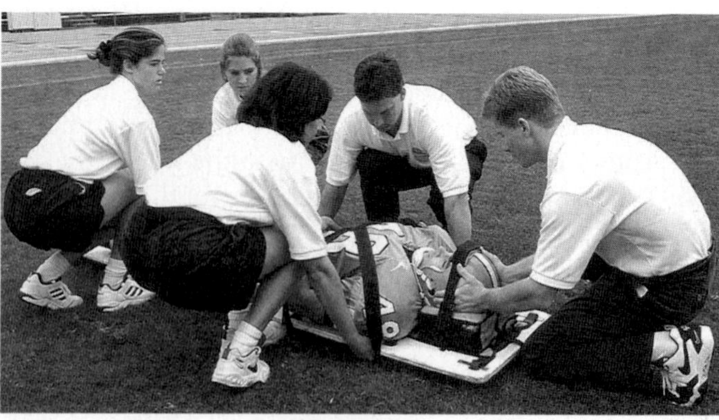

G

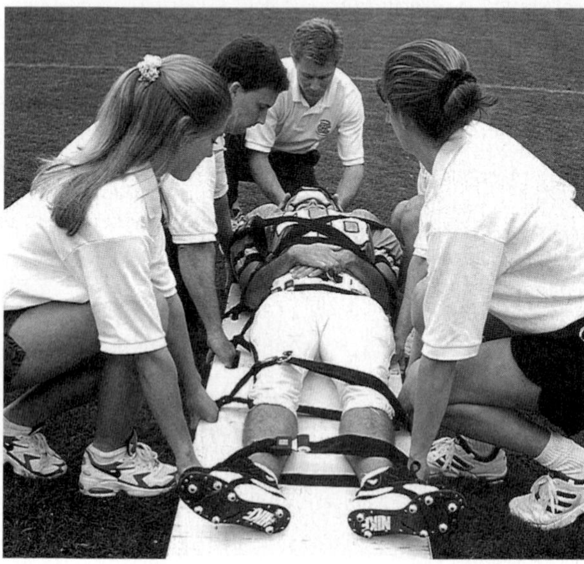

F

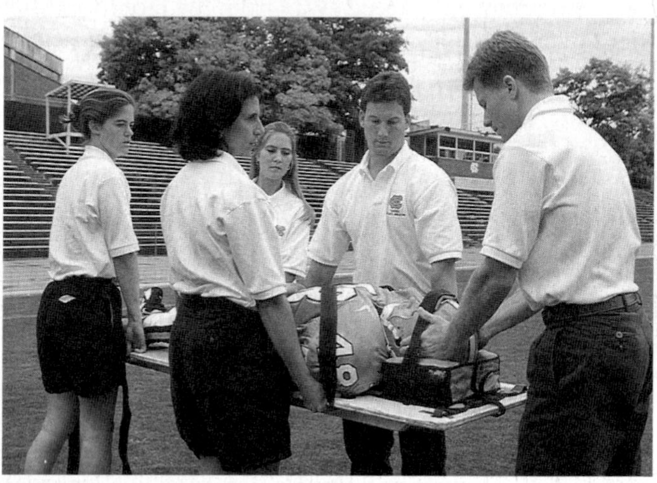

H

Figure 12-24—continued

E, The head and neck are stabilized onto the spine board by means of a chin strap secured to metal loops. **F,** The trunk and lower limbs are secured to the spine board by straps. **G,** All carriers assume a position to stand. **H,** Once the carriers are standing, the athlete may be transported.

7. Next, the head and neck are stabilized on the spine board by a chin strap secured to metal loops.[57] Finally, the trunk and lower limbs are secured to the spine board by straps (Figure 12-24E and F).
8. The rescuers place themselves in a position to stand, and then on the command of the person stabilizing the head, they collectively lift the athlete on the spine board (Figure 12-24G and H).

If the athlete is face up, the lift and slide technique can be used to move the athlete onto a spine board. Four or five persons are needed: a captain stationed at the athlete's head and three or four assistants. One assistant is in charge of lifting the athlete's trunk, one the hips, and one the legs. At the captain's lift command, the athlete is lifted while the fourth assistant slides a spine board under the athlete between the feet of the captain and the assistants (Figure 12-25A). The lift and slide technique has been shown to be more effective in restricting motion in the head, reducing both lateral flexion and axial rotation compared to the logroll technique.[9]

A scoop stretcher may also be used for transporting an athlete with a potential injury to the spine although it is not generally considered to be as safe as using a spine board (Figure 12-25B). A scoop stretcher has detachable hinges at each end, and thus

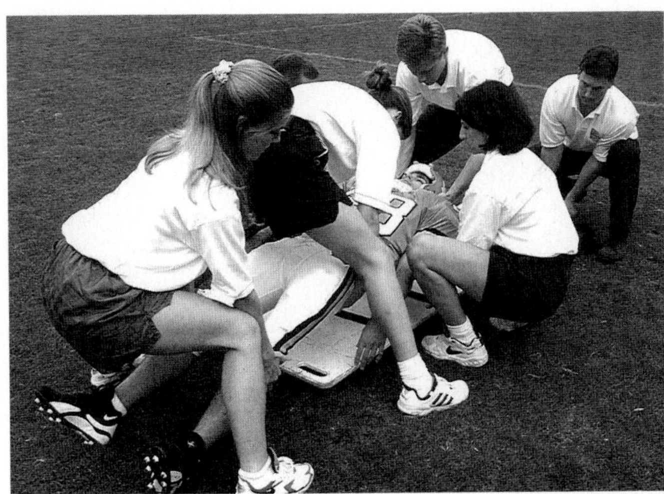

A

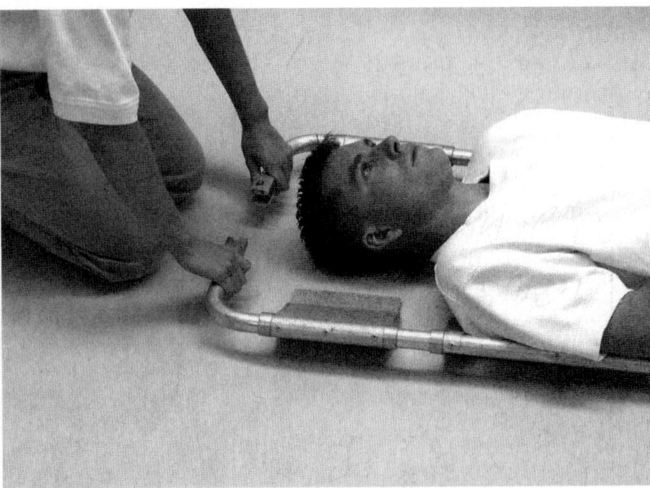

C

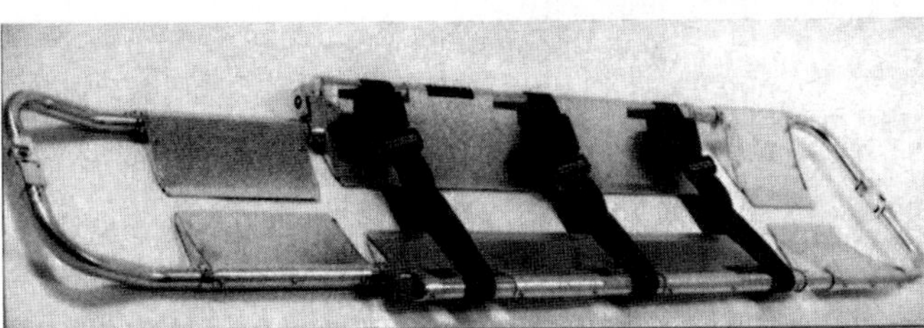

B

Figure 12-25

Alternative methods of placing the athlete on a spine board. **A,** The lift and slide technique. **B,** The scoop stretcher. **C,** Latching the top of the scoop stretcher.

can be split into two halves (Figure 12-25C). Each half of the stretcher is placed on either side of the prone athlete. The athletic trainer can easily slide each half of the stretcher under the athlete until the hinges are locked together, in effect "scooping" the athlete onto the stretcher. The advantage in using a scoop stretcher is that it is not necessary to roll the injured athlete onto his or her side to get the stretcher underneath.

Ambulatory Aid

Ambulatory aid is that support or assistance given to an injured athlete who is able to walk (Figure 12-26). Before the athlete is allowed to walk, he or she should be carefully scrutinized to make sure that the injuries are minor. Whenever serious injuries are suspected, walking should be prohibited. Complete support should be given on both sides of the athlete by two individuals who are approximately the same height. The athlete's arms are draped over the assistants' shoulders, and their arms encircle his or her back.

Manual Conveyance

Manual conveyance may be used to move a mildly injured individual a greater distance than could be walked with ease (Figure 12-27). Any decision to carry the athlete, like a decision to use ambulatory aid, must be made only after a complete examination to determine the existence of potentially serious conditions. The most convenient carry is performed by two assistants.

Stretcher Carrying

Whenever a serious injury is suspected, the best and safest mode of transportation for a short distance is by stretcher. With each segment of the body supported, the athlete is gently lifted and placed on the stretcher, which is carried adequately by a minimum of four assistants, two supporting either side (Figure 12-28). Any person with an injury serious enough to require the use of a stretcher must be carefully examined before being moved.

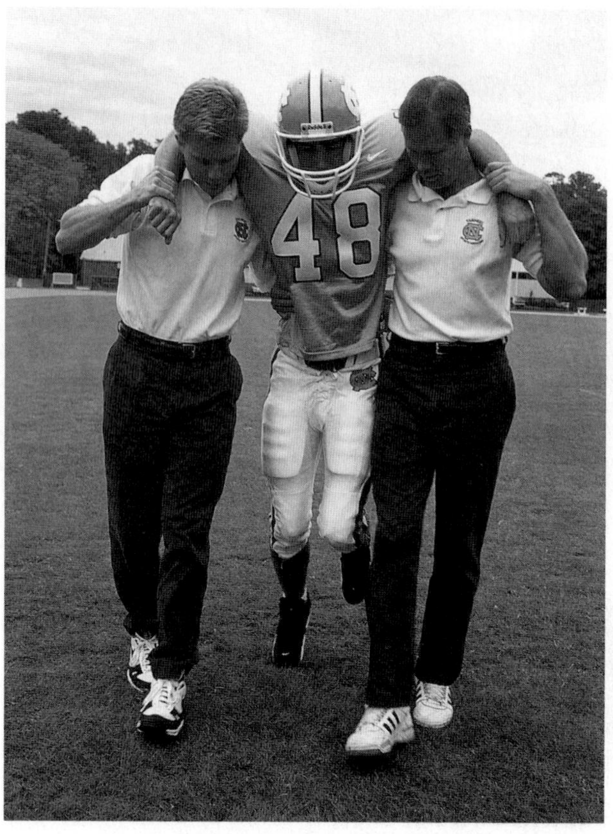

Figure 12-26

The ambulatory aid method of transporting a mildly injured athlete.

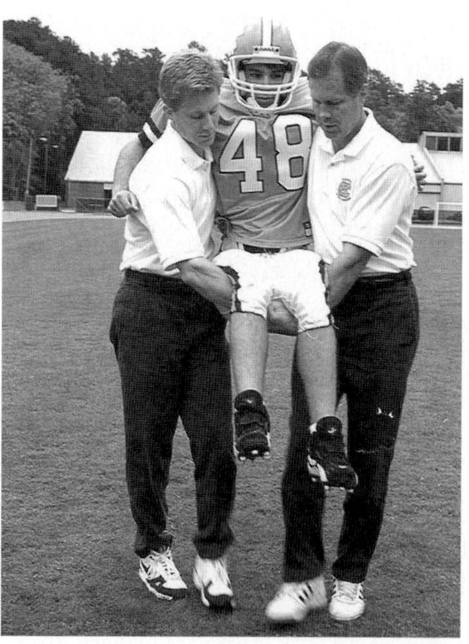

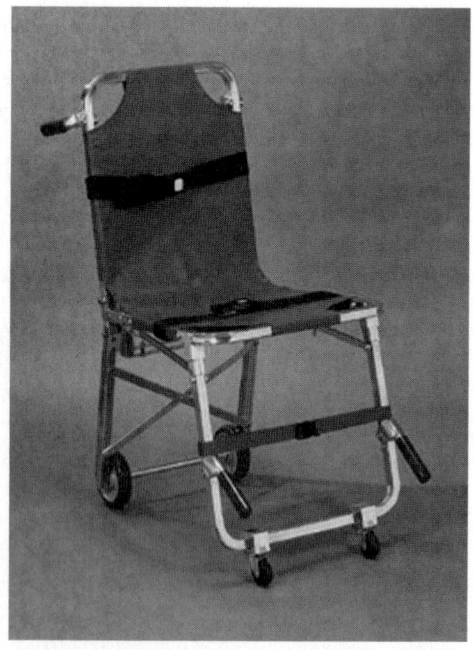

A

B

Figure 12-27

A, Manual conveyance method for transporting a mildly injured athlete. **B,** A stair chair can also be used if the athlete is too large for the athletic trainer to lift manually.

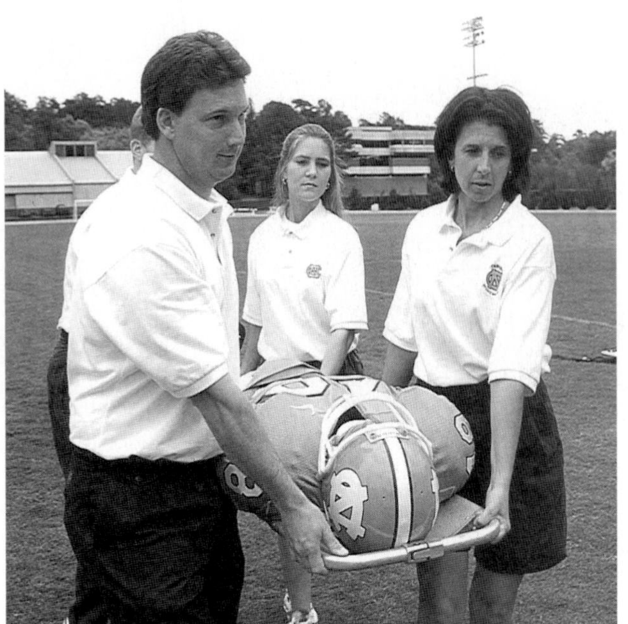

Figure 12-28

Whenever a serious injury is suspected, a stretcher is the safest method for transporting the athlete. A scoop stretcher makes it easy to get underneath the injured athlete.

A limb injury must be splinted properly before the athlete is transported. Athletes with shoulder injuries are more comfortably moved in a semisitting position, unless other injuries preclude such positioning. If injury to the upper extremity is such that flexion of the elbow is not possible, the individual should be transported on a stretcher with the limb properly splinted and carried at the side, with adequate padding placed between the arm and the body.

Pool Extraction

Removing an injured athlete from a swimming pool requires some special consideration on the part of the athletic trainer. Obviously an athletic trainer who is providing coverage for athletes training or competing in a pool must be able to swim and should have water safety or lifeguard training. The athletic trainer should routinely have immediate access to both a rescue tube and an aquatic spine board in case an athlete sustains an injury while in the pool. A rescue tube should always be used to extract an injured athlete from the pool.[3] The rescue tube will not only serve as a floatation device but also can help prevent an athlete who is distressed from grabbing the athletic trainer while in the water.

The following procedures are recommended for removing an injured athlete from a pool:

1. When dealing with an athlete who has sustained what appears to be a minor injury in the pool, if the athlete is close to the edge of the pool, the athletic trainer can reach out to the athlete with the rescue tube while standing on the pool deck and holding onto the shoulder strap with the other hand. Have the athlete grab the tube, then pull him or her to the edge of the pool (Figure 12-29A).[3]
2. If the athlete is too far away from the pool deck, the athletic trainer should get into the water, approach the athlete from the front, extend the rescue tube, have the athlete grab the tube and kick if possible, while the athletic trainer pulls them to the edge of the pool (Figure 12-29B).[3]

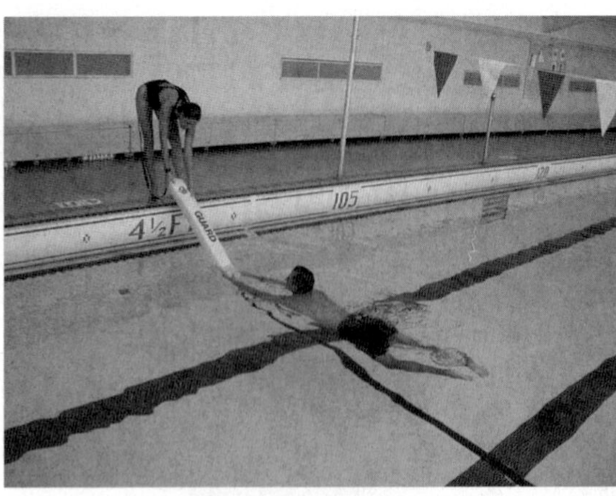

A

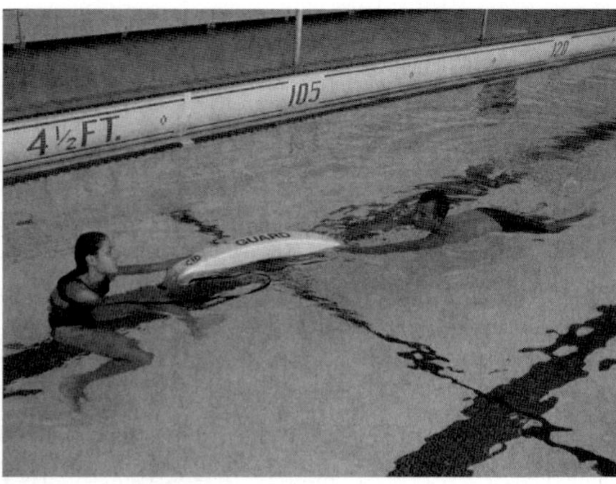

B

Figure 12-29

Techniques for pool rescue. **A,** Athlete is close to edge of pool. **B,** Athlete is in middle of pool.

12-7

***Critical Thinking* Exercise**

A diver, attempting a 2½ inward dive on a 3-meter board, hits her head on the end of the board. She lands on her face in the water, is briefly submerged, but floats quickly to the surface. She is conscious but disoriented; she has a bump on her forehead but is not bleeding. A teammate nearby jumps immediately in the water and, using a cross-chest technique, tows her about 10 feet to the side of the pool.

? The athletic trainer is concerned about both a head and neck injury. What precautions should be taken when removing the injured athlete from the pool?

3. If an athlete appears to be more severely injured, the athletic trainer should get into the water, approach the athlete from behind, reach under the armpits and grab the athlete's shoulders while putting the rescue tube between the athlete's back and the athletic trainer's chest. The athletic trainer should keep his or head to either side to avoid being hit by the athlete's head should it fall backwards. The athletic trainer should lean back pulling the athlete onto the rescue tube, which should support the athlete keeping the athlete's mouth and face out of the water; the athletic trainer should pull the athlete to the edge of the pool while attempting to keep him or her calm (Figure 12-30).[3]
4. Deciding to remove an injured athlete from the water depends on several factors including the athlete's condition, size, and the availability of help or how long until help arrives. For example, an injured athlete requiring CPR should be removed immediately from the water; rescue breathing should not be attempted in the water. A spine board should be used by two people to remove any athlete from the water who is unable to get out on his or her own, even if a spinal injury is not suspected. The primary rescuer brings the injured athlete to the side of the pool and turns him or her to face the pool deck. A second rescuer standing on the pool deck grabs the athlete's opposite wrists and pulls the athlete up, keeping the head above water and away from the edge of the pool (Figure 12-31A). The primary rescuer gets out of the water, grabs the spine board, then guides the spine board foot-end

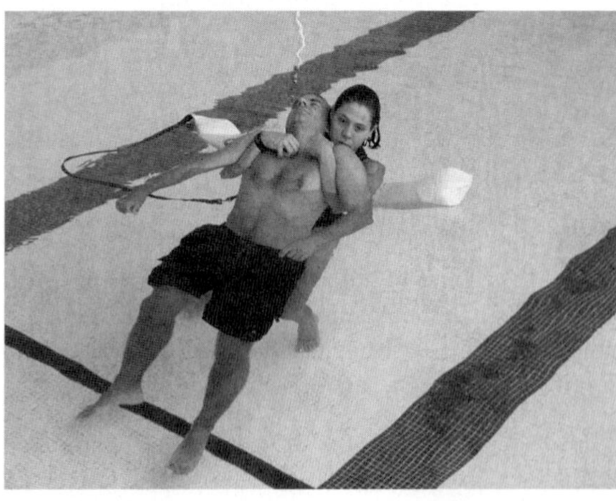

Figure 12-30

Technique for removing a severely injured athlete from the water.

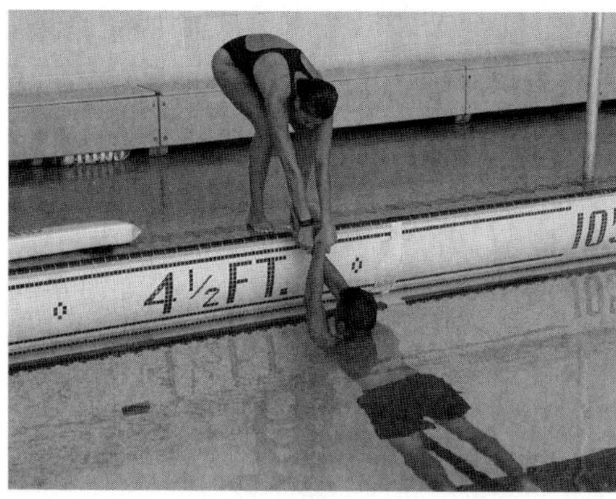

A

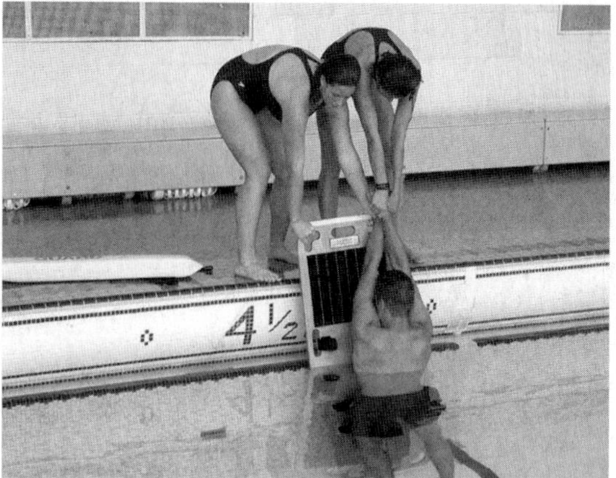

B

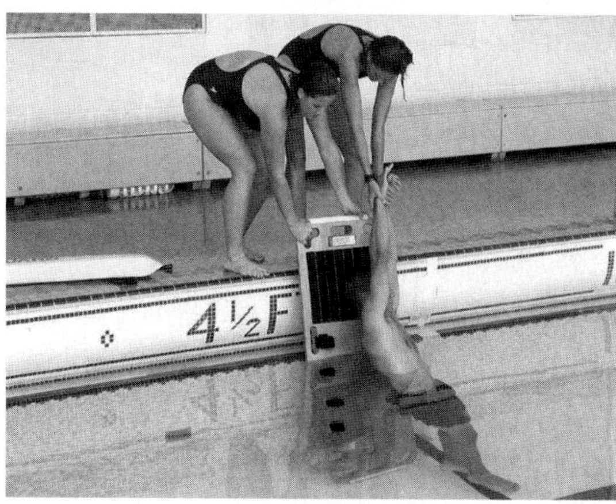

C

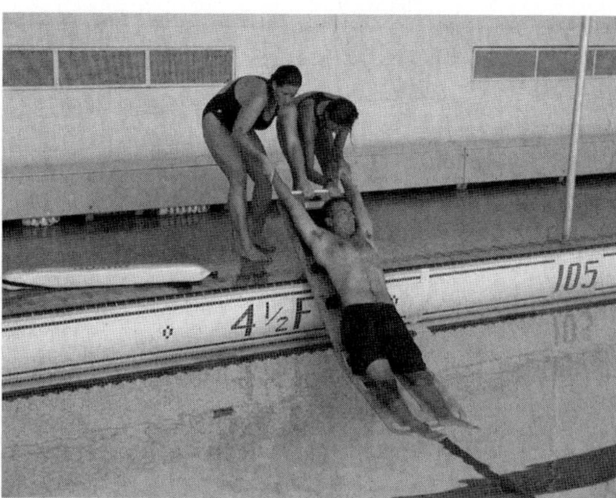

D

Figure 12-31

Technique for removing an athlete from the water who can't get out on their own.

first down into the water between the athlete and the edge of the pool (Figure 12-31B). The second rescuer then turns the athlete so his or her back rests against the spine board (Figure 12-31C). Each rescuer then grasps a wrist with one hand and the spine board with the other. The rescuers pull the spine board upward and backward leveraging the board onto the pool deck (Figure 12-31D).[3]

5. An athlete with a suspected head or cervical neck injury or an athlete who is unconscious requires special precaution. An athlete's cervical spine can be immobilized in the water by a single primary rescuer placing one forearm over the sternum and cupping the athlete's lower jaw while placing the other forearm over the athlete's spine and holding the back of his or her head. Squeezing the forearms together stabilizes the spine and head. The athlete may be held face-up in the water in this position until help arrives (Figure 12-32A). While the primary rescuer continues stabilizing the head and neck, a second rescuer submerges the spine board, positioning it appropriately under the athlete. The primary rescuer maintains stabilization of the athlete's chin while removing the other arm and repositioning it to support the back of the spine board (Figure 12-32B). Rescue tubes may be used to help float the spine board. The second rescuer moves to the athlete's head and, with the forearms resting against the sides of the spine board, assumes responsibility for stabilizing the athlete's head. The primary rescuer then securely straps the chest, hips, thighs, and finally immobilizes and secures the head to the spine board (Figure 12-32C). Both rescuers then remove the spine board from the pool, head first, by initially lifting the board onto the edge of the pool while still in the water. Then one rescuer gets on the pool deck while the other remains in the water to complete the pool extraction (Figure 12-32D).[3]

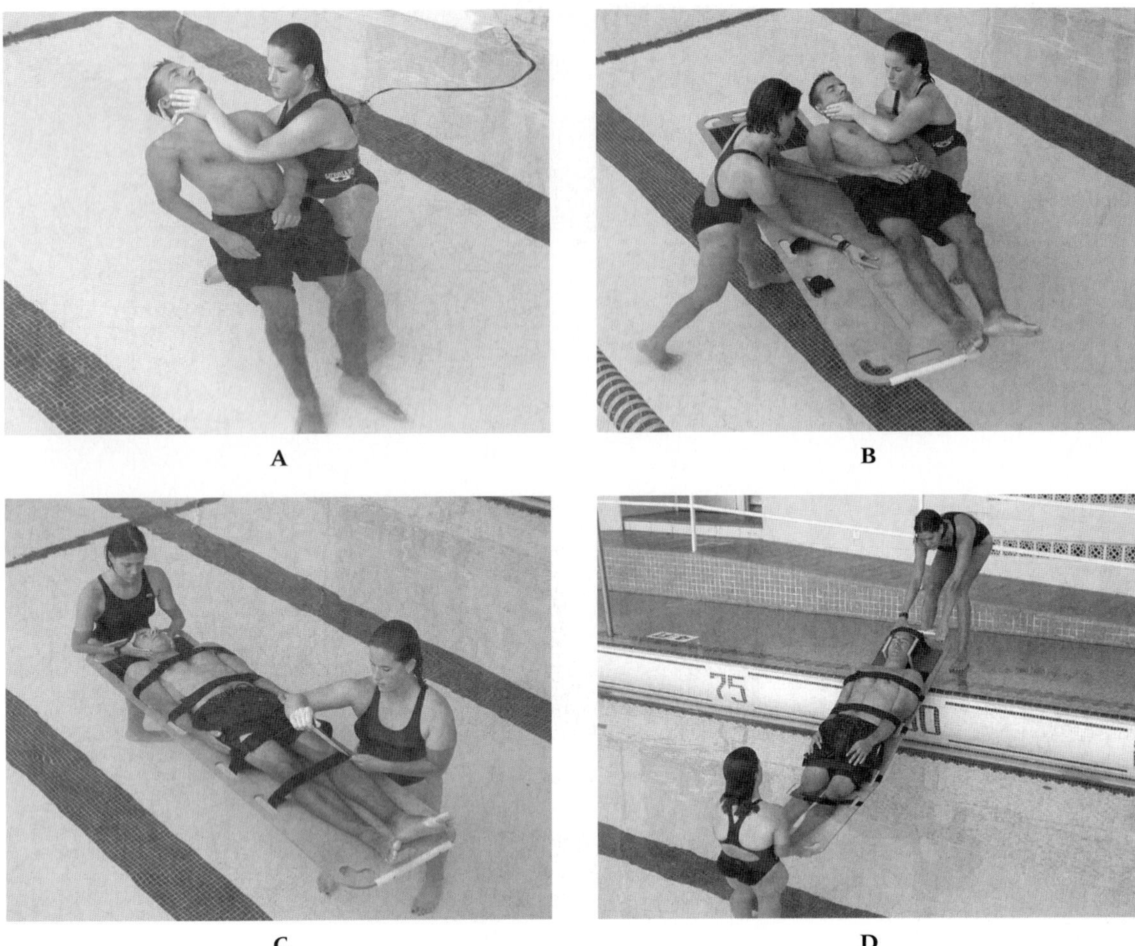

Figure 12-32

Technique for putting an athlete with a suspected spinal injury on a spine board and removing him or her from the pool.

PROPER FIT AND USE OF THE CRUTCH OR CANE

Weight bearing may be contraindicated for an athlete with a lower-limb injury, in which case a crutch or cane should be used for ambulation. The athletic trainer must be responsible for properly fitting the crutch or cane to the injured athlete and then for providing instruction in its use. If the crutch or cane is not properly fitted, the athlete may experience discomfort in the axilla from excessive pressure as well as pain in the low back. Faulty mechanics in the use of the crutch or cane when ambulating and particularly when ascending or descending stairs can cause the athlete to fall.

Fitting the Athlete

Properly fitting a crutch or cane is essential to avoid placing abnormal stresses on the body.

The adjustable wooden crutch is well suited to the athlete. For a correct fit, the athlete should wear low-heeled shoes and stand with good posture and the feet close together. The crutch length is determined first by placing the tip 6 inches (15 cm) from the outer margin of the shoe and 2 inches (5 cm) in front of the shoe. The underarm crutch brace is positioned 1 inch (2.5 cm) below the anterior fold of the axilla. Next, the hand brace is adjusted so that it is even with the athlete's hand when the elbow is flexed at approximately a 30-degree angle (Figure 12-33).

Fitting a cane to the athlete is relatively easy. Measurement is taken from the superior aspect of the greater trochanter of the femur to the floor while the athlete is wearing street shoes.

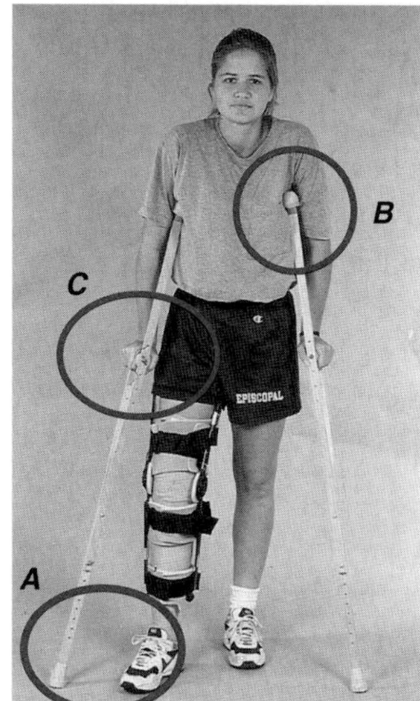

Figure 12-33

The crutch must be properly fitted to the athlete. **A,** The crutch tips are placed 6 inches (15 cm) from the outer margin of the shoe and 2 inches (5 cm) in front of the shoe. **B,** The underarm crutch brace is positioned 1 inch (2.5 cm) below the anterior fold of the axilla. **C,** The hand brace is placed even with the athlete's hand, with the elbow flexed approximately 30 degrees.

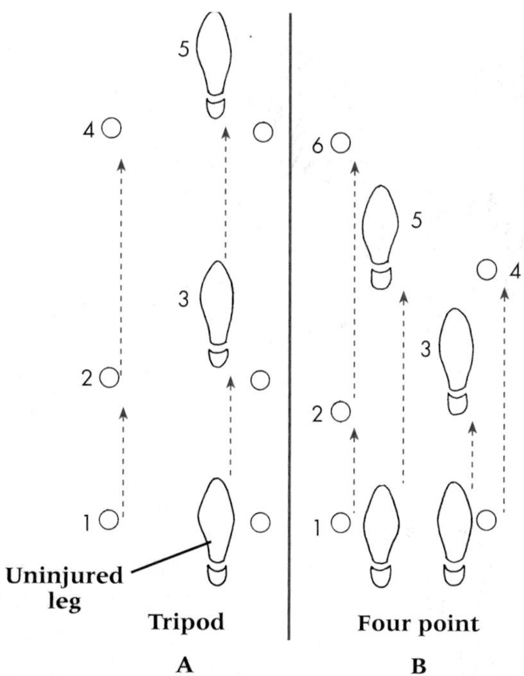

Figure 12-34

Crutch gait. **A,** Tripod method. **B,** Four-point gait.

Walking with the Crutch or Cane

Many elements of crutch walking correspond with normal walking. The technique commonly used in sports injuries is the tripod method. In this method, the athlete swings through the crutches without making any surface contact with the injured limb or by partially bearing weight with the injured limb. The following sequence is performed:

1. The athlete stands on the uninjured leg with no weight or partial weight on the injured leg.
2. Placing the crutch tips 12 to 15 inches (30 to 37.5 cm) ahead of the feet, the athlete leans forward, straightens the elbows, pulls the upper crosspiece firmly against the side of the chest, and swings or steps with the uninjured leg between the stationary crutches (Figure 12-34A). The athlete should avoid placing the major support in the axilla.
3. After moving through, the athlete recovers the crutches and again places the tips forward repeating the sequence. The crutches and the injured or non–weight-bearing leg always move together.

An alternative method is the four-point crutch gait. In this method, the athlete stands on both feet, moves one crutch forward, and steps forward with the opposite foot. The athlete moves the crutch on the same side as the foot that moved forward to just ahead of the foot, steps forward, using the opposite foot followed by the crutch on the same side, and so on (Figure 12-34B).

The tripod gait that is used for crutch walking on a level surface is also used on stairs. In going up stairs, the uninjured support leg moves up one step while the body weight is supported by the hands on the crutches. The full weight of the body is transferred to

12-8

Critical Thinking **Exercise**

A fencer has a grade 2 ankle sprain. After spending an hour in the training room applying ice, compression, and elevation, the athletic trainer decides that the athlete should be sent home on crutches. The athlete indicates some reluctance to use the crutches because he has never used them before.

? What instructions should the athletic trainer give the athlete so that he can correctly and safely ambulate on crutches?

the uninjured leg, and the crutch tips and injured leg are moved to that step. In going down stairs, the crutch tips and the injured leg move down one step, followed by the uninjured leg. If a handrail is available, the athlete uses the tripod gait holding both crutches with the outside hand.

Crutch walking will generally follow a progression from non–weight-bearing (NWB) to touch down weight bearing (TDWB) to partial weight bearing (PWB) to full weight bearing (FWB). The rate of progression will be dictated by limitations of the injury as well as capabilities of the athlete.

When the injured athlete needs to be partially weight bearing, a cane or perhaps a single crutch can be used to help with balance. In this case the athlete should hold the cane or crutch in the hand on the uninjured side and move the cane forward simultaneously with the injured leg. The athlete should avoid leaning too heavily on the cane or crutch. If this is a problem then the athlete should use two crutches.

SUMMARY

- An emergency is defined as "an unforeseen combination of circumstances and the resulting state that calls for immediate action."[24] The primary concern of emergency aid is to maintain cardiovascular function and, indirectly, central nervous system function. All sports programs should have an emergency action plan that is activated whenever an athlete is seriously injured.
- The athletic trainer must make a systematic assessment of the injured athlete to determine appropriate emergency care. A primary survey assesses and deals with life-threatening situations. Once the athlete is stabilized, the secondary survey makes a more detailed assessment of the injury.
- In adult CPR, the ratio of compression to breaths is 15 to 2, with 80 to 100 compressions per minute. An obstructed airway is relieved by using chest compressions, the finger sweep of the throat, or both.
- Hemorrhage can occur externally and internally. External bleeding can be controlled by direct pressure, by applying pressure at pressure points, and by elevation. Internal hemorrhage can occur subcutaneously, intramuscularly, or within a body cavity.
- Shock can occur from a variety of situations. Shock can be hypovolemic, respiratory, neurogenic, psychogenic, cardiogenic, septic, anaphylactic, and metabolic. Symptoms include pale skin, dilated eyes, weak and rapid pulse, and rapid, shallow breathing. Management includes maintaining normal body temperature and slightly elevating the feet.
- Rest, ice, compression, and elevation (RICE) should be used for the immediate care of a musculoskeletal injury. Ice should be applied for at least twenty minutes every 1 to 1½ hours, and compression and elevation should be continuous for at least seventy-two hours after injury.
- Any suspected fracture should be splinted before the athlete is moved. Commercial rapid form vacuum immobilizers and air splints are most often used as splints in an athletic training setting.
- Great care must be taken in moving the seriously injured athlete. The unconscious athlete must be handled as though he or she has a cervical fracture. Moving an athlete with a suspected serious neck injury must be performed only by persons specifically trained to do so. A spine board should be used for transport to avoid any movement of the cervical region.
- Athletes who are injured will respond emotionally to the situation. Their feelings must be understood and fully accepted by the coach and the athletic trainer.
- The athletic trainer should be responsible for the proper fitting and instruction in the use of crutches or a cane by an athlete with an injury to the lower extremity.
- When removing an injured athlete from a swimming pool, the athletic trainer should make every effort to minimize movement of the head and cervical spine while placing the athlete on a spine board in the water.

Websites

American Red Cross: http://www.redcross.org/what.html

The American Red Cross offers many emergency services and training. This site describes those services, introduces the information provided in various training opportunities, and explains how to obtain that training,

American Heart Association: http://www.amhrt.org

Cervical Spine Stabilization: http://www.trauma.org/spine/cspine-stab.html

This brief article describes the considerations with cervical spine stabilization.

The National Safety Council: http://www.nsc.org/

The National Safety Council is a membership organization with resources on safety, health and environmental topics, training, products, publications, news, and more.

First Aid with Parasol EMT: http://www.parasolemt.com.au

This site provides a comprehensive on-line first aid reference.

First Aid: http://www.mayohealth.org

This Website on first aid care is maintained by the Mayo Clinic.

Solutions to Critical Thinking EXERCISES

12-1 Because of the mechanism of injury, the athletic trainer should suspect that the athlete has a cervical neck injury, and the head should be stabilized throughout. Because the athlete is prone and breathing, the athletic trainer should do nothing until the athlete regains consciousness. An on-field exam should determine the athlete's neurological status. Then the player should be carefully logrolled onto a spine board because CPR could be necessary at any time. The face mask should be removed in case CPR is required. The helmet and shoulder pads should be left in place. The athlete should then be transported to an emergency facility. In this situation the worst mistake the athletic trainer can make is not exercising enough caution.

12-2 If the athletic trainer has been trained to do so and the appropriate equipment is available, supplemental oxygen can be administered using a bag-valve-mask and a pressurized oxygen cylinder to facilitate recovery.

12-3 The athletic trainer must first take precautions to protect against the transmission of bloodborne pathogens. The wound should be cleaned with soap and water. The athletic trainer should apply direct pressure using a gauze pad and should apply cold. If the athlete is not dizzy, he should remain in a sitting position. The athlete should be referred to a physician for suturing. Sterile strips or a butterfly bandage may also be applied, although sutures will generally leave a smaller scar. All blood-contaminated supplies should be disposed of in a clearly marked biohazard bag.

12-4 The athlete may be going into hypovolemic shock secondary to hemorrhage and trauma, which can be a life-threatening situation. The athletic trainer should first direct someone to dial 911 to access the emergency medical system. Next, the athletic trainer must control the bleeding by using direct pressure, elevation, and pressure points. If bleeding is controlled and the rescue squad has not arrived, the forearm should be immobilized in a rapid form vacuum immobilizer. The athlete should be supine, and his feet should be elevated in the shock position. His body temperature should be maintained.

12-5 The ankle should be wrapped with a wet elastic compression wrap. Ice should be applied to both sides of the joint over the compression wrap and secured. The ankle should be elevated so that the leg is above 45 degrees at a minimum. The compression wrap, ice, and elevation should be maintained initially for at least thirty minutes but not longer than an hour. The athletic trainer should also make some determination as to whether a fracture is suspected and make the appropriate referral.

12-6 A rapid form vacuum immobilizer will work well for this injury because of its ability to mold the splint to the joint without causing unnecessary movement. Therefore, the ankle can be immobilized in the current position before transporting the athlete.

12-7 The athletic trainer should place the athlete on a spine board and secure her before extracting her from the pool. Several people may be required to get the athlete appropriately positioned on the spine board while still in the water. The athlete should be given a brief neurological exam to determine the extent of the injury. The athlete should then be transported to an emergency facility in a rescue vehicle.

12-8 The athletic trainer should instruct the athlete in the tripod gait, in which the athlete swings through the crutches without making any surface contact with the injured limb. The tripod gait is also used on stairs. In negotiating stairs, the rule of thumb is go up with the good leg first, followed by crutches, and to go down with the crutches first, followed by the good leg. If the stairs have a handrail, the athlete can hold both crutches with his outside hand. Crutch walking will generally follow a progression: NWB to TDWB to PWB to FWB.

REVIEW QUESTIONS AND CLASS ACTIVITIES

1. What considerations are important in a well-planned system for handling emergency situations?
2. Discuss the rules for managing and moving an unconscious athlete.
3. What are the life-threatening conditions that should be evaluated in the primary survey?
4. What are the ABCs of life support?
5. Identify the major steps in giving CPR and managing an obstructed airway. When might these procedures be used in a sports setting?
6. List the basic steps in assessing a musculoskeletal injury.
7. What techniques should be used to stop external hemorrhage?
8. Numerous types of shock can occur from a sports injury or illness; list them and their management.
9. What first-aid procedures are used to decrease hemorrhage, inflammation, muscle spasm, and pain from a musculoskeletal injury?
10. Describe the basic concepts of emergency splinting.
11. How should an athlete with a suspected spinal injury be transported?
12. What techniques can be used to transport an athlete with a suspected musculoskeletal injury?
13. Discuss the methods for extracting an injured athlete from a swimming pool.
14. Explain how to properly fit crutches.
15. Describe methods that should be used when dealing with an injured athlete's emotional response to the injury.

REFERENCES

1. Almquist J: Spine injury management: a comprehensive plan for managing the cervical spine–injured football player, *Sports Med Update* 13(1):8, 1998.
2. American Red Cross: American Red Cross first aid/CPR/AED program instructors manual, Boston, 2001, American Red Cross.
3. American Red Cross: *Lifeguarding Instructors Manual training,* San Bruno, Calif., 2001, Staywell.
4. Andersen J, Courson R, Kleiner D: National Athletic Trainers' Association position statement: emergency planning in athletics, *J Ath Train* 37(1):99, 2002.
5. Brukner P, Kahn K, Hunte G: Sporting emergencies. In Brukner P, editor: *Clinical sports medicine,* ed 2, Sydney, 2002, McGraw-Hill.
6. Cartwright LA, Pitney WA: Extrication. In Cartwright LA, editor: *Athletic training for student assistants,* Champaign, Ill, 1999, Human Kinetics.
7. Delforge G: Sports injury assessment and problem identification. In Delforge G, editor: *Musculoskeletal trauma implications for sports injury management,* Champaign, IL, 2002, Human Kinetics.
8. Del Rossi G: Management of cervical-spine injuries. *Athletic Therapy Today* 7(2):46, 2002.
9. Del Rossi G, Horodyski M, Powers M: A comparison of spine-board transfer techniques and the effect of training on performance, *J Ath Train* 38(3), 2003.
10. Dick BH, Anderson JM: Emergency care of the injured athlete. In Zachazewski JE et al, editors: *Athletic injuries and rehabilitation,* Philadelphia, 1996, WB Saunders.
11. Farrell RN: AEDs and cardiac resuscitation: is prevention part of your plan? *Athletic Therapy Today* 6(3):46, 2001.
12. Feld F: Management of the critically injured football player, *J Ath Train* 28(3):206, 1993.
13. Feld F: Technology and emergency care, *Athletic Therapy Today* 2(5):28, 1997.
14. Fessey J: First aid for head and spinal injuries in sport, *Physiotherapy in Sport* 20(3):4, 1997.
15. Fincher AL: Managing medical emergencies, Part 1, *Athletic Therapy Today* 6(3):44, 2001.
16. Fuchs E: Face mask removal time of four face mask extrication devices. Master's thesis, San Jose State University, 1994.
17. Green BN: Important changes in the 2000 CPR guidelines, *J Sports Chiropractic & Rehabilitation* 15(2):80, 2001.
18. Hay JM: Taping, splinting, and fitting of athletic equipment. In Baker CL et al, editors: *The Hughston Clinic sports medicine book,* Baltimore, Md, 1995, Williams & Wilkins.
19. Helmet removal guidelines. In Schultz S, editor: *Sports medicine handbook,* Indianapolis, 2001, National Federation of State High School Athletic Associations.
20. Helmut removal guidelines, *Sports Med Update* 15(1):4, 2000.
21. Herbert D: Plan to save lives: create and rehearse an emergency response plan, *ACSM's Health & Fitness Journal* 1(5):34, 1997.
22. Herbert DL: Developing a comprehensive sports medicine emergency care plan, *Sports Med Stand Malprac Report* 7(4):49, 1995.
23. Jenkins H, Valovich T, Arnold B: Removal tools are faster and produce less force and torque on the helmet than cutting tools during face-mask retraction, *J Ath Train* 37(3):246, 2002.
24. Karren KJ, Hafen BQ: *First aid for colleges and universities,* Boston, 2003, Benjamin Cummings.
25. Kleiner D, Almquist J, Bailes J: *Prehospital care of the spine-injured athlete: a document from the Inter-Association Task Force for Appropriate Care of the Spine-Injured Athlete,* Dallas, 2001, National Athletic Trainers' Association.
26. Kleiner DM: 10 questions about football-helmet and face-mask removal: a review of the recent literature, *Athletic Therapy Today* 6(3):29, 2001.
27. Kleiner DM: Football helmet face mask removal, *Athletic Therapy Today* 1(1):11, 1996.
28. Knight K: *Cryotherapy in sport injury management,* Champaign, Ill, 1995, Human Kinetics.
29. Knox KE, Kleiner DM: The efficiency of tools used to retract a football helmet face mask, *J Ath Train* 32(3):211, 1997.
30. LaPrade RF, Schnetzler KA, Broxterman RJ: Cervical spine alignment in the immobilized ice hockey player: a computed tomographic analysis of the effects of helmet removal, *Am J Sports Med* 28(6):800, 2000.
31. Magee DL: *Orthopedic physical assessment,* Philadelphia, 2002, WB Saunders.
32. Martin DE: Emergency medicine and the underage athlete, *J Ath Train* 29(3):200, 1994.
33. Meredith RM, Butcher JD: Field splinting of suspected fractures: preparation, assessment, and application. *Physician Sportsmed* 25(10):29, 1997.
34. National Athletic Trainers' Association: *Position stand: helmet removal guidelines,* Dallas, 1998, National Athletic Trainers' Association.
35. National Collegiate Athletic Association: Guidelines for helmet fitting and removal. In Benson M, editor: *2003–2004 NCAA sports medicine handbook,* Indianapolis, Ind, 2003. National Collegiate Athletic Association.
36. National Safety Council: *First aid and CPR,* Boston, 2001, Jones & Bartlett.
37. Ortolani A: Helmets and face masks, *J Ath Train* 27(4):294, 1992 (letter).
38. Palumbo MA, Hulstyn MJ, Fadale PD: The effect of protective football equipment on alignment of the injured cervical spine: radiographic analysis in a cadaveric model, *Am J Sports Med* 24(4):446, 1996.
39. Patel M, Rund D: Emergency removal of football helmets, *Physician Sportsmed* 22(9):57, 1994.
40. Prentice WE: Considerations in designing a rehabilitation program, In Prentice WE: *Rehabilitation techniques in sports medicine and athletic training,* St. Louis, 2004, McGraw-Hill.
41. Prinsen R, Syrotuik D, Reid D: Position of the cervical vertebrae during helmet removal and cervical collar application in football and hockey, *Cl J Sports Med* 5(3):155, 1995.
42. Putman L: Alternative methods for football helmet face mask removal, *J Ath Train* 27(2):107, 1992.
43. Ransone J, Kersey R, Walsh K: The efficacy of the rapid form cervical vacuum immobilizer in cervical spine immobilization of the equipped football player, *J Ath Train* 35(1):65, 2000.
44. Ransone J, Dunn-Bennett LR: Assessment of first-aid knowledge and decision making of high school athletic coaches, *Journal Ath Train* 34(3): 267, 1999.
45. Ray R: Helmets and face masks, *J Ath Train* 27(4):294, 1992 (letter).
46. Ray R, Luchies C, Frens M: Cervical spine motion in football players during 3 airway-exposure techniques, *J Ath Train* 37(2):172, 2002.
47. Ray R, Luchies C, Bazuin D: Airway preparation techniques for the cervical spine–injured football player, *J Ath Train* 30(3):217, 1995.
48. Roberts WO: Helmet removal in head and neck trauma, *Physician Sportsmed* 26(7): 77, 1998.
49. Sailer SM, Lewis SB: Rehabilitation and splinting of common upper-extremity injuries in athletes, *Clin Sports Med* 14(2):411, 1995.
50. Schnirring L: AEDs gain foothold in sports medicine, *Physician Sportsmed* 29(4): 2001.
51. Segan RD, Cassidy C, Bentkowski J: A discussion of the issue of football helmet removal in suspected cervical spine injuries, *J Ath Train* 28(4):294, 1993.
52. Starkey C, Ryan J: *Evaluation of orthopedic and athletic injuries,* Philadelphia, 2002, FA Davis.
53. Swartz E, Armstrong C, Rankin J: A 3-dimensional analysis of face-mask removal tools in inducing helmet movement, *J Ath Train* 37(2):178, 2002.
54. Swartz E, Norkus S, Armstrong C: Face-mask removal: movement and time associated with cutting of the loop straps, *J Ath Train* 38(2):120, 2003.

55. *Taber's cyclopedic medical dictionary,* Philadelphia, 2002, FA Davis.
56. Terry G, Kyle J, Ellis J: Sudden cardiac arrest in athletic medicine, *J Ath Train* 36(2):205, 2001.
57. Tierney R, Mattacola C, Sitler M: Head position and football equipment influence cervical spinal-cord space during immobilization, *J Ath Train* 37(2):185, 2002.
58. United States Olympic Committee/American Red Cross: *Sport safety training: injury prevention and care handbook,* St Louis, 1997, Mosby Lifeline.
59. Veenema KR, Swenson EJ: Laryngeal trauma: securing the airway on the field, *Physician Sportsmed* 23(1):71, 1995.
60. Walsh K: Thinking proactively: the emergency action plan. *Athletic Therapy Today* 6(5):57, 2001.
61. Waninger KN: On-field management of potential cervical spine injury in helmeted football players: leave the helmet on, *Cl J Sports Med* 8(2):124, 1998.
62. Wilkerson GB: External compression for controlling traumatic edema, *Physician Sportsmed* 13:96, 1985.

ANNOTATED BIBLIOGRAPHY

American Red Cross: American Red Cross *First aid: responding to emergencies,* San Brunon, CA, 2001, Staywell, Co.

Karren KJ, Hafen BQ: *First aid for colleges and universities,* Boston, 2003, Benjamin Cummings.

A well-illustrated, simple approach to the treatment of emergency illness and injury.

Kleiner D, Almquist J, Bailes J: *Prehospital care of the spine-injured athlete: a document from the Inter-Association Task Force for Appropriate Care of the Spine-Injured Athlete,* Dallas, 2001, National Athletic Trainers' Association.

A well-referenced monograph that details consensus recommendations from NATA and a variety of other sports medicine organizations relative to the emergency care of an athlete with a suspected spinal injury from the time of injury until arrival at a medical care facility.

Leikin JB, Feldman BJ: *American Medical Association handbook of first aid and emergency care,* Philadelphia, 2000, Random House.

Covering urgent emergency situations as well as the common injuries and ailments that occur in every family, this AMA guide takes the reader step-by-step through basic first-aid techniques, the medical symptoms to recognize before an emergency occurs, and what to do when one does occur.

Magee DJ: *Orthopedic physical assessment,* Philadelphia, 2002, WB Saunders.

An extremely well-illustrated book, with excellent coverage. Its strength lies in its coverage of injuries commonly found during athletic training.

National Safety Council: *First aid and CPR,* Boston, 2001, Jones & Bartlett.

All three are standard, well-written, and extremely well-illustrated texts that deal with first aid and emergency procedures. Although most of the information is directed at the general population, the principles and techniques can certainly be applied to the injured athlete. Any one of the three will provide an excellent resource for the athletic trainer.

Chapter 13 Off-the-Field Injury Evaluation

When you finish this chapter you should be able to

- Differentiate between evaluation and diagnosis.
- Review terminology used in injury evaluation.
- Apply the HOPS off-the-field evaluation scheme.
- Organize the process for documenting the findings of an off-the-field or progress evaluation.
- Recognize additional diagnostic techniques available to the athletic trainer through the team physician.

EVALUATION OF SPORTS INJURIES

Injury evaluation is an essential skill for the athletic trainer. In athletic training, four distinct evaluations are routinely conducted: the (1) *preparticipation examination,* done prior to the start of preseason practice, was discussed in Chapter 2; the initial (2) *on-the-field injury assessment,* which was discussed in great detail in Chapter 12, is done immediately after acute injury to determine the immediate course of acute care, necessary first aid, and the handling of emergency situations; a more detailed (3) *off-the-field injury evaluation* is done in the athletic training room, clinic, emergency room, or physician's office after appropriate first aid has been rendered; and a (4) *progress evaluation* is done periodically throughout the rehabilitative process to determine the progress and effectiveness of a specific treatment regimen. This chapter concentrates on the off-the-field evaluation and the progress evaluation.

INJURY EVALUATION VERSUS DIAGNOSIS

Athletic trainers recognize and evaluate sports injuries, but by law they cannot make diagnoses.

A diagnosis denotes what disease, injury, or syndrome a person has or is believed to have. Making a diagnosis is usually reserved for individuals specifically licensed by a state to do so. Health professionals such as physicians are generally permitted to diagnose. Health professionals restricted to diagnosing one body area are dentists, who are limited to diagnosing mouth disorders; podiatrists, who are limited to diagnosing foot disorders; and optometrists, who are limited to determining refractory problems of the eyes and prescribing lenses to increase the efficiency of vision. Chiropractors usually base their diagnoses on the relationship of the body's structure to its overall function. In some states, nurse practitioners may make limited diagnoses.

There is a fine line between the evaluation of an injury and its diagnosis. Debating this difference serves no useful purpose other than to confound the distinction further. In situations in which time is of the essence, as is often the case in sports injuries, the ability to evaluate quickly, accurately, and decisively is vitally important. In such situations, the athletic trainer must remain within the limits of his or her ability and training and must act in full accord with professional ethics and state laws.

BASIC KNOWLEDGE REQUIREMENTS

To examine sports injuries the athletic trainer must have a thorough knowledge of human anatomy and its function and of the hazards inherent in sports.

The athletic trainer who is examining an athlete with a sports injury must have a general knowledge of normal human anatomy and biomechanics and an understanding of the major hazards inherent in a particular sport. Without this information, accurate assessment is impossible.

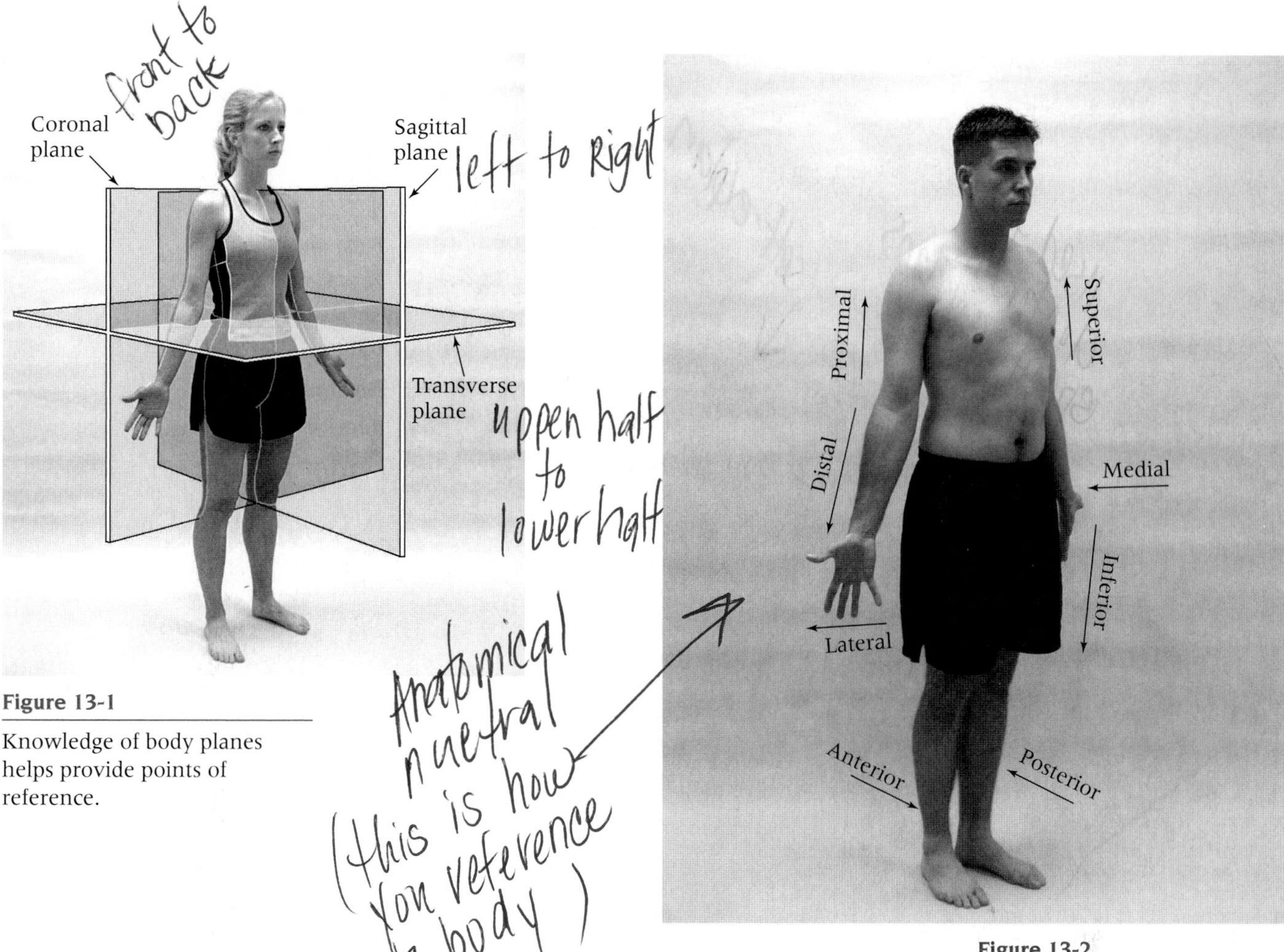

Figure 13-1

Knowledge of body planes helps provide points of reference.

Figure 13-2

Anatomical directions refer to the position of one body part in relation to another.

Normal Human Anatomy

Surface Anatomy

Understanding typical surface or topographical anatomy is essential when evaluating a possible injury. Key surface landmarks provide the examiner with indications of the normal or injured anatomical structures lying underneath the skin.[9]

Body planes and anatomical directions Associated with surface anatomy is the understanding of body planes and anatomical directions. Body planes are used as points of reference from which positions of body parts are indicated. The three most commonly mentioned planes are the midsagittal, transverse, and coronal (or frontal) planes (Figure 13-1). Anatomical directions refer to the position of one part in relation to another (Figure 13-2).

Abdominopelvic quadrants and regions The abdominopelvic *quadrants* are the four corresponding regions of the abdomen that are divided for evaluative and diagnostic purposes (Figure 13-3A). A second division system divides the abdominopelvic area into nine *regions* (Figure 13-3B). The quadrants and regions are used by clinicians as reference points for locating underlying organs or abdominopelvic pain or abnormality. The regions tend to be more specific relative to organ location, while the quadrants are simpler and generally more commonly used.

Musculoskeletal System Anatomy

Anyone examining the musculoskeletal system for sports injuries must have an in-depth knowledge of both structural and functional anatomy.[11] This knowledge encompasses the major joints and bony structures as well as skeletal musculature. A knowledge of neural anatomy is also of major importance, particularly that which is

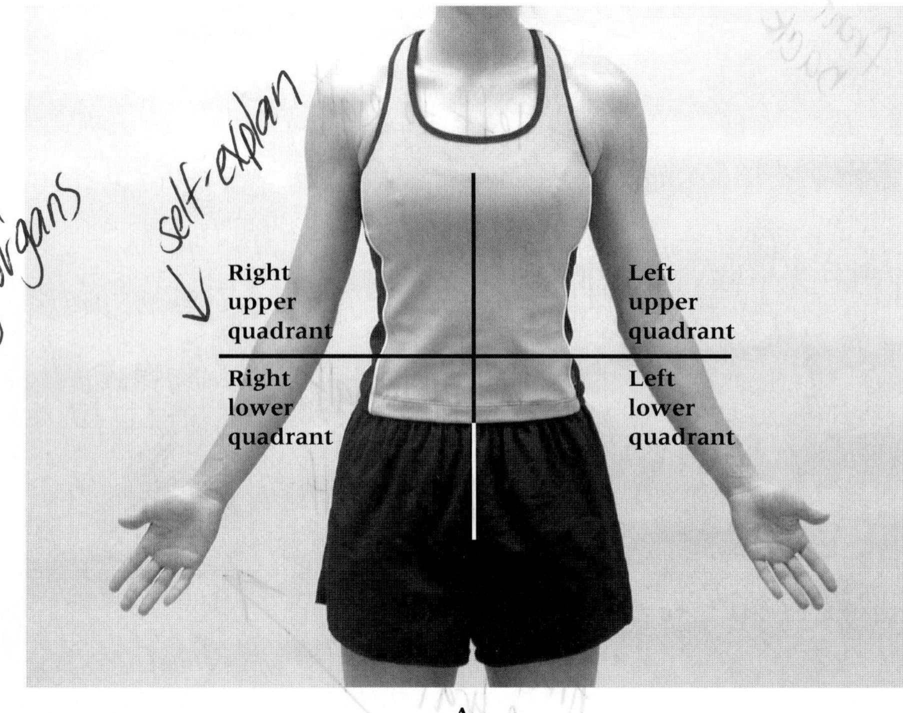

A

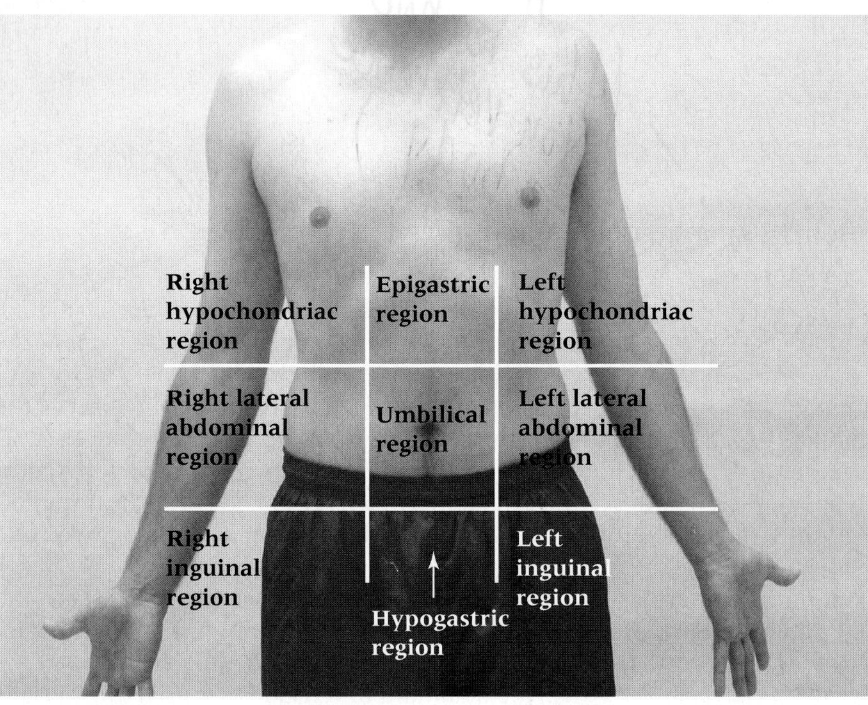

B

Figure 13-3

The division of the abdomen into quadrants and regions. **A,** Division into four quadrants. **B,** Division into nine regions.

13-1 Critical Thinking Exercise

A soccer player is taken down and lies on the field holding her knee. The athletic trainer comes onto the field and quickly examines the knee. There does not appear to be any major instability, so the athlete is moved to the sideline where the trainer does a more careful evaluation. The athletic trainer is fairly certain that the soccer player has sustained a minor grade 1 medial collateral ligament (MCL) sprain and elects not to refer the athlete to the physician. The next day the athlete comes into the training room with a very swollen knee. The athletic trainer now decides to refer the athlete to the physician. On examination, the physician determines that the athlete does have an MCL sprain but has also sustained a tear of the medial meniscus.

? How could the athletic trainer have handled this situation better?

involved in movement control and sensation, along with the neural factors that influence superficial and deep pain.

Standard musculoskeletal terminology for bodily positions and deviations When assessing the musculoskeletal system, a standard terminology must be used to convey precise information to others who may become professionally involved with the athlete. These terms are found in Table 13-1.

TABLE 13-1 Standard Orthopedic Definitions for Positions and Deviations

Term	Definition
Abduction	To draw away or deviate from the midline of the body
Adduction	To deviate toward or draw toward the midline of the body
Eversion	Turning outward
Extension	To straighten; when the part distal to a joint extends, it straightens; joint angle decreases toward 0 degrees
External rotation	Rotary motion in the transverse plane away from the midline
Flexion	To bend; when a joint is flexed, the part distal to the joint bends; joint angle increases toward 180 degrees
Internal rotation	Rotary motion in the transverse plane toward the midline
Inversion	Turning inward
Pronation	Applied to the foot and assuming the foot is in a prone position, it refers to a combination of eversion and abduction movements, resulting in a lowering of the medial margin of the foot; applied to the hand, it means the palm is turned downward
Supination	To assume a supine position; applied to the foot, it refers to raising the medial margin of the foot; applied to the hand, it refers to turning the palm upward
Valgus	Deviation of a part or portion of the extremity distal to a joint away from the midline of the body
Varus	Deviation of a part or portion of an extremity distal to a joint toward the midline of the body

Biomechanics

The understanding of biomechanics is the foundation for the assessment of musculoskeletal sports injuries. **Biomechanics** is the application of mechanical forces, which may stem from within or outside the body, to living organisms. Of major concern is pathomechanics, which may precede an injury. **Pathomechanics** refers to mechanical forces that are applied to the body because of a structural body deviation, leading to faulty alignment. Pathomechanics often cause overuse syndromes.

biomechanics Application of mechanical forces to living organisms.

pathomechanics Mechanical forces that are applied to a living organism and adversely change the body's structure and function.

Understanding the Sport

The more that the athletic trainer who examines sports injuries knows about how a sport is performed and its potential for trauma, the better his or her injury assessment can be.[28] To fully understand injuries that occur in a sport, the examiner needs a detailed knowledge of the correct kinesiological and biomechanical principles that should be applied. Violation of these principles can lead to repetitive and overuse syndromes. Understanding how an acute or chronic injury might occur helps the examiner focus more directly on tissues that have been affected.

Descriptive Assessment Terms

When evaluating sports injuries, examiners use selected terms to describe and characterize what is being learned about the condition. Students should become familiar with these terms.

Etiology refers to the cause of an injury or disease (for example, an athlete rolls the foot inward when landing after jumping). In sports medicine, the term *mechanism* is often used interchangeably with etiology. A **mechanism** refers to the mechanical description of the cause (for example, inversion and plantar flexion). **Pathology** refers to the structural and functional changes that result from the injury process.

After developing an understanding of an injury's etiology, the athletic trainer ascertains symptoms and signs. **Symptom** refers to a perceptible change in an athlete's body or its functions that indicates an injury or disease. Symptoms are subjective and

etiology Cause of disease.

mechanism Mechanical description of the cause.

pathology Structural and functional changes that result from injury.

symptom Change that indicates injury or disease.

sign
Indicator of a disease.

diagnosis
Name of a specific condition.

prognosis
Predicted outcome of an injury.

sequela
Condition resulting from disease or injury.

syndrome
Group of symptoms that indicate a condition or disease.

are described by the athlete to the coach, athletic trainer, or physician. In comparison, a **sign** is objective, a definitive and obvious indicator for a specific condition. Signs are often determined when the athlete is examined.

After it is inspected, an injury may be assigned a *grade.* Grade 1, 2, or 3 corresponds to an injury that is mild, moderate, or severe, respectively. Sometimes the term *degree* is used in place of grade, depending on the athletic trainer's preference.

Diagnosis denotes the name of a specific condition. To establish the diagnosis of an athlete's injury or illness, the athletic trainer must study all aspects of the condition. A *differential diagnosis* is a systematic method of diagnosing a disorder that lacks unique symptoms or signs. The differential diagnosis refers to a list of possible causes for an injury or condition. It involves a process of including, excluding, and prioritizing possibilities.[7] Prioritizing means to list the possible causes from the most likely to the least likely. Applying the differential diagnosis technique, the athletic trainer first develops a list of possible causes. By obtaining a history, observing, palpating, and conducting special tests, the clinician can include or exclude some of the possible causes. Occasionally, the terms *working diagnosis* or *hypothesis* are also used to refer to the differential diagnosis. These terms also suggest a process for determining the most likely diagnosis for that condition. Once all the possible information has been gathered about the athlete's condition, a **prognosis** is made. A prognosis is a prediction of the course of the condition. In other words, the athlete is told what to expect as the injury heals. The amount of pain, swelling, or loss of function is discussed. Prognosis also refers to the projected outcome of an illness or injury and to the length of time predicted for complete recovery. For the athlete, prognosis translates into "the length of time before I can compete."

Sequela refers to a condition following and resulting from a disease or injury. Sequela is the development of an additional condition as a complication of an existing disease or injury. For example, pneumonia might result from a bout with the flu, or osteoarthritis might follow a severe joint sprain.

The term **syndrome** is used throughout the text and refers to a group of symptoms and signs that, together, indicate a particular injury or disease.

THE OFF-THE-FIELD INJURY EVALUATION PROCESS

The on-the-field injury assessment discussed in detail in Chapter 12, is done on the field immediately after injury to rule out those injuries that may potentially become life threatening, to assess musculoskeletal injuries, and to determine how the athlete should be transported from the field. Once the athlete has been transported from the site of initial injury, away from the excitement and confusion inherent in an athletic arena, a more detailed off-the-field injury evaluation is performed. This detailed evaluation may be performed on the sideline, in the training room, in an emergency room, or in a sports medicine clinic. An injury may be evaluated immediately after the athlete has left the playing field when it is still in an acute phase, or it may take place several hours or perhaps even days following acute injury.

HOPS
- History
- Observation
- Palpation
- Special tests

The evaluation scheme is divided into four broad categories: history, observation, palpation, and a number of special tests that provide additional information about the extent of injuries. This evaluation scheme is sometimes referred to as the **HOPS** format (see *Focus Box:* "Off-the-field evaluation sequence"). The following discussion provides an overview of some of the steps and techniques that can be used in the evaluation process. (Chapters 18 through 27 provide the reader with specific injury assessment procedures.)

History

Taking a detailed history from the athlete is perhaps the most critical aspect of the off-the-field evaluation.

Obtaining as much information as possible about the history of the injury is perhaps the single most important aspect of the injury evaluation.[9] Understanding how the injury may have occurred and listening to the athlete's complaints and answers to key questions can provide important clues to the exact nature of the injury. The athletic

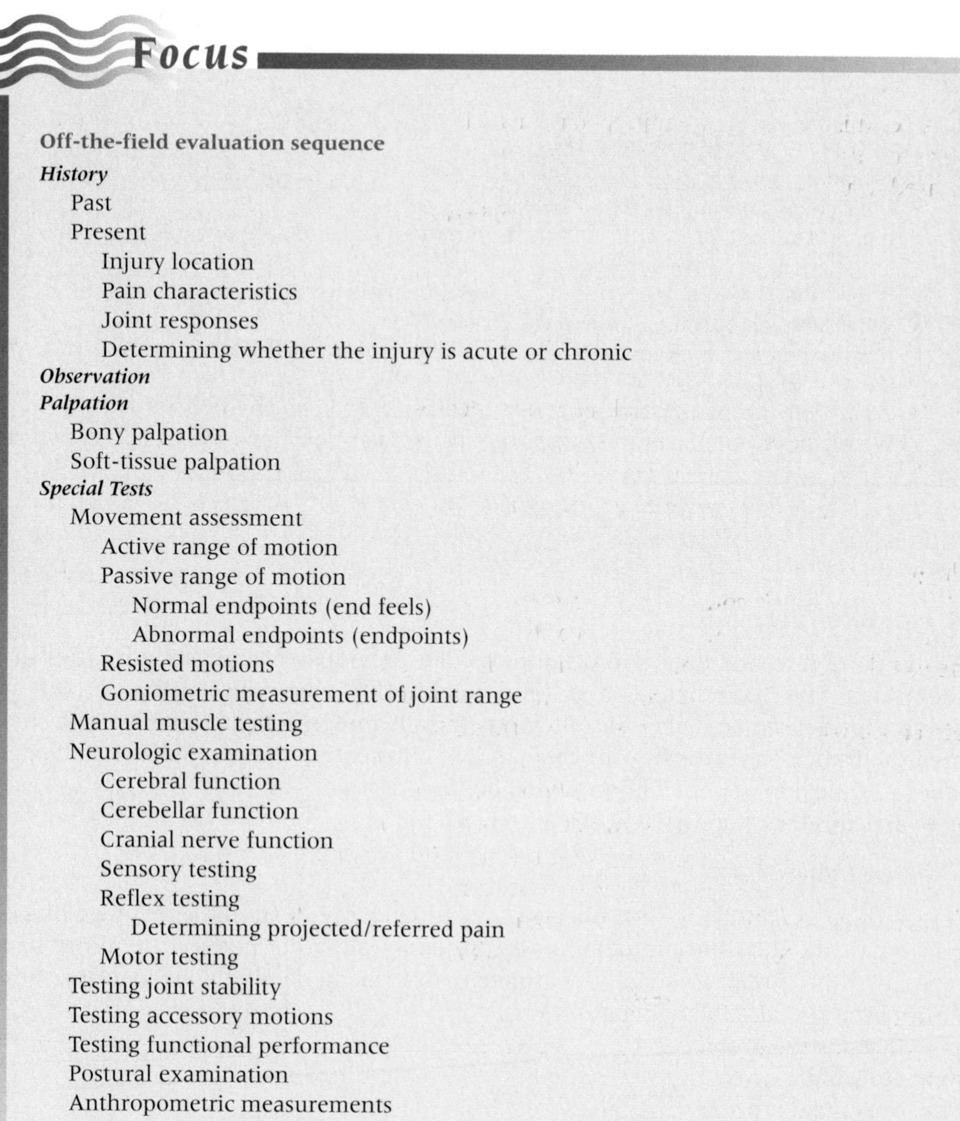

Focus

Off-the-field evaluation sequence

History
- Past
- Present
  - Injury location
  - Pain characteristics
  - Joint responses
  - Determining whether the injury is acute or chronic

Observation

Palpation
- Bony palpation
- Soft-tissue palpation

Special Tests
- Movement assessment
  - Active range of motion
  - Passive range of motion
    - Normal endpoints (end feels)
    - Abnormal endpoints (endpoints)
  - Resisted motions
  - Goniometric measurement of joint range
- Manual muscle testing
- Neurologic examination
  - Cerebral function
  - Cerebellar function
  - Cranial nerve function
  - Sensory testing
  - Reflex testing
    - Determining projected/referred pain
  - Motor testing
- Testing joint stability
- Testing accessory motions
- Testing functional performance
- Postural examination
- Anthropometric measurements
- Volumetric measurements

trainer becomes a detective in pursuit of as much accurate information as possible, which will lead to a determination of the true nature of the injury (see *Focus Box:* "History of musculoskeletal injuries"). From the history, the athletic trainer develops strategies for further examination and possible immediate and follow-up management.[3]

When obtaining a history, the athletic trainer should do the following:

- Be calm and reassuring.
- Express questions that are simple, not leading.
- Listen carefully to the athlete's complaints.
- Maintain eye contact to try and see what the athlete is feeling.
- Record exactly what the athlete says without interpretation.

Questions might be stated under specific headings in an attempt to get as complete a historical picture as possible. In many cases, a history becomes clear-cut because the mechanism, trauma, and pathology are obvious; in other situations, symptoms and signs may be obscured.

It is alright to observe the athlete when taking a history but there should be no palpation while the athlete is explaining what happened and what they are feeling.[8]

13-2

***Critical Thinking* Exercise**

A fencer comes into the training room complaining of pain in his shoulder that he has had for about a week. He indicates that he first hurt the shoulder when lifting weights but did not think it was a bad injury. During the past week he has not been able to lift because of pain. He has continued to fence during practice, but his shoulder seems to be getting worse instead of better.

? What is the standard evaluation scheme that the athletic trainer should use?

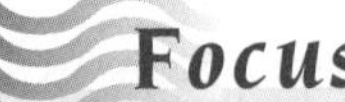

History of musculoskeletal injuries

Information to obtain:

- Chief complaints and present problems
- If pain is present, its location, character, duration, variation, aggravation, distribution or radiation, intensity, and course
- Is the pain increased or decreased by specific activities or stresses?
- What situation or trauma caused the problem?
- Has the problem occurred before? If so, when, and how was it treated? Was treatment successful?
- What were the existing environmental conditions when the injury occurred?
- What type of equipment was being worn at the time of the injury?

Past History of Injury

It is important to first obtain information about previous or preexisting injuries that the athlete may have had. The athletic trainer who is working with an athlete or group of athletes on a daily basis often has the advantage of being familiar with their medical history. Nevertheless, the first piece of information that should be obtained in an off-the-field injury evaluation would be

- Has this ever happened before? If so, when?

Present Injury

If the athlete is conscious and coherent, the athletic trainer should encourage him or her to describe the injury in detail. If the athletic trainer did not see the injury happen, he or she should try to get the athlete to describe in detail the mechanism of the injury by asking the following questions.

- What is the problem?
- How did it occur?
- When did it occur?
- Did you fall? How did you land?
- Which direction did your joint move?
- Did you hear or feel anything when it occurred?

If the athlete is unable to describe accurately how the injury occurred, perhaps a teammate or someone who observed the event can do so.

Injury location The athletic trainer should ask the athlete to locate the area of complaint by pointing to it with one finger only. If the athlete can point to a specific pain site, the injury is probably localized. If the exact pain site cannot be indicated, the injury may be generalized and nonspecific.

Pain characteristics The athlete should describe as accurately as possible exactly what the pain feels like.

- What type of pain is it? Nerve pain is sharp, bright, or burning. Bone pain tends to be localized and piercing. Pain in the vascular system tends to be poorly localized, aching, and referred from another area. Muscle pain is often dull, aching, and referred to another area.[21]
- Where is the pain? Determining pain origin makes the evaluation of musculoskeletal injuries difficult. The deeper the injury site, the more difficult it is to match the pain with the site of trauma. This factor often causes treatment to be performed at the wrong site. Conversely, the closer the injury is to the body surface, the better the elicited pain corresponds with the site of pain stimulation.[19]

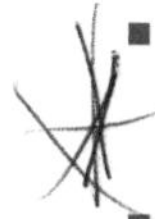

- Does the pain change at different times? Pain that subsides during activity usually indicates a chronic inflammation. Pain that increases in a joint throughout the day indicates a progressive increase in edema.
- Does the athlete feel sensations other than pain? Pressure on nerve roots can produce pain or a sensation of "pins and needles" (paresthesia). What movement, if any, causes pain or other sensations?

Joint responses

- If the injury is related to a joint, is there instability?
- Does the joint feel as though it will give way?
- Does the joint lock and unlock?

Positive responses may indicate that the joint has a loose body that is catching or that is inhibiting the normal muscular support in the area.

Determining whether the injury is acute or chronic The examiner should ask the athlete how long he or she has had the symptoms and how often they appear.

Observation

The examiner gains knowledge and understanding of the athlete's major complaint not only from a history but also through general observation, often done at the same time the history is taken. What is observed is commonly modified by the athlete's major complaints. The following are suggested as specific points to observe:

- How does the athlete move?
- Is there a limp?
- Are movements abnormally slow, jerky, and asynchronous?
- Is the athlete unable to move a body part?
- Is the athlete holding his or her body stiffly to protect against pain?
- Does the athlete's facial expression indicate pain or lack of sleep?
- Are there any obvious body asymmetries?
- Is there an obvious deformity?
- Does soft tissue appear swollen or wasted as a result of atrophy?
- Are there unnatural protrusions or lumps such as occur with a dislocation or fracture?
- Is there a postural malalignment?
- Are there abnormal sounds such as crepitus when the athlete moves?
- Does a body area appear inflamed?
- Is there swelling, heat, or redness?

Palpation

Some examiners use palpation in the beginning of the examination procedure, whereas others use it only when they believe they have identified the specific injury site by other assessment means.[6,20] In some cases, palpation would be beneficial at both the beginning and the end of the examination. The two areas of palpation are bony and soft tissue. Like all examination procedures, palpation must be performed systematically. The athletic trainer starts with very light pressure, followed by gradually deeper pressure, and usually begins away from the site of complaint and gradually moves toward it.

Bony Palpation

Both the injured and noninjured sites should be palpated and compared. The sense of touch might reveal an abnormal gap at a joint, swelling on a bone, joints that are misaligned, or abnormal protuberances associated with a joint or a bone.

Soft-Tissue Palpation

Through palpation, with the athlete as relaxed as possible, the athletic trainer can assess normal soft-tissue relationships. Tissue deviations such as swelling, lumps, gaps, abnormal muscle tension, and temperature variations can be detected. The palpation

13-3

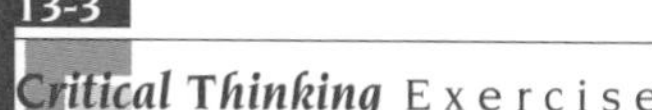

Critical Thinking Exercise

An athletic trainer is evaluating a volleyball player who complains of pain in her elbow. During the evaluation, manual muscle testing and active and passive range of motion tests reveal pain when the elbow is moved into extension both actively and passively. However, there is no pain when the elbow is moved actively into flexion.

? Does the injury more likely involve the ligament or the musculotendinous unit?

13-4

Critical Thinking Exercise

A baseball player complains of pain in his right shoulder. A resisted test for shoulder external rotation was weak and painful.

? What does this evaluation indicate about the tissue? If the result of the resisted motion test was weak and painless, what is a possible conclusion for this evaluation?

of soft tissue can detect where ligaments or tendons have torn. The athletic trainer can determine variations in the shape of structures, differences in tissue tightness and textures, differentiation of tissue that is pliable and soft from tissue that is more resilient. Involuntary muscle twitching or tremors may also be felt. Excessive skin dryness and moisture can also be noted. The athletic trainer can become aware of abnormal skin sensations such as diminished sensation (dysesthesia), numbness (anesthesia), or increased sensation (hyperesthesia). Like bony palpation, soft-tissue palpation must be performed on both sides of the body for comparison.

Special Tests

Special tests have been designed for almost every body region to detect specific pathologies. They are often used to substantiate what has been learned from the history, observation, and palpation portions of the evaluation process.[20]

Movement Assessment

Movement examination includes:

- Active movement
- Passive movement
- Resisted isometric movement

If a joint or soft-tissue lesion exists, the athlete is likely to complain of pain on movement. Cyriax has developed a method for locating and identifying a lesion by applying tension selectively to each of the structures that might produce this pain.[6] Tissues are classified as contractile or inert. Contractile tissues include muscles and their tendons; inert tissues include bones, ligaments, joint capsules, fascia, bursae, nerve roots, and dura mater.

If a lesion is present in contractile tissue, pain will occur on active motion in one direction and on passive motion in the opposite direction. Thus, a muscle strain would cause pain on both active contraction and passive stretch. Contractile tissues are tested through the midrange by an isometric contraction against maximum resistance. The specific location of the lesion within the musculotendinous unit cannot be identified by the isometric contraction.[5]

A lesion of inert tissue will elicit pain on active and passive movement in the same direction. A sprain of a ligament will result in pain whenever that ligament is stretched either through active contraction or passive stretching. It is not possible to identify a specific lesion of inert tissue by looking at movement patterns alone; other special tests must be done to identify injured structures.[3]

active range of motion Joint motion that occurs because of muscle contraction.

Active range of motion Movement assessment should begin with **active range of motion** (AROM). The athletic trainer should evaluate quality of movement, range of movement, motion in other planes, movement at varying speeds, and strength throughout the range but in particular at the endpoint. A complaint of pain on active motion will not distinguish contractile pain from inert pain, so the athletic trainer must proceed with an evaluation of both passive and resistive motion. An athlete who seems to be pain free in each of these tests throughout a full range should be tested by applying passive pressure at the endpoint.

passive range of motion Movement that is performed completely by the examiner.

Passive range of motion When **passive range of motion** (PROM) is being assessed, the athlete must relax completely and allow the athletic trainer to move the extremity to reduce the influence of the contractile elements. Particular attention should be directed toward the sensation of the athlete at the end of the passive range. Cyriax has described *normal endpoints* and *abnormal endpoints*. Normal endpoints have also referred to as *end feels* and are what the examiner is looking for in passive range of motion testing.[15] Abnormal end points, sometimes referred to simply as *endpoints* are what the examiner feels during ligamentous stress tests.[6] The athletic trainer should categorize the "feel" of the endpoints as described in the following sections.[6]

Normal endpoints (end feels) Normal endpoints include the following:[25]

- Soft-tissue approximation—soft and spongy, a gradual painless stop (e.g., knee flexion)
- Capsular feel—an abrupt, hard, firm endpoint with only a little give (e.g., endpoint of hip rotation)
- Bone to bone—a distinct and abrupt endpoint when two hard surfaces come in contact with one another (e.g., elbow in full extension)

- Muscular—a springy feel with some associated discomfort (e.g., end of shoulder abduction)

Abnormal endpoints (endpoints) Abnormal endpoints include the following:

- Empty feel—movement is definitely beyond the anatomical limit, and pain occurs before the end of the range (e.g., a complete ligament rupture)
- Spasm—involuntary muscle contraction that prevents motion because of pain; also called guarding (e.g., back spasms)
- Loose—occurs in extreme hypermobility (e.g., previously sprained ankle)
- Springy block—a rebound at the endpoint (e.g., meniscus tear)

Throughout the passive range of movement, the athletic trainer is looking for limitation in movement and the presence of pain. An athlete's report of pain before the end of the available range probably indicates acute inflammation in which stretching and manipulation are both contraindicated as treatments. Pain occurring synchronous with the end of the range indicates that the condition is subacute and has progressed to some inert tissue fibrosis. If no pain occurs at the end of the range, the condition is chronic and contractures have replaced inflammation.[29]

Resisted motions The purpose of resisted movement is to evaluate the status of the contractile tissues. The athlete is asked to perform an isometric contraction near the midrange of movement to avoid pinching other inert structures around the joint. Assessing resisted motion is different from manual muscle testing, in which muscle strength is evaluated throughout a full range of motion. Muscular contraction is under neural control; thus lesions of the nervous system may affect the strength of muscular contraction. Cyriax has designed the following system for differentiating lesions through assessment of muscular contraction.[6]

Resisted movement requires an isometric contraction at the midpoint in the range.

1. Strong and painless—normal muscle
2. Strong and painful—minor lesion in some part of the muscle or tendon
3. Weak and painless—complete rupture of muscle or tendon or some nervous system disorder
4. Weak and painful—a gross lesion of contractile tissue
5. Pain on repetition—a single contraction is strong and painless, but repetition produces pain as would exist in some vascular disorder
6. All muscles painful—may indicate a serious emotional or psychological problem

Goniometric measurement of joint range Goniometry, which measures joint range of motion, is an essential procedure during the early, intermediate, and late stages of injury. Full range of motion of an affected body part is a major criterion for an athlete to return to participation. Active and passive joint range of motion can be measured using goniometry (Figure 13-4).

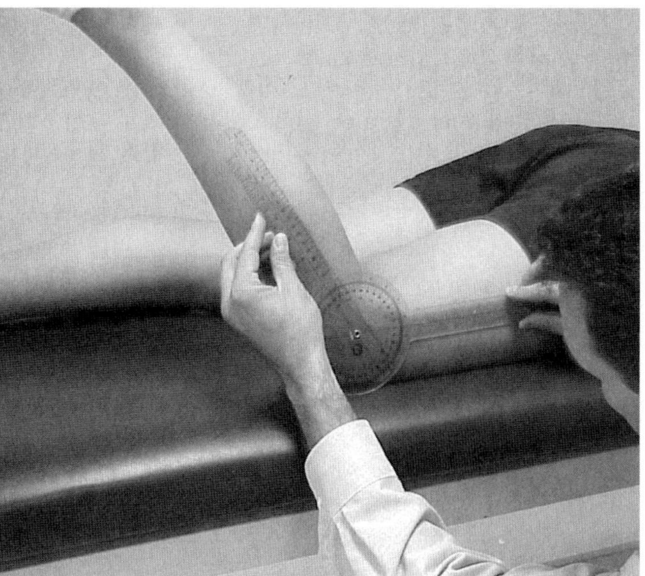

Figure 13-4

Goniometric measurement of knee joint flexion.

TABLE 13-2 Range of Joint Motion

Joint	Action	Degrees of Motion
Shoulder	Flexion	180
	Extension	50
	Adduction	40
	Abduction	180
	Medial rotation	90
	Lateral rotation	90
Elbow	Flexion	145
Forearm	Pronation	80
	Supination	85
Wrist	Flexion	80
	Extension	70
	Abduction	20
	Adduction	45
Hip	Flexion	125
	Extension	10
	Abduction	45
	Adduction	40
	Medial rotation	45
	Lateral rotation	45
Knee	Flexion	140
Ankle	Plantar flexion	45
	Dorsiflexion	20
Foot	Inversion	40
	Eversion	20

Although a number of different types of goniometers are on the market, the most commonly used are ones that measure 0 to 180 degrees in each direction. The arms of the instrument are usually 12 to 16 inches (30 to 40 cm) long, with one arm stationary and the other fully movable.[5,10]

When measuring joint range of motion, the goniometer should generally be placed along the lateral surface of the extremity being measured. The 0, or starting, position for any movement is identical to the standard anatomical position. The athlete should move the joint either actively or passively through the available range to the endpoint. The stationary arm of the goniometer should be placed parallel with the longitudinal axis of the fixed reference part. The movable arm should be placed along the longitudinal axis of the movable segment. (NOTE: The axis of rotation will change throughout the range as movement occurs. Thus the axis of rotation is located at the intersection of the stationary and movable arms.) A reading in degrees of motion should be taken and recorded as either active or passive range of motion for that specific movement. Accuracy and consistency in goniometric measurement require practice and repetition.

The normal available range of motion for specific movements at individual joints is indicated in Table 13-2. Specific goniometric measurement techniques for each joint are described in Chapters 18 through 25.

Manual Muscle Testing

Manual muscle testing is an integral part of the physical examination process.[14,16] The ability of the injured athlete to tolerate varying levels of resistance can indicate a great deal about the extent of the injury to the contractile units. For the athlete, the limitation in muscular strength is generally caused by pain. As pain diminishes and the healing process progresses, levels of muscular strength gradually return to normal. The development of isokinetic testing devices has enabled the athletic trainer to test levels of muscular strength objectively within the limitations of those devices.[13]

TABLE 13-3 Manual Muscle Strength Grading

Grade	Percentage (%)	Qualitative Value	Muscle Strength
5	100	Normal	Complete range of motion (ROM) against gravity with full resistance
4	75	Good	Complete ROM against gravity with some resistance
3	50	Fair	Complete ROM against gravity with no resistance
2	25	Poor	Complete ROM with gravity omitted
1	10	Trace	Evidence of slight contractility with no joint motion
0	0	Zero	No evidence of muscle contractility

Manual muscle testing is usually performed with the athlete positioned so that individual muscles or muscle groups can be isolated and tested through a full range of motion via the application of manual resistance. The ability of the athlete to move through a full range of motion or to offer resistance to movement is subjectively graded by the athletic trainer according to various classification systems and grading criteria that have been developed. Table 13-3 indicates a commonly used grading system for manual muscle testing.

Neurologic Examination

Neurological examination:
- Cerebral function
- Cranial nerve function
- Cerebellar function
- Sensory testing
- Reflex testing
- Motor testing

The neurologic examination usually follows manual muscle testing. Performing a detailed and accurate neurological exam is difficult for everyone, including physicians. The specialized training in neuroanatomy that is necessary to properly perform and interpret this exam is usually not available to the athletic trainer. Therefore, while the athletic trainer should have some knowledge of the process of performing a neurologic exam, the best course is to refer the athlete to a physician who has more experience and specific training. It consists of six major areas: cerebral function, cranial nerve function, cerebellar function, sensory testing, reflex testing, and motor testing. In cases of musculoskeletal injury that do not involve head injury, it is generally not necessary to assess cerebral function, cranial nerve function, and cerebellar function. The athletic trainer should concentrate instead on sensation testing, reflex testing, and motor testing to determine the involvement of the peripheral nervous system after injury.

Cerebral function Tests for general cerebral function include questions that assess general affect, level of consciousness, intellectual performance, emotional status, thought content, sensory interpretation (visual, auditory, tactile), and language skills.

Cranial nerve function The function of the twelve cranial nerves can be quickly determined by assessing the quality of the following: sense of smell, eye tracking, imitation of facial expressions, biting down, balance, swallowing, tongue protrusion, and strength of shoulder shrugs. Table 13-4 lists the cranial nerves and their specific functions.

Cerebellar function Because the cerebellum controls purposeful, coordinated movement, tests such as touching finger to nose, touching finger to finger of examiner, drawing alphabets in the air with the foot, heel-toe walking, and others will determine dysfunction.

Sensory testing A major component of musculoskeletal assessment is determining the distribution of peripheral nerves and dermatomes (Figure 13-5). A dermatome is an area of skin that is innervated by the cutaneous neurons of a single spinal nerve or cranial nerve. The term *dermatome* is sometimes confused with *myotomes,* which are found in developing embryos. Segmental myotomes eventually develop into groups of muscles that are innervated by a specific spinal nerve.

Although peripheral nerve distribution varies with individuals, it is more predictable than dermatome distribution.[13] As the dermatome examination progresses,

TABLE 13-4 Cranial Nerves and Their Function

I.	Olfactory	Smell
II.	Optic	Vision
III.	Oculomotor	Eye movement, opening of eyelid, constriction of pupil, focusing
IV.	Trochlear	Inferior and lateral movement of eye
V.	Trigeminal	Sensation to the face, mastication
VI.	Abducens	Lateral movement of eye
VII.	Facial	Motor nerve of facial expression; taste; control of tear, nasal, sublingual salivary, and submaxillary glands
VIII.	Vestibulocochlear	Hearing and equilibrium
IX.	Glossopharyngeal	Swallowing, salivation, gag reflex, sensation from tongue and ear
X.	Vagus	Swallowing; speech; regulation of pulmonary, cardiovascular, and gastrointestinal functions
XI.	Accessory	Swallowing, innervation of sternocleidomastoid muscle
XII.	Hypoglossal	Tongue movement, speech, swallowing

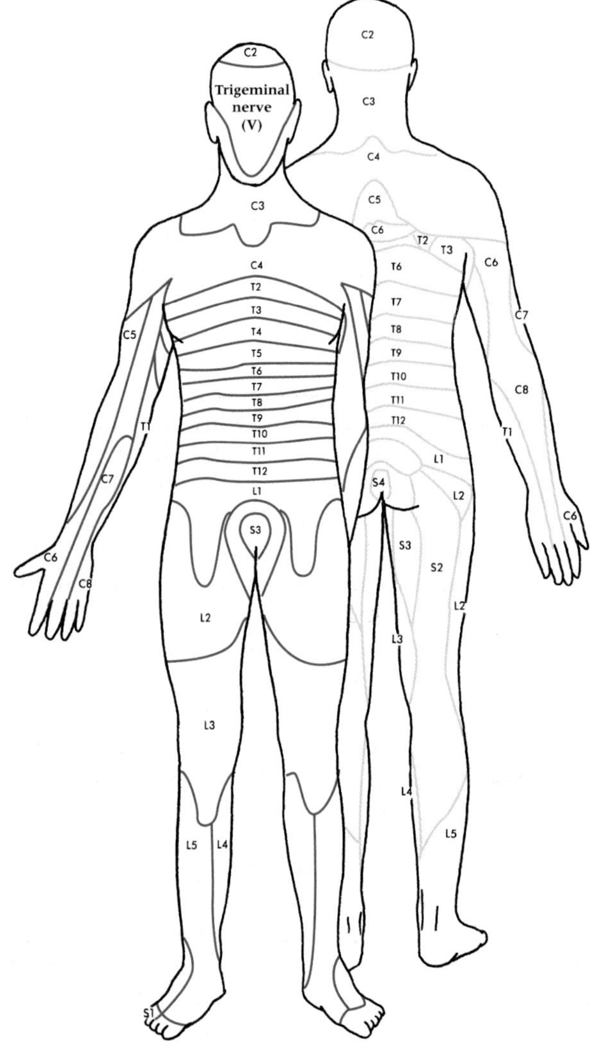

Figure 13-5

Numbness, referred pain, or other nerve involvements often follow the segmental distribution of spinal nerves on the skin's surface.

TABLE 13-5 **Reflex Grading**

	Grade	Definition
Absence of a reflex	0	Areflexia
Diminished reflex	1	Hyporeflexia
Average reflex	2	
Exaggerated reflex	3	Hyperreflexia (increased but not pathological)
Markedly hyperactive	4	Often associated with clonus, but clonus is not required for grade 4

the examiner compares sensation from one side of the body to the other using the following tests:

- Superficial sensation—touch dermatomes with cotton
- Superficial pain—touch dermatomes with a pin
- Deep pressure pain—squeeze a muscle (e.g., gastrocnemius)
- Sensitivity of temperature—touch dermatomes with ice cube
- Sensitivity of vibration—touch dermatomes with a tuning fork
- Position sense—move fingers or toes passively and ask athlete to indicate direction

Reflex testing The term *reflex* refers to an involuntary response to a stimulus. In terms of the neurological examination there are three types of reflexes: deep tendon (somatic) reflexes, superficial reflexes, and pathological reflexes.

A deep tendon reflex is caused by stimulation of the stretch reflex (see Chapter 4) and results in an involuntary contraction of a muscle when its tendon is stretched. Deep tendon reflexes can be elicited at the tendons of the biceps (C5), brachioradialis (C6), triceps (C7), patella (L4), and Achilles (S1). Table 13-5 shows a grading system for deep reflexes.[12]

Superficial reflexes are elicited by stimulation of the skin at specific sites, which produces a reflex muscle contraction. Superficial reflexes include upper abdominal (T7, 8, 9), lower abdominal (T11, 12), cremasteric (T12, L1), plantar (S1, 2), and gluteal (L4, S3). An absence of a superficial reflex is indicative of some lesion in the descending corticospinal tract.

Most, but not all, pathological reflexes are also superficial reflexes. The presence of a pathological reflex indicates a lesion in the descending upper motor neuron, including the spinal cord; an absence indicates integrity. Babinski's sign, in which stroking of the lateral plantar surface produces extension and splaying of the toes, is an example of a pathological reflex.[12] Chaddock's, Oppenheim's, and Gordon's are additional reflexes that are alternatives for eliciting a Babinski response.

In general, hyperactive reflexes, clonus, the Babinski sign and decreased superficial reflexes are all considered to be upper motor neuron signs and usually indicate a lesion somewhere in that tract as it courses through the brain, brain stem, and spinal cord.

Determining projected or referred pain As discussed in Chapter 10, a complaint of deep, burning pain, an ache that is diffused, or of a painful area with no signs of disorder or malfunctioning is most likely referred pain.[5] Cyriax considers that the common sites for pain referral are, in order of importance, joint capsule, tendon, muscle, ligament, and bursa.[6] Pressures from the dura mater or nerve sheath can also produce referred pain or other sensory responses. Palpation of what is thought to be the area at fault often is misleading. Detecting the selective tension of the tissue at fault is one of the best means for gathering correct data. Some musculoskeletal pain is caused by myofascial trigger points, which are not related to deep, referred pain. Palpation is used to determine the presence or absence of tense tissue bands and tender trigger points.

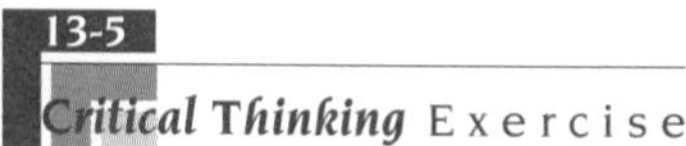

A receiver in football has his feet taken out from under him by a tackler and lands flat on his lower back with his legs above him. An on-the-field evaluation reveals unilateral decreased muscle strength, decreased sensation, and a decreased patellar tendon reflex in the right lower extremity.

? Based on the findings of the evaluation, how should the athletic trainer manage this injury?

Motor Testing The manual muscle tests discussed earlier in this chapter are used to test the function of the motor neurons in both the upper and lower extremities. Motor tests are done using evaluating strength in muscles that are innervated by a specific nerve root level to test neurologic function of that nerve root.

Testing Joint Stability

A number of specific tests for determining the integrity of the ligaments surrounding a particular joint are described in Chapters 18 through 25. Joint stability tests provide information about the grade of a sprain of a particular ligament and can determine the extent of the functional instability of the joint.

Testing Accessory Motions

Accessory motions refer to the manner in which one articulating joint surface moves relative to another.[2,27] Normal accessory component motions must occur for full-range movement to take place. Accessory motions are limited by tightness of the joint capsule and/or ligaments that surround a joint. It is critical for the athletic trainer to closely evaluate the injured joint to determine whether motion is limited by tightness of the musculotendinous units or by limitation in accessory motion involving the joint capsule and ligaments. If accessory motion is limited by some restriction of the joint capsule or the ligaments, joint mobilization techniques should be incorporated into the treatment program.[16] Joint mobilization is discussed in detail in Chapter 16.

Testing Functional Performance

Functional examination determines if the athlete has full strength, joint stability, and coordination, and if the part is pain free.

Functional performance testing may be done as part of an initial evaluation to determine if an injury is severe enough to keep the athlete out of practice or competition. It may also be used to evaluate progress during a rehabilitation program. Decisions about when an athlete is ready to return to full sports participation following injury should be based to a large extent on performance on functional tests. Functional testing should proceed gradually from minimal stress to tests that mimic the actual stress that would normally come from full sports participation. The major concern is whether the athlete has regained full strength, range of motion, speed, endurance, and neuromuscular control and is pain free.

Postural Examination

As will be discussed in Chapter 25, many cases of injuries in athletes can be attributed to body malalignments. Musculoskeletal assessment might be one area of a postural examination. It is designed to test for malalignments and asymmetries by viewing the body compared to a grid or plumb line (Figures 25-7 through 25-9).

Anthropometric Measurements

Anthropometry is the science of measuring the human body. Anthropometric measurements include osteometry (measurement of the dimensions of the skeletal system), craniometry (measurement of the bones of the skull), skin-fold measurements to determine body composition (see Chapter 5), and height and weight measurements (see Chapter 2). Limb girth measurements taken during a rehabilitation program would also be considered a type of anthropometric measurement. Anthropometric measurements are seldom used by athletic trainers in a sports medicine setting.

Volumetric Measurements

Volumetric measurements can be taken to determine changes in limb volume caused by swelling, which can be attributed to hemorrhage, edema, or inflammation.[26] Limb volume may be measured in a volumetric tank that essentially measures the amount of water displaced by immersion of the limb in the tank (Figure 13-6). *Focus Box:* "Constructing and using a volumetric tank" describes the tank and the procedure for measuring limb volume.

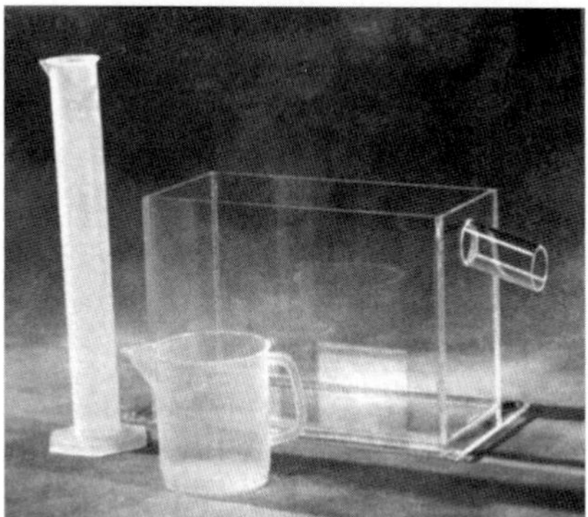

Figure 13-6

Tank for measuring limb volume.

PROGRESS EVALUATIONS

The athletic trainer who is overseeing a rehabilitation program must constantly monitor the progress of the athlete toward full recovery throughout the rehabilitative process. In many instances the athletic trainer will be able to treat the injured athlete on a daily basis. This close supervision affords the athletic trainer the luxury of being able to continuously adjust or adapt the treatment program based on the progress made by the athlete on a day-to-day basis.

13-6

***Critical Thinking* Exercise**

A gymnast is four months post-anterior cruciate ligament (ACL) reconstruction. She was last seen three months ago prior to leaving for summer vacation. She has returned for the beginning of classes and comes in to see the athletic trainer to see what kind of activities she should be doing in her rehabilitation program.

? To generate a progress note, what type of information does the athletic trainer need to know?

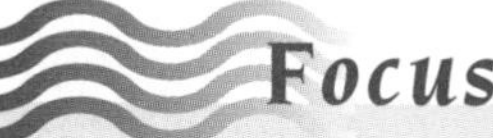

Focus

Constructing and using a volumetric tank

A volumetric tank (see Figure 13-6) is constructed of five 0.6-centimeter sheets of acrylic plastic molded together to form a container, which is mounted on a platform. The internal dimensions of the tank are: length = 35.6 centimeters, width = 17.8 centimeters, and depth = 20.3 centimeters. All the walls form right angles with each other as well as with the floor of the tank. The bottom of the tank has three adjustable leveling screws. Two of these screws are at one end of the tank base, while the third is centrally located on the opposite end. The end with one screw is classified as the front of the tank. A piece of acrylic plastic that measures 1.3 centimeters wide by 6 centimeters long is attached to the side of the tank, 4 centimeters from the back of the tank, to ensure consistent limb positioning in the tank.

A glass tube, 7.3 millimeters in diameter by 7.6 centimeters, passes through the front of the tank. The tube extends 3.2 centimeters outside the front wall of the tank. The tube is 5.1 centimeters from the top of the front wall and is perpendicular to the wall of the tank. A 10.2-centimeter piece of rubber tubing is attached to the end of the glass tube. This tubing combination allows for displaced water to be collected. A centimeter ruler, a skin thermometer, and a 500- and 1,000-milliliter graduated cylinder is used for all measurements. A water collection container is used to catch the runoff when the tubing is unclamped.

Procedure for measuring water displacement

The volumetric tank is placed on the floor and leveled using the adjusting screws. The tank is then filled to the 17-centimeter mark on the ruler with 33.5° C water. The subject places the limb against the back wall of the tank. The tank is then shaken gently to eliminate any air bubbles in the tank or on the surface of the limb. When the water is completely motionless, the tubing is unclamped and the runoff is collected in the container. Any water remaining in the tubing should be shaken out into the collection container. The amount of water collected in the runoff container is measured in the graduated cylinders and the measurements are noted.

The progress evaluation should be based on the athletic trainer's knowledge of exactly what is occurring in the healing process at any given time. The timelines of injury healing provide the framework that dictates the progress of the rehabilitation program. The athletic trainer must understand that the aggressive approach taken in rehabilitation of the injured athlete does little to speed up the healing process. Progression will be limited by the constraints of that process.

Progress evaluations will be more limited in scope than the detailed off-the-field evaluation sequence described in this chapter. The off-the-field evaluation should be thorough and comprehensive. The athletic trainer should take time to systematically rule out information that is not pertinent to the present injury. Once the extraneous information has been eliminated, the subsequent progress evaluation can focus specifically on how the injury appears today compared with yesterday. Is the athlete better or worse as a result of the treatment program rendered on the previous day?

To ensure that the progress evaluation will be complete, the athletic trainer still needs to go through certain aspects of history, observation, palpation, and special testing.

History

The athletic trainer should ask the athlete the following questions:

- How is the pain today compared to yesterday?
- Are you able to move better and with less pain?
- Do you think that the treatment done yesterday helped or made you more sore?

Observation

The athletic trainer should make the following observations:

- Is the swelling today more or less than it was yesterday?
- Is the athlete able to move better today?
- Is the athlete still guarding and protecting the injury?
- How is the athlete's affect? Is he or she upbeat and optimistic or depressed and negative?

Palpation

The athletic trainer should palpate the injured area to determine the following:

- Does the swelling have a different consistency today, and has the swelling pattern changed?
- Is the injured structure still as tender to the touch?
- Is there any deformity present today that was not obvious yesterday?

Special Tests

The athletic trainer should use special tests to make the following determinations:

- Does ligamentous stress testing cause as much pain? Has the athletic trainer's assessment of the grade of instability changed?
- How does a manual muscle test compare with yesterday?
- Has either active or passive range of motion changed?
- Does accessory movement appear to be limited?
- Can the athlete perform a specific functional test better today than yesterday?

DOCUMENTING INJURY EVALUATION INFORMATION

Complete and accurate documentation of findings from an evaluation is essential.[24] As stressed in Chapter 3, accurate documentation can be a strong ally should the athletic trainer become involved in litigation. For the athletic trainer working in a clinical setting, clear, concise, accurate record keeping is necessary for third-party reimbursement. Although the process may seem at times cumbersome and time consuming, the athletic trainer must develop proficiency not only in evaluation skills, but also in the ability to generate an accurate report of the findings from that evaluation.

In documenting medical information it is common practice for the clinician to use abbreviations for words that routinely appear in medical notes or evaluations. Table 13-6 provides many terms and their corresponding abbreviations that an athletic trainer might use in documenting injury information during an evaluation.

TABLE 13-6 Standard Abbreviations and Symbols Used in Medical Documentation

↑	increase	FWB	full weight bearing
↓	decrease	Fx	fracture
<	less than	G1–4	grades 1 to 4
>	greater than	GA	general appearance
Δ	change	H&P	history and physical
$\bar{c}$	with	H/O	history of
$\bar{p}$	after	HA	headache
$\bar{s}$ or w/o	without	HP	hot pack
1°	primary	HPI	history of present illness
2°	secondary	ht.	height; heart
+tive	positive	HTN	hypertension
A&O	alert & oriented	Hx	history
abnor.	abnormal	IN	inversion
AC	acromioclavicular or acute	IPPA	inspection, percussion, palpation, and auscultation
ADL	activities of daily living	L	left
ant.	anterior	LAT	lateral
ante	before	LBP	low back pain
AOAP	as often as possible	LE	lower extremity
AP	anterior-posterior; assessment and plans	MAEEW	moves all extremities equally well
AROM	active range of motion	MEDS	medications
ASAP	as soon as possible	mm	muscle; millimeter
ASIS	anterior superior iliac spine	MMT	manual muscle testing
AT	athletic training	MOD	moderate
B	bilateral	N	normal; never; no; not
BID or bid	twice a day	NC	neurologic check; no complaints; not completed
C/O	complained of; complaints; under care of	NEG	negative
CC	chief complaint; chronic complainer	NKA	no known allergies
ck.	check	NP	no pain
CP	cold pack; chronic pain	NPT	normal pressure and temperature
CPR	cardiopulmonary resuscitation	NSA	no significant abnormality
CWI	crutch walking instruction	NSAID	nonsteroidal antiinflammatory drug
D/C	discharge	NT	not tried
DF	dorsiflexion	NWB	non–weight bearing
DOB	date of birth	o	negative, without
DTR	deep tendon reflex	O	objective finding
DVT	deep vein thrombosis	OH	occupational history
Dx	diagnosis	ORIF	open reduction/internal fixation
E	edema	OT	occupational therapy
EENT	eyes, ears, nose, throat	P&A	percussion and auscultation
ELOP	estimated length of program	p.o.	postoperatively
EMS	emergency medical services	PA	posterior-anterior (x ray); physician assistant
EMT	emergency medical technician	PE	physical examination
EOA	examine, opinion, and advice	PF	plantar flexion
ES	electrical stimulation	PH	past history; poor health
EV	eversion	PMH	past medical history
exam.	examination	PNF	proprioceptive neuromuscular facilitation
FH	family history	PNS	peripheral nervous system
FROM	full range of movement	PPPBL	peripheral pulses palpable both legs

Continued

TABLE 13-6—continued

PRE	progressive resistance exercise	SLR	straight leg raises
pre-op	preoperatively	SOAP	subjective, objective, assessment, plan
prog.	prognosis	stat	immediately
PROM	passive range of motion	STG	short-term goals
PT	physical therapy	Sx	signs; symptom
Pt./pt.	patient	T	temperature
PWB	partial weight bearing	TENS	transcutaneous electrical nerve stimulation
Px	physical exam; pneumothorax	tid	three times a day
qd	once daily	TTWB	toe touch weight bearing
qid	four times a day	UE	upper extremity
R	right	UK	unknown
R/O	rule out	US	ultrasound
rehab	rehabilitation	WBAT	weight bearing as tolerated
ROM	range of motion	Whp	whirlpool
RROM	resistive range of motion	WNL	within normal limits
RTP	return to play	x	times
Rx	prescription, including therapy and treatment	y.o.	year old
S	subjective findings	Y/O	years old

SOAP Notes

SOAP note:
- Subjective
- Objective
- Assessment
- Plan

Documentation of acute athletic injury can be effectively accomplished through a system designed to record subjective and objective findings and to document the immediate and future treatment plan for the athlete. The SOAP note format (subjective, objective, assessment, and plan) provides a standard format for recording injury information obtained from either on-site, sideline, or clinical evaluations.[27] This method combines information provided by the athlete and observations of the examiner.[18] Figure 13-7 presents a recommended injury report form that includes these components of documentation. This form also includes a provision to document findings arising from more definitive evaluation or from the examiner's subsequent evaluation.

S (Subjective)

This component includes the subjective statements provided by the injured athlete. History taking is designed to elicit the subjective impressions of the athlete relative to time, mechanism, and site of injury. The type and course of the pain and the degree of disability experienced by the athlete are also noteworthy.

O (Objective)

Objective findings result from the athletic trainer's visual inspection, palpation, and assessment of active, passive, and resistive motion. Findings of special testing should also be noted here. Thus the objective report would include assessment of posture, presence of deformity or swelling, and location of point tenderness. Also, limitations of active motion and pain arising or disappearing during passive and resistive motion should be noted. Finally, the results of special tests relative to joint stability or apprehension are also included.

A (Assessment)

Assessment of the injury is the athletic trainer's professional judgment with regard to impression and nature of injury. Although the exact nature of the injury will not always be known initially, information pertaining to suspected site and anatomical structures involved is appropriate. A judgment of severity may be included but is not essential at the time of acute injury evaluation.

SUBJECTIVE: The patient is a ___________ -year-old athlete with the above diagnosis. The athlete notes a _________ onset on _________. Past history for this condition is remarkable for/unremarkable. Diagnostic testing of ________________. Medications include ______________________. The athletes' goals are to __________________________.
General medical history is remarkable for/unremarkable. The athlete will follow with MD on _________.

OBJECTIVE: Measurable, Reproducible, Observable findings—Be Objective
OBSERVATION: Be descriptive
ROM: AROM/PROM—Measure with goniometer
STRENGTH: Strength to MMT—Use grading system 1 to 5
FLEXIBILITY: Try to document with goniometer if possible
PALPATION:
SENSATION:
SPECIAL TEST:
GAIT:
FUNCTIONAL TESTS:
TREATMENT:

ASSESSMENT: Your professional opinion of the athlete's problem
The athlete presents with the following problems (1) ___________, (2) ___________,
(3) ___________, (4) ___________.

PLAN: Describe how you will manage the athlete regarding frequency of treatment, what the treatment will include (i.e., modalities, therapeutic exercise, home program, and follow up with you).
Short-term goals include (1) ___________, (2) ___________, (3) ___________,
(4) ___________.
Long-term goals include ____.

Signature ______________________________ ATC

Figure 13-7

SOAP note form.

P (Plan)

The plan should include the first aid treatment rendered to the athlete and the sports therapist's intentions relative to disposition. Disposition may include referral for more definitive evaluation or simply application of splint, wrap, or crutches and a request to report for reevaluation the next day. If the injury is chronic, the examiner's plan for treatment and therapeutic exercise would be appropriate. The treatment plan should establish specific short-term goals for the rehabilitation program and should provide criteria-based guidelines for accomplishing these goals. A specific long-term goal should also be clearly identified in the plan.

Progress Notes

Progress notes should be routinely written after each progress evaluation done throughout the course of the rehabilitation program. Progress notes can follow the SOAP format as indicated in the previous sections. They can be generated in the form of an expanded treatment note or done as a weekly summary. Information in the progress note should concentrate on the types of treatment received and the patient's response to that treatment, progress made toward the short-term goals established in the SOAP note, changes in the previous treatment plan and goals, and the course of treatment over the next several days.[1]

ADDITIONAL DIAGNOSTIC TESTS USED BY A PHYSICIAN

The physician, like the athletic trainer, often performs a detailed musculoskeletal examination on the injured athlete. Often the physician and the athletic trainer will

13-7 Critical Thinking Exercise

A field hockey player is tripped, twists her knee, and falls hard on artificial turf on that same knee. There is immediate swelling and pain. After evaluation, the athletic trainer is not sure what the injury is and sends the athlete directly to the physician for diagnosis. The physician decides that additional diagnostic tests are necessary to determine the exact pathology.

? What diagnostic tests is the physician likely to order to determine the exact nature and extent of the knee injury?

discuss and compare their individual findings. Because the physician is legally charged with determining a diagnosis and deciding on a course of treatment, he or she may have to acquire and compare additional information. This information can come from imaging techniques that may include plain film radiographs (X rays), arthrography, arthroscopy, myelography, computed tomography, bone scanning, magnetic resonance imaging, ultrasonography, and echocardiography.[23] Other tests might include electrocardiography, electroencephalography, electromyography, nerve conduction velocity, synovial fluid analysis, blood testing, and urinalysis.

Imaging Techniques

Plain Film Radiography (X rays)

An X-ray examination helps the physician to identify fractures and dislocations or any bone abnormality that may be present. It may also be used to rule out serious disease such as an infection or neoplasm. A trained radiologist can detect some soft-tissue factors, such as joint swelling and ectopic bone development in ligaments and tendons (Figure 13-8A).[4]

Arthrography

Arthrography is the visual study of a joint via X ray after injection of an opaque dye, air, or a combination of air and opaque dye into the joint space. This procedure can show the disruption of soft tissue and loose bodies in the joint.

Arthroscopy

Arthroscopy uses a fiber-optic arthroscope to view the inside of a joint.

The fiber-optic arthroscope is widely used by orthopedists in surgery. It is considered more accurate than the arthrogram but is more invasive, requiring anesthesia and a small incision for the introduction of the arthroscope (endoscope) into the joint space. While the arthroscope is in the joint, the surgeon can perform surgical procedures such as removing loose bodies and, in some cases, suturing torn tissues.[23]

Myelography

During myelography, an opaque dye is introduced into the spinal canal (epidural space) through a lumbar puncture. While the patient is tilted, the dye is allowed to flow to different levels of the spinal cord. Using this contrast medium, physicians can detect conditions such as tumors, nerve root compression, and disk disease as well as other diseases within the spinal cord.

Computed Tomography

Computed tomography (CT) penetrates the body with a thin, fan-shaped X-ray beam, producing a cross-sectional view of tissues. Unlike X-ray images, CT images allow the injured structure to be viewed from many angles. As the machine scans, a computer compares the many views; these electrical signals are then processed by a computer into a visual image (Figure 13-8B).

Bone Scanning

A bone scan involves the intravenous introduction of a radioactive tracer such as technetium-99. By imaging the entire skeleton or part of a skeleton, bony lesions in which there is some inflammation, such as stress fractures, can be detected (Figure 13-8C).

Magnetic Resonance Imaging

Magnetic resonance imaging (MRI) surrounds the body with powerful electromagnets, creating a field as much as 600,000 times as strong as that of the earth.[2] The magnetic current focuses on hydrogen atoms in water molecules and aligns them; when the current is shut off, the atoms continue to spin, emitting an energy that is detected by the computer. The hydrogen atoms in different tissue spin at different rates, thus producing different images. In many ways, MRI provides clearer images than

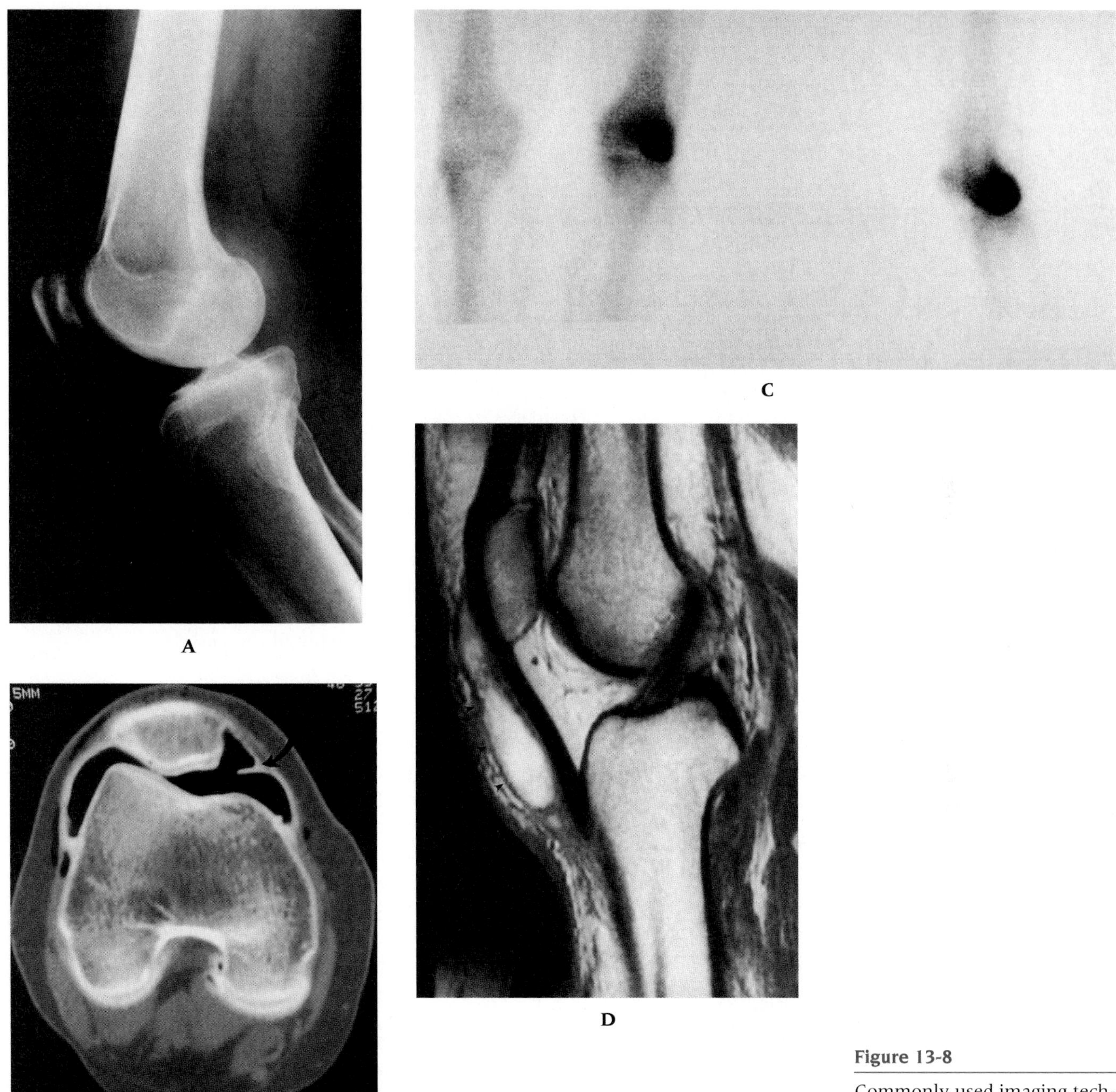

Figure 13-8

Commonly used imaging techniques for the knee. **A,** X ray. **B,** CT scan. **C,** Bone scan. **D,** MRI.

does CT scanning. Despite the expense of MRI, it is currently the test of choice by physicians for detecting soft-tissue lesions (Figure 13-8D).

Ultrasonography

Ultrasonography is the use of ultrasound to view location, measurement, or delineation of an organ or tissue by measuring the reflection or transmission of high-frequency ultrasound waves. A computer calculates the distance from the sound-reflecting or sound-absorbing surface and creates a two-dimensional image.

Echocardiography

Echocardiography uses ultrasound to produce a graphic record of internal cardiac structures. An echocardiogram is most often used to visualize the cardiac valves and to determine the dimensions of the left atrium and both ventricles.

Arteriogram

Arteriography is a procedure in which a catheter is inserted into a specific blood vessel, contrast material is injected, and radiographs are taken allowing the physician to see the vessel. An arteriogram can be used to examine almost any artery. In general, arteriograms give the best pictures of the body's blood vessels. Arteriograms are used to make specific diagnoses and to help determine the best treatment. Often the treatment itself can be performed using the same type of catheters used in the arteriogram, instead of requiring a more extensive surgery in an additional procedure (e.g., angioplasty).

Venogram

A venogram is a radiographic procedure used to image veins filled with a contrast medium. This imaging technique is most often used to detect thrombophlebitis. It provides a visual tracing of a venous pulse.

Doppler Ultrasonography

This test uses ultrasound to examine the blood flow in the major arteries and veins in the arms and legs. It is done as an alternative to arteriography and venography and may help diagnose a blood clot, venous insufficiency, arterial occlusion (closing), or abnormalities in the blood flow caused by a narrowing of the vessels.

Other Diagnostic Tests

Electrocardiography

An electrocardiogram (ECG) records the electrical activity of the heart to determine whether impulse formation, conduction, and depolarization and repolarization of the atria and ventricles follows a normal pattern. It is of value in diagnosing causes of abnormal cardiac rhythm and myocardial damage.

Electroencephalography

The electroencephalogram (EEG) records electrical potentials produced in the brain on an instrument called an electroencephalograph. It is used to detect changes or abnormalities in brain wave patterns.

Electromyography

Electromyography (EMG) involves the graphic recording of a muscle contraction and the amount of electrical activity generated in a muscle using either surface or needle electrodes. Motor unit potentials can be observed on an oscilloscope screen or from a graphic recording called an electromyogram. Various muscular conditions can be evaluated.

Nerve Conduction Velocity

Determining the conduction velocity of a nerve may provide key information to the physician about a number of neuromuscular conditions. After a stimulus is applied to a peripheral nerve, the speed with which a muscle action occurs is measured. Delays in conduction might indicate nerve compression or other muscular or nerve disease.

Synovial Fluid Analysis

Analysis of synovial fluid and blood can be used to detect musculoskeletal infections.

The primary purpose of synovial fluid analysis is to detect the presence of an infection in the joint. The test also confirms the diagnosis of gout and differentiates noninflammatory joint disease such as degenerative arthritis from inflammatory conditions such as rheumatoid arthritis.[4]

Blood Testing

The physician may decide to run a complete blood count (CBC) on the athlete for many different reasons. The most common reasons are to screen for anemia (too few red cells) or infection (too many white cells).[30] Samples may be taken in a syringe from a vein in the arm or from a needle stick in the finger. A routine CBC addresses the following:

- The red blood cell count looks at the number of cells per unit volume to detect anemias, prolonged infections, iron deficiencies, internal bleeding, and certain types of cancers.
- Hemoglobin levels are closely associated with red blood cell count and tend to reflect overall blood volume.
- The hematocrit measures how much of the total blood volume is made up of red blood cells. A low hematocrit indicates certain types of anemias.
- The white blood cell count is used to determine the presence of bacteria. Differentiation of white cell types microscopically can identify specific types of infection.
- A deficiency in the platelet count can lead to dangerous internal bleeding.
- Blood testing can also measure levels of serum cholesterol. The recommended desirable range is <200 mg/dL.

Normal laboratory values for the CBC are summarized in Table 13-7.

13-8

Critical Thinking Exercise

A female field hockey player complains of feeling tired and run down. The athletic trainer suspects that she may be anemic and sends her to the physician for a blood test. After getting the results the physician calls the athletic trainer and reports that her hematocrit was 36% and that her hemoglobin was 11 g/100 ml.

? Are these values normal and what should the athletic trainer conclude?

Urinalysis

Urinalysis is a common test that can yield a large quantity of information.[26] In most cases a sample of urine in a small, dry container is all that is needed. If the urine will not be analyzed within one hour, the sample should be refrigerated. A routine urinalysis addresses the following:[31]

- Specific gravity indicates the ability of the kidney to concentrate and dilute fluids.
- The pH refers to how acid or alkaline the urine is. It may be acidic in cases of diabetes or dehydration. Alkaline urine is present in urinary tract infections and kidney disease. Presence of glucose may indicate diabetes.
- The presence of ketones, a by-product of fat metabolism, may also indicate diabetes.
- Hemoglobin may appear in urine after intense exercise or from kidney disease.
- The presence of protein indicates kidney disease.
- The presence of nitrate indicates infection.
- A small amount of urine is examined under a microscope to find red blood cells, white blood cells, and bacteria.
- If bacteria are present, a urine culture may be necessary to determine the specific bacteria causing an infection.
- Many additional tests may also be done on urine, including electrolytes, hormones, and drug levels.

Normal laboratory values for a standard urinalysis are listed in Table 13-8.

TABLE 13-7 Normal Laboratory Values of a Complete Blood Count

Test	Normal Values
Red blood cell count	Males 5.4 million/mm^3 Females 4.8 million/mm^3
White blood cell count	5,000–9,000/mm^3
Platelet count	250,000–400,000/mm^3
Hematocrit	Male 40%–54% Female 38%–47%
Hemoglobin	Male 14–16.5 g/100 ml Female 12–15 g/100 ml
Cholesterol	<200 mg/dl

TABLE 13-8 Normal Laboratory Values of a Urinalysis

Test	Normal Values
Output	1,000–1,500 ml
Color	Yellow to amber and clear
Specific gravity	1.010–1.025
Osmolality	500–800 mosm/kg water
pH	4.6–4.8
Uric acid	0.6–1 g/24 hr
Urea	23–25 g/24 hr
Creatine	1–2 g/24 hr

Urinalysis using dip-and-read test strips (such as Chemstrips) can provide fast, accurate results for a wide range of test parameters such as specific gravity, leukocytes, nitrate, pH, protein, glucose, ketones, urobilinogen, bilirubin, and blood. Large test areas on each strip are impregnated with reagents that provide clear, easy-to-read color changes when dipped in urine. Color comparison charts are often located on the box.

SUMMARY

- Once the athlete has been transported from the site of initial injury, a detailed off-the-field injury evaluation may be performed on the sideline, in the training room, in an emergency room, or in a sports medicine clinic.
- Athletic trainers evaluate sports injuries, whereas physicians diagnose injuries.
- To accurately evaluate an injury, the athletic trainer must possess a thorough background in human anatomy, including surface anatomy, body planes, and anatomical directions. The athletic trainer also needs an in-depth understanding of the musculoskeletal system, with special focus on adverse biomechanical forces, which become pathomechanical. After they are assessed, sports injuries must be described using appropriate terminology.
- The off-the-field evaluation scheme is divided into four broad categories: history, observation, palpation, and a number of special tests that provide additional information about the extent of injuries.
- The progress evaluation focuses specifically on how the injury appears today compared with yesterday, and it is more limited in scope than the detailed off-the-field evaluation sequence is.
- The SOAP note (subjective, objective, assessment, and plan) provides a standard format for documenting and recording injury information. Progress notes may also be recorded in the SOAP format.
- To make an accurate diagnosis, the physician may need to use a particular imaging technique or one of several additional tests.

Websites

Cramer First Aider: http://www.cramersportsmed.com/first_aider.jsp

National Athletic Trainers' Association: http://www.nata.org

Solutions to Critical Thinking EXERCISES

13-1 The athletic trainer must realize that the physician has more training and is usually more skilled in injury diagnosis. Despite the fact that the athletic trainer correctly identified the MCL sprain, the meniscus tear was completely overlooked. Although the athletic trainer's actions were not inappropriate, it would have been better to refer the injured athlete to the physician for diagnosis. The injury evaluation done by the athletic trainer in most cases would hopefully reveal the same results as the physician diagnosis.

13-2 The athletic trainer should first take a subjective history from the injured athlete and follow that with an objective examination that includes observation, palpation, range-of-motion testing, manual muscle testing, a neurological examination, special tests, tests for joint stability, and a functional performance evaluation.

13-3 In this case, a ligamentous injury is more likely. A lesion of inert tissue will elicit pain on active and passive movement in the same direction. If a lesion is present in contractile tissue, pain will occur on active motion in one direction and on passive motion in the opposite direction. A sprain of a ligament will result in pain whenever that ligament is stretched either through active contraction or passive stretching.

13-4 A weak and painful action suggests there is a gross lesion of contractile tissue in the shoulder, such as the rotator cuff. A weak and painless contraction indicates there may be a complete rupture of the tissue or a potential nervous system disorder.

13-5 Generally, injury to the spinal cord would result in bilateral symptoms. Unilateral changes are more indicative of peripheral nerve injury. However, any change in the neurological status of the athlete is cause for great concern. The athletic trainer should remove the athlete from the playing field using a stretcher or, preferably, a spine board.

13-6 To ensure that the progress evaluation will be complete, the athletic trainer needs to go through history, observation, palpation, and special testing. The athlete should be asked pertinent questions such as "What types of exercises have you done for the past three months?" and "What type of pain, if any, are you still experiencing?" Observation of the symmetry to the other knee and palpation of the injured structures should be done. Range of motion, muscle strength, joint stability, and neuromuscular control should also be assessed.

13-7 Initially, it is likely that standard knee X-rays would be used to determine the presence of a fracture. An MRI is widely used by sports medicine physicians to determine injury to ligamentous, meniscal, or other soft tissues. On occasion, a diagnostic arthroscopy might be done to directly observe the injured structures.

13-8 Both the hematocrit and the hemoglobin levels are low and it is likely that the athlete does have anemia. However, depending on other signs and symptoms, the physician may need to order additional diagnostic tests to determine what may be causing this problem.

REVIEW QUESTIONS AND CLASS ACTIVITIES

1. Differentiate between injury evaluation and diagnosis.
2. What basic knowledge must the athletic trainer have before making an injury assessment?
3. Explain the key terminology needed to communicate the results of an assessment.
4. Identify the various descriptive assessment terms.
5. How should an athletic trainer take a history? What questions should be asked?
6. Describe palpation and when and how it should be performed.
7. What can be ascertained from active, passive, and resisted isometric movement?
8. Explain how muscle testing, reflex testing, and sensation testing are performed.
9. What part do special tests play in injury assessment?
10. When should a functional evaluation be given?
11. What information should be included in a SOAP note?
12. What insights can a physician gain by having special laboratory tests performed? Describe each test in detail.

REFERENCES

1. Arrigo C: Clinical documentation. In Konin J: *Clinical athletic training,* Thorofare, NJ, 1997, Slack.
2. Barak T, Rosen E, Sofer R: Mobility: passive orthopedic manual therapy. In Gould J, Davies G, editors: *Orthopedic and sports physical therapy,* St Louis, 1997, Mosby.
3. Bickley L, Bates B: *A guide to physical examination and history taking,* Philadelphia, 2002, Lippincott, Williams & Wilkins.
4. Birnbaum JS: *The musculoskeletal manual,* Orlando, 1986, Grune & Stratton.
5. Clarkson H, Gilewich G: *Musculoskeletal assessment: joint range of motion and manual muscle strength,* Philadelphia, 2000, Lippincott, Williams & Wilkins.
6. Cyriax J, Cyriax P: *Cyriax's illustrated manual of orthopaedic medicine,* London, 1996, Butterworth-Heinemann.
7. Delforge G: Sports injury assessment and problem identification. In Delforge G, editor, *Musculoskeletal trauma: implications for sports injury management,* Champaign, Ill, 2002, Human Kinetics.
8. DeMont R: The place for palpation. *Athletic Therapy Today* 8(2):42, 2003.
9. Evans R: *Illustrated orthopedic physical assessment,* St Louis, 2001, Mosby.
10. Gehring P: Physical assessment begins with a history, *RN* 54(11): 27, 1991.
11. Gross J, Fetto J, Rosen E: *Musculoskeletal examination,* Cambridge, Mass, 2001, Blackwell Scientific.
12. Hartley A: *Practical joint assessment,* St Louis, 1995, Mosby.
13. Hilsop H, Montgomery J: *Daniels and Worthingham muscle testing,* San Diego, 2002, Elsevier Science.
14. Hoppenfeld S: *Physical examination of the spine and extremities,* New York, 1976, Appleton-Century-Crofts.
15. Hurley W: Agreement of Clinical judgments of endfeel between 2 sample populations, *J Sport Rehabil* 11(3):209, 2002.
16. Kaltenborn F, Evjenth O, Kaltenborn T: *Manual mobilization of the joints: the Kaltenborn method of joint examination and treatment: the extremities,* Minneapolis, 1999, Orthopedic Physical Therapy Products.
17. Kendall F, Kendall E: *Muscles testing and function,* Philadelphia, 1993, Lippincott, Williams & Wilkins.
18. Kettenbach G: *Writing SOAP notes with patient/client management formats,* Philadelphia, 2003, FA Davis.
19. Lynch MK, Kessler RM: Pain. In Kessler RM, Hertling D, editors: *Management of common musculoskeletal disorders,* Baltimore, 1996, Lippincott, Williams & Wilkins.
20. Mattacola CG: Introduction to Clinical evaluation and testing, *Athletic Therapy Today* 8(2):24–25, 2003.
21. Magee DL: *Orthopedic physical assessment,* Little Rock, Ark, 2002, Elsevier Health Sciences.
22. McRae R: *Clinical orthopaedic examination,* Philadelphia, 1997, Churchill Livingstone.
23. Milbauer D: Principles of radiographic evaluation and imaging techniques. In Nicholas J, Hershman E: *The lower extremity and spine in sports medicine,* St Louis, 1995, Mosby.
24. Palmer ML, Epler MF, Adams M: *Fundamentals of musculoskeletal assessment techniques,* Philadelphia, 1998, Lippincott, Williams & Wilkins.
25. Petersen CM: Construct validity of Cyriax's selective tension examination: association of end-feels with pain at the knee and shoulder. *Journal of Orthopaedic and Sports Physical Therapy* 30(9)512, 2002.
26. Peterson EJ et al: Reliability of water volumetry and the figure of eight method on subjects with ankle joint swelling, *J Orthop Sports Phys Ther* 29(10):609, 1999.

27. Prentice W: *Rehabilitation techniques in sports medicine and athletic training*, St. Louis, 2004, McGraw-Hill.
28. Starkey C, Ryan J: *Evaluation of orthopedic and athletic injuries*, Philadelphia, 2001, FA Davis.
29. Wadsworth C: *Manual examination and treatment of the spine and extremities*, Baltimore, 1988, Williams & Wilkins.
30. Wurman R: *Medical access*, Los Angeles, 1985, Access Press.

ANNOTATED BIBLIOGRAPHY

Birnbaum JS: *The musculoskeletal manual*, Orlando, 1986, Grune & Stratton.

This text is written for medical professionals who require a direct and simple approach for recognizing and managing musculoskeletal problems. A great number of the conditions discussed relate to sports trauma.

Booher JM, Thibodeau GA: *Athletic injury assessment*, ed 4, St Louis, 2001, McGraw-Hill.

This outstanding text is addressed directly to the practitioner in sports medicine or athletic training. It considers all aspects of musculoskeletal and internal sports injuries.

Cyriax J, Cyriax P: *Cyriax's Illustrated manual of orthopaedic medicine*, London, 1996, Butterworth-Heinemann.

This beautifully color-illustrated text is designed for diagnosing and providing Cyriax management to musculoskeletal conditions.

Gross J, Fetto J, Rosen E: *Musculoskeletal examination*, Cambridge, Mass, 2002, Blackwell Publishers.

This evaluation text is written primarily for physicians.

Hoppenfeld S: *Physical examination of the spine and extremities*, New York, 1976, Appleton-Century-Crofts.

This classic text presents an easy-to-follow, methodical, and in-depth procedure for examining musculoskeletal conditions.

Konin J, Wiksten D, Isear J: *Special tests for orthopedic examination*, Stamford, CT, 2002, Thomson Learning.

This well-illustrated text details examination techniques used in evaluating musculoskeletal injuries.

Magee DJ: *Orthopedic physical assessment*, Little Rock, Ark, 2002, Elsevier-Health Sciences.

The strength of this extremely well-illustrated book with excellent depth of coverage lies in its coverage of injuries commonly found during athletic training.

Palmer ML, Epler MF, Adams M: *Fundamentals of Musculoskeletal assessment techniques*, Philadelphia, 1998, Lippincott, Williams & Wilkins.

This text contains contributions by many experts in the field of orthopedic examination. It covers each major joint in detail.

Starkey C, Ryan J: *Evaluation of orthopedic and athletic injuries*, Philadelphia, 2001, FA Davis.

This detailed, well-illustrated text addresses all aspects of injury assessment for the athletic trainer.

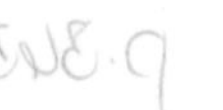

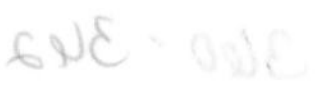

Bloodborne Pathogens

Chapter 14

When you finish this chapter you should be able to

- Explain what bloodborne pathogens are and how they can infect athletes and athletic trainers.
- Describe the transmission, symptoms, signs, and treatment of hepatitis B virus.
- Describe the transmission, symptoms, signs, and treatment of hepatitis C.
- Describe the transmission, symptoms, and signs of human immunodeficiency virus.
- Explain how human immunodeficiency virus is most often transmitted.
- List the pros and cons of athletes with hepatitis B virus, hepatitis C virus, or human immunodeficiency virus participating in sports.
- Evaluate universal precautions as mandated by the Occupational Safety and Health Administration and how they apply to the athletic trainer.

Bloodborne pathogens are transmitted through contact with blood or other bodily fluids. Hepatitis, especially the hepatitis B virus (HBV), the hepatitis C virus (HCV), and human immunodeficiency virus (HIV) are of special concern.[3] Despite the media attention given to bloodborne pathogens in recent years, many athletic trainers have only a moderate understanding of the magnitude of the problem.[10]

It has always been important for the athletic trainer as a health care provider to be concerned with maintaining an environment in the athletic training room that is as clean and sterile as possible.[1,18] In our society it has become critical for everyone to take measures to prevent the spread of infectious diseases.[12] Failure to do so may predispose any individual to life-threatening situations. The athletic trainer must take every precaution to minimize the potential for exposure to blood or other infectious materials (Figure 14-1).

VIRUS REPRODUCTION

A virus is a submicroscopic parasitic organism that is dependent on the nutrients within cells. A virus consists of a strand of either deoxyribonucleic acid (DNA) or ribonucleic acid (RNA). A virus contains one or the other, but not both. A virus consists

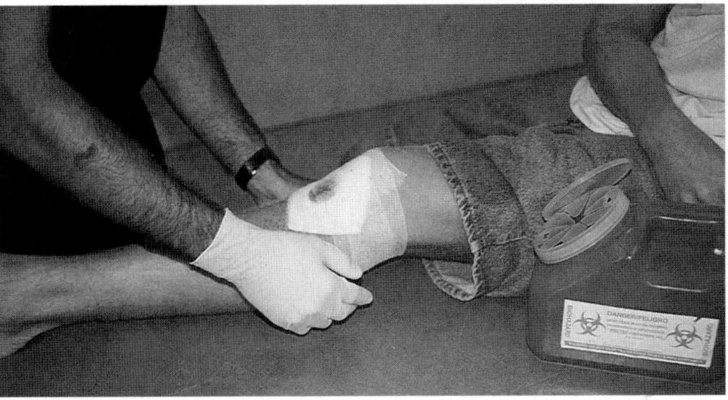

Figure 14-1

The athletic trainer must take precautions to prevent exposure to and transmission of bloodborne pathogens.

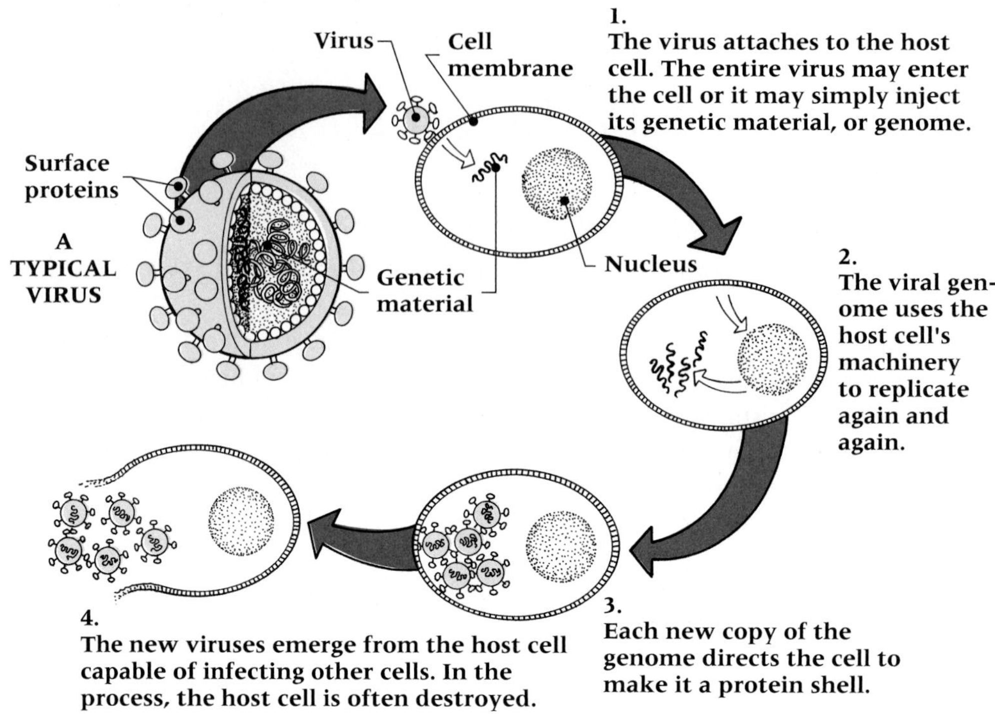

Figure 14-2

The reproducing virus.

of a shell of proteins surrounding genetic material. It is a parasite that depends on a host cell for metabolic and reproductive requirements. In general, viruses make their cell hosts ill by redirecting cellular activity to create more viruses (Figure 14-2).

BLOODBORNE PATHOGENS

Mode of transmission includes:
- Human blood
- Semen
- Vaginal secretions
- Cerebrospinal fluid
- Synovial fluid

Bloodborne pathogens are pathogenic microorganisms that can potentially cause disease and are present in human blood and other body fluids, including semen, vaginal secretions, cerebrospinal fluid, synovial fluid, and any other fluid contaminated with blood. The three most significant bloodborne pathogens are HBV, HCV, and HIV.

Although HIV has been widely addressed in the media, HBV and HCV have a higher possibility for spread than does HIV, and thus athletic trainers should be more concerned about contracting HBV and HCV.[14] Hepatitis B virus is stronger and more durable than HIV and can be spread more easily via sharp objects, open wounds, and bodily fluids.[20]

Bloodborne pathogens include:
- Hepatitis B virus (HBV)
- Hepatitis C virus (HCV)
- Human immunodeficiency virus (HIV)

Three additional viruses—hepatitis A, D, and E—exist, which, while related, are not generally considered to be bloodborne pathogens. Hepatitis A (HAV) is a virus that causes inflammation of the liver but does not lead to chronic disease of the liver. HAV is transmitted by the fecal or oral routes, through close personal contact, or through ingestion of contaminated food or water. For example it may be transmitted by an infected food preparer who doesn't wash his or her hands after going to the bathroom. HAV may show no outward symptoms or signs, but adults may have dark urine, light stools, fatigue, fever, and jaundice. Hepatitis D (HDV), like HAV, causes inflammation of the liver, but it will only infect those individuals who are already infected with HBV. It is transmitted through contact with infected blood or contaminated needles or through sexual contact. Hepatitis E (HEV) also causes inflammation of the liver, although it is rare in the United States. It is transmitted through the fecal or oral routes or through contaminated water supplies in foreign countries.[18]

Hepatitis B Virus

Hepatitis B virus is a major cause of viral infection; it results in swelling, soreness, and loss of normal liver function. The number of cases of HBV has risen dramatically during the last ten years. It has been estimated that 1.25 million people in the United States have chronic hepatitis and can potentially infect others. New cases are occurring at rates as high as 300,000 per year.[29]

Symptoms and Signs

The symptoms and signs in a person infected with HBV include flulike symptoms such as fatigue, weakness, and nausea; abdominal pain; headache; fever; and possibly jaundice. It is possible that an individual infected with HBV will exhibit no signs or symptoms, and the virus may go undetected. In these individuals, the HBV antigen will always be present. Thus the disease may be unknowingly transmitted to others through exposure to blood or other body fluids or through intimate contact. Cases of chronic active hepatitis may occur because of a problem with the immune system that prevents the complete destruction of virus-infected liver cells.

An infected person's blood may test positive for the HBV antigen within two to six weeks after the symptoms develop. Approximately 85 percent of those infected recover within six to eight weeks.

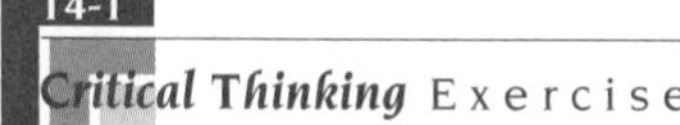

The athletic trainer is responsible for taking every precaution to prevent infection by bloodborne pathogens.

? How are bloodborne pathogen infections prevented from spreading from one athlete to another?

Prevention

Good personal hygiene and avoiding high-risk activities is the best way to avoid HBV.[13] Hepatitis B virus can survive for at least one week in dried blood or on contaminated surfaces and may be transmitted through contact with these surfaces. Caution must be taken to avoid contact with any blood or other fluid that potentially contains a bloodborne pathogen.[38]

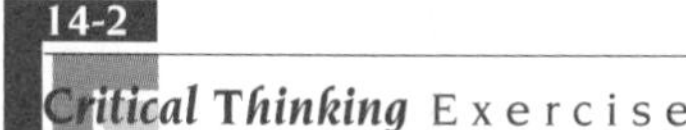

A wrestler has been diagnosed with hepatitis B virus.

? What are the symptoms and signs of HBV infection?

Management

Vaccination against HBV must be made available by employers at no cost to any individual who may be exposed to blood or other body fluids and may thus be at risk of contracting HBV.[40] All athletic trainers and any individual working in an allied health care profession should receive immunization. An estimated 8,700 health care workers contract HBV each year, and as many as 200 of these cases end in death.[29] The vaccine is given in three doses over a six-month period. Approximately 87 percent of those receiving the vaccine will be immune after the second dose, and 96 percent develop immunity after the third dose. Postexposure vaccination is available when individuals have come into direct contact with bodily fluids of an infected person.[7]

Hepatitis C

Originally referred to as non-A, non-B hepatitis, hepatitis C is both an acute and chronic form of liver disease caused by the hepatitis C virus (HCV). HCV is the most common chronic bloodborne infection in the United States. At least 85 percent of those infected acutely with HCV become chronically infected, and 67 percent develop chronic liver disease. It is the leading indication for liver transplant. Three percent of those with chronic liver disease die from cirrhosis or liver cancer. It is estimated that 3.9 million Americans have been infected with HCV, of whom 2.7 million are chronically infected. There were 25,000 new infections in 2001.[17]

Symptoms and Signs

Eighty percent of those infected with HCV have no signs or symptoms. Those who are symptomatic may be jaundiced and/or have mild abdominal pain, particularly in the upper right quadrant; loss of appetite; nausea, fatigue; muscle or joint pain; and/or dark urine.

Prevention

HCV is not spread by sneezing, hugging, coughing, food or water, sharing eating utensils or drinking glasses, or casual contact. It is rarely spread through sexual contact. It is spread by contact with the blood of an infected person.[38] It is most commonly transmitted by sharing needles or syringes. However it can also be transmitted by sharing personal care items that might have blood on them (razors, toothbrushes). Consider the risks of getting a tattoo or body piercing. Athletic trainers should always follow routine barrier precautions and safely handle needles and other sharp objects.

Management

Unlike for HBV, presently there is no vaccine for preventing HCV transmission. There are several blood tests that can be done to determine if a person has been infected with HCV. A physician may order just one or a combination of these tests. It is possible to find HCV within one to two weeks after being infected with the virus. A single positive test indicates infection with HCV. However a single negative test does not prove that a person is not infected. When hepatitis C is suspected, even though an initial test is negative, the test should be repeated.[17]

HCV-positive persons should be evaluated by their doctor for liver disease. Interferon and ribavirin are two drugs used in combination that appear to be the most effective for the treatment of persons with chronic hepatitis C. Drinking alcohol can make liver disease worse.

Human Immunodeficiency Virus

retrovirus
A virus that enters a host cell and changes its RNA to a proviral DNA replica.

Human immunodeficiency virus is a **retrovirus** that combines with a host cell. A number of cells in the immune system may be infected, such as T^4 blood cells, B cells, and monocytes (macrophages), which decreases their effectiveness in preventing disease. As of the end of 2003, an estimated 40 million people worldwide were living with HIV/AIDS. Worldwide, approximately 11 of every 1,000 adults ages 15 to 49 are infected with HIV. An estimated 5 million new HIV infections occurred worldwide during 2003. That is about 14,000 infections each day. In 2003 alone, HIV/AIDS-associated illnesses caused approximately 3 million deaths worldwide.[44]

Symptoms and Signs

As is the case with HBV, HIV is transmitted by exposure to infected blood or other body fluids or by intimate sexual contact.[45] Symptoms of HIV include fatigue, weight loss, muscle or joint pain, painful or swollen glands, night sweats, and fever. Antibodies to HIV can be detected in a blood test within one year after exposure. As with HBV, people with HIV may be unaware that they have contracted the virus and may go for eight to ten years before developing any signs or symptoms. Unfortunately most individuals who test positive for HIV will ultimately develop acquired immunodeficiency syndrome (AIDS). Table 14-1 summarizes information on HBV and HIV.

Acquired Immunodeficiency Syndrome A syndrome is a collection of signs and symptoms that are recognized as the effects of an infection. An individual with AIDS has no protection against even the simplest infections and thus is extremely vulnerable to developing a variety of illnesses, opportunistic infections, and cancers (such as Kaposi's sarcoma and non-Hodgkin's lymphoma) that cannot be stopped.[7,24]

According to the Centers for Disease Control (CDC), it is estimated that 850,000 to 950,000 U.S. residents are living with HIV infection, and that approximately 40,000 new HIV infections occur each year. As of the end of 2002, an estimated 384,906 people in the United States were living with AIDS, and an estimated 501,669 people with AIDS in the United States had died.[44]

A positive HIV test cannot predict when the individual will show the symptoms of AIDS.[32] About 50 percent of people develop AIDS within ten years of becoming HIV-infected. Those individuals who develop AIDS generally die within two years after the symptoms appear.

TABLE 14-1 Transmission of Hepatitis B and C Viruses and Human Immunodeficiency Virus

Disease	Symptoms and Signs	Mode of Transmission	Infectious Materials
Hepatitis B virus	Flulike symptoms, jaundice	Direct and indirect contact	Blood, saliva, semen, feces, food, water, and other products
Hepatitis C virus	Jaundice, upper right quadrant pain, loss of appetite, nausea, fatigue, dark urine	Direct and indirect contact with blood	Blood
Human immunodeficiency virus/acquired immunodeficiency syndrome	Fever, night sweats, weight loss, diarrhea, severe fatigue, swollen lymph nodes, lesions	Direct and indirect contact	Blood, semen, vaginal fluid

Management

Unlike HBV, there is no vaccine for HIV. Even though some drug therapy may extend their lives, there is currently no available treatment to cure patients with AIDS. Much research is being done to find a preventive vaccine and an effective treatment. Presently, the most effective treatment seems to be a therapy consisting of a combination of three drugs. One drug blocks the action of an enzyme that the virus needs to make some of the components for new virus cells. A second drug blocks the copying of viral genes that can enter the host cell's nucleus (a process called reverse transcription) and thus disables the synthesis of new viruses. A third drug helps protect the T cells and thus slows the progression of HIV.[32]

Although new treatments have extended the healthy life span of many people with AIDS, HIV prevalence has continued to increase. As the number of AIDS cases declines because of these new treatments, the number of people with HIV will increase, which means there will be a greater need for both prevention and treatment services.

Prevention

Athletes must understand that their greatest risk for contracting HIV is through intimate sexual contact with an infected partner.[23] Practicing safe sex is of major importance. The athlete must choose nonpromiscuous sex partners and use condoms for vaginal or anal intercourse. Latex condoms provide a barrier against both HBV and HIV. Male condoms should have reservoir tips to reduce the chance of ejaculate being released from the sides of the condom. Condoms that are prelubricated are less likely to tear. Water-based, greaseless spermicides or lubricants should be avoided.[39] If the condom tears, a vaginal spermicide should be used immediately. The condom should carefully be removed and discarded.[39] Additional ways to reduce the risk of HIV infection can be found in *Focus Box:* "HIV risk reduction."

Human immunodeficiency virus is most often transmitted through intimate sexual contact.

The use of latex condoms can reduce the chances of contracting HIV.

BLOODBORNE PATHOGENS IN ATHLETICS

In general the chances of transmitting HIV among athletes is low.[11,21,34,41] There is minimal risk of on-field transmission of HIV from one player to another in sports.[15,34] One study involving professional football estimated that the risk of transmission from player to player was less than 1 per 1 million games.[16] At this time there have been no validated reports of HIV transmission in sports.[27]

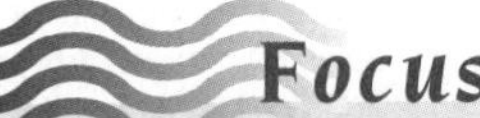

HIV risk reduction

- Avoid contact with others' bodily fluids, feces, and semen.
- Avoid sharing needles (e.g., when injecting anabolic steroids or human growth hormones).
- Choose nonpromiscuous sex partners.
- Limit sex partners.
- Consistently use condoms.
- Avoid drugs that impair judgment.
- Avoid sex with known HIV carriers.
- Get regular tests for sexually transmitted diseases.
- Practice good hygiene before and after sex.

Some sports may have a potentially higher risk for transmission because of close contact and the possibility of passing blood on to the other person.[15] Sports such as the martial arts, wrestling, and boxing have more theoretical potential for transmission (see *Focus Box:* "Risk categories for HIV transmission in sports").[27]

Policy Regulation

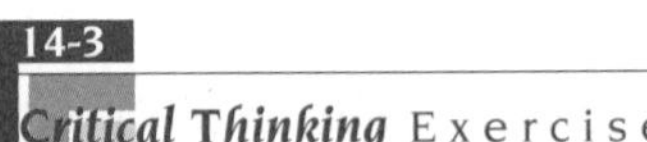

14-3 Critical Thinking Exercise

A wrestler comes into the training room very concerned that his wrestling partner got a bloody nose and that he came in contact with a few drops of that athlete's blood.

? What should the athletic trainer tell the athlete about the transmission of HIV from this type of contact?

Athletes participating in organized sports are subject to procedures and policies about the transmission of bloodborne pathogens.[37] The National Athletic Trainers' Association, U.S. Olympic Committee, National Collegiate Athletic Association, National Federation of State High School Athletic Associations, National Basketball Association, National Hockey League, National Football League, and Major League Baseball all have established policies to help prevent the transmission of bloodborne pathogens. These organizations have also initiated programs to help educate athletes under their control. The Centers for Disease Control and Prevention is another useful resource for the athletic trainer seeking information and guidelines for medical assistance on disease control, epidemic prevention, and notification.

All institutions should take responsibility for educating their student athletes about how bloodborne pathogens are transmitted.[37] In the case of a high school athlete, efforts should also be made to educate the parents.[6] Professional, collegiate, and high school athletes should be made aware that the greatest risk of contracting HBV or HIV is through their off-the-field activities, which may include unsafe sexual practices and sharing of needles, particularly in the use of steroids. Athletes, perhaps more than

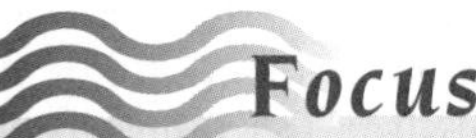

Risk categories for HIV transmission in sports[12]

Although the risk for HIV transmission in athletics is minimal, the following classifications of sports indicate risks relative to one another:

- Highest risk: boxing, martial arts, wrestling, rugby
- Moderate risk: basketball, field hockey, football, ice hockey, judo, soccer, team handball
- Lowest risk: archery, badminton, baseball, bowling, canoeing/kayaking, cycling, diving, equestrianism, fencing, figure skating, gymnastics, modern pentathlon, racquetball, rhythmic gymnastics, roller skating, rowing, shooting, softball, speed skating, skiing, swimming, synchronized swimming, table tennis, volleyball, water polo, weight lifting, yachting

other individuals in the population, think that they are immune and that infection will always happen to someone else. The athletic trainer should also assume the responsibility of educating and informing student trainers about exposure control policies.

Each institution should implement policies and procedures concerning bloodborne pathogens.[34] A recent survey of NCAA institutions found that a large number of athletic trainers and other health care providers at many colleges and universities demonstrated significant deficits in following the universal guidelines mandated by OSHA. Universal precautions in a sports medicine or other health care setting protect both the athlete and the health care provider.[25]

Human Immunodeficiency Virus and Athletic Participation

There is no definitive answer to whether asymptomatic HIV carriers should participate in sports.[42] Bodily fluid contact should be avoided, and the participant should also avoid engaging in exhaustive exercise that may lead to an increased susceptibility to infection.[42]

The Americans with Disabilities Act of 1991 says that athletes infected with HIV cannot be discriminated against and may be excluded from participation only on a medically sound basis.[27] Exclusion must be based on objective medical evidence and must take into consideration the extent of risk of infection to others, the potential harm to the athlete, and what means can be taken to reduce this risk.[19]

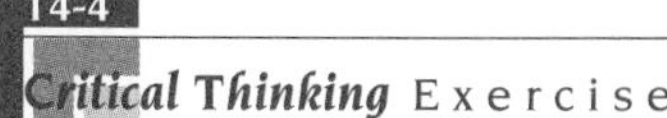

A female athlete has had unprotected sex with a male whom she has dated only once previously. She knows that she should be tested for HIV but is so worried and embarrassed that she has avoided going to a medical facility to have a test. Finally she goes to her athletic trainer and confides her concerns.

? What should the athletic trainer tell her about being tested for HIV?

Testing Athletes for Human Immunodeficiency Virus

Testing for HIV should not be used as a screening tool to determine if an athlete can participate in sports.[9,34] Mandatory testing for HIV may not be allowed because of legal reasons related to the Americans with Disabilities Act.[34] In terms of importance, mandatory testing should be secondary to education to prevent the transmission of HIV.[24] Neither the NCAA nor the Centers for Disease Control and Prevention recommends mandatory HIV testing for athletes.[34]

Athletes who engage in high-risk activities should be encouraged to seek voluntary anonymous testing for HIV.[36] A blood test analyzes serum using an enzyme-linked immunosorbent assay (ELISA) or an enzyme immunoassay (EIA). These tests detect antibodies to HIV proteins. Positive EIA or ELISA tests should be repeated to rule out false-positive results. A second positive test requires the Western blot examination, which is a more sensitive test.[7] Detectable antibodies may appear from three months to one year after exposure. Testing, therefore, should occur at six weeks, three months, and one year.[39]

Home testing kits are also available in which an individual can collect a sample for testing in the privacy of his or her home and then send it to a laboratory for analysis. There are more than a dozen different HIV home test kits being advertised on the market today. Only the Home Access test system is FDA approved and legally marketed in the United States. This approved system uses a simple finger prick process for home blood collection, which results in dried blood spots on special paper. The dried blood spots are mailed to a laboratory with a confidential and anonymous personal identification number (PIN). The sample is then analyzed by trained clinicians in a certified medical laboratory using the same procedures that are used for samples taken in a doctor's office. The purchaser obtains results by calling a toll-free telephone number and using the PIN; post-test counseling is provided by telephone when results are obtained.[4]

For additional information on HIV and AIDS care, contact the CDC National AIDS Hotline: 1 (800) 342-2437.

Many states have enacted laws that protect the confidentiality of the HIV-infected person. The athletic trainer should be familiar with state law and make every effort to guard the confidentiality and anonymity of HIV testing for athletes.

UNIVERSAL PRECAUTIONS IN AN ATHLETIC ENVIRONMENT

In 1991 the Occupational Safety and Health Administration **(OSHA)** established standards for an employer to follow that govern occupational exposure to bloodborne pathogens.[31]

OSHA
Occupational Safety and Health Administration.

Throughout the remainder of this text, whenever there is a discussion of an injury or a technique of care that requires universal precautions, the biohazard icon will appear in the margin.

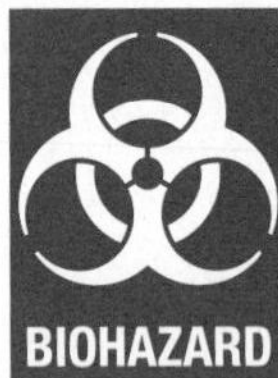

The guidelines instituted by OSHA were developed to protect the health care provider and the patient against bloodborne pathogens.[29] OSHA has mandated that training programs for dealing with bloodborne pathogens be repeated each year to provide the most current information. It is essential that every sports program develop and carry out a bloodborne pathogen exposure control plan.[35] NATA has established specific guidelines for athletic trainers.[22,28] (See Appendix H for NATA's policy statement.) This plan should include counseling, education, volunteer testing, and the management of bodily fluids.[34]

These guidelines should be followed by anyone coming into contact with blood or other bodily fluids.[4,43] Following are considerations specifically in the sports arena.

Preparing the Athlete

Before an athlete participates in practice or competition, all open skin wounds and lesions must be covered with a dressing that is fixed in place and does not allow for transmission to or from another athlete.[33] An occlusive dressing lessens the chances of cross-contamination. One example is the hydrocolloid dressing, which is considered a superior barrier. This type of dressing also reduces the chances that the wound will reopen because it keeps the wound moist and pliable.[33]

When Bleeding Occurs

14-5

Critical Thinking Exercise

A sports program must initiate and carry out a bloodborne pathogen exposure control plan.

? What are the universal precautions in an athletic environment as proposed by OSHA?

As mandated by the NCAA and the USOC, open wounds or other skin lesions considered a risk for disease transmission should be given aggressive treatment. Athletes with active bleeding must be removed from participation as soon as possible and can return only when it is deemed safe by the medical staff.[16] Uniforms containing blood must be evaluated for infectivity. A uniform that is saturated with blood must be removed and changed before the athlete can return to competition. All personnel managing potential infective wound exposure must follow universal precautions.[16,29]

Personal Precautions

Nonlatex gloves should be worn whenever the athletic trainer handles blood or bodily fluids.

The health care personnel working directly with bodily fluids on the field or in the athletic training facility must make use of the appropriate protective equipment in all situations in which there is potential contact with bloodborne pathogens. Protective equipment includes disposable nonlatex gloves, nonabsorbent gowns or aprons, masks and shields, eye protection, and disposable mouthpieces for resuscitation devices.[5] Equipment for dealing with bloodborne pathogens should be included in sideline emergency kits.[30] Disposable nonlatex gloves must be used when handling any potentially infectious material. Double gloving is suggested when there is heavy bleeding or sharp instruments are used. Gloves should always be removed carefully after use. In cases of emergency, heavy toweling may be used until gloves can be obtained[1] (see *Focus Box:* "Glove use and removal") (Figure 14-3).

Focus

Glove use and removal

1. Avoid touching personal items when wearing contaminated gloves.
2. Remove first glove, turn it inside out and, beginning at wrist, peel off second glove without touching skin.
3. Remove second glove, making sure not to touch soiled surfaces with ungloved hand.
4. Discard gloves that have been used, discolored, torn, or punctured.
5. Wash hands immediately after glove removal.

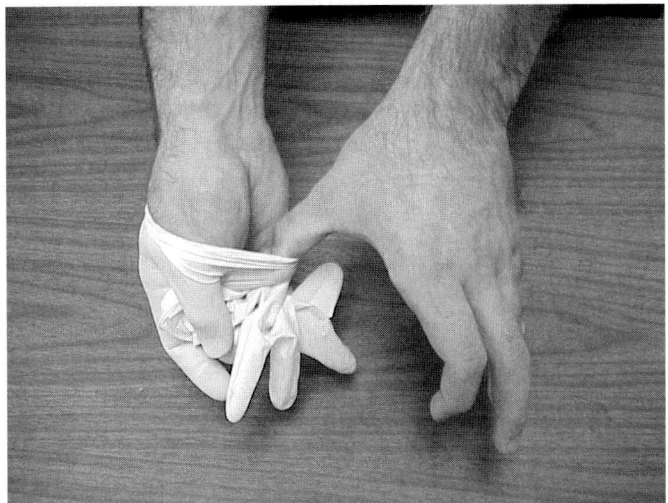

Figure 14-3

Technique for removing nonlatex gloves.

Hands and all skin surfaces that come in contact with blood or other bodily fluids should be washed immediately with soap and water or other antigermicidal agents. Hands should also be washed between each patient treatment. If there is the possibility of bodily fluids becoming splashed, spurted, or sprayed, the mouth, nose, and eyes should be protected. Aprons or nonabsorbent gowns should be worn to avoid clothing contamination.

First aid kits must contain protection for hands, face, and eyes and resuscitation mouthpieces. Kits should also contain towelettes for cleaning skin surfaces.[3]

14-6

Critical Thinking **Exercise**

During a basketball game, one of the players sustains a nosebleed. Blood is visible on the court and on the player's jersey and skin.

? What actions need to take place before the game can resume?

Latex Sensitivity and Using Nonlatex Gloves

It is recommended that athletic trainers use nonlatex gloves.[8] There are a number of manufacturers who produce nonlatex gloves. Latex, a sap from the rubber tree, is composed of compounds that may cause an allergic reaction of a severity that can range from a contact dermatitis to a systemic reaction. Recognizing the signs and symptoms associated with these reactions may help to prevent a more severe reaction from occurring. Some individuals are more at risk of latex allergies due to repetitive exposure to latex through their career paths, multiple surgeries, other allergies, or respiratory conditions. Management of an acute reaction involves removing the irritant, cleansing the affected area, monitoring vital signs for changes, and seeking additional medical assistance as warranted.[8]

Availability of Supplies and Equipment

In keeping with universal precautions, the sports program must also have available chlorine bleach, antiseptics, proper receptacles for soiled equipment and uniforms, wound care bandages, and a designated container for disposal of sharp objects such as needles, syringes, and scalpels.[16]

Universal precautions minimize the risk of exposure and transmission.

Biohazard warning labels should be affixed to containers for regulated wastes, refrigerators containing blood, and other containers used to store or ship potentially infectious materials (Figure 14-4). The labels are fluorescent orange or red. Red bags or containers should be used for the disposal of potentially infected materials.

Disinfectants

All contaminated surfaces such as treatment tables, taping tables, work areas, and floors should be cleaned immediately with a solution consisting of one part bleach to ten parts water (1:10) or with a disinfectant approved by the Environmental Protection Agency.[6] Disinfectants should inactivate the HIV virus. Towels or other linens that have been contaminated should be bagged and separated from other laundry. Soiled

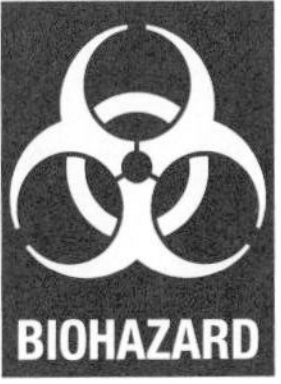

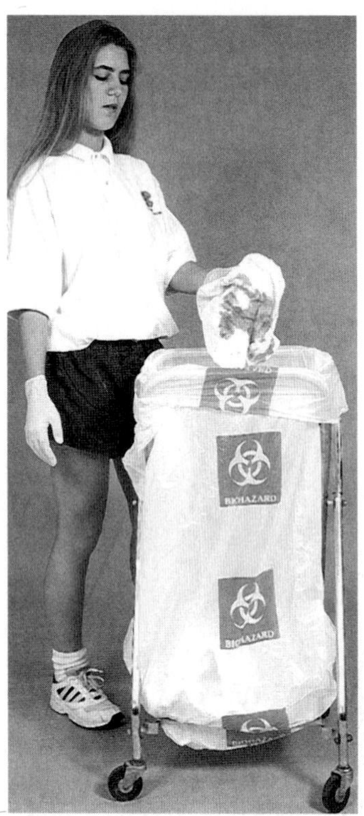

Figure 14-4

Soiled linens should be placed in a leakproof bag marked as a biohazard.

linen should be transported in red or orange containers or bags that prevent soaking or leaking and are labeled with biohazard warning labels (see Figure 14-4). Contaminated laundry should be washed in hot water (71° C/159.8° F for 25 minutes) using a detergent that deactivates the virus. Laundry done outside the institution should be sent to a facility that follows OSHA standards. Gloves must be worn during bagging and cleaning of contaminated laundry.

Sharps

Sharps refers to sharp objects used in athletic training, such as needles, razor blades, and scalpels. Extreme care should be taken when handling and disposing of sharps to minimize the risk of puncturing or cutting the skin. Athletic trainers rarely use needles, but it is not unusual for them to use scalpels or razor blades. Whenever needles are used, they should not be recapped, bent, or removed from a syringe. Sharps should be disposed of in a leakproof and puncture-resistant container.[6] The container should be red or orange and should be labeled as a biohazard (Figure 14-5). Scissors and tweezers are not as likely to cause injury as sharps are, but they should be sterilized with a disinfecting agent and stored in a clean place after use.

Sharps include:
- Scalpels
- Razor blades
- Needles

Protecting the Coach and Athletic Trainer

OSHA guidelines for bloodborne pathogens are intended to protect the coach, athletic trainer, and other employees and not the athlete.[31] Coaches do not usually come in contact with blood or other bodily fluids from an injured athlete, so their risk is considerably reduced. It is the responsibility of the high school, college, professional team, or clinic to ensure the safety of the athletic trainer as a health care provider by instituting and annually updating policies for education on the prevention of transmitting bloodborne pathogens through contact with athletes. The institution must provide the necessary supplies and equipment to carry out these recommendations.

The athletic trainer has the personal responsibility of adhering to these policies and guidelines and enforcing them in the training room. Athletic trainers may further minimize the risk of exposure in the athletic training setting by not eating, drinking, applying cosmetics or lip balm, handling contact lenses, or touching the face before washing hands. Food products should never be placed in a refrigerator containing contaminated blood.[2]

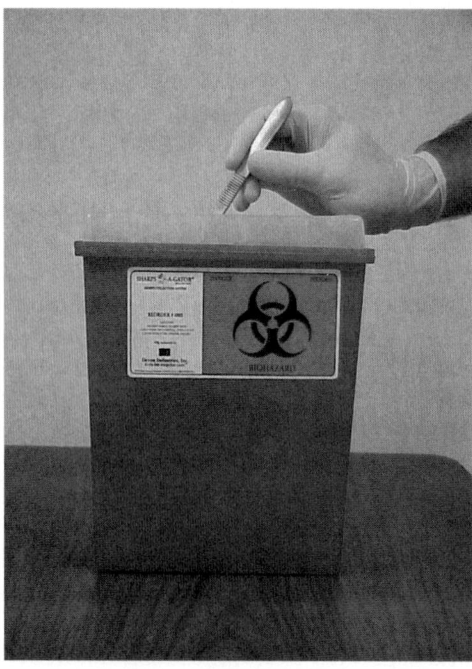

Figure 14-5

Sharps should be disposed of in a red or orange puncture-resistant plastic container marked as a biohazard.

Protecting the Athlete from Exposure

Several additional recommendations may further help to protect the athlete. The USOC supports the required use of mouthpieces in high-risk sports. It is also recommended that all athletes shower immediately after practice or competition. Athletes who may be exposed to HIV, HBV, or HCV should also be evaluated for immunization against HBV.

Postexposure Procedures

After a report of an exposure incident, the athletic trainer should have a confidential medical evaluation that includes documentation of the exposure route, identification of the source individual, a blood test, counseling, and an evaluation of reported illness. Again, the laws that pertain to reporting and confidentiality of test results notification vary from state to state.[31]

SUMMARY

- Bloodborne pathogens are microorganisms that can potentially cause disease and are present in human blood and other bodily fluids, including semen, vaginal secretions, cerebrospinal fluid, synovial fluid, and any other fluid contaminated with blood. Hepatitis B virus, hepatitis C virus, and HIV are bloodborne pathogens.
- A virus is a submicroscopic parasitic organism that contains either DNA or RNA, but not both. It is dependent on the host cell to function and reproduce.
- A vaccine is available to prevent HBV. Currently no effective vaccine exists for treating HCV or HIV.
- An individual infected with HIV may develop AIDS, which is fatal.
- The risks of contracting HBV, HCV, or HIV may be minimized by avoiding exposure to blood and other bodily fluids and by practicing safe sex.
- The risk of an athlete being exposed to bloodborne pathogens on the field is minimal. Off-field activities involving risky sexual behaviors pose the greatest threat for transmission.
- Various national medical and sports organizations have established policies and procedures for dealing with bloodborne pathogens in the athletic population.
- The Occupational Safety and Health Administration has established rules and regulations that protect the health care employee.
- Universal precautions must be taken to avoid bloodborne pathogen exposure. All sports programs must carry out a plan for counseling, education, volunteer testing, and the management of exposure.

Websites

Occupational Safety and Health Administration (OSHA): http://www.osha.gov

Department of Health and Human Services: http://www.os.dhhs.gov

HIV/AIDS Prevention: http://cdc.gov/nchstp/hiv_aids/dhap.htm

Centers for Disease Control and Prevention: http://www.cdc.gov

National Institutes of Health: http://www.nih.gov

Bloodborne Pathogens Self Study Module: http://www2.umdnj.edu/eohssweb/uhbbp/intro.htm

Solutions to Critical Thinking EXERCISES

14-1 During competition or practice the athlete should be most concerned about coming in contact with blood from another athlete. There should be little or no concern about exposure to sweat or saliva. The chances of contracting HIV during athletic participation are minimal. Certainly, the athlete is most likely to be exposed to HIV during unprotected intimate sexual contact.

14-2 The wrestler complained of flulike symptoms such as headache, fever, fatigue, weakness, nausea, and some abdominal pain. A blood test revealed the presence of the HBV antigen.

14-3 The greatest risk of contracting HIV is through intimate sexual contact with an infected partner. The athletic trainer should explain to the athlete that there is little chance of HIV transmission among athletes. There is a theoretical potential risk of transmission among athletes in close contact who pass blood from one to the other.

14-4 The athletic trainer should inform her that it is best if she waits for six weeks before being tested. The athletic trainer should strongly encourage her to seek testing and should explain to her that if she is uncomfortable with being tested in a medical care facility, there is a home test available that has been approved by the FDA and provides confidentiality. The athletic trainer should add that if the athlete were to test positive on the home test, it becomes imperative that she seek additional testing at a medical care facility.

14-5 Universal precautions should be practiced by anyone coming in contact with blood or other bodily fluids. This plan must include counseling, education, volunteer testing, and management of bodily fluids.

14-6 To prevent possible transmission of bloodborne pathogens, several precautions need to be followed. The athlete must be removed from the game until active bleeding has ceased and he or she has been cleared by the medical staff. The jersey must be removed and changed if the uniform is saturated with blood. Any blood on the skin must be cleaned off before the athlete can return to play. In addition, the basketball court needs to be properly cleaned and disinfected. The solution used to clean the court should be one part bleach to ten parts water or a solution approved by the Environmental Protective Agency. All contaminated products need to be properly disposed of according to OSHA standards.

REVIEW QUESTIONS AND CLASS ACTIVITIES

1. Define and identify the bloodborne pathogens.
2. Describe HBV and HCV transmission, symptoms, signs, prevention, and treatment.
3. Explain the pros and cons of allowing an athlete who is an HBV carrier to participate.
4. Describe HIV transmission, symptoms, signs, prevention, and treatment.
5. How is HIV transmitted, and why is it eventually fatal at this time?
6. Should an athlete who tests positive for HBV or HIV be allowed to participate in sports? Why or why not?
7. How can an athlete reduce the risk of HIV infection?
8. Define OSHA universal precautions for preventing bloodborne pathogen exposure.
9. What precautions would you, as an athletic trainer, take when caring for a bleeding wound on the field?

REFERENCES

1. American Academy of Pediatrics: Human immunodeficiency virus (acquired immunodeficiency syndrome [AIDS] virus) in athletic settings, *Pediatrics* 88:640, 1991.
2. American College Health Association: *General statement of institutional response to AIDS,* 1–6, Rockville, Md, 1988, Task Force on AIDS, American College Health Association.
3. American Medical Association Department of HIV, Division of Health Science: *Digest of HIV/AIDS policy,* 1–15, Chicago, Ill, 1993, Department of HIV, American Medical Association.
4. American Medical Society for Sports Medicine and the American Academy for Sports Medicine: Human immunodeficiency virus (HIV) and bloodborne pathogens in sport: joint position statement, *Am J Sports Med* 23:510, 1995.
5. American Red Cross: *Emergency response,* San Bruno, Calif, 2001, Staywell.
6. Arnold BL: A review of selected bloodborne pathogen position statements and federal regulations, *J Ath Train* 30(2):171, 1995.
7. Berkow R, editor: *The Merck manual diagnosis of therapy,* ed 16, Raway, NJ, 1992, Merck Sharp and Dohne Research Laboratories.
8. Binkley H, Schroyer T, Catalfano J: Latex Allergies: A review of recognition, evaluation, management, prevention, education, and alternative product use, *J Ath Train* 38(2):133, 2003.
9. Bitting LA, Trowbridge CA, Costello LE: A model for a policy on HIV/AIDS and athletics, *J Ath Train* 31(4):356, 1996.
10. Boyle M, Sitler M, Rogers K: Knowledge and attitudes of certified athletic trainers in Pennsylvania toward HIV/AIDS and treating HIV-positive athletes, *J Ath Train* 32(1):40, 1997.
11. Brown L, Dortman P: What is the risk of HIV infection in athletic competition? 19939:PO-C21-3102, International Conference on AIDS, 1993.
12. Brown LS, Phillips RY, Brown CL: HIV/AIDS policies and sports: the National Football League, *Med Sci Sports Exerc* 26(4):403, 1994.
13. Buxton BP et al: Prevention of hepatitis B virus in athletic training, *J Ath Train,* 29(2):107, 1994.
14. Coorts J, Michael T, Whitehill W: Hepatitis B immunization of athletic trainers in District IX, *J Ath Train* 32(4):315, 1997.
15. Deere R, Stopka C, Curran K, Bolger C: Universal precautions for bloodborne pathogens: a checklist for your program, *Strategies* 14(6):18, 2001.
16. Dick R: *National Collegiate Athletic Association 2002–2003 NCAA sports medicine handbook,* Indianapolis, Ind, 2002, National Collegiate Athletic Association.
17. Dolan M: *The hepatitis C handbook,* Berkeley, Calif, 1999, North Atlantic Books.
18. Hamann B: *Disease: identification, prevention, and control,* New York, 2001, McGraw-Hill.
19. Herbert DL: Mandatory testing for HIV and exclusion from athletic participation, *Sports Med Stand Malpract Report* 8(4):59, 1996.
20. Hunt BP, Pujol TJ: Athletic trainers as HIV/AIDS educators, *J Ath Train* 29(2):102, 1994.
21. Kleiner DM, Holcomb WR: Bloodborne pathogens: current information for the strength and conditioning professional, *Strength Cond* 17(4):42, 1995.
22. Knight K: Guidelines for preventing bloodborne pathogen diseases, *J Ath Train* 30:197, 1995.
23. Landry GL: HIV infection and athletes, *Sports Med Digest* 15(4):1, 1993.
24. LaPerriere A, Klimas N, Major P: Acquired immune deficiency syndrome. In American College of Sports Medicine: *ACSM's exercise management for persons with chronic disease and disabilities,* Champaign, Ill, 1997, Human Kinetics.
25. McGrew C: HIV and HBV in sports medicine. Part 2. *Sports Medicine in Primary Care* 1(4):29, 1995.
26. McGrew C, Dick R, Schneidewind K: Survey of NCAA institutions concerning HIV/AIDS policies and universal precautions, *Med Sci Sports Exerc* 25:917, 1993.
27. Mitten MJ: HIV-positive athletes, *Physician Sportsmed,* 22(10):63, 1994.
28. National Athletic Trainers' Association: Blood-borne pathogens guidelines for athletic trainers, *J Ath Train* 30(3):203, 1995.
29. National Safety Council: *Bloodborne pathogens,* Boston, 1998, Jones & Bartlett.
30. Nelson RC, Rinn TB: Sideline emergency kits and the need to include universal precautions against blood-borne pathogens, *J Sports Chiropractic & Rehabilitation* 10(1):32, 1996.
31. OSHA: The OSHA bloodborne pathogens standard, *Federal Register* 55(235):64175, 1991.
32. Payne W, Hahn D: *Understanding your health,* St. Louis, 2001, McGraw-Hill.
33. Rheinecker SB: Wound management: the occlusive dressing, *J Ath Train* 30(2):143, 1995.

34. Rogers KJ: Human immunodeficiency virus in sports. In Torg JS and Shephard RJ, editors: *Current therapy in sports medicine,* St Louis, 1995, Mosby.
35. Ross CM, Young SJ: Understanding the OSHA bloodborne pathogens standard and its impact upon recreational sports, *NIRSSA* J 19(2):12, 1999.
36. Sankaran G, Volkwein KAE, Bonsall DR: HIV infection: risk, right to know, and requirement to divulge, *Athletic Therapy Today* 1(3):49, 1996.
37. Sankaran G, editor: *HIV/AIDS in sport: impact, issues and challenges,* Champaign, Ill, 1999, Human Kinetics.
38. Schultz SJ: Preventing transmission of bloodborne pathogens. In Schultz SJ, editor, *Sports medicine handbook,* Indianapolis, Ind, 2001, National Federation of State High School Associations.
39. Seltzer DG: Educating athletes on HIV disease and AIDS, *Physician Sportsmed* 21(1):109, 1993.
40. Strikas RA: Immunizations: recommendations and resources for active patients. *Physician Sportsmed* 29(10):33, 2001.
41. Stringer WW: HIV and aerobic exercise: current recommendations, *Sports Med* 28(6):389, 1999.
42. Thomas CE: The HIV athlete: policy, obligations, and attitudes, *Sport Science Review* 5(2): 12, 1996.
43. Thygerson A: *First aid and CPR,* Boston, 2001, Jones & Bartlett.
44. United States Department of Health and Human Services: AIDS/HIV Statistics, http://www.niaid.nih.gov/factsheets/aidsstat.htm, 2004.
45. Zeigler T: *Management of bloodborne infections in sport,* Champaign, Ill, 1997, Human Kinetics.

ANNOTATED BIBLIOGRAPHY

Dick RA, editor: *National Collegiate Athletic Association 2002–2003 sports medicine handbook,* Indianapolis, Ind, 2002, National Collegiate Athletic Association.

This text offers a complete discussion of bloodborne pathogens and intercollegiate athletic policies and administration.

Berkow R, editor: *The Merck manual of diagnosis and therapy,* ed 16, Rahway, NJ, 1992, Merck Sharp and Dohne Research Laboratories.

This excellent guide discusses diagnosis, symptoms, signs, and treatment of bloodborne pathogens.

Bradley-Springer L, Fendrick RA: *AIDS/HIV instant instructor,* El Paso, Texas, 1994, Skidmore-Roth.

This excellent card system covers transmission, transmission prevention, occupational exposure prevention, testing, counseling, disease progression, and treatment of HIV and AIDS.

Dolan M: *The hepatitis C handbook,* Berkeley, Calif, 1999, North Atlantic Books.

This definitive guide outlines the course of the disease and associated symptoms. It discusses available treatments and lifestyle changes and contains an extensive section on herbs, vitamins, and nutritional supplements.

Hall K et al: *Bloodborne pathogens,* Boston, 1997, Jones & Bartlett.

This manual is dedicated to presenting OSHA regulations specific to bloodborne pathogens.

Hamann B: *Disease: identification, prevention, and control,* St Louis, 2000, McGraw-Hill.

This text is designed for health educators and covers AIDS and hepatitis in detail.

Neilson RP: *OSHA regulations and guidelines: a guide to health care providers,* Clifton Park, NY, 1998, Delmar Learning.

Presents OSHA standards with special emphasis on bloodborne pathogens and incident and injury reporting.

Zeigler T: *Management of bloodborne infections in sport,* Champaign, Ill, 1997, Human Kinetics.

Perhaps the most comprehensive single text available on dealing with bloodborne pathogens in an athletic population, this text contains procedure and policy statements from several different sport and health organizations on managing bloodborne pathogens in the athletic environment.

Chapter 15 Using Therapeutic Modalities

When you finish this chapter you should be able to

- Recognize the legal ramifications of treating the athlete with therapeutic modalities.
- Explain the relationship of most therapeutic modalities relative to electromagnetic energy.
- Describe the theoretical uses of the various types of modalities.
- Correctly demonstrate a variety of thermotherapy and cryotherapy techniques.
- Examine the use of ultrasound in an athletic training setting.
- Discuss the physiological basis and therapeutic uses of electrical stimulating currents.
- Describe how massage, traction, and intermittent compression can be used as therapeutic agents.

Most athletic trainers routinely incorporate the use of therapeutic modalities into their rehabilitation programs.[6] When used appropriately, therapeutic modalities can be an effective adjunct to various techniques of therapeutic exercise. Rehabilitation protocols and progressions must be based primarily on the physiological responses of the tissues to injury and on an understanding of how various tissues heal. The decisions the athletic trainer makes on how and when therapeutic modalities may best be used should be based on his or her recognition of signs and symptoms as well as some awareness of the time frames associated with the various phases of the healing process. This chapter is an introduction to the therapeutic modalities that may be used by an athletic trainer, including cryotherapy, thermotherapy, ultrasound, electrotherapy, massage, traction, intermittent compression, diathermy, lasers, and magnets.

LEGAL CONCERNS

The athletic trainer must carefully follow laws that prohibit him or her from use of certain therapeutic modalities.

Therapeutic modalities must be used in sports medicine with the greatest care possible; they should not be used indiscriminately. Specific laws governing the use of therapeutic modalities vary considerably from state to state. The athletic trainer must follow laws that specifically dictate how athletic trainers can use certain therapeutic modalities. An athletic trainer who uses any type of therapeutic modality must have a thorough understanding of the functions and the indications or contraindications for its use.[39]

The athletic trainer should avoid using a shotgun approach when deciding to incorporate therapeutic modalities into a treatment program. Selection of the appropriate modality should be based on an accurate evaluation of the injury and a decision about which modality can most effectively reach the desired target tissue to achieve specific results. The manufacturers of therapeutic modality equipment often provide recommended protocols for using their equipment in treating specific problems. The athletic trainer should certainly be familiar with these recommended treatment protocols. However, the athletic trainer does not necessarily have to follow the manufacturers' treatment protocols precisely. These are only recommendations. Decisions to alter recommended treatment protocols should be based on sound theory and previous experience. If used appropriately, modalities can be an integral part of a treatment and rehabilitation program.[39]

THE SCIENCE OF THERAPEUTIC MODALITIES: HOW ARE THEY RELATED?

Electrical stimulating currents, shortwave and microwave diathermy, the infrared modalities (e.g., hot packs, cold packs), ultraviolet therapy, and the low-powered laser are all therapeutic agents that emit or produce similar types of radiation and can be classified as *electromagnetic energy.* Ultrasound is a form of radiation that must be classified as *acoustic energy* rather than electromagnetic energy.[40]

The common characteristics of electromagnetic energy are as follows: it can be transmitted without a medium for support; all forms of electromagnetic energy travel at 300 million meters per second in a vacuum; energy waveforms travel in a straight line; and depending on the medium with which the waveform comes into contact, it may be reflected, refracted, absorbed, or transmitted. The electromagnetic radiation spectrum represents various regions classified according to specific wavelengths and frequencies. The lower the frequency, the longer the wavelength, and vice versa. Generally the longer the wavelength of the radiation, the greater the depth of penetration. In human tissue, the energy must be absorbed before any physiological changes can take place.[40]

TRANSMISSION OF THERMAL ENERGY

Thermal energy is transmitted through **conduction, convection, radiation,** and **conversion.**

conduction
Heating through direct contact with a hot medium.

convection
Heating indirectly through another medium such as air or liquid.

radiation
Transfer of heat through space from one object to another.

conversion
Heating through other forms of energy.

Conduction

Conduction occurs when heat is transferred from a warmer object to a cooler one. The ratio of this heat exchange depends on the temperature and the exposure time. Skin temperatures are influenced by the type of heat or cold medium, the conductivity of the tissue, the quantity of blood flow in the area, and the speed at which heat is being dissipated.[26] To avoid tissue damage, the temperature should never exceed 116.6° F (47° C). An exposure that includes close contact with a hot medium that has a temperature of 113° F (45° C) should not exceed thirty minutes. Examples of conductive therapeutic modalities are moist hot packs, paraffin baths, electric heating pads, ice packs, and cold packs.

Convection

Convection refers to the transference of heat through the movement of fluids or gases. Factors that influence convection heating are temperature, speed of movement, and the conductivity of the part.[41] The best example of a modality that uses convection is the whirlpool bath.

Radiation

Radiation is the process whereby heat energy is transferred from one object through space to another object. Shortwave and microwave diathermy, infrared heating, and ultraviolet therapy all rely on the process of radiation for energy transfer.

Conversion

Conversion refers to the generation of heat from another energy form such as sound, electricity, and chemical agents. The mechanical energy produced by high-frequency sound waves changes to heat energy at tissue interfaces (ultrasound therapy).[41] The deep heat of diathermy can be produced by applying electrical currents of specific wavelengths to the skin. Chemical agents such as liniments and balms create a heating sensation through counterirritation of sensory nerve endings.[41]

CRYOTHERAPY

The major therapeutic value of cold is its ability to produce anesthesia, allowing pain-free exercise.

The application of cold for the first aid of trauma to the musculoskeletal system is a widely used practice in sports medicine. When applied intermittently after injury, along with compression, elevation, and rest, it reduces many of the adverse conditions related to the inflammatory or reactive phase of an acute injury.[21,25,28] Depending on the severity of the injury, rest, ice, compression, and elevation (RICE) may be used from the first day to as long as two weeks after injury.

Physical Principles

Cold as a therapeutic agent is a type of electromagnetic energy classified specifically as infrared radiation. When a cold object is applied to a warmer object, heat is abstracted. In terms of cryotherapy, the most common method for cold transfer to tissue is through conduction. The extent to which tissue is cooled depends on the cold medium that is being applied, the length of cold exposure, and the conductivity of the area being cooled.[31] In most cases the longer the cold exposure, the deeper the cooling. At a temperature of 38.3° F (3.5° C), muscle temperatures can be reduced as deep as four centimeters. Cooling is dependent on the type of tissue. For example, tissue with a high water content, such as muscle, is an excellent cold conductor, whereas fat is a poor conductor. Because of fat's low cold conductivity, it acts as the body's insulator.[31] Tissue that has previously been cooled takes longer to return to a normal temperature than does tissue that has been heated.

The two most common means of delivering cold as therapy to the body are ice or cold packs and immersion in cool or cold water. The most effective type of pack contains wet ice rather than ice in a plastic container or in a commercial chemical pack (e.g., Cryogen).[41] Wet ice is a more effective coolant because of the extent of internal energy needed to melt the ice.[41] It has also been shown that ice that undergoes a phase change (i.e., ice melting to water) is more effective at lowering skin and intramuscular temperatures.[29]

Physiological Effects of Cold

When cold is applied to skin for fifteen minutes or less at a temperature of 50° F (10° C) or less, vasoconstriction of the arterioles and venules in the area occurs. This vasoconstriction is caused in part by the reflex action of the smooth muscles, which can result from stimulation of the sympathetic nervous system and adrenal medulla, causing a secretion of norepinephrine and epinephrine.[41] Cooled blood circulating to the anterior hypothalamus also causes vasoconstriction. If cold is continuously applied for fifteen to thirty minutes, an intermittent period of vasodilation occurs for four to six minutes. The **hunting response** involves a slight increase in temperature and not vasodilation as is often thought. This temperature increase is hypothesized to be a reaction against tissue damage from too much cold exposure.[25] When the hunting response occurs, the tissue temperature does not return to preapplication levels. This response has primarily been observed in the appendages. Cold during this period also causes an increase in blood viscosity and a decrease in vasodilator metabolites.[41]

hunting response
Causes a slight temperature increase during cooling.

Much of the damage done to cells after trauma is a result of compromised circulation, which decreases the amount of oxygen being delivered to the cells in the area of injury. The immediate use of ice after injury decreases the extent of ischemic injury to those cells on the periphery of the primary injury by slowing their metabolic rate.[28] This slowdown results in less damage to the tissues and thus decreases rehabilitation time.[25]

Because cold lowers the metabolic rate and produces vasoconstriction, swelling will be reduced in an acute inflammatory response. Cold does not reduce swelling that is already present.[25]

Cooling tissues can directly decrease a muscle spasm by slowing metabolism in the area, thus decreasing the waste products that may have accumulated—waste products that act as muscle irritants and cause spasm. A muscle spasm also can be decreased when cold is applied to decrease the gamma motor neuron activity and also to decrease afferent muscle spindle and GTO activity, as well as when cold increases the muscle's viscosity, slowing its ability to contract.[41]

TABLE 15-1 Skin Response to Cold

Stage	Response	Estimated Time after Initiation
1	Cold sensation	0 to 3 minutes
2	Mild burning, aching	2 to 7 minutes
3	Relative cutaneous anesthesia	5 to 12 minutes

TABLE 15-2 Physiological Variables of Cryotherapy

Variable	Response to Therapy
Muscle spasm	Decreases
Pain perception	Decreases
Blood flow	Decreases up to 10 minutes
Metabolic rate	Decreases
Collagen elasticity	Decreases
Joint stiffness	Increases
Capillary permeability	Increases
Edema	Controversial

Because the local application of cold can decrease an acute muscle spasm, the muscle becomes more amenable to stretch. A gentle stretch of a spastic muscle after an acute injury may be indicated; however, the stretching of long-standing contractures is contraindicated. The use of either cold or heat does not appear to help increase muscle length when used in combination with proprioceptive neuromuscular facilitation (PNF) stretching.[3] Cold tends to cause collagen stiffness.[41]

Cold decreases free nerve ending excitability as well as the excitability of peripheral nerves. Analgesia is caused by raising the nerve's threshold.[31] Nerve fiber response to cold depends mainly on the presence of myelination and the diameter of the fiber. For example, most sensitive to cold are the small, light-touch, cold, and gamma efferent myelinated fibers to the muscle spindles.[31] The next most sensitive to cold are the large myelinated fibers of the proprioceptors and alpha motor nerves.[31] The least sensitive to cold are the unmyelinated pain fibers and postganglionic sympathetic nerves.[31] Table 15-1 indicates the usual outward sequential response to cold application.

The extent of cooling depends on the thickness of the subcutaneous fat layer.

Cold, in general, is more penetrating than heat. Once a muscle has been cooled through the subcutaneous fat layer, cold's effects last longer than heat effects do because fat acts as an insulator against rewarming.[41] The major problem is to penetrate the fat layer initially so that muscle cooling occurs. In individuals with less than ½ inch (1.25 cm) of subcutaneous fat, significant muscle cooling can occur after ten minutes of cold application. In persons with more than ⅘ inch (2 cm) of subcutaneous fat, muscle temperatures barely drop after ten minutes (Table 15-2).[31]

Another unique quality of cooling is its ability to decrease muscle fatigue and increase and maintain muscular contraction. This ability is attributed to the decrease of the local metabolic rate and the tissue temperature.[41]

Special Considerations

Although adverse reactions to therapeutic cold application are uncommon, they do happen and are described as follows:

- Cooling for an hour at 30.2° to 15.8° F (−1° to −9° C) produces redness and edema that lasts for twenty hours after exposure.[17] Frostbite has been known to occur in subfreezing temperatures of 26.6° to 24.8° F (−3° to −4° C).[25]

- Immersion at 41° F (5° C) increases limb fluid volume by 15 percent due to placing the limb in the dependent position.
- Exposure for ninety minutes at 57.2° to 60.8° F (14° to 16° C) can delay resolution of swelling up to one week.[25]
- Some individuals are allergic to cold and react with hives and joint pain and swelling.[41]
- Icing through a towel or an elastic bandage limits the reduction in temperature, which could influence the effectiveness of the treatment.[52]

Raynaud's phenomenon Condition in which cold exposure causes vasospasm of digital arteries.

- **Raynaud's phenomenon** is a condition that causes vasospasm of digital arteries lasting for minutes to hours, which could lead to tissue death. The early signs of Raynaud's phenomenon are attacks of intermittent skin blanching or cyanosis of the fingers or toes, skin pallor followed by redness, and finally a return to normal color. Pain is uncommon, but numbness, tingling, or burning may occur during and shortly after an attack.
- Paroxysmal cold hemoglobinuria is a rare disease that occurs minutes after cold exposure and may lead to renal dysfunction, secondary hypertension, and coma. Early symptoms are severe pain in the back and legs, headache, vomiting, diarrhea, and dark brown urine.
- Although it is relatively uncommon, the application of ice can cause nerve palsy. Nerve palsy occurs when cold is applied to a part that has motor nerves close to the skin surface, such as the peroneal nerve at the fibular head. Usually the condition resolves spontaneously with no significant problem. As a general rule, ice should not be applied longer than twenty to thirty minutes at any one time.

Cryotherapy Techniques

A number of techniques of cold applications can be used therapeutically. The ones most commonly used in sports medicine are ice massage, cold or ice water immersion, ice packs, and vapocoolant sprays.

Ice Massage

Cold therapy can begin one to three days after injury.

Ice massage is a cryotherapeutic method that is performed on a small body area. It can be applied by the athletic trainer and the athlete alike.

Equipment Water is frozen in a foam cup, which forms a cylinder of ice. The foam is removed approximately an inch from the top of the cup. The remaining foam provides a handle for the athletic trainer to grasp while massaging. Another method is to fill a paper cup with water and insert a tongue depressor to act as a handle when the water is frozen. A towel should be present to absorb the water that is collected.

Indications Ice massage is commonly used over a small muscle area such as the tendons, the belly of the muscle, or the bursa or over myofascial trigger points.

Application Grasping the ice cylinder, the athletic trainer rubs the ice over the athlete's skin in overlapping circles in a ten- to fifteen-centimeter area for a period of five to ten minutes. The athlete should experience the sensations of cold, burning, aching, and numbness. When analgesia has been reached, the athlete can engage in stretching or exercise (Figure 15-1).

Special considerations In an athlete with normal circulation, tissue damage seldom occurs from cold application. The temperature of the tissue seldom goes below 59° F (15° C). However, when applying ice massage superficially, if an individual is going to have an adverse reaction to the cold, it tends to happen fairly early in the treatment.[25] The comfort of the athlete must be considered at all times.

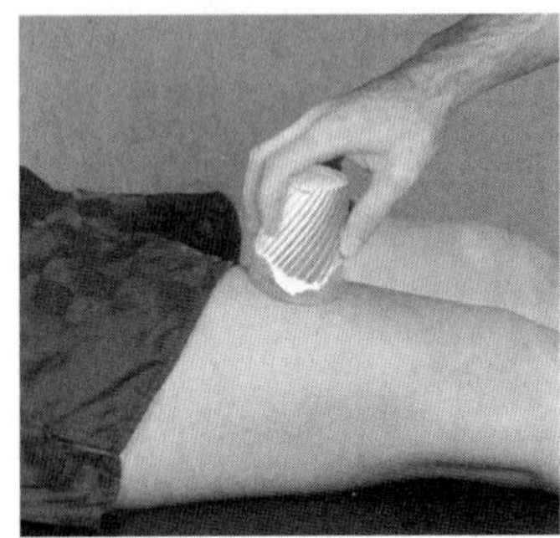

Figure 15-1

Ice massage can lead to an analgesia that can be followed by gentle muscle stretching.

Cold or Ice Water Immersion

Cold water immersion is a relatively simple means for treating a distal body part.

Equipment Depending on the body part to be immersed, a variety of containers or basins can be used. In some cases, a small whirlpool can be used. Water and crushed ice are mixed together to reach a temperature of 50° F (10° C) to 60° F (15° C). Towels must be available for drying.

Indications Where circumferential cooling of a body part is desired, cold or ice water immersion is preferred.

Application The athlete immerses the body part in the water and proceeds through the four stages of cold response. This process may take ten to fifteen minutes. When the pain cycle has been interrupted, the part is removed from the water, and normal movement patterns are conducted. When pain returns, the part is reimmersed. This procedure may be repeated three times. Cool water immersion used in combination with electrical stimulation has been shown to minimize edema formation.[5]

Special considerations Because cold makes collagen tissue brittle, caution should be taken in allowing the athlete to return to full sports performance after receiving cold treatment. Overcooling can lead to frostbite. Any allergic response to cold should also be noted.

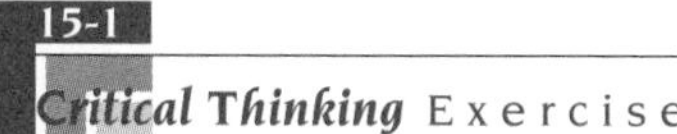
15-1 Critical Thinking Exercise

A soccer player has Achilles tendonitis.

? What different methods of cryotherapy can be used to control pain and inflammation for this condition? Describe the benefits for each application.

Ice Packs (Bags)

The use of ice packs is another way to apply cryotherapy.

Equipment There are a number of types of ice packs. Wet ice packs provide the best cooling properties. Flaked or crushed ice can be encased in a wet towel and placed on the body part to be treated. A pack can be made by placing crushed or chipped ice in a self-sealing plastic bag; this method is not as efficient but is less messy. If isopropyl alcohol is added at a two-to-one ratio, the packs can be put into a freezer and not completely frozen. When they are removed from the freezer, the packs easily fit the contour of the body part. These packs are useful for approximately fifteen or twenty minutes.[41] When the plastic packs are used, a wet towel should be placed between the skin and the pack. Besides toweling, an elastic wrap should be used to hold the pack firmly in place.

Two different types of chemical cold packs are available. One is a gel pack that may be refrozen after use and is hypoallergenic. The gel pack is commonly used in many athletic training settings. The other type is a liquid bag within a bag of crystals. When the inner bag is ruptured the chemicals mix, causing an endothermic reaction. If allowed contact with the skin, these chemicals can cause a chemical burn and a liability problem.[25]

Indications The athlete experiences the four stages of cold that were described earlier in this section and then proceeds with normal movement patterns (Figure 15-2).

Special considerations Excessive cold exposure must be avoided. With any indication of allergy to cold or of abnormal pain, the therapy should be discontinued.

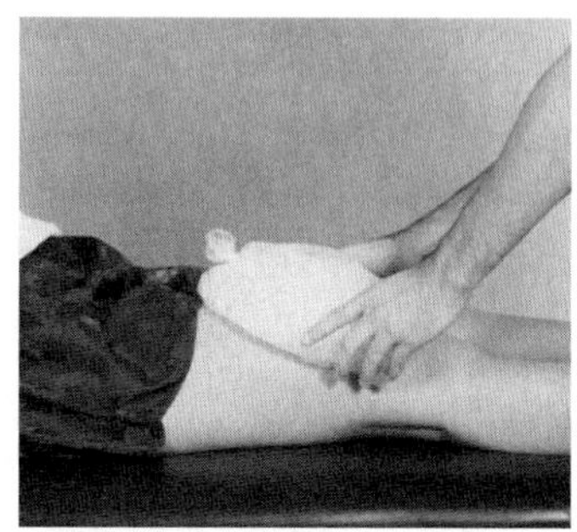
Figure 15-2

Ice packs can be another way to apply cryotherapy.

Vapocoolant Sprays

Increasingly, vapocoolant sprays are being used for the treatment of musculoskeletal conditions attributed to sports activity.

Fluori-methane spray is used in the spray and stretch technique.

Equipment Currently the most popular vapocoolant is fluori-methane, a nonflammable, nontoxic substance. Under pressure in a bottle, it gives off a fine spray when it is inverted and an emitter is pressed.

Indications The major value of a vapocoolant spray is its ability to reduce muscle spasm and increase range of motion. It is also a major treatment for myofascial pain and trigger points.[41] Care must be taken, however, to avoid frostbite.

Application When vapocoolant spray is used to increase the athlete's range of motion in an area in which there is no trigger point, the following procedure is performed:

1. Hold the vapocoolant at a 30-degree angle, 12 to 18 inches (30 to 47 cm) from the skin.
2. Spray the entire length of the muscle from its proximal attachment to its distal attachment.
3. Cover the skin at a rate of approximately four inches (10 cm) per second; apply the spray two or three times as a gradual stretch is applied.

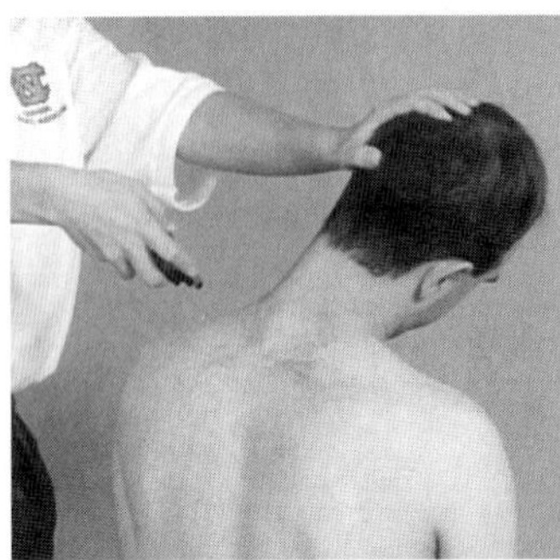

Figure 15-3

A vapocoolant spray such as fluori-methane can assist in reducing muscle spasm.

When dealing with a possible trigger point, the procedure is first to determine its presence, then to alleviate it. One method by which the athletic trainer can determine an active trigger point is to reproduce the injured athlete's major pain complaint by pressing firmly on the site for five to ten seconds. Another assessment technique used by the athletic trainer is to elicit a jump response by placing the athlete's muscle under moderate tension, applying firm pressure, and briskly pulling a finger across the tight band of muscle. This procedure causes the tight band of muscle to contract and the athlete to wince or cry out.[31]

The spray and stretch method for treating trigger points and myofascial pain (Figure 15-3) is performed as follows:[31]

1. Position the athlete in a relaxed but well-supported position. The muscle that contains the trigger point is stretched (an exception to this is the sternocleidomastoid muscle).
2. Alert the athlete that the spray will feel cool.
3. Hold the fluori-methane bottle approximately 12 inches (30 cm) away from the skin to be sprayed.
4. Direct the spray at an acute angle in one direction toward the reference zone of pain.
5. Direct the spray to the full length of the muscle, including the reference zone of pain.
6. Begin firm stretching that is within the athlete's pain tolerance.
7. Continue spraying in parallel sweeps that are approximately ¼ inch (0.6 cm) apart at a speed of approximately four inches (10 cm) every second.
8. Cover the skin area one or two times.
9. Continue passive stretching while spraying. Do not force the stretch; allow time for the muscle to let go.
10. After the first session of spraying and stretching, warm the muscle with a hot pack or by vigorous massage.
11. If necessary, perform a second session after step 10.
12. When a stretch has been completed, have the athlete actively but gently move the part in a full range of motion.
13. Do not overload a muscle with strenuous exercise immediately after a stretch.
14. After an initial spraying and stretching session, instruct the athlete about stretch exercises that should be performed at home on a daily basis.

Cryokinetics

cryokinetics
Combines cryotherapy with exercise.

Cryokinetics is a technique that combines cryotherapy, or the application of cold, with exercise.[25] The goal of cryokinetics is to numb the injured part to the point of analgesia and then work toward achieving normal range of motion through progressive active exercise.

The technique begins by numbing the body part via ice immersion, cold packs, or ice massage. Most athletes report a feeling of numbness within twelve to twenty minutes. If numbness is not perceived within twenty minutes, the athletic trainer should proceed with exercise regardless. The numbness usually lasts for three to five minutes, at which point ice should be reapplied for an additional three to five minutes until numbness returns. This sequence should be repeated five times (see *Focus Box:* "Summary of cryokinetics").

Exercises are performed during the periods of numbness. The exercises selected should be pain free and progressive in intensity; the athlete should concentrate on both flexibility and strength.[45] Changes in the intensity of the activity should be limited by both the nature of the healing process and by individual patient differences in perception of pain. However, progression always should be encouraged within the framework of those limiting factors; the ultimate goal is to return the athlete to full sport activities.[25]

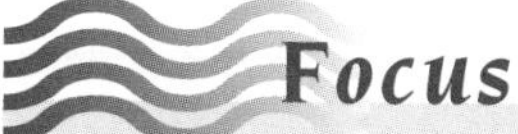

Summary of cryokinetics

1. Immerse ankle in ice water until numb (12 to 20 min).
2. Exercise within limits of pain (see progression in step 6 below) (3 to 5 min).
3. Renumb ankle by immersion (3 to 5 min).
4. Exercise within limits of pain (3 to 5 min).
5. Repeat steps 3 and 4 three more times.
6. Principles of exercising:
   a. All exercise should be active, that is, performed totally by the patient.
   b. All exercise must be pain free.
   c. All exercise must be performed smoothly, without limping, twitching, or any other abnormal motion.
   d. The exercise must be aggressively progressive; that is, it must progress to more complex and difficult levels as quickly as possible (remember—*no pain*).

THERMOTHERAPY

The application of heat to treat disease and traumatic injuries has been used for centuries. Recently, however, its use in the immediate treatment phase of musculoskeletal injury has been replaced with cold application. Heat is an energy form that increases molecular activity by conduction, convection, conversion, and radiation.[41] Thermotherapy modes are moist, dry, superficial, and deep.

Physiological Effects of Heat

The body's response to heat depends on the type of heat energy applied, the intensity of the heat energy, the duration of application, and the unique tissue response to heat. For a physiological response to occur, heat must be absorbed into the tissue, causing an increase in molecular activity. After the tissue's absorption of heat energy, heat is spread to adjacent tissue. To effect a therapeutic change that results in normal function of the absorbing tissue, the correct amount of heat must be applied. With too little, no change occurs; with too much, the tissue is damaged further.

There are still many unanswered questions about how heat produces therapeutic responses and what types of thermotherapy are most appropriate for a given condition. The desirable therapeutic effects of heat include increasing the extensibility of collagen tissues; decreasing joint stiffness; reducing pain; relieving muscle spasm; reducing inflammation, edema, and exudates in the postacute phase of healing; and increasing blood flow.[41]

Heat affects the extensibility of collagen tissue by increasing the viscous flow of collagen fibers and subsequently relaxing the tension. From a therapeutic point of view, heating contracted connective tissue permits an increase in extensibility through stretching. Muscle fibrosis, a contracted joint capsule, and scars can be effectively stretched while being heated or just after the heat is removed.[41] An increase in extensibility does not occur unless heat treatment is associated with stretching exercises.

Heat has the capacity to increase the extensibility of collagen tissue.

Both heat and cold relieve pain, stimulating the free nerve endings and peripheral nerves by a gating mechanism or secretion of endorphins (see Chapter 10). Muscle spasm caused by **ischemia** can be relieved by heat, which increases blood flow to the area of injury. Heat is also believed to assist inflammation and swelling by a number of related factors such as raising temperature, increasing metabolism, reducing oxygen tension, lowering the pH level, increasing capillary permeability, and releasing histamine and bradykinin, which cause vasodilation. Histamine and bradykinin are released from some cells during acute and chronic inflammation. Heat is also produced

ischemia Lack of blood supply to a body part.

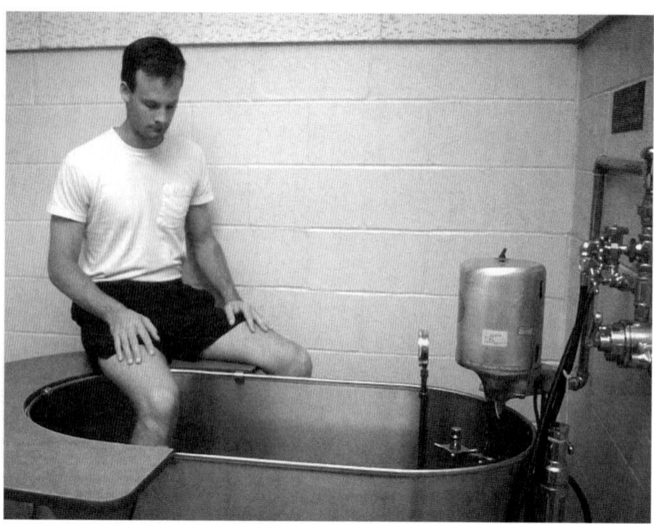

Figure 15-5

A whirlpool bath provides therapy through heat conduction and convection.

TABLE 15-4 Whirlpool Temperatures

Descriptive Terms	Temperature
Very cold	>55° F (12.8° C)
Cold	55°–65° F (12.8°–18.3° C)
Tepid	80°–90° F (27°–33.5° C)
Neutral	92°–96° F (33.5°–35.5° C)
Warm	96°–98° F (35.5°–36.5° C)
Hot	98°–104° F (36.5°–40° C)

This medium assists the body part by reducing swelling, muscle spasm, and pain. Because of the buoyancy of the water, active movement of the part is also assisted.

Application

1. The water temperature should be set according to Table 15-4. Some athletic trainers prefer to perform only cold water treatments, whereas others prefer to increase the temperature according to the healing phase of an acute injury. Chronic conditions normally require a higher water temperature.
2. Once the tank has been filled with water at the desired temperature, the athlete is comfortably positioned so that the body part to be treated can be easily reached by the agitated water. In many cases, the water jet should not be placed directly on the body part but to the side of the tank. This placement is particularly relevant in the early stages of the acute injury. In cases in which the stream is concentrated directly toward the injury site, the site should be at least eight to ten inches from the jet.
3. The duration of treatment is of major concern for the athletic trainer. The maximum length of treatment time for acute injuries should not exceed twenty minutes. In the early stages of acute injury treatment, a graduated program should be implemented. Treatment time should be increased slowly on a daily basis—to five minutes, ten minutes, fifteen minutes, and finally to twenty minutes. A duration of twenty minutes is usually recommended for treatment of chronic injuries.

Special considerations

1. Caution should be taken when an athlete undergoes full-body immersion because of the possibility that the athlete will experience light-headedness.[54]
2. Proper whirlpool maintenance is necessary to avoid infection. The following procedures should be adhered to:
   a. Empty tank after use.
   b. Scrub inside of tank with a commercial disinfectant, rinse with clean water, and dry.

c. Polish external surface of tank with a commercial stainless steel polish.

3. Safety is of major importance in the use of the whirlpool. All electrical outlets should have a ground fault circuit interrupter. At no time should the athlete turn the motor on or off. Ideally, the on/off switch should be a considerable distance from the machine.[54]

Paraffin Bath

Paraffin is a popular method for applying heat to the distal extremities.

Paraffin bath therapy is particularly effective for injuries to the more angular body areas.

Equipment The commercial paraffin bath is a thermostatically controlled unit that maintains a temperature of 126° to 130° F (52° to 54° C). The paraffin mixture consists of a ratio of twenty-five kilograms of paraffin wax to one liter of mineral oil. Slats at the bottom of the container protect the athlete from burns and collect the settling dirt. Also required for treatment are plastic bags, paper towels, and towels.

Indications The mineral oil acts to lower the melting point of the paraffin and thus the specific heat. Consequently, the ability to tolerate the heat from the paraffin is greater than it would be from water at the same temperature.

This therapy is especially effective in treating chronic injuries occurring to the more angular areas of the body such as the hands, wrists, elbows, ankles, and feet.

Application Therapy by means of the paraffin bath can be delivered in several ways. The body part can be dipped and wrapped in a plastic bag, or it can be dipped and reimmersed to form eight to ten layers. The paraffin can be painted on in several layers, or the body part can be soaked in the paraffin.

Before therapy, the body part to be treated is thoroughly cleaned and dried. Then the athlete dips the affected part into the paraffin bath and quickly pulls it out, allowing the accumulated wax to dry and form a solid covering. The process of dipping and withdrawing is repeated six to twelve times until the wax coating is ¼ to ½ inch (0.6 to 1.25 cm) thick.

If the dip and wrap technique is used, the accumulated wax is allowed to solidify on the last withdrawal; then the wax is completely wrapped in a plastic material that in turn is wrapped with a towel. The packed body part is placed in a position of rest for approximately thirty minutes or until heat is no longer generated. The covering is then removed and the paraffin is scraped back into the container.

If the soak technique is selected, the athlete is instructed to soak the wax-coated part in the hot wax container for twenty to thirty minutes without moving it, after which the part is removed from the container and the paraffin on it is allowed to solidify. The part can be packed in towels following the soak, or the paraffin coating can be scraped back into the container immediately after it hardens. Once the paraffin has been removed from the part, an oily residue remains that provides an excellent surface for massage (Figure 15-6).

Special considerations Avoid paraffin bath therapy on body areas that have hemorrhaging or a decrease in normal circulation.

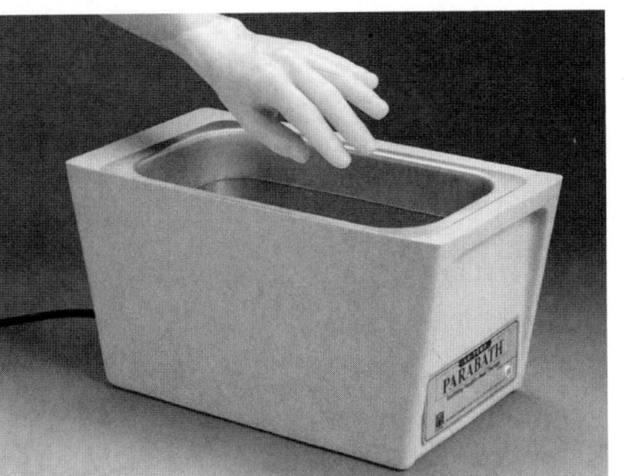

Figure 15-6

A paraffin bath is an excellent form of therapeutic heat for the distal extremities. After paraffin coating has been accomplished, the part is covered by a plastic material. When heat is no longer generated, the paraffin is scraped back into the container.

contrast bath procedure Technique that uses immersion in ice slush, followed by immersion in tepid water (93° to 98° F [33.9° to 37.7° C]).

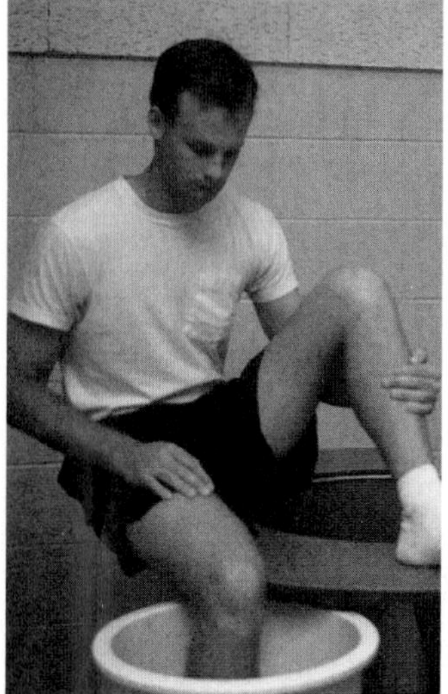

Figure 15-7

A contrast bath, which uses alternating cold water immersion and hot water immersion, is a popular therapy with many athletic trainers.

Contrast baths do not appear to produce alternating vasodilation and vasoconstriction.

It is essential that the athlete clean the body part thoroughly before therapy to avoid contaminating the mixture. In most cases, if this rule is closely adhered to, the mixture will only have to be replaced approximately every six months.[41]

Contrast Bath

Contrasting hot and cold water is primarily used in the treatment of the extremities.

Equipment The **contrast bath procedure** requires the use of two containers—one to hold hot water at 105° to 110° F (40.6° to 43.3° C) and one to hold cold water at 50° to 65° F (10° to 18° C). A whirlpool can be used for the hot container, and a basin or bucket can be used for the cold.

Indications Contrast baths are used when changing the treatment modality from cold to heat to facilitate a mild tissue temperature increase. The use of contrast baths allows for a transitional period during which a slight rise in temperature may be effective for increasing blood flow to an injured area without causing accumulation of additional edema. Only a slight temperature change occurs superficially using the contrast technique.[32] The theory that contrast baths induce a type of pumping action by alternating vasoconstriction with vasodilation has little or no credibility.[41] Likewise, the use of hot and cold packs to produce a contrast effect has also proven to be ineffective.[33]

Application During the initial stages of contrast bath treatment, the ratio of heat to cold treatment begins with a relatively brief exposure to heat; this exposure is gradually increased in subsequent treatments. Recommendations of specific ratios vary. However, it appears that a 3:1 ratio (3 minutes in heat, 1 minute in cold) or 4:1 for nineteen or twenty minutes is fairly well accepted (Figure 15-7).[41] The ratio may be modified as the transition from cold to heat progresses.

Special considerations

- Care must be taken to keep the water temperature constant.
- The athlete should be kept as comfortable as possible throughout the procedure.

Alternative method A second method of contrast that has become popular in sports medicine uses the concept of alternatively submerging the limb in an ice slush bath for two minutes and then in tepid water at 93° to 98° F (33.9° to 37.7° C) for thirty seconds. The baths are alternated for fifteen minutes, beginning and ending with cold immersion.

Fluidotherapy

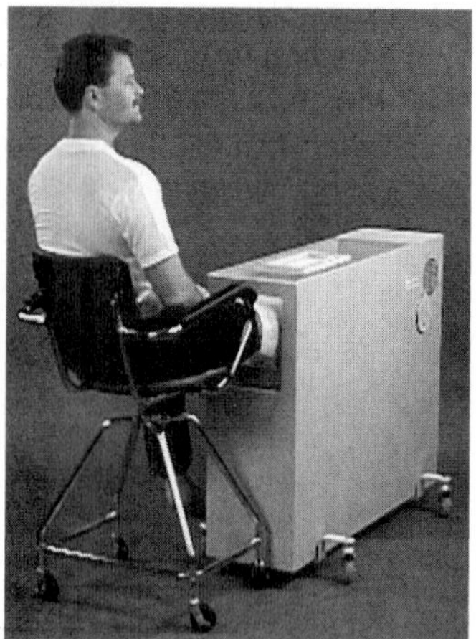

Figure 15-8

Fluidotherapy units contain fine cellulose particles in which warm air is circulated.

Fluidotherapy creates a therapeutic environment with dry heat and forced convection through a suspended airstream.

Equipment Fluidotherapy units come in a variety of sizes, ranging from ones that treat distal extremities to ones that treat large body areas. The unit contains fine cellulose particles in which warm air is circulated. As the air is circulated, the cellulose particles become suspended, giving them properties that are similar to liquid.[41] Fluidotherapy allows the athlete to tolerate much greater temperatures than would be possible using water or paraffin heat (Figure 15-8).

Indications Fluidotherapy is successful, resulting in decreased pain, increased joint range of motion, and decreased spasm and swelling.

Application

- Treatment temperature usually ranges from 100° to 113° F (37.8° to 45° C).
- Particle agitation should be controlled for comfort.
- Exercise can be performed while the athlete is in the cabinet.
- The athlete should be positioned for comfort.
- Treatment duration is fifteen to twenty minutes.

ULTRASOUND THERAPY

Ultrasound is another widely used modality in athletic training. It is a valuable therapeutic tool in the rehabilitation of many different injuries because it stimulates the repair of soft-tissue injuries and relieves pain.[12] Ultrasound is a deep-heating modality and is used primarily for elevating tissue temperatures. Ultrasound is a form of acoustic rather than electromagnetic energy. Ultrasound is defined as inaudible, acoustic vibrations of high frequency that may produce either thermal or nonthermal physiological effects.[9] The use of ultrasound as a therapeutic agent may be extremely effective if the athletic trainer has an adequate understanding of its effects on biological tissues and of the physical mechanisms by which these effects are produced.[9]

Ultrasound can be applied either to the skin or through a water medium.

The number of movements, or oscillations, in one second is referred to as the frequency of a sound wave and is known as a hertz (Hz) unit. More commonly, 1 Hz equals one cycle per second, 1 kHz equals one thousand cycles per second, and 1 MHz equals one million cycles per second.[42] The human ear cannot detect sound greater than 20,000 Hz; therefore inaudible sound is considered ultrasound. When sound scatters and absorbs as it penetrates tissue, its energy is decreased **(attenuation).** Absorption of sound increases with an increase in frequency.

attenuation
A decrease in intensity as the sound enters deeper tissues.

Tissue penetration depends on impedance or acoustical properties of the media that are proportional to tissue density.[12] Sound reflection occurs when adjacent tissues have different impedance. The greater the impedance, the greater the reflection, and the more heat produced. The greatest heat is developed between bone and the adjacent soft-tissue interface.

Equipment The main piece of equipment for delivering therapeutic ultrasound is a high-frequency generator, which provides an electrical current through a coaxial cable to a transducer contained within an applicator. In the applicator or transducer are synthetic crystals such as barium titanate or lead zirconate titanate that possess the property of piezoelectricity. These crystals are in disks 2 to 3 mm thick and 1 to 3 cm in diameter.[9] The **piezoelectric effect** causes expansion and contraction of the crystals, which produce oscillation voltage at the same frequency as the sound wave.[7]

piezoelectric effect
Electrical current produced by applying pressure to certain crystals such as quartz.

Frequency Therapeutic ultrasound has a frequency range between 0.75 and 3.0 MHz (megahertz). The majority of ultrasound generators are set at a frequency between 1 and 3 MHz. A generator that can be set between 1 and 3 MHz affords the athletic trainer the greatest treatment flexibility. Ultrasound energy generated at 1 MHz is transmitted through the more superficial tissues and absorbed primarily in the deeper tissues at depths of 3 to 5 cm. A 1 MHz frequency is most useful in individuals with high percent body fat cutaneously and whenever the desired effects are in the deeper structures.[9,27] At 3 MHz the energy is absorbed in the more superficial tissues with a depth of penetration between 1 and 2 cm (⅓ and ¾ inch).[10]

Ultrasound beam The portion of the surface of the ultrasound transducer that produces the sound wave is referred to as the **effective radiating area.** Energy is delivered to the tissues in a collimated cylindrical beam. The beam from ultrasound generated at 1 MHz is more divergent than at 3 MHz. Within this beam, the distribution of ultrasound energy is nonuniform. The amount of variability of intensity in the beam is indicated by the **beam nonuniformity ratio (BNR).** The lower the BNR, the more uniform the energy output. Optimally the BNR would be 1:1.

effective radiating area
That portion of the transducer that produces sound energy.

beam nonuniformity ratio (BNR)
The amount of variability in intensity of the ultrasound beam.

Intensity The intensity of the ultrasound beam is determined by the amount of energy delivered to the sound head (applicator). It is expressed in the number of watts per square centimeter (W/cm^2). As a therapeutic modality used in sports medicine, the intensity ranges from 0.1 to 3 W/cm^2.

Pulsed versus continuous ultrasound Virtually all therapeutic ultrasound generators can emit either continuous or pulsed ultrasound waves. If continuous ultrasound is used, the sound intensity remains constant throughout the treatment and the ultrasound energy is being produced 100 percent of the time. With pulsed ultrasound, the intensity is periodically interrupted and no ultrasound energy is produced during the off period. The percentage of time that ultrasound is being generated is referred to as the *duty cycle.* If the pulse duration is one millisecond and the total pulse period is five milliseconds, the duty cycle would be 20 percent. Therefore the total amount of energy being delivered to the tissues would be only 20 percent of the energy delivered if a continuous wave were being used.

Ultrasound can be pulsed or continuous.

Duty cycle indicates the percentage of time that ultrasound is being generated.

Continuous ultrasound is most commonly used to produce thermal effects. The use of pulsed ultrasound results in a reduced average heating of the tissues. Pulsed ultrasound or continuous ultrasound at a low intensity will produce nonthermal or mechanical effects, which may be associated with soft-tissue healing.[9]

Indications

Ultrasound produces effects that are thermal or nonthermal.

Thermal versus nonthermal effects Therapeutic ultrasound produces both *thermal and nonthermal effects.*[9] Traditionally, ultrasound has been used primarily to produce a tissue temperature increase. The clinical effects of using ultrasound to heat the tissues are similar to those of other forms of superficial heat discussed in earlier sections. For the majority of these effects to occur, the tissue temperature must be raised to a level of 104° to 113° F (40° to 45° C) for a minimum of five minutes. Temperatures below this range will be ineffective, and temperatures above 113° F (45° C) may be potentially damaging.[9] Ultrasound at 1 MHz with an intensity of 1 W/cm^2 can raise soft-tissue temperature by 0.2° C per minute, and at 3 MHz, by as much as 0.6° C per minute.[9,15]

Nonthermal effects include cavitation and microstreaming.

Whenever ultrasound is used to produce thermal changes, nonthermal changes also occur. However, if appropriate treatment parameters are selected, nonthermal effects can occur with minimal thermal effects. The nonthermal effects of therapeutic ultrasound include *cavitation* and acoustic *microstreaming*. Cavitation is the formation of gas-filled bubbles that expand and compress because of ultrasonically induced pressure changes in tissue fluids.[11] Cavitation results in an increased flow in the fluid around these vibrating bubbles. Microstreaming is the unidirectional movement of fluids along the boundaries of cell membranes resulting from the mechanical pressure wave in an ultrasonic field.[11] Microstreaming can alter cell membrane structure and function because of changes in cell membrane permeability to sodium and calcium ions important in the healing process. As long as the cell membrane is not damaged, microstreaming can be of therapeutic value in accelerating the healing process.[9] These nonthermal effects have been reported to alter membrane properties, alter cellular proliferation, and produce increases in proteins associated with inflammation and injury repair, implying that ultrasound can modify the inflammatory response.[22]

The nonthermal effects of therapeutic ultrasound in the treatment of injured tissues may be as important as the thermal effects and perhaps are even more important. The nonthermal effects of cavitation and microstreaming can be maximized and the thermal effects minimized by using an intensity of 0.1 to 0.2 W/cm^2 with continuous ultrasound or 1.0 W/cm^2 at a duty cycle of 20 percent.

Acute conditions require more frequent treatments over a shorter period of time, whereas chronic conditions require fewer treatments over a longer period of time.[9] Ultrasound treatments should begin as soon as possible after injury, ideally within hours but definitely within forty-eight hours to maximize effects on the healing process.[9] Acute conditions may be treated using low-intensity ultrasound once or twice daily for six to eight days until acute symptoms such as pain and swelling subside. In chronic conditions, when acute symptoms have subsided, treatment may be done on alternating days for a total of ten to twelve treatments.

Application There are a number of options for using ultrasound in sports medicine.

coupling medium
Used to facilitate the transmission of ultrasound into the tissues.

Direct skin application Because acoustic energy cannot travel through air and is reflected by the skin, there must be a **coupling medium** applied to the skin.[9] Coupling mediums include a variety of materials, such as mineral oil or water-soluble creams or gels. The purpose of a coupling medium is to provide an airtight contact with the skin and a slick, low-friction surface. When a water-soluble material is used, the skin should first be washed and dried to prevent air bubbles from hampering the flow of mechanical energy into the skin (Figure 15-9). The use of topical analgesics as a coupling medium has also been recommended, although evidence regarding their effectiveness has not been clearly demonstrated.[34]

Underwater application Underwater ultrasound is suggested for such irregular body parts as the wrist, hand, elbow, knee, ankle, and foot. The part is fully submerged in water; then the ultrasound head is submerged and positioned approximately 1 inch (2.5 cm) from the body part to be treated. The water medium provides an airtight coupling and allows sound waves to travel at a constant velocity. To ensure uninterrupted therapy, air bubbles that form on the skin must be continually wiped away. The sound head is moved slowly in a circular or longitudinal pattern.[9]

Underwater application should be done in a plastic or rubber nonmetal container to avoid reflection of energy off the metal walls.

Bladder technique If, for some reason, the treatment area cannot be immersed in water, a bladder technique can be used. In this technique, a balloon is filled with water, and the ultrasound energy is transmitted from the transducer to the treatment surface through this bladder. Both sides of the balloon should be coated with gel to ensure good contact.[9] Athletic trainers rarely use this technique.

Moving the transducer Moving the transducer during treatment leads to a more even distribution of energy within the treatment area and can reduce the likelihood of developing hot spots. The transducer should be moved slowly at approximately 1½ inches (4 cm) per second. The transducer should be kept in maximum contact with the skin via some coupling agent throughout the treatment.

Movement of the transducer can be in a circular pattern or a stroking pattern. In the circular pattern, the transducer is applied in small overlapping circles. In the stroking pattern, the transducer is moved back and forth, overlapping the preceding stroke by half. Both techniques are performed slowly and deliberately. The field covered should not exceed three to four inches (7.5 to 10 cm). The pattern is determined mainly by the skin area to be treated. For example, the circular pattern is best for highly localized areas such as the shoulder, whereas in larger, more diffuse injury areas, the stroking pattern is best used. When a highly irregular surface area is to be given therapy, the underwater method should be used.[57]

Dosage and treatment time Dosage of ultrasound varies according to the depth of the tissue treated and the state of injury, such as subacute or chronic.[4] Basically, 0.1 to 0.3 W/cm^2 is regarded as low intensity, 0.4 to 1.5 W/cm^2 is medium intensity, and 1.5 to 3 W/cm^2 is high intensity. The duration of treatment ranges from five to ten minutes.

Special considerations Although ultrasound is a relatively safe modality, certain precautions must be taken, and in some situations ultrasound should never be used. Great care must be taken when treating anesthetized areas because the sensation of pain is one of the best indicators of overdosage. Great precautions must be used in areas that have reduced circulation. In general, ultrasound must not be applied to highly fluid areas of the body such as the eyes, ears, testes, brain, spinal cord, and heart. Reproductive organs and women who are pregnant must not receive ultrasound. Acute injuries should not be treated with ultrasound. Epiphyseal areas in children should have only minimum ultrasound exposure.[57]

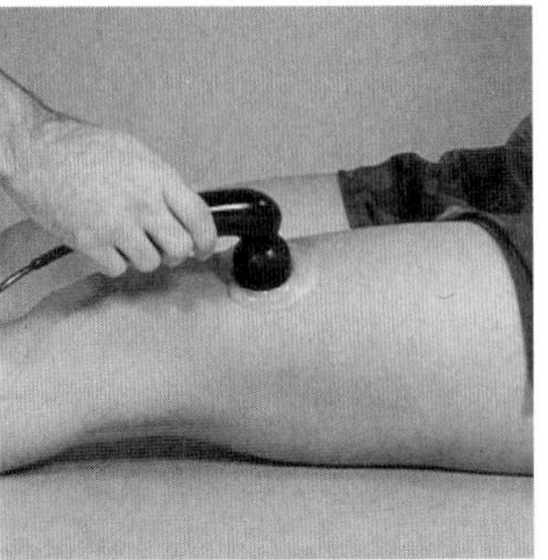

Figure 15-9

Ultrasound therapy, when applied directly to the skin, must be performed over a coupling medium because acoustical energy cannot travel through air.

15-3 Critical Thinking Exercise

A field hockey player has a three-week-old deep quadriceps contusion. She has returned to full practice. There is still a palpable swollen area present and some remaining purplish-yellow discoloration. The injury is no longer tender to the touch, but the athlete does not have full range of motion in flexion.

? At this point in the process of healing, what modalities would be most appropriate?

Ultrasound in Combination with Other Modalities

Ultrasound is commonly used in conjunction with other modalities.

In an athletic training environment, it is not uncommon to combine modalities to accomplish a specific treatment goal. Ultrasound is frequently used with other modalities, including hot packs, cold packs, and electrical stimulating currents.

Hot packs and ultrasound are a useful combination because of the relaxing effects of hot packs in muscle spasm or muscle guarding. Hot packs produce more superficial heating while ultrasound produces heating in the deeper tissues. The use of a hotpack and 1-MHz ultrasound treatments appears to have an additive effect on muscle temperature.[7]

Cold packs are frequently used before ultrasound application. However, if the treatment goal is an increase in deep tissue temperature, the use of a cold pack before ultrasound interferes with heating and is not recommended.[11,44]

Ultrasound is often used with electrical stimulating currents and is thought to be particularly effective in treating trigger points and acupuncture points. Ultrasound

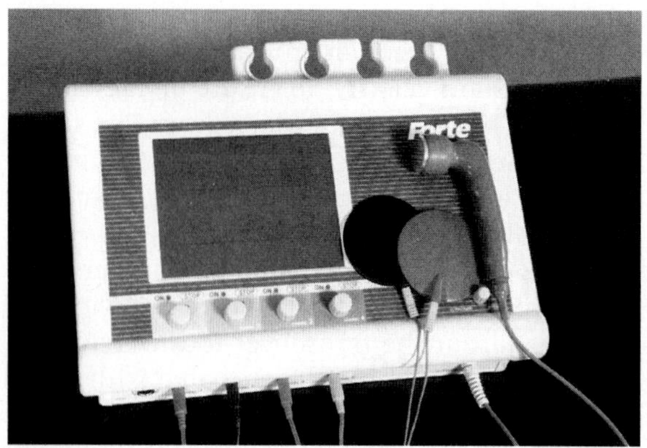

Figure 15-10

Combination ultrasound and electrical stimulator unit.

increases the blood flow to the deep tissues while the electrical currents produce a muscle contraction or modulate pain associated with an injury (Figure 15-10).[9]

Phonophoresis

Phonophoresis is a method of driving molecules through the skin with ultrasound.

Phonophoresis is a method of transporting molecules through the skin using the mechanical vibration of the ultrasound.[57] The techniques of phonophoresis and *iontophoresis* are often confused, and occasionally the two terms are erroneously interchanged. Both techniques are used to deliver chemicals to various biologic tissues. Phonophoresis involves the use of acoustic energy in the form of ultrasound to transport whole molecules across the skin into the tissues, while iontophoresis uses an electrical current to transport ions into the tissues.

Phonophoresis is designed to move medication into injured tissues. Some sports medicine personnel prefer this method to iontophoresis, indicating that it is less hazardous to the skin and that there is greater penetration.[57] As with iontophoresis, phonophoresis is predominantly used to introduce hydrocortisone and an anesthetic into the tissues. This method has been proposed for treating painful trigger points, tendinitis, and bursitis.[35] The effectiveness of phonophoresis as a treatment technique is questionable and needs further research.[35]

Many clinicians prefer to use a 10 percent hydrocortisone ointment.[35] Sometimes lidocaine is added to the cortisone to provide a local anesthetic effect. This medicine is massaged into the skin over an area of tendinitis, bursitis, or other chronic soft-tissue condition. The coupling gel is then spread over the medication, and the ultrasound is applied.

Chem-pads are commercially produced pads that are impregnated with medication; they may be used instead of the traditional medicated ointment application.

ELECTROTHERAPY

The use of electrotherapy is commonplace in the athletic training setting.[16]

Physical Principles

In general, electricity is a form of energy that displays magnetic, chemical, mechanical, and thermal effects on tissue. It implies a flow of electrons between two points. Electrons are particles of matter that have a negative electrical charge and revolve around the core, or nucleus, of an atom.

ampere
Volume or amount of electrical energy.

ohm
Resistance.

voltage
Force.

An electrical current refers to a string of electrons that pass along a conductor such as a nerve or wire. The volume or amount of the current is measured in **amperes** (A); 1 A equals the rate of flow of 1 coulomb (C) per second. A coulomb is a unit of electrical charge and is defined as the quantity of an electrical charge that can be transferred by 1 A in one second.

Resistance to the passing of an electrical current along a conductor is measured in **ohms** (Ω), and the force that moves the current along is called **voltage** (V). One volt is the amount of electrical force required to send a current of 1 A through a resistance of 1 Ω. In terms of electrotherapy, currents of 0 to 150 V are considered low-voltage currents, and currents above 150 V are considered high voltage. The intensity of a current varies directly with the voltage and inversely with the resistance. Electrical power is measured in **watts** (amps × volts).[49]

watt
Power.

An electrical current applied to nerve tissue at a sufficient intensity and duration to reach that tissue's excitability threshold will result in a membrane depolarization or firing of that nerve. There are three major types of nerve fibers: sensory, motor, and pain. As current intensity or duration is increased, the threshold for depolarization will be reached first for sensory fibers, then for motor fibers, and then for pain fibers. Thus it is possible to produce different physiological responses by adjusting the treatment parameters.[17]

Electrical Stimulating Units

Electrotherapeutic devices generate three different types of current, which, when introduced into biological tissue, are capable of producing specific physiological changes. These three types of current are biphasic (AC), monophasic (DC), and polyphasic (pulsatile).[37]

Electrical currents include monophasic (DC), biphasic (AC), and polyphasic (pulsatile).

A great deal of confusion has developed about the terminology used to describe electrotherapeutic currents. All therapeutic electrical generators, regardless of whether they deliver biphasic, monophasic, or polyphasic or pulsatile currents through electrodes attached to the skin, are *transcutaneous electrical stimulators.* The majority of these generators are used to stimulate peripheral nerves and are correctly called *transcutaneous electrical nerve stimulators (TENS)* (Figure 15-11). Occasionally the terms *neuromuscular electrical stimulator (NMES)* or *electrical muscle stimulator (EMS)* are used; however, these terms are appropriate only when the electrical current is being used to stimulate muscle directly, as would be the case with denervated muscle in which peripheral nerves are not functioning. In recent years, a new type of transcutaneous electrical stimulator has gained popularity that uses current intensities too small to excite peripheral nerves. In the past these devices have been called *microcurrent electrical nerve stimulators (MENS),* although they are currently being referred to as *low-intensity stimulators (LIS).*[37]

Current parameters:
- Waveform
- Modulation
- Intensity
- Duration
- Frequency
- Polarity
- Electrode setup

Monophasic (Direct) Current

Monophasic current, also called direct or galvanic current, flows in one direction only from the positive pole to the negative pole. Direct current may be used for pain modulation or muscle contraction or to produce ion movement. Specific physiological effects are determined by how the treatment parameters are set on the stimulating unit. Most electrical stimulators currently used in athletic training settings are DC units.

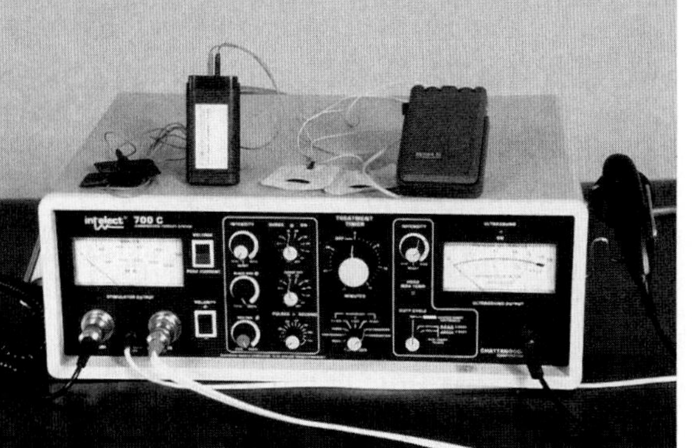

Figure 15-11
Many therapeutic electrical generators are transcutaneous electrical nerve stimulators (TENS) units.

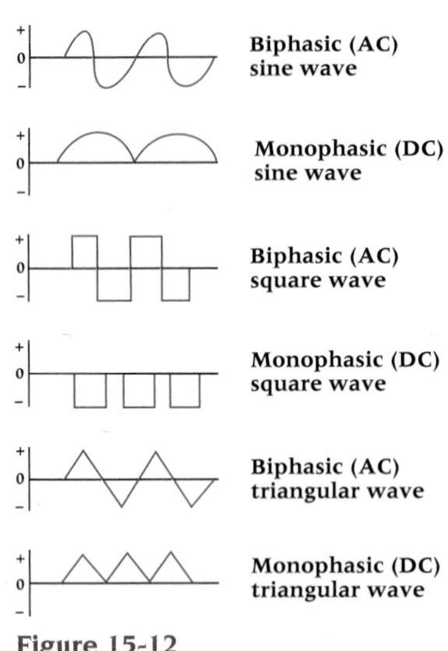

Figure 15-12

Waveforms can be either sine, square, or triangular for both monophasic (DC) and biphasic (AC) currents.

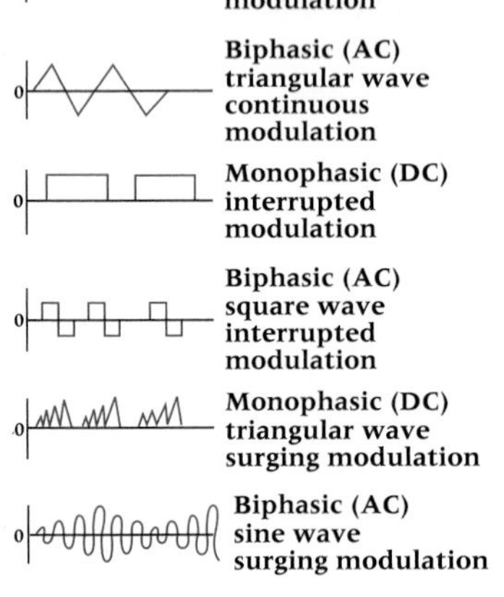

Figure 15-13

Modulation may be continuous, surged, or interrupted for either monophasic (DC) or biphasic (AC) currents.

frequency
Measured in hertz (Hz), cycles per second (CPS), or pulses per second (PPS).

Biphasic (Alternating) Current

With biphasic or AC current, the direction of current flow reverses itself once during each cycle. Alternating current may be used for pain modulation or muscle contraction.

Polyphasic (Pulsatile) Current

Polyphasic or pulsatile currents usually contain three or more pulses grouped together. These groups of pulses are interrupted for short periods of time and repeat themselves at regular intervals. Pulsatile currents are used in interferential and so-called Russian currents.

Current Parameters

Waveforms

Electrical stimulating units can take on various waveforms depending on the capability of the generator. A waveform is a graphic representation of the shape, direction, amplitude, and direction of a particular electrical current. Both AC and DC units can produce currents with waveforms that are either sine, square, or triangular in shape (Figure 15-12).

Modulation

Current modulation refers to the ability of the electrical stimulating unit to change the magnitude or duration of a waveform. Modulation may be continuous, interrupted, or surged for both AC and DC currents (Figure 15-13).

Intensity

Current intensity refers to the voltage output of the stimulating unit. Generators that produce voltage outputs of up to 150 V are low-voltage generators. Those that produce up to 500 V are high-voltage generators. Low-voltage generators are almost always DC; high-voltage generators may be either AC or DC. The majority of the electrical stimulators used in athletic training settings are high-voltage DC generators.

Duration

Duration refers to the length of time that current is flowing. It is also referred to as pulse width or pulse duration. Duration is preset on most of the high-voltage DC stimulators.

Frequency

Frequency refers to the number of waveforms being emitted by the electrical stimulating unit in one second. Frequency is identified in pulses per second (PPS), cycles per second (CPS), or hertz. Frequencies may range from one PPS to several thousand PPS.

Polarity

Polarity refers to the direction of current flow. It may move toward either a positive or a negative pole.

Electrode Setup

In electrotherapy, moist electrode pads are fixed directly to the skin. Electrodes may be of different sizes. Using a large *(dispersive)* electrode remote from the treatment area while placing a smaller *(active)* electrode as close as possible to the nerve or muscle motor point will give the greatest effect at the small electrode. The large electrode disperses the current over a large area; the small electrode concentrates the current in the area of the motor point. The physiological effects can occur anywhere between the two pads, but they usually occur at the active electrode, because current density is greater at this point.[17] Many newer electrical stimulating units have pads that are of equal size, and thus both electrodes would be considered active electrodes.

Indications

Monophasic, biphasic, and pulsatile currents can be used to modulate pain and to induce muscle contraction.[37] Monophasic current may also be used to produce ion movement (iontophoresis).[17]

Pain Modulation

Electrical stimulating currents can reduce pain associated with injury.[17] The neurophysiological mechanisms associated with pain modulation—including gate control, descending pain control (central biasing), and opiate pain control—were discussed in Chapter 10.

Gate control Electrical stimulation of sensory nerves will evoke the gate control mechanism and diminish awareness of painful stimuli. As long as the stimulation is causing the sensory nerves to fire, the gate to pain should be closed. If the stimulus stops, the gate is then open, and pain returns to perception. The following parameters can be used for gate control: intensity should be adjusted to create a tingling sensation but should not cause a muscular contraction; both pulse duration and frequency should be at the maximum setting on the machine.[17]

Descending pain control Intense electrical stimulation of the smaller pain fibers at trigger and acupuncture points for short time periods causes stimulation of descending neurons, which then affect the transmission of pain information by closing the gate at the spinal cord level. Current intensity should be very high, approaching a noxious level; pulse duration should be 10 msec; frequency should be 80 pulses per second.[17]

Opiate pain control theory Electrical stimulation of sensory nerves stimulates the release of enkephalin from local sites throughout the central nervous system and the release of β-endorphins from the pituitary gland into the cerebrospinal fluid. Pain modulation is caused by applying an electrical current to areas close to the site of pain or to acupuncture or trigger points both local to and distant from the pain area. A point stimulator can be used, with current intensity set as high as tolerable; pulse duration should be set at the maximum possible on the machine; frequency should be set at 1 to 5 PPS.[17]

Muscle Contraction

The quality of a muscle contraction will change according to the changes in current parameters. As the frequency of stimulation increases, the muscle will develop more tension because of progressive shortening of the muscle until a tetanic contraction is achieved.[20] Tetany will occur for virtually all muscles at approximately 50 PPS. Increases in intensity spread the current over a larger area and increase the number of motor units activated by the current. Increases in current duration also cause more motor units to be activated. A variety of therapeutic gains can be made by electrically stimulating a muscle contraction; these gains include muscle pumping contractions, muscle strengthening, retardation of atrophy, and muscle reeducation.

A muscle contraction can be used for:
- Muscle pumping
- Muscle strengthening
- Retardation of atrophy
- Muscle reeducation

Muscle pumping This type of contraction is used to help stimulate circulation by pumping fluid and blood through the venous and lymphatic channels back to the heart. High-voltage monophasic current is recommended. Intensity should be increased to elicit a muscle contraction at a frequency of 20 to 40 PPS, using a surged mode with on/off times set at five seconds each. The injured body part should be elevated, and active contraction should be encouraged. Treatment time is twenty to thirty minutes.[17]

Muscle strengthening Electrical stimulation can be used to facilitate strength gains. High-frequency biphasic current is recommended. Intensity should be increased at a frequency of 50 to 60 PPS to elicit a tetanic muscle contraction using surging current set at 15 seconds on and 50 seconds off. Treatment should include ten repetitions three times per week. For best results, the athlete should combine this electrically induced tetanic contraction with maximal active contraction against some resistance.[17]

Retardation of atrophy Electrically induced muscle contraction can be used to minimize atrophy and loss of muscle function that typically occurs with immobilization after injury. High-frequency biphasic current is recommended. Intensity should be increased to 30 to 60 PPS to elicit a tetanic contraction using interrupted current mode. The athlete should incorporate voluntary isometric contraction. Treatment time should be fifteen to twenty minutes.[17]

Muscle reeducation Muscular inhibition after surgery or injury can be reduced by electrically stimulating a muscle. Intensity should be increased to a level necessary for a comfortable contraction at 30 to 50 PPS using either interrupted or surged current. The athlete should watch and feel the contraction and attempt to initiate a voluntary contraction. Treatment time is fifteen to twenty minutes; treatment is repeated several times daily.[17]

Iontophoresis

Iontophoresis uses electrical current to drive ions.

Iontophoresis is a technique in which chemical ions are transported through the intact skin using electrical current for the purpose of treating skin infections or for a counterirritating effect.[49] The type of current used is always a low-voltage direct current set on a continuous mode because the pulse duration must be long enough to allow for migration of ions.

There are three techniques of application: an active pad is applied over gauze that is saturated with a solution containing the ions (this pad is positioned as close as possible to the involved tissue); the active electrode is suspended in a container of the ion solution, and then the body part to be treated is immersed in the container; or a special stimulator with a specially adapted electrode containing the treatment ions is positioned as close to the involved tissue as possible. In all cases, a large dispersive pad is applied to the patient and the proper polarity of the active electrode is selected based on the polarity of the ions in the solution.

Positive ions require an active electrode that is positive; negative ions require an active electrode that is negative. Treatment time will vary. A more comprehensive source dealing with iontophoresis should be consulted before using this technique.[49]

Interferential Currents

Interferential currents make use of two separate electrical generators that emit currents at two slightly different frequencies. Two pairs of electrodes are arranged in a square pattern such that the currents cross one another, creating an interference pattern at a central point of stimulation. The interference pattern creates a broader area of stimulation (Figure 15-14).[17]

Low-Intensity Stimulators

Low-intensity stimulators (LIS) are among the newest of the electrical stimulators available to the athletic trainer. *Low-intensity stimulator* is the latest term for what used

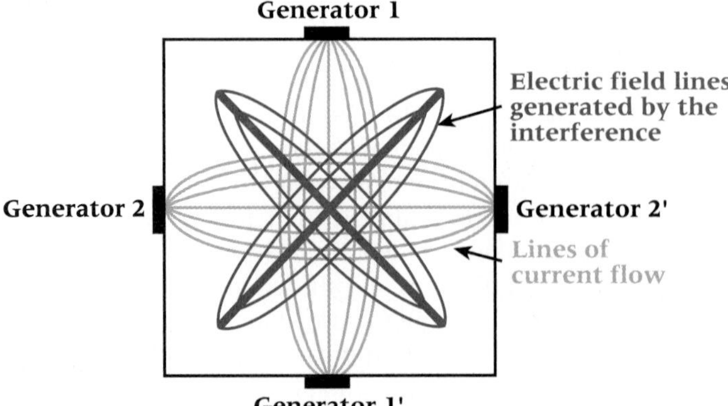

Figure 15-14

Pattern created by interferential current.

to be called microcurrent electrical nerve stimulator, or MENS. Low-intensity stimulators deliver current to the athlete at very low frequencies (1 PPS) and at extremely low intensities that are subsensory. This type of current is used to stimulate the healing process in both soft tissue and bone by altering the electrical activity of individual cells. The effectiveness of LIS therapy is currently based primarily on theory; there is little research information to support its use.[17]

Biofeedback

Biofeedback is a therapeutic procedure that uses electronic or electromechanical instruments to accurately measure, process, and feed back reinforcing information via auditory or visual signals. Perhaps the biggest advantage of biofeedback is that it provides the athlete with a chance to make small changes in performance that are immediately noted and rewarded so that eventually larger changes or improvements in performance can be accomplished.[38]

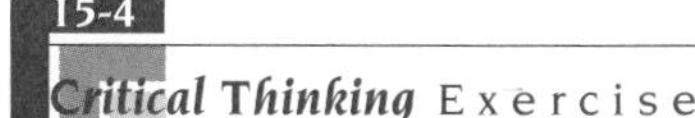
15-4 *Critical Thinking* Exercise

A soccer player is having difficulty contracting her quadriceps muscle on the second day after a surgical reconstruction of her knee. She has some swelling in the vastus medialis, and she is still experiencing some pain.

? What modality can the athletic trainer use to help her achieve a quadriceps contraction?

Several different types of biofeedback modalities are available for use in rehabilitation; EMG biofeedback is the most widely used in a clinical setting.[38] An EMG biofeedback unit measures the electrical activity produced by depolarization of a muscle fiber as an indicator of the quality of a muscle contraction. The EMG biofeedback unit receives small amounts of electrical energy generated during muscle contraction through active electrodes, then separates or filters extraneous electrical energy via a differential amplifier before the signal is processed and subsequently converted to some type of information that has meaning to the user. Biofeedback information is displayed either visually using lights or meters, or auditorily using tones, beeps, buzzes, or clicks. High sensitivity levels should be used during relaxation training, whereas comparatively lower sensitivity levels would be more useful in muscle reeducation.

In athletic training, biofeedback is most typically used for muscle reeducation, to decrease muscle guarding, or for pain reduction.[38]

MASSAGE

Massage is defined as the systematic manipulation of the soft tissues of the body. The movements of gliding, compressing, stretching, percussing, and vibrating are regulated to produce specific responses in the athlete.[13]

Therapeutic Effects of Massage

Historically, wherever sports have been seriously undertaken, massage has been used in some form. Today sports massage seems to be regaining popularity among athletic trainers as a treatment modality. Manipulation of soft tissue by massage is a useful adjunct to other modalities.[2] Sports massage causes mechanical, physiological, and psychological responses.[43]

Mechanical Responses

Mechanical responses to massage occur as a direct result of the graded pressures and movements of the hand on the body. Such actions encourage venous and lymphatic drainage and mildly stretch superficial and scar tissue.[56] Connective tissue can be effectively stretched by friction massage, which helps prevent rigidity in scar formation. When an athlete is forced to remain inactive while an injury heals or when edema surrounds a joint, the stagnation of circulation may be prevented by using certain massage techniques.[14]

Physiological Responses

Possible physiological responses of massage include:
- Reflex effects
- Relaxation
- Stimulation
- Increased circulation

Massage can increase circulation and, as a result, increase metabolism to the musculature and aid in the removal of metabolites such as lactic acid.[13] It also helps overcome venostasis and edema by increasing circulation at and around the injury site, assisting in the normal venous blood return to the heart.

15-5

Critical Thinking Exercise

A javelin thrower has a muscle strain in his back. He comes into the training room on the sixth day after the initial injury complaining of pain. He asks the athletic trainer if anything can be done to help modulate his pain.

? What modalities can the athletic trainer use to modulate pain?

The reflex effects of massage are processes that, in response to nerve impulses initiated through rubbing the body, are transmitted to one organ by afferent nerve fibers and then back to another organ by efferent fibers. Reflex responses elicit a variety of organ reactions such as body relaxation, stimulation, and increased circulation.[43]

Relaxation can be induced by slow, superficial stroking of the skin. It is a type of massage that is beneficial for tense, anxious athletes who may require gentle treatment.

Stimulation is attained by quick, brisk action that causes a contraction of superficial tissue. The benefits derived by the athlete are predominantly psychological. He or she feels invigorated after intense manipulation of the tissue. In the early days of American sports, stimulation massage was given as a warm-up procedure, but it has gradually lost popularity because of the time involved and the recognition that it is relatively ineffectual physiologically.[43]

Increased circulation is accomplished by mechanical and reflex stimuli. Together they cause the capillaries to dilate and be drained of fluid as a result of firm outside pressure, thus stimulating cell metabolism, eliminating toxins, and increasing lymphatic and venous circulation. In this way the healing process is aided.

Psychological Responses

The tactile system is one of the most sensitive systems in the human organism. From earliest infancy, humans respond psychologically to being touched. Because massage is the act of laying on of hands, it can be an important means for creating a bond of confidence between the athletic trainer and the athlete.

Massage Strokes

Massage strokes can be separated into five basic categories: effleurage, petrissage, friction, tapotement, and vibration.

Effleurage

effleurage (**eff** flu raj) Stroking.

Effleurage, or stroking (Figure 15-15), is divided into light and deep methods. Light stroking is designed primarily to be sedative. It is also used in the early stages of injury treatment. Deep stroking is a therapeutic compression of soft tissue, which encourages venous and lymphatic drainage. A different application of effleurage may be used for a specific body part.

Stroking variations There are many variations in effleurage massage; some that are of particular value to sports injuries are pressure variations, the hand-over-hand method, and the cross-body method.[13] Pressure variations range from very light to deep and vigorous stroking. Light stroking, as discussed previously, can induce relaxation or may be used when an area is especially sensitive to touch; on the other hand, deep massage is designed to bring about definite physiological responses. Light and deep effleurage can be used alternately when both features are desired. The hand-over-hand stroking method is of special benefit to those surface areas that are particularly unyielding. It is performed by an alternate stroke in which one hand strokes, followed immediately by the other hand, somewhat like shingles on a roof (Figure 15-16). The cross-body effleurage technique is an excellent massage for the low back region. The operator places a hand on each side of the athlete's spine. Both hands first stroke simultaneously away from the spine, then both hands at the same time stroke toward the spine (Figure 15-17).

Petrissage

petrissage (**pet** tris saj) Kneading.

Kneading, or **petrissage** (Figure 15-18), is a technique adaptable primarily to loose and heavy tissue areas such as the trapezius, the latissimus dorsi, or the triceps muscles. The procedure consists of picking up the muscle and skin tissue between the thumb and forefinger of each hand and rolling and twisting it in opposite directions. As one hand is rolling and twisting, the other begins to pick up the adjacent tissue.

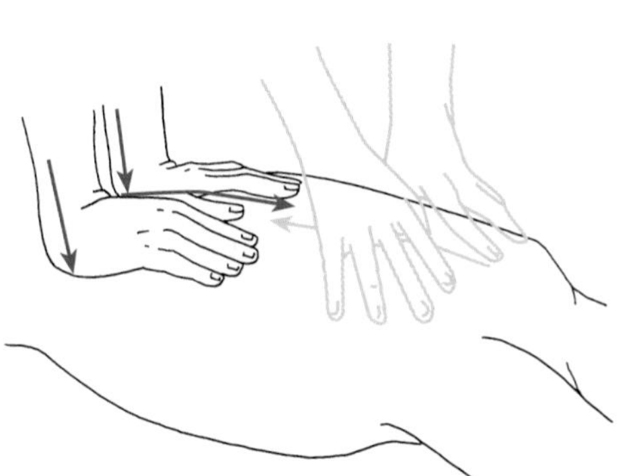

Figure 15-15

Effleurage.

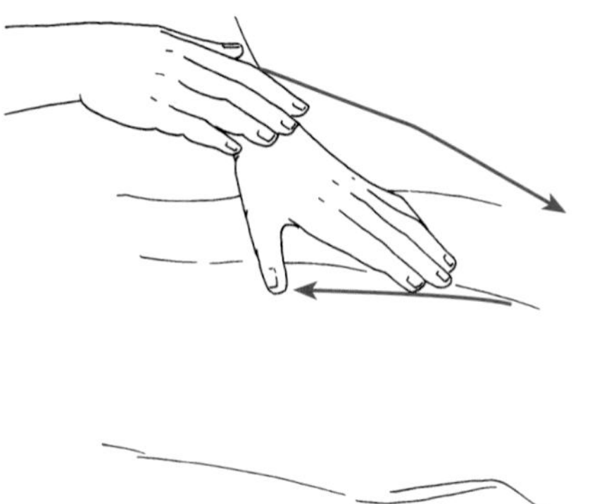

Figure 15-16

Hand-over-hand effleurage.

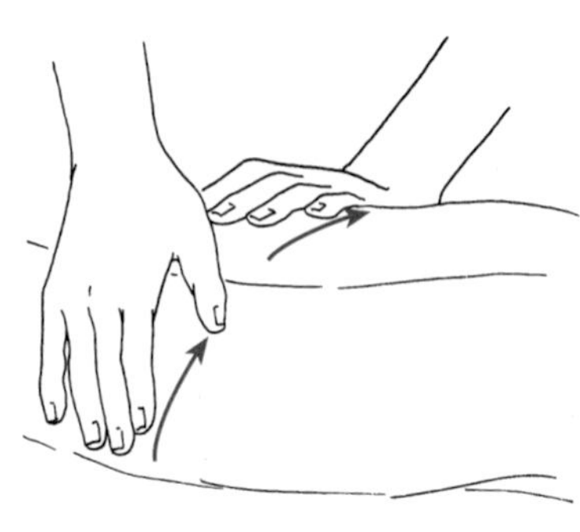

Figure 15-17

Cross-body effleurage.

The kneading action wrings out the muscle, thus loosening adhesions and squeezing congestive materials into the general circulation. Picking up skin may cause an irritating pinch. Whenever possible, deep muscle tissue should be gathered and lifted.

Friction

The **friction** massage (Figure 15-19) is used often around joints and other areas where tissue is thin and is used on tissues that are especially unyielding such as scars, adhesions, muscle spasms, and fascia. The action is initiated by bracing with the heels of the hands, then either holding the thumbs steady and moving the fingers in a circular motion or holding the fingers steady and moving the thumbs in a circular motion. Each method is adaptable to the type of area or articulation that is being massaged. The motion is started at a central point, and then a circular movement is initiated, with the hands moving in opposite directions away from the center point. The purpose is to stretch the underlying tissue, develop friction in the area, and increase circulation around the joint.

friction
Heat producing.

Tapotement

The most popular methods of **tapotement,** or percussion, are cupping, hacking, and pincerlike or pincing movements.

tapotement (ta **pote** *ment*)
Percussion.

Cupping The cupping action produces an invigorating and stimulating sensation. It is a series of percussion movements rapidly duplicated at a constant tempo. The hands are cupped to such an extent that the beat emits a dull and hollow sound, unlike the sound of the slap of the open hand. The hands move alternately, from the wrist, with the elbow flexed and the upper arm stabilized (Figure 15-20A). The cupping action should be executed until the skin in the area develops a pinkish coloration.

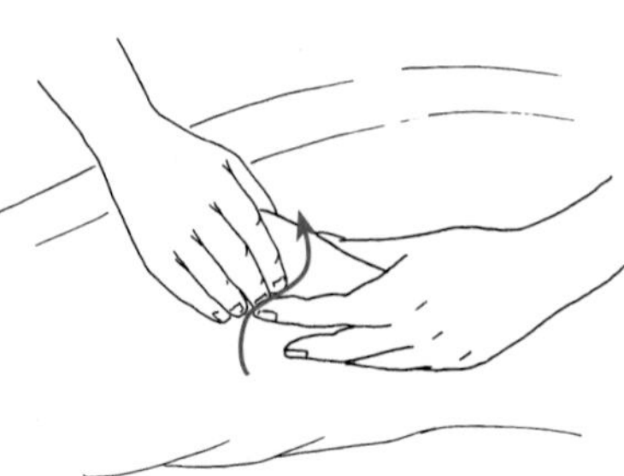

Figure 15-18

Petrissage.

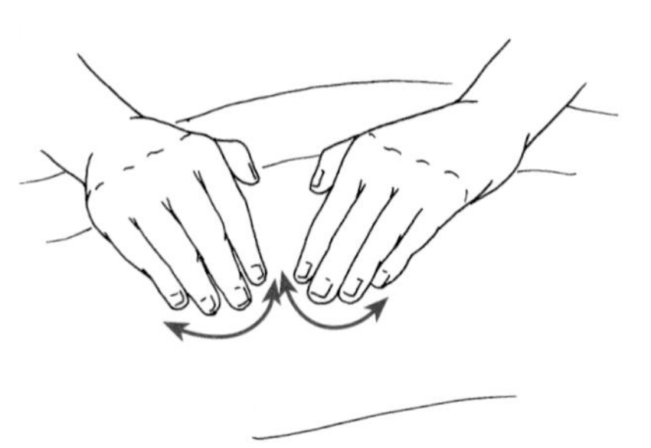

Figure 15-19

Friction massage.

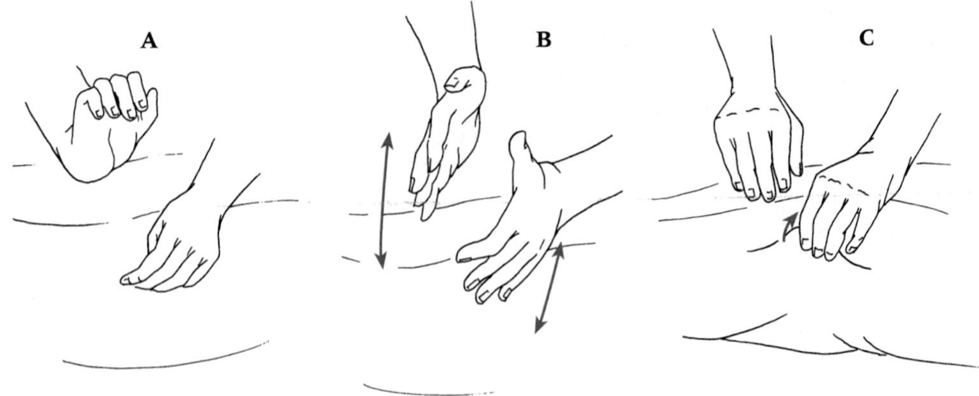

Figure 15-20

Tapotement. **A,** Cupping. **B,** Hacking. **C,** Pincing.

Hacking Hacking can be used in conjunction with cupping to bring about a varied stimulation of the sensory nerves (Figure 15-20B). Hacking is similar to cupping except that the hands are rotated externally and the ulnar, or little finger, border of the hand is the striking surface. Only the heavy muscle areas should be treated in this manner.

Pincing Although pincing is not in the strictest sense percussive, it is categorized under tapotement because of the vigor with which it is applied. Alternating hands lift small amounts of tissue between the first finger and thumb in quick, gentle pinching movements (Figure 15-20C).

Vibration

vibration Rapid shaking.

Vibration is rapid movement that produces a quivering or trembling effect. It is used in sports because of its ability to relax and soothe. Although vibration can be done manually, the machine vibrator is usually the preferred modality.

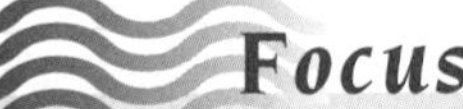

Focus

Guidelines for an effective massage

Besides knowing the different kinds of massage, the athletic trainer should understand how to give the most effective massage. The following rules should be used whenever possible:

1. Make the athlete comfortable.
   a. Place the body in the proper position on the table.
   b. Place a pad under the areas of the body that are to be massaged.
   c. Keep the training room at a constant 72° F (22.2° C) temperature.
   d. Respect the athlete's privacy by draping him or her with a blanket or towel, exposing only the body parts to be massaged.
2. Develop a confident, gentle approach when massaging.
   a. Assume a position that is easy both on you and on the athlete.
   b. Avoid using too harsh a stroke, or further injury may result.
3. To ensure proper lymphatic and venous drainage, stroke toward the heart whenever possible.
4. Know when not to use massage.
   a. Never give a massage if the athlete may have a local or general infection. To do so may encourage the infection's spread or may aggravate the condition.
   b. Never apply massage directly over a recent injury; limit stroking to the periphery. Massaging over recent injuries may dislodge the clot organization and start bleeding.

Sports Massage

Massage in sports is usually confined to a specific area and is seldom given to the full body.[2] The time required for giving an adequate and complete body massage is excessive in athletics. It is not usually feasible to devote this much time to one athlete; five minutes is usually all that is required for massaging a given area. The *Focus Box:* "Guidelines for an effective massage" provides suggestions for giving an effective massage.

Massage Lubricants

To enable the hands to slide easily over the body, a friction-reducing medium must be used. Rubbing the dry body can cause gross skin irritation by tearing and breaking off the hair. Many mediums (e.g., fine powders, oil liniments, or almost any substance having a petroleum base) can be used as a lubricant.

Positioning of the Athlete

It is important to position an athlete properly for a massage. The injured body part must be easily accessible, the athlete must be comfortable, and the part to be massaged must be relaxed.

Confidence

If the person doing the massage lacks confidence, this is easily transmitted through inexperienced hands. Every effort should be made to think out the procedure to be used and to present a confident appearance to the athlete.

Ensuring Athlete Privacy and Athletic Trainer Integrity

As is the case with a number of other therapeutic techniques, massage involves direct physical contact between the athletic trainer and the athlete. It is critical that the athletic trainer be aware of and, if necessary, take necessary precautions to ensure that this physical contact can in no way be construed or misinterpreted as being of a sexual nature. This is particularly important when dealing with an athlete of the opposite sex or with athletes who are under legal age. The athletic trainer should always make certain that only the body part or body region being treated is exposed and that the rest of the body is appropriately covered or draped. It is also advisable to perform the massage with another athlete or athletic trainer physically present in the same room or to do the massage in plain view of others in the athletic training room. There is no good reason not to take these precautions, and failure to do so may create situations that unnecessarily threaten the athletic trainer's professional and personal integrity.

Deep Transverse Friction Massage

The transverse, or Cyriax, method of deep friction massage is a specific technique for treating muscles, tendons, ligaments, and joint capsules. The major purpose of transverse massage is to move transversely across a ligament or tendon to mobilize it as much as possible. This technique often precedes active exercise. Deep transverse friction massage restores mobility to a muscle in the same way that mobilization frees a joint.[13]

Transverse massage is a method of deep transverse friction massage.

The position of the athletic trainer's hands is important in gaining maximum strength and control. Four positions are suggested: index finger crossed over the middle finger, middle finger crossed over the index finger, two fingers side by side, and an opposed finger and thumb (Figure 15-21).

The massage must be directly over the site of lesion and pain. The fingers move with the skin and do not slide over it. Massage must be across the grain of the affected tissue. The thicker the structure, the more friction is given.[13] The technique is to sweep back and forth over the full width of the tissue. Massage should not be given to acute injuries or over highly swollen tissues. A few minutes of this method will produce a numbness in the area, and exercise or mobilization can be instituted.

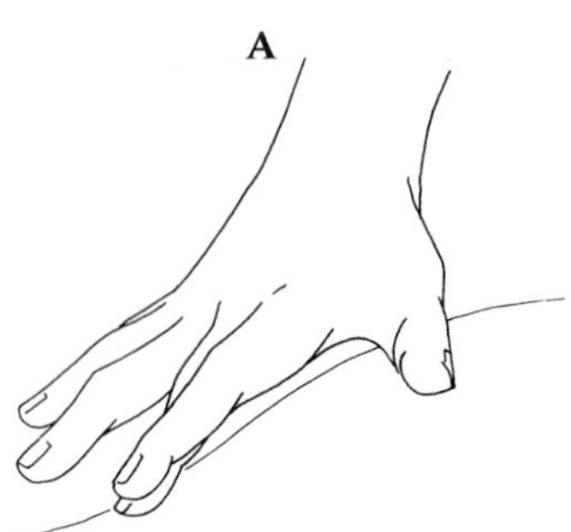
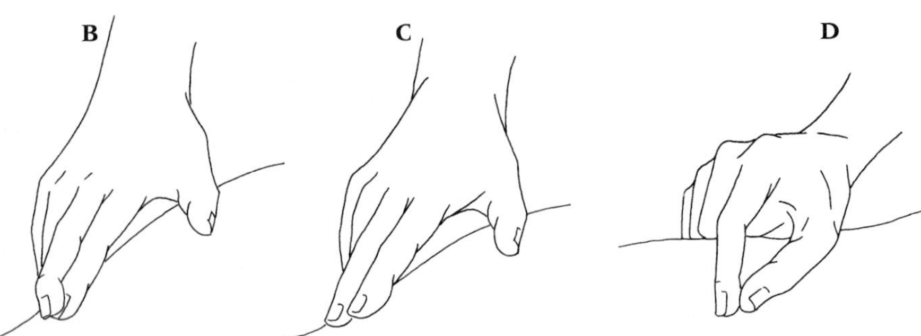

Figure 15-21

Cyriax massage is a specific technique for muscle, tendons, ligaments, and joint capsules using a variety of hand positions. **A,** Index finger crossed over the middle finger. **B,** Middle finger crossed over the index finger. **C,** Two fingers side by side. **D,** Opposed finger and thumb.

Acupressure Massage

Acupressure is a type of massage based on the ancient Chinese art of acupuncture, which was discussed in Chapter 10. Physiological explanations of the effectiveness of acupressure massage may likely be attributed to some interaction of the various mechanisms of pain modulation.

The athletic trainer uses acupuncture charts to select specific points that are described in the literature as having some relationship to the area of pain. The charts provide the athletic trainer with a general idea of where these points are located. Two techniques may be used to specifically locate acupressure points. Because it is known that electrical impedance is reduced at acupuncture points, an ohmmeter may be used to locate the points. Perhaps the easiest technique is for the athletic trainer simply to palpate the area until he or she feels either a small fibrous nodule or a strip of tense muscle tissue that is tender to the touch.

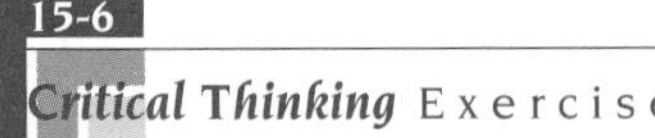

A track and field athlete complains of pain in his left knee. The athletic trainer assesses the injury as patellar tendinitis.

? What type of massage may be indicated for this condition in the acute stage? What type of massage may be indicated for this condition after a few days?

Once the point is located, the athletic trainer begins massage with the index or middle fingers, the thumb, or the elbow, using small circular motions on the point. The amount of pressure applied to these acupressure points should be determined by patient tolerance; however, the pressure must be intense and will likely be painful to the patient. Generally, the more pressure the patient can tolerate, the more effective the treatment is.

Effective treatment times range from one to five minutes at a single point per treatment. It may be necessary to massage several points during the treatment to obtain the greatest effects. If so, the athletic trainer should work distal points first and move proximally.

During the massage, the patient will report a dulling or numbing effect and will frequently indicate that the pain has diminished or subsided totally during the massage. The lingering effects of acupressure massage vary tremendously from patient to patient. The effects may last for only a few minutes in some but may persist in others for several hours.

TRACTION

Traction is commonly used in the cervical and lumbar spine.

Traction can be defined as a drawing tension applied to a body segment. It is most commonly used in the cervical and lumbar regions of the spine.[19]

Physiological Effects

Traction is used to produce separation of the vertebral bodies and in so doing can effect stretching of the ligaments and joint capsules of the spine, stretching of spinal and paraspinal muscles, increased separation of the articular facet joints, relief in pressure on nerves and nerve roots, decrease in the central pressure of the intervertebral disks allowing for the movement of herniated disk material back into the center of the disk, increases of and changes in joint proprioception, and relief of the compressive effects of normal posture.[19]

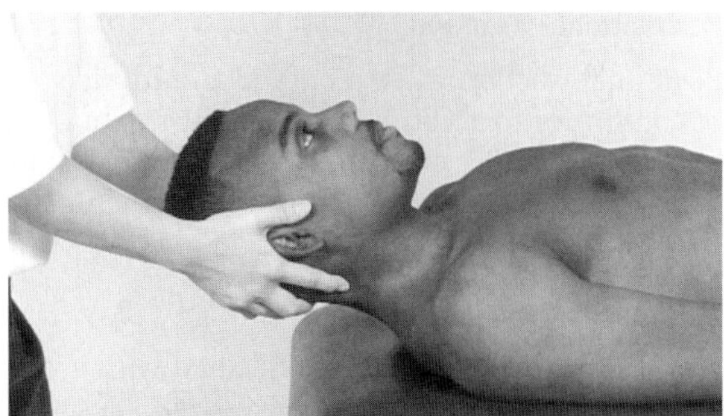

Figure 15-22

Manual cervical traction.

Indications

Traction is most commonly used for the treatment of spinal nerve root impingement, which may result from many causes, including vertebral disk herniation or prolapse and spondylolisthesis. It may also be used to decrease muscle guarding, to treat muscle strain, to treat sprain of the spinal ligaments, and to relax discomfort resulting from normal spinal compression.

Application

Traction may be applied to the spine through the use of manual techniques or traction machines, including table traction units, wall-mounted traction units, and inverted traction techniques.

Manual Traction

Manual traction is infinitely more adaptable and offers greater flexibility than mechanical traction. Changes in force, direction, duration, and patient position can be made instantaneously as the athletic trainer senses relaxation or resistance (Figure 15-22).

Mechanical Traction

For mechanical lumbar traction, a split table with a movable section to eliminate friction must be used to allow for smooth, nonrestricted traction. A nonslip traction harness applied directly to the skin is needed to transfer the traction force comfortably to the athlete and to stabilize the trunk while the lumbar spine is placed under traction (Figure 15-23). For cervical traction, the athlete may be either in the supine or sitting position. A nonslip cervical harness should be secured under the chin and back of the head.

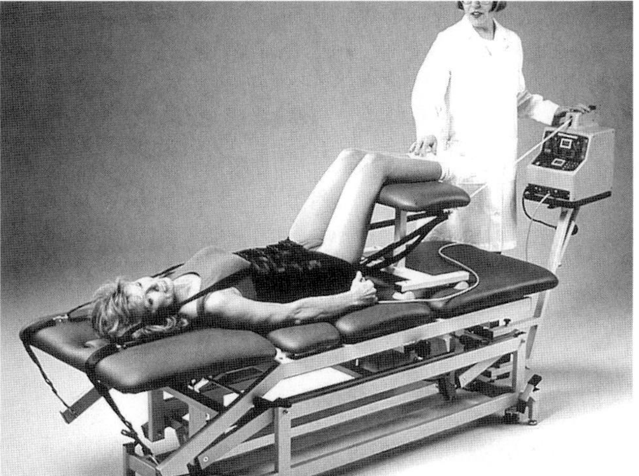

Figure 15-23

Lumbar traction using a split table and a traction machine.

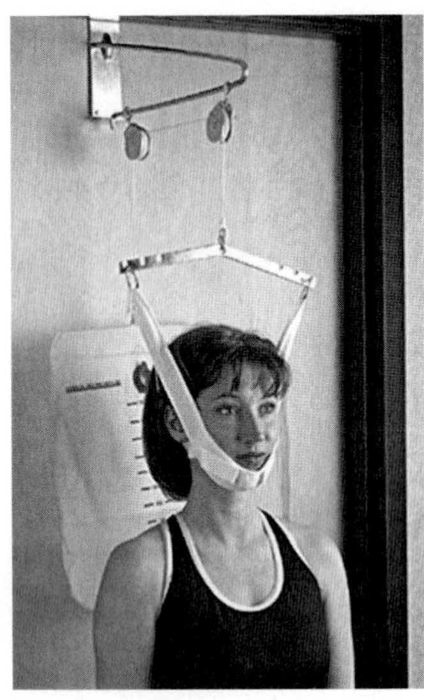

Figure 15-24

Cervical traction using a wall-mounted unit.

Positional Traction

Positional traction is used on a trial-and-error basis to determine maximum position of comfort or to accomplish a specific treatment goal. For example, placing an athlete with a lumbar disc problem in a backlying position with the hips and knees flexed and supported at 90 degrees increases the opening of the foramen and takes pressure off the disk, thus minimizing pain and making the athlete more comfortable.

Wall-Mounted Traction

Cervical traction can be accomplished with a wall-mounted system. Plates, sand bags, or water bags can be used for weights. These units are relatively inexpensive and effective (Figure 15-24).

Inverted Traction

Specialized equipment or simply hanging upside down will place the person in an inverted position. The spine is lengthened because of the stretch provided by the weight of the trunk (Figure 15-25).

Special Considerations

- Good results have been achieved using both intermittent and sustained traction. In most cases of lumbar disk problems, sustained traction seems to be the treatment of choice. Intermittent traction is considered to be more comfortable.[19]
- Progressive traction increases the traction force gradually in a preselected number of steps, which allows the athlete to adapt slowly to the traction and helps him or her to stay relaxed.
- Recommendations on length of treatment and on/off times vary depending on the specific problem to be treated.
- For the lumbar spine, a traction force equal to one half the athlete's body weight is a good guideline to use in selecting a force high enough to cause vertebral separation. Cervical traction forces can be adjusted from 20 to 50 pounds depending on patient comfort and response.

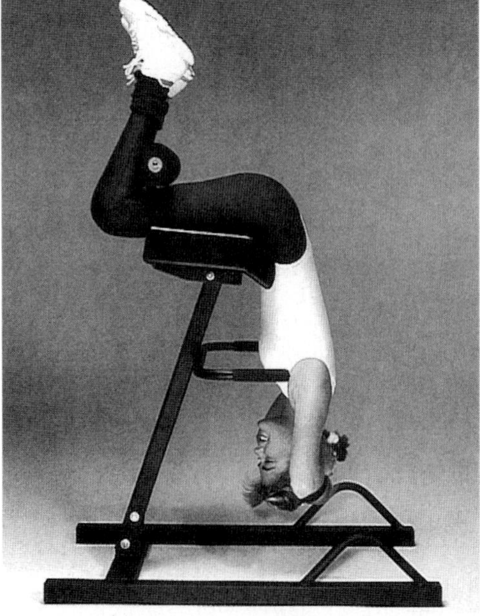

Figure 15-25

Inversion traction apparatus.

INTERMITTENT COMPRESSION UNITS

Intermittent compression units are used for controlling or reducing swelling after acute injury or for pitting edema, which tends to develop in the injured area several hours after injury.[18]

Equipment

Intermittent compression makes use of a nylon pneumatic inflatable sleeve applied around the injured extremity (Figure 15-26). The sleeve can be inflated to a specific pressure that forces excessive fluid accumulated in the interstitial spaces into vascular and lymphatic channels through which it is removed from the area of injury.[53] Compression facilitates the movement of lymphatic fluid, which helps eliminate the by-products of the injury process.[46] The extremity should be elevated during treatment.

Treatment Parameters

Intermittent compression devices have three parameters that may be adjusted: on/off time, inflation pressures, and treatment time. Recommended treatment protocols have been established through clinical trial and error with little experimental data currently available to support any protocol.[18]

On/off times are variable, including 1 minute on, 2 minutes off; 2 minutes on, 1 minute off; and 4 minutes on, 1 minute off. Again, these recommendations are not research based. Patient comfort should be the primary guide.

Recommended inflation pressures have been loosely correlated with blood pressures. The Jobst Institute recommends that pressure be set at 30 to 50 mm Hg for the upper extremity and at 30 to 60 mm Hg for the lower extremity. Because arterial capillary pressures are approximately 30 mm Hg, any pressure that exceeds this level should encourage the absorption of edema and the flow of lymphatic fluid.[46]

Clinical studies have demonstrated a significant reduction in limb volume after thirty minutes of compression.[1,46] Thus a thirty-minute treatment time seems to be efficient in reducing edema.

Some intermittent compression units have the capability of combining cold along with compression. Compression when combined with cold is more effective in reducing edema.[1,46] It is also common to use electrical stimulating currents to produce muscle pumping, thus facilitating lymphatic flow.

Cryo-Cuff

The Cryo-Cuff is a device that uses both cold and compression simultaneously (Figure 15-27A). The Cryo-Cuff is used both acutely following injury and post surgically. Originally developed by Aircast, it is made of a nylon sleeve that connects via a tube to a one gallon cooler/jug. Cold water flows into the sleeve from the cooler. As the

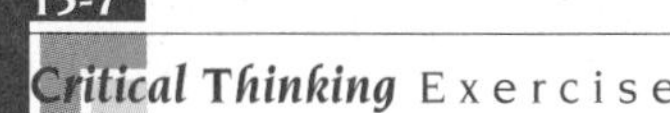

15-7 Critical Thinking Exercise

A gymnast has been told by a physician that she has a sprain of a ligament between two lumbar vertebrae in her low back. He tells her that it is important to stretch her low back. Because she was extremely flexible before her injury, she does not feel that the stretching she has been doing is effectively stretching the injured ligament.

? The gymnast comes to the athletic trainer and asks if any other therapeutic technique will help her stretch the injured ligament.

15-8 Critical Thinking Exercise

A basketball player has a two-day-old postacute ankle sprain. The initial injury was not managed appropriately, and as a result, the athlete has a considerable amount of swelling. He has little range of motion and is capable of only touch down weight bearing.

? The athlete will have a difficult time regaining function until the swelling is reduced. What therapeutic modalities can reduce this postacute lymphedema?

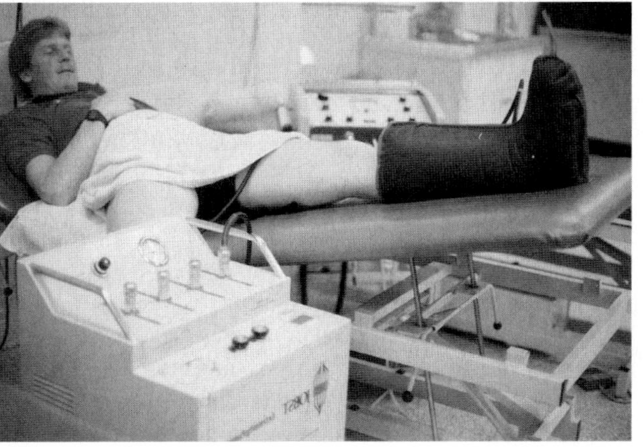

Figure 15-26

Intermittent compressive devices are designed to reduce edema after injury.

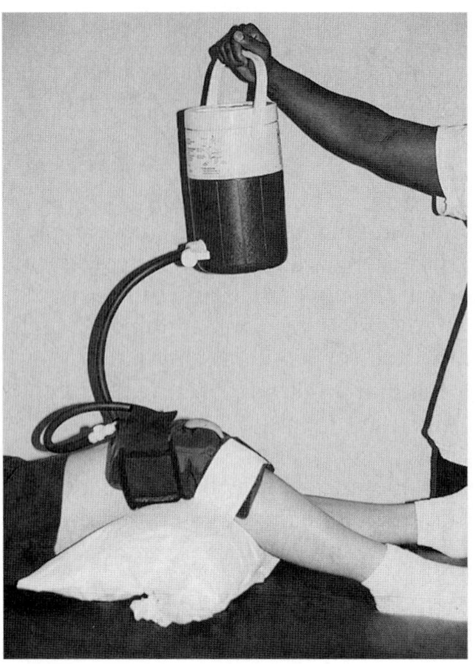

A

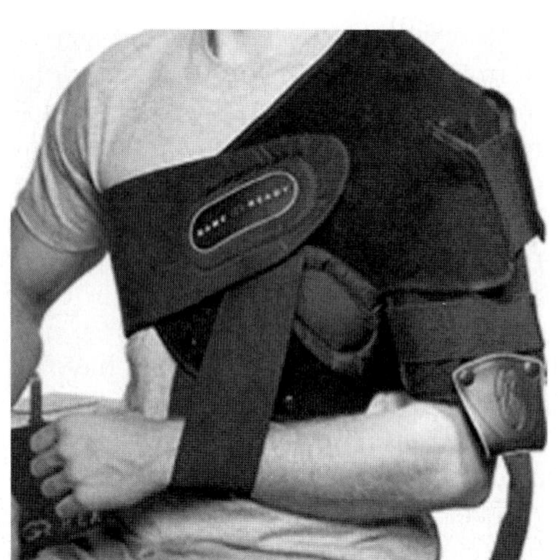

B

Figure 15-27

Portable compression and cold systems. **A,** Cryo-Cuff. **B,** Game Ready Accelerated Recovery System.

cooler is raised the pressure in the cuff is increased. During the treatment the water warms and can be rechilled by lowering the cooler to drain the cuff, mixing the warmer water with the colder water, and then again raising the jug to increase pressure in the cuff. The only drawback to this simple yet effective piece of equipment is that the water in the cuff must be continually rechilled. However the Cryo-Cuff is portable, easy to use, and inexpensive.

Game Ready System

The Game Ready Accelerated Recovery System consists of various soft wraps and a control unit designed to simultaneously deliver cold therapy and intermittent compression (Figure 15-27B). The wraps are made from flexible fabric designed to fit various body parts. The wraps fit snugly to apply consistent cooling and intermittent pressure to an injury. To operate the system, the control unit reservoir is filled with ice and water, which is circulated through the wraps over the course of a standard treatment program that can be customized for various time, temperature, and compression settings.

SHORTWAVE AND MICROWAVE DIATHERMY

Shortwave and microwave diathermy are two modalities that emit electromagnetic energy that is capable of producing temperature increases in the deeper tissues. Tissues with a higher water content (e.g., muscle) selectively absorb the heat delivered by shortwave and microwave diathermies.[24] The extent of muscle heating depends on the thickness of the subcutaneous fat layer. Both shortwave and microwave diathermies provide less heat penetration than does ultrasound. In contrast to shortwave and microwave diathermies, ultrasonic vibration is not absorbed by fat and is therefore not influenced by its thickness.[24]

Shortwave Diathermy

Shortwave diathermy heats deeper tissues by introducing a high-frequency electrical current. Shortwave diathermy is in essence a radio transmitter; the Federal Communications Commission (FCC) has assigned a wavelength of 7.5 to 22 meters and a frequency of 13.56 or 27.12 megacycles per second for therapeutic purposes.[42]

Shortwave diathermy can be used in two ways: through a condenser that uses electrostatic field heating or through electromagnetic or induction field heating.[41] In electrostatic field heating, the patient is a part of the circuit. Heating is uneven because of

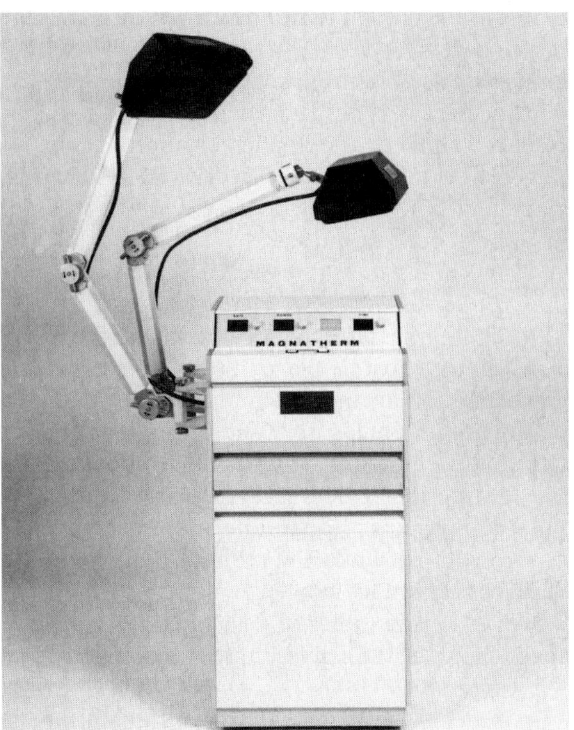

Figure 15-28

The Magnatherm is an example of a currently used shortwave diathermy unit.

different tissue resistance to energy flow, an application of Joule's law, which states that the greater the resistance or impedance, the more heat will develop. In electromagnetic field heating, the patient is not part of the circuit but is heated by an electromagnetic field.[42]

Pulsed shortwave diathermy is a relatively new form of diathermy.[33] Pulsed diathermy is created by simply interrupting the output of continuous shortwave diathermy at consistent intervals. Pulsing reduces the likelihood of any significant tissue temperature increase and reduces the patient's perception of heat. Generators that deliver pulsed shortwave diathermy typically use a drum type of electrode. Pulsed diathermy is claimed to have therapeutic value and to produce nonthermal effects with minimal thermal physiological effects, depending on the intensity of the application. When pulsed diathermy is used in intensities that create an increase in tissue temperature, its effects are no different from those of continuous shortwave diathermy.

Equipment In general, the shortwave diathermy unit consists of a power supply to a power amplifier and a frequency generator. It has an oscillator that produces high frequency (either 13.56 or 27.12 megacycles) and a power amplifier that converts alternating current (AC) to direct current (DC).[26] It also has a circuit that tunes in the patient automatically or manually as part of the circuitry (Figure 15-28).

The shortwave diathermy treatment applicators are either condensor or inductive types.[42] With the condensor, or field heating, the patient is a natural part of the circuit. The condensor applicator consists of electrodes that are formed by sheets of flexible or rigid metal covered by heavy insulation.

There are two types of inductive electrodes: the coil and the single drum unit. The inductive coil is a cable electrode that ranges from 6 to 16 feet (2 to 5 meters) long and is wound around the patient's injured part. Whereas the coil can heat generally, the single drum unit is designed to treat a more specific area.[24] Tissues with high water content such as blood and muscle are the most easily heated.

Indications Shortwave diathermy is highly effective for bursitis, capsulitis, osteoarthritis, deep muscle spasm, and strains. The depth of the inductive technique can be as much as two inches (5 cm). The condensor technique penetrates from one to two inches (2.5 to 5 cm). Tissue temperature can reach 107° F (41.7° C). Although shortwave diathermy has been used in connection with stretching, it is not clear whether using both diathermy and stretching increases flexibility more than stretching alone.[8,36]

Application If more superficial heating is desired, a condensor plate is used; when deeper therapy is desired, the induction coil should be used. A double-layered towel is placed between the applicator and the skin. When the patient is as comfortable as possible, he or she is tuned in with the oscillating circuit of the unit. In most cases the treatment times range from twenty to thirty minutes.

Special considerations

- It is difficult to treat localized body areas.
- Dosage is subjective.
- There is less heating of skin and more chance for deep tissue burns.
- Towels must be placed between the applicator and the skin. Towels absorb perspiration during treatment.
- When there is loss of sensation, shortwave diathermy should not be used.
- When metal objects such as implants, pacemakers, jewelry, a metal table, intrauterine devices (IUDs), zippers on clothing, or glasses are present, shortwave diathermy should not be administered.
- Avoid use when the athlete is hemorrhaging, is pregnant, has open wounds, or wears contact lenses.
- Diathermy cables or coils must not touch one another or any metal.
- Avoid heating eyes, testicles, ovaries, bony prominences, and bone-growth areas.
- A deep, aching sensation during treatment may indicate overheating.
- In 2002 the FDA issued an advisory warning that shortwave and microwave diathermy in both heating and nonheating modes can result in serious injury to an individual who has any type of implanted device or leads.

15-9

Critical Thinking Exercise

An athletic trainer is treating a gymnast who has painful muscle spasms and guarding of the entire low back on both sides.

? How can the athletic trainer use ultrasound to treat this problem?

Microwave Diathermy

Clinical microwave diathermy generally has a wavelength of 12 cm to 33 cm and an FCC-assigned frequency of 915 to 2,450 megacycles. Lower microwave frequencies (e.g., 915 megacycles per second) cause less conversion of energy into the subcutaneous tissue and, as a result, produce more uniform muscle heating.[30] Microwave diathermy heats deeper tissue by conversion. It is more easily absorbed in tissue with higher water content such as muscle and blood than is shortwave diathermy.[24]

Equipment In the microwave diathermy unit, AC is changed into DC. The unit consists of a magnetron oscillator, which is a tube that incorporates a complete oscillator circuit capable of generating a radio frequency. A *coaxial cable* transports the energy from the magnetron oscillator to the applicator head. Within the delivery head is an antenna that radiates energy to the athlete. A commonly used spaced applicator is contained within a rectangular metallic reflector. It is suggested for use on flat or concave body surfaces.[24] The further away the reflector is from the skin, the greater the body coverage will be with a proportional increase in wattage.

A coaxial cable consists of an insulated central conductor with tubular stranded conductors, which are separated by layers of insulation laid concentrically over the central conductor.

Indications Microwave diathermy is highly effective in treating conditions such as fibrositis, myositis, osteoarthritis, bursitis, calcific tendinitis, sprains, strains, and posttraumatic joint stiffness.[26] In an athlete with a subcutaneous fat thickness of 0.5 cm or less, microwave diathermy can penetrate tissue as much as 5 cm (2 inches) thick.[42]

Application The athlete is made comfortable, and the microwave diathermy director is positioned at right angles to the part to be treated. The athlete's subjective heat sensation is the major guide to dosage. The therapeutic heat range for microwave diathermy, as for shortwave diathermy, is 104° to 113° F (40° to 45° C).[41] The length of treatment does not usually exceed thirty minutes. A dosage scheme has been suggested that can be used for both shortwave diathermy and microwave diathermy (Table 15-5).[24,32] A towel must be placed over the skin to absorb any perspiration that accumulates.

TABLE 15-5 Sample Shortwave Diathermy and Microwave Diathermy Dosage

Dosage	Effect	Application
Lowest dose (I)	Just below the point of any sensation of heat (acute inflammatory process)	2 to 5 minutes daily for 2 weeks
Low dose (II)	Mild heat sensation, barely felt (subacute, resolving inflammatory process)	2 to 5 minutes daily for 2 weeks
Medium dose (III)	Moderate but pleasant heat sensation (subacute, resolving inflammatory process)	2 to 30 minutes from 2 to 3 times weekly for 1 to 4 weeks
Heavy dose (IV)	Vigorous heating that causes a sensation that is well tolerated (chronic conditions); pain threshold should not be exceeded	5 to 30 minutes from 2 to 3 times weekly for 1 to 4 weeks

Special considerations The same considerations given to shortwave diathermy must also be given to microwave diathermy. The applicator should never come in contact with the skin. At no time should heating exceed the athlete's pain threshold.[42]

Comparing Microwave Diathermy and Shortwave Diathermy

In general, shortwave and microwave diathermies penetrate the body to approximately the same depth; however, microwave diathermy provides deeper muscle heating and comparatively more skin heating than does shortwave diathermy.[23] Microwave diathermy heating is more localized than is shortwave diathermy heating.

LOW-LEVEL LASER THERAPY

laser Light amplification by stimulated emission of radiation.

Laser is an acronym that stands for light amplification by stimulated emission of radiation.[47] The low-level laser is a relatively new device whose proposed applications in an athletic training setting include acceleration of collagen synthesis, control of microorganisms, increased vascularization, and reduction of pain and inflammation.[47]

The helium-neon (HeNe) and the gallium-arsenide (GaAs) lasers are two low-level lasers currently being investigated by the Food and Drug Administration (FDA) for potential use in physical medicine.[23] In the United States the lower-level laser is considered an investigational device by the FDA and is not available for general use except in the treatment of carpal tunnel syndrome, for which the FDA has approved its use (Figure 15-29).

EXTRACORPOREAL SHOCK WAVE THERAPY (ESWT)

Shock wave therapy was first used for kidney stone fragmentation in early 1980s. Extracorporeal shock wave therapy (ESWT) is a pulsed, high-pressure, short-duration (< 1 ms) acoustical sound wave that is produced by a generator and transmitted through a coupling medium over a large skin area to a specific target region with little attenuation.[50] This acoustic energy is concentrated in a focal area 2 to 8 mm in diameter. The treatment uses a sequence of 1,000 to 4,000 shock wave pulses at 1 to 4 pps. Focusing is checked every 200 to 400 shocks. Treatment lasts for fifteen to thirty minutes.

Currently, because of its high cost, this modality is most likely to be found in a hospital, although there are a few athletic training facilities that have EWST available. Imaging devices (e.g., ultrasound, X ray) are sometimes used to target energy precisely but are not necessary in extremities. Shock waves are applied to the point of maximal tenderness at the lowest energy setting. With direct patient feedback the exact site of

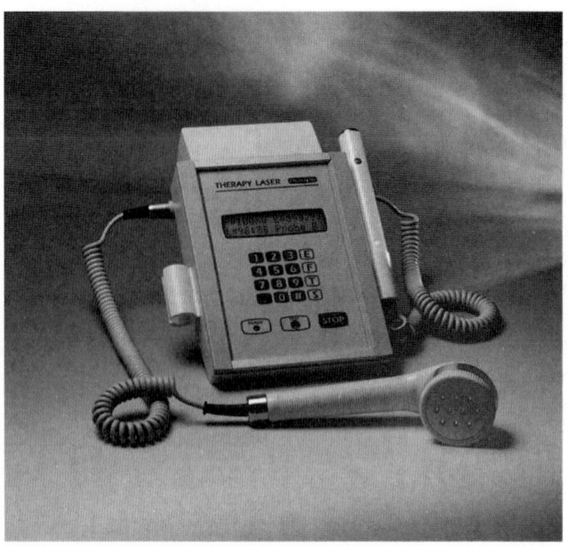

Figure 15-29

Low-level laser unit.

pain and pathology is identified. The intensity is slowly increased within the patient's level of tolerance. Anesthesia is sometimes used to minimize the pain associated with the treatment. However anesthesia is not only unnecessary, but undesirable since only the patient can verify that the correct site has been targeted. If the pain is not reproduced by the shock wave, the condition is unlikely to respond. Since the mid 1990s, ESWT has been approved for use in treating tennis elbow, plantar fasciitis, and nonunion fractures as well as for its analgesic effects. The mechanism of action is not well understood, but the healing that occurs with EWST has been attributed to enhanced metabolism, circulation, and revascularization.[55]

Since this is a relatively new modality, techniques for using ESWT have not yet been standardized. Precise dosages and optimal frequency of application have not been studied extensively. It has not been demonstrated whether shock waves should be directed to the target area by radiological or ultrasound imaging. Also it is not yet clear whether local anesthetic injections should be used in the target area prior to treatment to reduce pain.

MAGNET THERAPY

Recently, magnet therapy has become popular among both competitive and recreational athletes. An increasing number of athletic trainers are using magnets as a treatment modality for athletes who complain of a variety of musculoskeletal ailments. Although a wealth of anecdotal information on magnet therapy can be found in the popular literature, a careful review of the medical literature indicates few data-based research articles on the efficacy or potential therapeutic benefits of using magnets.

Magnet therapy may be defined as the application of a magnetic field to the human body. A magnet is a natural ferrous material with inseparable positively and negatively charged poles that characteristically attract particles of opposite charge and repel particles of similar charge. The strength of a magnetic field is measured in Gauss units. Most therapeutic magnets range between 300 and 1,000 Gauss. The explanations of the potential beneficial physiological effects of magnets include changes in polarity within a damaged cell, increased blood flow and thus increased oxygen saturation, increased muscle strength, increased hormone secretions, increased cell division rate, increased enzyme activity, increased lymphatic flow, and changes in blood pH. It has been shown that magnets do not appear to cause a local increase in tissue temperature.[51]

Although magnet therapy appears to be a relatively safe treatment modality, it should be used with caution by athletic trainers until some definitive basis for use has been determined scientifically.

Patient's Name ____________ Sport ____________

Diagnosis ____________ Date of Injury ____________

Athletic Trainer ____________

Therapeutic Modality ____________

Treatment Parameters

Intensity/Output ____________

Frequency ____________

Duty Cycle ____________

Temperature ____________

Duration of Treatment ____________

Electrode Placement ____________

Special Instructions:

Month/Year ____________

Date Administered:

12345678910111213141516171819202122232425262728293031

Figure 15-30

Therapeutic modalities treatment log.

RECORDING THERAPEUTIC MODALITY TREATMENTS

Athletic trainers who use a therapeutic modality in treatment need to record the procedure. The specifics of the modality treatment should be recorded on the original SOAP note, on the progress note, and on a therapeutic modalities treatment log like the one shown in Figure 15-30. Changes in the treatment parameters should be noted on the treatment log so that anyone administering a modality treatment can consult the log to determine the appropriate treatment parameters.

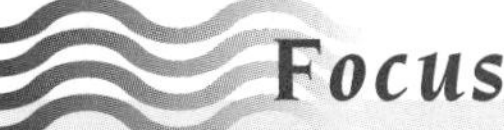

Focus

Safe use of therapeutic modalities

Regardless of the type of therapeutic modality being used, the following safety practices should be considered when using any type of electrical modality:

- The entire electrical system of the building or training room should be designed or evaluated by a qualified electrician. Problems with the electrical system may exist in older buildings or in situations where rooms have been modified to accommodate therapeutic devices (e.g., putting a whirlpool in a locker room where the concrete floor is always wet or damp).
- It should not be assumed that all three-pronged wall outlets are grounded. The ground must be checked.
- The athletic trainer should become very familiar with the equipment being used and with any potential problems that may exist or develop. Any defective equipment should be immediately removed from the clinic.
- The plug should not be jerked out of the wall by pulling on the cable.
- Extension cords or multiple adapters should never be used.
- Equipment should be reevaluated yearly and should conform to National Electrical Code guidelines. If a clinic or training room is not in compliance with this code, then there is no legal protection in a lawsuit.
- Common sense should always be exercised when using electrotherapeutic devices. A situation that appears to be potentially dangerous may in fact result in injury or death.

SAFETY IN USING THERAPEUTIC MODALITIES

When using any type of therapeutic modality, the athletic trainer must ensure that the equipment is used and maintained in an appropriate manner.[37] Manufacturers of therapeutic modality equipment usually provide written guidelines and recommendations for appropriate care and maintenance in the manuals that accompany new equipment. There is usually a regular maintenance schedule for each piece of equipment that is designed to discover any defects or breakdowns that may occur due to normal wear and tear. The athletic trainer should be familiar with and closely follow the manufacturer's recommendations for equipment maintenance. Failure to do so may make the athletic trainer legally negligent should an incident occur that results in an unnecessary injury to a patient. The athletic trainer should arrange to have the maintenance done either by the manufacturer or by some other qualified agency. *Focus Box:* "Safe use of therapeutic modalities" lists recommended safety practices for using and maintaining therapeutic equipment.

SUMMARY

- To avoid legal problems, athletic trainers must use therapeutic modalities with extreme care. Athletic trainers must be familiar with the laws of their state regarding therapeutic modality use. Before using any modality, the athletic trainer must have a thorough understanding of its function and when it should and should not be used.
- Heat energy is transmitted through conduction, convection, radiation, and conversion. Conduction occurs when heat is transferred from a warmer object to a cooler one. Convection heating occurs by means of fluid or gas movement. Radiation is heat energy that is transmitted through empty space. Conversion is heat that is generated when one type of energy is changed to another.
- The use of cold for therapeutic purposes and as part of an emergency procedure is extremely popular in sports medicine. Cold penetrates more deeply than superficial heat. Therapy is usually performed when the tissue has reached a state of relative anesthesia. Cryotherapy decreases muscle spasm, pain perception, and blood flow. It increases the inelasticity of collagen fibers, joint stiffness, and capillary permeability. Common cryotherapy procedures are cold water immersion, ice massage, ice packs, and the use of vapocoolant sprays.
- Thermotherapy increases blood flow, increases collagen viscosity, decreases joint stiffness, and reduces pain and muscle spasm. When the body's temperature is raised, tissue metabolism is increased, vascular permeability is increased, and chemicals such as histamine, bradykinin, and serotonin are released.
- Superficial therapeutic heat should not be applied under the following circumstances: when there is a loss of sensation; immediately after an acute injury; or when there is decreased arterial bleeding. Superficial therapeutic heat should not be used over the eyes or genitals or over the abdomen of a pregnant woman. Types of superficial heat are moist heat packs, whirlpool baths, paraffin baths, fluidotherapy, and contrast baths.
- Ultrasound is a form of acoustic energy. It creates a mechanical vibration that is converted to heat energy within the body. Heating occurs in the denser tissues such as bone and connective tissue. More heat is built up at tissue interfaces. Ultrasound has both thermal and nonthermal physiological effects. It can be combined with electrical stimulation or used to transport molecules through the skin with the method known as phonophoresis.
- The use of electrical stimulating currents is popular in sports medicine. Electrical stimulating units produce either alternating current (AC), direct current (DC), or pulsed current. Both AC and DC can be used for pain modulation and muscle contraction. Direct current can also be used for iontophoresis. The physiological effects of electrical current are determined by the treatment parameters and equipment selected. Current parameters include waveforms, modulation, intensity, duration,

frequency, polarity, and electrode placement. Interferential currents and LIS are two of the newest electrical stimulating currents available to the athletic trainer.

- The low-level laser may be used to stimulate the healing process or to modulate pain. It has been approved as an investigational device by the FDA for limited use in the United States.
- Massage is a useful modality for many sport-related injuries. Techniques include effleurage, petrissage, friction, tapotement, and vibration. Deep transverse massage is used on connective tissue.
- Traction is used to produce separation of the vertebrae, most commonly for the treatment of spinal nerve root impingement and associated abnormalities. It is typically used in the cervical and lumbar spine and may involve either manual or machine-assisted traction.
- Intermittent compression devices are used to control swelling after acute injury or to reduce pitting edema.
- Both shortwave and microwave diathermies produce heat through electromagnetic energy, whereas ultrasound produces heat through acoustical energy. The contraindications for the use of shortwave diathermy and microwave diathermy are the same as for superficial heating, with the additional restrictions of no implants, jewelry, or intrauterine devices. Care must be taken not to cross the cables.

Websites

National Athletic Trainers' Association: http://www.nata.org

Cramer First Aider:
http://www.cramersportsmed.com/first_aider.jsp

Solutions to Critical Thinking EXERCISES

15-1 Ice massage may be used for Achilles tendinitis and is beneficial since this area of the body is small. Cold water immersion is an alternative for cryotherapy. Ice water immersion is indicated because the injury is in a distal area and the entire area can be iced easily. The athlete is also able to perform cryokinetics simultaneously with the cryotherapy. Another alternative for cryotherapy is the use of ice packs, which can be formed around the ankle.

15-2 The decision is to some extent subjective. The athletic trainer must understand what is going on with the healing process. By the fifth day, the inflammatory process is ending and the fibroblastic stage is establishing itself. At this point it is still advisable to avoid any treatment that may increase swelling, which can interfere with healing. Heat would increase circulation, which might increase swelling. The athletic trainer would not likely exacerbate the injury by using heat, but it is recommended that cold be used during this time. A rule of thumb is that when the tenderness is gone, it is safe to change to some form of heat.

15-3 At this point, some form of heat to increase blood and lymphatic flow to the injured area is warranted. Increased blood flow will help facilitate the process of healing, and an increased lymphatic flow will help remove the by-products of the inflammatory process. Hot packs provide superficial heat and would not be effective in this case. Both diathermics and ultrasound would be recommended because they all have a depth of penetration great enough to affect the injured area; ultrasound would be somewhat more effective. For best results, stretching and strengthening exercises should always be used along with modalities.

15-4 A biofeedback unit can help the athlete relearn how to fire the quadriceps muscle. The biofeedback unit can provide both visual and auditory feedback to indicate the strength of a contraction as well as the timing of a contraction. Biofeedback can be used almost immediately following surgery.

15-5 The athletic trainer can use cryotherapy, heat, or electrical stimulating currents to help reduce pain. Electrical stimulating currents may be the most useful if the athletic trainer also wants to elicit a muscle contraction to help decrease muscle guarding. Massage also is useful for modulating pain and for relaxing muscles. Regardless of the modality chosen, the athlete should engage in some stretching and strengthening exercises after the modality treatment.

15-6 Effleurage massage strokes are ideal during the initial stages of injury to help encourage venous and lymphatic drainage, especially if swelling is present. This method also is sedative for the athlete. Friction massage is beneficial for patellar tendonitis to increase circulation in the area and to develop friction.

15-7 The athletic trainer should try using manual lumbar traction techniques, which, if done properly, can be effective in isolating a specific ligament between two lumbar vertebrae. If the athletic trainer cannot manually generate enough traction force to stretch the ligament, a table traction unit or an inverted traction technique may prove to be more useful.

15-8 Proper initial management of the injury could have prevented a great deal of the swelling that has occurred. At this point, the athletic trainer should make use of ice to modulate pain; intermittent compression and electrical stimulating current to induce a muscle pumping contraction (both of which can help the lymphatic system remove the swelling); and low-intensity ultrasound (>0.2 W/cm^2), which can help facilitate the healing process. In addition, the athlete should continually wear a compressive elastic wrap. He must also progress to full weight bearing, concentrating on regaining a normal gait as soon as it can be tolerated.

15-9 In this case, the best treatment is not to use ultrasound at all. A better decision would be to use either hydrocollator packs or diathermy, both of which are more useful in treating larger areas. If depth of penetration is a concern, then shortwave diathermy would be the treatment modality of choice.

REVIEW QUESTIONS AND CLASS ACTIVITIES

1. Explain the legal factors that a coach or athletic trainer should consider before using a therapeutic modality.
2. Give examples of modalities that heat through conduction, convection, radiation, and conversion.
3. What physiological changes occur when heat is applied to the body?
4. Discuss the physiological effects of using cryotherapy.
5. Demonstrate the proper technique for a variety of cryotherapeutic approaches.
6. Compare therapy delivered through heat to that delivered through cold. When would you use each?
7. What are shortwave and microwave diathermy used for?
8. Discuss how ultrasound can be used during a rehabilitation program.
9. Compare phonophoresis with iontophoresis.
10. What is a TENS unit?
11. Identify the potential treatment goals of an electrically stimulated muscle contraction.
12. How is massage best used in a sports medicine setting?
13. List the mechanical effects of cervical and lumbar traction.
14. Explain when and how intermittent compression can best be used as a treatment modality.

REFERENCES

1. Angus J, Prentice W, Hooker D: A comparison of two external intermittent compression devices and their effect on post acute ankle edema, *J Ath Train* 29(2):178, 1994.
2. Archer PA: Three clinical sports massage approaches for treating injured athletes. *Athletic Therapy Today* 6(3):14, 2001.
3. Burke D, Holt L, Rasmussen R: The effect of hot or cold water immersion and proprioceptive neuromuscular facilitation on hip joint range of motion, *J Ath Train* 36(1):16, 2001.
4. Castel C, Draper D, Castel D: Rate of temperature increase during ultrasound treatments: are traditional times long enough? *J Ath Train* 29(2):156, 1994.
5. Dolan M, Mychaskiw A, Mendel F: Cool-water immersion and high-voltage electric stimulation curb edema formation in rats, *J Ath Train* 38(3), 2003.
6. Draper D: Are certified athletic trainers qualified to use therapeutic modalities?, *J Ath Train* 37(1):11, 2002.
7. Draper DO, Harris ST, Schulthies S et al: Hot-pack and 1-MHz ultrasound treatments have an additive effect on muscle temperature, *J Ath Train* 33(1):21, 1998.
8. Draper D, Miner L, Knight K: The carry-over effects of diathermy and stretching in developing hamstring flexibility, *J Ath Train* 37(1):37, 2002.
9. Draper D, Prentice W: Therapeutic ultrasound. In Prentice W, editor: *Therapeutic modalities in sports medicine and athletic training,* ed 5, St Louis, 2003, McGraw-Hill.
10. Draper DO, Ricard M: Rate of temperature decay in human muscle following 3-Mhz ultrasound: the stretching window revealed, *J Ath Train* 30(4):304, 1995.
11. Draper D, Schulthies S, Sorvisto P: The effect of cooling the tissue prior to ultrasound treatment, *J Ath Train* 29(2):154, 1994.
12. Draper D, Sunderland S: Examination of the law of Grotthus-Draper: does ultrasound penetrate subcutaneous fat? *J Ath Train* 28(3):246, 1993.
13. Fritz S: *Mosby's fundamentals of therapeutic massage,* St Louis, 1999, Mosby Year Book.
14. Gazzillo LM: Therapeutic massage techniques for three common injuries. *Athletic Therapy Today* 6(3):5, 2001.
15. Holcomb W: A practical guide to electrical therapy, *J Sport Rehabil* 6(3):272, 1997.
16. Holcomb W, Joyce C: A comparison of temperature increases produced by 2 commonly used ultrasound units, *J Ath Train* 38(1):24, 2003.
17. Hooker D: Electrical stimulating currents. In Prentice W, editor: *Therapeutic modalities in sports medicine and athletic training,* ed 5, St Louis, 2003, McGraw-Hill.
18. Hooker D: Intermittent compression devices. In Prentice W, editor: *Therapeutic modalities in sports medicine and athletic training,* ed 5, St Louis, 2003, McGraw-Hill.
19. Hooker D: Traction as a specialized modality. In Prentice W, editor: *Therapeutic modalities in sports medicine and athletic training,* ed 5, St Louis, 2003, McGraw-Hill.
20. Hopkins J, Ingersoll C, Edwards J: Cryotherapy and transcutaneous electric neuromuscular stimulation decrease arthrogenic muscle inhibition of the vastus medialis after knee joint effusion, *J Ath Train* 37(1):25, 2002.
21. Hubbard T, Aronson S, Denegar C: Does cryotherapy hasten return to participation? A systematic review, *J Ath Train* 39(1):88, 2004.
22. Johns L: Nonthermal effects of therapeutic ultrasound, *J Ath Train* 37(3):293, 299, 2002.
23. Johnson DS: Low-level laser therapy in the treatment of carpal tunnel syndrome, *Athletic Therapy Today* 8(2):30–31, 2003.
24. Kloth L: Shortwave and microwave diathermy. In Michlovitz SL, editor: *Thermal agents in rehabilitation,* Philadelphia, 1996, Davis.
25. Knight K: *Cryotherapy in sport injury management,* Champaign, Ill, 1995, Human Kinetics.
26. Krumholz A, Gelfand B, O'Conner P: Therapeutic modalities. In Nicholas J, Hershman EB, editors: *The lower extremity and spine in sports medicine,* vol 1, St Louis, 1995, Mosby.
27. Merrick M: Does 1-MHz ultrasound really work? *Athletic Therapy Today* 6(6):48, 2001.
28. Merrick M: Secondary injury after musculoskeletal trauma: a review and update. *J Ath Train* 37(2):209, 2002
29. Merrick M, Jutte L, Smith M: Cold modalities with different thermodynamic properties produce different surface and intramuscular temperatures, *J Ath Train* 38(1):28–33, 2003.
30. Michlovitz SL: Biophysical principles of heating and superficial heat agents. In Michlovitz SL, editor: *Thermal agents in rehabilitation,* Philadelphia, 1996, Davis.
31. Michlovitz SL: Cryotherapy: the use of cold as a therapeutic agent. In Michlovitz SL, editor: *Thermal agents in rehabilitation,* Philadelphia, 1996, Davis.
32. Myrer J, Draper D, Durrant E: Contrast therapy and intramuscular temperature in the leg, *J Ath Train* 29(4):318, 1994.
33. Myrer JW, Measom G, Durrant E, et al: Cold- and hot-pack contrast therapy: subcutaneous and intramuscular temperature change, *J Ath Train* 32(3):238, 1997.
34. Myrer J, Measom G, Fellingham G: Intramuscular temperature rises with topical analgesics used as coupling agents during therapeutic ultrasound, *J Ath Train* 36(1):20, 2001.
35. Penderghest C, Kimura I, Gulick D: Double-blind clinical efficacy study of pulsed phonophoresis on perceived pain associated with symptomatic tendinitis, *J Sport Rehabil* 7(1):9, 1998.
36. Peres S, Draper D, Knight K: Pulsed shortwave diathermy and long-duration stretching increase dorsiflexion range of motion more than identical stretching without diathermy, *J Ath Train* 37(1):43, 2002.

37. Prentice W: Basic principles of electricity. In Prentice W, editor: *Therapeutic modalities in sports medicine and athletic training,* ed 5, St Louis, 2003, McGraw-Hill.
38. Prentice W: Biofeedback. In Prentice W, editor: *Therapeutic modalities in sports medicine and athletic training,* ed 5, St Louis, 2003, McGraw-Hill.
39. Prentice W: Preface. In Prentice W, editor: *Therapeutic modalities in sports medicine and athletic training,* ed 5, St Louis, 2003, McGraw-Hill.
40. Prentice W: The science of therapeutic modalities. In Prentice W, editor: *Therapeutic modalities in sports medicine and athletic training,* ed 5, St Louis, 2003, McGraw-Hill.
41. Prentice W, Bell G: Infrared modalities. In Prentice W, editor: *Therapeutic modalities in sports medicine and athletic training,* ed 5, St Louis, 2003, McGraw-Hill.
42. Prentice W, Draper, D, Donley P: Shortwave and microwave diathermy. In Prentice W, editor: *Therapeutic modalities in sports medicine and athletic training,* ed 5, St Louis, 2003, McGraw-Hill.
43. Prentice W, Lehn C: Therapeutic massage. In Prentice W, editor: *Therapeutic modalities in sports medicine and athletic training,* ed 5, St Louis, 2003, McGraw-Hill.
44. Rimington S, Draper D, Durrant E: Temperature changes during therapeutic ultrasound in the precooled human gastrocnemius muscle, *J Ath Train* 29(4):325, 1994.
45. Rubley M, Denegar C, Buckley W: Cryotherapy, sensation, and isometric-force variability, *J Ath Train* 38(2):113, 2003.
46. Rucinski T, Hooker D, Prentice W: The effects of intermittent compression on edema in postacute ankle sprains, *J Orthop Sports Phys Ther* 13(8):65, 1991.
47. Saliba E, Saliba S: Low-power laser. In Prentice W, editor: *Therapeutic modalities in sports medicine and athletic training,* ed 5, St Louis, 2003, McGraw-Hill.
48. Schliephakle E: Carrying out treatment. In Throm H, editor: *Introduction to shortwave and microwave therapy,* ed 3, Springfield, Ill, 1966, Charles C Thomas.
49. Snyder-Mackler L, Robinson A: *Clinical electrophysiology: electrotherapy and electrophysiology,* Baltimore, 1995, Lippincott, Williams & Wilkins.
50. Stemmans C: Low-energy extracorporeal shock-wave therapy. *Athletic Therapy Today* 8(2):44, 2003.
51. Sweeney K, Merrick M, Ingersoll C: Therapeutic magnets do not affect tissue temperature, *J Ath Train* 36(1):27–31, 2001.
52. Tsang K et al: The effects of cryotherapy applied through various barriers, *J Sport Rehabil* 6(4):343, 1997.
53. Tsang K, Hertel J, Denegar C: Volume decreases after elevation and intermittent compression are negated by gravity-dependent positioning. *J Ath Train* 38(4):320, 2003.
54. Walsh M: Hydrotherapy: the use of water as a therapeutic agent. In Michlovitz SL, editor: *Thermal agents in rehabilitation,* Philadelphia, 1996, Davis.
55. Wang, CJ, Chen HS: Shock wave therapy for patients with lateral epicondylitis of the elbow: a one- to two-year follow-up study. *Am J Sports Med* 30(3):422, 2002.
56. Whitehill W: Massage and skin conditions: indications and contraindications. *Athletic Therapy Today* 7(3):24, 2002.
57. Ziskin MC, Michlovitz SL: Therapeutic ultrasound. In Michlovitz SL, editor: *Thermal agents in rehabilitation,* Philadelphia, 1996, Davis.

ANNOTATED BIBLIOGRAPHY

Cameron M: *Physical agents in rehabilitation: from research to practice.* Philadelphia, 2003, W.B. Saunders.

A guide for the physical therapist using therapeutic modalities.

Denegar C: *Therapeutic modalities for athletic injuries,* Champaign, Ill, 2000, Human Kinetics.

This text focuses on the neurophysiologic mechanisms of pain control as medicated by a variety of different therapeutic modalities.

Knight KL: *Cryotherapy in sports injury management,* Champaign, Ill, 1995, Human Kinetics.

This text presents excellent coverage, both theoretical and practical, of one of the most widely used therapeutic approaches in sports medicine and athletic training—cryotherapy. The text is clearly written and easily applied.

Michlovitz SL, editor: *Thermal agents in rehabilitation,* Philadelphia, 1996, Davis.

This excellent text is about understanding the foundations and use of thermal agents in sports medicine and athletic training. It provides detailed discussions of inflammation, pain, superficial heat and cold, and the therapeutic use of ultrasound and shortwave and microwave diathermies.

Prentice W: *Therapeutic modalities in rehabilitation,* New York, 2005, McGraw-Hill.

A comprehensive guide to using therapeutic modalities in treating a variety of patient populations. This text contains pertinent case studies and laboratory activities.

Prentice W: *Therapeutic modalities for sports medicine and athletic training,* ed 5, St Louis, 2003, McGraw-Hill.

This text is a complete and comprehensive guide to the use of therapeutic modalities in the sports medicine setting. It addresses all aspects of modality use, including massage, traction, and intermittent compression. The text is an excellent blend of theory and practical application.

Starkey C: *Therapeutic modalities for athletic trainers,* Philadelphia, 2004, Davis.

This text discusses many of the modalities used by athletic trainers in a clinical setting.

Travell JG, Simons DG: *Myofascial pain and dysfunction,* Baltimore, 1983, Williams & Wilkins.

This valuable text about myofascial trigger points provides a clear understanding of trigger-point evaluation in the upper body and the treatment of choice; it also covers muscle stretch after the application of a vapocoolant.

Chapter 16

Using Therapeutic Exercise in Rehabilitation

When you finish this chapter you should be able to

- Explain how the athletic trainer approaches rehabilitation.
- Contrast therapeutic exercise and conditioning exercise.
- Describe the consequences of sudden inactivity and injury immobilization.
- Recognize the primary components of a rehabilitation program.
- Discuss the concept of open versus closed kinetic chain exercises.
- Explain the importance of incorporating core stabilization training into a rehabilitation program.
- Evaluate the value of aquatic exercise in rehabilitation.
- Identify the techniques and principles of proprioceptive neuromuscular facilitation.
- Demonstrate the use of mobilization and traction techniques for improving accessory joint motions.
- Discuss how muscle energy, myofascial release, strain/counterstrain, positional release, and active release techniques can be incorporated into a rehabilitation program.

One of the primary goals of both the coach and the athletic trainer is to create a playing environment for the athlete that is as safe as it can possibly be. In spite of that effort, the nature of athletic participation dictates that injuries will eventually occur. When injuries do occur, the focus of the athletic trainer shifts from injury prevention to injury treatment and rehabilitation.

THE ATHLETIC TRAINER'S APPROACH TO REHABILITATION

The athletic trainer is responsible for design, implementation, and supervision of the rehabilitation program.

The process of rehabilitation begins immediately after injury. Initial first aid and management techniques can have a substantial impact on the course and ultimate outcome of the rehabilitative process. Thus, in addition to possessing a sound understanding of how injuries can be prevented, the athletic trainer must also be competent in providing correct and appropriate initial care when injury occurs. In a sports medicine setting, the athletic trainer generally assumes the primary responsibility for design, implementation, and supervision of the rehabilitation program for the injured athlete.

The long-term goal is to return the injured athlete to practice or competition as quickly and safely as possible.

Designing programs for rehabilitation is relatively simple and involves several basic short-term goals: controlling pain, maintaining or improving flexibility, restoring or increasing strength, reestablishing neuromuscular control, and maintaining levels of cardiorespiratory fitness. The long-term goal is to return the injured athlete to practice or competition as quickly and safely as possible. The design is the easy part of supervising a rehabilitation program. The difficult part comes in knowing exactly when and how to change the rehabilitation protocols to most effectively accomplish both long- and short-term goals. Progression during the rehabilitation program should be based on specific criteria, and return to competition must be based on level of function and patient outcomes.

The approach to rehabilitation in an athletic training environment is considerably different than in most other rehabilitation settings. The competitive nature of athletics necessitates an aggressive approach to rehabilitation. Because the competitive season in most sports is relatively short, the athlete does not have the luxury of simply sitting around and doing nothing until the injury heals. The goal is for the athlete to return to activity as soon as safely possible. Thus, the athletic trainer who is supervising the rehabilitation program must perform a balancing act between not pushing the athlete hard enough and being overly aggressive. In either case, a mistake in judgment on the part of the athletic trainer may hinder the athlete's return to activity.

Decisions as to when and how to alter and progress a rehabilitation program should be based within the framework of the healing process. The athletic trainer must possess a sound understanding of both the sequence and time frames for the various phases of healing and must realize that certain physiological events must occur during each of the phases. Any actions taken during a rehabilitation program that interfere with this healing process will likely increase the length of time required for rehabilitation and will slow the athlete's return to full activity. The healing process must have an opportunity to accomplish what it is supposed to. At best, the athletic trainer can only try to create an environment that is conducive to the healing process. Little can be done to speed up the process physiologically, but many things can be done during rehabilitation to impede healing.

Athletic trainers have many tools at their disposal that can facilitate the rehabilitative process. How the athletic trainer chooses to use those tools is often a matter of individual preference and experience. Additionally, each individual patient is different, and the responses to various treatment protocols vary. Thus, a cookbook approach to rehabilitation, with specific protocols that can be followed like a recipe, is impossible. In fact, the use of rehabilitation recipes is strongly discouraged. Instead, the athletic trainer must develop a broad theoretical knowledge base from which he or she can select and apply specific rehabilitation techniques to each individual athlete.

RAMP is an acronym for **r**ehabilitation goals: management of the **a**cute responses to injury, restoration of **m**obility, and successful completion of **p**erformance goals.[49] The RAMP system of rehabilitation has been proposed to provide a systematic format to help less-experienced clinicians progress injured athletes through the phases of recovery. Daily reassessment of an injury allows the rehabilitation plan to be current and appropriate. The goal-based progression of the system ensures maximum resolution of each rehabilitation objective, contributing to the athletes' optimal return to sport or activity. The RAMP system designates the current highest-priority rehabilitation goal as the primary objective and any other goals as secondary, thus ensuring that the pursuit of one rehabilitation goal is not at the expense of another, more currently relevant goal.[49]

16-1

Critical Thinking Exercise

A soccer player has been diagnosed as having a grade 2 sprain of the medial collateral ligament in her knee. The team physician has referred the athlete to the athletic trainer, who is responsible for overseeing the rehabilitation program.

? What are the short-term goals of a rehabilitation program, and how can the athletic trainer best achieve these goals?

THERAPEUTIC EXERCISE VERSUS CONDITIONING EXERCISE

Exercise is an essential factor in fitness conditioning, injury prevention, and injury rehabilitation. To compete successfully at a high level, the athlete must be fit. An athlete who is not fit is more likely to sustain an injury. Coaches and athletic trainers both recognize that improper conditioning is one of the major causes of sports injuries. It is essential that the athlete engage in training and conditioning exercises that minimize the possibility of injury while maximizing performance.

The basic principles of training and conditioning that were discussed in Chapter 4 also apply to therapeutic, rehabilitative, or reconditioning exercises for restoring normal body function following injury. The term *therapeutic exercise* is perhaps most widely used to indicate exercises that are used in a rehabilitation program.

Therapeutic exercises are concerned with restoring normal body function after injury.

SUDDEN PHYSICAL INACTIVITY AND INJURY IMMOBILIZATION

The human body is a dynamic, moving entity that requires physical activity to maintain proper physical function. When an injury occurs, two problems immediately arise that must be addressed. First is the generalized loss of physical fitness that occurs when activity is stopped, and second is the specific inactivity of the injured part, resulting from protective splinting of the soft tissue and, in some cases, immobilization by some external means.

Effects of General Inactivity

A sudden loss of physical activity leads to a generalized loss of physical fitness.

An athlete who is highly conditioned will experience a rapid, generalized loss of fitness when exercise is suddenly stopped.[31] This sudden lack of activity causes a loss of muscle strength, endurance, and coordination. Whenever possible, the athlete, without aggravating the injury, must continue to exercise the entire body.

Effects of Immobilization

An injured body part that is immobilized for a period of time causes a number of disuse problems that adversely affect muscle, joints, ligaments, bone, neuromuscular efficiency, and the cardiorespiratory system.

Muscle and Immobilization

When a body part is immobilized for as short a period as twenty-four hours, definite adverse muscular changes occur.

Immobilization of a part causes atrophy of slow-twitch muscle fibers.

Atrophy and fiber-type conversion Disuse of a body part quickly leads to a loss of muscle mass. The greatest atrophy occurs in the type I (slow-twitch) fibers. Over time, the slow-twitch fibers develop fast-twitch characteristics. Slow-twitch fibers also diminish in number without type II (fast-twitch) fibers lessening in number.[53] A muscle that is immobilized in a lengthened or neutral position tends to atrophy less. In contrast, immobilizing a muscle in a shortened position encourages atrophy and greater loss of contractile function.[31] Atrophy can also be prevented through isometric contraction and electrical stimulation of the muscles. As the unused muscle decreases in size because of atrophy, protein is also lost. When activity is resumed, normal protein synthesis is reestablished.

Decreased neuromuscular efficiency Immobilization causes motor nerves to become less efficient in recruiting and stimulating individual muscle fibers within a given motor unit.[2] Once immobilization ends, the original motor neuron discharge returns within about one week.

Joints and Immobilization

Joint immobilization decreases normal lubrication.

The immobilization of joints causes a loss of normal compression, which in turn leads to a decrease in lubrication within the joint that subsequently causes degeneration. This degeneration occurs because the articular cartilage is deprived of its normal nutrition. The use of continuous passive motion, electrical muscle stimulation, or hinged casts has in some cases retarded loss of articular cartilage.[2]

Ligament and Bone and Immobilization

Both ligaments and bones adapt to normal stress by maintaining their strength or becoming stronger. However, when stress is eliminated or decreased, ligament and bone become weaker.[31] Once immobilization has been removed, high-frequency, short-duration endurance exercise positively enhances the mechanical properties of ligaments. Endurance activities tend to increase both the production and the hypertrophy of the collagen fibers. Full remodeling of ligaments after immobilization may take as long as twelve months or more.

Cardiorespiratory System and Immobilization

Like other structures, the cardiorespiratory system is adversely affected by immobilization. The resting heart rate increases approximately one-half beat per minute each day of immobilization. The stroke volume, maximum oxygen uptake, and vital capacity decrease concurrently with the increase in heart rate.

MAJOR COMPONENTS OF A REHABILITATION PROGRAM

A well-designed rehabilitation program should routinely address several key components before an injured athlete can return to preinjury competitive levels. Those components include minimizing swelling through appropriate first aid and management of initial injury, controlling pain, restoring full range of motion, restoring or increasing strength, reestablishing neuromuscular control, regaining balance, maintaining levels of cardiorespiratory fitness, and incorporating functional progressions.[44]

Components of a rehabilitation program include:

- Minimizing swelling
- Controlling pain
- Restoring full range of motion
- Restoring muscle strength and endurance
- Reestablishing neuromuscular control
- Regaining balance
- Maintaining cardiorespiratory fitness
- Incorporating functional progressions

Minimizing Initial Swelling

The process of rehabilitation begins immediately after injury. The manner in which the injury is first managed unquestionably has a significant impact on the course of the rehabilitative process. The one problem all injuries, regardless of type, have in common is swelling. Swelling may be caused by any number of factors, including bleeding, the production of synovial fluid, an accumulation of inflammatory by-products, edema, or a combination of several factors. Once swelling has occurred, the healing process is significantly retarded. The injured area cannot return to normal until all the swelling is gone. Therefore, all first aid management of these conditions should be directed toward controlling the swelling.[44] If the swelling can be controlled initially in the acute stage of injury, the time required for rehabilitation is likely to be significantly reduced. To control and significantly limit the amount of swelling, the RICE principle—rest, ice, compression, and elevation—should be applied (see Chapter 12).

Controlling Pain

When an injury occurs, the athletic trainer must realize that the athlete will experience some degree of pain (see Chapter 10). The extent of the pain will be determined by the severity of the injury, the athlete's individual response to and perception of pain, and the circumstances under which the injury occurred. The athletic trainer can modulate acute pain by using the RICE technique immediately after injury.[44] A physician may also make use of various medications to help ease pain.

Persistent pain can make strengthening or flexibility exercises more difficult and thus interfere with the rehabilitation process. The athletic trainer should routinely address pain during each treatment session. Making use of appropriate therapeutic modalities, including various techniques of cryotherapy, thermotherapy, and electrical stimulating currents, will help modulate pain throughout the rehabilitation process (see Chapter 15).[47]

Restoring Range of Motion

Injury to a joint will always be associated with some loss of motion. That loss of movement may be attributed to contracture of connective tissue (i.e., ligaments, joint capsules), resistance to stretch of the musculotendinous unit (i.e., muscle, tendon, and fascia), or some combination of the two.

Physiological versus Accessory Movements

Two types of movement govern range of motion about a joint. *Physiological movements* result from an active muscle contraction that moves an extremity through flexion, extension, abduction, adduction, and rotation. *Accessory motions* refer to the manner in which one articulating joint surface moves relative to another; such motions include *spin, roll, and glide.*[25] Physiological movement is voluntary, and accessory movements normally accompany physiological movement. The two occur simultaneously. Normal accessory motions must occur for full-range physiological movement to take place. If any of the accessory component motions are restricted, normal physiological cardinal plane movement will not occur.[65]

Accessory motions:

- Spin
- Roll
- Glide

Traditionally, rehabilitation programs tend to concentrate more on passive physiological movements and do not pay much attention to accessory motions. It is critical for

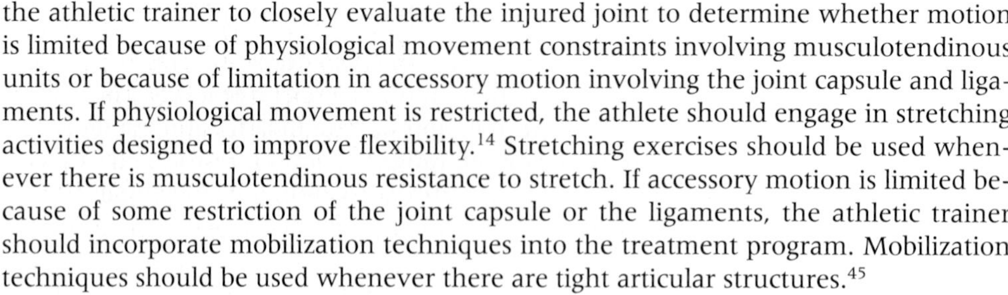

the athletic trainer to closely evaluate the injured joint to determine whether motion is limited because of physiological movement constraints involving musculotendinous units or because of limitation in accessory motion involving the joint capsule and ligaments. If physiological movement is restricted, the athlete should engage in stretching activities designed to improve flexibility.[14] Stretching exercises should be used whenever there is musculotendinous resistance to stretch. If accessory motion is limited because of some restriction of the joint capsule or the ligaments, the athletic trainer should incorporate mobilization techniques into the treatment program. Mobilization techniques should be used whenever there are tight articular structures.[45]

Restricted physiological movement = stretching.

Restricted accessory motion = joint mobilization.

Restoring Muscular Strength, Endurance, and Power

Muscular strength is one of the most essential factors in restoring the function of a body part to preinjury status. Isometric, isotonic, isokinetic, and plyometric exercises can benefit rehabilitation. A major goal in performing strengthening exercises is for the athlete to work through a full pain-free range of motion.

Isometric Exercise

Isometric exercises are commonly performed in the early phase of rehabilitation when a joint is immobilized for a period of time. They are useful when resistance training through a full range of motion may make the injury worse. Isometrics increase static strength and assist in decreasing the amount of atrophy. Isometrics also can lessen swelling by causing a muscle pumping action to remove fluid and edema.

Strength gains are limited primarily to the angle at which the joint is exercised. No functional force or eccentric work is developed. Other major difficulties are motivation and measuring the force that is being applied.

Progressive Resistance Exercise

Progressive resistance exercise is the most commonly used strengthening technique in a reconditioning program. This exercise may be done using free weights, exercise machines, rubber tubing, or manual resistance (Figure 16-1).[62] Progressive resistance exercise uses isotonic contractions in which force is generated while the muscle is changing in length.

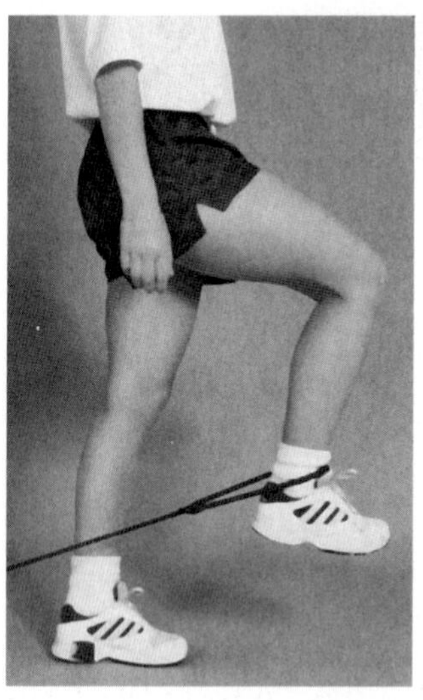

Figure 16-1

Exercises using rubber tubing are used for strengthening.

Concentric and eccentric muscle contractions Isotonic contractions may be either concentric or eccentric. Traditionally, athletes engaging in progressive resistance exercise have concentrated primarily on the concentric component without paying much attention to the importance of the eccentric component. The use of eccentric contractions, particularly in the rehabilitation of various injuries related to sport, has received considerable emphasis in recent years.[40] Eccentric contractions are critical for deceleration of limb motion, especially during high-velocity dynamic activities. For example, a baseball pitcher relies on an eccentric contraction of the external rotators at the glenohumeral joint to decelerate the humerus, which may be internally rotating at speeds as high as 8,000 degrees per second. Strength deficits or the inability of a muscle to tolerate these eccentric forces can predispose an athlete to injury. Eccentric contractions are used to facilitate concentric contractions in plyometric exercises and may also be incorporated with functional proprioceptive neuromuscular facilitation strengthening exercises. Thus, the athletic trainer should incorporate both eccentric and concentric strengthening exercises in a rehabilitation program.

Both concentric and eccentric contractions are possible with free weights, with most isotonic exercise machines, and with rubber tubing or an elastic band. A disadvantage of machines and free weights is that they do not allow exercises to be performed in diagonal or functional planes. It is also difficult to exercise at functional velocities without producing additional injuries. Conversely, resistance exercise using rubber tubing allows both concentric and eccentric resistance and is not encumbered by the design of an exercise machine. It offers a wide range of usefulness at an extremely low cost.

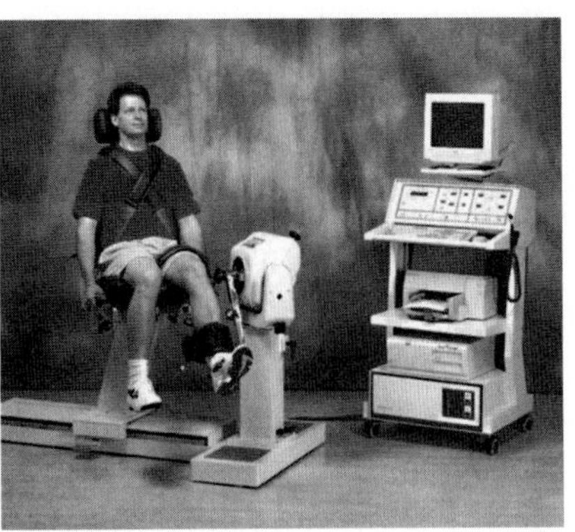

Figure 16-2

Isokinetics are primarily used as a diagnostic tool to determine levels of strength.

Isokinetic Exercise

If isokinetic exercise is used in the rehabilitative process, it is most often incorporated during the later phases of a rehabilitation program.[40] Isokinetics uses a fixed speed with accommodating resistance to provide maximal resistance throughout the range of motion (Figure 16-2). Isokinetic devices are generally capable of calculating measures of torque, average power, and total work and ratios of torque to body weight, each of which may be used diagnostically by the athletic trainer. Isokinetic measures are commonly used as a criterion for return of the athlete to functional activity after injury.

The speed of movement can be altered in isokinetic exercise. Gains in strength from training at slower speeds are fairly specific to the angular velocity used in training. Isokinetic machines allow the athlete to exercise at speeds that are somewhat more functional. Training at faster speeds seems to produce more general improvement because increases in torque values can be seen at both fast and slow speeds. Isokinetic exercise performed at high speeds tends to decrease the joint's compressive forces. Fast-speed exercises produce fewer negative effects on joints than do slow-speed exercises. Short-arc submaximal isokinetics exercise spreads out synovial fluid that helps to nourish the articular cartilage and therefore to prevent deterioration.[40] It also develops neuromuscular patterning for functional speed and movements demanded by specific sports.

Testing Strength, Endurance, and Power

Testing for improvement in muscular strength, endurance, or power can be accomplished through manual muscle tests, isotonic resistance exercises, or isokinetic dynamometers. Isokinetic testing generally provides the most reliable objective measure of changes in strength.

16-2 Critical Thinking Exercise

After an ankle sprain, a basketball player is placed in an ankle immobilizer and given crutches with instructions to begin totally non–weight bearing and progress to full weight bearing without crutches as soon as possible. After four days, the athlete is out of the immobilizer and can walk without crutches but still has a significant limp.

? What should the athletic trainer do to help the athlete regain a normal gait pattern, and why is it important to do so as soon as possible?

Reestablishing Neuromuscular Control, Proprioception, Kinesthesia, and Joint Position Sense

After injury and subsequent rest and immobilization, the central nervous system "forgets" how to put together information coming from muscle and joint mechanoreceptors and from cutaneous, visual, and vestibular input.[19] *Neuromuscular control* is the mind's attempt to teach the body conscious control of a specific movement.[30] Successful repetition of a patterned movement makes its performance progressively less difficult and thus requires less concentration; eventually the movement becomes automatic. Reestablishing neuromuscular control requires many repetitions of the same movement through a step-by-step progression from simple to more complex movements. Strengthening exercises, particularly those that tend to be more functional, such as closed kinetic chain exercises, are essential for reestablishing neuromuscular control.[63]

Regaining neuromuscular control means regaining the ability to follow some previously established sensory pattern.[38] The central nervous system compares the intent and production of a specific movement with stored information, continually adjusting until any discrepancy in movement is corrected.[63] Four elements are critical for reestablishing neuromuscular control: (1) proprioceptive and kinesthetic awareness, (2) dynamic stability, (3) preparatory and reactive muscle characteristics, and (4) conscious and unconscious functional motor patterns.[60]

Relearning normal functional movement and timing after injury to a joint may require several months. Addressing neuromuscular control is critical throughout the recovery process but may be most critical during the early stages of rehabilitation to avoid reinjury.[63]

proprioception
The ability to determine the position of a joint in space.

kinesthesia
The ability to detect movement.

Neuromuscular control produces coordinated movements.

Reestablishing proprioception and kinesthesia should also be of primary concern to the athletic trainer in all rehabilitation programs.[30] **Proprioception** is the ability to determine the position of a joint in space; **kinesthesia** refers to the ability to detect movement.[17] The ability to sense the position of a joint in space is mediated by mechanoreceptors found in both muscle and joints and by cutaneous, visual, and vestibular input. Neuromuscular control relies on the central nervous system to interpret and integrate proprioceptive and kinesthetic information and then to control individual muscles and joints to produce coordinated movement.[61,63]

Joint Mechanoreceptors

Joint mechanoreceptors include Ruffini's endings, Pacinian corpuscles, and free nerve endings.

Joint mechanoreceptors are found in ligaments, capsules, menisci, labra, and fat pads. They include Ruffini's endings, Pacinian corpuscles, and free nerve endings. These receptors are sensitive to changes in the shape of various joint structures and to the rate and direction of movement of the joint. They are most active in the end ranges of motion.[51]

Muscle Mechanoreceptors

Muscle mechanoreceptors include muscle spindles and Golgi tendon organs.

The receptors found in muscles and tendons are the muscle spindles and the Golgi tendon organs. The muscle spindles are sensitive to changes in the length of the muscle, and Golgi tendon organs are sensitive to changes in tension. The actions of these receptors are discussed in detail in Chapter 4.[51]

Regaining Postural Stability and Balance

Postural stability involves the integration of muscular, neurological, and biomechanical information.

Balance involves the complex integration of muscular forces, neurological sensory information received from the mechanoreceptors, and biomechanical information.[23] Achieving postural stability involves positioning the body's center of gravity within the base of support. When the center of gravity extends beyond the base of support, the limits of stability have been exceeded even though the base of support has not changed, and a corrective step or stumble is necessary to prevent a fall. Even when an individual appears to be motionless, the body is undergoing constant postural sway caused by reflexive muscle contractions, which correct and maintain dynamic equilibrium in an upright posture.[12] When balance is disrupted, the response to correct it is primarily reflexive and automatic.[3] The primary mechanisms for controlling postural stability occur in the joints of the lower extremity.[63]

The ability to balance and maintain postural stability is essential to an athlete who is acquiring or reacquiring complex motor skills.[63] Athletes who show a decreased sense of balance or lack of postural stability after injury may lack sufficient proprioceptive and kinesthetic information or muscular strength, either of which may limit the athlete's ability to generate an effective correction response to disequilibrium. A rehabilitation program must include functional exercises that incorporate balance and proprioceptive training to prepare the athlete for return to activity. Failure to address balance problems may predispose the athlete to reinjury (Figure 16-3).

Maintaining Cardiorespiratory Fitness

Although strength and flexibility are commonly regarded as essential components in any injury rehabilitation program, relatively little consideration is given to maintaining

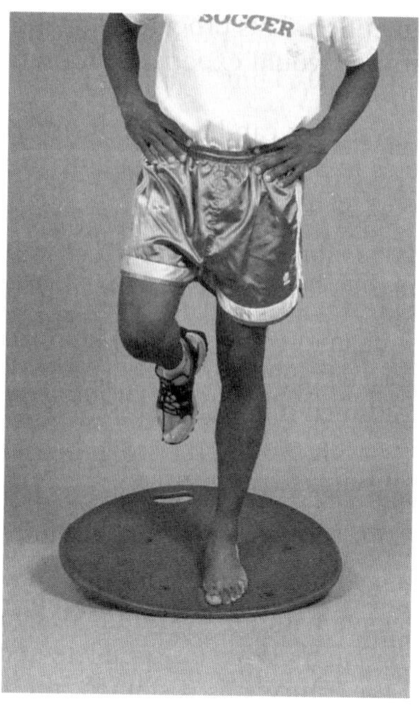

A

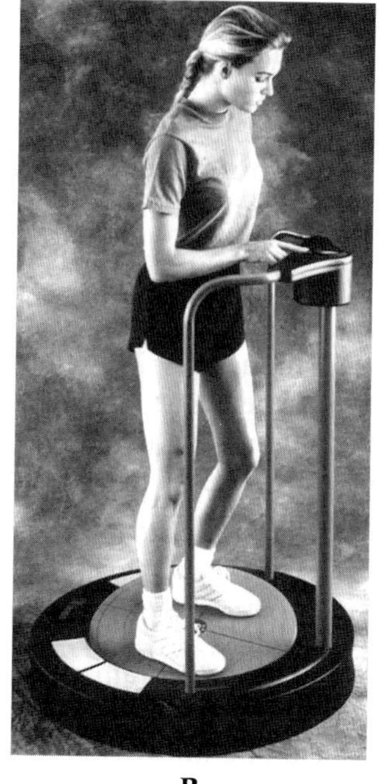

B

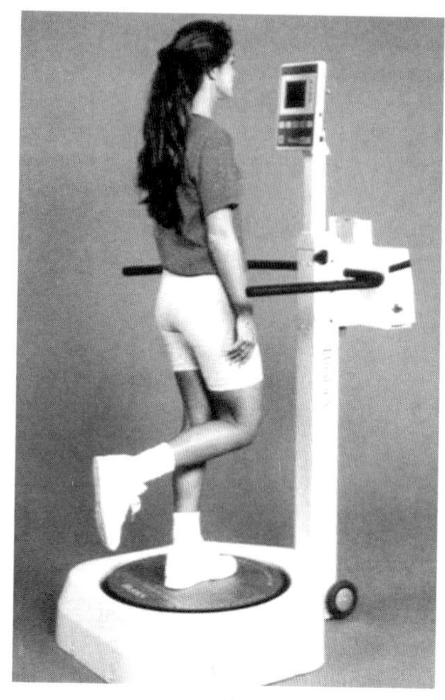

C

Figure 16-3

Balance training is essential in the rehabilitation program. Many balance training products are available. **A,** BAPS Board. **B,** Kinesthetic Awareness Trainer. **C,** Biodex Balance System.

levels of cardiorespiratory fitness. An athlete spends a considerable amount of time preparing the cardiorespiratory system to be able to handle the increased demands made on it during a competitive season. When injury occurs and the athlete is forced to miss training time, levels of cardiorespiratory endurance may decrease rapidly. Thus the athletic trainer must design or substitute alternative activities that allow the individual to maintain existing levels of cardiorespiratory fitness during the rehabilitation period.

Depending on the nature of the injury, a number of possible activities are open to the athlete. For a lower-extremity injury, non–weight bearing activities should be incorporated. Pool activities provide an excellent means for injury rehabilitation. Cycling also can positively stress the cardiorespiratory system (Figure 16-4).

Incorporating Functional Progressions

Functional progressions incorporate sport-specific skills into the rehabilitation program.

The purpose of any rehabilitation program is to restore normal function after injury. Functional progressions involve a series of gradually progressive activities designed to prepare the individual for return to a specific sport.[63] Functional progressions should be incorporated into the treatment program as early as possible. Well-designed functional progressions will gradually assist the injured athlete in achieving normal, pain-free range of motion, restoring adequate strength levels, and regaining neuromuscular control throughout the rehabilitation program. Ultimately, the focus becomes a safe return to competition. Those skills necessary for successful participation in a given sport are broken down into component parts, and the athlete gradually reacquires those skills within the limitations of his or her individual progress.[63]

Functional activities follow a consistent progression from simple to complex skills, slow to fast speeds, short to longer distances, or light to heavy activities. The athletic trainer must monitor every new activity introduced to determine the athlete's ability to perform as well as his or her physical tolerance. If an activity does not produce additional pain or swelling, the level should be advanced; new activities should be introduced as quickly as possible. Thus the injured athlete would be gradually introduced to the stresses imposed by a particular demand until function is adequate for the athlete to return to *sport-specific activity.*[63]

The optimal functional progression program would be designed such that the athlete would have an opportunity to practice every possible skill that is required in a

16-3

Critical Thinking **Exercise**

A runner complains of anterior knee pain. She has greatly cut back on the distance of her training runs and indicates that she has been taking antiinflammatory medication to help her continue to train. However, she is frustrated because her knee seems to be getting worse instead of better.

? What can the athletic trainer recommend to most effectively help the athlete deal with her knee pain?

the likelihood of swelling. Electrical stimulating currents can help control pain and improve strength and range of motion.[47]

Phase 3: The Maturation-Remodeling Phase

The maturation-remodeling phase is the longest of the three phases and may last for several years, depending on the severity of the injury. The ultimate goal during this maturation stage of the healing process is return to activity. The injury is no longer painful to the touch, although some progressively decreasing pain may still be felt on motion. The collagen fibers must be realigned according to tensile stresses and strains placed on them during functional sport-specific exercises.[44]

The focus during this phase should be on regaining sport-specific skills. Dynamic functional activities related to individual sport performance should be incorporated into the rehabilitation program. Functional training involves the repeated performance of an athletic skill for the purpose of perfecting that skill. Strengthening exercises should progressively place on the injured structures stresses and strains that would normally be encountered during that sport. Plyometric strengthening exercises can be used to improve muscle power and explosiveness.[30] Functional testing should be done to determine specific skill weaknesses that need to be addressed before full return to activity.

At this point, some type of heating modality is beneficial to the healing process. The deep-heating modalities, ultrasound, or the diathermies should be used to increase circulation to the deeper tissues. Massage and gentle mobilization may also be used to reduce spasm, increase circulation, and reduce pain. Increased blood flow delivers the essential nutrients to the injured area to promote healing, and increased lymphatic flow assists in the breakdown and removal of waste products.[47] As the maturation-remodeling phase begins, aggressive, active range-of-motion and strengthening exercises should be incorporated to facilitate tissue remodeling and realignment.

Engaging in exercise that is too intense or too prolonged can be detrimental to the progress of rehabilitation. Any increase in the amount of swelling, an increase in pain, a loss or a plateau in strength, a loss or a plateau in range of motion, an increase in the laxity of a healing ligament, or exacerbation of other clinical symptoms during or after a particular exercise or activity indicates that the load is too great for the level of tissue repair or remodeling.[63]

Adherence to a Rehabilitation Program

For a rehabilitation program to be successful, the injured athlete must comply with and adhere to the plan of rehabilitation.[5] In the field of athletic injury, compliance is the biggest deterrent to successful rehabilitation.[18] The athletic trainer can take several steps to enhance adherence.

- The athletic trainer can provide the encouragement and positive reinforcement necessary for the athlete to make a commitment. Athletes who are committed to the rehabilitation program work harder and thus return to competition more quickly with better results than those who are not committed.[18,52]
- The athletic trainer can be creative in designing and varying the exercise routine to keep the athlete interested and motivated.[42]
- Support from peers, coaches, and rehabilitation staff is important in influencing compliance. Those athletes with support show a greater effort to fit the rehabilitation effort into their schedules.[7]
- The athletic trainer's attitude is another important consideration when dealing with injured athletes. An athletic trainer who feels that an athlete is not going to adhere to the treatment program is less likely to motivate the athlete to comply with the program.
- The athlete is more likely to follow treatment plan instructions that are clearly explained verbally and then written down.[41,66]
- The coach must support the rehabilitation concept and must discipline the athlete if he or she does not participate in the rehabilitation process.

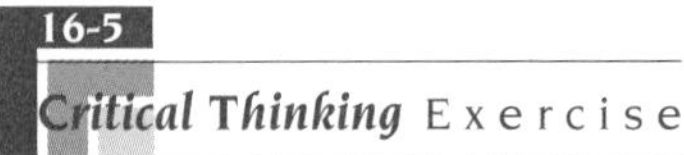

Following a recurrent shoulder injury, a lacrosse player seems to have developed a bad attitude toward doing his injury rehabilitation.

? What can the athletic trainer do to help this athlete be more compliant and adhere to his rehabilitation program?

- The athletic trainer can make an effort to fit the rehabilitation program into the athlete's schedule rather than the reverse.[15]
- Almost all rehabilitation should be pain free. Painful exercise not only is harmful but also reduces compliance, especially in the nonadherent athlete. The athletic trainer should examine rehabilitation programs to determine the aspects that may be painful.[7]

Criteria for Full Return to Activity

All exercise rehabilitation plans must determine what is meant by complete recovery from an injury. Often it means that the athlete is fully reconditioned and has achieved full range of movement, strength, neuromuscular control, cardiovascular fitness, and sport-specific functional skills. Besides physical well-being, the athlete must also have regained full confidence to return to his or her sport.

The decision to release an athlete recovering from injury to a full return to athletic activity is the final stage of the rehabilitation and recovery process. The decision should be carefully considered by each member of the sports medicine team involved in the rehabilitation process. The team physician should be ultimately responsible for deciding that the athlete is ready to return to practice or competition. The decision to return an athlete to activity should address the following concerns:

- *Physiological healing constraints*—Has rehabilitation progressed to the later stages of the healing process?
- *Pain status*—Has pain disappeared, or is the athlete able to play within his or her own levels of pain tolerance?
- *Swelling*—Is there still a chance that swelling may be exacerbated by a return to activity?
- *Range of motion*—Is the athlete's range of motion adequate to allow him or her to perform both effectively and with minimized risk of reinjury?
- *Strength*—Is strength, endurance, or power great enough to protect the injured structure from reinjury?
- *Neuromuscular control/Proprioception/Kinesthesia*—Has the athlete relearned how to use the injured body part?
- *Cardiorespiratory fitness*—Has the athlete been able to maintain cardiorespiratory fitness at or near the level necessary for competition?
- *Sport-specific demands*—Are the demands of the sport or a specific position such that the athlete will not be at risk of reinjury?
- *Functional testing*—Does the athlete's performance on appropriate functional tests indicate that his or her extent of recovery is sufficient to allow successful performance?
- *Prophylactic strapping, bracing, padding*—Are any additional supports necessary for the injured athlete to return to activity?
- *Responsibility of the athlete*—Is the athlete capable of listening to his or her body and recognizing a potential reinjury situation?
- *Predisposition to injury*—Is this athlete prone to reinjury or to a new injury when he or she is not fully recovered?
- *Psychological factors*—Is the athlete capable of returning to activity and competing at a high level without fear of reinjury?
- *Athlete education and preventive maintenance program*—Does the athlete understand the importance of continuing to engage in conditioning exercises that can greatly reduce the chances of reinjury?

ADDITIONAL APPROACHES TO THERAPEUTIC EXERCISE IN REHABILITATION

Open versus Closed Kinetic Chain Exercises

The concept of the kinetic chain deals with the functional anatomical relationships that exist in the upper and lower extremities. In a weight-bearing position, the lower extremity kinetic chain involves the transmission of forces among the foot, ankle,

A closed kinetic chain occurs when the foot or hand is on the ground.

An open kinetic chain occurs when the foot or hand is off the ground.

lower leg, knee, thigh, and hip. In the upper extremity, the hand as a weight-bearing surface transmits forces to the wrist, forearm, elbow, upper arm, and shoulder girdle.[45]

An open kinetic chain exists when the foot or hand is not in contact with the ground or some other surface.[45] In a closed kinetic chain, the foot or hand is weight bearing. Movements of the more proximal anatomical segments are affected by open and closed kinetic chain positions.[6] For example, the rotational components of the ankle, knee, and hip reverse direction when changing from an open to closed kinetic chain activity. In a closed kinetic chain, the forces begin at the ground and work their way up through each joint. In a closed kinetic chain, forces must be absorbed by various tissues and anatomical structures rather than simply dissipating as would occur in an open chain.[50]

16-6

Critical Thinking Exercise

A racquetball player twists his knee during a match and sprains his anterior cruciate ligament. Knee movement is limited because of the pain, and full weight bearing is extremely painful. He has a weekend-long racquetball tournament in two weeks and is concerned about regaining his knee motion while being able to maintain the fitness levels necessary to compete for two consecutive days.

? What type of rehabilitative technique could the athletic trainer recommend that would allow the athlete to address both his range of motion and fitness concerns even though he is unable to bear weight?

The use of closed chain strengthening techniques has become the rehabilitation treatment of choice for many athletic trainers.[29] Because most sports activities involve some aspect of weight bearing with the foot in contact with the ground or with the hand in a weight-bearing position, closed kinetic chain strengthening activities are more functional than are open chain activities. Closed kinetic chain exercises are more sport or activity specific, involving exercise that more closely approximates the desired activity. Specificity of training must be emphasized to athletes for them to maximize carryover to functional activities on the playing field.[43] Therefore, the treatment program should incorporate rehabilitative exercises that emphasize strengthening the entire kinetic chain rather than an isolated body segment.

Closed kinetic chain exercises use varying combinations of isometric, concentric, and eccentric contractions, which must occur simultaneously in different muscle groups within the chain. Isolation exercises typically make use of one specific type of muscular contraction to produce or control movement.[20] Consequently, there must be some neuromuscular adaptation to this type of strengthening exercise.

In the athletic training setting, several different closed kinetic chain exercises have gained popularity and have been incorporated into rehabilitation protocols.[22] Exercises commonly used for the lower extremity are minisquats, leg presses, forward and lateral step-ups, terminal knee extensions using tubing, and exercises that use equipment such as stair climbing or stepping machines, slide boards, and stationary bicycles.[43] Push-ups and weight-shifting exercises on a medicine ball are two of the more typically used upper extremity exercises (Figure 16-6).[36,57,61,64]

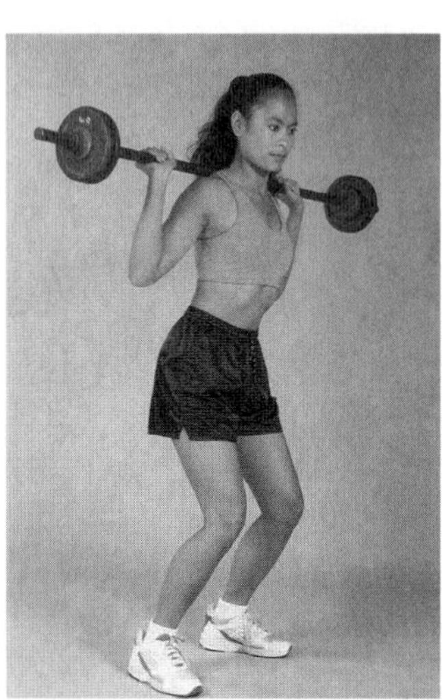

A

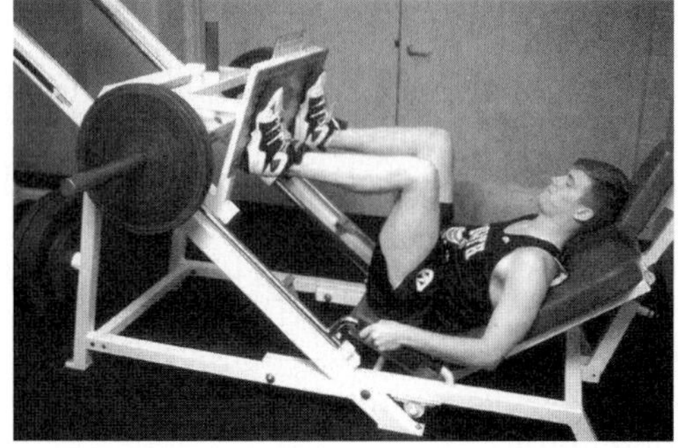

B

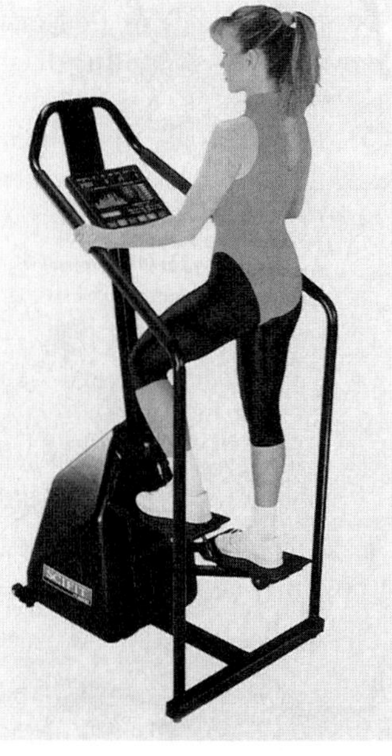

C

Figure 16-6

Closed kinetic chain exercises. **A,** Minisquats. **B,** Leg press. **C,** Stepping machines.

Continued

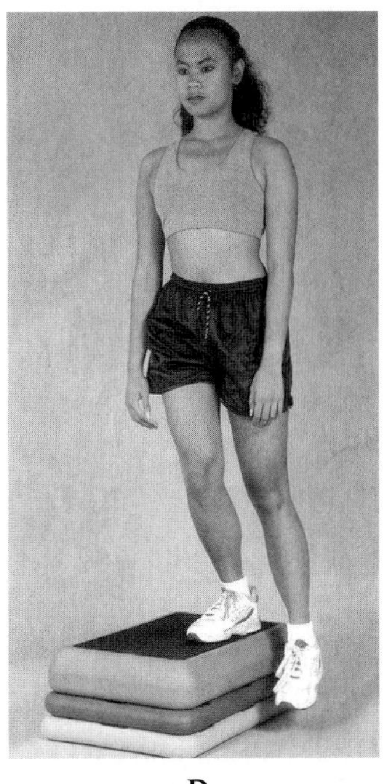

D

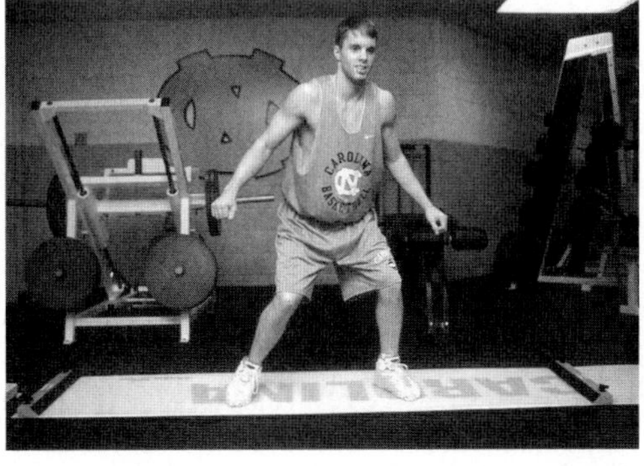

E

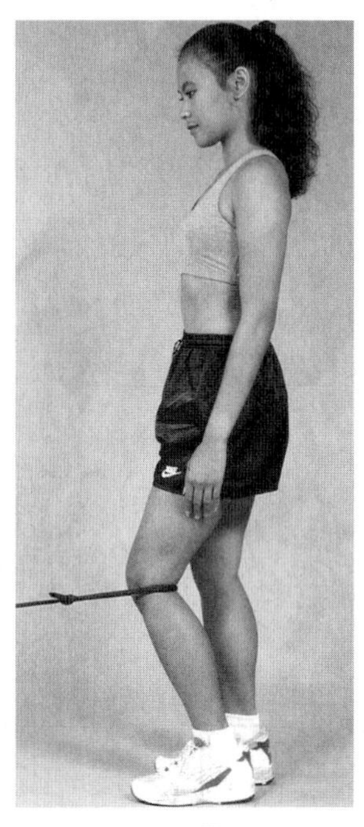

F

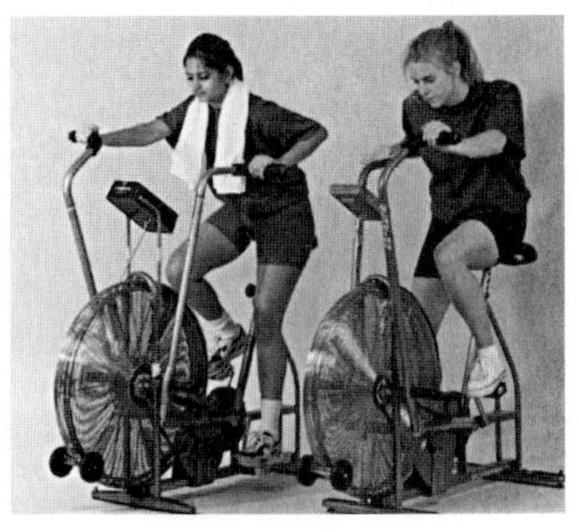

G

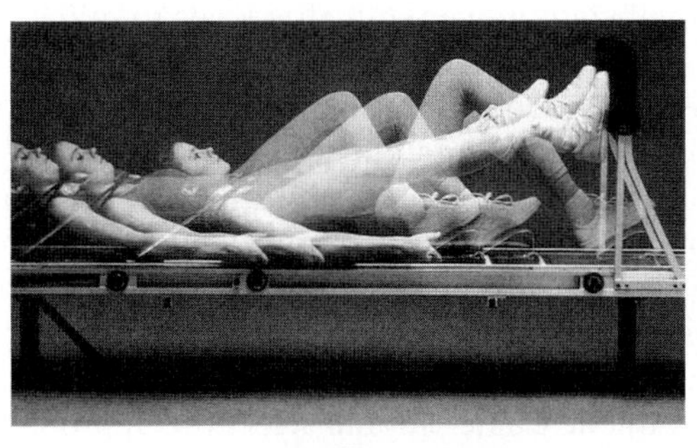

H

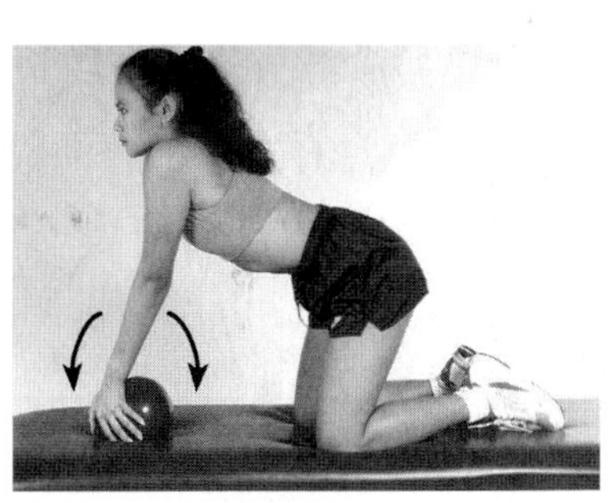

I

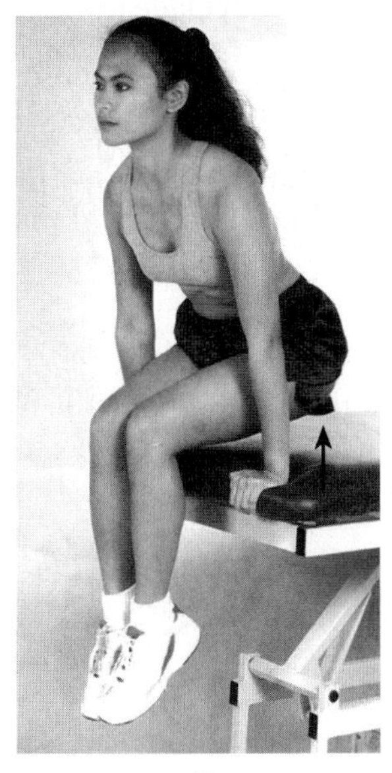

J

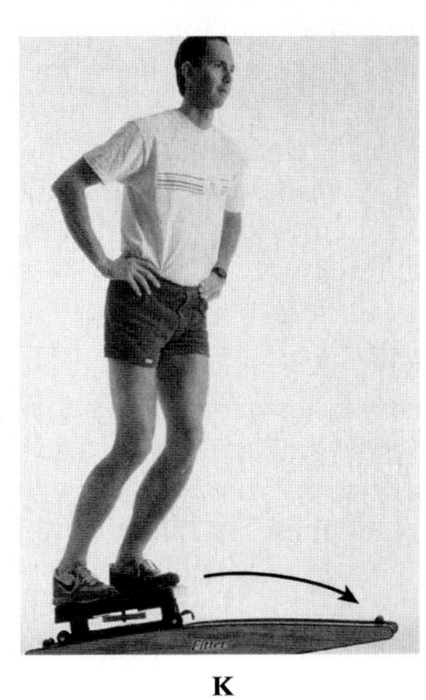

K

Figure 16-6—continued

D, Lateral step-ups. **E,** Slide boards. **F,** Terminal knee extensions using tubing. **G,** Stationary bicycling. **H,** Shuttle 2000. **I,** Weight shifting. **J,** Push-ups. **K,** Fitter.

Core Stabilization Training

A dynamic core stabilization training program should be an important component of all comprehensive strengthening and injury rehabilitation programs.[27] The *core* is defined as the lumbo-pelvic-hip complex. The core is where the center of gravity is located and where all movement begins. There are twenty-nine muscles that have their attachment to the lumbo-pelvic-hip complex. The key lumbar spine muscles include the transversospinalis group, erector spinae, quadratus lumborum, and latissimus dorsi. The key abdominal muscles include the rectus abdominus, external oblique, internal oblique, and transverse abdominus. The key hip musculature includes the gluteus maximus, gluteus medius, and psoas.[11]

A core stabilization program improves dynamic postural control, ensures appropriate muscular balance and joint movement around the lumbo-pelvic-hip complex, allows for the expression of dynamic functional strength, and improves neuromuscular efficiency throughout the entire body.[11] This permits optimal acceleration, deceleration, and dynamic stabilization of the entire kinetic chain during functional movements. It also provides proximal stability for efficient lower extremity movements.

Many athletes have developed the functional strength, power, neuromuscular control, and muscular endurance in specific muscles that enable them to perform functional activities. However, relatively few athletes have developed the muscles required for stabilization of the spine (see Chapter 25). The body's stabilization system has to be functioning optimally to effectively use the strength, power, neuromuscular control, and muscular endurance that athletes have developed in their prime movers. If the extremity muscles are strong and the core is weak, then there will not be enough force created to produce efficient movements. A weak core is a fundamental problem of inefficient movements that leads to injury.

A core stabilization training program is designed to help an individual gain strength, neuromuscular control, power, and muscle endurance in the lumbo-pelvic-hip complex.[27] This approach facilitates a balanced muscular functioning of the entire kinetic chain. Greater neuromuscular control and stabilization strength will offer a more biomechanically efficient position for the entire kinetic chain, therefore allowing optimal neuromuscular efficiency throughout the kinetic chain.

A comprehensive core stabilization training program should be systematic, progressive and functional. When designing a functional core stabilization training program, the athletic trainer should select the appropriate exercises to elicit a maximal training response. The exercises must be safe, challenging, stress multiple planes, incorporate a variety of resistance equipment (physioball, medicine ball, bodyblade, weight vest, dumbbells, tubing, etc.), derive from fundamental movement skills, and be activity specific (Figure 16-7). The athletic trainer should follow a progressive functional continuum to allow optimal adaptations. The athlete starts with the exercises at the highest level at which he or she can maintain stability and optimal neuromuscular control. Athletes then progress through the program as they achieve mastery of the exercises in each level.[11]

Aquatic Exercise

Aquatic exercise provides an excellent means for rehabilitation.

Aquatic exercise has become popular as a rehabilitative tool in sports medicine.[1] An athletic trainer who has access to a swimming pool is fortunate. Water submersion offers an excellent environment for beginning a program of exercise therapy, and it can complement all phases of rehabilitation.[48]

Because of buoyancy and hydrostatic pressure, submersion in a pool presents a versatile exercise environment that can be varied easily according to individual needs.[21] With the proper technique, the athlete can reduce muscle guarding; relax tense muscles; increase the range of joint motion; reestablish correct movement patterns; and above all, increase strength, power, and muscular endurance.[21]

Aquatic exercise uses the water's buoyancy and pressure; it can be described as assistive, supportive, and resistive. As an assistive medium, the water's buoyancy can increase range of motion, strength, and control. The athlete starts by placing the body

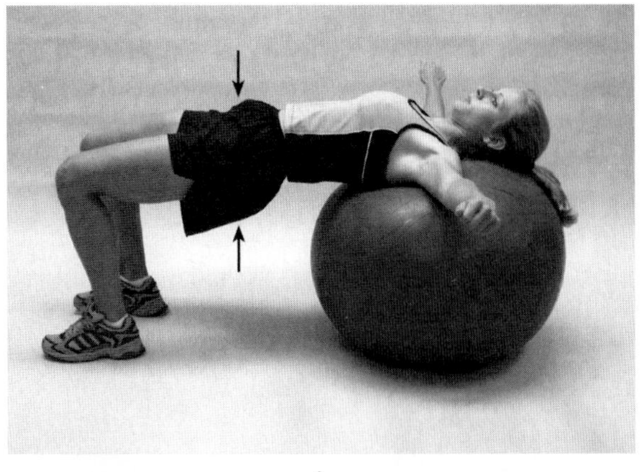
A

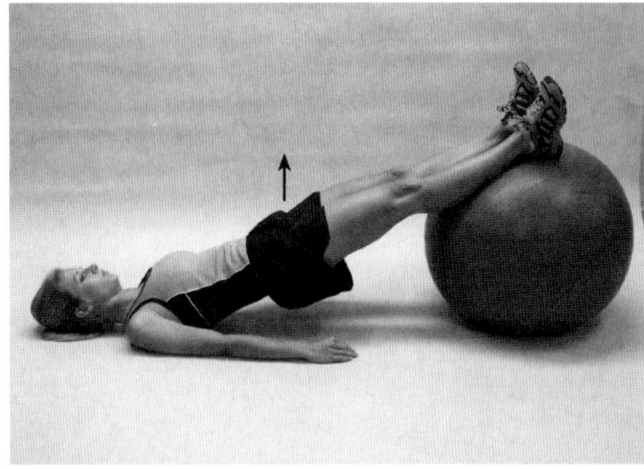
B

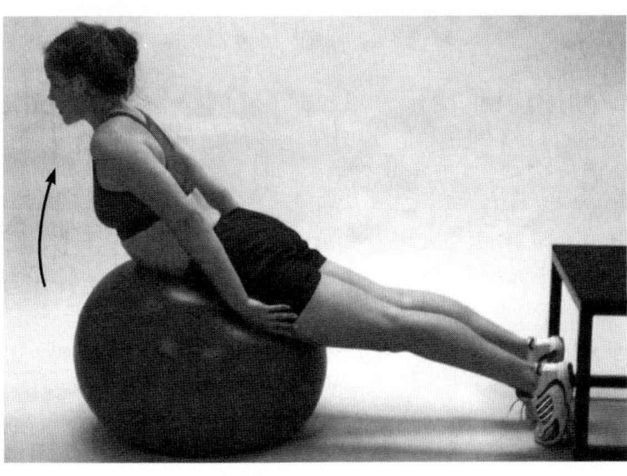
C

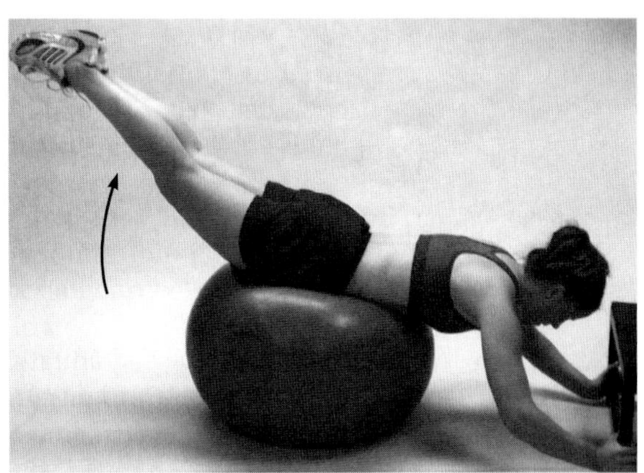
D

Figure 16-7

Core stabilization training exercises using a physioball to increase strength and control in the lumbo-pelvic-hip complex.

part below the water level and allows the part to be carried passively upward, keeping within pain-free limits. As the athlete gains strength, he or she actively engages in movement, again assisted by the buoyancy of the water. Progression of the movement can be initiated by increasing speed and by using the water above the body part as a resistive medium[39] (Figure 16-8).

A second use of water buoyancy is support. The limb normally will float just below the water's surface. In this position the limb is parallel to the surface of the water. An increase in speed will make movement more difficult. Progression also can be accomplished if the part is less streamlined. In exercising the arm, for example, the athlete can increase the difficulty by moving across the water with the flat of the hand or by using a hand paddle or webbed glove. Flippers can increase resistance to the leg.

Resistance is the third use of water buoyancy. The injured body part is moved downward against the upward thrust of the water. Maximum resistance is attained by keeping the limb at a right angle to the water's surface. Like the supportive technique, the resistive technique can be made progressively more difficult by the use of different devices. Extra resistance is added by pushing or dragging flotation devices down into the water.[4]

Besides engaging in specific exercises, the athlete can practice sports skills, using the water's buoyancy and resistance to his or her advantage. For example, locomotor or throwing skills can be practiced to regain normal movement patterns.[37] The swimming pool can also be an excellent medium for retaining or restoring functional capacities as well as restoring cardiovascular endurance. Wearing a flotation device around the waist, the athlete can perform a variety of upper- and lower-limb movement patterns (Figure 16-9). Movements of straight-ahead running, backward running, side stepping, figure eights, and carioca can be performed by an athlete bearing full weight while in three to five feet of water.

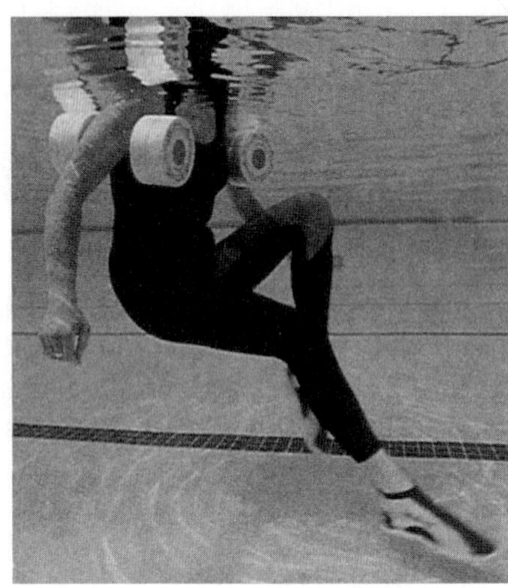

A

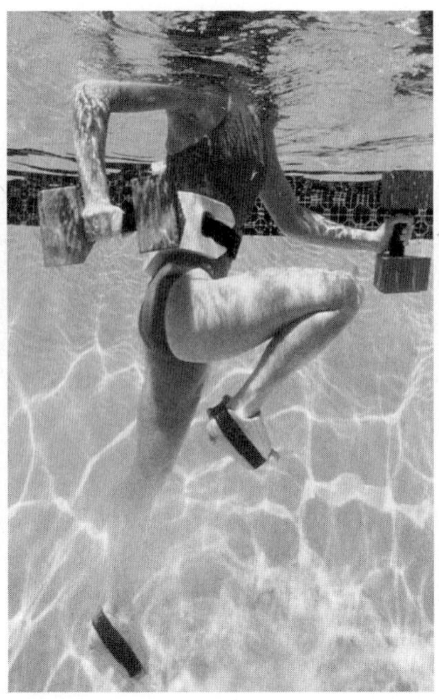

B

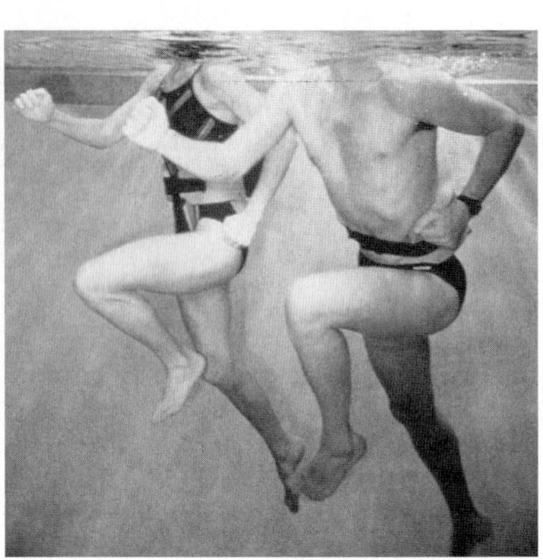

C

Figure 16-8

Use of the water's buoyancy and pressure for progressive exercise. **A,** Several buoyancy and resistive devices may be used in aquatic exercise. **B,** Using the water for buoyancy. **C,** Using the water for resistance.

Focus Box: "Suggested aquatic workouts" suggests aquatic workouts using a swim program and a kickboard program.

Proprioceptive Neuromuscular Facilitation Techniques

Proprioceptive neuromuscular facilitation (PNF) is an approach to therapeutic exercise that uses proprioceptive, cutaneous, and auditory input to produce functional improvement in motor output and can be a vital element in the rehabilitation process of many sports-related injuries. These techniques have been recommended and are widely used in sports medicine for increasing strength, flexibility, and coordination as well as decreasing deficits in kinesthetic sense in response to demands placed on the

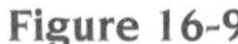

Figure 16-9

A wet vest can facilitate exercise programs in the water by making the athlete more buoyant.

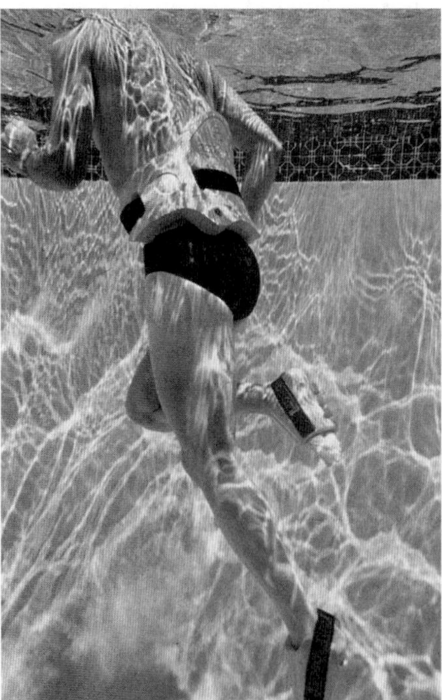

Focus

Suggested aquatic workouts

Swim Workout*

Activity	*Time*
Warm up (jog in place)	5 minutes
Scissors (abduction/adduction)	1 minute
Kicking	1 minute
(Standing position with toes dorsiflexed—increase difficulty by plantar flexing toes)	
High knees	1 minute
Heels to butt	1 minute
Rest (passive)	45 seconds
Repeat sequence three times	
Running in place (sprinting)	10 times—30 seconds on, 15 seconds off
Active cool down	3:30 minutes
Total Time:	30 minutes

Kick workout with a kickboard

Use flutter kick for this workout (prone to work hip flexors/knee extensors or supine to work hip extensors/knee flexors using a kickboard).

Activity	*Time*
Warm up	5 minutes
Prone	20 seconds hard, 10 seconds easy for 5 minutes
Rest (passive)	1 minutes
Supine	20 seconds hard, 10 seconds easy for 5 minutes
Rest (passive)	1 minute
Sprint the middle 15 yards**	5 minutes
Active cool down	5 minutes
Total Time:	27 minutes

*Increase difficulty by adding arm and leg buoys.

Scissors and kicking should focus on both speed and a medium range of motion.

Athlete needs to be suspended in the water by a waist belt or tethered to the side of the Swim-Ex. Athlete should not worry about treading during the workout.

**Each lane is 25 yards. Have athlete kick easy for the first 5 yards of the lap, kick hard for the middle 15 yards, and kick easy for the final 5 yards. Repeat for 5 minutes.

neuromuscular system.[58] The principles and techniques of PNF are based primarily on the neurophysiological mechanisms involving the stretch reflex (see Chapter 4).[46]

Techniques of PNF

The PNF techniques are generally used in rehabilitation for the purposes of facilitating strength and increasing range of motion. Flexibility is increased by the techniques of contract-relax, hold-relax, and slow-reversal-hold-relax. In contrast, strength can be facilitated by repeated contraction and the slow-reversal, rhythmic initiation, and rhythmic stabilization techniques.[46]

Strengthening techniques To assist the athlete in developing muscle strength, muscle endurance, and coordination, use the following techniques.

PNF strengthening techniques:
- Rhythmic initiation
- Repeated contraction
- Slow reversal
- Slow-reversal-hold
- Rhythmic stabilization

Rhythmic initiation Rhythmic initiation consists of a progressive series, first of passive movement, then of active assistive movement, followed by an active movement through an agonist pattern. This approach helps athletes with limited movement progressively regain strength through the range of motion.

Repeated contraction Repeated contraction of a muscle or a muscle group is used for general weakness or weakness at one specific point. The athlete moves isotonically against the maximum resistance of the athletic trainer until he or she experiences fatigue. At the time fatigue is felt, stretch is applied to the muscle at that point in the range to facilitate greater strength production. All resistance must be carefully accommodated to the strength of the athlete. Because the athlete is resisting as much as possible, this technique may be contraindicated for some injuries.

Slow reversal The athlete moves through a complete range of motion against maximum resistance. Resistance is applied to facilitate antagonist and agonist muscle groups and to ensure smooth and rhythmic movement. It is important that reversals of the movement pattern be instituted before the previous pattern has been fully completed. The major benefit of this PNF technique is that it promotes normal reciprocal coordination of agonist and antagonist muscles.

Slow-reversal-hold In this technique the athlete moves a body part isotonically using agonist muscles and immediately follows that movement with an isometric contraction. The athlete is instructed to hold at the end of each isotonic movement. The primary purpose of this technique is to develop strength at a specific point in the range of movement.

Rhythmic stabilization Rhythmic stabilization uses an isometric contraction of the agonists, followed by an isometric contraction of the antagonist muscles. With repeated contraction of these muscles, strength is maximum at this point.

PNF stretching techniques:
- Contract-relax
- Hold-relax
- Slow-reversal-hold-relax

Stretching techniques To produce muscle relaxation through an inhibitory response for purposes of increasing range of motion, the following PNF techniques may be used.

Contract-relax The affected body part is passively moved until resistance is felt. The athlete is then told to contract the antagonistic muscle isotonically. The movement is resisted by the athletic trainer for ten seconds or until the athlete feels fatigued. The athlete is instructed to relax for ten seconds. The athletic trainer passively moves the limb to a new stretch position, and the exercise is repeated three times.

Hold-relax The hold-relax technique is similar to contract-relax except that an isometric contraction is used. The athlete moves the body part to the point of resistance and is told to hold that position. The muscles are isometrically resisted by the athletic trainer for ten seconds. The athlete is then told to relax for ten seconds, and the body part is moved to a new range, either actively by the athlete or passively by the athletic trainer. This exercise is repeated three times.

Slow-reversal-hold-relax The athlete moves the body part to the point of resistance and is told to hold that position. The muscles are isometrically resisted by the athletic trainer for ten seconds. The athlete is then told to relax for ten seconds, thus relaxing the antagonist while the agonist is contracted, moving the part to a new limited range (Figure 16-10).

16-7 Critical Thinking Exercise

A wrestler was immobilized in a cast for six weeks after a fracture of the olecranon process of the ulna. The cast was removed three weeks ago, and the athlete has been working hard on stretching exercises to regain elbow extension. At this point he is still lacking 16 degrees of extension and does not seem to be gaining any additional motion.

? Because the stretching seems to be ineffective at this point, what can the athletic trainer do to help the athlete regain range of motion?

Basic Principles for Using PNF Techniques

These principles are the basis of PNF and must be used with any specific techniques. Application of the following principles may assist in promoting a desired response in the individual being treated.[28]

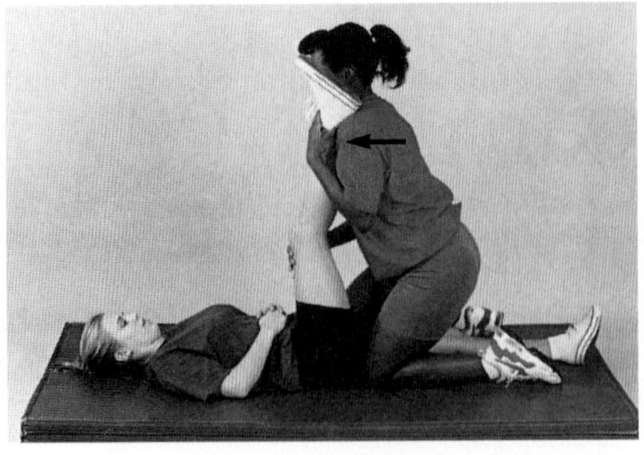

Figure 16-10

The slow-reversal-hold-relax stretching technique for the hamstring muscle.

1. The athlete must be taught through brief, simple descriptions the PNF patterns for sequential movements from starting position to terminal positions.
2. When learning the patterns, the athlete should look at the moving limb for feedback on directional and positional control.
3. Verbal commands should be firm and simple—push, pull, or hold.
4. Manual contact with the hands can facilitate a movement response.
5. The athletic trainer must use correct body mechanics when providing resistance.
6. The amount of resistance given should facilitate a maximal response that allows smooth, coordinated motion.
7. Rotational movement is a critical component in all the PNF patterns.
8. The distal movements of the patterns should occur first and should be completed by no later than halfway through the pattern.
9. The stronger components are emphasized to facilitate the weaker components of a movement pattern.
10. Pressing the joint together causes increased stability, whereas traction pulls the joint apart and facilitates movement.
11. Giving a quick stretch causes a reflex contraction of that muscle.

PNF Patterns

The PNF exercise patterns involve three component movements: flexion-extension, abduction-adduction, and internal-external rotation. Human movement is patterned and rarely involves straight motion because all muscles are spiral in nature and lie in diagonal directions.[28]

The PNF patterns involve distinct diagonal and rotational movements of upper extremity, lower extremity, upper trunk, lower trunk, and neck. The exercise pattern is initiated with the muscle groups in the lengthened or stretched position. The muscle group is then contracted, moving the body part through the range of motion to a shortened position.

The upper and lower extremities each have two separate patterns of diagonal movement for each part of the body, which are referred to as the diagonal 1 (D1) and diagonal 2 (D2) patterns. These two diagonal patterns are subdivided into D1 moving into flexion, D1 moving into extension, D2 moving into flexion, and D2 moving into extension. The patterns are named according to the movement occurring at either the shoulder or the hip.

Figures 16-11 and 16-12 are examples of PNF patterns that may be used for rehabilitating some sports injuries. PNF techniques for specific joints will be discussed in Chapters 18 through 24.

Muscle Energy Techniques

Muscle energy is a technique that has been established to treat complex kinetic chain dysfunction.[16] *Muscle energy techniques (MET)* are manually applied stretching techniques that use principles of neurophysiology to relax overactive muscles and/or stretch chronically shortened muscles.[9] Muscle energy is a manual therapy technique that is a variation of the PNF contract-relax and hold-relax techniques. Like the PNF techniques, the muscle energy techniques are based on the same neurophysiologic mechanisms involving the stretch reflex discussed in Chapter 4. Muscle energy techniques involve the voluntary contraction of a muscle in a specifically controlled direction at varied levels of intensity against a distinctly executed counterforce applied by the athletic trainer.[54] The athlete provides the corrective *intrinsic* forces and controls the intensity of the muscular contractions, while the athletic trainer controls the precision and localization of the procedure. The amount of effort by the athlete can vary from a minimal muscle twitch to a maximal muscle contraction.

Five components are needed to make muscle energy techniques effective:

1. Active muscle contraction by the athlete
2. A muscle contraction oriented in a specific direction
3. Some control by the athlete of contraction intensity

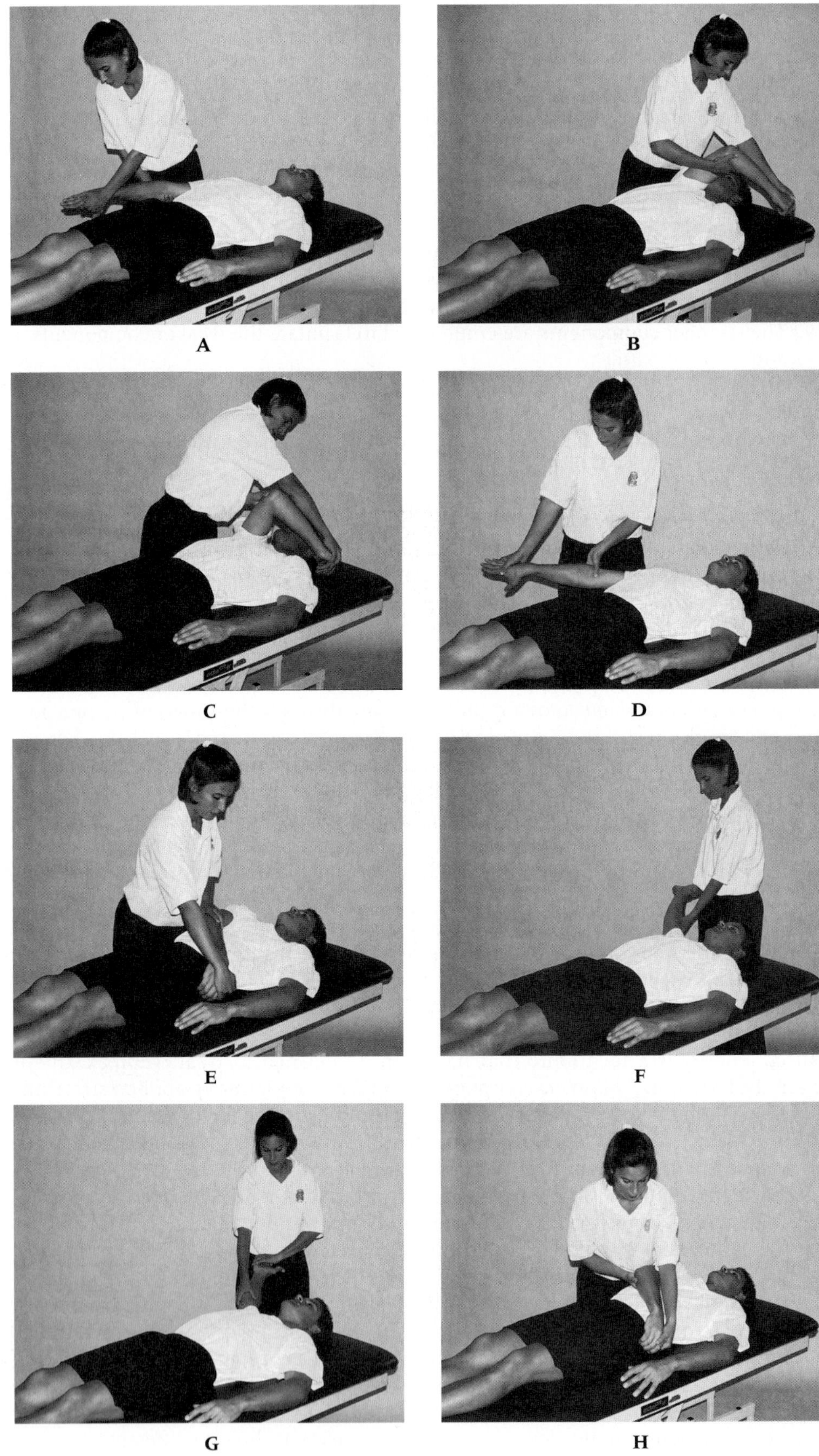

Figure 16-11

Upper Extremity PNF Patterns. **A & B,** D1 moving into flexion. **C & D,** D1 moving into extension. **E & F,** D2 moving in flexion. **G & H,** D2 moving into extension.

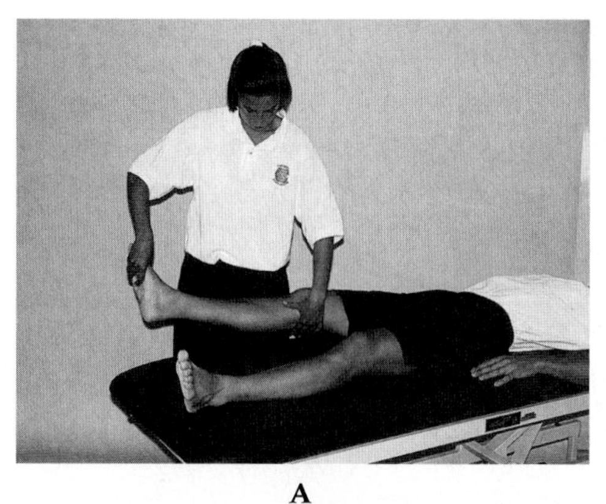
A

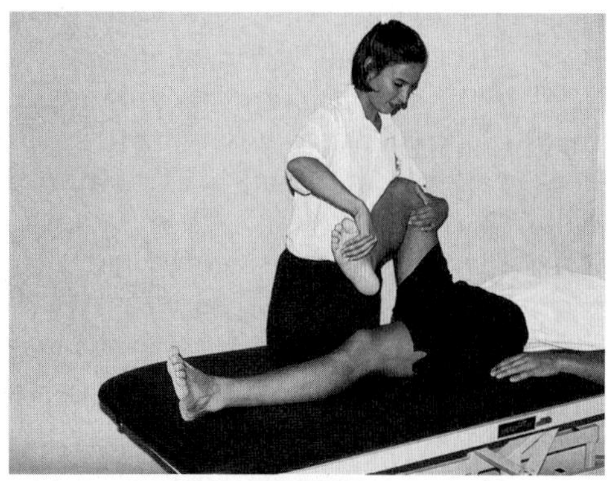
B

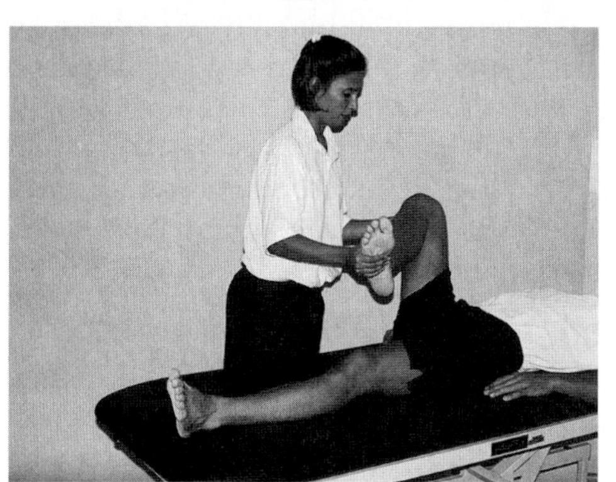
C

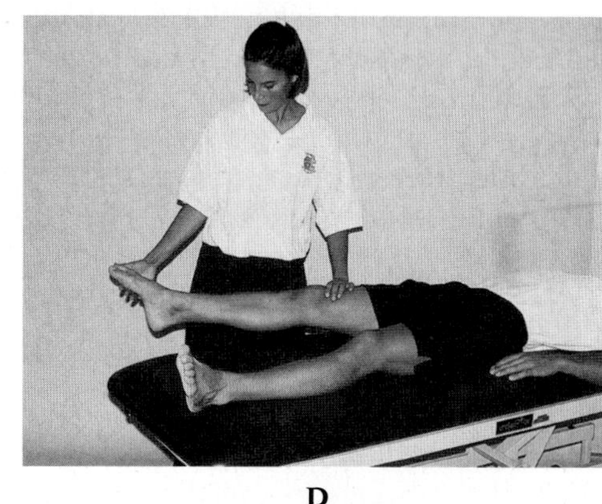
D

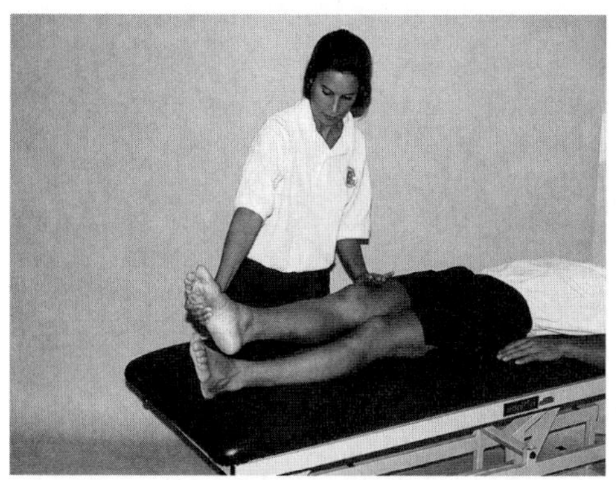
E

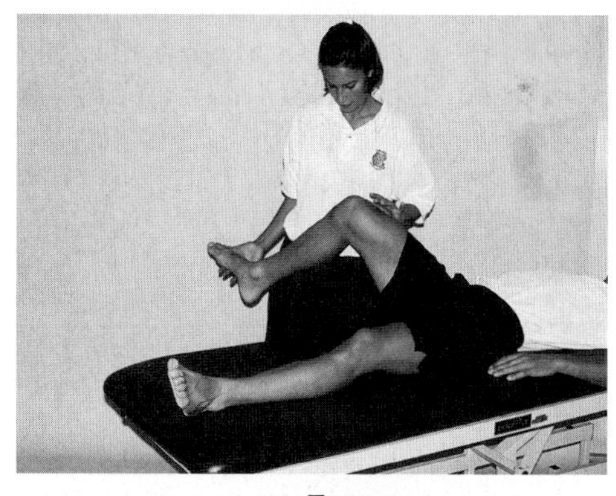
F

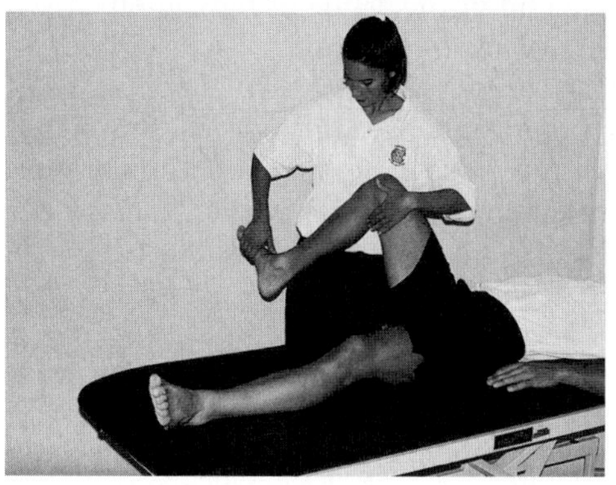
G

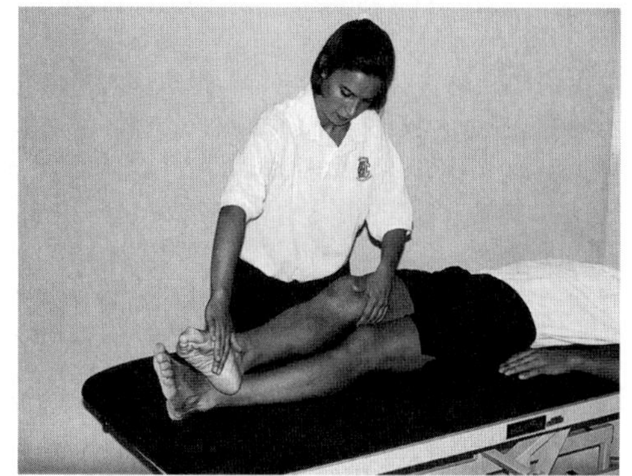
H

Figure 16-12

Lower Extremity PNF Patterns. **A & B,** D1 moving into flexion. **C & D,** D1 moving into extension. **E & F,** D2 moving into flexion. **G & H,** D2 moving into extension.

4. Control of the joint position by the athletic trainer
5. Appropriate counterforce applied by the athletic trainer

The specific muscle energy technique begins by locating a point of resistance to stretch that is referred to as a *resistance barrier.* This is not necessarily a pathological barrier but does represent the point in the range of motion at which movement will not occur without some degree of passive assistance. Beginning at that resistance barrier, the athlete is asked to contract the antagonist (muscle to be stretched) isometrically for ten seconds. At this point the athlete is asked to relax completely and to inhale and exhale maximally. As the athlete exhales, the athletic trainer moves the body part to the new resistance barrier. This process should be repeated three to five times or until there is no further gain in range of motion.[9]

Joint Mobilization and Traction

The techniques of joint mobilization are used to improve joint mobility or to decrease joint pain by restoring accessory movements to the joint, thus allowing for full, nonrestricted, pain-free range of motion.[45] Mobilization techniques may be used to attain a variety of treatment goals such as the following: reducing pain; decreasing muscle guarding; stretching or lengthening tissue surrounding a joint, especially capsular and ligamentous tissue; reflexogenic effects that either inhibit or facilitate muscle tone or the stretch reflex; and proprioceptive effects that improve postural and kinesthetic awareness.

Mobilization Techniques

Mobilization works to improve accessory motions.

Mobilization techniques are used to increase the accessory motions about a joint.[45] Treatment techniques designed to improve accessory motion involve small-amplitude oscillating movements called *glides* within a specific part of the range.[31] Mobilization should be done with both the athlete and the athletic trainer in comfortable and relaxed positions. The athletic trainer should mobilize one joint at a time. The joint should be stabilized as near one articulating surface as possible; the other surface should be held with a firm, confident grasp.[45]

Maitland has categorized mobilization techniques into five grades as follows:[32]

- Grade I—a small-amplitude glide at the beginning of the range of movement. Used when pain and spasm limit movement early in the range of motion.
- Grade II—a large-amplitude glide within the midrange of movement. Used when spasm limits movement sooner with a quick oscillation than with a slow one, or when slowly increasing pain restricts movement halfway into the range.
- Grade III—a large-amplitude glide up to the pathological limit in the range of movement. Used when pain and resistance from spasm, inert tissue tension, or tissue compression limit movement near the end of the range.
- Grade IV—a small-amplitude glide at the end of the range of movement. Used when resistance limits movement in the absence of pain and spasm.
- Grade V—a small-amplitude, quick thrust delivered at the end of the range of movement, usually accompanied by a popping sound that is called a manipulation. Used when minimal resistance limits the end of the range. Manipulation is most effectively accomplished by the velocity of the thrust rather than by the force of the thrust. Most authorities agree that manipulation should be used only by individuals trained specifically in these techniques because a great deal of skill and judgment is necessary for safe and effective treatment.

In Maitland's system, grades I and II are used primarily for the treatment of pain, and grades III and IV are used for treating stiffness. It is necessary to treat pain first and stiffness second.[32] Figure 16-13 shows the various grades of oscillation that are used in a joint with some limitation of motion.

The shape of the articulating surfaces usually dictates the direction of the mobilization being performed.[45] Generally one articulating surface may be considered to be concave and the other to be convex. When the concave surface is stationary and the

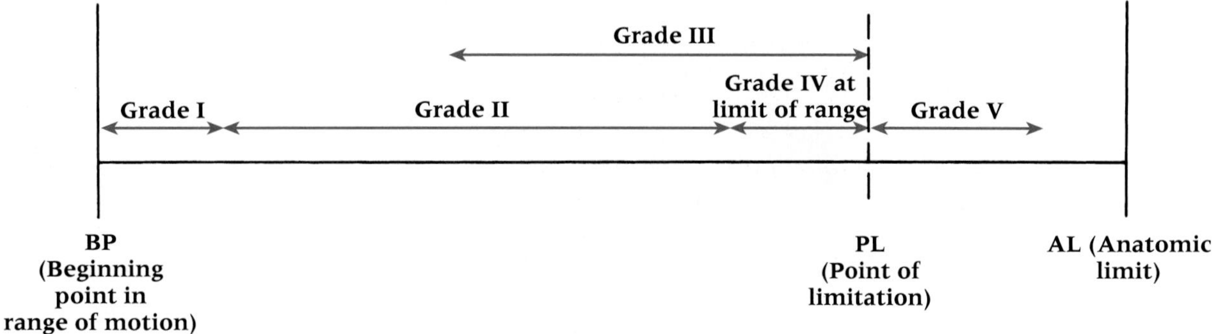

Figure 16-13

Maitland's five grades of motion.

convex surface is moving, the glide should be done in the opposite direction of the bone movement. If the convex surface is stationary and the concave surface is moving, the glide should be done in the same direction as the bone movement. If mobilization in the appropriate direction exacerbates complaints of pain or stiffness, the athletic trainer should apply the technique in the opposite direction until the patient can tolerate the application of the technique in the appropriate direction.

In many cases, traction can be combined with mobilization.[25] *Traction* refers to a technique in which one articulating segment is pulled to produce some separation of the two joint surfaces. Both mobilization and traction techniques use a translational movement of one joint surface relative to the other. This translation may be in one of two directions: it may be either perpendicular or parallel to the *treatment plane.* The treatment plane falls perpendicular to, or at a right angle to, a line running from the axis of rotation in the convex surface to the center of the concave articular surface (Figure 16-14). Mobilization techniques use glides that translate one articulating surface along a line parallel with the treatment plane. Traction techniques translate one of the articulating surfaces in a perpendicular direction to the treatment plane. Mobilization glides are done parallel to the treatment plane; traction is performed perpendicular to the treatment plane. Like mobilization techniques, traction may be used either to decrease pain or to reduce joint hypomobility.[25,33]

Figure 16-15 shows examples of joint mobilization techniques for some joints and body segments. Mobilizations for specific joints are discussed further in Chapters 18 through 24.

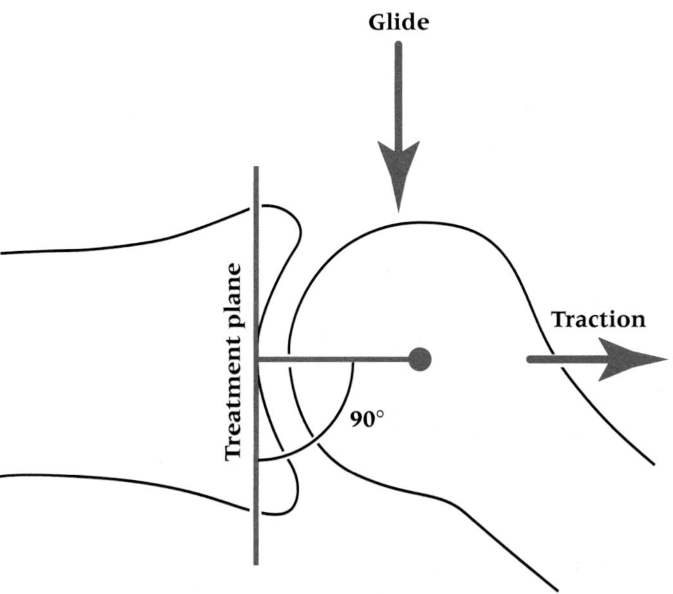

Figure 16-14

The treatment plane is perpendicular to a line drawn from the axis of rotation to the center of the articulating surface of the concave segment.

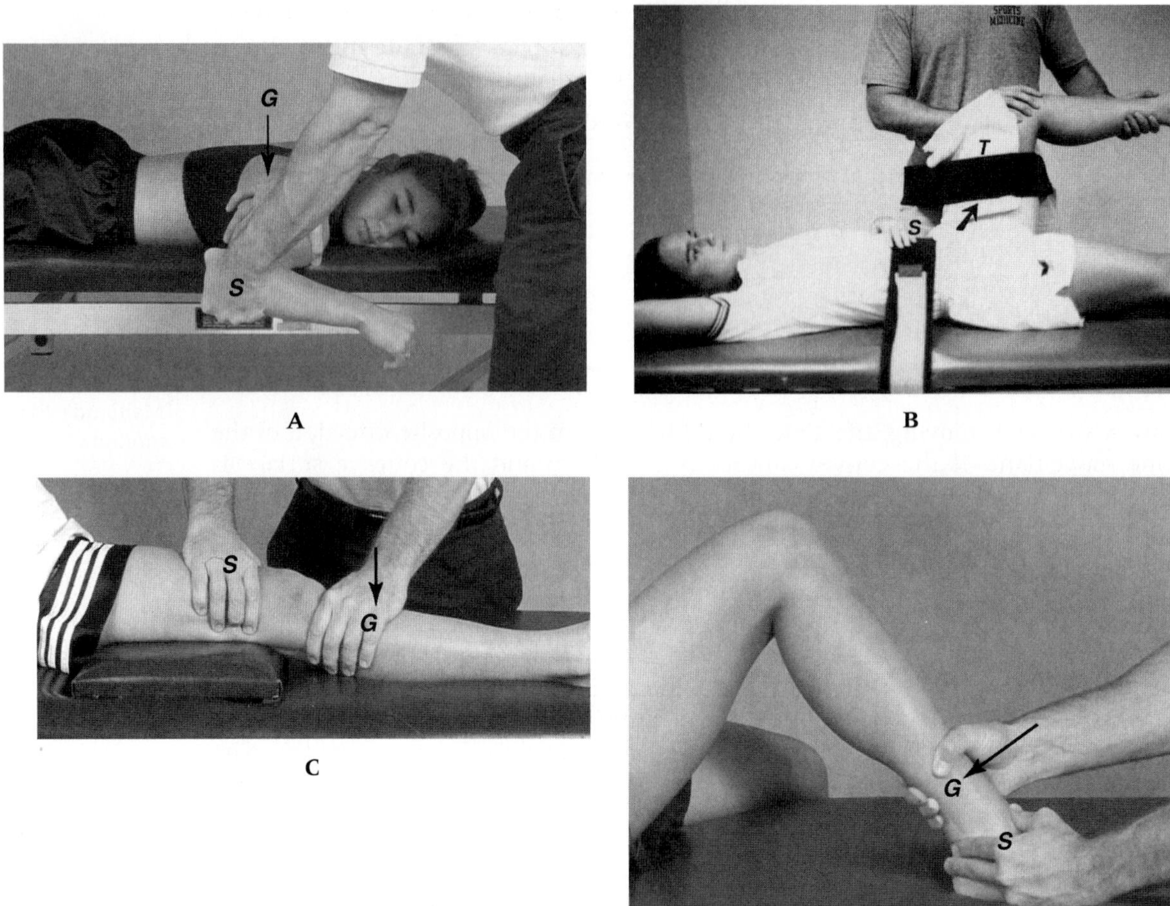

Figure 16-15

A, Anterior humeral glide (for increasing extension and lateral rotation). **B,** Inferior femoral glide (for increasing abduction and flexion). **C,** Posterior tibial glide (for increasing flexion). **D,** Posterior tibial glide (for increasing plantar flexion). (S = stabilize, G = glide, T = traction)

Myofascial Release

Myofascial release is a term that refers to a group of techniques used for the purpose of relieving soft tissue from the abnormal grip of tight fascia.[26] It is essentially a form of stretching that has been reported to have significant impact in treating a variety of conditions. Some specialized training is necessary for the athletic trainer to understand specific techniques of myofascial release. It is also essential to have an in-depth understanding of the fascial system.

Fascia is a type of connective tissue that surrounds muscles, tendons, nerves, bones, and organs. It is essentially continuous from head to toe and is interconnected in various sheaths or planes. Fascia is composed primarily of collagen along with some elastic fibers. During movement the fascia must stretch and move freely. If there is damage to the fascia from injury, disease, or inflammation, it will not only affect local adjacent structures but also may affect areas far removed from the site of the injury. Thus it may be necessary to release tightness in both the area of injury and in distant areas. Tightness in these areas will tend to soften and release in response to gentle pressure over a relatively long period of time.[34]

Myofascial release has also been referred to as *soft-tissue mobilization,* although technically all forms of massage involve the mobilization of soft tissue. Soft-tissue mobilization should not be confused with joint mobilization, although it must be emphasized that the two are closely related. Joint mobilization is used to restore normal joint arthrokinematics, and specific rules exist regarding direction of movement and joint position based on the shape of the articulating surfaces. Myofascial restrictions are considerably more unpredictable and may occur in many different planes and directions. Myofascial treatment is based on localizing the restriction and moving into the direction of the restriction, regardless of whether that follows the arthrokinematics of a nearby joint.[55] Thus, myofascial manipulation is considerably more subjective and relies heavily on the experience of the clinician.

Myofascial manipulation focuses on large treatment areas, while joint mobilization focuses on a specific joint. Releasing myofascial restrictions over a large treatment area can have a significant impact on joint mobility.[34] Once a myofascial restriction is located, the massage should be directly through the restriction. The progression of the technique is from superficial to deep. Once more superficial restrictions are released, the deep restrictions can be located and released without causing any damage to superficial tissues. Joint mobilization should follow myofascial release and will likely be more effective once soft-tissue restrictions are eliminated.

As the extensibility is improved in the myofascia, elongation and stretching of the musculotendinous unit should be incorporated. In addition, strengthening exercises are recommended to enhance neuromuscular reeducation, which helps promote new, more efficient movement patterns.[55] As freedom of movement improves, postural reeducation may help to ensure the maintenance of the less restricted movement patterns.

Generally, acute cases tend to resolve in just a few treatments. The longer a condition has been present, the longer it will take to resolve. Occasionally, dramatic results will occur immediately after treatment. It is usually recommended that treatment be done at least three times per week.

Strain/Counterstrain

Strain/counterstrain is an approach to decreasing muscle tension and guarding that may be used to normalize muscle function. It is a passive technique that places the body in a position of greatest comfort, thereby relieving pain.[24]

In this technique, the athletic trainer locates "tender points" on the athlete's body that correspond to areas of dysfunction in specific joints or muscles that are in need of treatment. These tender points are not located in or just beneath the skin as are many acupuncture points, but deeper in muscle, tendon, ligament, or fascia. They are characterized by tense, tender, edematous spots on the body; they are 1 cm or less in diameter, with the most acute point 3 mm in diameter, although they may be a few centimeters long within a muscle; there may be multiple points for one specific joint dysfunction; they may be arranged in a chain; points are often found in a painless area opposite the site of pain and/or weakness.[24]

The athletic trainer monitors the tension and level of pain elicited by the tender point as he or she moves the patient into a position of ease or comfort. This is accomplished by markedly shortening the muscle.[56] When this position of ease is found, the tender point is no longer tense or tender. When this position is maintained for a minimum of ninety seconds, the tension in the tender point and in the corresponding joint or muscle is reduced or cleared. By slowly returning to a neutral position, the tender point and the corresponding joint or muscle remains pain free with normal tension. For example with neck pain and/or tension headaches, the tender points may be found on either the front or back of the athlete's neck and shoulders. The athletic trainer will have the athlete lay on his or her back and will gently and slowly bend the athlete's neck until that tender point is no longer tender. After holding that position for ninety seconds, the athletic trainer gently and slowly returns the athlete's neck to its resting position. Upon pressing that tender point again, the athlete should notice a significant decrease in pain at that tender point (Figure 16-16).[56]

The physiological rationale for the effectiveness of the strain-counterstrain technique can be explained by the stretch reflex. The stretch reflex was discussed in detail in Chapter 4. When a muscle is placed in a stretched position, impulses from the muscle spindles create a reflex contraction of the muscle in response to stretch. With strain/counterstrain, the joint or muscle is not placed in a position of stretch but rather

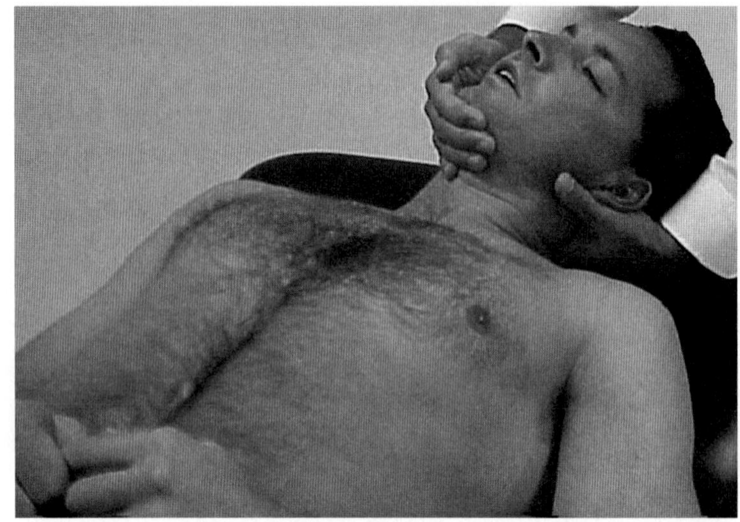

Figure 16-16

Strain and counterstrain technique. The body part is placed in a position of ease for 90 seconds and then slowly moved back to neutral position.

a slack position. Thus muscle spindle input is reduced and the muscle is relaxed, allowing for a decrease in tension and pain.

16-8

Critical Thinking Exercise

A sprinter on the track team is complaining of pain in her right hamstring. She says that she doesn't feel like she has "torn" the muscle but it feels very tight and she is afraid to go all out for fear of making the injury worse. On palpation the athletic trainer finds two or three tender points in the muscle.

? What manual therapy techniques could the athletic trainer use to help alleviate this problem?

Positional Release Therapy

Positional release therapy (PRT), is based on the strain/counterstrain technique. The primary difference between the two is the use of a facilitating force (compression) to enhance the effect of the positioning.[10]

Like strain/counterstrain, PRT is an osteopathic mobilization technique in which the body is brought into a position of greatest relaxation.[13] The athletic trainer finds the position of greatest comfort and muscle relaxation for each joint with the help of movement tests and diagnostic tender points. Once located, the tender point is maintained with the palpating finger at a subthreshold pressure. The patient is then passively placed in a position that reduces the tension under the palpating finger and causes a subjective reduction in tenderness as reported by the patient. This specific position is adjusted throughout the ninety-second treatment period. It has been suggested that maintaining contact with the tender point during the treatment period exerts a therapeutic effect.[10] This technique is one of the most effective and most gentle methods for the treatment of acute and chronic musculoskeletal dysfunction (Figure 16-17).[59]

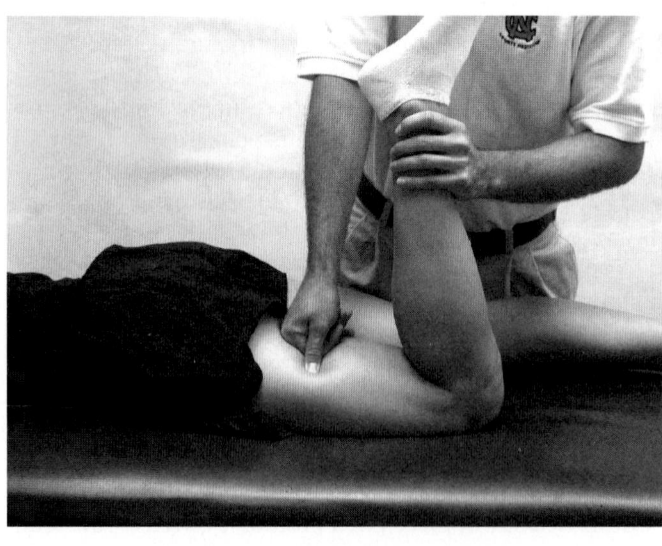

Figure 16-17

Positional release therapy uses a position of comfort with the finger or thumb exerting submaximal pressure on a tender point.

Active Release Technique

Active release technique (ART®) is a relatively new type of manual therapy that has been developed to correct soft tissue problems in muscle, tendon, and fascia caused by the formation of fibrotic adhesions as a result of acute injury, repetitive or overuse injuries, or constant pressure or tension injuries.[29] When a muscle, tendon, fascia, or ligament is torn (strained or sprained) or a nerve is damaged, the tissues heal with adhesions or scar tissue formation rather than the formation of brand new tissue. Scar tissue is weaker, less elastic, less pliable, and more pain sensitive than healthy tissue. These fibrotic adhesions disrupt the normal muscle function, which in turn affects the biomechanics of the joint complex and can lead to pain and dysfunction. Active release technique provides a way to diagnose and treat the underlying causes of cumulative trauma disorders that, left uncorrected, can lead to inflammation, adhesions/fibrosis, muscle imbalances resulting in weak and tense tissues, decreased circulation, hypoxia, and symptoms of peripheral nerve entrapment, including numbness, tingling, burning, and aching.[29]

Active release technique is a deep tissue technique used for breaking down scar tissue/adhesions and restoring function and movement.[29] In the active release technique, the athletic trainer should first locate through palpation those adhesions in the muscle, tendon, or fascia that are causing the problem. Once these are located, the athletic trainer traps the affected muscle by applying pressure or tension with the thumb or finger over these lesions in the direction of the fibers. Then the athlete is asked to actively move the body part so that the musculature is elongated from a shortened position while the athletic trainer continues to apply tension to the lesion (Figure 16-18). This should be repeated three to five times per treatment session. By breaking up the adhesions, the technique improves the athlete's condition by softening and stretching the scar tissue, resulting in increased range of motion, increased strength, and improved circulation, which optimizes healing. Treatments tend to be uncomfortable during the movement phases as the scar tissue or adhesions tear apart. This is temporary and subsides almost immediately after the treatment. An important part of active release technique is for the athlete to heed the athletic trainer's recommendations regarding activity modification, stretching, and exercise.

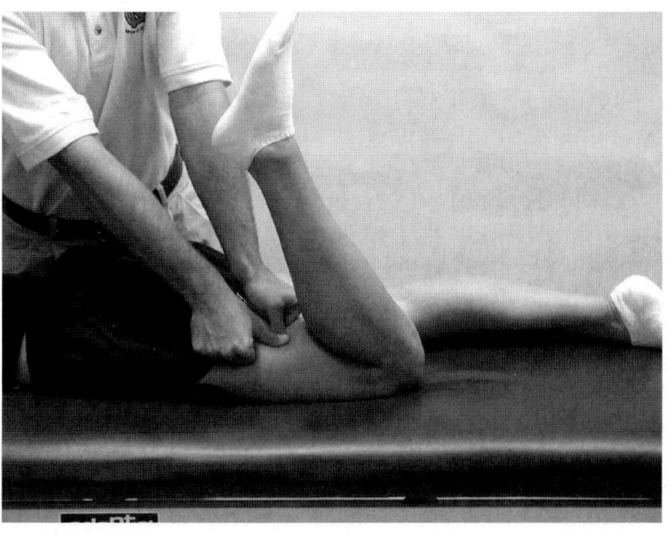

A

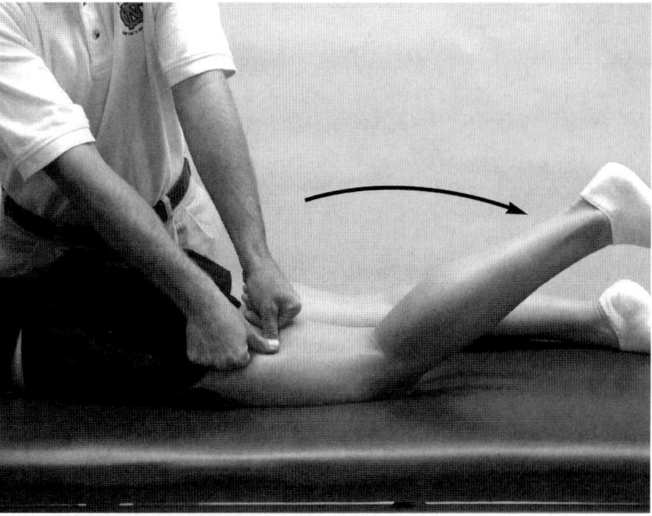

B

Figure 16-18

Active release technique. **A,** Starting position. **B,** Muscle is elongated from a shortened position while static pressure is applied to the lesion.

PURCHASING AND MAINTAINING THERAPEUTIC EXERCISE EQUIPMENT

The extent and variety of therapeutic exercise equipment available to use in injury rehabilitation can at times be overwhelming. Prices of rehabilitation equipment can range from $2 for a piece of surgical tubing, to $4,000 for an electrical stimulating unit, to $80,000 for certain computer-driven isokinetic or balance devices. It is certainly not necessary to purchase expensive exercise equipment to see good results. It is likely that an injured athlete can achieve many of the same physiological benefits from using a $2 piece of surgical tubing that would result from exercising on an $80,000 isokinetic device. Many athletic trainers would argue that the most useful pieces of rehabilitation equipment available are the hands of a well-trained and experienced clinician. Others maintain that the greater the extent and variety of rehabilitation equipment available, the more flexibility the athletic trainer has in devising rehabilitation programs.

For almost everyone, budgetary constraints, at least to some extent, will limit the pieces of rehabilitation equipment that can be purchased. Decisions to purchase pieces of rehabilitation equipment should be based on a realistic assessment of the usefulness and functionality of that piece of equipment, the extent to which it will be used, and its durability. Perhaps the most important question that should be asked when purchasing a new piece of equipment is whether this piece of equipment will help the athlete to reach the goals of the rehabilitation program.

Once rehabilitation equipment has been purchased, the athletic trainer should assume the responsibility of making sure that it is being used correctly and for the intended purpose as stated in the manufacturer's instructions for use. It is also essential that the athletic trainer apply the manufacturer's guidelines for the periodic inspection and maintenance of therapeutic exercise equipment to ensure that it is operating safely.

SUMMARY

- When injuries occur in sports medicine, the focus of the athletic trainer shifts from injury prevention to injury treatment and rehabilitation. The athletic trainer usually assumes the primary responsibility for the design, implementation, and supervision of the rehabilitation program for the injured athlete. Two major goals of rehabilitation are to prevent deconditioning and to restore the injured part to a preinjury state. Besides the physical aspect, the mental and emotional aspects of rehabilitation must always be considered.
- When an injured body part is immobilized for a period of time, a number of disuse problems adversely affect muscle, joints, ligaments, bone, cartilage, neuromuscular efficiency, and the cardiorespiratory system.
- Designing programs for rehabilitation is relatively simple and involves several basic components: minimizing swelling, controlling pain, maintaining or improving flexibility, restoring or increasing strength, reestablishing neuromuscular control, regaining balance, maintaining levels of cardiorespiratory fitness, and incorporating functional progressions. The long-term goal is to return the injured athlete to practice or competition as quickly and safely as possible.
- Rehabilitation programs in sports medicine can be subdivided into three phases, based primarily on the three stages of the healing process: phase 1, the acute inflammatory response phase; phase 2, the fibroblastic repair phase; and phase 3, the maturation-remodeling phase. If surgery is necessary, a fourth phase, the preoperative phase, must also be considered.
- The decision to release an athlete recovering from injury to a full return to athletic activity is the final stage of the rehabilitation and recovery process. The decision should be carefully considered by each member of the sports medicine team involved in the rehabilitation process.

- An open kinetic chain exists when the foot or hand is not in contact with the ground or some other surface. In a closed kinetic chain, the foot or hand is weight bearing. The use of closed chain strengthening techniques has become the rehabilitation treatment of choice for many athletic trainers. Closed kinetic chain strengthening activities are more functional than are open kinetic chain activities.
- Aquatic exercises can be an important rehabilitative tool for the athletic trainer, particularly with injuries involving the lower extremity. Aquatic exercises allow for resistance with motion without weight bearing.
- Proprioceptive neuromuscular facilitation is a manual therapy technique that can be used for strengthening muscle or increasing range of motion. The PNF movement patterns involve a sequential series of specific movements for the lower extremity, lower trunk, upper trunk, and upper extremity.
- Mobilization and traction are manual therapy techniques used to improve joint mobility or to decrease joint pain by restoring accessory movements to the injured joint, which allows full, pain-free range of motion.
- A variety of manual therapy techniques, including muscle energy, myofascial release, strain/counterstrain, positional release, and active release techniques, can be effectively incorporated into a rehabilitation program.

Websites

Cramer First Aider:
http://www.cramersportsmed.com/first_aider.jsp

National Athletic Trainers' Association: http://www.nata.org
Accesses rehabilitation in the athletic training journals.

The Physician and Sportsmedicine:
http://www.physsportsmed.com
Search back issues and access the ones specifically geared toward weight training and rehabilitation.

Archives of Physical Medicine and Rehabilitation:
http://www.archives-pmr.org/

The AOSSN Online Media Kit: http://www.sportsmed.org/

Journal of Sport Rehabilitation:
http://www.humankinetics.com/product/journals/journal.cfm?id=JSR

Solutions to Critical Thinking EXERCISES

16-1 The short-term goals in any sports medicine rehabilitation program should include controlling pain, regaining range of motion, regaining strength, reestablishing neuromuscular control, and maintaining levels of cardiorespiratory fitness. The approach to rehabilitation should be aggressive, and decisions as to when and how to alter and progress specific components within a rehabilitation program should be based on and are limited by the healing process. The long-term goal is to return the athlete to full activity as soon as safely possible.

16-2 After injury and subsequent rest and immobilization, it is not unusual for the athlete to "forget" how to walk. The athletic trainer must help the athlete relearn neuromuscular control, which means regaining the ability to follow some previously established motor and sensory pattern by regaining conscious control of a specific movement until that movement becomes automatic. Strengthening exercises, particularly those that tend to be more functional, such as closed kinetic chain exercises, are essential for reestablishing neuromuscular control. Addressing neuromuscular control is critical throughout the recovery process but may be most critical during the early stages of rehabilitation to avoid reinjury or overuse injuries to additional structures.

16-3 Anterior knee pain can result from many different causes. Strengthening the quadriceps can be helpful. If full range of motion strengthening exercises increase pain, the athlete should begin with positional isometric exercises done at different points in the range, progressing to full-range concentric and eccentric exercise as tolerated. Closed kinetic chain exercises such as minisquats, stepping exercises, or leg presses are excellent quadriceps-strengthening exercises and tend to be more functional in nature than are traditional open kinetic chain exercises.

16-4 The athlete should have minimal signs of inflammation, such as pain and swelling. The appropriate healing time frame should also be reached before the athlete progresses.

16-5 The athletic trainer can provide the encouragement and positive reinforcement necessary for the athlete to make a commitment. Support from peers, coaches, and rehabilitation staff is important. The athletic trainer should clearly explain the instructions verbally to the athlete and then write them down. The rehabilitation program should fit into the athlete's schedule. The athletic trainer must be creative in designing and varying the exercise routine. The rehabilitation program should be as pain free as possible. The coach needs to support the rehabilitation process.

16-6 Perhaps the best recommendation would be to have the athlete engage in an aquatic exercise program. In the water, the athlete would not be weight bearing and could exercise the injured knee through a pain-free range of motion while simultaneously working on maintaining levels of fitness by engaging in water-resisted conditioning exercises.

16-7 To achieve a full physiological range of movement, the joint must have normal accessory motions. Stretching techniques address motion restriction caused by tightness of the musculotendinous unit. The athletic trainer should incorporate joint mobilization techniques that address restriction of motion caused by some tightness of capsular and ligamentous structures that surround the affected joint.

16-8 To some extent the answer depends on exactly what is causing her pain. In general, the athletic trainer may choose to use one of several or a combination of manual therapy techniques, including myofascial release, strain/counterstrain, positional release, or active release technique.

REVIEW QUESTIONS AND CLASS ACTIVITIES

1. What occurs physiologically when an athlete is suddenly forced to stop physical activity?
2. Discuss the physiological effects of immobilization on muscles, ligaments, joints, neuromuscular efficiency, and the cardiovascular system.
3. Discuss the similarities and differences between training and conditioning exercises and therapeutic exercise.
4. Why must an athlete condition the entire body while an injury heals?
5. Why is it important to modulate pain during a rehabilitation program?
6. How is range of motion restored after an injury?
7. Critically compare the use of isometric, isotonic, and isokinetic exercises in rehabilitation.
8. Discuss the difference between proprioception and kinesthesia, and explain how they are related to neuromuscular control.
9. How and when should functional progressions be incorporated into the rehabilitation program?
10. Describe how to determine if an athlete is ready to return to activity after injury.
11. What is the importance of developing a rehabilitation plan? Include the criteria for moving to various phases.
12. What are the important considerations during each of the three phases of rehabilitation?
13. Why are closed kinetic chain exercises more useful than open kinetic chain exercises in the rehabilitation of sports injuries?
14. What is the significance of having the athlete engage in core stabilization training during a rehabilitation program?
15. How may aquatic exercise be incorporated into a rehabilitation program?
16. Proprioceptive neuromuscular facilitation includes stretching, strengthening, and movement-patterning techniques. How can these techniques apply to sports injuries?
17. How can a muscle energy technique be used to increase range of motion?
18. Explain why it is necessary to use stretching techniques to increase physiological movement and to use mobilization techniques to improve accessory motions.
19. How are the strain/counterstrain technique and positional release therapy related to one another?

REFERENCES

1. Arrigo C: Aquatic rehabilitation, *Sports Med Update* 7(2):1, 1992.
2. Barak T, Rosen E, Sofer R: Mobility: passive orthopedic manual therapy. In Gould J, Davies G, editors: *Orthopedic and sports physical therapy,* St Louis, 1990, Mosby.
3. Bernier MR: Perturbation and agility training in the rehabilitation of soccer athletes. *Athletic Therapy Today* 8(3):20, 2003.
4. Binkley H: Aquatic therapy in the treatment of upper extremity injuries. *Athletic Therapy Today* 7(1):49, 2002.
5. Brewer B, Avondoglio J, Cornelius A: Construct validity and interrater agreement of the sport injury rehabilitation adherence scale, *J Sport Rehab* 11(3):170, 2002.
6. Bunton E, Pitney W, Kane A: The role of limb torque muscle action and proprioception during closed kinetic chain rehabilitation of the lower extremity, *J Ath Train* 28(1):11, 1993.
7. Byerly P, Worrell T, Gahimer J et al: Rehabilitation compliance in an athletic training environment, *J Ath Train* 29(4):352, 1994.
8. Carter A et al: Proprioceptive neuromuscular facilitation decreases muscle activity during the stretch reflex in selected posterior thigh muscles, *J Sport Rehabil* 9(4):268, 2000.
9. Chaitlow L: *Muscle energy techniques,* Philadelphia, 2001, Churchill Livingstone.
10. Chaitlow L: *Positional release techniques,* Philadelphia, 2002, Elsevier Science.
11. Clark M: Core stabilization training in rehabilitation. In Prentice W, editor: *Rehabilitation techniques in sports medicine and athletic training,* St Louis, 2004, McGraw-Hill.
12. Cox E, Lephart S, Irrgang J: Unilateral balance training of noninjured individuals and the effects on postural sway, *J Sport Rehabil* 2(2):87, 1993.
13. D'Ambrogio K, Roth G: *Positional release therapy: assessment and treatment of musculoskeletal dysfunction,* Philadelphia, 1997, Elsevier Science.
14. De Deyne PG: Application of passive stretch and its implications for muscle fibers. *Phys Ther* 81:819, 2001.
15. Fields J et al: Factors associated with adherence to sport injury rehabilitation in college age recreational athletes, *J Sport Rehabil* 4(3):172, 1995.
16. Giammetto T, Giammetto S: Integrative manual therapy: for biomechanics application of muscle energy and beyond technique, vol 3, Berkley, CA, 2003, North Atlantic Books.
17. Grigg P: Peripheral neural mechanisms in proprioception, *J Sport Rehabil* 3(1):2, 1994.
18. Hedgepath E, Gieck J: Psychological considerations for rehabilitating the injured athlete. In Prentice W, editor: *Rehabilitation techniques in sports medicine and athletic training,* St Louis, 2004, McGraw-Hill.
19. Hertel J, Denegar C: A rehabilitation paradigm for restoring neuromuscular control following athletic injury, *Athletic Therapy Today* 3(5):12, 1998.
20. Hillman S: Principles and techniques of open kinetic chain rehabilitation, *J Sport Rehabil* 3(4):319, 1994.
21. Hoogenboom B, Lomax N: Aquatic therapy in rehabilitation. In Prentice W, editor: *Rehabilitation techniques in sports medicine and athletic training,* St Louis, 2004, McGraw-Hill.
22. Hopkins JT et al: An electromyographic comparison of 4 closed chain exercises, *J Ath Train* 34(4):353, 1999.
23. Irrgang J, Whitney S, Cox E: Balance and proprioceptive training for rehabilitation of the lower extremity, *J Sport Rehabil* 3(1):68, 1994.
24. Jones L: *Strain-counterstrain,* Boise, Idaho, 1995, Jones Strain-CounterStrain, Inc.
25. Kaltenborn F, Evjenth O, Kaltenborn B: *Manual mobilization of the joints: the Kaltenborn method of joint examination and treatment: the extremities,* vol 1 and *The spine,* vol 2, Minneapolis, 2003, Orthopedic Physical Therapy Products.
26. Keirns M, editor: *Myofascial release in sports medicine,* Champaign, Ill, 2000, Human Kinetics.
27. King M: Core stability: creating a foundation for functional rehabilitation, *Athletic Therapy Today* 5(2):6, 2000.
28. Knott M, Voss EE: *Proprioceptive neuromuscular facilitation: patterns and techniques,* ed 2, Philadelphia, 1968, Harper & Row.
29. Leahy M: Improved treatments for carpal tunnel and related syndromes, *Chiropractic Sports Medicine* 9(1):6, 1995.
30. Lephart S, Swanik C, Fu F: Reestablishing neuromuscular control. In Prentice W, editor: *Rehabilitation techniques in sports medicine and athletic training,* St Louis, 2004, McGraw-Hill.

31. Magnusson P, McHugh M: Current concepts on rehabilitation in sports medicine. In Nicholas J, Hirschman E, editors: *The lower extremity and spine in sports medicine,* St Louis, 1995, Mosby.
32. Maitland G: *Extremity manipulation,* London, 1977, Butterworth.
33. Mangus BC: Basic principles of extremity joint mobilization using a Kaltenborn approach. *Sport Rehabil* 11(4):235, 2002.
34. Manheim C: *Myofascial release manual,* Thorofare, NJ, 2001, Slack.
35. McGee M: Functional progressions and functional testing in rehabilitation. In Prentice W, editor: *Rehabilitation techniques in sports medicine and athletic training,* St Louis, 2004, McGraw-Hill.
36. McMullen J, Uhl TL: A kinetic chain approach for shoulder rehabilitation, *J Ath Train* 35(3):329, 2000.
37. Miller M, Berry D, Bullard S: Comparisons of land-based and aquatic-based plyometric programs during an 8-week training period, *J Sport Rehabil* 11(4):268, 2002.
38. Myers JB et al: Proprioception and neuromuscular control of the shoulder after muscle fatigue, *J Ath Train* 34(4):362, 1999.
39. O'Neill DF: Return to function through aquatic therapy, *Athletic Therapy Today* 5(2):14, 2000.
40. Perrin D: *Isokinetic exercise and assessment,* Champaign, Ill, 1993, Human Kinetics.
41. Piccininni J, Drover J: Athlete-patient education in rehabilitation: developing a self-directed program, *Athletic Therapy Today* 4(6):51, 1999.
42. Pitney W, Bunton E: Improving rehabilitation effectiveness by enhancing the creative process, *J Ath Train* 30(3):261, 1995.
43. Prentice W: Closed kinetic chain exercise. In Prentice W, editor: *Rehabilitation techniques in sports medicine and athletic training,* St Louis, 2004, McGraw-Hill.
44. Prentice W: The healing process and pathophysiology of musculoskeletal injury. In Prentice W, editor: *Rehabilitation techniques in sports medicine and athletic training,* St Louis, 2004, McGraw-Hill.
45. Prentice W: Mobilization and traction techniques in rehabilitation. In Prentice W, editor: *Rehabilitation techniques in sports medicine and athletic training,* St Louis, 2004, McGraw-Hill.
46. Prentice W: Proprioceptive neuromuscular facilitation techniques. In Prentice W, editor: *Rehabilitation techniques in sports medicine and athletic training,* St Louis, 2004, McGraw-Hill.
47. Prentice W: *Therapeutic modalities in sports medicine and athletic training,* ed 5, St Louis, 2003, McGraw-Hill.
48. Prins J, Cutner D: Aquatic therapy in the rehabilitation of athletic injuries, *Clin Sports Med* 18(2):447, 1999.
49. Ralston D: The RAMP system: a template for the progression of athletic-injury rehabilitation, *J Sport Rehabil* 12(3):280, 2003.
50. Rivera J: Open vs closed kinetic chain rehabilitation of the lower extremity, *J Sport Rehabil* 3(2):154, 1994.
51. Rowinski M: Afferent neurobiology of the joint. In Gould J, Davies G: *Orthopedic and sports physical therapy,* St Louis, 1990, Mosby.
52. Scherzer C, Brewer B, Cornelius A: Psychological skills and adherence to rehabilitation after reconstruction of the anterior cruciate ligament, *J Sport Rehabil* 10(3):165, 2001.
53. Smith MJ: Muscle fiber types: their relationship to athletic training and rehabilitation. In Garron GW, editor: *Gymnastics: Clinics in sports medicine,* vol 4, no 1, Philadelphia, 1985, Saunders.
54. Stone J: Muscle energy technique, *Athletic Therapy Today* 5(5):25, 2000.
55. Stone J: Myofascial release, *Athletic Therapy Today* 5(4):34, 2000.
56. Stone J: Strain-counterstrain, *Athletic Therapy Today* 5(6):30, 2000.
57. Stone J, Partin N, Lueken J: Upper extremity proprioceptive training, *J Ath Train* 2(1):15, 1994.
58. Surburg PR, Schrader JW. Proprioceptive neuromuscular facilitation technique in sports medicine: a reassessment, *J Ath Train* 32(1):34, 1997.
59. Swann E: Uses of manual-therapy techniques in pain management. *Athletic Therapy Today* 7(4):14, 2002.
60. Swanik C et al: Reestablishing proprioception and neuromuscular control in the ACL-injured athlete, *J Sport Rehabil* 6(2):182, 1997.
61. Swanson K: Improving proprioception and neuromuscular control following shoulder injury, *Athletic Therapy Today* 3(5):30, 1998.
62. Thomas M, Müller T, Busse M: Comparison of tension in thera-band and cando tubing, *J Orthop Sports Phys Ther* 32(11):576, 2002.
63. Tippett S, Voight M: *Functional progressions for sport rehabilitation,* Champaign, Ill, 1995, Human Kinetics.
64. Ubinger M, Prentice W, Guskiewicz K: Effect of closed kinetic chain training on neuromuscular control in the upper extremity, *J Sport Rehabil* 8(3):184, 1999.
65. Wadsworth C: *Manual examination and treatment of the spine and extremities,* Baltimore, 1988, Williams & Wilkins.
66. Webburn A, Carbon R, Miller B: Injury rehabilitation programs: what are we talking about? *J Sport Rehabil* 6(1):54, 1997.

ANNOTATED BIBLIOGRAPHY

Buschbacher R, Braddom R: *Sports medicine and rehabilitation: a sport specific approach,* Philadelphia, 1994, Hanley & Belfus.

This text discusses the rehabilitation of injuries that occur in specific sports.

Chaitlow L: *Muscle energy techniques,* Philadelphia, 2001, Churchill Livingstone.

This text discusses muscle energy techniques (manipulative treatments in which a patient engages a muscle against a counterforce) for osteopaths, chiropractors, athletic trainers, physical therapists, and massage therapists.

D'Ambrogio K, Roth G: *Positional release therapy: assessment & treatment of musculoskeletal dysfunction,* St Louis, 1997, Mosby-Year Book.

This text organizes the concept of strain/counterstrain into a systemic approach that is easy to use and document. It contains pictures demonstrating each release position with an awareness of the clinician's body mechanics.

Edmond S: *Manipulation and mobilization: extremity and spinal techniques,* St Louis, 1993, Mosby.

This text provides the entry-level student and the practicing clinician with a comprehensive text on mobilization and manipulation techniques.

Kisner C, Colby A: *Therapeutic exercise: foundations and techniques,* Philadelphia, 2002, Davis.

This clear, concise presentation of the field of therapeutic exercise is well suited to sports medicine. It covers exercise for increasing range of motion and for treating soft tissue, bone, and postsurgical problems extremely well.

Prentice W: *Mobilization and traction: principles and techniques* (video, 33 minutes), St Louis, 1993, Mosby/McGraw-Hill.

This videotape presents a thorough overview of mobilization and traction and includes detailed demonstrations of various techniques.

Prentice W: *Proprioceptive neuromuscular facilitation: principles and techniques* (video, 26 minutes), St Louis, 1993, Mosby/McGraw-Hill.

This videotape presents an introduction to PNF stretching and strengthening exercises complete with detailed hands-on demonstration of specific techniques.

Prentice W: *Rehabilitation techniques in sports medicine and athletic training,* ed 4, St Louis, 2004, McGraw-Hill.

This comprehensive text deals with all aspects of rehabilitation used in a sports medicine setting.

Tippett S, Voight M: *Functional progressions for sport rehabilitation,* Champaign, Ill, 1995, Human Kinetics.

This text presents scientific principles and practical applications for using functional exercise to rehabilitate athletic injuries.

Zachazewski J, Magee D, Quillen W: *Athletic injuries and rehabilitation,* Philadelphia, 1996, Saunders.

This extremely detailed, scientifically based, advanced text deals with athletic injury rehabilitation.

Chapter 17 Pharmacology, Drugs, and Sports

When you finish this chapter you should be able to

- Define the term *drug*.
- Identify the various methods by which drugs can be administered.
- Analyze pharmacokinetics relative to absorption, distribution, metabolism, and excretion.
- Explain the difference between administering and dispensing medications.
- Express legal concerns for administering medications to the athletic population.
- Apply the various protocols that the athletic trainer should follow for administering over-the-counter medications to athletes.
- Categorize the various drugs that can be used to treat infection, reduce pain and inflammation, relax muscles, treat gastrointestinal disorders, treat symptoms of colds and congestion, and control bleeding.
- Recognize the problem of substance abuse in the athletic population.
- Describe the ergogenic aids used by athletes to improve performance.
- Discuss the use of alcohol, drugs, and tobacco by athletes.
- Evaluate the drug testing policies and procedures, and list the different types of banned drugs.

pharmacology The study of drugs and their origin, nature, properties, and effects on living organisms.

Pharmacology is the branch of science that deals with the actions of drugs on biological systems, especially drugs that are used in medicine for diagnostic and therapeutic purposes. Pharmaceutical care is the direct provision of medication-related care for the purpose of achieving definite outcomes that improve quality of life.[20] Medications of all types, both prescription and over-the-counter, are commonly used by athletes as they are by others in the population.[1]

Unfortunately, the abuse of various drugs and other substances for performance enhancement or for recreational mood alteration is also widespread among athletes. Thus the athletic trainer must be knowledgeable about drug use and substance abuse within the athletic population.

WHAT IS A DRUG?

drug A chemical agent used in the prevention, treatment, or diagnosis of disease.

A **drug** is a chemical agent used in the prevention, treatment, or diagnosis of disease.[37] The use of substances for the express purpose of treating some infirmity or disease dates back to early history. The ancient Egyptians were highly skilled in making and using medications, treating a wide range of external and internal conditions.

Many of our common drugs, such as aspirin and penicillin, are derived from natural sources. Historically, medications were composed of roots, herbs, leaves, or other natural materials that were identified as having or believed to have medicinal properties. Today many medications that originally came from nature are produced synthetically.

PHARMACOKINETICS

pharmacokinetics The method by which drugs are absorbed, distributed, metabolized, and eliminated.

Pharmacokinetics refers to the method by which drugs are absorbed, distributed, metabolized, and eliminated or excreted by the body. The term *pharmacodynamics* is often confused with pharmacokinetics. Pharmacodynamics refers to the actions or the effects of a drug on the body.[25,37]

Administration of Drugs

To be effective therapeutically, a drug must first enter the system and then reach a receptor in a target tissue. The administration of medications in athletes, as in any individual, can be either internal or external and is based on the type of local or general response desired.

Drugs can be administered internally or externally.

Internal Administration

Drugs and medications can be taken internally through inhalation, or they may be administered intradermally, intramuscularly, intranasally, intraspinally, intravaginally, intravenously, orally, rectally, or sublingually.

Inhalation is a means of bringing medication or substances to the respiratory tract. This method is most often used in sports to relieve the athlete of the symptoms of respiratory illnesses such as asthma. The vehicle for inhalation is normally water vapor, oxygen, or highly aromatic medications.

Intradermal (into the skin) or *subcutaneous* (under the cutaneous tissues) administration is usually accomplished through a hypodermic needle injection. Such introduction of medication is initiated when a rapid response is needed, but this method does not produce as rapid a response as intravenous injection offers.

Intramuscular injection means that the medication is given directly into the muscle tissue. The site for such an injection is usually the gluteal area or the deltoid muscle of the upper arm.

Intranasal application varies according to the condition that is to be treated. The introduction of a decongestant intranasal solution by using a dropper or an atomizer may relieve the discomfort of head colds and allergies.

Intraspinal injection may be indicated for any of the following purposes: introduction of drugs to combat specific organisms that have entered the spinal cord, injection of a substance such as procaine to anesthetize the lower limbs, or withdrawal of spinal fluid to be studied.

Intravaginal administration involves placement of a drug or drug-containing device inside the vagina. Drugs are readily absorbed through the vaginal mucosa.

Intravenous injection (into a vein) is given when an immediate reaction to the medication is desired. The drug enters the venous circulation and is spread rapidly throughout the body.

Oral administration of medicines is the most common method of all. Forms such as tablets, capsules, powders, and liquids are easily administered orally.

Rectal administration of drugs is limited. In the past some medications have been introduced through the rectum to be absorbed by its mucous lining. Such methods have proved undesirable because of difficulties in regulating dosage.

Sublingual and *buccal* introductions of medicines usually consist of placing easily dissolved agents such as troches (lozenges) or tablets under the tongue. They dissolve slowly and are absorbed by the mucous lining.

External Administration

Medications administered externally include inunctions, ointments, pastes, plasters, transdermal patches, and solutions.

Inunctions are oily or medicated substances that are rubbed into the skin and result in a local or systemic reaction. Oil-based liniments and petroleum analgesic balms used as massage lubricants are examples of inunctions.

Ointments consisting of oil, petroleum jelly, or lanolin combined with drugs are applied for long-lasting topical medication.

Pastes are ointments with a nonfat base. They are spread on cloth and usually produce a cooling effect on the skin.

Plasters are thicker than ointments and are spread either on cloth or paper or directly on the skin. They usually contain an irritant, are applied as a counterirritant, and are used for relieving pain, increasing circulation, and decreasing inflammation.

TABLE 17-1 Drug Vehicles

Liquid preparations	
Aqueous solution	Sterile water containing a drug substance
Elixir	Alcohol, sugar, and flavoring with a drug dissolved in solution, designed for internal consumption
Liniment	Alcohol or oil containing a dissolved drug, designed for external massage
Spirit	A drug dissolved in water and alcohol or in alcohol alone
Suspension	Undissolved powder in a fluid medium; must be mixed well by shaking before use
Syrup	A mixture of sugar and water containing a drug
Solid preparations	
Ampule	A closed glass receptacle containing a drug
Capsule	A gelatin receptacle containing a drug
Ointment (emollient)	A semisolid preparation for external application of such consistency that it may be applied to the skin by inunction
Paste	An inert powder combined with water
Tablet	A solid pharmaceutical dosage compressed into a small oval, circle, square, or other form
Plaster	A substance intended for external application, made of such materials and of such consistency as to adhere to the skin and thereby attach a dressing
Powder	Finely ground drug plus vehicle or effervescent granules
Suppository	A medicated gelatin molded into a cone for placement in a body orifice (e.g., the anal canal)

Transdermal patches are patches resembling adhesive bandages that contain various types of slow-release medications that are absorbed gradually through the skin. They may be left in place for several days.

Solutions can be administered externally and are extremely varied, consisting principally of bacteriostatics. Antiseptics, disinfectants, vasoconstrictors, and liquid rubefacients are examples.

Drug Vehicles

drug vehicle
The substance in which a drug is transported.

A **drug vehicle** is a therapeutically inactive substance that transports a drug. A drug is housed in a vehicle that may be either a solid or a liquid. Some of the more common drug vehicles are listed in Table 17-1.

Absorption of Drugs

Once a drug is in the system, it must be dissolved before it can be absorbed. The rate and extent of absorption is determined by the chemical characteristics of the drug, the dosage form (i.e., tablet or solution), and the gastric-emptying time. Solutions in which the drug is already dissolved have the fastest absorption rate, and time-release medications have the slowest rate.[37]

bioavailability
How completely a particular drug is absorbed by the system.

Bioavailability refers to how completely a particular drug is absorbed by the system. Bioavailability is most dependent on the characteristics of the drug and not on the dosage form, whereas absorption rate is largely determined by dosage form.

volume of distribution
The volume of plasma in which a drug is dissolved.

Distribution

efficacy
A drug's capability of producing a specific therapeutic effect.

Once absorbed, the drug is transported through the blood to a specific target tissue. The drug will be distributed to other parts of the body as well. **The volume of distribution** is the volume of fluid or plasma in which the drug is dissolved and indicates the extent of distribution of that drug. The **efficacy** of a drug is its capability of producing a specific therapeutic effect once it reaches a particular receptor site in a target tissue. **Potency** is the dose of the drug that is required to produce a desired therapeutic effect.[37]

potency
The dose of a drug required to produce a desired therapeutic effect.

Metabolism

The **biotransformation** of drugs into water-soluble compounds that can be excreted is referred to as **metabolism.** Most of the metabolism takes place in the liver, with some occurring in the kidneys and blood. Metabolism of drugs in the liver transforms most active drugs into inactive compounds. Occasionally, when an active drug is metabolized, the metabolites may be toxic.[37]

biotransformation
Transforming a drug so it can be metabolized.

metabolism
Changing a drug into a water-soluble compound that can be excreted.

Excretion

Excretion of a drug or its metabolites is controlled by the kidneys. Drugs are filtered through the kidneys and are usually excreted in the urine, although some may be reabsorbed. Some drugs may also be excreted in saliva, sweat, and feces.[37]

Drug Half-Life

The rate at which a drug disappears from the body, either through metabolism or excretion or a combination of the two, is called the **half-life.** This rate is the amount of time required for the plasma drug level to be reduced by one-half. For most drugs, the half-life is measured in hours, but for some it is measured in minutes or days. Knowing the half-life of a drug is critical in determining how often and in what dosage a drug must be administered to achieve and maintain therapeutic levels of concentration. The dosage interval, or time between administration of individual doses, may be equal to the half-life of that particular drug.[37]

half-life
The rate at which a drug disappears from the body through metabolism, excretion, or both.

How often a drug will be administered is determined in part by the drug's **steady-state,** which is reached when the amount that is taken is equal to the amount that is excreted. A steady-state is usually reached after five half-lives of the drug have occurred. Drugs with long half-lives may take several days to weeks to reach a steady-state.[37]

steady-state
When the amount of the drug taken is equal to the amount that is excreted.

Effects of Physical Activity on Pharmacokinetics

In general, exercise decreases the absorption after oral administration of a drug, whereas exercise increases absorption after intramuscular or subcutaneous administration because of an increased blood flow in the muscle.[47] Thus, exercise has an influence on the amount of a drug that reaches a receptor site, which significantly affects the pharmacodynamic activity of that drug.[47]

LEGAL CONCERNS IN ADMINISTERING VERSUS DISPENSING DRUGS

Administering a drug is defined as providing a single dose of medication for immediate use by the patient. Dispensing refers to providing the patient with a drug in a quantity sufficient to be used for multiple doses.

Dispensing Prescription Drugs

At no time can anyone other than a person licensed by law legally prescribe or dispense prescription drugs for an athlete. An athletic trainer, unless specifically allowed by state licensure, is not permitted to dispense a prescription drug.[5] Failure to heed this fact can be a violation of federal laws and state statutes. Table 17-2 lists information about how medication dispensing is controlled. A violation of these laws could mean legal problems for the physician, athletic trainer, school, school district, or even the league.[23]

At no time can anyone other than a person licensed by law legally prescribe or dispense prescription drugs for an athlete.

Administering Over-the-Counter Drugs

The situation is not so clear-cut for nonprescription drugs. Basically, the athletic trainer may be allowed to administer a single dose of a nonprescription medication. For example, most secondary schools do not allow the athletic trainer to administer nonprescription (over-the-counter [OTC]) drugs that are to be taken internally by the

TABLE 17-2 Agencies and Regulations that Govern the Provision of Pharmaceutical Care

Regulation	Enforced/Administered by	Purpose
Federal Food, Drug, and Cosmetic Act (FDCA) of 1938	Food and Drug Administration	Regulates the quality, strength, bioequivalence, and labeling of prescription and nonprescription drugs
Durham-Humphrey Amendment of 1951	Food and Drug Administration	Separates prescription from nonprescription drugs
Current Good Manufacturing Practice Regulations of 1962	Food and Drug Administration	Mandates standards for repackaging of medications
Federal Controlled Substances Act of 1970	Food and Drug Administration	Regulates controlled substances (drugs that have potential for abuse)
Poison Prevention Packaging Act (PPPA) of 1970	Food and Drug Administration	Regulates packaging of prescription and nonprescription drugs in child-resistant safety containers
Medical Device Act of 1976	Food and Drug Administration	Regulates classification and performance standards of medical devices.
Federal Anti-Tampering Act of 1983	Food and Drug Administration	Mandates tamper-resistant packaging on all nonprescription drugs
Fair Packaging and Labeling Act	Food and Drug Administration	Mandates labeling of the contents of nonprescription drugs to assist consumers in identifying similar products
Prescription Drug Marketing Act of 1987	Food and Drug Administration	Mandates accountability of sample drugs from receiving through administering or dispensing
Anti–Drug Abuse Act of 1988	Drug Enforcement Authority	Regulates anabolic steroids as controlled substances
Omnibus Reconciliation Act of 1990 (OBRA '90)	Food and Drug Administration	Mandates drug review, patient medication records, and verbal patient education as part of dispensing of prescription medications
State Pharmacy Practice Acts	Individual State Boards of Pharmacy	Regulates the provision of pharmaceutical care within each state. Laws and regulations may vary considerably between states
State Medical Acts	Individual State Boards of Medicine	Regulates the practice within each state
Health Insurance Portability-Accountability Act of 1996 (HIPAA)	Department of Health and Human Services	Provides national standards to protect the privacy of personal health information

athlete, including aspirin and OTC cold remedies. The application of nonprescription wound medications is allowed by some secondary schools under the category of first aid. On the other hand, some high school athletic trainers in the United States are not allowed to apply even a wound medication in the name of first aid but can only clean the wound with soap and water. The athlete must then be sent to the school nurse for medication. The dispensing of vitamins and even dextrose may be specifically disallowed by some school districts. At the college or professional level, minors are not usually involved, and the administration of nonprescription medications may be less restrictive. It is assumed that athletes who are of legal age have the right to use whatever nonprescription drugs they choose. However, this right does not preclude the fact that the athletic trainer must be reasonable and prudent about the types of nonprescription drugs offered to the athlete.

A 2003 study indicated that nine years after a National Collegiate Athletic Association (NCAA) drug-distribution study of university athletic programs, many problem areas persisted, including unqualified personnel dispensing medications, inappropriately packaged and labeled medications, and a lack of record keeping.[24] In most athletic training rooms, athletic trainers (55.9 percent) and students (13.3 percent) still dispensed prescription drugs. In addition, in most athletic training rooms athletic trainers (53.8 percent) administered any amount of over-the-counter medication necessary, and many did not record the transaction (46.2 percent). In virtually every state

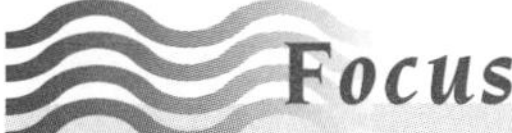

General guidelines for administering medications to athletes

- Medications should only be taken as directed.
- Medications should not be used in combination before consulting a physician/pharmacist.
- Labels should not be removed from medications' bottles or containers.
- Medications should not be used past the expiration date marked on the container.
- Oral medications should be taken with a full glass of water unless directed otherwise.
- Medications should be taken with food or on an empty stomach according to instructions.
- Specifically marked measuring spoons or caps should be used when measuring liquid medications.
- Containers should be childproof.
- Always consult individual states for rules and regulations governing the use of therapeutic medications.
- Check the banned substance status of all medications taken by athletes (according to the NCAA, IOC, and other governing bodies).
- Provide both verbal and written instructions for the use of medications.
- Make sure the athlete reads the label information prior to taking a medication.
- Make sure the athlete knows the dose schedule for the medications he or she is taking.
- Advise athletes not to share medications with other people.
- Be aware of interactions between medications and exercise.
- NSAIDs are commonly used among athletes for their analgesic and antiinflammatory effects. Make sure athletes understand the potential side effects and possible addiction to these medications. They should be taken as prescribed.

From NATA Research and Education Foundation: *Guidelines for the use of therapeutic medications in sports,* Dallas, 2000, NATA.

this practice is against the law. Athletic trainers should work in conjunction with members of the sports medicine team to review federal and state laws and revise institutional drug policies and procedures to comply with regulations to provide the best health care to student athletes in a legal and safe manner.[24]

Generally, the administration of single doses of nonprescription medicines by a member of the athletic staff to any athlete depends on the philosophy of the school district and must be under the direction of the team physician.[42] In this area, as in all other areas of sports medicine and athletic training, the athletic trainer is obligated to act reasonably and prudently. See the *Focus Box:* "General guidelines for administering medications to athletes."

Record Keeping

Those involved in any health care profession are acutely aware of the necessity of maintaining complete, up-to-date medical records. The athletic training setting is no exception. The athletic trainer who administers medications must realize that maintaining accurate records of the types of medications administered is just as important as recording progress notes, treatments given, and rehabilitation plans. The athletic trainer may be dealing with a number of different patients simultaneously while trying to get a team ready for practice or competition. Situations may become hectic, and stopping to record each time a medication is administered is difficult. Nevertheless, the athletic trainer should include the following information on the medication administration log:

1. name of the athlete,
2. complaint or symptoms,
3. current medications,

4. any known drug allergies,
5. name of medication given,
6. lot number if available,
7. expiration date,
8. quantity of medication given,
9. method of administration,
10. date and time of administration.[23,56]

Each athletic trainer should be aware of state regulations and laws that pertain to the ordering, prescribing, distributing, storing, and dispensing or administering of medications. Obtaining legal counsel, working with the state board of pharmacy or a student health clinic, working in cooperation with a team physician, and establishing strict written policies are all actions that can minimize the chances of violating state laws that regulate the use of medications.[23,56]

Labeling Requirements

OTC drugs are required to have directions for use and precautions that are adequate and readable. The federal eight-point label for nonprescription drugs requires the following information:

1. The name of the product
2. The name and address of the manufacturer, packer, or distributor
3. The net contents of the package
4. The established name of all active ingredients and the quantity of certain other ingredients whether active or not
5. The name of any habit-forming drug contained in the preparation
6. Cautions and warnings to protect the consumer
7. Adequate directions for safe and effective use
8. Expiration date and lot number

Nonprescription drugs may not be repackaged without meeting labeling criteria. All drugs dispensed from the athletic training room must be properly labeled. Legal violations may occur if a portion of a nonprescription drug is removed from an original, properly labeled package and dispensed to an athlete. This practice carries the same liability as does dispensing prescription drugs, because the athlete is not given the opportunity to review the label for name, contents, precautions, directions, and other information considered essential for the safe use of the product. Liability for any adverse patient outcome is therefore transferred to the dispenser of the improperly labeled OTC drug.[23]

17-1 *Critical Thinking* Exercise

A college-age softball player comes into the training room complaining of a sore throat and stuffy head and asks the athletic trainer to give her some "drugs" to get rid of her problem.

? Is the athletic trainer legally allowed to give her any type of medication, and if so, how should the athletic trainer give it to the athlete?

Safety in the Use of Pharmaceuticals

No drug can be considered completely safe and harmless. If a drug is potent enough to effect some physiological action, it is also strong enough, under some conditions, to be dangerous. All persons react individually to any drug. A given amount of a specific medication may produce no adverse reaction in one athlete and a pronounced adverse response in another. Both the athlete and the athletic trainer should be fully aware of any untoward effect a drug may have. It is essential that the athlete be instructed clearly about when specifically to take medications, with meals or not, and what not to combine with the drug, such as other drugs or specific foods. Some drugs can nullify the effect of another drug or can cause a serious antagonistic reaction. For example, calcium, which is found in a variety of foods and in some medications, can nullify the effects of the antibiotic tetracycline.

Drug Responses

Individuals react differently to the same medication, and different conditions may alter the effect of a drug on the athlete. Drugs themselves can be changed through age or improper preservation, as well as through the manner in which they are administered. Response variations also result from differences in each individual's size or age.

Alcohol should not be ingested with a wide variety of drugs, both prescription and nonprescription. Alcohol is a central nervous system depressant and can increase or decrease the effects of other drugs. Alcohol may intensify drowsiness if used in combination with another depressant. It is also important to realize that alcohol is used in many liquid preparations that are being used as medications. Warnings concerning the use of alcohol should be listed on the drug label.

Medications can potentially effect certain physiologic functions that are related to dehydration, such as sweating, urination, and the ability to control and regulate body temperature. Some medications can cause fluid depletion that results in dehydration, which can increase the risk of heat illness. Other medications can make an individual more sensitive to sunlight, increasing the risk of sunburn or allergic reactions to sunlight. A fatty diet may decrease a drug's effectiveness by interfering with its absorption. Excessively acid foods such as fruits, carbonated drinks, or vegetable juice may cause adverse drug reactions.[7] Athletic trainers must thoroughly know the athletes with whom they work. The possibility of an adverse drug reaction is ever present and requires continual education and vigilance.

Table 17-3 is a list of general body responses sometimes produced by drugs and medications.

TABLE 17-3 General Responses Produced by Drugs and Medications

Addiction	Body response to certain types of drugs that produces both a physiological need and a psychological craving for the substance
Antagonistic action	Result observed when medications, used together, have adverse effects or counteract one another
Cumulative effect	Exaggerated drug effects, which occur when the body is unable to metabolize a drug as rapidly as it is administered; the accumulated, unmetabolized drug may cause unfavorable reactions
Depressive action	Effect from drugs that slow down cell function
Habituation	Individual's development of a psychological need for a specific medication
Hypersensitivity	Allergic response to a specific drug; such allergies may be demonstrated by a mild skin irritation, itching, a rash, or a severe anaphylactic reaction, which could be fatal
Idiosyncrasy	Unusual reaction to a drug; a distinctive response
Irritation	Process, as well as effect, caused by substances that result in a cellular change; mild irritation may stimulate cell activity, whereas moderate or severe irritation by a drug may decrease cell activity
Paradoxical reaction	A drug-induced effect that is the exact opposite of that which is therapeutically intended
Potentiating agent	A pharmaceutical that increases the effect of another; for example, codeine is potentiated by aspirin, and therefore less of it is required to relieve pain
Specific effect	Action usually produced by a drug in a select tissue or organ system
Side effect	The result of a medication that is given for a particular condition but affects other body areas or has effects other than those sought
Stimulation	Effect caused by drugs that speed up cell activity
Synergistic effect	Result that occurs when drugs given together produce a greater reaction than when given alone
Tolerance	Condition existing when a certain drug dosage is no longer able to give a therapeutic action and must therefore be increased

Buying Medications

One of the athletic department's best friends is the local pharmacist. The pharmacist can assist in the selection and purchase of nonprescription drugs, can save money by suggesting the lower-priced generic drugs, and can act as a general advisor on the effectiveness of drugs, the dose of a medicine, and even the inherent dangers in a specific drug.

All pharmaceuticals must be properly labeled, indicating clearly the content, expiration date, and any dangers or contraindications for use. Pharmaceutical manufacturers place the expiration date on drugs, and athletic trainers should locate this date on the package. When storing medications:

1. Always keep both prescription and over-the-counter medications in a locked cabinet or secured place.
2. Keep them in the original container.
3. Store them away from heat, direct light, damp places, and extreme cold.
4. Keep over-the-counter medications in single-dose packs.[44]

Traveling with Medications

When traveling with a team or individually, the athlete should be advised to do the following with regard to medications:

1. Medication should not be stored in a bag or luggage but carried by the athlete taking it.
2. A sufficient supply of medication should be packaged in case of emergency.
3. Make sure there is a source of medication while traveling.
4. Take copies of written prescriptions.
5. Keep medications in their original containers and in a secure place.
6. When traveling internationally, understand the restrictions of individual jurisdictions.

SELECTED THERAPEUTIC DRUGS USED TO TREAT THE ATHLETE

in vitro = in a laboratory
in vivo = in the body

The use of drugs and medicine is widespread in the athletic population, as it is in society in general. Thousands of drugs, both prescription and nonprescription, are available for physicians and consumers to choose from, and new drugs are being constantly developed. Pharmaceutical laboratories develop compounds *in vitro*, and then test, retest, and refine the drug *in vivo* before submitting it for Food and Drug Administration (FDA) approval.

bioequivalence Having a similar biological effect.

A number of texts and databases are available (i.e., *Physician's Desk Reference* and *Drug Facts and Comparisons*) and are widely used as references for comparison of **bioequivalent drugs** (drugs that produce similar biological effects) relative to their appropriateness and effectiveness in treating a specific condition or illness.[35] Table 17-4 summarizes the various classifications of drugs available.

The following sections discuss the most common pharmaceutical practices in athletic training to date and the specific drugs that are in use (see also Table 17-5). The discussions include both prescription and nonprescription drugs, with emphases on what should most concern the athletic trainer and what the medications or materials are designed to accomplish.

Drugs to Combat Infection

Drugs used to combat infection include local antiseptics and disinfectants, antifungal agents, and antibiotics.

Combating infection, especially skin infection, is of major importance in sports. Serious infection can cause countless hours of lost time and has even been the indirect cause of death.

Local Antiseptics and Disinfectants

Antiseptics are substances that can be placed on living tissue for the express purpose of either killing bacteria or inhibiting their growth. Disinfectants are substances that combat microorganisms but should be applied only to nonliving objects. Other general

TABLE 17-4 **List of Drug Classifications and Definitions**

Analgesics	Pain-relieving drugs
Anesthetics	Agents that produce local or general numbness to touch, pain, or stimulation
Antacids	Substances that neutralize acidity; commonly used in the digestive tract
Anticoagulants	Agents that prevent coagulation of blood
Antidotes	Substances that prevent or counteract the action of a poison
Antipruritics	Agents that relieve itching
Antiseptics	Agents that kill bacteria or inhibit their growth and can be applied to living tissue
Antispasmodics	Agents that relieve muscle spasm
Antitussives	Agents that inhibit or prevent coughing
Astringents	Agents that cause contraction or puckering action
Bacteriostatics and fungistatics	Agents that retard or inhibit the growth of bacteria or fungi
Carminatives	Agents that relieve flatulence (caused by gases) in the intestinal tract
Cathartics	Agents used to evacuate substances from the bowels; active purgatives
Caustics	Burning agents, capable of destroying living tissue
Counterirritants	Agents applied locally to produce an inflammatory reaction for the relief of a deeper inflammation
Depressants	Agents that diminish body functions or nerve activity
Disinfectants	Agents that kill or inhibit the growth of microorganisms; should be applied only to nonliving materials
Diuretics	Agents that increase the excretion of urine
Emetics	Agents that cause vomiting
Expectorants	Agents that suppress coughing
Hemostatics	Substances that either slow down or stop bleeding or hemorrhage
Irritants	Agents that cause irritation
Narcotics	Drugs that produce analgesic and hypnotic effects
Sedatives	Agents that relieve anxiety
Skeletal muscle relaxants	Drugs that depress neural activity within skeletal muscles
Stimulants	Agents that excite the central nervous system
Vasoconstrictors and vasodilators	Drugs that, respectively, constrict or dilate blood vessels

names given to antiseptics and disinfectants are germicides, which are designed to destroy bacteria; fungicides, which kill fungi; sporicides, which destroy spores; and sanitizers, which minimize contamination by microorganisms.

Antiseptics and disinfectants include alcohol, phenol, halogens, and oxidizing agents.

In sports many agents are used to combat infection. It is critical that agents have a broad spectrum of activity against infective organisms, including the human immunodeficiency virus (HIV).

Alcohol Alcohol is one of the most widely used skin disinfectants. Ethyl alcohol (70% by weight) and isopropyl alcohol (70%) are equally effective. They are inexpensive and nonirritating; they kill bacteria immediately, with the exception of spores. However, they have no long-lasting germicidal action. Besides being directly combined with other agents to form tinctures, alcohol acts independently on the skin as an antiseptic and astringent. In a 70 percent solution, alcohol can be used for disinfecting instruments. Because of alcohol's rapid rate of evaporation, it produces a mild

TABLE 17-5 Athletic Trainers' Guide to Medications Frequently Used in Sports Medicine

Generic Name	Trade Name	Primary Use of Drug/Prescription	Sports Medicine Consideration
Analgesics, antipyretics, and antinflammatories (NSAIDs)			
Aspirin	Many trade names	Analgesic, antipyretic, antiinflammatory.	Gastric irritation, nausea, tinnitus, prolonged bleeding if injured in contact sports
Acetaminophen	Tylenol, Datril, others	Analgesic, antipyretic.	Do not combine with alcohol
Flurbiprofen	Ansaid*	All are analgesic, antipyretic, antiinflammatory (NSAIDs). Notify doctor immediately for skin rash, itching, visual disturbances, weight gain, edema, black stools, dark urine, or persistent headache. *Drug interactions:* salicylates, other NSAIDs, probenecid, cimetidine, diuretics, lithium, phenytoin, beta blockers, ACE inhibitors, anticoagulants, digoxin	Gastric irritation less common than with aspirin except for indomethacin. These medications should be used for reducing pain and inflammation; they should not be substituted for acetaminophen in cases of mild headache or low fever. Adequate hydration reduces the risk of adverse effects in the renal system. *NSAID hypersensitivity:* Because of cross sensitivity to aspirin and all other NSAIDs do not give these agents to athletes in whom aspirin, iodides, or other NSAIDs have caused symptoms of asthma, rhinitis, rash, nasal polyps, bronchospasm, or other symptoms of allergic reactions.
Ketoprofen	Orudis*		
Indomethacin	Indocin*		
Ibuprofen	Advil, Motrin,* Nuprin		
Naproxen	Naprosyn,* Anaprox,* Aleve		
Diflunisal	Dolobid*		
Piroxicam	Feldene*		
Tolmetin	Tolectin*		
Fenoprofen	Nalfon*		
Meclofenamate	Meclomen*		
Diclofenac	Voltaren,* Cataflam*		
Ketorolac	Toradol*		
Etodolac	Lodine*		
Mefenamic acid	Ponstel*		
Nabumetone	Relafen*		
Meloxicam	Mobic*		
Oxaprozin	Daypro*		
Sulindac	Clinoril*		
Celecoxib	Celebrex*		
Valdecoxib	Bextra*		
Antifungal agents			
Ketoconazole	Nizoral*	Systemic (oral) antifungal drug. Drug has been associated with hepatic toxicity including fatalities. Notify doctor immediately for unusual fatigue, anorexia, nausea, jaundice, dark urine, pale stools, abdominal pain, fever, or diarrhea.	Should not be taken within two hours of antacids. May cause dizziness or drowsiness. *Hypersensitivity:* Anaphylaxis has been reported.
Griseofulvin	Fulvicin P/G,* Gris-Peg*	Oral antifungal agent. Notify doctor immediately for fever, sore throat, or skin rash. Reduces the effectiveness of oral contraceptives.	Photosensitivity may occur: Patient should avoid prolonged exposure to sunlight or sunlamps.
Fluconazole	Diflucan*	Oral antifungal agent. Warnings: hepatic injury, anaphylaxis, dermatologic changes have been reported. Notify doctor immediately for skin rash. *Drug interactions:* cimetidine, rifampin, nonsedating antihistamines, phenytoin, theophylline, zidovudine	

*Requires a prescription.

Generic Name	Trade Name	Primary Use of Drug/Prescription	Sports Medicine Consideration
Terbinafine	Lamisil*	Oral antifungal agent for treatment of toenails or fingernails, scalp, body, groin, or feet. Notify doctor immediately for skin rash, itching, aching joints, dark urine, difficulty swallowing, fever, chills, pale skin, pale stool, redness, blistering, peeling or loosening of skin, unusual tiredness and yellowing of skin or eyes *Drug interactions:* cimetidine, rifampin, terfenadine, caffeine	Weeks to months may be required to resolve infection. Alcohol consumption during treatment increases risk of liver toxicity.
Antibiotics			
Penicillins	V-Cillin-K,* Pen Vee K,* Trimox*	*Drug interactions:* beta blockers, oral contraceptives, erythromycin, tetracycline	If diarrhea occurs, do not give Imodium AD.
Cephalosporins	Keflex,* Ceftin*	*Drug interactions:* oral contraceptives, alcohol, probenecid	Patients allergic to penicillin may have cross sensitivity to cephalosporins.
Macrolides	Ery-Tab,* Zithromax,* Biaxin,* Dynabac*	*Drug interactions:* fluconazole, zidovudine, theophylline, nonsedating antihistamines, oral contraceptives, carbamazepine, ergot alkaloids, penicillins	
Fluoroquinolones	Cipro,* Noroxin,* Floxin,* Penetrex,* Maxaquin,* Zagam,* Levaquin*	Notify doctor immediately for agitation, confusion, tremors, fever, skin rash. *Drug interactions:* antacids, sucralfate, Pepto-Bismol, cimetidine, caffeine, probenecid, phenytoin, theophylline, oral contraceptives	Photosensitivity; avoid overexposure to sunlight or sunlamps. May cause dizziness. Rarely associated with pain, inflammation, or rupture of a tendon.
Tetracyclines	Sumycin,* Vibramycin*	*Drug interactions:* antacids, anticoagulants, cimetidine, insulin, lithium, oral contraceptives, penicillins, sodium bicarbonate.	Should not be taken with milk, antacids, or minerals because of reduced absorption. Photosensitivity may occur.
Drugs that affect the respiratory tract			
Chlorpheniramine	Chlor-Trimeton	Antihistamine for allergies	Used primarily for treatment of allergic rhinitis. Causes drowsiness, decreased coordination.
Cromolyn	Nasalcrom	Nasal allergy symptom controller; prevents and relieves nasal allergy symptoms.	Allergic rhinitis, seasonal allergies
Oxymetazoline	Afrin, Dristan Long Lasting, Neosynephrine 12 Hour, Allerest	Adrenergic decongestant applied topically as spray or nose drops.	Do not exceed recommended duration of treatment because of rebound congestion; may cause sneezing, dryness of nasal mucosa, and headache.
Pseudoephedrine	Sudafed, Cenafed, Oranyl, others	Adrenergic decongestant used orally.	Produces stimulation of the central nervous system; topically applied decongestants work faster, but oral decongestants are preferred for long-term use.
Diphenhydramine	Benadryl, Benylin cough syrup	Antihistamine used primarily for allergic reaction; also used for sleep.	Produces drowsiness and dry mouth; found in over-the-counter sleeping medications.

*Requires a prescription.

TABLE 17-5 Athletic Trainers' Guide to Medications Frequently Used in Sports Medicine—continued

Dextromethorphan	Robitussin DM, Benylin DMO, Sucrets Lozenges	Nonnarcotic antitussive used for cough suppression. Drug interaction: newer antidepressants	Very effective in cases of unproductive cough; rarely produces drowsiness and other side effects.
Cetirizine	Zyrtec*	Antihistamine; effective for some allergic reactions.	May cause some sedation but less than traditional antihistamines.
Fexofenadine Loratidine	Allegra* Claritin	Antihistamines.	Nonsedating.
Benzonatate	Tessalon*	Peripherally acting antitussive that acts as an anesthetic.	May cause dizziness; should not be chewed.
Codeine	Robitussin AC*	Narcotic antitussive that depresses the central cough mechanism.	Used in combination with expectorant; can produce sedation, dizziness, constipation, or nausea.
Guaifenesin	Robitussin, Glyate	Expectorant used for symptomatic relief of unproductive cough.	Used for treating dry or sore throat; good hydration maximizes effects.
Drugs that affect the gastrointestinal tract			
Sodium bicarbonate	Soda Mint	Antacid used for quick relief of upset stomach.	Produces gas, belching; overuse may cause systemic alkalinity.
Aluminum hydroxide	Amphogel, Dialume	Antacid used for upset stomach.	May produce constipation: moderate acid neutralizer.
Calcium carbonate	Titralac, Mallamint	Antacid used for upset stomach and for calcium supplementation.	May produce constipation and acid rebound; high acid neutralizing capacity.
Magnesium hydroxide	Milk of Magnesia	Laxative used for constipation.	May cause diarrhea.
Cimetidine	Tagamet HB	Histamine-2 antagonist used for relief of upset stomach, heartburn, acid indigestion.	Numerous drug interactions.
Nizatidine	Axid AR	Histamine-2 antagonist used for relief of upset stomach, heartburn, acid indigestion.	
Ranitidine Famotidine	Zantac 75 Pepcid AC		
Combination antacids	Alka-Seltzer, Digel, Gaviscon, Gelusil, Maalox, Mylanta, Wingel, others	Combination drugs for controlling gastric upset.	May produce either diarrhea or constipation.
Promethazine	Phenergan*	Antiemetic used for preventing motion sickness, nausea, and vomiting.	Produces sedation and drowsiness.
Diphenoxylate HCL	Lomotil,* Uni-Lom*	Narcotic antidiarrheal.	Causes dry mouth, nausea, drowsiness.
Loperamide	Imodium AD	Nonnarcotic systemic antidiarrheal.	Abdominal discomfort, drowsiness with large doses.
Combination antidiarrheals	Donnagel, Kaopectate	Relief of diarrhea.	All are relatively safe with few side effects; effectiveness is questionable.
	Pepto-Bismol		Effective for traveler's diarrhea.
Proton pump inhibitor	Prilosec	Relief of heartburn.	Used in preventing NSAID-induced ulcers.

*Requires a prescription.

anesthetic action. Combined with 20 percent benzoin, it is used in athletics as a topical skin dressing to provide a protective skin coating and astringent action.

Phenol Phenol was one of the earliest antiseptics and disinfectants used by the medical profession. From its inception to the present, phenol has been used to control disease organisms, both as an antiseptic and as a disinfectant. It is available in liquids of varying concentrations and in emollients. Substances that are derived from phenol and that cause less irritation are now used more extensively. Some of these derivatives are resorcinol, thymol, and the common household disinfectant Lysol.

Halogens Halogens are chemical substances (chlorine, fluoride, and bromine) that are used for their antiseptic and disinfectant qualities. Iodophors, or halogenated compounds, a combination of iodine and a carrier, create a much less irritating preparation than tincture of iodine is. A popular iodophor is povidone-iodine complex (Betadine), which is an excellent germicide commonly used as a surgical scrub by surgeons. Betadine as an antiseptic and germicide in athletic training has proved extremely effective on skin lesions such as lacerations, abrasions, and floor burns.

Oxidizing agents Oxidizing agents, as represented by hydrogen peroxide (3%), are commonly used in athletic training. Hydrogen peroxide is an antiseptic that, because of its oxidation, affects bacteria but readily decomposes in the presence of organic substances such as blood and pus. For this reason it has little effect as an antiseptic. Contact with organic material produces an effervescence, during which no great destruction of bacteria takes place. The chief value of hydrogen peroxide in the care of wounds is its ability to cleanse the infected cutaneous and mucous membranes. Application of hydrogen peroxide to wounds results in the formation of an active effervescent gas that dislodges particles of wound material and debris and, by removing degenerated tissue, eliminates the wound as a likely environment for bacterial breeding. Hydrogen peroxide also possesses compounds that are widely used as antiseptics. Because it is nontoxic, hydrogen peroxide may be used for cleansing mucous membranes. A diluted solution (50% water and 50% hydrogen peroxide) can be used for treating inflammatory conditions of the mouth and throat.

Antifungal Agents

Many medicinal agents on the market are designed to treat fungi, which are commonly found in and around athletic facilities. The three most common fungi are *Epidermophyton, Trichophyton,* and *Candida albicans.*

In recent years, there has been successful development and use of antifungal agents such as Terbinafine (Lamisil), ketoconazole (Nizoral), amphotericin B (Fungizone), and griseofulvin. Both ketoconazole and amphotericin B seem to be effective against deep-seated fungus infections such as those caused by *Candida albicans.* Ketoconazole, fluconazole, and griseofulvin, all of which can be administered orally, produce an effective fungistatic action against the specific fungus species of *Microsporum, Trichophyton,* and *Epidermophyton,* all of which are associated with common athlete's foot.[3] Given over a long period of time, griseofulvin becomes a functioning part of the cutaneous tissues, especially the skin, hair, and nails, producing a prolonged and continuous fungistatic action. Any patient taking an oral antifungal agent must be carefully monitored by a clinician. Terbinafine (Lamisil), miconazole (Micatin), clotrimazole (Lotrimin), and tolnaftate (Tinactin, which does not treat *Candida* infections) are topical medications for a superficial fungus infection caused by *Trichophyton* and other fungi.

Mechanical antiseptics, usually soaps that provide a cleansing and detergent action, remove pathogens from the skin.

Antibiotics

Antibiotics are bacteriostatic or bacteriocidal. Their useful action is primarily a result of their interfering with the necessary metabolic processes of pathogenic microorganisms.

In sports antibiotics are used by the physician as either topical dressings or systemic medications. The indiscriminate use of antibiotics can produce extreme hypersensitivity or idiosyncrasies and can prevent the development of natural immunity or resistance to subsequent infections. The use of any antibiotic must be carefully controlled by the physician, who selects the drug on the basis of the most desirable type of administration and the least amount of toxicity to the patient.

Antibiotics include penicillin, bacitracin, tetracycline, erythromycin, sulfonamides, and quinolones.

The antibiotics mentioned here are just a few of the many available. New types continue to be developed, mainly because, over a period of time, microorganisms often become resistant to a particular antibiotic, especially if it is indiscriminately used. Some of the more common antibiotics are penicillin, ephalosporins, bacitracin, quinolones, tetracycline, erythromycin, and the sulfonamides.[7]

Penicillins and Cephalosporins Penicillins and cephalosporins as prescription medications are probably the most important of the antibiotics; they are useful in a variety of skin and systemic infections. In general, penicillins and cephalosporins interfere with the metabolism of the bacteria.

Bacitracin Bacitracin has a broad spectrum of effectiveness as an antibacterial agent. Bacitracin plus polymixin (Polysporin) also has a broad spectrum of effectiveness as an antibacterial agent. Adding neomycin to the product (Neosporin) does not increase effectiveness, and some individuals are allergic to neomycin.

Tetracycline Tetracyclines consist of a wide group of antibiotics that have a broad antibacterial spectrum. Their application, which is usually oral, modifies the infection rather than eradicating it completely.

Erythromycin Erythromycin is most often used for streptococcal infection and Mycoplasma pneumoniae. It has the same general spectrum as penicillin and is a useful alternative in the penicillin-allergic patient.

Sulfonamides Sulfonamides are a group of synthetic antibiotics. In general, sulfonamides make pathogens vulnerable to phagocytes by inhibiting certain enzymatic actions.

Quinolones Quinolones are a relatively new group of antibiotics. They have a broad spectrum of activity. Patients taking these antibiotics must be carefully monitored for adverse effects.

Drugs for Asthma

17-2 *Critical Thinking* Exercise

A field hockey player has a recurrent breathing problem, especially during high-intensity fitness training. Since the weather has gotten warmer, her symptoms have gotten worse.

? What should the athletic trainer expect is wrong with this athlete, and how should her condition be managed?

Asthma is a chronic inflammatory lung disorder that is characterized by obstruction of the airways as a result of complex inflammatory processes, smooth muscle spasm, and hyperresponsiveness to a variety of stimuli.[31] Asthma triggers may include exercise, viral infection, animal exposure, dust mites, mold, air pollutants, weather, and NSAIDs as well as other drugs. The National Asthma Education and Prevention Program (NAEPP) has established international guidelines for the diagnosis and management of asthma.[32,45] The goals of asthma therapy are to prevent chronic and troublesome symptoms, maintain normal lung function and activity levels, prevent asthma exacerbations, provide optimal pharmacotherapy with minimal adverse effects, and meet athletes' expectation of and satisfaction with asthma care.[21]

Exercise-induced bronchospasm (EIB) is a limiting and disruptive experience. Any asthma patient may be subject to EIB. A bronchospastic event caused by loss of heat, water, or both from lungs during exercise or exertion, EIB results from hyperventilation of air that is cooler and dryer than that in the respiratory tract.[2] EIB may occur during or minutes after physical activity, reaches its peak in five to ten minutes after stopping the activity, and usually resolves in twenty to thirty minutes. In some asthma patients, exercise may be the only precipitating factor.

The athlete who has asthma must be monitored carefully. The NAEPP recommends measurements of the following: asthma signs and symptoms, pulmonary function (peak flow or spirometry), quality of life/functional status, history of asthma exacerbations, and pharmacotherapy. Table 17-6 identifies medications recommended in asthma management.

TABLE 17-6 Medications Recommended for the Management of Asthma

Long-Term Control	Quick Relief Medications
Inhaled corticosteroids	Short-acting beta 2 agonists
Beclomethasone (Beclovent, Vanceril)	Albuterol (Proventil, Ventolin)
Fluticasone propionate (Flovent)	Pirbuterol (Maxair)
Flunisolide (Aero-Bid)	Terbutaline (Brethaire)
Triamcinolone acetonide (Azmacort)	Anticholinergics
Budesanide (Pulmicort)	Ipratropium bromide (Atrovent)
Cromolyn (Intal)	Oral corticosteroids
Nedocromil (Tilade)	Methylprednisolone (Medrol)
Long-acting beta 2 agonists	Prednisolone (various generics)
Salmeterol (Serevent)	Prednisone (various generics)
Albuterol sustained-release (Proventil Repetabs)	
Formoterol (Foradil Aerolizer)	
Theophyllin (Theodur, Theolair-SR)	
Leukotriene modifiers	
Zafirlukast (Accolate)	
Zileuton (Zyflo)	
Montelukast (Singulair)	

Using an Inhaler

The use of inhalers by athletes who have asthma and/or exercise-induced bronchospasm is common. Portable, handheld inhalers are convenient in that they deliver medicine directly to the lungs very rapidly. A variety of inhalers have been developed to relieve or control asthma symptoms. The two most common devices used to deliver inhaled medication are *metered-dose inhalers* and *dry powder inhalers.* A metered-dose inhaler includes a pressurized canister with measured doses of medication inside. The athlete squeezes the top of the canister. The pressure within the canister converts the medication into a fine powder. The athlete places his or her lips on or near the inhaler's mouthpiece to inhale the mist. Using a metered-dose inhaler calls for coordinating two actions: squeezing the canister and inhaling the medication (Figure 17-1). Many individuals who use the metered-dose inhaler use it improperly; however, with careful and repeated instruction, more than 90 percent of people can use it correctly. Metered dose inhalers can use a spacer, which is a tube four to eight inches long that attaches to the inhaler that allows time to inhale more slowly. The spacer acts as a holding chamber that keeps medication from escaping into the air.

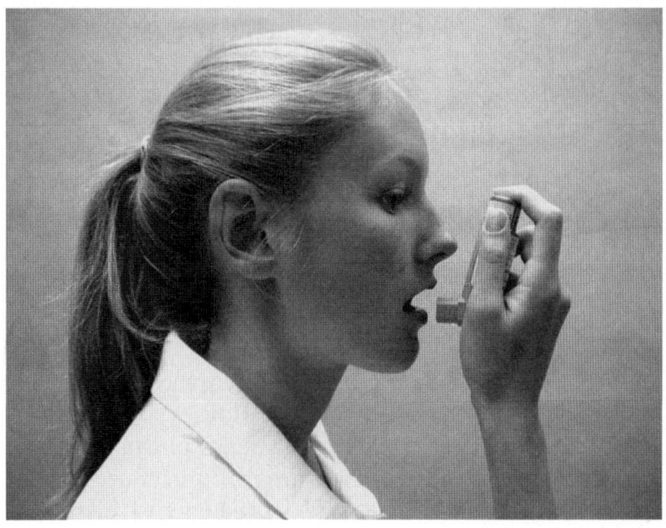

Figure 17-1

Inhalers are commonly used by athletes who have asthma.

Dry powder inhalers are not pressurized but rather release medication by rapidly inhaling. This type of inhaler requires the athlete to place the lips on the mouthpiece and inhale more rapidly than with a traditional metered-dose inhaler. Generally, dry powder inhalers are easier to use than the conventional pressurized metered-dose inhalers because hand-lung coordination is not required. Spacers can't be used with dry powder inhalers. A third device called a *nebulizer* is a compressor-driven pump that converts medication into a mist and is used by individuals who are not able to use an inhaler.

People with asthma can rely too much on inhaled bronchodilators. Because these fast-acting medications can relieve symptoms quickly, there is a tendency particularly among athletes to use them too often, leading to an overdose.

Using an inhaler is just one part of an asthma treatment plan. The treatment plan may also include checking lung function with a peak flow meter, eliminating asthma triggers, or exercising.

Drugs that Inhibit Pain and Inflammation

Pain Relievers

Drugs used to inhibit pain or inflammation include counterirritants and local anesthetics, narcotic analgesics, and nonnarcotic analgesics and antipyretics.

Controlling pain in an athlete can involve innumerable drugs and procedures, depending on the beliefs of the athletic trainer, coach, or physician. As discussed in Chapter 9, why pain is positively affected by certain methods is not clearly understood; however, some of the possible reasons are as follows:

- The excitatory effect of an individual impulse is depressed.
- An individual impulse is inhibited.
- The perceived impulse is decreased.
- Anxiety created by the pain or impending pain is decreased.

Counterirritants and Local Anesthetics

Counterirritants include spray coolants, alcohol, cold, menthol, and local anesthetics.

Analgesics give relief by causing a systemic and topical analgesia. Many chemical reactions on the skin can inhibit pain sensations by rapid evaporation, which causes a cooling action, or by counterirritating the skin. Irritating and counterirritating substances used in sports act as rubefacients (skin reddeners) and skin stimulants, although their popularity has decreased in recent years. Their application causes local increase in blood circulation, redness, and rise in skin temperature. Frequently mild pain can be reduced by a counterirritant, which produces a stimulus to the skin of such intensity that the athlete is no longer aware of the pain. Some examples of counterirritants include liniments, analgesic balms, heat, and cold.

Spray coolants Spray coolants, because of their rapid evaporation, act as topical anesthetics to the skin. Several commercial coolants are presently on the market. Chloromethane is one of the most popular spray coolants currently used in sports. Cooling results so quickly that superficial freezing takes place, inhibiting pain impulses for a short time. Athletic trainers disagree on the effectiveness of spray coolants. Some athletic trainers use them extensively for strains, sprains, and contusions. In most cases, spray coolants are useful only when other analgesics are not available.

Alcohol Alcohol evaporates rapidly when applied to the skin, causing a refreshingly cool effect that gives a temporary analgesia.

Menthol Menthol is an alcohol taken from mint oils and is principally used as a local analgesic, counterirritant, and antiseptic. In sports, menthol is used most often with a petroleum base for treating cold symptoms and in analgesic balms.

Cold Cold applications also immediately act to constrict blood vessels and to numb sensory nerve endings. Applications of ice packs or submersion of a part in ice water may completely anesthetize an area. If extreme cold is used, caution must be taken that tissue damage does not result.

Local anesthetics Local anesthetics are usually injected by a physician in and around injury sites for minor surgical procedures or to alleviate the pain of movement. Lydocaine hydrochloride is used extensively as a local anesthetic.

Narcotic Analgesics

Most narcotics used in medicine are derived directly from opium or are synthetic opiates. They depress pain impulses and the individual's respiratory center. The two most often used derivatives are codeine and morphine.

Narcotic analgesics include codeine, propoxyphene hydrochloride, morphine, and meperidine.

Codeine Codeine resembles morphine in its action but is less potent. Codeine is effective in combination with nonnarcotic analgesics. In small doses it is a cough suppressant found in many cough medicines.

Propoxyphene hydrochloride Propoxyphene hydrochloride (Darvon) is a mild analgesic narcotic that is slightly stronger than aspirin in its pain relief. It is not an antiinflammatory drug. It is addictive, and when combined with alcohol, tranquilizers, or other sedatives or depressants, it can be fatal.

Morphine Morphine depresses pain sensations to a greater extent than any other drug. It is also the most dangerous drug because of its ability to depress respiration and because of its habit-forming qualities. Morphine is never used in the following situations: before a diagnosis has been made by the physician; when the subject is unconscious; when there is a head injury; or when there is a decreased rate of breathing. It is never repeated within two hours.

Meperidine Meperidine (Demerol) is used as a substitute for morphine for the relief of mild or moderate pain and is effective only when given intravenously or intramuscularly.

Nonnarcotic Analgesics and Antipyretics

Nonnarcotic analgesics are those drugs designed to suppress all but the most severe pain, without the patient's losing consciousness. In most cases these drugs also act as antipyretics, regulating the temperature control centers.

Nonnarcotic analgesics include acetaminophen.

Acetaminophen Acetaminophen (Tylenol) is an effective analgesic and antipyretic but has no antiinflammatory activity. Because it does not irritate the gastrointestinal system, it is often a replacement for aspirin in noninflammatory conditions. Overingestion could lead to liver damage. Chronic heavy alcohol users may be at risk for liver damage when taking more than the recommended dose of acetaminophen.

Drugs to Reduce Inflammation

Sports physicians have a wide choice of drugs at their disposal for the treatment of inflammation. A great variety of OTC drugs also claim to deal effectively with inflammation of the musculoskeletal system. The problem of proper drug selection is tenuous, even for a physician, because new drugs are continually coming to the forefront. The situation is compounded by highly advertised OTC preparations. Any drug selection, especially drugs designed to treat the inflammatory process, must be effective, must be appropriate for the highly physical athlete, and must not create any adverse reactions.[4] These points are addressed by the following discussions of the more generally accepted antiinflammatory drugs.

Antiinflammatories include acetylsalicylic acid (aspirin), NSAIDs, and corticosteroids.

Acetylsalicylic Acid (Aspirin)

Aspirin is one of the most widely used analgesics, antiinflammatories, and antipyretics. It is also one of the most abused drugs in use today. A number of medications that have salicylates act in reducing pain, fever, and inflammation. Aspirin has been associated with various adverse reactions that are primarily centered in the gastrointestinal region. Those reactions include difficulty in food digestion (dyspepsia), nausea, vomiting, and gastric bleeding.

Overingestion of aspirin can lead to serious side effects. Adverse reactions to aspirin, especially in high doses, are ear ringing or buzzing (tinnitus) and dizziness. A major problem that can arise in individuals under eighteen years of age is Reye's syndrome. The administration of aspirin to a child during chicken pox or influenza can induce Reye's syndrome. Its etiology is unknown.

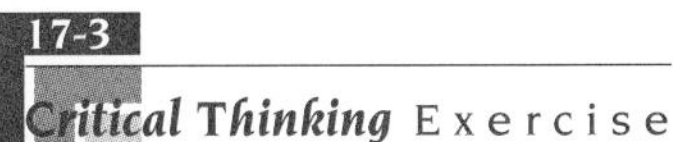

A golfer has an inflamed knee due to patellar tendonitis. He asks his athletic trainer what medication he should take for the pain.

? What medication should the athlete take for this purpose?

Severe allergic response resulting in an anaphylactic reaction can occur in individuals who have an intolerance to aspirin. Asthmatic patients may be at greater risk for allergic reactions to aspirin. Aspirin use should be avoided by athletes in contact sports since it prolongs blood clotting time.

Nonsteroidal Antiinflammatory Drugs

Nonsteroidal drugs have antiinflammatory, antipyretic, and analgesic properties.[46] They are strong inhibitors of prostaglandin synthesis and are effective for such chronic problems as rheumatoid arthritis and osteoarthritis.[3] Nonsteroidal antiinflammatory drugs (NSAIDs) are used primarily for reducing the pain, stiffness, swelling, redness, and fever associated with localized inflammation.[22] Their antiinflammatory capabilities are thought to be equal to those of aspirin; their advantages are fewer side effects and relatively longer duration of action. NSAIDs are effective for patients who cannot tolerate aspirin because of gastrointestinal distress associated with aspirin use. Even though NSAIDs have analgesic and antipyretic capabilities, they should not be used in place of aspirin or acetaminophen in cases of mild headache or increased body temperature. However, they can be used to relieve many other mild to moderately painful somatic conditions, such as menstrual cramps and soft-tissue injury. Table 17-7 lists the NSAIDs commonly used in treating athletes.

The NSAIDs can produce adverse reactions and should be used cautiously.[28a,54] Athletes who have aspirin allergy triad of nasal polyps, associated bronchospasm or asthma, and history of anaphylaxis should not receive any NSAID. The NSAIDs can cause gastrointestinal tract reactions, headache, dizziness, depression, tinnitus, and a variety of other systemic reactions. Taking ibuprofen with heavy alcohol use may increase the risk of stomach bleeding.

17-4

***Critical Thinking* Exercise**

A college-age softball player comes into the training room complaining of a headache and asks the athletic trainer to give her some ibuprofen to get rid of her headache.

? Is ibuprofen the most appropriate medication to use in this case?

TABLE 17-7 NSAIDs Frequently Used among Athletes

Drug/ Trade Name	Dosage Range (mg) and Frequency	Maximum Daily Dose (mg)
Celebrex	100–200 mg twice a day	200
Aspirin	325–650 mg every 4 hours	4,000
Voltaren	50–75 mg twice a day	200
Cataflam	50–75 mg twice a day	200
Dolobid	500–1,000 mg followed by 250–500 mg 2 to 3 times a day	1,500
Nalfon	300–600 mg 3 to 4 times a day	3,200
Motrin	400–800 mg 3 to 4 times a day	3,200
Indocin	5–150 mg a day in 3 to 4 divided doses	200
Orudis	75 mg 3 times a day or 50 mg 4 times a day	300
Ponstel	500 mg followed by 250 mg every 6 hours	1,000
Naprosyn	250–500 mg twice a day	1,250
Anaprox	550 mg followed by 275 mg every 6 to 8 hours	1,375
Feldene	20 mg per day	20
Clinoril	200 mg twice a day	400
Tolectin	400 mg 3 to 4 times a day	1,800
Relafen	1,000 mg once or twice a day	2,000
Ansaid	50–100 mg 2 to 3 times a day	300
Toradol	10 mg every 4 to 6 hours for pain; *Not to be used for more than 5 days*	40
Lodine	200–400 mg every 6 to 8 hours for pain	1,200
Mobic	7.5 mg once per day	15
Daypro	1,200 mg once per day	1,800
Bextra	10 mg once per day	40

Note: Prescription required for all except aspirin.

Corticosteroids

Corticosteroids, of which cortisone is the most common, are used primarily for chronic inflammation of musculoskeletal and joint regions. Cortisone is a synthetic glucocorticoid that is usually given orally or by injection. More caution is taken in the use of corticosteroids than was practiced in the past. Prolonged use of corticosteroids can produce the following serious complications:

- Fluid and electrolyte disturbances (e.g., water retention caused by excess sodium levels)
- Musculoskeletal and joint impairments (e.g., bone thinning and muscle and tendon weakness)
- Dermatological problems (e.g., delayed wound healing)
- Neurological impairments (e.g., vertigo, headache, convulsions)
- Endocrine dysfunctions (e.g., menstrual irregularities)
- Ophthalmic conditions (e.g., glaucoma)
- Metabolic impairments (e.g., negative nitrogen balance, muscle wasting)

Cortisone is primarily administered by injection. Other methods of administration are iontophoresis and phonophoresis (see Chapter 15). Studies have indicated that cortisone injected directly into tendons, ligaments, and joint spaces can lead to weakness and degeneration. Strenuous activity may predispose the treated part to rupturing. Tennis elbow and plantar fasciitis have benefited from corticosteroid treatment.

Drugs that Produce Skeletal Muscle Relaxation

Drugs that produce skeletal muscle relaxation include methocarbamol (Robaxin), and carisoprodol (Soma). There is growing speculation among physicians that, because centrally acting muscle relaxants also act as sedatives or tranquilizers on the higher brain centers, these drugs are less specific to muscle relaxation than was once believed. Another major side effect is that they cause drowsiness.

Muscle spasm and guarding accompany many musculoskeletal injuries. Elimination of spasm and guarding should facilitate programs of rehabilitation. In many situations, centrally acting oral muscle relaxants are used to reduce spasm and guarding. However, to date the efficacy of using muscle relaxants has not been substantiated, and they do not appear to be superior to analgesics or sedatives in either acute or chronic conditions.

Drugs Used to Treat Gastrointestinal Disorders

Disorders of the gastrointestinal tract include upset stomach or formation of gas because of food incompatibilities and acute or chronic hyperacidity, which leads to inflammation of the mucous membrane of the intestinal tract. Poor eating habits may lead to digestive tract problems such as diarrhea or constipation. Drugs that elicit responses within the gastrointestinal tract include antacids, antiemetics, carminatives, cathartics or laxatives, antidiarrheals, and histamine-2 blockers.

Drugs used to treat gastrointestinal disorders include antacids, antiemetics, carminatives, cathartics or laxatives, antidiarrheals and histamine-2 blockers.

Antacids

The primary function of an antacid is to neutralize acidity in the upper gastrointestinal tract by raising the pH and inhibiting the activity of the digestive enzyme pepsin, thus reducing its action on the gastric mucosal nerve endings. Antacids are effective not only for the relief of acid indigestion and heartburn but also in the treatment of peptic ulcer. Antacids available in the market possess a wide range of acid-neutralizing capabilities and side effects.

One of the most commonly used antacid preparations is sodium bicarbonate, or baking soda. Other antacids include alkaline salts, which again neutralize hyperacidity but are not easily absorbed in the blood. Ingestion of antacids containing magnesium tends to have a laxative effect. Those containing aluminum or calcium seem to

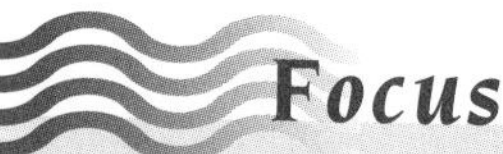

Protocols for the use of over-the-counter drugs for athletic trainers

The athletic trainer is often responsible for the initial screening of athletes who have various illnesses or injuries. Frequently, the athletic trainer must make decisions regarding the appropriate use of over-the-counter medications for athletes. Subjective findings such as onset, duration, medication taken, and known allergies must be included in the screening evaluation.

The following protocols should be viewed as guidelines to the disposition of the athlete. The protocols are aimed at clarifying the use of over-the-counter drugs in the treatment of common problems encountered by the athletic trainer while covering or traveling with a team. These guidelines do not cover every situation the athletic trainer encounters in assessing and managing the athlete's physical problems. Therefore, physician consultation is recommended wherever there is uncertainty in making a decision regarding the appropriate care of the athlete.

Existing Illness or Injury	Appropriate Treatment Protocol
Temperature	
Greater than or equal to 102° F orally	Consult physician ASAP.
Less than 102° F but more than 99.5° F orally	Patient may be given acetaminophen. *See Acetaminophen Administration Protocol.* Limit exercise of athlete. Do not allow participation in practice. If fever decreases to less than 99.5° the athlete may participate in practice. If athlete is to be involved in an intercollegiate event, consult with a physician concerning participation.
Less than or equal to 99.5° F orally	Follow management guidelines for fever less than 102° but allow athlete to practice and/or compete.
Throat	
History Sore throat No fever No chills	Advise saline gargles (½ tsp. salt in a glass of warm water). Patient may also be given Cepastat®/Chloraseptic® throat lozenges. Before administering determine: Is the patient allergic to Cepastat®/Chloraseptic® (phenol containing) lozenges? If yes, do not administer.
Sore throat Fever	Determine temperature. If fever, manage as outlined in temperature protocol and consult physician ASAP.
Sore throat and/or fever and/or swollen glands	Consult physician ASAP.
Nose	
Watery discharge	Patient may be given pseudoephedrine (Sudafed®) tablets. *See Pseudoephedrine Administration Protocol.*
Nasal congestion	Patient may be given oxymetazoline HCl (Afrin®) nasal spray. *See Oxymetazoline Administration Protocol.*
Chest	
Cough Dry hacking or clear mucoid sputum	You may administer Robitussin DMR® (generic guaifenesin with dextromethorphan). Before administering determine: Is the patient going to be involved in practice or game within 4 hours from administration of medication? If yes, do not give Robitussin DM®. If indicated, you may administer one dose, 10 ml (2 teaspoonfuls). Inform the patient that drowsiness may occur. Repeat doses may be administered every 6 hours. Push fluids, encourage patient to drink as much as possible.

Continued

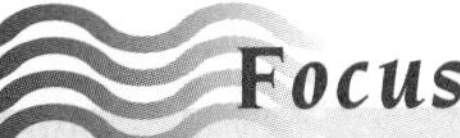

Protocols for the use of over-the-counter drugs for athletic trainers—continued

Chest—continued	
Green or rusty sputum	Consult physician ASAP.
Severe, persistent cough	Consult physician ASAP.
Ears	
Discomfort due to ears popping	Patient may be given pseudoephedrine (Sudafed®) tablets and/or oxymetazoline HCl (Afrin®) nasal spray. *See Pseudoephedrine Administration Protocol and/or Oxymetazoline Protocol*
Earache (or external otitis)	Patient may be given acetaminophen. Consult physician ASAP. *See Acetaminophen Administration Protocol.*
Recurrent earache	Consult physician ASAP.
Prevention of Motion Sickness	
Complaint: History of nausea, dizziness, and/or vomiting associated with travel	Patient may be given dimenhydrinate (Dramamine®) or diphenhydramine (Benadryl®). Before administering, determine: Is the patient sensitive or allergic to Dramamine®, Benadryl® or any other antihistamine? If yes, do not administer. Has the patient taken any other antihistamines (e.g. Actifed®, Chlor-Trimeton®, various cold medications) or other medications that cause sedation, within the last 6 hours? If yes, do not administer. Does the patient have asthma, glaucoma, or enlargement of the prostate gland? If yes, do not administer. Is the patient going to be involved in practice or game within 4 hours from administration of medication? If yes, do not administer. Administer Dramamine® or Benadryl® dose based on body weight, 30 to 60 minutes before departure time: Under 125 lbs: one Dramamine® 50 mg tablet. Over 125 lbs: two Dramamine 50 mg tablets Benadryl® dose: Under 125 lbs: one 25 mg capsule. Over 125 lbs: two 25 mg capsules. Inform the patient that drowsiness may occur for 4–6 hours after taking this medication. Avoid alcoholic beverages. Avoid driving for 6 hours after taking. If travelling time is extended, another dose may be administered 6 hours after the first dose.
Nausea, Vomiting	
Prolonged and severe	Consult physician ASAP.
Nausea, Gastric Upset, Heartburn, Butterflies in the Stomach, Acid Indigestion	
Associated with dietary indiscretion or tension	You may administer an antacid as a single dose, as defined by label of particular antacid (e.g. Riopan®, Gelusil®, Maalox®, Pepto Bismol®, Titralac®), or a histamine (H_2) antagonist (Pepcid AC®, Tagamet HB®, Axid A®, Zantac 75®). *See histamine H2 antagonist protocol. Pepto Bismol® warning: Contains salicylates. Do not give to children or teenagers who have or are recovering from chicken pox or flu because of the risk of Reye's syndrome. Do not use this product with aspirin.*

Continued

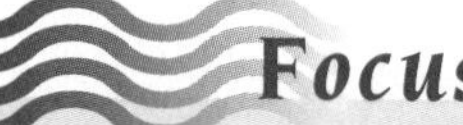

Protocols for the use of over-the-counter drugs for athletic trainers—continued

Nausea, Gastric Upset, Heartburn, Butterflies in the Stomach, Acid Indigestion—continued

Associated with abdominal or chest pain	Consult physician ASAP.
Vomiting, nausea—no severe distress	Monitor symptoms. Patient may be given dimenhydrinate (Dramamine®) or diphenhydramine (Benadryl®) orally. Same as instructions and precautions under motion sickness.
Vomiting: projectile, coffee ground, febrile	Consult physician ASAP.
Diarrhea	
Associated with abdominal pain or tenderness and/or dehydration, bloody stools, febrile, recurrent diarrhea	Consult physician ASAP.
Frequent loose stools not associated with any of the above signs or symptoms	Encourage clear liquid diet. Encourage avoidance of dairy products and high-fat foods for 24 hours. (BART diet—bananas, apples, rice, toast). If it persists consult physician ASAP. Patient may be given loperamide (Imodium A-D®). Before administering, determine: How long has patient had diarrhea? If longer than 24 hours, see physician. You may administer one dose (2 caplets) of loperamide (Immodium A-D® 2 mg per caplet). One caplet may be administered after each loose stool not to exceed 8 mg (4 caplets) per 24 hours. Inform the patient that dizziness or drowsiness may occur within 12 hours after taking this medication. Avoid alcoholic beverages. Use caution while driving or performing tasks requiring alertness.
Constipation	
Prolonged or severe abdominal pain or tenderness, nausea or vomiting	Consult physician ASAP.
Discomfort associated with dietary change or decreased fluid intake	You may administer milk of magnesia 30 ml as a single dose. Before administering determine: Does the patient have chronic renal disease? If yes, do not administer. Recommend increased fluid intake, increased intake of fruits, bulk vegetables, or cereals.
Headache	
Pain associated with elevated BP, temperature elevation, blurred vision, nausea, vomiting, or history of migraine	Consult physician ASAP.
Pain across forehead (Mild headache)	Patient may be given acetaminophen or NSAID. *See Acetaminophen Administration or NSAID Administration Protocols.*

Continued

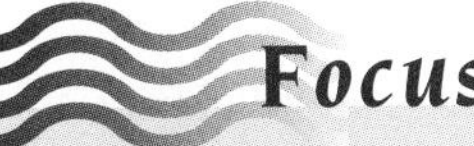

Protocols for the use of over-the-counter drugs for athletic trainers—continued

Headache—continued	
Tension headache, occipital pain	Patient may be given acetaminophen. *See Acetaminophen Administration Protocol.*
Pain in antrum or forehead associated with sinus or nasal congestion	Patient may be given pseudoephedrine (Sudafed®) tablets and acetaminophen. *See protocols for Pseudoephedrine and Acetaminophen Administration.*
Musculoskeletal Injuries	
Deformity	Consult physician ASAP.
Localized pain and tenderness, impaired range of motion	First aid to part as soon as possible: Ice Compression—Ace bandage Elevation Protection—crutches or sling and/or splint
Pain with swelling discoloration, no impaired movement or localized tenderness	If this injury interferes with the patient's normal activities, consult a physician within 24 hours. Patient may be given acetaminophen or NSAID. *See Acetaminophen Administration or NSAID Administration Protocols.*
Skin	
Localized or generalized rash accompanied by elevated temperature, enlarged lymph nodes, sore throat, stiff neck, infected skin lesion, dyspnea, wheezing	Consult physician ASAP.
Mild, localized, nonvesicular skin eruptions accompanied by pruritis	Hydrocortisone 1.0% cream may be applied. Before administering, determine: Is the patient taking any medication? If yes, do not administer. Refer to physician. Are eyes or any large area of the body involved? If yes, do not administer. Refer to physician. Is there any evidence of lice infestation? The cream may be repeated every 6 hours if needed. Do not use more than 3 times daily.
Abrasions	Control bleeding. Clean with antibacterial soap and water. Apply appropriate dressing and antibiotic ointment. Monitor for signs of infection. Dressing may be changed 2–3 times a day if needed.
Localized erythema due to ultraviolet rays	Advise application of compresses soaked in a solution of cold water.

Continued

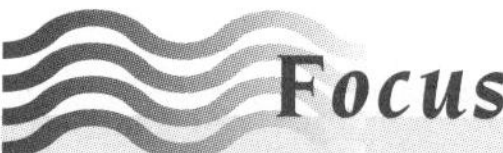

Protocols for the use of over-the-counter drugs for athletic trainers—continued

Skin—continued

Jock itch or athlete's foot	Advise 10–15 minute application of compresses soaked in cool water to relieve intense itching. Patient may be given terbinafine (Lomisil) or miconazole (Micatin®) cream topically. Before administering, determine: Is the patient sensitive or allergic to miconazole or terbinafine? If yes, do not administer. Consult physician ASAP. Is the patient receiving other types of treatment for rash in same area? If yes, do not administer. Consult physician ASAP. Instruct patient to wash and dry area of rash, and then apply ¼–½ inch ribbon of cream. Give patient the cream on a clean gauze pad and rub gently on the infected area. Spread evenly and thinly over rash. The dose may be repeated in 8–12 hours (twice a day). Consult physician within 24 hours.
Skin Wounds	
Lacerations	Control bleeding. Cleanse area with antibacterial soap and water. Apply steristrips. Consult physician immediately if there is any question about the necessity for suturing.
Extensive lacerations or other severe skin wounds	Control bleeding. Protect area with dressing. Refer to physician immediately.
Wound Infection	
Febrile, marked cellulitis, red streaks, tender or enlarged nodes	Consult physician ASAP.
Localized inflammation, afebrile, absence of nodes and streaks	Warm soaks to affected area. Consult physician ASAP.
Burns	
1st degree erythema of skin, limited area	Apply cold compresses to affected area. Dressing is not necessary on 1st degree burns. If less than 45 minutes have elapsed since burn injury, clean gently with soap and water. Patient may be given acetaminophen. *See Acetaminophen Administration Protocol.*
1st degree with extensive involvement over body	Consult physician ASAP.
2nd degree erythema with blistering	Consult physician ASAP.
3rd degree pearly white appearance of affected area, no pain	Consult physician ASAP.

Continued

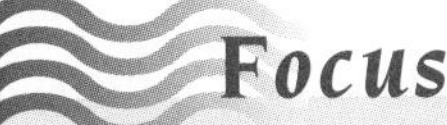

Protocols for the use of over-the-counter drugs for athletic trainers—continued

Allergies

Athlete with known seasonal allergies who forgot to bring own medication	Patient may be given 10 mg tablet of loratidine (Claritin). Before administering determine: Is the patient sensitive to loratidine? If yes, do not administer. Consult physician ASAP. Does the patient have liver or kidney disease? If yes, do not administer. Consult physician ASAP. Has the patient taken any other antihistamines (e.g. Chlorpheniramine, Dramamine®, various cold medications) or other medications that cause drowsiness within the last 6 hours? If yes, do not administer. Consult physician ASAP. You may administer l dose of loratidine (10 mg) every 24 hours. Avoid alcoholic beverages. Contact physician if symptoms do not abate.

Contact Lens Care

Note: There are 3 types of contact lenses: hard, gas permeable, soft

Solutions are labeled for use with a particular type of lens and should not be used for any other type of lens.

Do not use solutions preserved with thimersol or chlorhexidine because of possible allergy or irritation.

Lens needs rinsing/wetting before insertion	Hard lens: use all-purpose wetting/soaking solution (e.g., Wet-N-Soak®). Gas permeable lens: use all-purpose wetting/soaking solution (e.g., Wet-N-Soak®). Soft lens: use rinsing/soaking solution (e.g., Soft Mate ps®).
Lens needs soaking/storage	Hard lens: use all-purpose wetting/soaking solution (e.g., Wet-N-Soak®). Gas permeable lens: use all-purpose wetting/soaking solution (e.g., Wet-N-Soak®). Soft lens: use rinsing/soaking solution (e.g., Soft Mate ps®).
Lens needs cleaning	Hard lens: use cleaning solution (e.g., EasyClean®). Gas permeable lens: use cleaning solution (e.g., Easy Clean®). Soft lens: use cleaning solution (e.g., Lens Plus Daily Cleaner®).

Eye Care

Foreign body—minor: sand, eyelash, etc.	Use eye wash irrigation solution (Dacriose®).
Irritation—minor	Use artificial tears. Do not use with contact lens in eye.
Severe irritation, foreign body not easily removed, trauma	Consult physician ASAP.

Red Eye

Only one eye affected	Consult physician ASAP.
Change in vision	Consult physician ASAP.

Continued

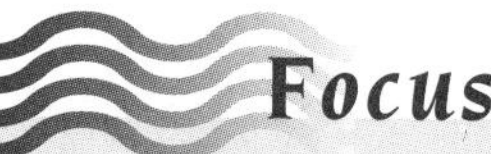

Protocols for the use of over-the-counter drugs for athletic trainers—continued

Red Eye—continued

Pain in eye	Consult physician ASAP.
Sensitivity to light	Consult physician ASAP.
Thick discharge from eye, especially with lids sealed shut in morning	Consult physician ASAP.
Patient wears contacts	Consult physician ASAP.
Redness, tearing, both eyes itch	1. Apply cold compresses. 2. Instill 1–2 drops of antihistamine/decongestant eye drop (e.g., Vasocon-A®) into each eye 4 times a day. (Do not use one bottle for more than one patient.) 3. If condition does not improve or worsens, consult physician ASAP. 4. If condition has not improved in 24 hours or persists for more than 48 hours, consult physician ASAP.
Redness, tearing, both eyes itch in patient with known allergies who forgot to bring own medication	1. Apply cold compresses. 2. Instill 1–2 drops of antihistamine/decongestant eye drop (e.g., Vasocon-A®) into each eye 4 times a day. (Do not use one bottle for more than one patient.) 3. See also Allergies Treatment Protocol 4. See #4 above.

Administration protocols for common over-the-counter drugs used in sports medicine

Acetaminophen protocol (Tylenol®)

Before *administering,* determine:

Is the patient allergic to acetaminophen? If yes, do not give acetaminophen.

You may *administer* acetaminophen 325 mg, two tablets. Repeat doses may be *administered* every 4 hours if needed. If *dispensing* occurs, use labeled 2/pack only. Patient instructions must accompany *dispensing.* The maximum dose must not exceed 4 gms (4,000 mg) in 24 hours.

Pseudoephedrine protocol (Sudafed®)

Before *administering,* determine:

Is the patient allergic or sensitive to pseudoephedrine? If yes, do not give pseudoephedrine.

Does the patient have high blood pressure, heart disease, diabetes, urinary retention, glaucoma, or thyroid disease? If yes, do not give pseudoephedrine.

Does the patient have problems with sweating? If yes, do not give pseudoephedrine.

Do not administer 4 hours before practice or game.

Do not administer if patient is involved in postseason play.

You may *administer* pseudoephedrine (Sudafed®) 30 mg, two tablets. Repeat doses may be *administered* every 6 hours up to 4 times a day. If *dispensing* occurs, use labeled 2/pack only. Patient instructions must accompany *dispensing.*

Oxymetazoline protocol (Afrin®)

Before *administering,* determine:

Is the patient allergic or sensitive to Afrin® or Otrivin®? If yes, do not administer.

Does the patient react unusually to nose sprays or drops? If yes, do not administer.

You may *administer* 2–3 sprays of oxymetazoline (Afrin®) 0.05% nasal spray into each nostril. Repeat doses may be administered every 12 hours. (The container can be marked with the patient's name and maintained by the trainer for repeat administration or dispensed to the patient. Patient instructions must accompany *dispensing.*)

Continued

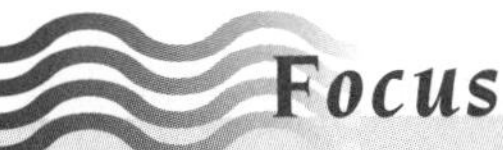

Protocols for the use of over-the-counter drugs for athletic trainers—continued

Oxymetazoline protocol (Afrin®)—continued

Do not use the same container for different patients.

Do not use for more than three days without MD supervision.

Use small package sizes to reduce risk of overuse/rebound congestion.

NSAID Protocol (ibuprofen: Advil®, naproxen sodium: Aleve®, ketoprofen: Orudis KT®, Actron®)

Before *administering,* determine:

Is the patient allergic to aspirin, e.g. asthma, swelling, shock or hives associated with aspirin use? If yes, do not give ibuprofen because even though ibuprofen contains no aspirin or salicylates, cross reactions may occur in patients allergic to aspirin.

Does the patient have renal disease or gastrointestinal ulcerations? If yes, do not administer ibuprofen.

You may *administer* ibuprofen 200 mg (Advil®) one or two tablets. Repeat doses may be *administered* every 6 hours if needed. Do not exceed 6 tablets in a 24-hour period without consulting an MD. Do not administer if patient is less than 12 years of age.

or

You may *administer* naproxen sodium 220 mg (Aleve®) one tablet every 8 to 12 hours or two tablets to start followed by 1 tablet 12 hours later. Do not exceed 3 tablets in a 24-hour period without consulting a physician. Do not administer if patient is less than 12 years of age.

or

You may *administer* ketoprofen 12.5 mg (Orutis KT®, Actron®) one tablet or caplet every 4 to 6 hours if needed. If pain or fever persists after one hour, one more 12.5 mg tablet or caplet may be given. Do not exceed 6 tablets or caplets in a 24-hour period without consulting a physician. Do not administer if the patient is less than 16 years of age.

The patient should take the NSAID with a full glass of water and food if occasional and mild heartburn, upset stomach, or mild stomach pain occurs. Consult MD if these symptoms are more than mild or persist. Discontinue drug if patient experiences skin rash, itching, dark, tarry stools, visual disturbances, dark urine, or persistent headache. Instruct patient to avoid concurrent aspirin or alcoholic beverages.

Histamine H2 Antagonist Protocol (ranitidine: Zantac 75®, nizatidine: Axid AR®, famotidine: Pepsid AC®, cimetidine: Tagamet-HB®)

Before *administering,* determine:

Is the patient less than 12 years of age? If yes, do not give H_2 antagonist.

Does the patient have difficulty swallowing or persistent abdominal pain? If yes, do not give H_2 antagonist.

You may *administer* ranitidine (Zantac 75®) one 75 mg tablet with water up to two times a day. Do not administer more than 2 tablets in a 24-hour period.

or

You may *administer* nizatidine (Axid AR®) one 75 mg tablet with water up to two times a day. Do not administer more that two tablets in a 24-hour period.

or

You may *administer* famotidine (Pepsid AC®) one 10 mg tablet with water up to two times a day. Do not administer more than 2 tablets in a 24-hour period.

or

You may *administer* cimetidine (Tagamet-HB®) one 10 mg tablet with water up to two times a day. Do not administer more than two tablets in a 24-hour period. Do not administer cimetidine if the patient is taking phenytoin (Dilantin®) or theophyllin (Theodur®).

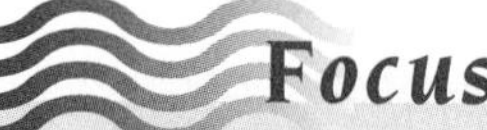

Identifying the substance abuser

- The following are signs of drug abuse:
- Sudden personality changes
- Severe mood swings
- Changing peer groups
- Decreased interest in extracurricular and leisure activities
- Worsening grades
- Disregard for household chores and curfews
- Feeling of depression most of the time
- Breakdown in personal hygiene habits
- Increased sleep and decreased eating
- Smell of alcohol or marijuana on clothes and skin
- Sudden weight loss
- Lying, cheating, stealing
- Arrests for drunk driving or for possessing illegal substances
- Truancies from school
- Frequent loss or change of jobs
- Defensiveness at the mention of drugs or alcohol
- Increased isolation (spends time in room)
- Deteriorating family relationship
- Drug paraphernalia (needles, empty bottles, etc.)
- Observations by others about negative behavior
- Signs of intoxication
- Missed appointments
- Falling asleep in class or at work
- Financial problems
- Missed assignments or deadlines
- Diminished productivity

substance abuse in the athletic population and should be able to recognize signs that may indicate when an athlete is engaging in substance abuse (*Focus Box:* "Identifying the substance abuser").

Performance-Enhancing Substances (Ergogenic Aids)

Ergogenic aid is a term used to describe any method, legal or illegal, used to enhance athletic performance.[55] Athletic trainers should have a primary concern about the use of various pharmacological agents by athletes for enhancing performance. NATA has prepared an official statement on this topic (*Focus Box:* "NATA Official Statement on Drug and Performance Enhancement Supplement Use in Athletics").

Stimulants

The intention of the athlete when he or she ingests a stimulant may be to increase alertness, reduce fatigue, or in some instances, increase competitiveness and even hostility. Some athletes respond to stimulants with a loss of judgment that may lead to personal injury or injury to others.

Two major categories of stimulants are psychomotor-stimulant drugs and adrenergic (sympathomimetic) drugs. Psychomotor stimulants are of two general types: amphetamines (e.g., methamphetamine) and nonamphetamines (e.g., methylphenidate and cocaine). The major actions of psychomotor stimulants result from the rapid turnover of catecholamines, which have a strong effect on the nervous and cardiovascular systems, metabolic rates, temperature, and smooth muscle.

Sympathomimetic drugs act directly on adrenergic receptors, or those that release catecholamines (i.e., epinephrine and norepinephrine) from nerve endings, and thus act indirectly on catecholamines. Ephedrine is an example of this type of drug and

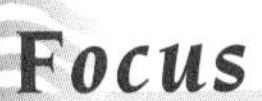

NATA Official Statement on Drug and Performance Enhancement Supplement Use in Athletics

Members of the National Athletic Trainers' Association are on the front line in the battle against drug use and abuse in athletics. Athletic trainers know first hand the negative effects steroids and performance enhancing drugs can have on healthy athletes. Certified athletic trainers (ATCs) are medical professionals who specialize in the prevention, assessment, treatment and rehabilitation of injuries and illnesses that occur to athletes and physically active people. Athletic trainers in the professional, college/university and high school settings often are the first to identify athletes with potential drug abuse problems. ATCs are involved in research on the effects of steroids and performance enhancing drugs. In addition, they provide drug education and are involved in the drug testing process.

The National Athletic Trainers' Association and its members are working to eliminate drug use and abuse from athletics and schools.

can, in high doses, cause mental stimulation and increased blood flow. As a result, it may also cause elevated blood pressure and headache, increased and irregular heartbeat, anxiety, and tremors.

Amphetamines and cocaine are the psychomotor drugs most commonly used in sports. Cocaine is discussed in the section on recreational drug abuse in this chapter. Sympathomimetic drugs present an extremely difficult problem in sports medicine because they are commonly found in cold remedies.[14] The U.S. Olympic Committee (USOC) has approved some substances to be used by asthmatics who develop exercise-induced bronchospasms. These substances are selective B_2 agonists and consist ofalbuterol (Proventil), salbutamol (Serevent), and terbutaline (in its aerosol form). Before an athlete engages in Olympic competition, his or her team physician must notify the USOC Medical Subcommission in writing about the athlete's use of these drugs.[14]

Common ergogenic aids include stimulants, beta blockers, narcotic analgesics, diuretics, anabolic steroids, human growth hormone, and blood doping.

Amphetamines Amphetamines are synthetic alkaloids that are extremely powerful and dangerous drugs. They may be injected, inhaled, or taken as tablets. Amphetamines are among the most abused of those drugs used for the goal of enhancing sports performance. In ordinary doses, amphetamines can produce euphoria, with an increased sense of well-being and heightened mental activity, until fatigue sets in (from lack of sleep), accompanied by nervousness, insomnia, and anorexia. In high doses, amphetamines reduce mental activity and impair the performance of complicated motor skills. The athlete's behavior may become irrational. The chronic user may be "hung up," that is, stuck in a repetitious behavioral sequence. This perseveration may last for hours and become increasingly more irrational. The long-term or even short-term use of amphetamines can lead to amphetamine psychosis, manifested by auditory and visual hallucinations and paranoid delusions. Physiologically, high doses of amphetamines can cause mydriasis (abnormal pupillary dilation), increased blood pressure, hyperreflexia (increased reflex action), and hyperthermia.

Athletes believe that amphetamines improve sports performance by promoting quickness and endurance, delaying fatigue, and increasing confidence, thereby causing increased aggressiveness. Studies indicate that there is no improvement in performance but there is an increased risk of injury, exhaustion, and circulatory collapse.[12]

17-5

Critical Thinking **Exercise**

A lacrosse player comes into the athletic trainer's office very concerned over the fact that she has been chosen for a random drug test later that afternoon. She met her boyfriend for lunch and she drank a large cup of espresso. Now she is concerned that she will test positive for a performance-enhancing drug.

? What should the athletic trainer tell the athlete to reduce her anxiety about the drug test?

Caffeine Caffeine is found in coffee, tea, cocoa, and cola and is readily absorbed into the body (Table 17-9).[36] Caffeine is a central nervous system stimulant and diuretic and also stimulates gastric secretion. One cup of coffee can contain from 100 to 150 milligrams of caffeine. In moderation, caffeine causes stimulation of the cerebral cortex and medullar centers, resulting in wakefulness and mental alertness. In larger amounts and in individuals who ingest caffeine daily, it raises blood pressure,

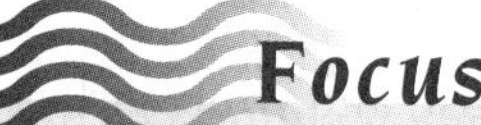

Contacting the poison control center

Each state has at least one and usually several poison control centers located in different regions of the state. The number of the poison control center is usually clearly accessible in the front of the phone book. The rescue squad can also contact the poison control center directly. The following information is necessary when communicating with the poison control center:

- Name and location of the person making the call
- Name and age of the person who has taken the medication
- Name and amount of the drug taken (if known)
- Time the drug was taken
- Signs and symptoms associated with the overdose, including vital signs

The experts at the poison control center will provide instructions for immediate care of the individual until the rescue squad arrives.

A website at Fast Health, http://www.fasthealth.com/poison/nc.php provides a list of phone numbers for all the poison control centers in each state.

The athletic trainer should immediately insist that the rescue squad be called by dialing 911. In cases of suspected drug overdose, the athletic trainer should also insist that the poison control center be contacted. *Focus Box:* "Contacting the poison control center" tells how the poison control center can be contacted. It is imperative that the athletic trainer follow up to make certain that the right steps have been taken either by telephone or by actually going to deal with the athlete in person.

DRUG TESTING IN ATHLETES

Both the NCAA and the USOC conduct drug testing programs.

Drug testing of athletes for the purpose of identifying individuals who may have some problems with drug abuse is commonplace.[14] Both the NCAA and the USOC routinely conduct drug testing.[32,53] The legality and ethics of testing only those individuals involved with sports are still open to debate.[19,30] The pattern of drug usage among athletes may simply reflect that of our society in general. Great care must be taken that an athlete's personal rights are not violated.[48]

Drug testing began with the 1968 Olympic Games. In 1985 the USOC began drug testing athletes involved in both national and international competitions. In January 1986 the member institutions of the NCAA voted overwhelmingly to expand the NCAA drug education program to include mandatory random drug testing in specific sports throughout the year and during and after NCAA championship events.[32] The major goals of both organizations are to protect the health of athletes and to help ensure that competition is fair and equitable.[14]

Most professional teams and many individual colleges and universities have initiated drug testing programs for their athletes.[43] Unfortunately, drug testing is rarely done at the high school level because of cost constraints.

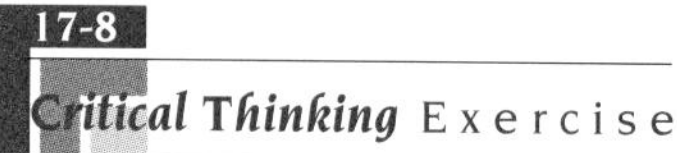

17-8 Critical Thinking Exercise

A university has recently implemented a drug testing program for athletes in all sports. The athletic director has decided that the athletic trainer is perhaps the best individual to supervise the program.

? Should the athletic trainer be willing to take on the additional responsibilities of overseeing the drug testing program for the athletes?

The Drug Test

There are some slight differences between NCAA and USOC drug testing procedures and protocols. Most of these differences have to do with how the athletes are selected for random tests. The NCAA requires all athletes to sign a consent form agreeing to participate in the drug testing program throughout the year. The USOC tests athletes on a random basis throughout the year and tests all athletes before a USOC-sanctioned competition.[14]

During the drug test, the athlete must first provide positive identification. Then, under direct observation, the athlete must urinate into two separate specimen bottles (labeled A and B), which are sealed and submitted to an official NCAA or USOC testing laboratory for analysis. In the laboratory, specimen A is used for both screening and confirmation tests. A confirmation test uses analysis techniques that are more sensitive and accurate should a positive test result occur during the screening test. Specimen B is used only when a reconfirmation is needed for a positive test of specimen A. The athlete is then notified of a positive test result and becomes subject to sanctions from either the NCAA or the USOC.[14]

Sanctions for Positive Tests

For a first-time positive test, the NCAA will declare the athlete ineligible for all regular and postseason competitions for a minimum of one year. During that year the athlete may be retested at any time. The athlete must be retested with a negative result and have eligibility restored before he or she may return to competition. Additional positive tests can result in a lifetime disqualification from NCAA competition.[32]

The USOC sanctions range from three to twenty-four months of disqualification, depending on the drug, for a first-time violation, and a minimum of two years to a lifetime ban for subsequent positive tests.[53]

Banned Substances

Both the NCAA and the USOC have established lists of substances that are banned from use by athletes. The lists include performance-enhancing drugs and street, or recreational, drugs as well as many OTC and prescription drugs.

The list of drugs banned by either the NCAA or the USOC or by both is extensive and includes approximately 4,600 separate medications.[14] The list of drugs banned by the USOC is considerably more extensive than the NCAA list because the USOC is subject to internationally used drugs banned by the International Olympic Committee (IOC). *Focus Box:* "Banned drugs—common ground" summarizes the various categories of drugs that appear on the banned lists for the NCAA and the USOC.[14]

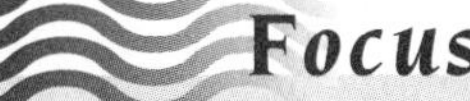

Focus

Banned drugs—common ground

Drugs banned by both NCAA and USOC

Anabolic steroids
Diuretics
Beta blockers (used to lower blood pressure, decrease heart rate, decrease cardiac arrythmias)
Peptide hormones (human growth hormone, corticotropin, erythropoietin, human chorionic gonadotropin, etc.)
Stimulants* (amphetamines, cocaine, and anorexiants)
Caffeine (limited ingestion permits up to 12 μg/ml USOC and 15 μg/ml NCAA)
Blood doping

Drugs banned by USOC only

Narcotic analgesics (codeine is permitted)
Skeletal muscle relaxants (banned for modern pentathlon and biathlon events only)
Cough and cold decongestants (sympathomimetic drugs)
Injectable anesthetics (acceptable with prior written permission)
Corticosteroids (intramuscular, intravenous, rectal, and oral use is banned; most topical and inhaled use is permitted with written permission)

Drugs banned by NCAA only†

Substances that contain alcohol (banned for riflery)
Street drugs (heroin and marijuana)

Modified from Fuentes R: *Athletic drug reference,* Durham, NC, 1996, Galaxo.

*USOC permits inhaled albuterol and terbutaline with prior written permission; NCAA permits all inhalants.

†USOC reserves the right to test for alcohol and street drugs with possible sanctions for positive tests.

The athletic trainer working with athletes who may be tested for drug use by the NCAA or with world-class or Olympic athletes governed by the USOC should be thoroughly familiar with the list of banned drugs.[12] Having an athlete disqualified because of the indiscriminate use of some prescription or OTC medication would be most unfortunate. Table 17-10 list those drugs currently banned by the NCAA.

TABLE 17-10 NCAA Banned Drug Classes

The following is a list of banned drug classes, with examples of substances under each class:

(a) Stimulants:

amiphenazole
amphetamine
bemigride
benzphetamine
bromantan
Caffeine[1] (guarana)
chlorphentermine
cocaine
cropropamide
crothetamide
diethylpropion
dimethylamphetamine
doxapram
ephedrine (ephedra, ma huang)
ethamivan
ethylamphetamine
fencamfamine
meclofenoxate
methamphetamine
methylene-dioxymethamphetamine (MDMA, Ecstasy)
methylphenidate
nikethamide
pemoline
pentetrazol
phendimetrazine
phenmetrazine
phentermine
phenylephrine
phenylpropanolamine (ppa) effective August 2003
picrotoxine
pipradol
prolintane
strychnine
synephrine (citrus, aurantium, zhi shi, bitter orange) and related compounds

(b) Anabolic Agents:

anabolic steroids
androstenediol
androstenedione
boldenone
clenbuterol
clostebol
dehydrochlormethyl-testosterone
dehydroepiandrosterone (DHEA)
dihydrotestosterone (DHT)
dromostanolone
fluoxymesterone
mesterolone
methandienone
methenolone
methyltestosterone
nandrolone
norandrostenediol
norandrostenedione
norethandrolone
oxandrolone
oxymesterone
oxymetholone
stanozolol
testosterone[2] and related compounds
other anabolic agents

(c) Substances Banned for Specific Sports:

Rifle:
alcohol
atenolol
metoprolol
nadolol
pindolol
propranolol
timolol
and related compounds

(d) Diuretics:

acetazolamide
bendroflumethiazide
benzthiazide
bumetanide
chlorothiazide
chlorthalidone
ethacrynic acid
flumethiazide
furosemide
hydrochlorothiazide
hydroflumethiazide
methyclothiazide
metolazone
polythiazide
quinethazone
spironolactone
triamterene
trichlormethiazide
and related compounds

(e) Street Drugs:

heroin
marijuana[3]
THC (tetrahydrocannabinol)[3]

(f) Peptide Hormones and Analogues

chorionic gonadotrophin (HCG—human chorionic gonadotrophin)
corticotrophin (ACTH)
growth hormone (HGH, somatotrophin)
All the respective releasing factors of the above-mentioned substances also are banned.
erythropoietin (EPO)
sermorelin

(g) Definitions of positive depend on the following:

[1]for caffeine—if the concentration in the urine exceeds 15 micrograms/ml.

[2]for testosterone—if the administration of testosterone or the use of any other manipulation has the result of increasing the ratio of the total concentration of testosterone to that of epitestosterone in the urine to greater than 6:1, unless there is evidence that this ratio is due to a physiological or pathological condition.

[3]for marijuana and THC—if the concentration in the urine of THC metabolite exceeds 15 nanograms/ml.

Supplements

Many nutritional/dietary supplements contain HCAA-banned substances. In addition, the U.S. Food and Drug Administration (FDA) does not strictly regulate the supplement industry; therefore purity and safety of nutritional/dietary supplements cannot be guaranteed. Impure supplements may lead to a positive NCAA drug test. The student-athlete is at his or her own risk when using supplements. Student-athletes should contact their institution's team physician or athletic trainer for further information.

SUMMARY

- A drug is a chemical agent used in the prevention, treatment, or diagnosis of disease that may be administered either internally or externally. It is transported in an inactive substance called a vehicle.
- Pharmacokinetics refers to the method by which drugs are absorbed, distributed, metabolized, and eliminated or excreted by the body.
- Administering a drug is defined as providing a single dose of medication for immediate use by the athlete. Dispensing refers to providing the athlete with a drug in a quantity sufficient to be used for multiple doses. At no time can anyone other than a person licensed by law legally prescribe or dispense drugs for an athlete. In certain situations, the athletic trainer may be allowed to administer a single dose of a nonprescription medication.
- Drugs used to combat infection include local antiseptics and disinfectants, antifungal agents, and antibiotics.
- Drugs used to inhibit pain or inflammation include counterirritants and local anesthetics, narcotic analgesics, nonnarcotic analgesics and antipyretics, acetylsalicylic acid (aspirin), nonsteroidal antiinflammatory drugs, and corticosteroids.
- Drugs used to treat gastrointestinal disorders include antacids, antiemetics, carminatives, cathartics or laxatives, and antidiarrheals.
- Drugs used to treat colds and allergies include nasal decongestants, antihistamines, cough suppressants, and asthma drugs.
- Drugs used to control bleeding include vasoconstrictors, hemostatic agents, and anticoagulants.
- The athletic trainer is often responsible for the initial screening of athletes who have various illnesses or injuries. Frequently, the athletic trainer must make decisions regarding the appropriate use of over-the-counter medications for athletes. Specific protocols have been established that can serve as a guide for the use of these medications by the athletic trainer.
- Substance abuse involves the use of performance-enhancing drugs and the widespread use of recreational drugs, or street drugs. The athletic trainer must be knowledgeable about substance abuse in the athletic population and should be able to recognize signs that an athlete is engaging in substance abuse. Substance abuse has no place in the athletic population.
- The use of performance-enhancing drugs (ergogenic aids) by athletes must be discouraged because of potential health risks and to ensure equal competition. Among the more common ergogenic aids used by athletes are stimulants, beta blockers, narcotic analgesics, diuretics, anabolic steroids, human growth hormone, and blood doping.
- Recreational drug abuse among athletes is of major concern. It can lead to serious psychological and physical health problems. The most prevalent substances that are abused are tobacco, alcohol, cocaine, and marijuana.
- Drug testing of athletes for the purpose of identifying individuals who may have some problems with drug abuse is done routinely by the NCAA and the USOC. The major goals of drug testing are to protect the health of athletes and to help ensure that competition is fair and equitable. Most professional teams and many individual colleges and universities have initiated drug testing programs for their athletes. Unfortunately, drug testing is rarely done at the high school level because of cost constraints.
- Both the NCAA and USOC have established lists of drugs that are banned for use by athletes competing in either NCAA- or USOC-sanctioned events.

Websites

Wheeless' Textbook of Orthopaedics: http://www.wheelessonline.com

Clicking on "medications" at this website allows the reader to search for information on dosages, indications, contraindications, and so on.

Online Pharmacology: http://www.pharmacology.com/phatyme.htm

This site allows the reader to search for various medications; it gives information about warnings, recent studies, and so on.

NCAA Drug Testing Program http://www.ncaa.org/membership/ed_outreach/health-safety/drug_testing/index.html

Provides an updated list of banned drugs and drug testing information.

www.usantidoping.org/

This organization is dedicated to eliminating the practice of doping in sport.

www.olympic-usa.org/

Contains information about drug testing from the USOC.

www.wada-ama.org/en/t3asp?p.41627

A comprehensive list of all medicines (over 5,000) showing which are prohibited or permitted in international sport.

www.substanceabuse.about.com

Information on basic questions concerning drugs and addiction.

Solutions to Critical Thinking EXERCISES

17-1 At no time can anyone other than a person licensed by law legally prescribe or dispense drugs for an athlete. An athletic trainer is not permitted to administer or dispense a prescription drug. However, the athletic trainer may be allowed to administer a single dose of a nonprescription medication. The athletic trainer must be reasonable and prudent about the types of nonprescription drugs offered to the athlete. If medications are administered by an athletic trainer, he or she must maintain accurate records of the types of medications administered. Each athletic trainer should be aware of state regulations and laws that pertain to the use of medications.

17-2 It is possible that this athlete has exercise-induced bronchospasm (EIB). EIB may be caused by loss of heat, water, or both from lungs during exercise or exertion, resulting from hyperventilation of air that is cooler and dryer than that in the respiratory tract. The goals of asthma therapy are to prevent chronic and troublesome symptoms, maintain normal lung function and activity levels, prevent asthma exacerbations, provide optimal pharmacotherapy with minimal adverse effects, and meet athletes' expectations of and satisfaction with asthma care.

17-3 The athlete should use a nonsteriodal antiinflammatory drug, such as ibuprofen or naprosyn. Although acetaminophen is a drug with analgesic qualities, a nonsteriodal antiinflammatory drug (NSAID) is advantageous because of its analgesic and antiinflammatory capabilities. Aspirin is also an analgesic and antiinflammatory drug, however, aspirin is associated with more frequent side effects and adverse reactions compared with an NSAID.

17-4 Ibuprofen is an NSAID. The NSAIDs are most effective for reducing pain, stiffness, swelling, redness, and fever associated with localized inflammation. Even though NSAIDs have analgesic and antipyretic capabilities, they should not be used in cases of mild headache or increased body temperature in place of aspirin or acetaminophen. However, they can be used to relieve many other mild to moderately painful somatic conditions, such as menstrual cramps and soft-tissue injury.

17-5 The athletic trainer should let the athlete know that her drug test is designed to screen for recreational drugs rather than for performance-enhancing drugs, and so this should not be a problem. Additionally, even if the test was screening for performance-enhancing drugs, it is highly unlikely that one cup of espresso would contain enough caffeine for her to test positive.

17-6 The visible signs of steroid abuse include male pattern baldness, acne, voice deepening, mood swings, aggressive behavior, gynecomastia, reduction in the size of a testicle, and changes in libido. Because the athlete denies steroid abuse, the athletic trainer might suspect that human growth hormone has been used to achieve these results.

17-7 The athletic trainer should first point out the potential long-term effects of using smokeless tobacco, which include bad breath, stained teeth, tooth sensitivity to heat and cold, cavities (with tooth loss), gum recession, periodontal destruction, and oral and throat cancer. The trainer may also try to give the players a substitute for the tobacco, such as gum or sunflower seeds, so that their habitual need to chew on something and spit while playing baseball is satisfied.

17-8 In this particular case, the issue of added responsibility is irrelevant. The athletic trainer should be more concerned with how this responsibility would affect his or her ability to perform normal job functions. Athletic trainers work hard to develop a sense of trust in the athletes for whom they must provide health care. Being forced to assume a role as a police officer or enforcer can only serve to undermine that trust. Thus, this athletic trainer should be adamant in recommending to the athletic director that some other individual assume the responsibility of overseeing the drug testing program.

REVIEW QUESTIONS AND CLASS ACTIVITIES

1. What is the branch of science known as pharmacology, and what is the difference between a prescription and a nonprescription drug?
2. What is a drug vehicle? Give some examples of drug vehicles.
3. By what methods can drugs be administered to an individual?
4. Describe the pharmacokinetics of how a drug is handled by the body.
5. List procedures that should be followed in the selection, purchase, storage, record keeping, and safety precautions of over-the-counter drugs.
6. What are the legal implications if an athletic trainer administers prescription and nonprescription drugs?
7. List the responses that an athlete may experience to a drug.
8. List examples of common drugs used by athletes to combat infection, to reduce pain and inflammation, to treat colds and allergies, to treat gastrointestinal disorders, to treat muscle dysfunctions, and to control bleeding.
9. Describe the specific protocols for administering over-the-counter medications to athletes.
10. Discuss the use of performance-enhancing drugs by athletes.

11. How do stimulants enhance an athlete's performance?
12. What are the purposes of narcotic analgesic drugs in sports? How do they affect performance?
13. What type of athlete would use beta blockers? Why are they used?
14. Describe why athletes use anabolic steroids, diuretics, and growth hormone. What are their physiological effects on the athlete?
15. Describe blood doping in sports. Why is it used? What are its dangers?
16. Contrast psychological and physical dependence, tolerance, and withdrawal syndromes.
17. List the dangers of smokeless tobacco. List the effects of nicotine on the body.
18. Why is cocaine use a danger to the athlete?
19. Select a recreational drug to research. What are the physiological responses to it, and what dangers does it pose to the athlete?
20. How can an athlete who is abusing drugs be identified? Describe behavioral identification as well as drug testing.
21. Debate the issue of drug testing in athletics.

REFERENCES

1. Almekinders L: Athletic injuries and the use of medication. In Torg J, Shephard R, editors: *Current therapy in sports medicine,* St Louis, 1995, Mosby.
2. Barnes P: Is immunotherapy for asthma worthwhile? *N Eng J Med* 334:531, 1996.
3. Blood K: Nonmedical substance use among athletes at a small liberal arts college, *Ath Train* 25(4):335, 1990.
4. Boissonnault W, Meek P: Risk Factors for Anti–inflammatory-Drug- or aspirin-induced gastrointestinal complications in individuals receiving outpatient physical therapy services, *J Orthop Sports Phys Ther* 32(10), 2002.
5. Burkholder R: Needed: a system of dispensing prescription medication, *Athletic Therapy Today* 3(2):25, 1998.
6. Cassisi NJ: Smokeless tobacco: is it worth the risk? *NCAA Sports Sciences Education Newsletter,* Spring 2000.
7. Clark W: *Goth's medical pharmacology,* ed 13, St Louis, 1992, Mosby.
8. Connolly G: Use of smokeless tobacco in major league baseball, *N Engl J Med* 318:1281, 1988.
9. Cooper J, Ellison J, Walsh M: Spit (smokeless)-tobacco use by baseball players entering the professional ranks, *J Ath Train* 38(2):126, 2003.
10. DuRant R: Use of multiple drugs among adolescents who use anabolic steroids, *N Engl J Med* 328:922, 1993.
11. Earnest CP: Dietary androgen 'supplements:' separating substance from hype, *Physician Sportsmed* 29(5):63, 2001.
12. Edwards S et al: The effects of smokeless tobacco on heart rates and neuromuscular reactivity, *Physician Sportsmed* 15(7):141, 1987.
13. Erlich N: The athletic trainer's role in drug testing, *Ath Train* 21:225, 1986.
14. Fuentes R: *Athletic drug reference '96: complies with NCAA and USOC rules,* Durham, NC, 1996, Galaxo.
15. Gledhill N: Control of drug abuse in sports. In Torg J, Shephard R, editors: *Current therapy in sports medicine,* St Louis, 1995, Mosby.
16. Gordon NF et al: Effect of beta-blockers on exercise physiology: implication for exercise training, *Med Sci Sports Exerc* 23(6):668, 1991.
17. Green GA, Uryasz FD, Petr TA, Bray CD: NCAA study of substance use and abuse habits of college student-athletes, *Clinic J Sports Med* 11(1):51, 2001.
18. Hartgens F, Van Marken Lichtenbelt WD, Ebbing S: Androgenic-anabolic steroid-induced body changes in strength athletes, *Physician Sportsmed* 29(1):49, 2001.
19. Heck J: Drug testing, *J Ath Train* 28(3):197, 1993.
20. Hillman S: Pharmacology: the study of drugs, *Athletic Therapy Today* 3(2):7, 1998.
21. Houglum JE: Asthma medications: basic pharmacology, *J Ath Train* 35(2):179, 2000.
22. Houglum JE: Pharmacologic considerations in the treatment of injured athletes with nonsteroidal anti-inflammatory drugs, *J Ath Train* 33(3):259, 1998.
23. Huff P: Drug distribution in the training room, *Clin Sports Med* 17(2):214, 1998.
24. Kahanov L, Furst D, Johnson S: Adherence to drug-dispensation and drug-administration laws and guidelines in collegiate athletic training rooms, *J Ath Train* 38(3), 2003.
25. Kersey RD: What athletic trainers and therapists should know about androstenedione, *Athletic Therapy Today* 6(1):59, 2001.
26. Koda-Kimble MA, Young LL: *Applied therapeutics: the clinical use of drugs,* Philadelphia, 2003, Lippencott Williams & Wilkins.
27. Koziris L: Anabolic-androgenic steroid abuse, *Physician Sportsmed* 28(12):67, 2000.
28. Koziris L: Reducing alcohol abuse in active patients, *Physician Sportsmed* 28(12):65, 2000.

28a. Kraemer W, Gomez A, Ratamess H: Effects of vicoprofen and ibuprofen on anaerobic performance after muscle damage, *J Sport Rehabil* 11(2):104, 2002.

29. Laster J, Russell J: Anabolic steroid–induced tendon pathology: a review of literature, *Med Sci Sports Exerc* 23(1):81, 1991.
30. Mazur AF: Substance abuse and NCAA drug testing: are we being fair? *NCAA Sports Sciences Education Newsletter,* Spring 2001.
31. National Asthma Education and Prevention Coordinating Committee; National Heart, Lung, and Blood Institute; and World Health Organization: *Global initiative for asthma,* Bethesda, Md, 1995, National Institutes of Health, Publication No. NIH-95-3659.
32. National Collegiate Athletic Association: 2003–04, *NCAA drug testing: education programs,* Indianapolis, 2003, NCAA.
33. National Collegiate Athletic Association: Ergogenic drug use down: binge-drinking on the rise according to a national study, *NCAA Sport Sciences Education Newsletter,* Winter 4:1, 1993.
34. O'Brien C: Alcohol and sport: impact of social drinking on recreational and competitive sports performance, *Sports Med* 15:71, 1993.
35. Orr E: Sources of drug information for the athletic therapist, *Athletic Therapy Today* 3(2):18, 1998.
36. Partin P: Effects of caffeine on athletes, *Ath Train* 23(4):12, 1988.
37. Poe TE: Pharmacology. In Malone T: *Physical and occupational therapy: drug implications for practice,* Philadelphia, 1989, JB Lippencott.
38. Potteiger J, Stilger V: Anabolic steroid use in the adolescent athlete, *J Ath Train* 29(1):60, 1994.
39. Powers M: The safety and efficacy of anabolic steroid precursors: what is the scientific evidence?, *J Ath Train* 37(3):300, 2002.
40. Randall T: Cocaine and alcohol mix in the body to form even longer lasting, more lethal drug, *JAMA* 267:1943, 1992.
41. Reents S, editor: *Sport and exercise pharmacology,* Champaign, Ill, 2000, Human Kinetics.
42. Rich B: Drugs: a common link between physicians and athletic therapists, *Athletic Therapy Today* 3(2):13, 1998.
43. Schneider D, Morris J: College athletes and drug testing: attitudes and behaviors, by gender and sport, *J Ath Train* 28(2):146, 1993.
44. Schnirring L: Growth hormone doping: the search for a test, *Physician and Sportsmedicine* 28(4):16, 2000.
45. Second Expert Panel on the Management of Asthma; National Heart, Lung, and Blood Institute: *Highlights of Expert Panel Report 2: guidelines for the diagnosis and management of asthma,* Bethesda, Md, 1997, National Institutes of Health, Publication No. NIH 97-4051A.
46. Smith M: NSAIDs: the most common drug in sports healthcare, *Athletic Therapy Today* 3(2):30, 1998.
47. Somani SM, Kamimori GH: The effects of exercise on absorption, distribution, metabolism, excretion, and pharmacokinetics of drugs. In Somani SM: *Pharmacology in exercises and sports,* Boca Raton, Fla, 1996, CRC Press.
48. Starkey C, Abdenour T, Finnane D: Athletic trainers' attitudes toward drug screening of intercollegiate athletes, *J Ath Train* 29(2):120, 1994.

49. Stewart C: Acute hyperthermia: the spectrum of heat emergencies. *Emergency Medicine Reports* 14(16):133, 1993.
50. Stilger V: Androstenedione and anabolic-androgenic steroids: what you need to know, Athletic Therapy Today 5(1):56, 2000.
51. Terney R, McLain L: The use of anabolic steroids in high school students, *Am J Dis Child* 144:99, 1990.
52. Trulock SC: Drug use in athletics: abuse of the human growth hormone in amateur athletes, *Sports Med Update,* 14(4):18, 2000.
53. US Olympic Committee: *Drug education handbook 1993–1996,* Colorado Springs, Colo, 1993, USOC.
54. VanHeest J, Stoppani J, Scheett, T: Effects of ibuprofen and vicoprofen on physical performance after exercise-induced muscle damage, *J Sport Rehabil* 11(3):224, 2004.
55. Wagner J: Enhancement of sport performance with drugs: an overview, *Sports Ed* 12:250, 1991.
56. Whitehill W, Wright K, Robinson J: Guidelines for dispensing medications, *J Ath Train* 27(1):20, 1992.
57. Wilson W, editor: Doping in elite sport: the politics of drugs in the Olympic movement, Champaign, Ill, 2001, Human Kinetics.
58. Windsor R, Dumitru D: Prevalence of anabolic steroid use by male and female adolescents, *Med Sci Sports Exerc* 21(5):494, 1989.
59. Yesalis CE, editor: Anabolic steroids in sport and exercise, ed 2, Champaign, Ill, 2000, Human Kinetics.

ANNOTATED BIBLIOGRAPHY

Clark WG: *Goth's medical pharmacology,* ed 13, St Louis, 1992, Mosby.

This text presents modern pharmacology in a readable and easily understood manner.

Fuentes R, Rosenberg J, Davis A: *Athletic drug reference,* Durham, NC, 1996, Galaxo.

This text is perhaps the most complete resource for the use of medications, substance abuse, and drug testing in the athletic population; it has a comprehensive listing of all drugs banned by the NCAA and USOC.

Gauwitz D, Bayt P: *Administering medications: pharmacology for health careers,* New York, 2000, McGraw-Hill.

Provides the fundamentals of drug administration, drug laws, principles of pharmacology, drug handling procedures, physician's orders, routes of administration, dosage calculation, and drug actions related to specific body systems and disorders.

Griffith HW: *Complete guide to prescription and nonprescription drugs,* New York, 2003, Perigee.

User-friendly reference text listing dosage and usage information, actions in the body, generic equivalents, potential adverse interactions (including those with foods and other drugs), overdose symptoms, precautions, side effects from prolonged use, and guidelines for usage.

Houglum, J: Pharmacology: a textbook for Athletic Trainers, Thorofare, NJ, 2004, Slack.

Provides athletic trainers with guidance for using medications in the athletic training room.

Martin M, Yates W: *Therapeutic medications in sports medicine,* Baltimore, 1998, Williams & Wilkens.

This guide serves as a quick reference to therapeutic medications used in the treatment of common injuries and illnesses of the physically active population.

Reents S: *Sport and exercise pharmacology,* Champaign, Ill, 2000, Human Kinetics.

This book provides physicians and sports medicine specialists with information on how various commonly used drugs and supplements can affect exercise performance in their patients and athletes, and how exercise activities can drastically change the effects of drugs.

Williams M: *The ergogenics edge: pushing the limits of sports performance,* Champaign, Ill, 1997, Human Kinetics.

This text for athletes, coaches, and personal trainers provides the most recent information on a wide variety of ergogenics and analyzes their positive and negative effects on sports performance factors.

Somani SM: *Pharmacology in exercise and sports,* Boca Raton, Fla, 1996 CRC Press.

This book describes the pharmacological interaction of drugs and exercise with organ systems at molecular and cellular levels.

Pharmacology for athletic trainers—performance enhancement and social drugs, Champaign, Ill, 1998, Human Kinetics.

This book is written on an extremely basic level by the staff at Human Kinetics.

The Foot

Chapter 18

When you finish this chapter you should be able to

- Identify the major anatomical and functional features of the foot.
- Discuss how foot injuries may be prevented.
- Explain the process for evaluating injuries to the foot.
- Identify specific injuries that occur in the foot, and discuss plans for management.
- Design rehabilitation techniques for the injured foot.

Many sport activities involve some elements of running, jumping, and changing direction. The foot is in direct contact with the ground, and the forces created by these athletic movements place a great deal of stress on the structures of the foot. Consequently, the foot has a high incidence of injury.[7,32,52]

The function of the foot is critical in running, jumping, and changing direction. In one instant, the foot must act as a shock absorber to dissipate the ground reaction forces. In the next instant, it must become a rigid lever that functions to propel the body forward, backward, or to the side.

Because of the stress that these movements place on the foot and because of the complex nature of the anatomical structures of this body part, recognition and management of injuries to the foot present a major challenge to the athletic trainer.

FOOT ANATOMY

Bones

The foot consists of 26 bones: 14 phalangeal, 5 metatarsal, and 7 tarsal (Figure 18-1). Additionally, there are two sesamoid bones beneath the first metatarsal.

Toes

The toes are somewhat similar to the fingers in appearance but are much shorter and serve a different function. The toes are designed to give a wider base both for balance and for propelling the body forward. The first toe, or hallux, has two phalanges, and the other toes each have three phalanges.

Two sesamoid bones are located beneath the first metatarsophalangeal joint. Their functions are to assist in reducing pressure in weight bearing, to increase the mechanical advantage of the flexor tendons of the great toe, and to act as sliding pulleys for tendons.

Metatarsals

The metatarsals are the five bones that lie between and articulate with the tarsals and the phalanges, thus forming the semimovable tarsometatarsal and metatarsophalangeal joints. Although there is little movement permitted, the ligamentous arrangement gives elasticity to the foot in weight bearing. The metatarsophalangeal joints permit hinge action of the phalanges, which is similar to the action found between the hand and fingers. The first metatarsal is the largest and strongest and functions as the main weight-bearing support during walking and running.

The medial and lateral sesamoid bones are located on the plantar aspect of the metatarsophalangeal joint of the great toe within the flexor hallucis tendon. Their

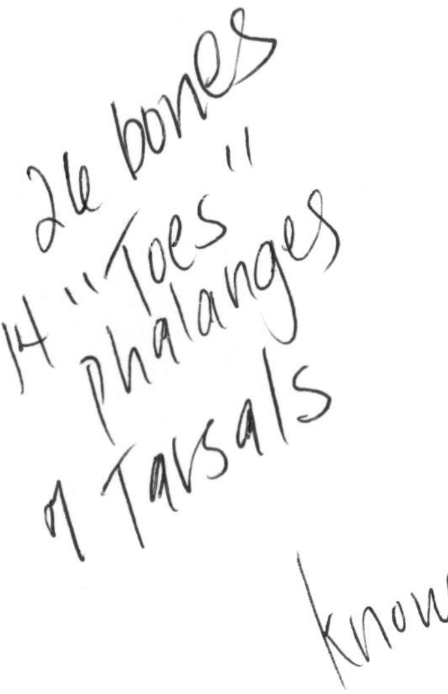

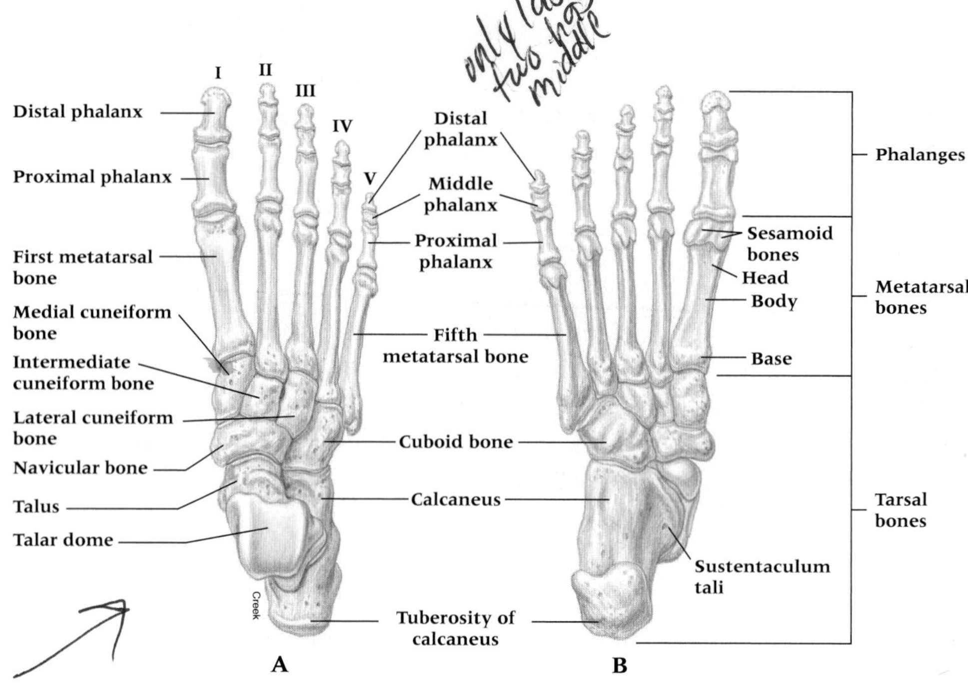

Figure 18-1

Bony structure of the foot. **A,** Dorsal aspect. **B,** Plantar aspect.

purpose is (1) to increase the mechanical efficiency of the tendon, and (2) to decrease frictional stress as the tendon passes over bony prominances.

Tarsal Bones

The foot has seven tarsal bones, which are located between the bones of the lower leg and the metatarsals. These bones are important for support of the body and its locomotion. They consist of the calcaneus, talus, cuboid, navicular, and the first, second, and third cuneiform bones.

Calcaneus The calcaneus is the largest tarsal bone. It supports the talus and shapes the heel; its main functions are to convey the body weight to the ground and to serve as an attachment for both the Achilles tendon and several structures on the plantar surface of the foot.

The wider portion on the posterior calcaneus is called the tuberosity of the calcaneus. The medial and lateral tubercles are located on the inferior lateral and medial aspects and are the only parts of this bone that normally touch the ground.

Talus The irregularly shaped talus is the most superior of the tarsal bones. It is situated above the calcaneus over a bony projection called the sustentaculum tali. The talus consists of a body, neck, and head. The uppermost part of the talus is the trochlea, which articulates with the medial and lateral malleoli to form the ankle joint. The talus is broader anteriorly than posteriorly, thus preventing forward slipping of the tibia during locomotion.

Because the talus fits principally into the space formed by the malleoli, lateral movement is restricted by the stabilizing ligaments of the ankle. Because the uppermost articular surface of the talus is narrower posteriorly than anteriorly, dorsiflexion is limited. At a position of full dorsiflexion, the anterior aspect of the medial collateral ligaments is taut; whereas in plantar flexion, internal rotation occurs because of the shape of the talus. The average range of motion is 10 degrees in dorsiflexion and 23 degrees in plantar flexion.[59]

Navicular The navicular bone is positioned anterior to the talus on the medial aspect of the foot. Anteriorly the navicular bone articulates with the three cuneiform bones.

Cuboid The cuboid is positioned on the lateral aspect of the foot. It articulates posteriorly with the calcaneus and anteriorly with the fourth and fifth metatarsals.

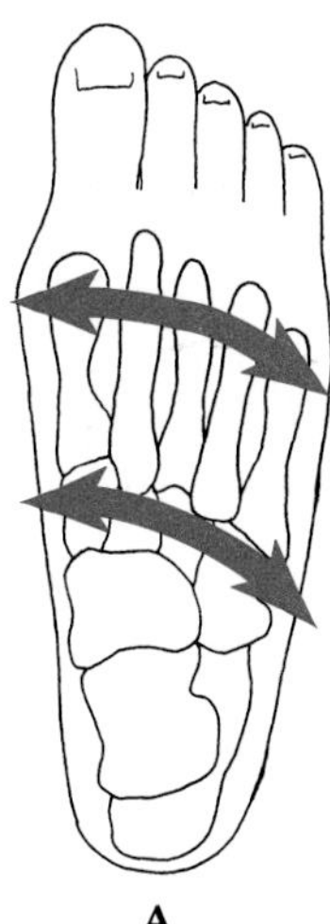

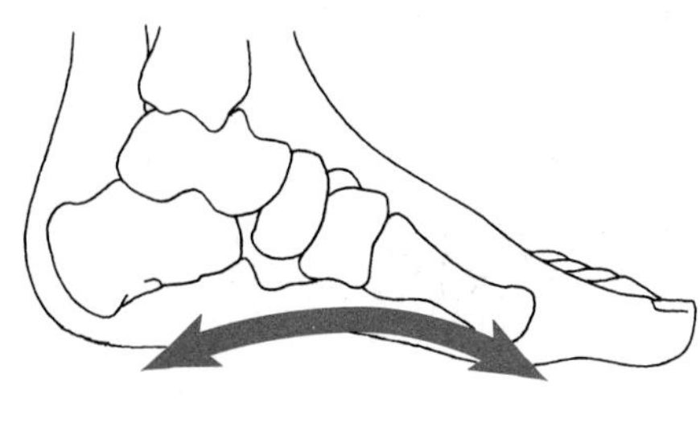

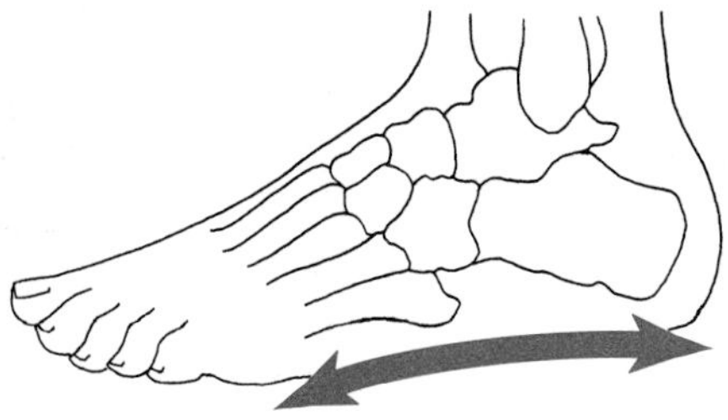

Figure 18-2

The arches of the foot. **A,** Anterior metatarsal and transverse arches. **B,** Medial longitudinal arch. **C,** Lateral longitudinal arch.

Cuneiforms The three cuneiform bones are located between the navicular and the base of the three metatarsals on the medial aspect of the foot.

Arches of the Foot

The foot is structured, by means of ligamentous and bony arrangements, to form several arches. The arches assist the foot in supporting the body weight; in absorbing the shock of weight bearing; and in providing a space on the plantar aspect of the foot for the blood vessels, nerves, and muscles.[25] There are four arches: the anterior metatarsal, the transverse, the medial longitudinal, and the lateral longitudinal (Figure 18-2).

Anterior Metatarsal Arch

The anterior metatarsal arch is shaped by the distal heads of the metatarsals. The arch has a semiovoid appearance, stretching from the first to the fifth metatarsal.

Transverse Arch

The transverse arch extends across the transverse tarsal bones, primarily the cuboid and the internal cuneiform, and forms a half dome. It gives protection to soft tissue and increases the foot's mobility.

Medial Longitudinal Arch

The medial longitudinal arch originates along the medial border of the calcaneus and extends forward to the distal head of the first metatarsal. Bony support is provided by the calcaneus, talus, navicular, first cuneiform, and first metatarsal. The main supporting ligament of the longitudinal arch is the plantar calcaneonavicular ligament, which acts as a spring by returning the arch to its normal position after it has been stretched. The tendon of the posterior tibialis muscle helps to reinforce the plantar calcaneonavicular ligament.

Lateral Longitudinal Arch

The lateral longitudinal arch is on the outer aspect of the foot and follows the same pattern as that of the medial longitudinal arch. It is formed by the calcaneus, cuboid, and fifth metatarsal bones. It is much lower and less flexible than the inner longitudinal arch.

Plantar Fascia (Plantar Aponeurosis)

The plantar fascia is a thick white band of fibrous tissue originating from the medial tuberosity of the calcaneus and ending at the proximal heads of the metatarsals. Along

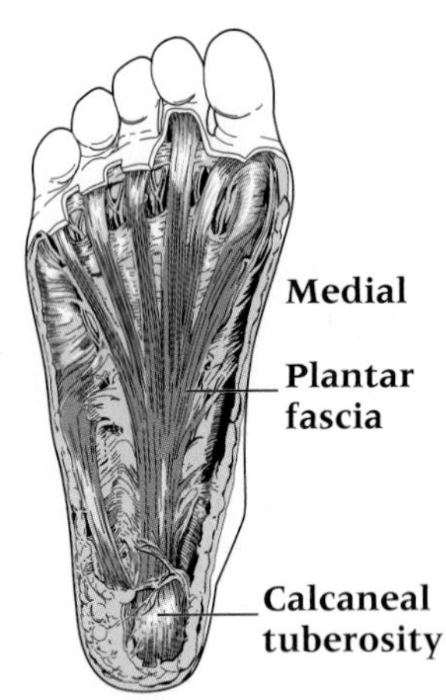

Figure 18-3

Plantar fascia.

with ligaments, the plantar fascia supports the foot against downward forces (Figure 18-3). The plantar fascia is a distal continuation of fascia that runs posteriorly from the muscles of the thigh to the muscles of the calf and continues under the calcaneus, where it thickens to become the plantar fascia.

Articulations

Joints of the foot are categorized into five regions: interphalangeal, metatarsophalangeal, intermetatarsal, tarsometatarsal, subtalar, and midtarsal.

Interphalangeal Joint

The interphalangeal joints are located at the distal extremities of the proximal and middle phalanges at the bases of the adjacent middle and distal phalanges. These joints are designed only for flexion and extension. All interphalangeal joints have reinforcing collateral ligaments on their medial and lateral sides. Also located between the collateral ligaments on the plantar and dorsal surfaces are interphalangeal ligaments (Figure 18-4).

Metatarsophalangeal Joint

The metatarsophalangeal joints are the condyloid type, which permits flexion, extension, adduction, and abduction. Each of these joints has collateral ligaments as well as plantar and dorsal metatarsophalangeal ligaments.

Intermetatarsal Joint

The intermetatarsal joints are sliding joints. They include two sets of articulations. One set consists of an articulation on each side of the base of the metatarsal bones, and the second articulations are on each side of the heads of the metatarsal bone. Each of these articulations permits only slight gliding movements. Shafts of the metatarsals are connected by interosseous ligaments. The bases are connected by plantar and dorsal ligaments, and the heads are attached by transverse metatarsal ligaments.

Tarsometatarsal Joint

The tarsometatarsal joint is formed by the junction of the bases of the metatarsal bones with the cuboid and all three cuneiforms. The slight saddle shape of this joint allows for some gliding and thus for a restricted amount of flexion, extension, adduction, and abduction. Metatarsal bones are attached to the tarsal bones by the dorsal and plantar tarsometatarsal ligaments. Interosseous ligaments connect the three cuneiforms to the metatarsals. The tarsometatarsal joint is also known as Lisfranc's joint.

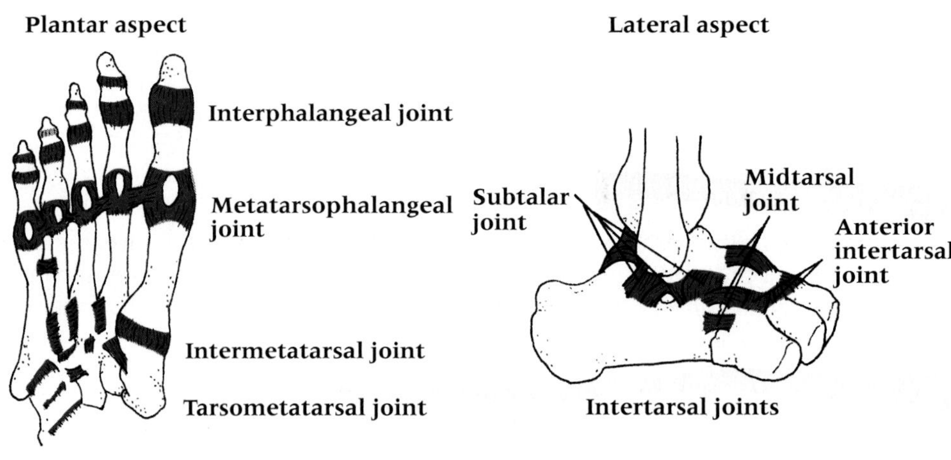

Figure 18-4

A, Ligaments of the interphalangeal, metatarsophalangeal, intermetatarsal, and tarsometatarsal joints. **B,** Ligaments of the intertarsal joints.

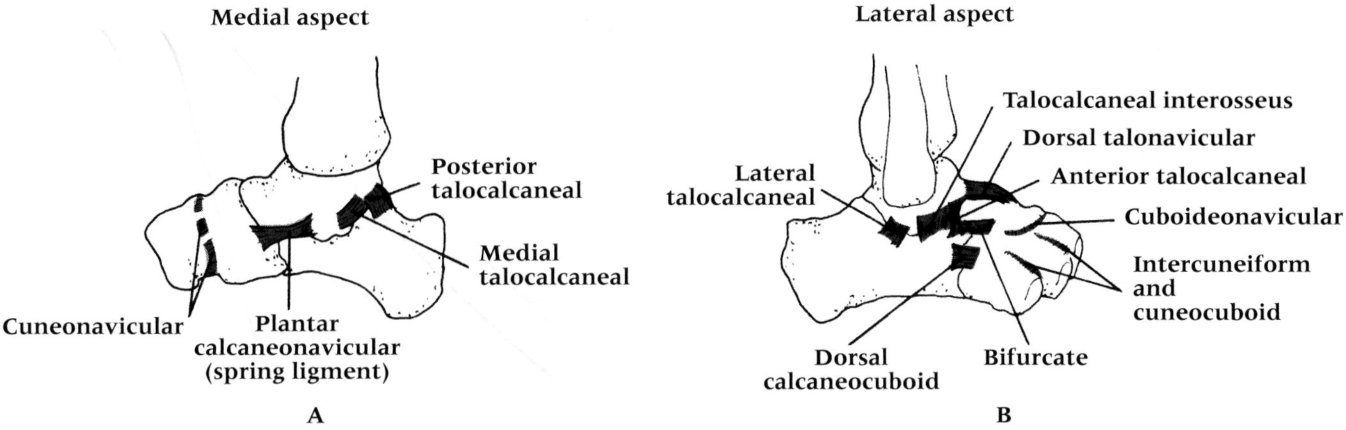

Figure 18-5

Ligaments of the subtalar joint. **A,** Medial aspect. **B,** Lateral aspect.

Subtalar Joint

The subtalar joint is the articulation between the talus and the calcaneus. *Inversion, eversion, pronation,* and *supination* are normal movements that occur at the subtalar joint. Inversion refers to a movement of the calcaneus such that the sole of the foot turns inward or medially. Eversion refers to a movement of the calcaneus such that the sole of the foot turns outward or laterally.

In weight bearing, foot pronation refers to the combined movements of talar plantar flexion and adduction and calcaneal eversion. In contrast, foot supination is the combined movements of talar dorsiflexion and abduction and calcaneal inversion.[18] These movements, which occur at the subtalar joint, are triplanar movements, that is, movements that occur in all three planes simultaneously.[31] The movements of the talus during pronation and supination have profound effects on the lower extremity, both proximally and distally.

Midtarsal Joint

The midtarsal joint consists of two distinct joints: the calcaneocuboid and the talonavicular joint. The midtarsal joint depends mainly on ligamentous and muscular tension to maintain position and integrity. Midtarsal joint stability is directly related to the position of the subtalar joint. If the subtalar joint is pronated, the talonavicular and calcaneocuboid joints become hypermobile. If the subtalar joint is supinated, the midtarsal joint becomes hypomobile. As the midtarsal joint becomes more or less mobile, it affects the distal portion of the foot because of the articulations at the tarsometatarsal joint.[31]

Stabilizing Ligaments

The subtalar ligaments are the talocalcaneal interosseus and the anterior, posterior, lateral, and medial talocalcaneal (Figure 18-5). A major ligament is the plantar calcaneonavicular, which passes from the medial longitudinal arch. Because of its relatively large number of elastic fibers and its primary purpose of providing shock absorption, the plantar calcaneonavicular is commonly called the spring ligament.

The primary ligaments of the midtarsal joint are the dorsal talonavicular, bifurcate, and dorsal calcaneocuboid. The midtarsal joint is given added strength in its plantar aspect by the long plantar ligaments.

Ligaments of the anterior tarsal joints are divided into those of the cuneonavicular, cuboideonavicular, intercuneiform, and cuneocuboid joints. Each of these joints has both dorsal and plantar ligaments. The intercuneiform ligaments have three transverse bands; one band connects the first cuneiform with the second and the second with the third. A ligament also connects the third cuneiform with the cuboid bone.

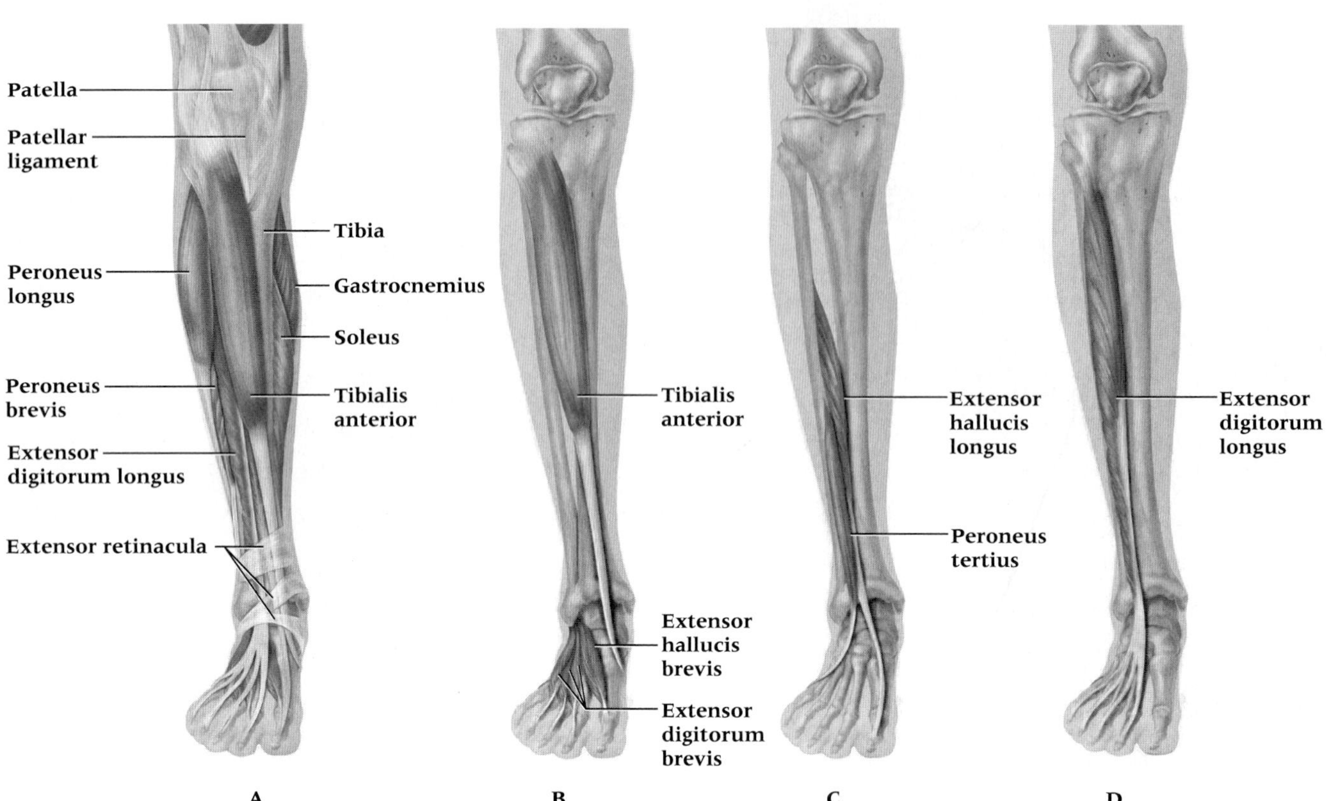

Figure 18-6

Muscles and tendons of the anterior aspect of the ankle and foot.

Muscles and Movement

The movements of the foot are produced by numerous muscles (Figures 18-6 and 18-7; Table 18-1).

Dorsiflexion and Plantar Flexion

Dorsiflexion and plantar flexion of the foot take place at the ankle joint and will be discussed in greater detail in Chapter 19. The gastrocnemius, soleus, plantaris, peroneus longus, peroneus brevis, tibialis posterior, flexor hallucis longus, and flexor digitorum longus muscles are the plantar flexors. Dorsiflexion is accomplished by the tibialis anterior, extensor digitorum longus, extensor hallucis longus, and peroneus tertius muscles (see Figure 18-6).

Inversion, Adduction, and Supination

The medial movements of the foot are produced by the same muscles as inversion, adduction (medial movement of the forefoot), and supination (a combination of inversion and adduction). Muscles that produce these movements pass behind and in front of the medial malleolus. Muscles passing behind are the tibialis posterior(see Figure 19-5B), flexor digitorum longus, and flexor hallucis longus (see Figure 19-5D). Muscles passing in front of the medial malleolus are the tibialis anterior (see Figure 19-5A) and the extensor hallucis longus (see Figure 18-6C).

Eversion, Abduction, and Pronation

The lateral movements of the foot are caused by the same muscles that produce eversion, abduction (lateral movement of the forefoot), and pronation (a combination of eversion and abduction). Muscles passing behind the lateral malleolus are the peroneus longus and the peroneus brevis. Muscles passing in front of the lateral malleolus are the peroneus tertius and extensor digitorum longus (see Figure 18-6C and D).

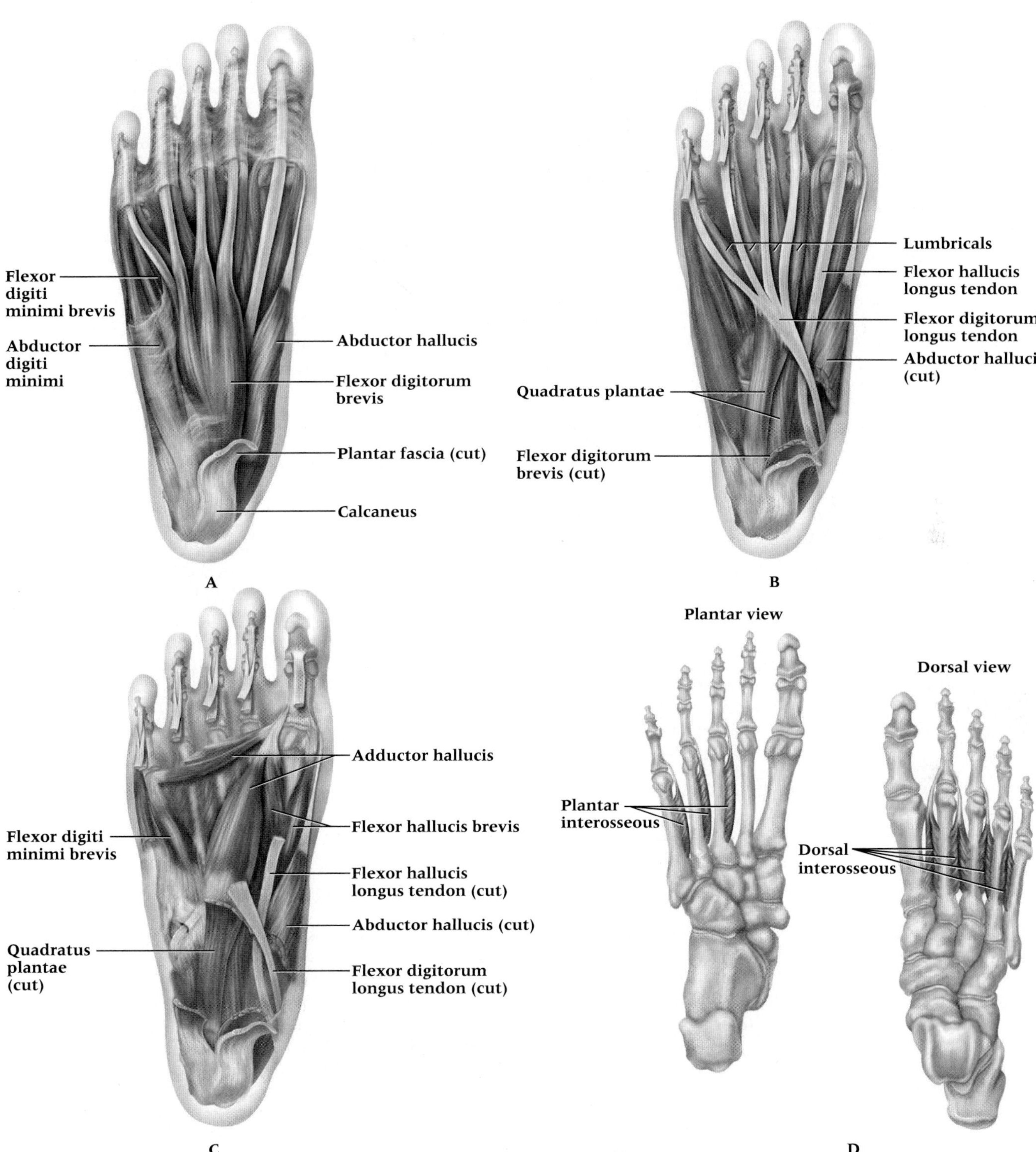

Figure 18-7

Intrinsic muscles of the foot. **A,** First layer. **B,** Second layer. **C,** Third layer. **D,** Fourth layer.

Movement of the Phalanges

The movements of the phalanges are flexion, extension, abduction, and adduction. Flexion of the second, third, fourth, and fifth distal phalanges is executed by the flexor digitorum longus and the quadratus plantar muscles. Flexion of the middle phalanges is performed by the flexor digitorum brevis, and flexion of the proximal phalanges is performed by the lumbricales and the interossei. The great toe is flexed by the flexor hallucis longus. The extension of all the middle phalanges is done by the abductor

TABLE 18-1 Intrinsic Muscles of the Foot

Muscle	Origin	Insertion	Action	Nerve
Dorsal Muscle				
Extensor digitorum brevis	Lateral surface of the calcaneus	Tendon of the extensor digitorum longus	Extends the second through fifth toes	Deep peroneal
Plantar Muscles				
First Layer				
Abductor hallucis	Calcaneus	Proximal phalanx of the great toe (with the tendon of the flexor hallucis brevis)	Abducts the great toe	Medial plantar
Flexor digitorum brevis	Calcaneus and plantar aponeurosis	Middle phalanx of the second through fifth toes	Flexes the second through fifth toes	Medial plantar
Abductor digiti minimi	Calcaneus and plantar aponeurosis	Proximal phalanx of the small toe	Abducts the small toe	Lateral plantar
Second Layer				
Quadratus plantae	Calcaneus	Into tendons of the flexor digitorum longus	Aids in flexing the second through fifth toes by straightening the pull of the flexor digitorum longus	Lateral plantar
Lumbricales	From tendons of the flexor digitorum longus	Into tendons of the extensor digitorum longus	Flexes the second through fifth toes	Medial and lateral plantar
Third Layer				
Flexor hallucis brevis	Cuboid and lateral cuneiform	Proximal phalanx of the great toe	Flexes the great toe	Medial plantar
Adductor hallucis	*Oblique head:* second, third, and fourth metatarsals; *Transverse head:* ligaments of the metatarsophalangeal joints	Proximal phalanx of the small toe	Adducts the great toe	Lateral plantar
Flexor digiti minimi brevis	Fifth metatarsal	Proximal phalanx of the small toe	Flexes the small toe	Lateral plantar
Fourth Layer				
Plantar interossei	Third, fourth, and fifth metatarsals	Proximal phalanx of the same toe	Adducts the toes toward the second toe	Lateral plantar
Dorsal interossei	Bases of the adjacent metatarsals	Proximal phalanges; both sides of the second toe; lateral side of the third and fourth toes	Abducts the toes from the second toe; moves the second toe medially and laterally	Lateral plantar

hallucis and abductor digiti quanti, the lumbricales, and the interossei. Extension of all distal phalanges is effected by the lumbricales, extensor digitorum longus, the extensor hallucis longus, and the extensor digitorum brevis. The adduction of the foot is performed by the interossei plantares and adductor hallucis; abduction is performed by the interossei dorsalis, the abductor hallucis, and the abductor digiti quanti.

Nerve Supply and Blood Supply

Nerve Supply

The tibial nerve, the largest division of the sciatic nerve, supplies the muscles of the back of the leg and the plantar aspect of the foot. The common peroneal nerve is a

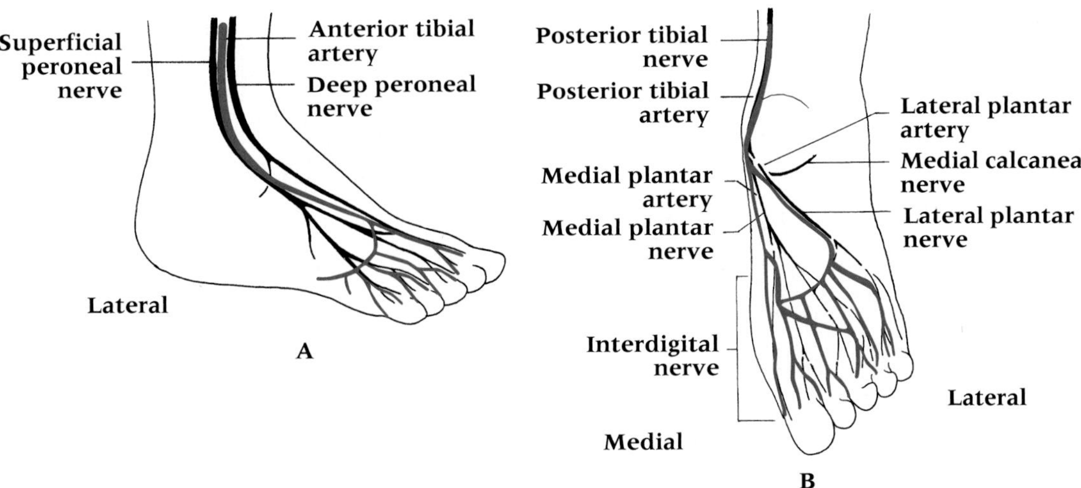

Figure 18-8

The major nerves and arteries of the foot. **A,** Dorsal aspect. **B,** Plantar aspect.

smaller division of the sciatic nerve and, with its branches, supplies the front of the leg and the foot (Figure 18-8).

Blood Supply

The major portion of the blood is supplied to the foot by the anterior and posterior tibial arteries. The dorsal venous arch and digital veins and the dorsal digital vein stem from the short and long saphenous veins.

FUNCTIONAL ANATOMY AND FOOT BIOMECHANICS

Most people will at some time in their lives develop foot problems.

Athletic trainers must realize, when considering foot, ankle, and leg injuries, that these segments are joined together to form a kinetic chain. Each movement of a body segment has a direct effect on proximal and distal body segments.[16] A study of lower-extremity chronic and overuse injuries related to sports participation must include some understanding of the biomechanics of the foot, especially in the act of walking and running. A number of biomechanical factors may be related to injuries of the lower leg region.

Normal Gait

The action of the lower extremity during a complete gait cycle in walking can be divided into two primary phases (Figure 18-9). The **stance phase** starts with initial contact of the heel on the ground and ends when the toe breaks contact with the ground (toe-off). This phase accounts for about 60 percent of the total gait cycle. The stance phase involves weight bearing in a closed kinetic chain. The stance phase can be further subdivided into five periods: *initial contact, loading response, mid stance, terminal stance,* and *pre swing.* At mid stance and terminal stance, the body is supported by a single limb while at initial contact and in the early portion of the loading response period there is double support with both feet on the ground. [28,44]

stance phase From initial contact to toe-off.

The time between toe-off and the subsequent initial contact is termed the **swing phase,** which is a period of non–weight bearing. The swing phase can be subdivided into three periods: *initial swing, mid swing,* and *terminal swing.* In normal gait, while one leg is in the stance phase, the other is in the swing phase.

swing phase Period of non–weight bearing.

As in the walking gait, a running gait has both stance and swing phases. However there are several differences. In running, the loading response and mid stance periods occur more rapidly. There is also a period after toe-off in which neither foot is in contact with the ground and there is no time when both feet contact the ground

Figure 18-9

The stance and swing phases of a normal gait cycle.

Stance Phase (60% of total)					Swing Phase		
Initial Contact (heel contact)	Loading Response	Mid Stance	Terminal Stance	Pre Swing (toe off)	Initial Swing	Mid Swing	Terminal Swing
External Rotation of Tibia	Internal Rotation of Tibia			External Rotation of Tibia			
Supination	Pronation			Supination			

simultaneously. In running the stance phase accounts for only one-third of the gait cycle.

The foot's function during the stance phase of running is twofold. At heel strike, the foot acts as a shock absorber to the impact forces and then adapts to the uneven surfaces. At toe-off, the foot functions as a rigid lever to transmit the explosive force from the lower extremity to the running surface. In a heel-strike running gait, initial contact of the foot is on the lateral aspect of the calcaneus with the subtalar joint in supination. It is estimated that 80 percent of distance runners use this heel-strike pattern and the remainder are either midfoot or forefoot strikers.[59] Sprinters tend to be forefoot strikers, whereas a number of joggers are midfoot strikers.

At initial contact, the subtalar joint is supinated (Figure 18-10). Associated with this supination of the subtalar joint is an obligatory external rotation of the tibia.[44] As the foot is loaded, the subtalar joint moves into a pronated position until the forefoot is in contact with the running surface. The change in subtalar motion occurs between initial heel strike and 20 percent into the support phase of running.[44] As pronation occurs at the subtalar joint, there is obligatory internal rotation of the tibia. Transverse plane rotation occurs at the knee joint because of this tibial rotation. Pronation of the foot unlocks the midtarsal joint and allows the foot to assist in shock absorption and to adapt to uneven surfaces. It is important during initial impact to reduce the ground reaction forces and to distribute the load evenly on many different anatomical structures throughout the foot and leg. Pronation is normal and allows for this distribution of forces on as many structures as possible to avoid excessive loading on just a few structures. The subtalar joint remains in a pronated position through 55 percent to 85 percent of the stance phase, with maximum pronation being concurrent with the body's center of gravity passing over the base of support.[14]

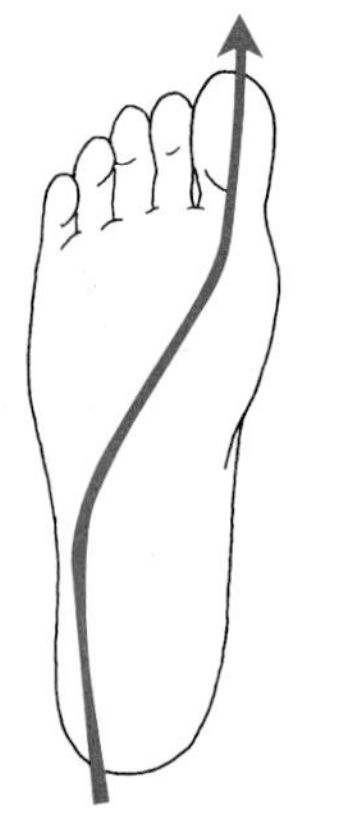

Figure 18-10

Foot bearing weight in walking as it moves from heel strike to toe off.

The foot begins to resupinate and will approach the neutral subtalar position at 70 percent to 90 percent of the stance phase.[14] In supination, the midtarsal joints are locked and the foot becomes stable and rigid to prepare for toe-off. This rigid position allows the foot to exert a great amount of force from the lower extremity to the running surface.

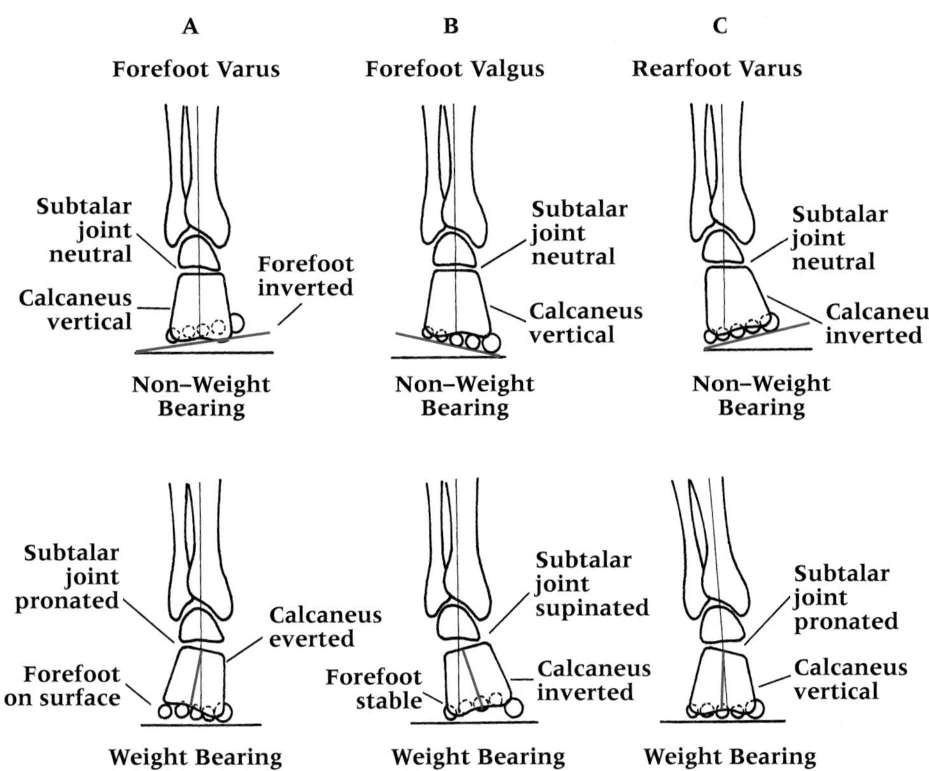

Figure 18-11

Structural foot deformities in non–weight bearing and compensations in weight bearing. **A,** Forefoot varus. **B,** Forefoot valgus. **C,** Rearfoot varus.

Subtalar Joint Pronation and Supination

Pronation and supination of the foot and subtalar joint are normal during the stance phase of running. However, excessive or prolonged pronation or supination will often cause or contribute to overuse injuries. When structural or functional deformities exist in the foot or leg, compensation is likely to occur at the subtalar joint. The subtalar joint compensates in a manner that allows the foot to make stable contact with the ground and get into a weight-bearing position (Figure 18-11). This excessive motion compensates for an existing structural deformity.[31]

Structural Deformities The most typical structural deformities of the foot that produce excessive pronation or supination include forefoot varus, forefoot valgus, and rearfoot varus (Figure 18-11).[44] These structural deformities exist in a non–weight bearing position. Structural forefoot varus and structural rearfoot varus deformities are usually associated with excessive pronation. A structural forefoot valgus causes excessive supination. The deformities usually exist in one plane, but the subtalar joint will interfere with the normal functions of the foot and make it more difficult for the joint to act as a shock absorber, to adapt to uneven surfaces, and to act as a rigid lever for toe-off. The compensation, which occurs when the foot goes into weight bearing, rather than the deformity itself, usually causes overuse injuries.[31]

Excessive Pronation Excessive or prolonged pronation during running is one of the major causes of stress injuries. Overload of specific structures results when excessive pronation is produced in the stance phase or when pronation is prolonged into the propulsive phase of running.[11] Excessive pronation during the stance phase will cause compensatory subtalar joint motion such that the midtarsal joint remains unlocked, resulting in an excessively loose foot.[26] As more motion occurs at the midtarsal joint, the first metatarsal and first cuneiform become more mobile. These bones comprise a functional unit known as the *first ray.* With pronation of the midtarsal joint, the first ray is more mobile because of its articulations with that joint. The first ray is also stabilized by the attachment of the peroneus longus tendon, which attaches to the base of the first metatarsal.[21]

18-1

Critical Thinking **Exercise**

An athletic trainer observes a forefoot valgus deformity in a soccer player during a preseason screening.

? Why might this deformity be a problem? What can be done to manage this condition?

The peroneus longus tendon passes posteriorly around the base of the lateral malleolus and then through a notch in the cuboid to cross the foot to the first metatarsal. The cuboid functions as a pulley to increase the mechanical advantage of the peroneal tendon. Stability of the cuboid is essential in this process. In the pronated position, the cuboid loses much of its mechanical advantage as a pulley; therefore the peroneus longus tendon no longer stabilizes the first ray effectively. This condition creates hypermobility of the first ray and increased pressure on the other metatarsals. There is also an increase in tibial rotation, which forces the knee joint to absorb more transverse rotation motion.[31]

Prolonged pronation of the subtalar joint will not allow the foot to resupinate in time to provide a rigid lever for toe-off, resulting in a less powerful and efficient force. Thus various foot and leg problems will occur with excessive or prolonged pronation during the stance phase; these problems include stress fractures of the second metatarsal, plantar fasciitis, posterior tibial tendinitis, Achilles tendinitis, tibial stress syndrome, and medial knee pain.[30]

Excessive Supination At heel strike in prolonged or excessive supination, compensatory movement at the subtalar joint will not allow the midtarsal joint to unlock, which causes the foot to remain excessively rigid. Because less movement occurs at the calcaneocuboid joint, the cuboid becomes hypomobile. The peroneus longus tendon has a greater amount of tension because the cuboid has less mobility and thus will not allow mobility of the first ray. In this case, the majority of the weight is borne by the first and fifth metatarsals. Thus the foot cannot absorb the ground reaction forces as efficiently.[29]

Excessive supination limits tibial internal rotation. Injuries typically associated with excessive supination include inversion ankle sprains, tibial stress syndrome, peroneal tendinitis, iliotibial band friction syndrome, and trochanteric bursitis.[30]

PREVENTION OF FOOT INJURIES

Certainly the foot is highly vulnerable to a variety of injuries. The repetitive stresses and strains incurred by the foot during athletic activities are unquestionably sufficient to cause both acute traumatic and overuse injuries. Foot injuries can best be prevented by selecting appropriate footwear, by correcting biomechanical structural deformities through the use of appropriate orthotics, and by paying attention to appropriate foot hygiene and care.[43,55]

Selecting Appropriate Footwear

The athletic and fitness shoe manufacturing industry has become extremely sophisticated and offers a number of options when it comes to purchasing shoes for different athletic activities. Selecting an appropriate shoe is one of the most critical considerations in preventing a foot problem. Before a shoe is selected, the athletic trainer should evaluate the athlete's foot to determine the existence of a structural deformity such as a forefoot valgus or varus or a rearfoot varus. The type of shoe selected should depend on the existing structural deformity.

As noted earlier, pronation is a problem of hypermobility. Individuals who excessively pronate need stability and firmness to reduce this excess movement. Research indicates that shoe compression, compared to a barefoot condition, may actually increase pronation.[13] The ideal shoe for a pronated foot is one that is less flexible and has good rearfoot control. Conversely, supinated feet are usually very rigid. Increased cushioning and flexibility benefit this type of foot.

Several construction factors may influence the firmness and stability of a shoe. The basic form upon which a shoe is built is called the last. The upper is fitted onto a last in several ways. Each method has its own flexibility and control characteristics. A slip-lasted shoe is sewn together like a moccasin and is very flexible. A board-lasted shoe contains a piece of fiberboard to which the upper is attached, which provides a very firm, inflexible base for the shoe. A combination-lasted shoe is boarded in the back half of the shoe and slip lasted in the front, which provides rearfoot stability with forefoot mobility.

The shape of the last may also determine shoe selection. Most athletes with excessive pronation perform better in a straight-lasted shoe, that is, a shoe in which the forefoot does not curve inward in relation to the rearfoot. Midsole design also affects the stability of a shoe. The midsole separates the upper from the outsole.[19] More dense, less yielding material is often used under the medial aspect of the foot to control pronation.

In an effort to control rearfoot movement, many shoe manufacturers have reinforced the heel counter both internally and externally, often in the form of extra plastic along the outside of the heel counter. Other factors that may affect the performance of a shoe are the outsole contour and composition, lacing systems, and forefoot wedges.[31]

Using a Shoe Orthotic

Many injuries to the foot can be prevented by using an orthotic device to correct biomechanical problems that may exist in the foot and that can potentially cause an injury.[17] The orthotic is a plastic, rubber, or leather support that is placed in the shoe as a replacement for the existing insert. Ready-made orthotics can be purchased in sporting goods or shoe stores. Some athletes will need to have orthotics that are custom fitted or made by the athletic trainer.[54]

The use of orthotics for correcting specific problems will be discussed in the section on rehabilitation at the end of this chapter.

Foot Hygiene

Athletes who perform simple tasks such as keeping their toenails trimmed correctly; shaving down excessive calluses; keeping their feet clean; wearing clean, correctly fitted socks; and keeping their feet as dry as possible to prevent the development of athlete's foot (see Chapter 28) can separately and collectively reduce a number of potential problems that can cause them to unnecessarily miss days of practice or competition.

FOOT ASSESSMENT

When assessing foot injuries, athletic trainers must clearly understand that the foot is part of a kinetic chain that includes both the ankle and the lower leg. Acute injuries must be differentiated from those injuries that had a relatively slow onset.[47]

History

An athletic trainer making a decision about how to manage a foot injury must perform a quick assessment to determine the type of injury and its history. He or she should ask the following questions:[47]

- Is this the first time this condition has occurred? If it has happened before, when, how often, and under what circumstances did it occur?
- How did the injury occur?
- Did it occur suddenly or come on slowly?
- Was the mechanism a sudden strain, twist, or blow to the foot?
- Where is the pain (ankle, heel, arches, toes)?
- What type of pain is the athlete experiencing?
- Is there muscle weakness?
- Is there any snapping, popping, or crepitus during movement?
- Is there any alteration in sensation?
- Can the athlete point to the exact site of the pain?
- When is the pain or other symptoms more or less severe?

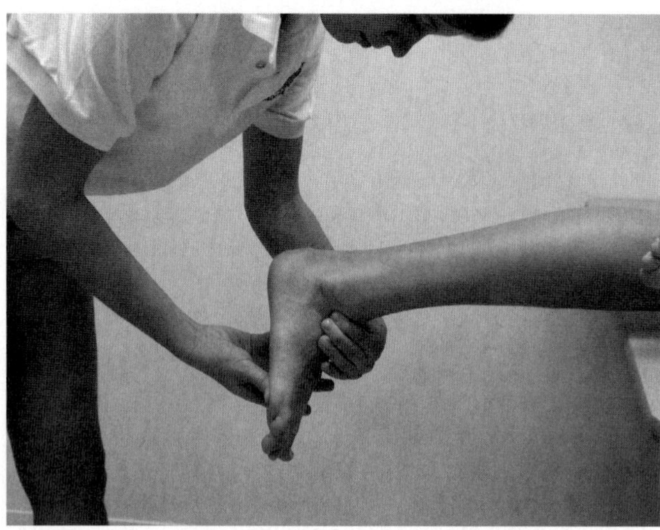

Figure 18-12

Position for assessing existing structural deformities.

- On what type of surface has the athlete been training?
- What type of footwear was worn during training? Is it appropriate for the type of training? Is discomfort increased when footwear is worn?

Observation

The athletic trainer should observe the athlete determine the following:

- Is the athlete favoring the foot, walking with a limp, or unable to bear weight?
- Is the injured part deformed, swollen, or discolored?
- Does the foot change color when weight bearing and not weight bearing (changing rapidly from a darker to lighter pink when not weight bearing)?
- Is there pes planus (a flatfoot) or pes cavus (a high arch)?
- Is the foot well aligned? Does it maintain its shape on weight bearing?
- Do any abnormalities exist in the toes (e.g., hammer toes, mallet toes, claw toes, Morton's toe, hallux valgus, corns, bunions, plantar warts)?

Looking for Structural Deformities

The first step in looking for structural deformities is to establish a position of subtalar neutral. The athlete should be prone with the distal third of the leg hanging off the end of the table (Figure 18-12). A line should be drawn bisecting the leg from the start of the musculotendinous junction of the gastrocnemius to the distal portion of the calcaneus. With the athlete still prone, the athletic trainer should palpate the talus while the forefoot is inverted and everted. One finger should palpate the talus at the anterior aspect of the fibula and another finger at the anterior portion of the medial malleolus. The position at which the talus is equally prominent on both sides is considered a neutral subtalar position in which the subtalar joint is neither pronated or supinated.

Once the subtalar joint is placed in a neutral position, the athletic trainer should apply mild dorsiflexion while observing the metatarsal heads in relation to the plantar surface of the calcaneus. Forefoot varus is an osseous deformity in which the medial metatarsal heads are inverted in relation to the plane of the calcaneus. Forefoot varus is the most common cause of excessive pronation (see Figure 18-11A, page 529). Forefoot valgus is a position in which the lateral metatarsals are everted in relation to the rearfoot (see Figure 18-11B, page 529).

These forefoot deformities are benign in a non–weight bearing position, but during weight bearing, the metatarsal heads must somehow make contact with the surface to bear weight. To accomplish this movement for a forefoot varus, the talus plantar flexes and adducts and the calcaneus everts. For the forefoot valgus, the calcaneus inverts and the talus abducts and dorsiflexes. A forefoot valgus is the most common forefoot deformity.

In a rearfoot varus deformity, when the foot is in a subtalar neutral position and non–weight bearing, the medial metatarsal heads are elevated, as in a forefoot varus, and the calcaneus is also in an inverted position (see Figure 18-11C, page 529). For the foot to bear weight, the subtalar joint must pronate.

An equine foot, and particularly a rigid equinus foot, is another structural deformity that is thought to be associated with poor shock absorption during running. In an equinus foot, the forefoot is plantar flexed relative to the rearfoot when the ankle is at 90 degrees of flexion. A similar condition in which only the first metatarsal is plantar flexed relative to the rearfoot is referred to as a plantar flexed first ray.[25]

Shoe Wear Patterns

Athletes with excessive pronation often wear out the front of the running shoe under the second metatarsal. Shoe wear patterns are commonly misinterpreted by athletes who think they must be pronators because they wear out the back outside edges of their heels. However, most people wear out the back outside edges of their shoes. Just before heel strike, the anterior tibialis fires to prevent the foot from slapping forward. The anterior tibialis not only dorsiflexes the foot but also slightly inverts it; hence the wear pattern on the back edge of the shoe. An athlete who excessively supinates tends to show a wear pattern on the lateral border of the shoe. The key to inspection of wear patterns on shoes is observation of the heel counter and the forefoot.[30]

Palpation

Besides determining pain sites, swelling, and deformities, palpation is used to determine and evaluate circulation.

Bony Palpation

The following bony landmarks should be palpated:

Medial Aspect
- Medial calcaneus
- Calcaneal dome
- Medial malleolus
- Sustentaculum tali (plantar aspect of medial calcaneus)
- Talar head
- Navicular tubercle
- First cuneiform
- First metatarsal
- First metatarsophalangeal joint
- First phalanx

Dorsal Aspect
- Second, third, fourth metatarsals
- Second, third, fourth metatarso-phalangeal joints
- Second, third, fourth phalanges
- Third and fourth cuneiform bones

Lateral Aspect
- Lateral calcaneus
- Lateral malleolus
- Sinus tarsi
- Peroneal tubercle
- Cuboid bone
- Styloid process (proximal head of the fifth metatarsal)
- Fifth metatarsal
- Fifth metatarsophalangeal joint
- Fifth phalanx

Plantar Aspect
- Metatarsal heads
- Medial calcaneal tubercle
- Sesamoid bones

Soft-Tissue Palpation

The following soft-tissue structures should be palpated:

Medial and Plantar Aspect
- Tibialis posterior tendon
- Flexor hallucis longus tendon
- Flexor digitorum longus tendon
- Deltoid ligament
- Calcaneonavicular ligament (spring ligament)
- Medial longitudinal arch
- Plantar fascia
- Transverse arch

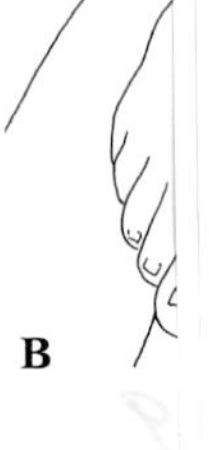

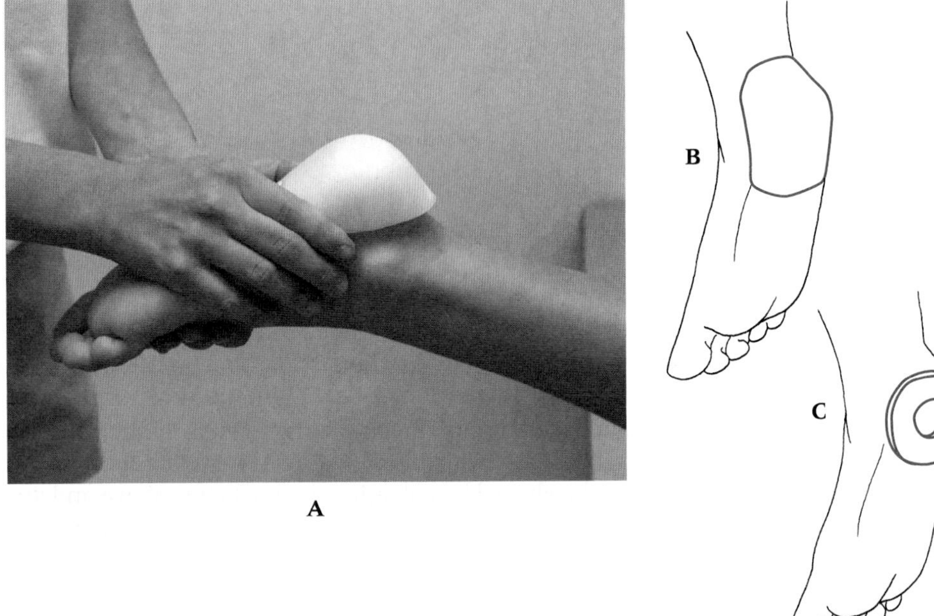

Figure 18-18

A & B, Heel protection achieved through the use of a heel cup. **C,** Protective heel doughnut.

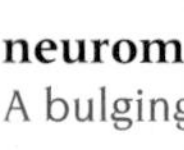

Symptoms and signs This displacement of the cuboid causes pain along the fourth and fifth metatarsals as well as over the cuboid. This problem often refers pain to the heel area as well. Many times this pain is increased when the athlete rises after a prolonged non–weight bearing period.

Management Dramatic treatment results may be obtained by manipulating to restore the cuboid to its natural position (Figure 18-19). Once the cuboid is manipulated, an orthotic often helps to support it in its proper position. If manipulation is successful, quite often the athlete can return to play immediately with little or no pain. The athlete should wear an appropriately constructed orthotic when practicing or competing to reduce the chances of recurrence.

Tarsal Tunnel Syndrome

Etiology The tarsal tunnel is a loosely defined area behind the medial malleolus that forms a tunnel with an osseous floor and the roof composed of the flexor retinaculum. Through this tunnel pass the tibialis posterior, flexor hallucis longus, and

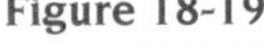

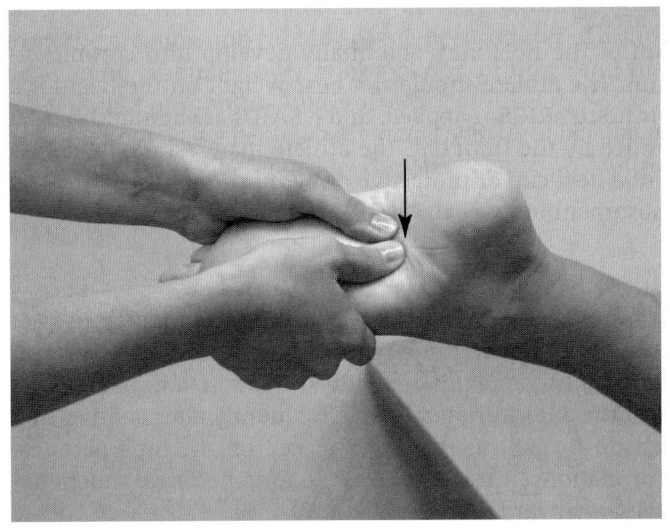

Figure 18-19

A cuboid manipulation is done with the athlete prone. The lateral plantar aspect of the forefoot is grasped by the thumbs, with the fingers supporting the dorsum of the foot. The thumbs should be over the cuboid. The manipulation should be a thrust downward to move the cuboid into its more dorsal position. Often, a pop is felt as the cuboid moves back into place.

flexor digitorum muscles with their surrounding synovial sheaths and the tibial nerve artery and vein. Any condition that compromises the structures within this tunnel can cause tarsal tunnel syndrome, including tenosynovitis, previous fractures, excessive pronation, or any acute trauma.[33]

Symptoms and signs Complaints of pain and paresthesia are typical, particularly along the medial and plantar aspects of the foot.[31] Complaints of increased pain at night are also common. Tinel's sign will be positive in cases of tarsal tunnel syndrome (see Figure 18-14). If the condition persists, motor weakness and atrophy may gradually appear, following the course of the tibial nerve.

Management Initial conservative management includes the use of antiinflammatory medication and other antiinflammatory modalities. The use of an appropriate orthotic to correct excessive pronation may effectively reduce the symptoms. Surgery may be necessary if the symptoms become recurrent.[33]

Tarsometatarsal Fracture/Dislocation (Lisfranc Injury)

Etiology Named after a French surgeon who described amputations at the tarsometatarsal joint, this is an uncommon injury that can cause long-term disability. The ankle is plantar flexed with the rearfoot locked, and there is a sudden forceful hyper–plantar flexion of the forefoot that results in dorsal displacement of the proximal end of the metatarsals. The dorsum of the foot rolls forward with the body weight providing the force to displace the base of the metatarsals dorsally.[58]

Symptoms and signs In the athlete, the symptoms may be relatively subtle. The athlete complains of pain and an inability to bear weight. Swelling and tenderness are localized over the dorsum of the foot. There may be a fracture of the metatarsals. Sprain of the fourth and fifth proximal metatarsals causes ongoing pain. It is not uncommon to overlook the serious disruption of the supporting ligaments because attention is often focused on a metatarsal fracture.

Management If the athletic trainer suspects this injury, the athlete should be referred to the physician for evaluation. The key to treatment is first recognizing the injury, then restoring alignment, and finally maintaining stability. Closed reduction often fails, and most likely it will be necessary to do an open reduction with internal fixation to stabilize the dislocation. Potential complications include metatarsalgia, limited motion of the metatarsophalangeal joints, and long-term disability.[58]

Injuries to the Metatarsal Region

Pes Planus Foot (Flatfoot)

Etiology The term *pes planus* refers to a type of foot in which the medial longitudinal arch appears to be flat and is sometimes said to be fallen (Figure 18-20). In general,

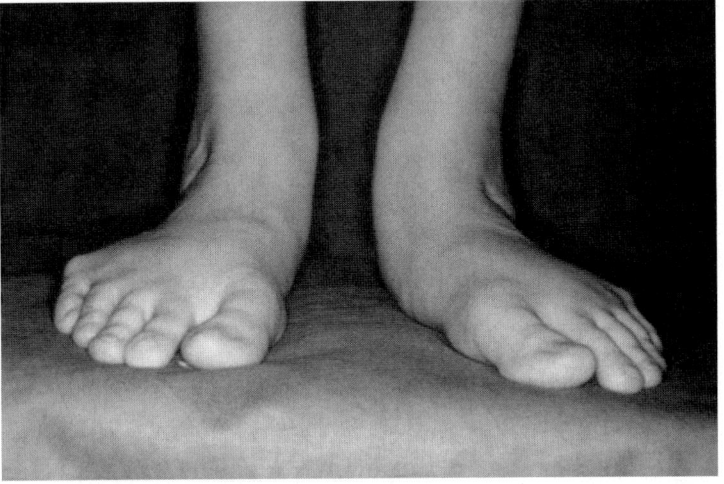

Figure 18-20

Fallen medial longitudinal arch.

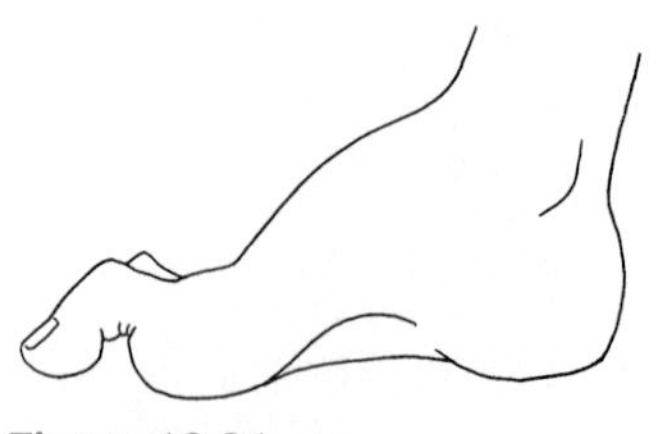

Figure 18-21

Pes cavus.

pes planus is associated with excessive foot pronation and may be caused by a number of factors, including a structural forefoot varus deformity, wearing shoes that are too tight, trauma that weakens supportive structures such as muscles and ligaments, overweight, or excessive exercise that repeatedly subjects the arch to severe pounding on an unyielding surface.[49]

Symptoms and signs The athlete may complain of pain and a feeling of weakness or fatigue in the medial longitudinal arch. There may be calcaneal eversion, a bulging of the navicular bone, a flattening of the medial longitudinal arch, and dorsiflexing with lateral splaying of the first metatarsal.

Management Regardless of how flattened the medial longitudinal arch appears to be, if it is not causing the athlete any pain or related symptoms, then absolutely nothing should be done to try to correct the apparent problem. Attempts to do so may in fact create an unnecessary problem. However, if the athlete is experiencing pain, an appropriately constructed orthotic designed to correct excessive pronation by using a medial wedge will most likely alleviate symptoms. In certain cases, incorporating an arch support into the orthotic or taping the arch for support may be helpful (see Figures 8-14 through 8-17).

18-3 Critical Thinking Exercise

An athlete enters the athletic training room complaining of her flat feet and that she has pain in her knees and a big callus under her second metatarsal.

? What is likely causing this problem, and how can it usually be corrected?

Pes Cavus Foot (High Arch Foot)

Etiology The term *pes cavus* refers to a type of foot that has an arch that is higher than normal (Figure 18-21). Sometimes called *clawfoot* or *hollow foot,* pes cavus is not as common as pes planus. A pes cavus is generally associated with excessive supination. The accentuated high medial longitudinal arch may be congenital or may indicate a neurological disorder.[33]

Symptoms and signs In cases of pes cavus, shock absorption is poor, and thus problems such as general foot pain, metatarsalgia, and clawed or hammer toes are seen. Commonly associated with this condition are a structural forefoot valgus deformity and an abnormal shortening of the Achilles tendon. The Achilles tendon is directly linked with the plantar fascia (Figure 18-22). Also, because of the abnormal distribution of body weight, heavy calluses develop on the ball and heel of the foot.[49]

Management As is the case with pes planus, pes cavus may be asymptomatic, in which case no attempt should be made to correct the problem. If there are associated problems, then an orthotic should be constructed using a lateral wedge to correct a

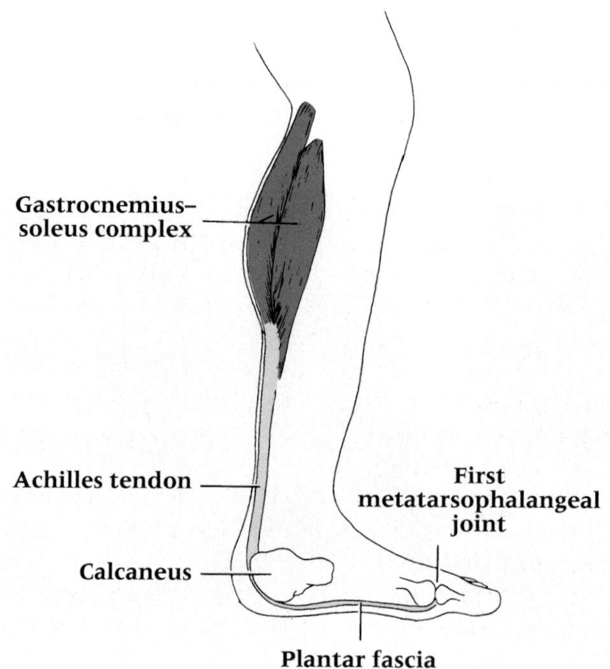

Figure 18-22

The Achilles tendon is directly linked with the plantar fascia. Achilles tendon stretching releases a tight medial longitudinal arch.

structural forefoot valgus deformity. Stretching of the Achilles tendon and the plantar fascia may also be helpful.

Longitudinal Arch Strain

Etiology Longitudinal arch strain is usually an early-season injury caused by subjecting the musculature of the foot to increased stress produced by repetitive contact with hard playing surfaces. In this condition, there is a flattening or depression of the longitudinal arch while the foot is in the midsupport phase, resulting in a strain to the arch. Such a strain may appear suddenly, or it may develop slowly over a considerable length of time.

Symptoms and signs As a rule, pain is experienced only during running or jumping. The pain usually appears just below the posterior tibialis tendon and is accompanied by swelling and tenderness along the medial aspects of the foot. This injury may also be associated with a sprain of the calcaneonavicular ligament as well as a strain of the flexor hallucis longus tendon.

Management The management of a longitudinal arch strain involves immediate care, consisting of RICE, followed by appropriate therapy and reduction of weight bearing. Weight bearing must be performed pain free. Arch taping technique no. 1 or 2 might be used to allow earlier pain-free weight bearing (see Figures 8-15 through 8-18).

18-4

***Critical Thinking* Exercise**

A distance runner is experiencing pain in the left arch. There is palpable tenderness in the left foot's aponeurosis, primarily in the epicondyle region of the calcaneus.

? What condition does this scenario describe, and how should it be managed?

Plantar Fasciitis

Heel pain is a very common problem in the athletic and nonathletic population. This phenomenon has been attributed to several etiologies, including heel spurs, plantar fascia irritation, and bursitis.[16] *Plantar fasciitis* is a catchall term that is commonly used to describe pain in the proximal arch and heel. The plantar fascia (plantar aponeurosis) runs the length of the sole of the foot (see Figure 18-3). It is a broad band of dense connective tissue that is attached proximally to the medial surface of the calcaneus. It fans out distally, with fibers and their various small branches attaching to the metatarsophalangeal articulations and merging into the capsular ligaments. The function of the plantar fascia is to assist in maintaining the stability of the foot and in securing or bracing the longitudinal arch.[34]

Etiology Tension develops in the plantar fascia both during extension of the toes and during depression of the longitudinal arch as the result of weight bearing.[1] When the weight is principally on the heel, as in ordinary standing, the tension exerted on the fascia is negligible. However, when the weight is shifted to the ball of the foot (on the heads of the metatarsals), fascial tension is increased. In running, because the toe-off phase involves both a forceful extension of the toes and a powerful thrust by the ball of the foot (on the heads of the metatarsals), fascial tension is increased to approximately twice the body weight.[12] Tightening of the plantar fascia during dorsiflexion, thus shortening the longitudinal arch, has been described as the "windlass" mechanism.[6]

Plantar fasciitis can occur in athletes with high arches in which case the foot has too little motion or in those with a low arch in which case there is too much motion.[6]

Street shoes, by nature of their design, take on the characteristics of splints and tend to restrict foot action to such an extent that the arch may become somewhat rigid. This rigidity occurs because of shortening of the ligaments and other mild abnormalities. The athlete, changing from such footwear into a flexible gymnastic slipper or soft track shoe, often experiences trauma when the foot is subjected to stress. Trauma may also result from poor running technique.

A number of anatomical and biomechanical conditions have been studied as possible causes of plantar fasciitis. Those conditions include leg length discrepancy, excessive pronation of the subtalar joint, inflexibility of the longitudinal arch, and tightness of the gastrocnemius-soleus unit.[42] Wearing shoes without sufficient arch support, running with a lengthened stride, and running on soft surfaces are also potential causes of plantar fasciitis.[57]

Signs & Symptoms
Management Plan
Therapy
Exercise Rehabilitation

Management PLAN

Plantar Fasciitis

Injury Situation A male cross-country runner injured the proximal arch and heel when he stepped into a hole during a meet. The athlete continued to run and work out for a week before reporting his injury to the athletic trainer.

Symptoms and Signs The athlete complained of early pain in the medial arch and medial distal heel that tended to move centrally as the week progressed. He complained of severe pain when rising in the morning and after sitting for a long period. The area appeared slightly swollen with a severe sharp pain on palpation at the plantar fascia insertion and medial aspect of the calcaneus. Pain increased with passive dorsiflexion of the great toe. An X ray showed the beginning of a heel spur. The athlete was found to have a cavus foot.

Management Plan The athlete was diagnosed as having plantar fasciitis (heel spur syndrome), and a conservative plan was chosen.

Phase 1 Acute Injury

GOALS: Minimize inflammation and pain.
ESTIMATED LENGTH OF TIME (ELT): 1 week.

■ **Therapy** RICE plus NSAID as needed to reduce pain and inflammation. Injection therapy consisting of a steroid and anesthetic for trigger points.

■ **Exercise rehabilitation** Toe touch crutch walking. Begin heel cord stretching and rolling pin exercise to increase fascia flexibility.

Phase 2 Repair

GOALS: Gain full weight bearing and walking pattern.
ELT: 1 to 3 weeks.

■ **Therapy** Ultrasound to increase blood flow. Cross friction massage over injury site. Apply shock absorption shoe insert with cutout (3 to 5 cm) in the tender area. Apply arch taping.

■ **Exercise rehabilitation** Continue heel cord stretching and rolling pin exercise to stretch the plantar fascia. Begin a program of gradual pain-free weight bearing. Begin a program of foot flexor strengthening.

Phase 3 Remodeling

GOALS: Focus on full pain-free weight bearing while engaged in running.
ELT: 2 weeks.

■ **Therapy** Ultrasound as warranted. Continue cross friction massage. Use of a heel cup and arch taping when athlete is supporting weight.

■ **Exercise rehabilitation** Continue heel cord and plantar fascia stretching. Use shoes with a reinforced heel counter for heel control. Initiate foot flexor strengthening against tubular resistance. Perform general exercise to the lower leg. Begin a running program that is pain free.

Criteria for Return to Competitive Cross-Country Running

1. Proximal arch and heel are pain free.
2. Heel cord and plantar fascia are stretched.
3. Lower leg has maximum strength.
4. Athlete is able to run competitively without pain.
5. Athlete is psychologically ready for competition.

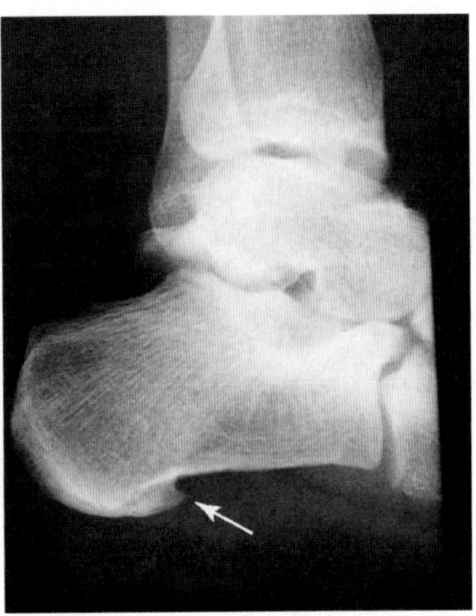

Figure 18-23

X ray of a large plantar calcaneal exostotic spur.

Symptoms and signs The athlete complains of pain in the anterior medial heel, usually at the attachment of the plantar fascia to the calcaneus. The pain eventually moves into the central portion of the plantar fascia. This pain is increased when the athlete rises in the morning or bears weight after sitting for a long period. However, the pain lessens after a few steps. Pain also will be intensified when the toes and forefoot are forcibly dorsiflexed. If irritation persists, a painful heel spur will probably develop at the attachment of the plantar fascia to the medial aspect of the calcaneus; the heel spur will be visible on an X ray (Figure 18-23).

Management Management of plantar fasciitis will generally require an extended period of treatment.[53] It is not uncommon for symptoms to persist for as long as eight to twelve weeks. Orthotic therapy is very useful in the treatment of this problem. A soft orthotic works better than a hard orthotic. An extra-deep heel cup should be built into the orthotic. The orthotic should be worn at all times, especially when the athlete rises from bed in the morning.[31] Use of a heel cup compresses the fat pad under the calcaneus, providing a cushion under the area of irritation. When soft orthotics are not feasible, taping may reduce the symptoms. A simple arch taping or alternative taping often allows pain-free ambulation.[16] The use of a night splint to maintain a position of static stretch has also been recommended. In some cases, the athlete may need to use a short leg walking cast for four to six weeks.

The athlete should engage in vigorous heel cord stretching and in exercises that stretch the plantar fascia in the arch.[51] Exercises that increase dorsiflexion of the great toe also may be of benefit to this problem. Stretching should be done at least three times a day. Antiinflammatory medications are recommended. Steroidal injection may be warranted at some point if symptoms fail to resolve.

18-5

Critical Thinking Exercise

A basketball player sustains a grade 2 lateral sprain of the left ankle.

? What metatarsal fracture may be associated with this type of sprain?

Jones Fracture

Etiology Fractures may occur to any of the metatarsals and can be caused by inversion and plantar flexion of the foot; by direct force, such as being stepped on by another player; or by repetitive stress. By far the most common acute fracture is to the diaphysis at the base of the fifth metatarsal, which is referred to specifically as a Jones fracture (Figure 18-24).[56]

Symptoms and signs A Jones fracture is characterized by immediate swelling and pain over the fifth metatarsal. Healing of a Jones fracture is slow and frustrating for the athlete. This injury has a high nonunion rate, and the course of healing is unpredictable.[9]

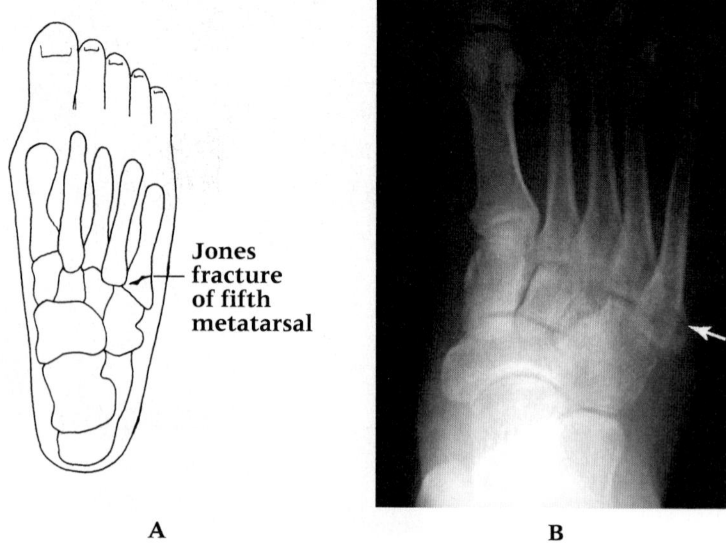

Figure 18-24

A, Jones fracture occurs at the neck of the fifth metatarsal.
B, Jones fracture X-ray.

Management Treatment for a Jones fracture is controversial but it appears that the use of crutches with no immobilization, gradually progressing to full weight bearing as pain subsides, may allow the athlete to return to activity in about six weeks. However, nonunion may cause a refracture to occur. It has been recommended that athletes be treated more aggressively using early internal fixation.[22] It has also been suggested that an ultrasonic bone-growth stimulator will promote healing in a Jones fracture.[10]

18-6 Critical Thinking Exercise

A cross-country runner changes her running patterns by increasing distance and performing more hill work. She complains to the athletic trainer of a gradually worsening pain in her forefoot. Inspection reveals point tenderness in the region of the fourth metatarsal bone. X-ray reveals a stress fracture.

? How should this condition be managed?

Metatarsal Stress Fractures

Etiology The most common metatarsal stress fracture in the foot involves the shaft of the second metatarsal and is often referred to as a *march fracture.* It occurs in the runner who has suddenly changed patterns of training, such as increasing mileage, running hills, or running on a harder surface. An athlete who has an atypical condition such as a structural forefoot varus, hallux valgus, flatfoot, or a short first metatarsal is more predisposed to a second metatarsal stress fracture.[20,40]

An athlete can also experience a stress fracture of the fifth metatarsal at the insertion of the peroneus brevis tendon, but this injury should not be confused with a Jones fracture.[3]

Management A bone scan is the best way to detect the presence of a stress fracture. Management of a metatarsal stress fracture usually consists of three or four days of partial weight bearing followed by two weeks of rest. Return to running should be very gradual. An orthotic that corrects excessive pronation can help take stress off the second metatarsal.[8]

18-7 Critical Thinking Exercise

A field hockey player complains to the athletic trainer of swelling, tenderness, and aching in the head of the first metatarsophalangeal joint of her left foot. On inspection, the athletic trainer observes that the great toe is deviated laterally.

? What is this condition commonly called, and why does it occur?

Bunion (Hallux Valgus Deformity) and Bunionettes (Tailor's Bunions)

Etiology A bunion, one of the most frequent painful deformities, occurs at the head of the first metatarsal (Figure 18-25). The term *bunion* is often used to refer to an exostosis. Commonly, a bunion is associated with a structural forefoot varus in which the first ray tends to splay outward, putting pressure on the first metatarsal head. Bunions are often caused by shoes that are pointed, too narrow, or too short. It is generally believed that women's shoes play a predominant role in the development of a hallux valgus deformity.[36]

The bursa over the first metatarsophalangeal joint becomes inflamed and eventually thickens. Tendinitis may develop in the flexor tendons of the great toe.[41] The joint becomes enlarged and the great toe becomes malaligned, moving laterally toward the second toe, sometimes to such an extent that it eventually overlaps the second toe.

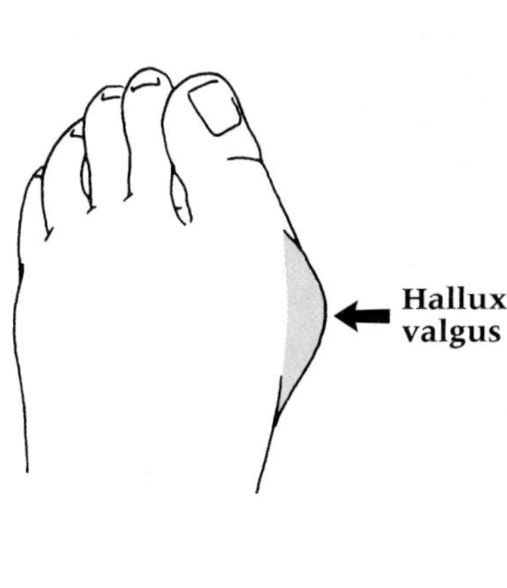

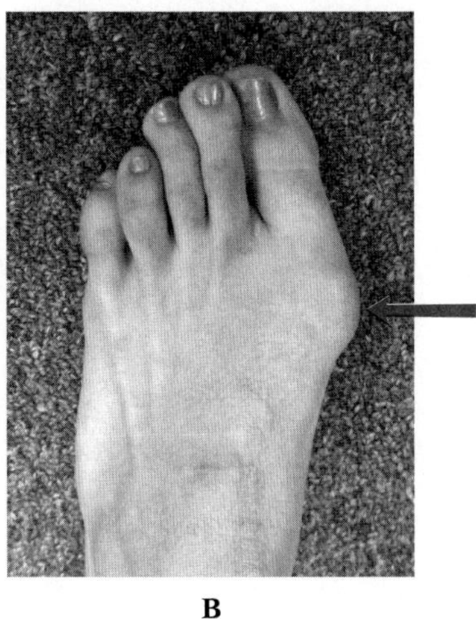

Figure 18-25

Bunion with hallux valgus deformity.

This type of bunion is also associated with a depressed or flattened transverse arch and a pronated foot.

The bunionette, or tailor's bunion, is much less common than hallux valgus and affects the fifth metatarsophalangeal joint. In this case, the little toe angulates toward the fourth toe, causing an enlarged metatarsal head.[13]

In all bunions, both the flexor and extensor tendons are malaligned, creating more angular stress on the joint. NOTE: Sesamoid fractures and sesamoiditis could be secondary to hallux valgus.

Symptoms and signs In the beginning of bunion formation, there is tenderness, swelling, and enlargement of the joint. Poorly fitting shoes increase the irritation and pain. As the inflammation continues, angulation of the toe progresses, eventually leading to painful ambulation.

Management Each bunion has unique characteristics. Early recognition and care can often prevent increased irritation and deformity. Following are some management procedures:

1. Wear correctly fitting shoes with a wide toe box.
2. Wear an appropriate orthotic to correct a structural forefoot varus deformity.
3. Place a felt or sponge rubber doughnut pad over the first and/or fifth metatarsophalangeal joint.
4. Wear a tape splint along with a resilient wedge placed between the great toe and the second toe (see Figure 8-20, page 539).
5. Engage in daily foot exercises to strengthen the extensor and flexor muscles.

Ultimately, a surgical procedure called a bunionectomy may be necessary to correct the problem.

Sesamoiditis

Etiology Two sesamoid bones lie within the flexors and adductor tendons of the great toe. These sesamoids function to transmit forces from the ground to the head of the first metatarsal. Sesamoiditis is caused by repetitive hyperextension of the great toe that eventually results in inflammation. Sesamoiditis is most common in dancing and basketball. It is estimated that 30 percent of sesamoid injuries are sesamoiditis.[45] Fractures of the sesamoids are also common.

Symptoms and signs The athlete complains of pain under the great toe, especially during a push-off. There is palpable tenderness under the first metatarsal head.

Management Sesamoiditis is treated with a variety of orthotic devices, including metatarsal pads, arch supports, and most often, a metatarsal bar (Figure 18-26). Activity should be decreased to allow inflammation to subside.

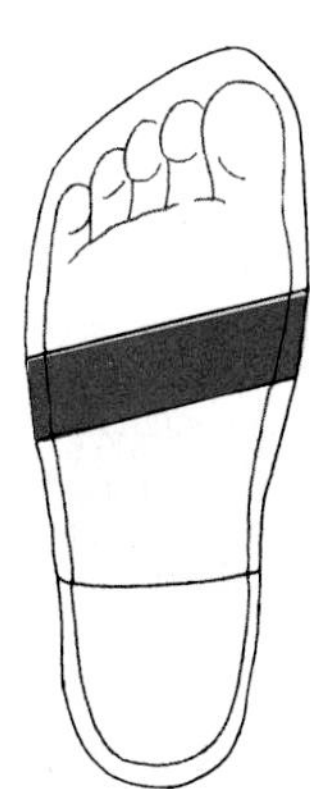

Figure 18-26

Metatarsal bar to treat both metatarsalgia and sesamoiditis.

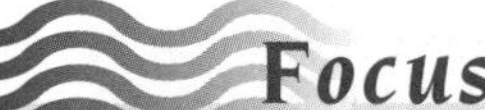

Metatarsal pad support

The purpose of the metatarsal pad is to reestablish the normal relationships of the metatarsal bones. It can be purchased commercially or constructed out of felt or sponge rubber (see Figure 18-30).

Materials needed

One roll of 1-inch (2.5 cm) tape, a ⅛-inch (0.3 cm) adhesive felt oval cut to a 2-inch (5 cm) circumference, and tape adherent.

Position of the athlete

The athlete sits on a table or chair with the plantar surface of the affected foot turned upward.

Position of the operator

The operator stands facing the plantar aspect of the athlete's foot.

Procedure

1. The circular pad is placed just behind the metatarsal heads.
2. Approximately two or three circular strips of tape are placed loosely around the pad and foot.

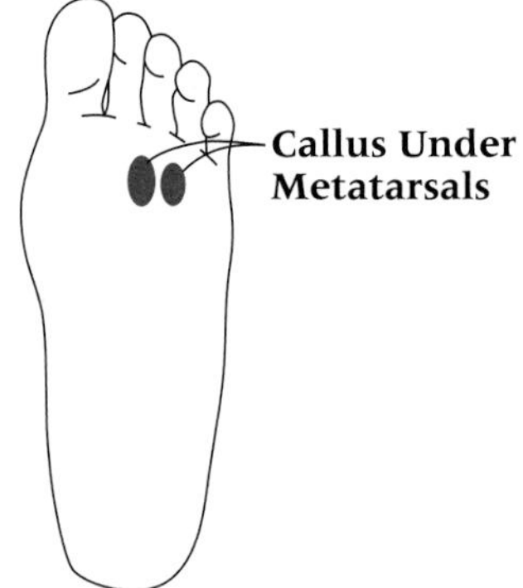

Figure 18-27

A heavy callus often forms under the metatarsal heads in metatarsalgia.

Metatarsalgia

Etiology Although *metatarsalgia* is a general term used to describe pain in the ball of the foot, it is more commonly associated with pain under the second and sometimes the third metatarsal head. A heavy callus often forms in the area of pain (Figure 18-27).[60]

One of the causes of metatarsalgia is restricted extensibility of the gastrocnemius-soleus complex. Because of this restriction, the athlete shortens the midstance phase of the gait and emphasizes the toe-off phase, causing excessive pressure under the forefoot. This excess pressure over time causes a heavy callus to form in this region. As the forefoot bears weight, normal skin becomes pinched against the inelastic callus and produces pain.[45]

Another cause of metatarsalgia is a fallen metatarsal arch.

Symptoms and signs As the transverse arch becomes flattened and the heads of the second, third, and fourth metatarsal bones become depressed, pain can result. A cavus deformity can also cause metatarsalgia.

Management Management of metatarsalgia usually consists of applying a pad to elevate the depressed metatarsal heads. See *Focus Box:* "Metatarsal pad support." NOTE: The bar is placed behind and not under the metatarsal heads (see Figure 18-26). Abnormal callus buildup should be removed by paring or filing. An athlete for whom the etiology of metatarsalgia is primarily a gastrocnemius-soleus contracture should perform a regimen of static stretching several times per day. An athlete whose metatarsal arch is depressed as a result of weakness should practice a daily regimen of exercise, concentrating on strengthening flexor and intrinsic muscles and stretching the Achilles tendon. A Thomas heel (Figure 18-28), which elevates the medial aspect of the heel from ⅛ to 3⁄16 inch (0.3 to 0.47 cm), also could prove beneficial.

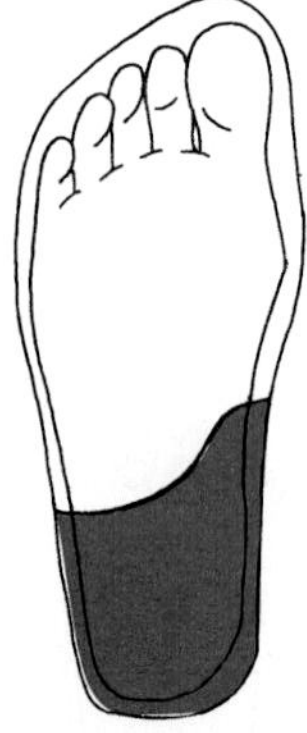

Figure 18-28

The Thomas heel elevates the medial aspect of the calcaneus ⅛ to 3⁄16 inch (0.3 to 0.47 cm), which can help relieve pronation and metatarsalgia.

Metatarsal Arch Strain

Etiology The athlete who has a fallen metatarsal arch or who has a pes cavus is susceptible to strain.[8] Normally, the heads of the first and fifth metatarsal bones bear slightly more weight than the heads of the second, third, and fourth metatarsal bones. The first metatarsal head bears two-sixths of the body weight, the fifth bears slightly more than one-sixth, and the second, third, and fourth each bear approximately one-sixth. If the foot tends to excessively pronate or if the intermetatarsal ligaments are weak, allowing the foot to spread abnormally (splayed foot), a fallen metatarsal arch may result (Figure 18-29).

Symptoms and signs The athlete has pain or cramping in the metatarsal region. There is **point tenderness** and weakness in the area. Morton's test may produce pain in the metatarsals (see Figure 18-15).

point tenderness Pain produced when an injury site is palpated.

Management Treatment of a metatarsal arch strain usually consists of applying a pad to elevate the depressed metatarsal heads. The pad is placed in the center and just behind the ball of the foot (metatarsal heads) (Figure 18-30).

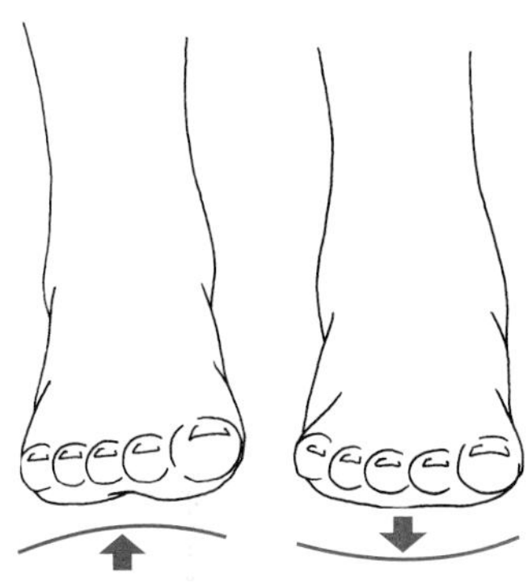

Figure 18-29

Normal and fallen metatarsal arch.

Morton's Neuroma

Etiology A neuroma is a mass that occurs about the nerve sheath of the common plantar nerve at the point at which it divides into the two digital branches to adjacent toes. A neuroma usually occurs between the metatarsal heads and is the most common nerve problem of the lower extremity.[58] A Morton's neuroma is located between the third and fourth metatarsal heads where the nerve is the thickest because it receives branches from both the medial and lateral plantar nerves (Figure 18-31).

Irritation increases with the collapse of the transverse arch of the foot, which puts the transverse metatarsal ligaments under stretch and thus compresses the common digital nerve and vessels. Excessive foot pronation can also be a predisposing factor, because more metatarsal shearing forces occur with the prolonged forefoot abduction.

Symptoms and signs The athlete complains of a burning paresthesia and severe intermittent pain in the forefoot that is often localized to the third web space and radiating to the toes. The pain is often relieved with non–weight bearing.[31] Hyperextension of the toes on weight bearing, as in squatting, stair climbing, or running, can increase the symptoms. Wearing shoes with a narrow toe box or high heels can increase the symptoms. If there is prolonged nerve irritation, the pain can become constant.[24]

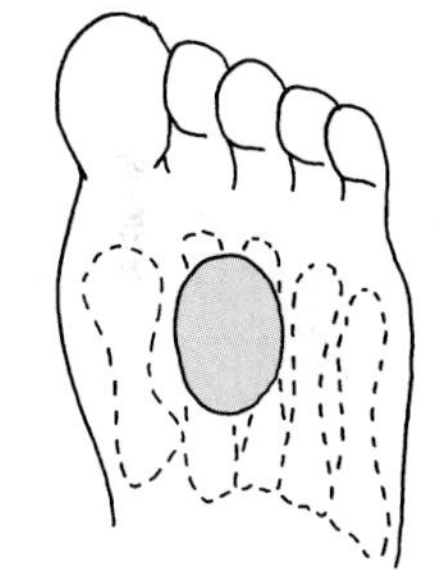

Figure 18-30

Metatarsal pad.

Management A bone scan is often necessary to rule out a metatarsal stress fracture. A teardrop-shaped pad is placed between the heads of the third and fourth metatarsals in an attempt to splay the metatarsals apart during weight bearing, which decreases pressure on the neuroma. Often this teardrop pad will markedly reduce pain, and the athlete can continue to play despite this condition. Shoe selection also plays an important role in the treatment of neuromas. Narrow shoes, particularly women's shoes that are pointed in the toe area and certain men's boots, may squeeze the metatarsal heads together and exacerbate the problem. A shoe that is wide in the toe box area should be selected. A straight-laced shoe often provides increased space in the toe box.[58] On rare occasions, surgical excision may be required.

Injuries to the Toes

Sprained Toes

Etiology Sprains of the phalangeal joints of the toes are caused most often by kicking some nonyielding object. Sprains result from a considerable force applied in such a manner as to extend the joint beyond its normal range of motion (jamming it) or to impart a twisting motion to the toe, thereby twisting and tearing the ligaments and joint capsule.

Symptoms and signs Pain is immediate and intense but is generally short lived. There is immediate swelling with discoloration appearing during the first or second day. There will be stiffness and residual pain that may last for several weeks.

Management RICE must be applied immediately to minimize swelling. Casting or splinting of the small toes is difficult. Thus, buddy taping the injured toe to the adjacent toes is an effective technique of immobilization. The athlete may begin weight bearing as soon as tolerated and may not need to be on crutches at all.

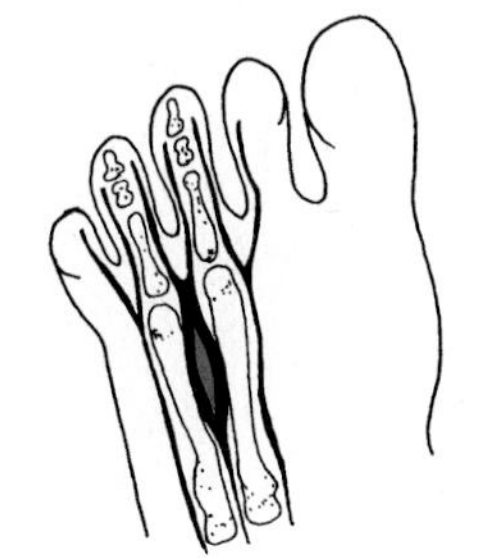

Figure 18-31

Morton's neuroma.

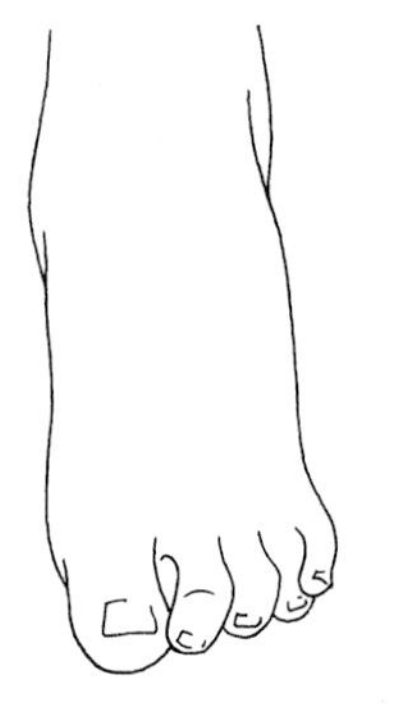

Figure 18-34

Overlapping toes.

may also help to reduce skin irritation. Once the deformities become fixed, it is likely that surgical procedures that involve straightening the toes and then maintaining positioning by using K-wire (Kirshner wire) inserted longitudinally through the phalanges into the metacarpals becomes necessary.[13]

Overlapping Toes

Etiology Overlapping of the toes (Figure 18-34) may be congenital or may be brought about by improperly fitting footwear, particularly shoes that are too narrow.

Symptoms and signs At times, the condition indicates an outward projection of the great toe articulation or a drop in the longitudinal or metatarsal arch.

Management As in the case of hammertoes, surgery is the only cure, but some therapeutic modalities such as a whirlpool bath can assist in alleviating inflammation. Taping may prevent some of the contractural tension within the sport shoe.

Blood under the Toenail (Subungual Hematoma)

Etiology Blood can accumulate under a toenail as a result of the toe being stepped on, of dropping an object on the toe, or of kicking another object. Repetitive shearing forces on toenails, as may occur in the shoe of a long-distance runner, may also cause bleeding into the nail bed. In any case, blood that accumulates in a confined space underneath the nail is likely to produce extreme pain and can ultimately cause loss of the nail[1] (Figure 18-35).

Symptoms and signs Bleeding into the nail bed may be either immediate or slow, producing considerable pain. The area under the toenail assumes a bluish-purple color and gentle pressure on the nail greatly exacerbates pain.

Management An ice pack should be applied immediately, and the foot should be elevated to decrease bleeding. Within the next 12 to 24 hours, the pressure of the blood under the nail should be released by drilling a small hole through the nail into the nail bed. This drilling must be done under sterile conditions and is best done by either a physician or an athletic trainer. It is not uncommon to have to drill the nail a second time because more blood is likely to accumulate.

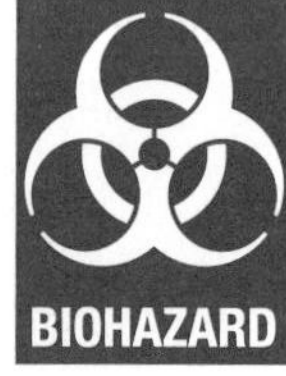

FOOT REHABILITATION

It is critical that the athletic trainer incorporate appropriate rehabilitation techniques in managing injuries of the foot. The foot is the base of support for the entire kinetic chain. Thus, injuries to the foot can affect the biomechanics of not only the foot, but also the ankle, knee, hip, and spine.

General Body Conditioning

Rehabilitation techniques for managing injuries to the lower extremity in general and to the foot in particular often require that the athlete be non–weight bearing for some period of time. Even if weight bearing is allowed, the injured athlete will not be able

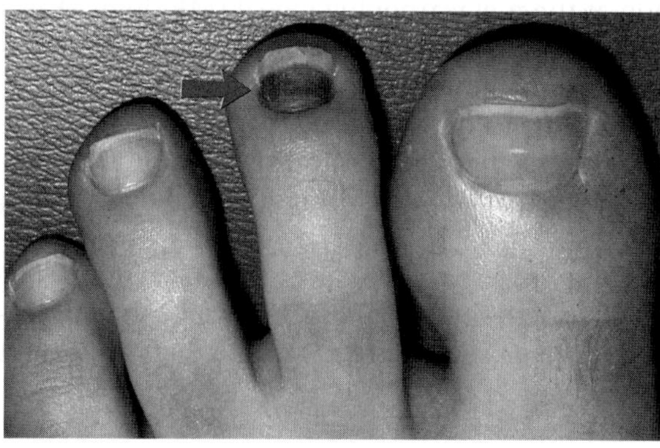

Figure 18-35

A subungual hematoma is blood accumulating under the nail.

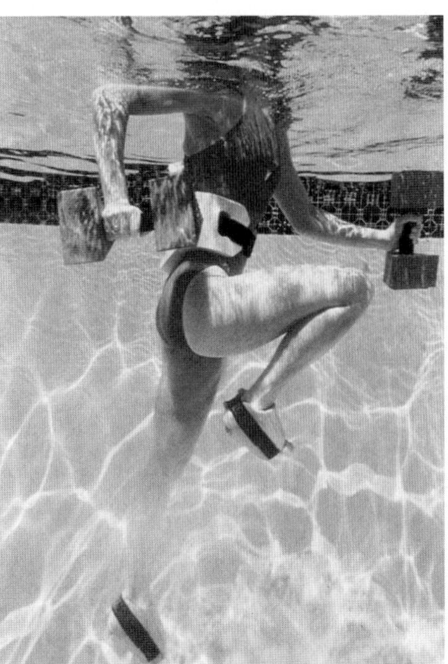

Figure 18-36

Pool exercises are useful in maintaining fitness while non–weight bearing.

to maintain his or her level of fitness by engaging in running activities. Thus it becomes necessary to substitute alternative conditioning activities such as running in a pool or working on an upper extremity ergometer (Figure 18-36).[15] The athlete should certainly continue to engage in strengthening and flexibility exercises as allowed by the constraints of the injury.

18-11

***Critical Thinking* Exercise**

A tennis player complains of pain in the ball of the right foot. Inspection reveals a heavy callus formation under the second metatarsal head. This condition produces a metatarsalgia.

? What is this probable cause of this condition?

Weight Bearing

If the athlete is unable to walk without a limp, non–weight bearing or limited weight-bearing crutch walking might be employed. Using incorrect gait mechanics will certainly affect other joints within the kinetic chain, causing unnecessary pain, and tends to do more harm than good. Progressing to full weight bearing as soon as it may be tolerated is generally recommended.

Joint Mobilization

Manual joint mobilization techniques are useful in maintaining or normalizing joint motions (Figure 18-37). The following joint mobilization techniques can be used in the foot:

- Anterior/posterior calcaneocuboid glides are used for increasing adduction and abduction. The calcaneus should be stabilized while the cuboid is mobilized.
- Anterior/posterior cuboidmetatarsal glides are done with one hand stabilizing the cuboid and the other gliding the base of the fifth metatarsal. These glides are used for increasing mobility of the fifth metatarsal.
- Anterior/posterior tarsometatarsal glides decrease hypomobility of the metatarsals.
- Anterior/posterior talonavicular glides also increase adduction and abduction. One hand stabilizes the talus while the other mobilizes the navicular bone.
- With anterior/posterior metatarsophalangeal glides, the anterior glides increase extension and the posterior glides increase flexion. Mobilizations are accomplished by isolating individual segments.

Flexibility

Maintaining normal flexibility is critical in the foot. Restoring full range of motion following various injuries to the phalanges is particularly important. It is also critical to engage in stretching activities in the case of plantar fasciitis (Figure 18-38). Stretching

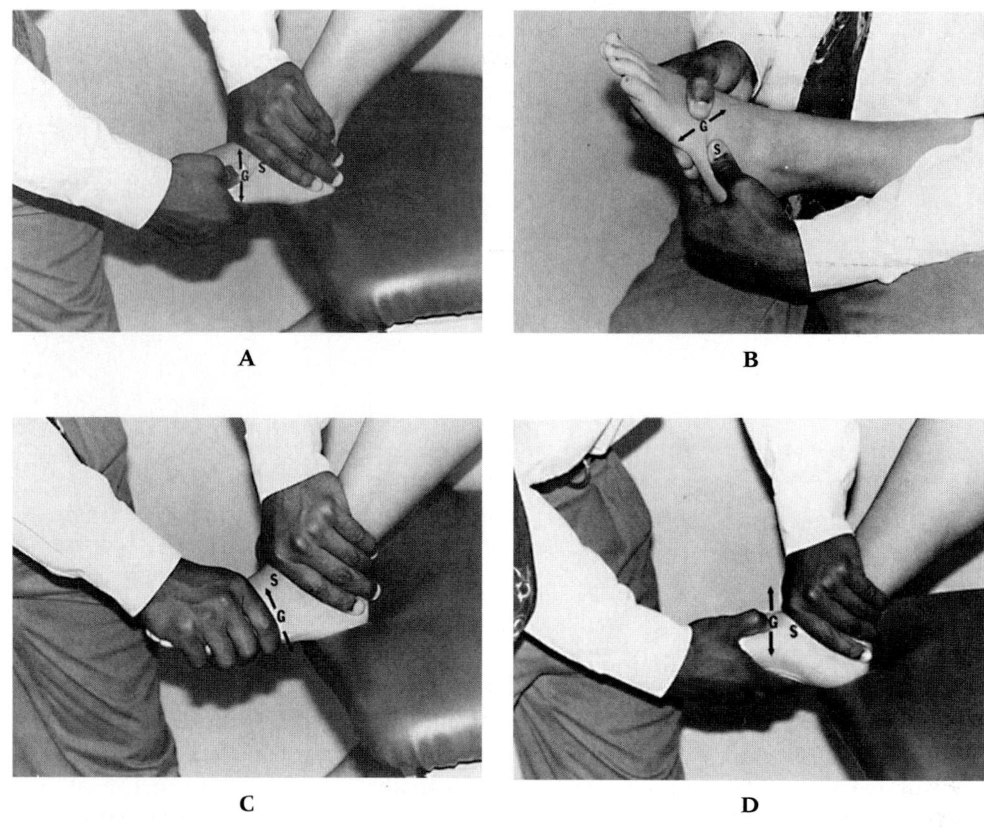

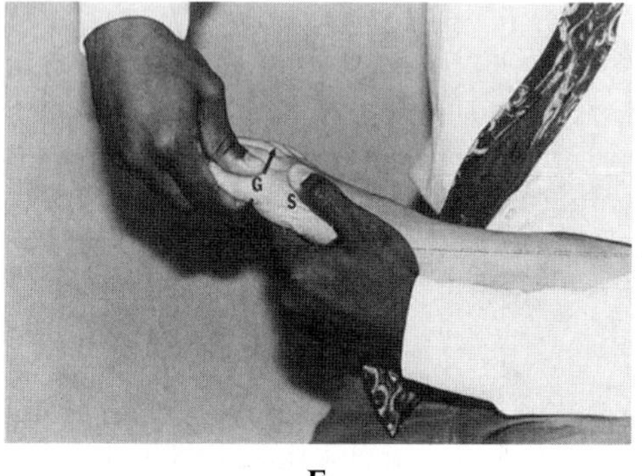

Figure 18-37

A, Anterior/posterior calcaneocuboid glides. **B,** Anterior/posterior cuboidmetatarsal glides. **C,** Anterior/posterior tarsometatarsal glides. **D,** Anterior/posterior talonavicular glides. **E,** Anterior/posterior metatarsophalangeal glides.

18-12

***Critical Thinking* Exercise**

A defensive lineman on a college football team complains of severe intermittent pain in the region between the third and fourth toes of the left foot. Inspection reveals that the pain radiates from the base to the tip of the toes. There is numbness of the skin between the toes.

? What is this condition, and how should it be conservatively managed?

of the gastrocnemius-soleus complex is also important for a number of injuries (see Figure 19-33B and C).

Muscular Strength

Strength exercises for the foot can be done using a variety of resistance methods, including rubber tubing, towel exercises, and manual resistance.

Exercises commonly used in strengthening the muscles involved in foot motion include:

- Writing the alphabet—With the toes pointed, the athlete writes the complete alphabet in the air three times.
- Picking up objects—The athlete picks up small objects such as marbles with the toes and places them in a container.
- Ankle circumduction—The ankle is circumducted in as extreme a range of motion as possible (ten circles in one direction and ten circles in the other).

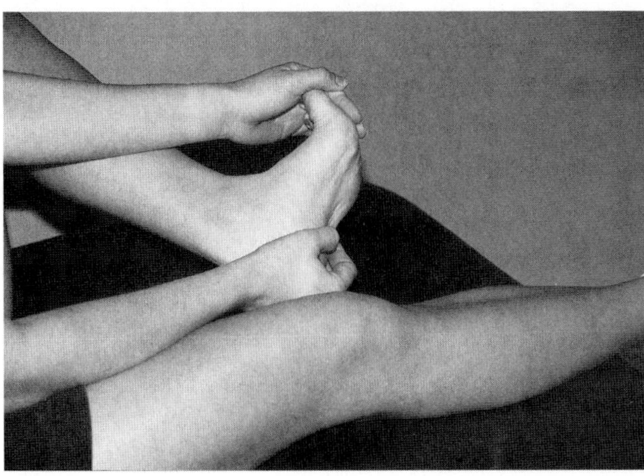
A

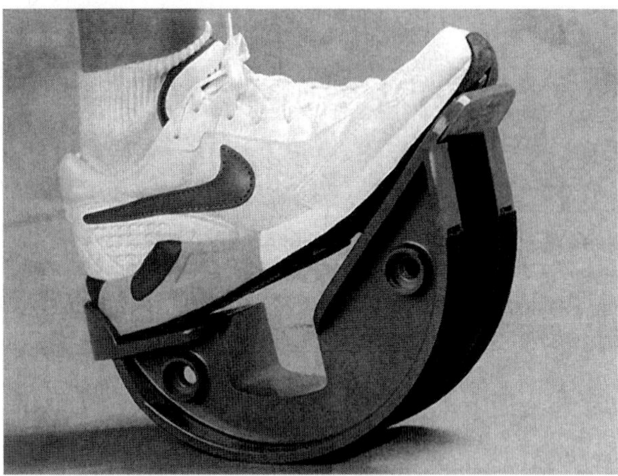
B

Figure 18-38

Plantar fascia stretches.

- Gripping and spreading of the toes— Gripping and spreading is repeated for up to ten repetitions (Figure 18-39).
- Towel gathering—A towel is extended in front of the feet. The heels are firmly planted on the floor with the forefoot on the end of the towel. The athlete then attempts to pull the towel with the feet without lifting the heels from the floor. As execution becomes easier, a weight can be placed at the other end of the towel for added resistance. Each exercise should be performed ten times (Figure 18-40A). This exercise can also be used for exercising the foot in abduction and adduction.
- Towel scoop—A towel is folded in half and placed sideways on the floor. The athlete places the heel firmly on the floor and the forefoot on the end of the towel. To ensure the greatest stability of the exercising foot, it is backed up with the other foot. Without lifting the heel from the floor, the athlete scoops the towel forward with the forefoot. Again, a weight resistance can be added to the end of the towel. The exercise should be repeated up to ten times (Figure 18-40B).

Neuromuscular Control

Reestablishing neuromuscular control following foot injury is a critical component in the rehabilitative process and should not be overlooked. Although maintaining neuromuscular control while weight bearing may appear to be a rather simple motor skill for uninjured athletes, neuromuscular control is compromised when injuries occur. Muscular weakness, proprioceptive deficits, and range of motion deficits may

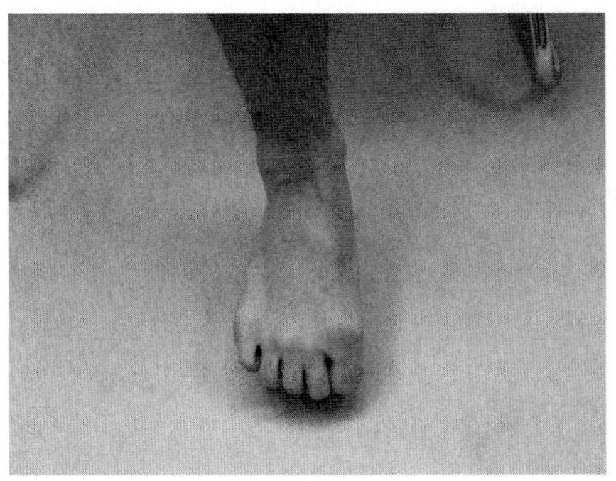
A

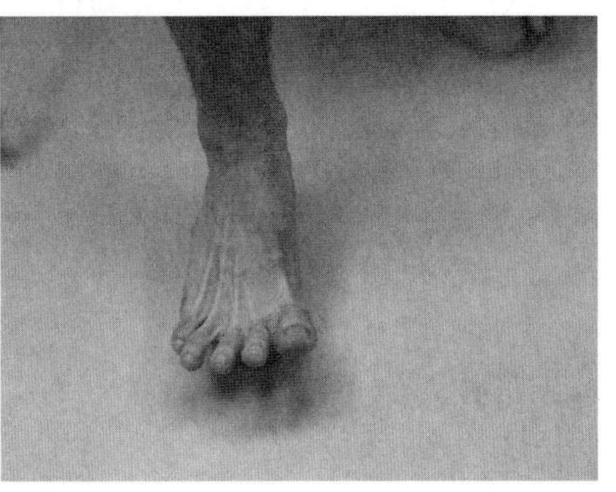
B

Figure 18-39

A, Gripping and **B,** spreading of the toes can be an excellent rehabilitation exercise for the injured foot.

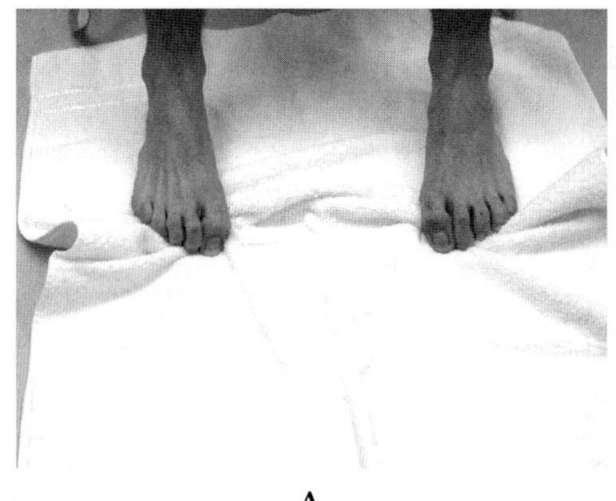

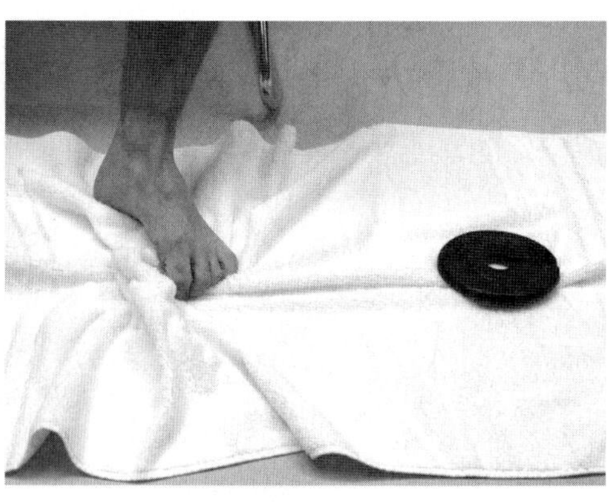

A B

Figure 18-40

A, The towel gathering exercise. **B,** The towel scoop exercise.

challenge an athlete's ability to maintain a center of gravity within the body's base of support, causing the athlete to lose balance. Neuromuscular control in the foot is the single most important element dictating movement strategies within the closed kinetic chain. The capability of adjusting and adapting to changing surfaces while creating a stable base of support is perhaps the single most important function of the foot in weight bearing.[31]

Neuromuscular control involves a highly integrative, dynamic process involving multiple neurological pathways. Neuromuscular control relative to joint position sense, proprioception, and kinesthesia is essential to all athletic performance but is particularly important to those athletic activities that require weight bearing. Current rehabilitation protocols are therefore focusing more on closed kinetic chain exercises, and neuromuscular control is receiving more attention in the sports medicine community.

Exercises for reestablishing neuromuscular control in the foot should expose the injured athlete to a variety of walking, running, and hopping exercises involving directional changes performed on varying surfaces. Balance board or wobble exercises can be useful to establish a dynamic base of support (Figure 18-41).

Figure 18-41

BAPS board exercises.

Exercise sandals can be incorporated into rehabilitation as a closed-kinetic-chain functional exercise that places increased proprioceptive demands on the athlete. The exercise sandals are wooden sandals with a rubber hemisphere located centrally on the plantar surface (Figure 18-42A). The athlete can progress into the exercise sandals once he or she demonstrates proficiency in barefoot single-leg stance. Prior to using the exercise sandals the athlete is instructed in the short-foot concept—a shortening of the foot in an anterior/posterior direction while the long toe flexors are relaxed, thus activating the short toe flexors and foot the intrinsics. Clinically the short foot appears to enhance the longitudinal and transverse arches of the foot. Once the athlete can perform the short-foot concept in the sandals, he or she progresses to walking in place and forward walking with short steps (Figure 18-42B). The exercise sandals are excellent for increasing muscle activation in the foot and lower leg.[5]

Foot Orthotics and Taping

Throughout this chapter, references have been made to taping techniques and to the use of orthotics as means of providing additional support or correcting biomechanical abnormalities. Taping techniques have been thoroughly discussed in Chapter 8, and the use of orthotics was discussed briefly earlier in this chapter. This section expands on the discussion of orthotic use relative to the various injuries discussed in this chapter.

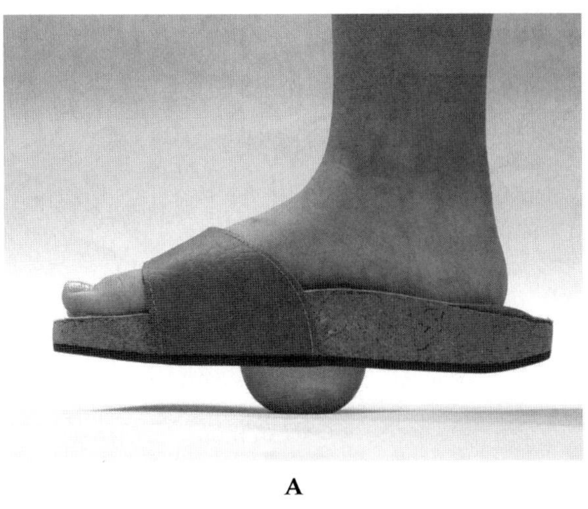

A

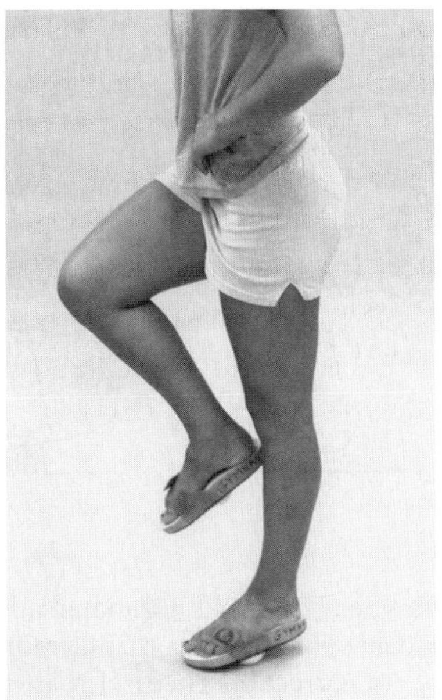

B

Figure 18-42

Exercise sandals are used to increase muscle activation and neuromuscular control in the foot. (OPTP Minneapolis)

The use of orthotics to correct foot deformities is a common practice in athletic training. The normal foot functions most efficiently when no deformities are present that predispose it to injury or exacerbate existing injuries. Orthotics are used to control abnormal compensatory movements of the foot by "bringing the floor up to meet the foot."[30]

The foot functions most efficiently in a neutral position. By providing support so that the foot does not have to move abnormally, an orthotic should help prevent compensatory problems.[19] For problems that have already occurred, the orthotic provides a platform of support so that soft tissues can heal properly without undue stress.[48]

Basically, there are three types of orthotics:[30]

1. Pads and flexible felt supports, referred to as *soft orthotics.* These soft inserts are readily fabricated and are advocated for mild overuse syndromes. Pads are particularly useful in shoes, such as spikes and ski boots, that are too narrow to hold orthotics.
2. *Semirigid orthotics* made of flexible thermoplastics, rubber, or leather.[39] These orthotics are prescribed for athletes who have increased symptoms. These orthotics are molded from a neutral cast. They are well tolerated by athletes whose sports require speed or jumping.[23]
3. Functional or *rigid orthotics* are made from hard plastic and also require neutral casting.[39] These orthotics allow control for most overuse symptoms.

Many athletic trainers make a neutral mold, put it in a box, mail it to an orthotic laboratory, and several weeks later, receive an orthotic back in the mail. Others like to construct the entire orthotic from start to finish, which requires a more skilled technician than does the mail-in method.[27]

Orthotics for Correcting Excessive Pronation and Supination

To correct a structural forefoot varus deformity in which the foot excessively pronates, the orthotic should be the rigid type and should have a medial wedge under the head of the first metatarsal. It is also advisable to add a small wedge under the medial calcaneus to make the orthotic more comfortable (Figure 18-43A).

Conversely, to correct a structural forefoot valgus deformity in which the foot excessively supinates, the orthotic should be semirigid and have a lateral wedge under

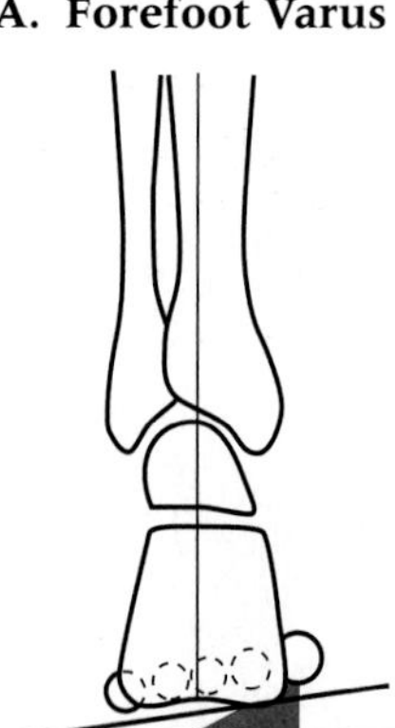

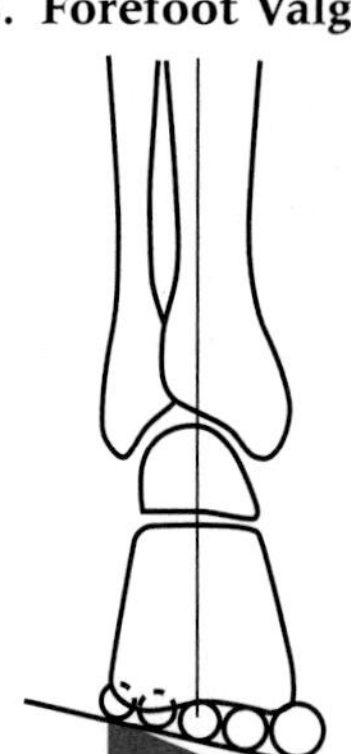

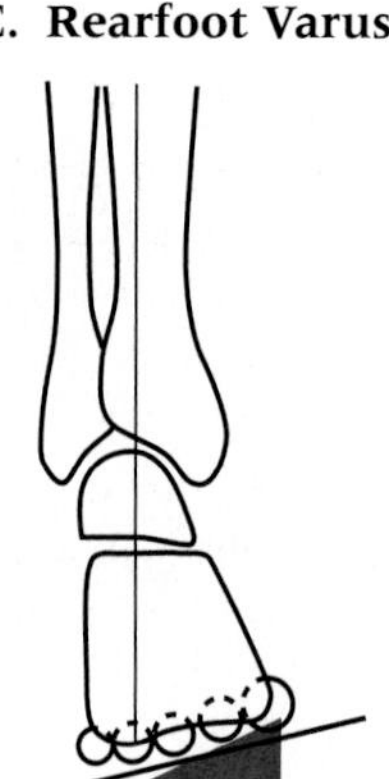

Figure 18-43

A, Medial wedge for forefoot varus. **B,** Lateral wedge for forefoot valgus. **C,** Medial wedge for rearfoot varus.

the head of the fifth metatarsal. Again, adding a small wedge under the lateral calcaneus will make the orthotic more comfortable (Figure 18-43B).

To correct a structural rearfoot varus deformity, the orthotic should be semirigid and have a wedge under the medial calcaneus and a small wedge under the head of the first metatarsal (Figure 18-43C).[50]

Functional Progressions

Athletes engage in functional progression following injury to the foot in order to gradually regain the ability to walk, jog, run, change directions, and hop.[37] *Focus Box:* "Functional progression for the foot" details an appropriate functional progression for an injury to the foot.

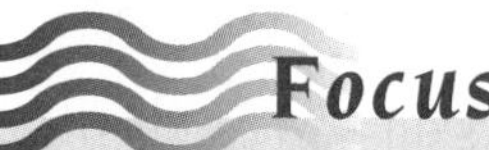

Functional progression for the foot

- Non–weight bearing
- Partial weight bearing
- Full weight bearing
- Walking
  - Normal
  - Heel
  - Toe
  - Side Step/Shuffle Slides
- Jogging
  - Straightaways on track
  - Walk turns
  - Jog complete oval of track
- Short sprints
- Acceleration/deceleration sprints
- Carioca
- Hopping
  - Two feet
  - One foot
  - Alternate
- Cutting, jumping, hopping on command

SUMMARY

- The function of the foot is critical in running, jumping, or changing direction, and the complex nature of the anatomical structures of this body part makes recognition and management of foot injuries a major challenge to the athletic trainer.
- Many chronic and overuse injuries to the lower extremity can be related to faulty biomechanics of the foot because the foot is the part of the kinetic chain that is in direct contact with the ground.
- Essential movements that occur in the foot include pronation and supination, dorsiflexion and plantar flexion, adduction and abduction, and inversion and eversion.
- Foot injuries can best be prevented by selecting appropriate footwear, by correcting biomechanical structural deformities through the use of appropriate orthotics, and by paying attention to appropriate foot hygiene and care.
- Assessment of an injury to the foot includes a history and a palpation of soft-tissue and bony structures. In addition, observation should include a check for existing structural deformities including forefoot varus, which might cause excessive pronation, forefoot valgus, which causes excessive supination, and rearfoot varus, which contributes to excessive pronation.
- Injuries to the foot can best be classified into three categories: injuries to the tarsal region; injuries to the metatarsal region, including the arches; and injuries to the toes.
- An athlete engaging in rehabilitation of an injury to the foot should maintain general body conditioning and should engage in exercises designed to regain essential joint mobility, strength, flexibility, and neuromuscular control through a series of functional progressions that gradually increase stress to the injured structures.
- The use of orthotics and taping techniques can be essential in treating many foot injuries.

Websites

Foot and Ankle Web Index: http://www.footandankle.com

The foot and ankle link library of this site is very helpful.

Premiere Medical Search Engine: http://www.medsite.com

This site allows the reader to enter any medical condition and it will search the Internet to find relevant articles.

Dr. Pribut's Running Injuries Page: http://www.drpribut.com/sports/spsport.html

This page lists common running injuries to the foot, ankle, knee, and hip.

Wheeless' Textbook of Orthopaedics: http://www.wheelessonline.com

This Web page is great for injuries, anatomy, and X rays.

North Shore Podiatry Foot Care Center: http://www.bunionbusters.com

This site provides information about foot care and includes surgical care and abnormalities of the foot.

American College of Foot and Ankle Surgeons: http://www.acfas.org

Podiatric physicians and surgeons provide information on topics related to foot health.

Medline Plus: Foot & Ankle Disorders http://www.nlm.nih. gov/medlineplus/footinjuriesanddisorders.html

A resource for many athletes related to foot injuries.

Solutions to Critical Thinking EXERCISES

18-1 A forefoot valgus deformity can cause excessive or prolonged supination. This condition may limit the ability of the foot and lower extremity to absorb ground reaction forces, resulting in injury. These injuries may include inversion ankle sprains, tibial stress syndrome, peroneal tendinitis, iliotibial band friction syndrome, and trochanteric bursitis. The athlete can use an orthotic to correct this biomechanical problem or wear proper footwear with extra cushioning and flexibility.

18-2 Sever's disease is a traction injury to the apophysis of the calcaneal tubercle where the Achilles tendon attaches. The circulation becomes disrupted, resulting in a degeneration of the epiphyseal region.

18-3 It is likely that this athlete has a forefoot varus. To correct a structural forefoot varus deformity where the foot excessively pronates, the orthotic should be the rigid type and should have a medial wedge under the head of the first metatarsal. It is also advisable to add a small wedge under the medial calcaneus to make the orthotic more comfortable. The athletic trainer should also recommend that this athlete purchase a board-lasted shoe with a medial heel wedge and a firm heel counter.

18-4 This condition is characteristic of a plantar fascial strain. It should be managed symptomatically. A doughnut placed over the epicondyle region, a heel lift, and a shoe with a stiff shank may relieve some pain. The athlete should stretch the plantar muscles and gastrocnemius and perform arch exercises. Application of LowDye taping for pronation can also relieve pain.

18-5 A lateral sprain can produce an avulsion fracture of the proximal head of the fifth metatarsal bone.

18-6 Management of this stress fracture usually consists of three or four days' partial weight bearing followed by two weeks of rest. Return to running should be very gradual. An orthotic that corrects excessive pronation can help take stress off the second metatarsal.

18-7 This condition is a bunion, or hallux valgus deformity. It is associated with wearing shoes that are too pointed, narrow, or short. It may begin with an inflamed bursa over the metatarsophalangeal joint. It can be associated with a depressed transverse arch or a pronated foot.

18-8 A sprain of the first metatarsophalangeal joint (turf toe) stems from hyperextension, usually because of the unyielding surface of artificial turf. This injury is a tear of the joint capsule from the metatarsal head.

18-9 Kicking the locker with the great toe could cause a fracture of the proximal or distal phalanx. This injury may develop swelling, discoloration, and point tenderness.

18-10 This condition could be either hammertoes, mallet toes, or claw toes. It is likely that this condition developed from years of wearing shoes that were too tight or small. The athletic trainer could try padding the toes and recommend that the player wear a pair of shoes that has a larger toebox for the rest of the season. It is likely that to permanently correct this problem the soccer player will have to have surgery after the season.

18-11 Metatarsalgia can be caused by a restricted gastrocnemius-soleus complex that produces a pes cavus. It can also be caused by a fallen metatarsal arch that abnormally depresses the second or third metatarsal heads and causes a heavy callus to develop.

18-12 The defensive lineman has a Morton's neuroma. Conservatively, it is treated by having the athlete wear a broad-toed shoe, a transverse arch support, and a metatarsal bar or teardrop pad.

REVIEW QUESTIONS AND CLASS ACTIVITIES

1. Describe the anatomy of the foot.
2. How does the foot function during the gait cycle?
3. How can an injury on the plantar surface of the foot cause soreness and pain in the knee?
4. Demonstrate an appropriate procedure for assessing injuries of the foot.
5. How does a structural forefoot varus deformity cause an individual to excessively pronate?
6. Identify the types of acute strains that occur in the region of the foot. How can they be prevented? How can they be managed?
7. What are the common fractures that occur in the foot, and how can they be managed?
8. How does plantar fasciitis occur, and what measures should be taken to treat it?
9. Where are the two most likely places for an exostosis to occur in the foot?
10. What is the difference between a pes cavus and a pes planus foot?
11. What is the difference between a Morton's toe and a Morton's neuroma?
12. How is a hallux valgus deformity related to excessive pronation?
13. Why does a Jones fracture often take such a long time to heal?
14. How would you construct the most appropriate orthotic for an athlete who excessively supinates? Why?

REFERENCES

1. Allen R, Gross M: Toe flexors strength and passive extension range of motion of the first metatarsophalangeal joint in individuals with plantar fasciitis, *J Orthop Sports Phys Ther* 33(8):468, 2003.
2. Baker C, Deese M: Diagnostic and operative ankle arthroscopy. In Baxter DE: *The foot and ankle in sports,* St Louis, 1995, Mosby.
3. Bender J: Fifth metatarsal fractures: diagnosis and management, *Sports Medicine Alert,* 6(3):18, 2000.
4. Bender J: Turf toe injuries: correctly diagnosing an uncommon injury, *Sports Medicine Alert,* 6(4):28, 2000.
5. Blackburn T, Hirth C, Guskiewicz K: Exercise sandals increase lower extremity electromyographic activity during functional activities, *J Ath Train* 38(3):198, 2003.
6. Bolgla L, Malone T: Plantar fasciitis and the windlass mechanism: a biomechanical link to clinical practice, *J Ath Train* 39(1):77, 2004.
7. Bruckner P: Foot pain. In Bruckner P, editor: *Clinical sports medicine,* Sydney, 2002, McGraw-Hill.
8. Candelora PD, Hunter SC: Overuse foot injuries. In Baker CL et al, editors: *The Hughston Clinic sports medicine book,* Baltimore, Md, 1995, Williams & Wilkins.
9. Collins KS, Streitz W: Bilateral Jones fractures in a high school football player, *J Ath Train* 31(3):253, 1996.
10. Conner C: Use of an ultrasonic bone-growth stimulator to promote healing of a Jones fracture, *Athletic Therapy Today* 8(1):37, 2003.
11. Cornwall M: Common pathomechanics of the foot, *Athletic Therapy Today* 5(1):10, 2000.
12. Cornwall MW, McPoil TG: Plantar fasciitis: etiology and treatment, *J Orthop Sports Phys Ther* 29(12):756, 2000.
13. Coughlin MJ: Forefoot disorders. In Baxter DE, editor: *The foot and ankle in sports,* St Louis, 1995, Mosby.
14. Craik R, Oatis C: *Gait analysis: theory and application,* St Louis, 1995, Mosby.
15. Davis P et al: Rehabilitation strategies and protocols for the athlete. In Sammarco GJ, editor: *Rehabilitation of the foot and ankle,* St Louis, 1995, Mosby.
16. Denegar CR, Siple B: Bilateral foot pain in a collegiate distance runner, *J Ath Train* 31(1):61, 1996.
17. Dolan MG: The use of foot orthotic devices in clinical practice, *Athletic Therapy Today* 5(1):17, 2000.
18. Fair J: Turf toe injuries: continuing to increase despite decline in artificial surfaces, *Sports Med Update* 15(1):8, 2000.
19. Genova JM, Gross MT: Effect of foot orthotics on calcaneal eversion during standing and treadmill walking for subjects with abnormal pronation, *J Orthop Sports Phys Ther* 30(11):664, 2000.
20. Glasoe W, Allen M, Kepros T: Dorsal first ray mobility in women athletes with a history of stress fracture of the second or third metatarsal, *J Orthop Sports Phys Ther* 32(11):560, 2002.
21. Glasoe WM, Allen MK, Ludewig PM: Comparison of first ray dorsal mobility among different forefoot alignments, *J Orthop Sports Phys Ther* 30(10):612, 2000.
22. Glick J, Sampson T: Ankle and foot fractures in athletics. In Nicholas J, Herschman E: *The lower extremity and spine in sports medicine,* St Louis, 1995, Mosby.

23. Gross M, Byers J, Krafft J: The impact of custom semirigid foot orthotics on pain and disability for individuals with plantar fasciitis, *J Orthop Sports Phys Ther* 32(4):149, 2002.
24. Gulick DT: Differential diagnosis of Morton's neuroma, *Athletic Therapy Today* 7(1):38, 2002.
25. Hamill J et al: Biomechanics of the foot and ankle. In Sammarco GJ, editor: *Rehabilitation of the foot and ankle,* St Louis, 1995, Mosby.
26. Hargrave M, Carcia C, Gansneder B: Subtalar pronation does not influence impact forces or rate of loading during a single-leg landing, *J Ath Train* 38(1):18, 2003.
27. Henry T, Cohen L: Fabricating foot orthotics, *Athletic Therapy Today* 5(1):22, 2000.
28. Hertel J, Gay J, Denegar C: Differences in postural control during single-leg stance among healthy individuals with different foot types, *J Ath Train* 37(2):129, 132, 2002.
29. Hunter S, Burnett G: Subtalar joint neutral and orthotic fitting, *Athletic Therapy Today* 5(1):6, 2000.
30. Hunter S, Dolan M, Davis M: *Foot orthotics in therapy and sport,* Champaign, Ill, 1996, Human Kinetics.
31. Hunter S, Prentice W: Rehabilitation of foot injuries. In Prentice WE, editor: *Rehabilitation techniques in sports medicine and athletic training,* ed 4, St Louis, 2004, McGraw-Hill.
32. Jaivin JS: Foot injuries and arthroscopy in sport, *Sports Med* 29(1):65, 2000.
33. Jones D, Singer K: Soft tissue conditions of the foot and ankle. In Nicholas J, Herschman E: *The lower extremity and spine in sports medicine,* St Louis, 1995, Mosby.
34. Kaya R: Plantar fasciitis in athletes, *J Sport Rehabil* 5(4):305, 1996.
35. Mancuso J, Cuskiewicz K, Petschauer M: Posterior foot pain in a collegiate field-hockey player, *J Sport Rehabil* 11(1):67, 2002.
36. Mann RA: Great toe disorders. In Baxter DE, editor: *The foot and ankle in sports,* St Louis, 1995, Mosby.
37. McGee M: Functional progressions and functional testing in rehabilitation. In Prentice WE, editor: *Rehabilitation techniques in sports medicine and athletic training,* ed 4, St Louis, 2004, McGraw-Hill.
38. Meyer J, Kulig K, Landel R: Differential diagnosis and treatment of subcalcaneal heel pain: a case report, *J Orthop Sports Phys Ther* 32(3):114, 2002.
39. Minert D: Foot orthoses: materials and manufacturers, *Athletic Therapy Today* 5(1):27, 2000.
40. Moul J, Massey A: Recurrent metatarsal stress fractures in a college football lineman, *J Ath Train* 30(1):72, 1994.
41. Nachazel KMJ: Mechanism and treatment of tendinitis of the flexor hallucis longus in classical ballet dancers, *Athletic Therapy Today* 7(2):13, 2002.
42. Patla CE, Abbott JH: Tibialis posterior myofascial tightness as a source of heel pain: diagnosis and treatment, *J Orthop Sports Phys Ther* 30(10):624, 2000.
43. Peterson, J: 10 steps for preventing and treating foot problems, *ACSM's Health and Fitness Journal,* 6(2):44, 2002.
44. Perry J: *Gait analysis: normal and pathological function,* Thorofare, NJ, 1992, Slack Inc.
45. Petrizzi MJ: Foot injuries. In Birrer RB, editor: *Sports medicine for the primary care physician,* ed 3, Boca Raton, Fla, 2004, CRC Press.
46. Pfeffer GB: Plantar heel pain. In Baxter DE, editor: *The foot and ankle in sports,* St Louis, 1995, Mosby.
47. Reynolds JC: Functional examination of the foot and ankle. In Sammarco GJ, editor: *Rehabilitation of the foot and ankle,* St Louis, 1995, Mosby.
48. Rose J, Shultz S, Arnold B: Acute orthotic intervention does not affect muscular response times and activation patterns at the knee, *J Ath Train* 37(2):133, 2002.
49. Sammarco GJ: Soft tissue injuries. In Torg JS, Shephard RJ, editors: *Current therapy in sports medicine,* ed 3, St Louis, 1995, Mosby.
50. Sandrey J, Zebas C, Bast J: Rear-foot motion in soccer players with excessive pronation under 4 experimental conditions, *J Sport Rehab* 10(2):143, 2001.
51. Shea M: Plantar fasciitis: describing effective treatments, *Physician Sportsmed* 30(7):21, 2002.
52. Sherman KP: The foot in sport, *British Journal of Sports Medicine* 33(1):6, 1999.
53. Schnirring L, Mees PD: New treatment for plantar fasciitis, *Physician Sportsmed* 29(3):16, 2001.
54. Swanik C: Orthotics in sports medicine, *Athletic Therapy Today* 5(1):5, 2000.
55. Tiller R: Prevention of common pes problems, *Athletic Therapy Today* 7(6):52, 2002.
56. Torg JS: Jones fractures. In Torg JS, Shephard RJ, editors: *Current therapy in sports medicine,* ed 3, St Louis, 1995, Mosby.
57. Torg JS: Plantar fasciitis. In Torg JS, Shephard RJ, editors: *Current therapy in sports medicine,* ed 3, St Louis, 1995, Mosby.
58. Turco V: Injuries to the foot and ankle. In Nicholas J, Herschman E: *The lower extremity and spine in sports medicine,* St Louis, 1995, Mosby.
59. Valmassy R: *Clinical biomechanics of the lower extremities,* St Louis, 1996, Mosby.
60. Welsh RP: Metatarsalgia problems. In Torg JS, Shephard RJ, editors: *Current therapy in sports medicine,* ed 3, St Louis, 1995, Mosby.

ANNOTATED BIBLIOGRAPHY

Alexander I: *The foot: examination and diagnosis,* New York, 1997, Churchill-Livingston.

This practical guide to clinical care of the foot and ankle presents anatomy, biomechanics, and a systematic approach to evaluation and discusses common complaints.

Baxter DE: *The foot and ankle in sport,* St Louis, 1995, Mosby.

This complete medical text addresses all aspects of the foot and ankle. It covers common sports syndromes, anatomical disorders in sports, unique problems, athletic shoes, orthoses, and rehabilitation.

Donatelli R: *The biomechanics of the foot and ankle,* Philadelphia, 1995, F.A. Davis.

This practical book is for the therapist working directly with the patient.

Tremaine MD, Elias M: *The foot and ankle source book: everything you need to know,* New York, 1998, Contemporary Books.

This book discusses common problems affecting feet and ankles, from bunions and corns to flat feet and sports injuries. It surveys the range of problems, preventative treatments, orthopedic inserts, and other health solutions to foot ailments, providing an uncommon range of disorders and treatments ranging from self-help to surgery.

Chapter 19

The Ankle and Lower Leg

When you finish this chapter you should be able to

- Identify the major anatomical components of the ankle and lower leg that are commonly injured in sports.
- Accurately assess ankle and lower leg injuries.
- Discuss the etiology, symptoms and signs, and management of injuries occurring to the ankle and lower leg.
- Develop a rehabilitation plan for various injuries to the ankle and lower leg.

Like the foot, the ankle and lower leg are common sites of injury in the athletic population.[3] Ankle injuries, especially to the stabilizing ligaments, are the most frequent injuries in sports. This chapter focuses on acute and chronic sports injuries in the ankle and lower leg (Figure 19-1).

ANATOMY OF THE LOWER LEG AND ANKLE

Bones

The portion of the lower extremity that lies between the knee and the ankle is defined as the lower leg and contains two bones, the tibia and the fibula. The bones that form the ankle joint are the distal portion of the tibia, the distal portion of the fibula, and the talus. The calcaneus also plays a critical role in the function of the ankle joint.

Tibia

With the exception of the femur, the tibia is the longest bone in the body. It serves as the principal weight-bearing bone of the leg. It is located on the medial side of the lower leg. The tibia is triangularly shaped in its upper two-thirds but is rounded and more constricted in the lower third. The most pronounced change occurs in the lower third of the shaft and produces an anatomical weakness that establishes this area as

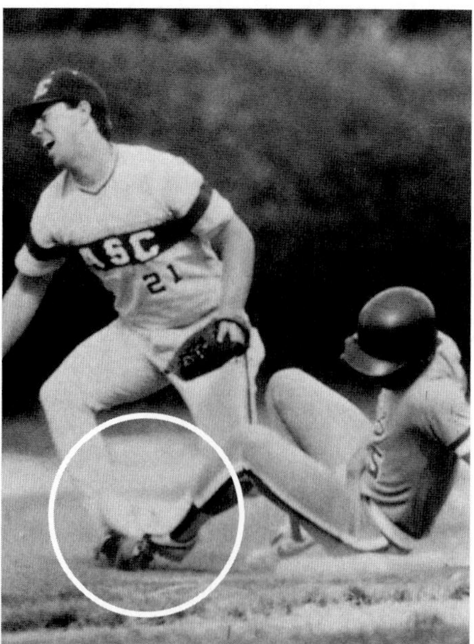

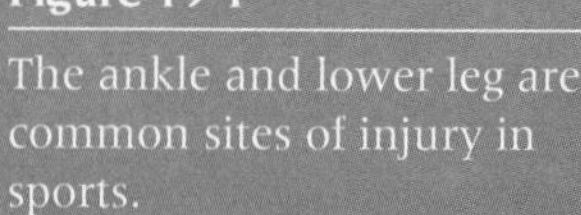

Figure 19-1

The ankle and lower leg are common sites of injury in sports.

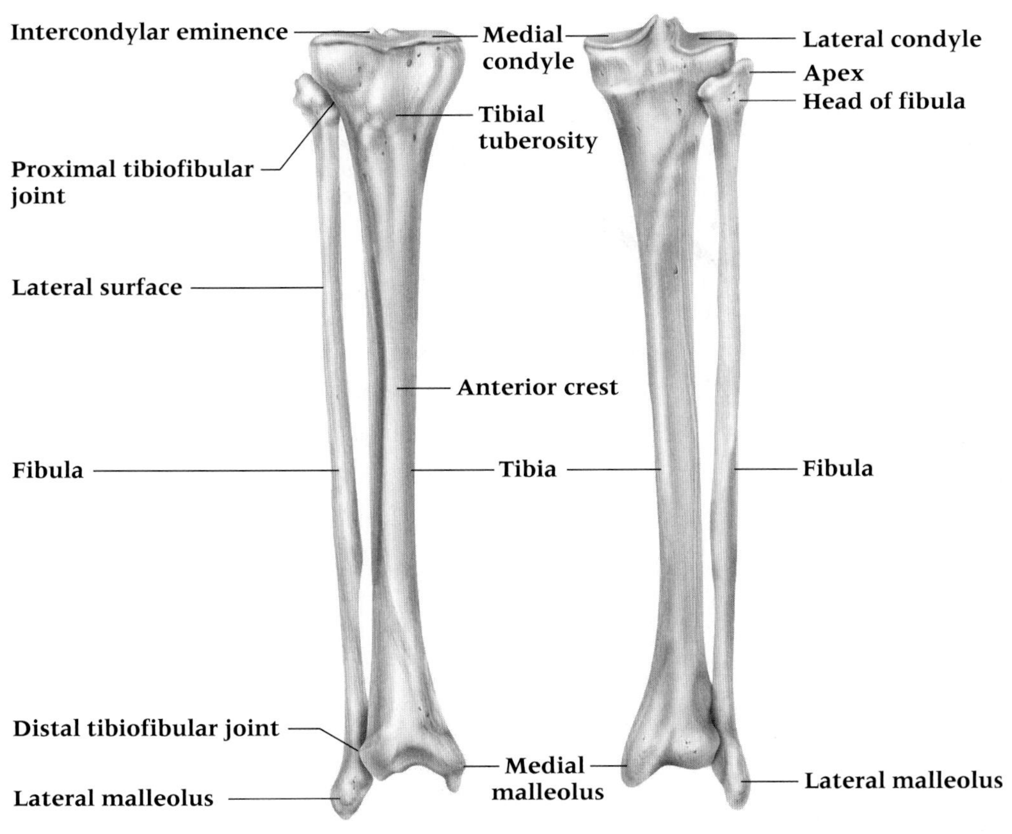

Figure 19-2

Bones of the lower leg.
A, Anterior view.
B, Posterior view.

the site of most fractures occurring to the leg. The shaft of the tibia has three surfaces: posterior, medial, and lateral. The posterior and lateral surfaces are covered by muscle; the medial surface is subcutaneous and, as a result, is vulnerable to outside trauma (Figure 19-2).

Fibula

The fibula is long and slender and is located along the lateral aspect of the tibia, joining it in an arthrodial articulation at the upper end, just below the knee joint, and as a syndesmotic joint at the lower end. Both the upper and the lower tibiofibular joints are held in position by strong anterior and posterior ligaments. The main function of the fibula is to provide for the attachment of muscles.

Tibial and fibular malleoli The thickened distal ends of both the tibia and the fibula are referred to, respectively, as the medial malleolus and lateral malleolus. The lateral malleolus of the fibula extends further distally so that the stability created by the bony arrangement at the ankle joint is greater on the lateral aspect of the ankle than on the medial aspect (Figure 19-2).

Talus

The talus, the second largest tarsal and the main weight-bearing bone of the articulation, rests on the calcaneus and receives the articulating surfaces of the lateral and medial malleoli. The talus forms a link between the lower leg and the foot, or tarsus (Figure 18-1).

Calcaneus

The calcaneus is one of the tarsal bones and was discussed in Chapter 18. The calcaneus is the bone that forms the heel and to which many of the supporting ligaments of the ankle joint as well as the Achilles tendon attach (see Figure 18-1).

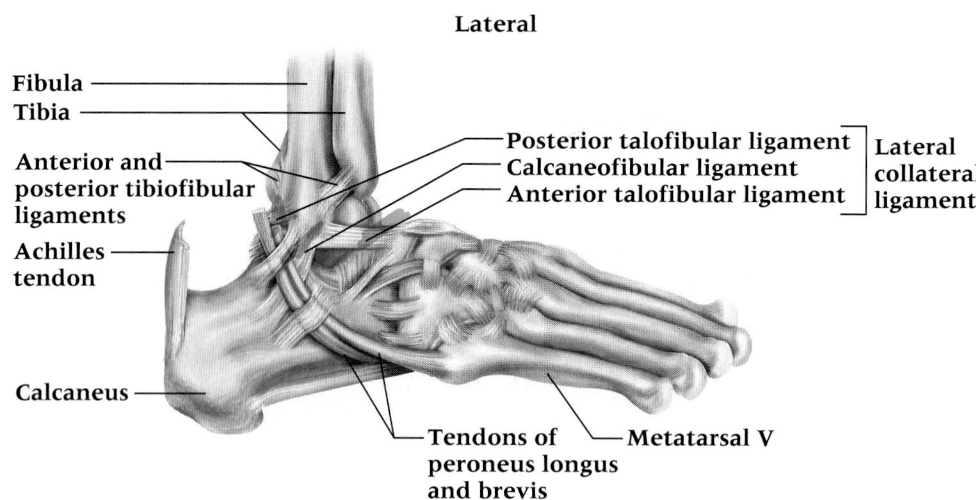

Figure 19-3

Lateral ligaments of the ankle.

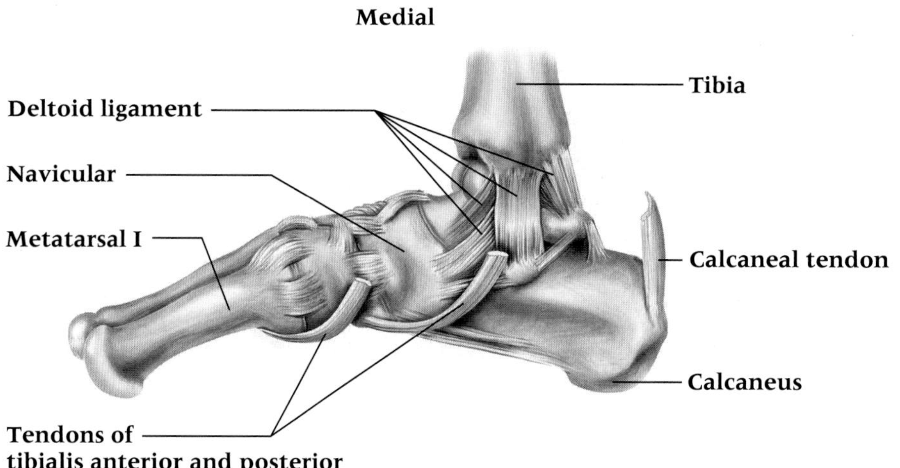

Figure 19-4

Medial ligaments of the ankle.

Articulations

Superior and Inferior Tibiofibular Joints

The tibia and fibula articulate with one another superiorly and inferiorly (tibiofibular joints). The superior tibiofibular joint is diarthrotic, allowing some gliding movements. The articulation is formed by the tibia's lateral condyle and the head of the fibula. It is surrounded by a fibrous capsule reinforced with anterior and posterior ligaments. The superior tibiofibular joint is stronger in front than in back (Figure 19-2).

The inferior tibiofibular joint is a fibrous articulation. The articulation is between the lateral malleolus and the distal end of the tibia. The joint is reinforced by the ankle ligaments (Figures 19-3, 19-4).

Talocrural Joint

The ankle joint, or talocrural joint, is a hinge joint (ginglymus) that is formed by the articular facet on the distal portion of the tibia, which articulates with the superior articular surface (trochlea) of the talus; the medial malleolus, which articulates with the medial surface of the trochlea of the talus; and the lateral malleolus, which articulates with the lateral surface of the trochlea (see Figure 19-2, Figure 19-3). This bony arrangement is typically referred to as the *ankle mortise.* Ankle movements that occur at the talocrural joint include plantar flexion and dorsiflexion.

Subtalar Joint

The anatomy and function of the subtalar joint were discussed in Chapter 18. The subtalar joint consists of the articulation between the talus and the calcaneus. Ankle movements that occur at the subtalar joint include inversion, eversion, pronation, and supination.

Stabilizing Ligaments

Tibiofibular Ligaments

Joining the tibia and fibula is a strong interosseous membrane. The fibers display an oblique downward and outward pattern. The oblique arrangement aids in diffusing the forces placed on the leg. The membrane completely fills the tibiofibular space except for a small area at the superior aspect that is provided for the passage of the anterior tibial vessels. The anterior and posterior tibiofibular ligaments, which hold the tibia and fibula together and form the distal portion of the interosseous membrane, are sometimes referred to as the syndesmotic ligaments.

Ankle Ligaments

In addition to the tibiofibular ligaments, the ligamentous support of the ankle consists of three lateral ligaments and the medial, or deltoid, ligament (Figure 19-3, Figure 19-4).

Lateral ligaments The three lateral ligaments include the anterior talofibular, the posterior talofibular, and the calcaneofibular (Table 19-1).

Medial ligaments The deltoid ligament is triangular. It attaches superiorly to the borders of the medial malleolus; it attaches inferiorly to the medial surface of the talus, to the sustentaculum tali of the calcaneus, and to the posterior margin of the navicular bone. The deltoid ligament is the primary resistance to foot eversion. It, along with the plantar calcaneonavicular (spring) ligament, also helps maintain the inner longitudinal arch. Although it should be considered one ligament, the deltoid ligament includes both superficial and deep fibers (Figure 19-4). Anteriorly are the anterior tibiotalar part and the tibionavicular part. Medially is the tibiocalcaneal part, and posteriorly is the posterior tibiotalar part.

Joint Capsule

A thin articular capsule encases the ankle joint and attaches to the borders of the bone involved. It is somewhat different from most other capsules in that it is thick on the medial aspects of the joint but becomes a thin, gauzelike membrane at the back.

Ankle Musculature

The movements of the talocrural joint are dorsiflexion (flexion) and plantar flexion (extension). Inversion and eversion occur at the subtalar joint. Tendons of muscles passing posterior to the malleoli will produce ankle plantar flexion along with toe flexion in the foot. Muscles and their tendons passing anterior to the talocrural joint function to dorsiflex the foot and to produce toe extension. The muscles that cross the ankle joint laterally cause eversion, while the muscles that cross the ankle joint medially cause inversion (Figure 19-5).

TABLE 19-1 Function of Key Ankle Ligaments

Ligament	Primary Function
Anterior talofibular	Restrains anterior displacement of talus
Calcaneofibular	Restrains inversion of calcaneus
Posterior talofibular	Restrains posterior displacement of talus
Deltoid	Prevents abduction and eversion of ankle and subtalar joint Prevents eversion, pronation, and anterior displacement of talus

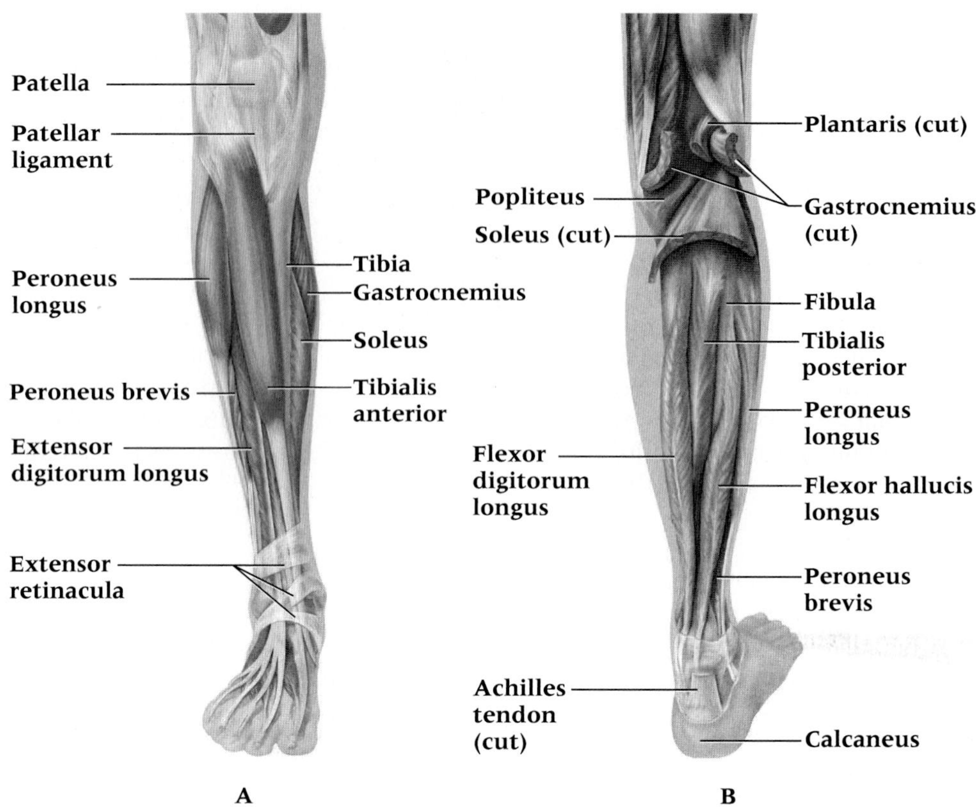

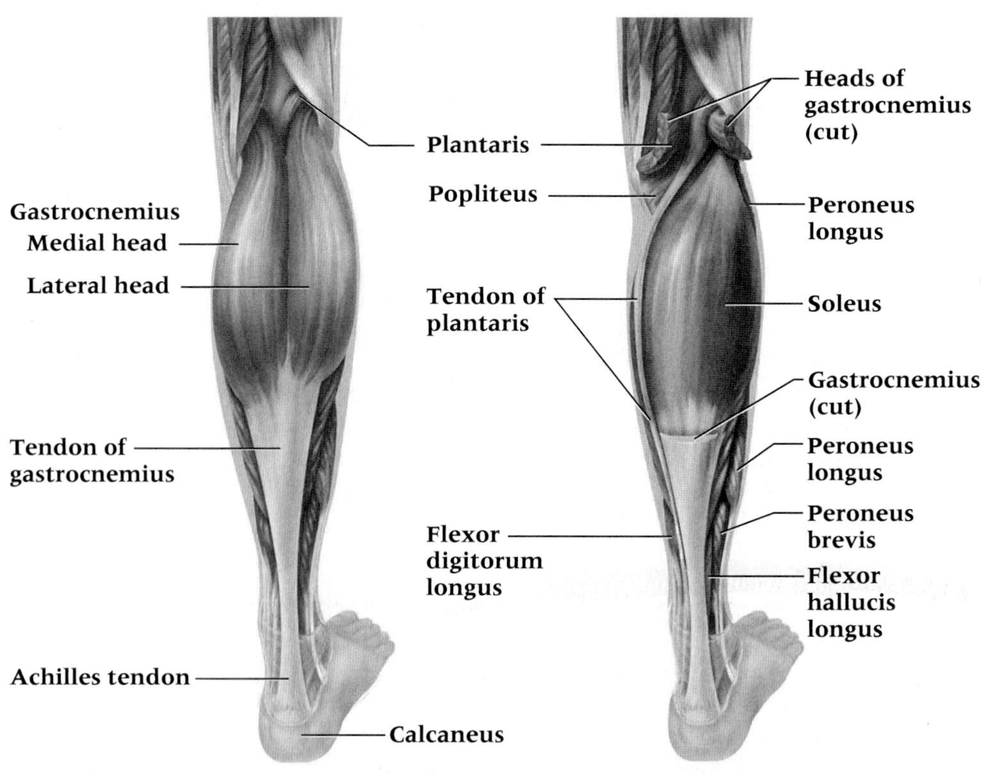

Figure 19-5

Muscles of the ankle and lower leg. **A,** Anterior, **B,** Lateral, **C,** Superficial posterior, **D,** Deep posterior.

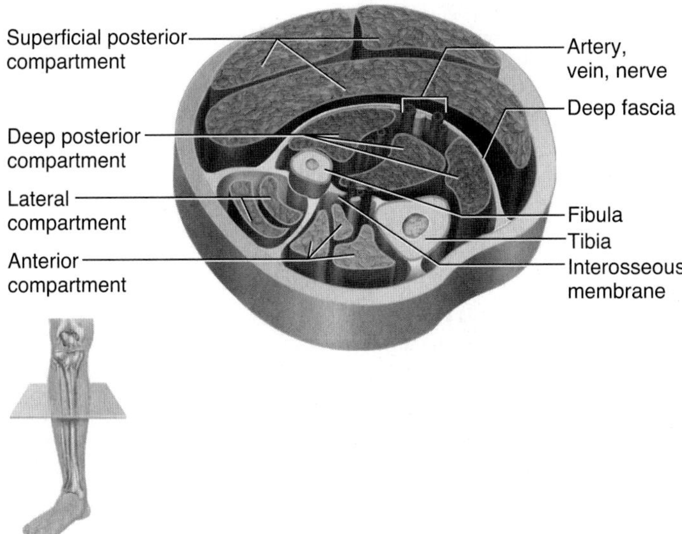

Figure 19-6

The four compartments of the lower leg.

Muscle Compartments

The musculature of the lower leg is contained within four distinct compartments, which are bounded by heavy fascia (Figure 19-6). Acute or chronic trauma to any of these compartments can lead to swelling and neurological motor and sensory deficits.

The *anterior compartment* contains those muscles that dorsiflex the ankle and extend the toes—the tibialis anterior, extensor hallucis longus, and extensor digitorum longus muscles—and contains the anterior tibial nerve and the tibial artery.

The *lateral compartment* contains the peroneus longus and brevis, which evert the ankle; the peroneus tertius muscle, which assists in dorsiflexion; and the superficial branch of the peroneal nerve.

The *superficial posterior compartment* contains the gastrocnemius muscle and the soleus muscle. These muscles plantar flex the ankle.

The *deep posterior compartment* contains the tibialis posterior, flexor digitorum longus, and flexor hallucis longus muscles, which invert the ankle, and the posterior tibial artery.

Table 19-2 summarizes the muscles in the lower leg and ankle and their actions.

Nerve and Blood Supply

The major nerves of the lower leg are the tibial and common peroneal, stemming from the large sciatic nerve. The major arteries often accompany the nerves and are the posterior and anterior tibial arteries (Figure 19-7). The primary veins consist of the popliteal peroneal and the anterior and posterior tibial veins.

FUNCTIONAL ANATOMY

The biomechanical motions occurring at the ankle and rear foot are complex. Anatomically, the ankle is a stable hinge joint in which the dome of the talus articulates with the distal ends of the tibia and fibula. Medial or lateral displacement of the talus is prevented by the malleoli. The arrangement of the ankle ligaments permits flexion and extension at the talocrural joint and limits inversion and eversion at the subtalar joint (see Chapter 18).[50]

The square shape of the talus contributes to ankle stability. Because the talus is wider anteriorly than posteriorly, the most stable position of the ankle is with the foot in dorsiflexion. In this position, the wider anterior aspect of the talus comes in contact with the narrower portion lying between the malleoli, gripping it tightly. By contrast, as the ankle moves into plantar flexion, the wider portion of the tibia is brought in

Because the talus is wider anteriorly than posteriorly, the most stable position of the ankle is with the foot in dorsiflexion.

TABLE 19-2 Muscles of the Lower Leg and Ankle

Muscle	Origin	Insertion	Muscle Action	Nerve
Anterior Compartment				
Tibialis anterior	Lateral condyle and proximal two-thirds of the shaft of the tibia and the interosseous membrane	Medial surface of first cuneiform and first metatarsal	Dorsiflexes and inverts foot	Deep peroneal
Extensor hallucis longus	Anterior surface of the middle of the fibula and the interosseous membrane	Dorsal surface of the distal phalanx of the great toe	Dorsiflexes and inverts foot; extends the great toe	Deep peroneal
Extensor digitorum longus	Lateral condyle of the tibia, proximal three-fourths of the anterior surface of the fibula, and the interosseous membrane	Dorsal surface of the phalanges of the second through fifth toes	Dorsiflexes and everts the foot; extends the toes	Deep peroneal
Peroneus tertius	Distal third of the anterior surface of the fibula and the interosseous membrane	Dorsal surface of the fifth metatarsal	Dorsiflexes and everts the foot	Deep peroneal
Lateral Compartment				
Peroneus longus	Proximal two-thirds of the lateral surface of the fibula	Ventral surface of the first metatarsal and the medial cuneiform	Plantar flexes and everts the foot	Superficial peroneal
Peroneus brevis	Distal two-thirds of the fibula	Lateral side of the fifth metatarsal	Plantar flexes and everts the foot	Superficial peroneal
Superficial Posterior Compartment				
Gastrocnemius	Medial and lateral condyles of the femur	Calcaneus, via the Achilles tendon	Flexes the leg; plantar flexes the foot	Tibial
Soleus	Posterior surface of the proximal third of the fibula and the middle third of the tibia	Calcaneus, via the Achilles tendon	Plantar flexes the foot	Tibial
Plantaris	Posterior surface of the femur above the lateral condyle	Calcaneus, via the Achilles tendon	Flexes the leg; plantar flexes the foot	Tibial
Deep Posterior Compartment				
Popliteus	Lateral condyle of the femur	Proximal portion of the tibia	Flexes and rotates the leg medially	Tibial
Flexor hallucis longus	Lower two-thirds of the fibula	Distal phalanx of the great toe	Plantar flexes and inverts the foot; flexes the great toe	Tibial
Flexor digitorum longus	Posterior surface of the tibia	Distal phalanx of the second through fifth toes	Plantar flexes and inverts the foot; flexes the toes	Tibial
Tibialis posterior	Posterior surface of the interosseous membrane, the tibia, and the fibula	Navicular, cuneiforms, cuboid; second through fourth metatarsals	Plantar flexes and inverts the foot	Tibial

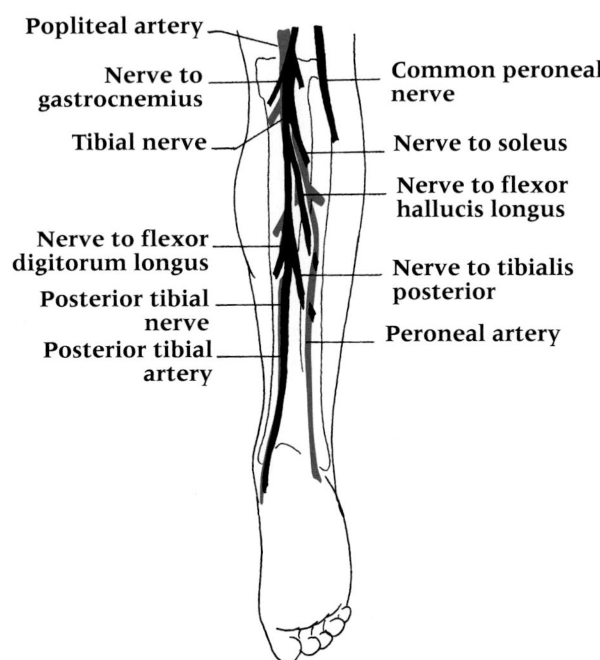

Figure 19-7

Blood and nerve supply of the lower leg (posterior view).

contact with the narrower posterior aspect of the talus, which makes plantar flexion a much less stable position than dorsiflexion.

The degree of motion for the ankle joint ranges from 10 degrees of dorsiflexion to 50 degrees of plantar flexion. Normal gait mechanics require at least 20 degrees of plantar flexion and 10 degrees of dorsiflexion with the knee extended.[33]

Normal ankle function depends on the joints of the rearfoot, the most important of which is the subtalar joint. The movements of the talus during pronation and supination have profound effects on the lower extremity both proximally and distally.

PREVENTING INJURY TO THE LOWER LEG AND ANKLE

Many lower leg and ankle conditions, especially sprains, can be reduced if the athlete engages in the following: stretching the Achilles tendon, strengthening key muscles, learning neuromuscular and proprioceptive control, wearing proper footwear, and in some cases, being properly taped.[69]

Preventing ankle sprains is achieved by:
- Stretching the Achilles tendon
- Strengthening key muscles
- Obtaining proprioceptive training
- Wearing proper footwear
- Taping when appropriate

Achilles Tendon Stretching

It is critical for normal gait that the ankle dorsiflex at least 10 degrees or more. A tight heel cord may limit dorsiflexion and may predispose the athlete to ankle injury. The athlete, especially one with tight Achilles tendons, should routinely stretch before and after practice (see Figure 19-34B, C, D, page 592).[51] To adequately stretch the Achilles tendon complex, stretching should be performed both with the knee extended and then with it flexed 15 to 30 degrees.

Strength Training

Of major importance in ankle injury prevention is the achievement of both static and dynamic joint stability (see Figure 19-36, page 593). A normal range of motion must be maintained, and the muscles and tendons that surround the talocrural joint must be kept strong.

Neuromuscular Control Training

Athletes must develop neuromuscular control at the ankle joint. Neuromuscular control involves adapting to uneven surfaces by controlling motion at the ankle joint.

Athletes can enhance ankle neuromuscular control by training in controlled activities on uneven surfaces or by spending time each day on a BAPS board, Bosu Balance Trainer, rocker board, or Dynadisc (Figure 19-36, page 593).

Footwear

As discussed in Chapter 7, proper footwear can be an important factor in reducing injuries to both the foot and the ankle. Shoes should not be used in activities for which they were not intended—for example, running shoes designed for straight-ahead activity should not be used to play tennis, a sport that demands a great deal of lateral movement. Cleats on a shoe should not be centered in the middle of the sole but should be placed far enough on the border to avoid ankle sprains. High-top shoes, when worn by athletes with a history of ankle sprain, can offer greater support than low-top shoes do.[60]

Preventive Ankle Taping and Orthoses

Chapter 8 discussed the controversy surrounding the benefits of routinely taping ankles that have no history of sprain. There is some indication that tape, properly applied, can provide some prophylactic protection.[22,59] However, tape that constricts soft tissue or disrupts normal biomechanical function can create unnecessary injuries. Lace-up supports and semirigid ankle braces are increasingly being used in place of tape.[9] The sport-stirrup orthosis has been found to be superior to taping in preventing recurrent ankle sprains (see Figure 7-24).[42]

ASSESSING THE LOWER LEG AND ANKLE

History

The athlete's history may vary depending on whether the problem is the result of sudden trauma or is chronic. The athletic trainer should ask the athlete with an acute injury to the lower leg or ankle the following questions:[8,44]

- Have you ever hurt your ankle before?
- How did you hurt your ankle?
- What did you hear when the injury occurred—a crack, snap, or pop?
- How bad was the pain and how long did it last?
- Is there any sense of muscle weakness or difficulty in walking?
- How disabling was the injury? Could you walk right away, or were you not able to bear weight for a period of time?
- Has a similar injury occurred before?
- Was there immediate swelling, or did the swelling occur later (or at all)?
- Where did the swelling occur?

The athlete with a chronic painful condition might be asked the following:

- How much does it hurt?
- Where does it hurt?
- Under what circumstances does pain occur—when bearing weight, after activity, or when arising after a night's sleep?
- What past ankle injuries have occurred?
- What first aid and therapy, if any, were given for these previous injuries?

Observation

In looking initially at the ankle, the athletic trainer should determine the following:[8, 44]

- Are there any postural deviations? (Toeing in may indicate tibial torsion or genu valgum or varum; foot pronation should also be noted.)
- Is there any difficulty in walking?
- Is there an obvious deformity or swelling?
- Are the bony contours of the ankle normal and symmetrical, or is there a deviation such as a bony deformity?
- Are the color and texture of the skin normal?

- Is there crepitus or abnormal sound in the ankle joint?
- Is heat, swelling, or redness present?
- Is the athlete in obvious pain?
- Does the athlete have a normal ankle range of motion?
- If the athlete is able to walk, is there a normal walking pattern?

Palpation

The area of injury should be palpated to determine obvious structural deformities, areas of swelling, or points of tenderness.

Bony Palpation

The following bony landmarks should be palpated:

Anterior Aspect

- Fibular head
- Fibular shaft
- Lateral malleolus
- Tibial plateau
- Tibial shaft
- Medial malleolus
- Dome of the talus
- Posterior aspect
- Medial malleolus
- Lateral malleolus

Posterior Aspect

- Medial malleolus
- Lateral malleolus
- Dome of the talus
- Calcaneus

Soft-Tissue Palpation

The following soft tissue structures should be palpated:

Lateral Aspect

- Lateral compartment
  —Peroneus longus muscle
  —Peroneus brevis muscle
  —Peroneus tertius muscle
- Peroneus longus tendon
- Peroneus brevis tendon
- Anterior talofibular ligament
- Calcaneofibular ligament
- Posterior talofibular ligament

Anterior Aspect

- Anterior compartment
  —Anterior tibialis muscle
  —Extensor hallucis longus muscle
  —Extensor digitorum longus muscle
- Anterior tibialis tendon
- Extensor hallucis longus tendon
- Extensor digitorum longus tendon
- Peroneus tertius tendon
- Anterior tibiofibular ligament

Medial Aspect

- Deep posterior muscles
  —Posterior tibialis muscle
  —Flexor digitorum longus muscle
  —Flexor hallucis muscle
- Flexor digitorum longus tendon
- Posterior tibialis tendon
- Flexor hallucis tendon
- Deltoid ligament

Posterior Aspect

- Superficial posterior compartment
  —Gastrocnemius muscle
  —Soleus muscle
- Achilles tendon
- Posterior tibiofibular ligament

Special Tests

Lower Leg

Lower leg alignment tests Determining malalignment of the lower leg can reveal the causes of abnormal stresses applied to the foot, ankle, and lower leg as well as the knees and hip. In normal alignment of the lower extremity, anteriorly, a straight line can be drawn from the anterior superior iliac spine of the pelvis, through the patella, and to the web between the first and second toes. Laterally, a straight line can be drawn from the greater trochanter of the femur, through the center of the patella, and

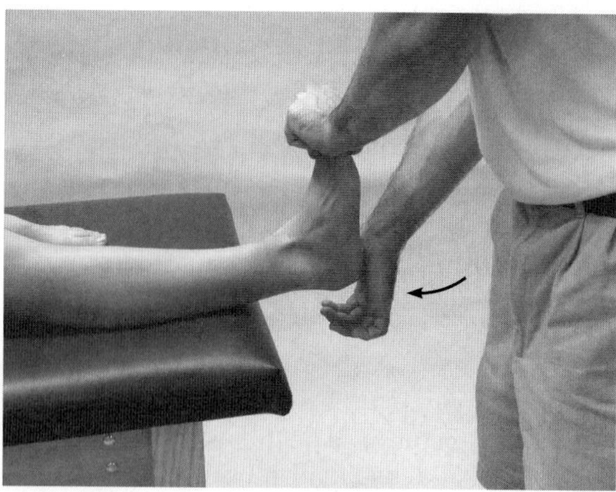

Figure 19-8

Percussion test to check for fractures of the ankle or lower leg.

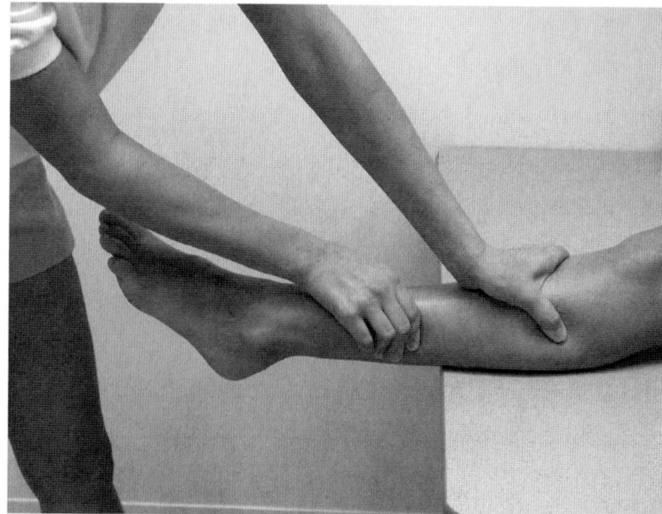

Figure 19-9

Compression test to check for fractures of the tibia or fibula.

to just behind the lateral malleolus. Posteriorly, a straight line can be drawn from the center of the lower leg to the midline of the Achilles tendon and calcaneus.[10] A common malalignment of the lower leg is internal or external tibial torsion.

Percussion and compression tests When fracture is suspected, a gentle percussive blow can be given to the tibia or fibula below or above the suspected site. Percussion can also be applied upward on the bottom of the heel. Such blows set up a vibratory force that resonates at the fracture, causing pain (Figure 19-8).

In a compression test, the tibia and fibula are compressed either above or below the fracture site (Figure 19-9). Increased pain over the area of point tenderness may be indicative of a fracture, and referral should be made for X rays.

Thompson test The Thompson test (Figure 19-10) is performed by squeezing the calf muscle while the leg is extended and the foot is hanging over the edge of the table. A positive Thompson sign is one in which squeezing the calf muscle does not cause the heel to move or pull upward or causes the heel to move less when compared with the uninjured leg.

Homan's sign The test for Homan's sign gives some indication of the presence of a deep vein thrombophlebitis. With the athlete in a supine position with the knee fully extended, the ankle is passively dorsiflexed so that the calf muscles are stretched. Pain in the calf is a positive sign (Figure 19-11). The athlete should be referred immediately to a physician for further diagnosis.

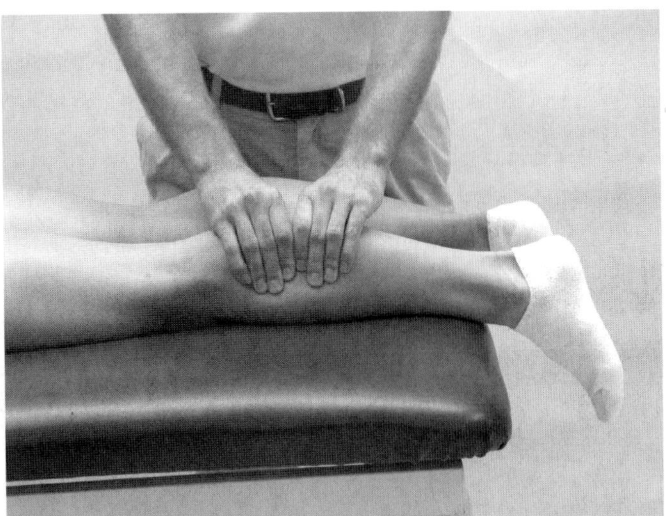

Figure 19-10

The Thompson test to determine an Achilles tendon rupture by squeezing the calf muscle. A positive result to the test is one in which there is no plantar flexion of the foot.

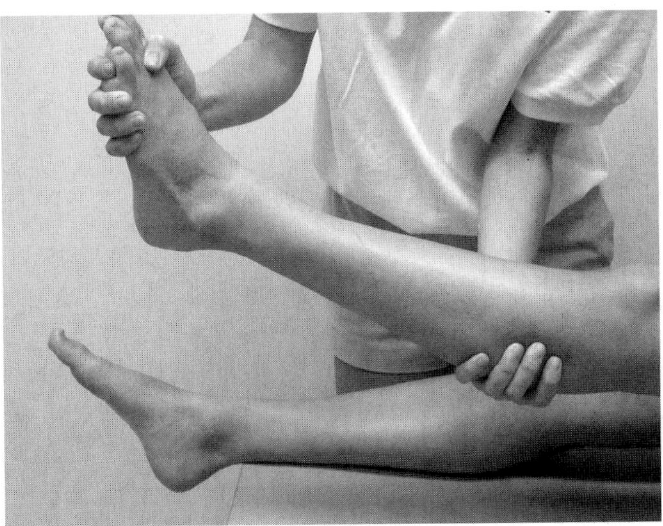

Figure 19-11

Homan's sign may indicate a deep vein thrombophlebitis.

Ankle Stability Tests

Anterior drawer test The anterior drawer test is used to determine the extent of injury to the anterior talofibular ligament primarily and to the other lateral ligaments secondarily (Figure 19-12). The athlete sits on the edge of a treatment table with legs and feet relaxed. The athletic trainer grasps the lower tibia in one hand and the calcaneus in the palm of the other hand. The tibia is then pushed backward as the calcaneus is pulled forward. A positive anterior drawer sign occurs when the foot slides forward, sometimes making a clunking sound as it reaches its end point, and generally indicates a tear in the anterior talofibular ligament. An ankle arthrometer has been used to determine subtalar joint ligament complex laxity.[30,39]

A positive anterior drawer sign of ankle stability is when the foot slides forward, sometimes making a clunking sound as it reaches its end point.

A positive talar tilt occurs when the calcaneofibular ligament is sprained.

Talar tilt test Talar tilt tests are used to determine the extent of inversion or eversion injuries. With the foot positioned at 90 degrees to the lower leg and stabilized, the calcaneus is inverted. Excessive motion of the talus indicates injury to the calcaneofibular and possibly the anterior and posterior talofibular ligaments as well (Figure 19-13).

The deltoid ligament can be tested in the same manner except that the calcaneus is everted.

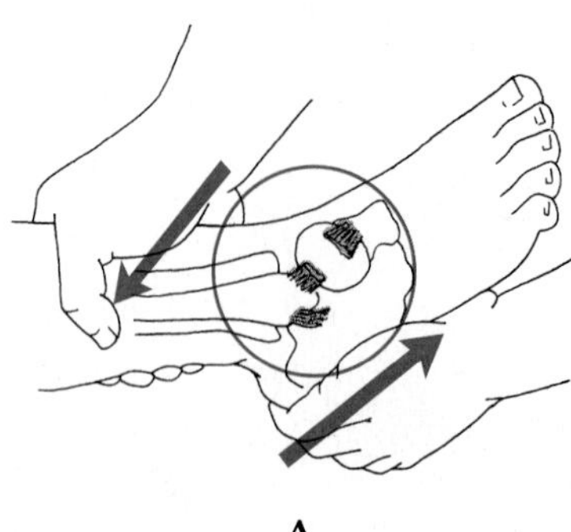

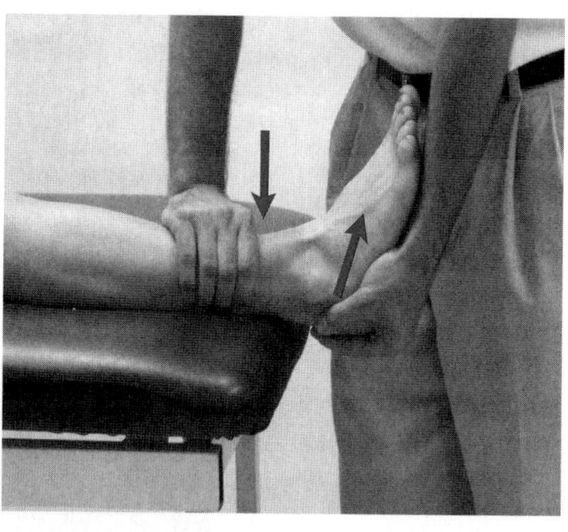

Figure 19-12

Anterior drawer test for ankle ligament instability.

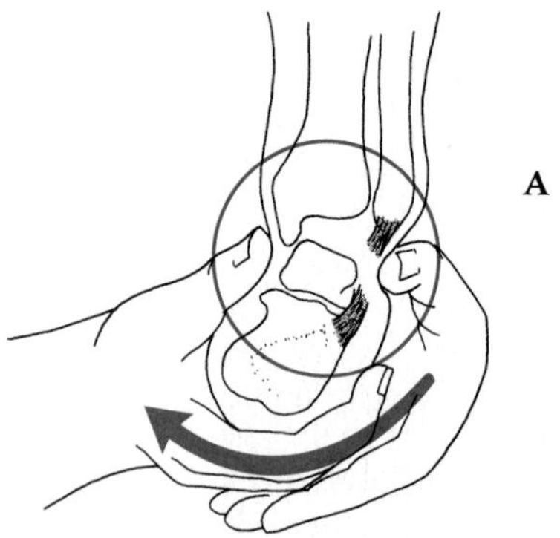

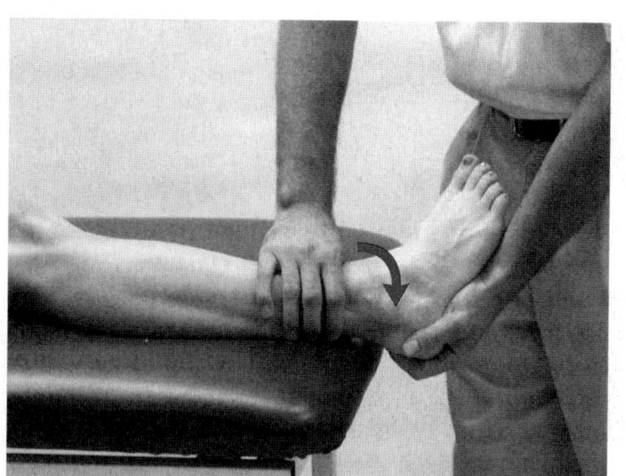

Figure 19-13

Talar tilt testing for lateral ankle instability.

Kleiger's test Kleiger's test is used primarily to determine injury to the deltoid ligament. It can also indicate injury to the structures that support the distal ankle syndesmosis, including the anterior tibiofibular ligament, the posterior tibiofibular ligament, and the interosseous membrane. The athlete should be seated with his or her legs over the end of the table. The athletic trainer uses one hand to stabilize the lower leg and the other to hold the medial aspect of the foot and rotate it laterally (Figure 19-14). Pain over the deltoid ligament indicates injury to that structure, while pain over the lateral malleolus would likely indicate injury to the syndesmosis.

Medial subtalar glide test The medial subtalar glide test is done to determine the presence of excessive medial translation of the calcaneus on the talus in the transverse plane.[26] The athletic trainer uses one hand to hold the talus in subtalar neutral then glides the calcaneus in a medial direction on the fixed talus (Figure 19-15). In a positive test there is excessive movement, indicating injury to the lateral ligaments.

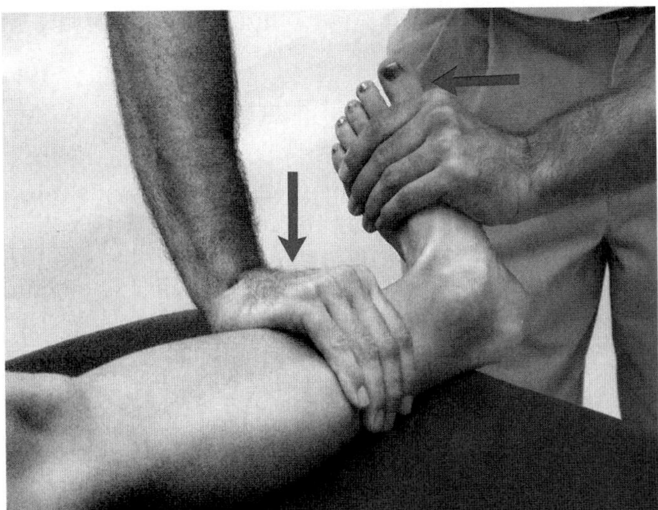

Figure 19-14

Kleiger's test to determine sprain at the deltoid ligament or injury to the syndesmosis.

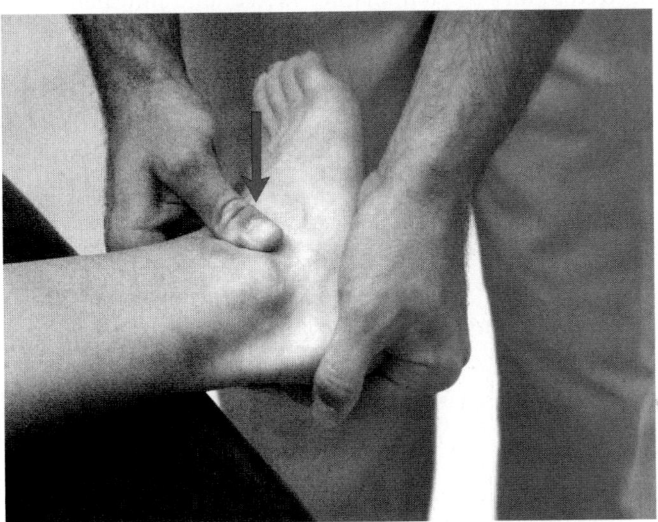

Figure 19-15

The medial subtalar glide test looks for excessive medial translation of the calcaneus relative to the talus, indicating injury to the lateral ligaments.

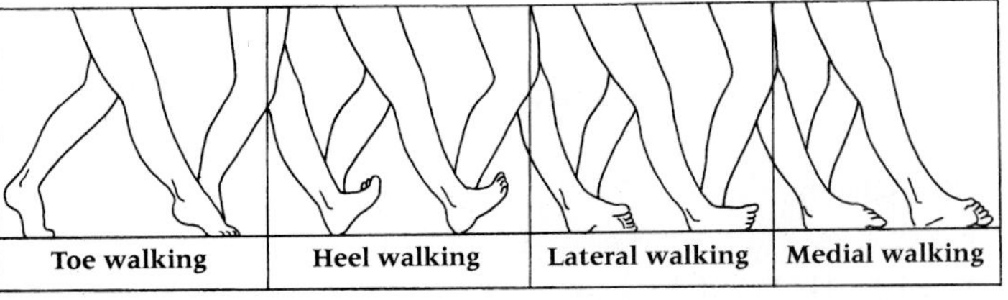

Figure 19-16

Evaluating ankle function during walking.

Functional Tests

Muscle function is important in evaluating the ankle injury (Figure 19-16). *If the following movements aggravate a recent injury, they should be avoided.* While bearing weight on both feet, the athlete should do the following:

- Walk on toes (tests plantar flexion)
- Walk on heels (tests dorsiflexion)
- Walk on lateral border of feet (tests inversion)
- Walk on medial border of feet (tests eversion)
- Hop on the injured ankle

Passive, active, and resistive movements should be manually applied to determine joint integrity and muscle function.

RECOGNITION OF SPECIFIC INJURIES

Ankle Injuries

Ankle sprains are perhaps the single most common injury in the athletic population. Appreciation of the anatomy and mechanics of the ankle joint and the pathomechanics and patholphysiology related to acute and chronic ankle instability is integral to the process of effectively evaluating and treating ankle injuries.[24] Ankle sprains are generally caused by sudden inversion or eversion, often in combination with plantar flexion or dorsiflexion (Table 19-3). Injuries may be classified according to either location or mechanism of injury.

Inversion Sprains

Inversion ankle sprains are the most common and result in injury to the lateral ligaments (Figure 19-17). The anterior talofibular ligament is the weakest of the three lateral ligaments. Its major function is to stop forward subluxation of the talus. It is injured in an inverted, plantar flexed, and internally rotated position (Figure 19-18). The calcaneofibular and posterior talofibular ligaments may also be injured in inversion sprains as the force of inversion is increased.

TABLE 19-3 Mechanisms of Ankle Sprain and Ligament Injury

Mechanisms	Area Injured
Plantar flexion or inversion	Anterior talofibular ligament Calcaneofibular ligament Posterior talofibular ligament Tibiofibular ligament (severe injury)
Inversion	Calcaneofibular ligament (along with anterior or posterior talofibular ligament)
Dorsiflexion	Tibiofibular ligament
Eversion	Deltoid ligament Tibiofibular ligament (severe injury) Interosseous membrane (as external rotation increases) Possible fibular fracture (proximal or distal)

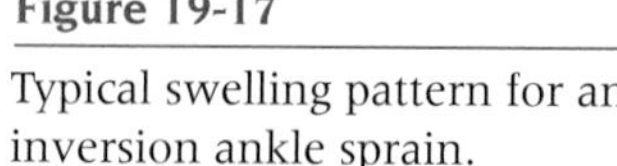

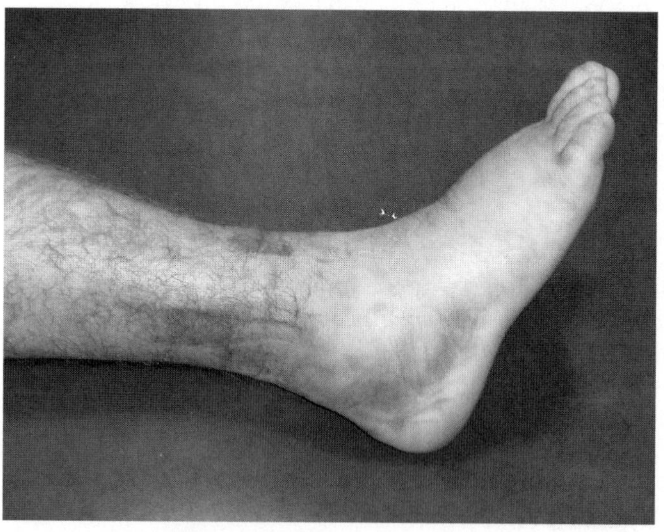

Figure 19-17

Typical swelling pattern for an inversion ankle sprain.

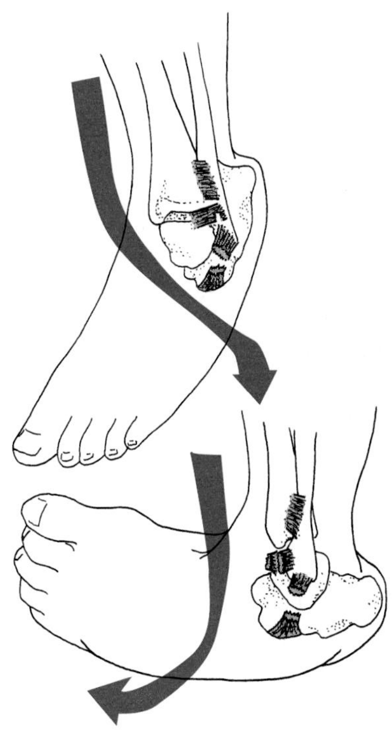

Figure 19-18

The mechanism of an inversion ankle sprain involves plantar flexion and/or inversion.

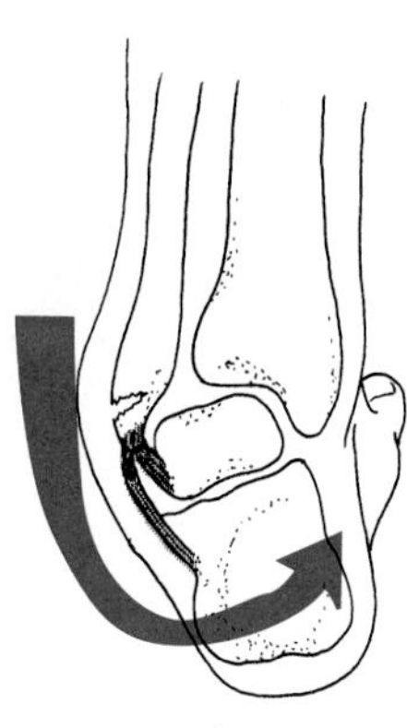

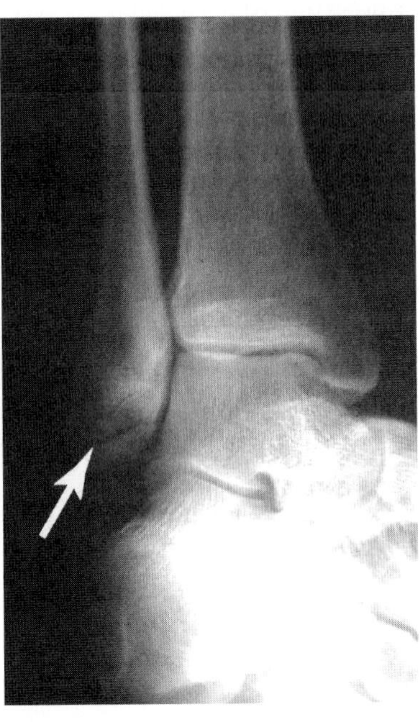

A B

Figure 19-19

A, The same mechanism that produces an ankle sprain can also cause an avulsion fracture of the malleolus. **B,** X-ray view of distal fibular avulsion fracture.

Occasionally an inversion force could be of sufficient magnitude to cause a portion of bone to be avulsed from the lateral malleolus (Figure 19-19).[3] It is also possible that inversion can cause both an avulsion of the lateral malleolus and a fracture of the medial malleolus. This injury is known as a *bimalleolar fracture* (Pott's fracture).[3]

The severity of lateral ankle sprains is classified according to grades. A grade 1 sprain usually involves the anterior talofibular ligament; a grade 2, the anterior talofibular and calcaneofibular ligaments; and a grade 3, the anterior talofibular, calcaneofibular, posterior talofibular, and frequently the anterior tibiofibular ligaments. In each instance, the foot is forcefully inverted such as when a basketball player jumps and comes down on the foot of another player. Inversion sprains can also occur when an individual is walking or running on an uneven surface or suddenly steps into a hole.

Gender does not appear to be a risk factor for suffering an ankle sprain. Athletes who have suffered a previous sprain have a decreased risk of reinjury if a brace is worn, and the consensus is that generalized joint laxity and anatomical foot type are not risk factors for ankle sprains. However, the literature is divided on whether or not height, weight, limb dominance, ankle-joint laxity, and anatomical alignment, muscle strength, muscle-reaction time, and postural sway are risk factors for ankle sprains.[5]

Grade I inversion ankle sprain The grade 1 ankle sprain is the most common type of sprain. Lateral sprains are probably the most frequent injury in sports in which running and jumping occur.[6]

Etiology The inversion sprain occurs with the foot in inversion, plantar flexion, and adduction with a mild stretching of the anterior talofibular ligament.

Symptoms and signs Mild pain and disability occur. Weight bearing is minimally impaired. Signs are point tenderness and swelling over the ligament with no joint laxity.[22]

Management Rest, ice, compression, and elevation (RICE) are used for twenty minutes every few hours for one to two days. The application of a horseshoe pad provides

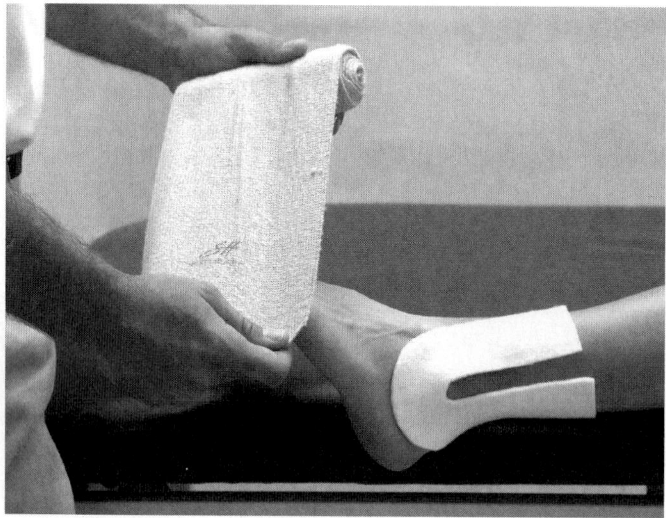

Figure 19-20

A horseshoe-shaped pad provides excellent focal compression when held in place by an elastic wrap.

focal compression and may also help control hemorrhage (Figure 19-20).[72] It may be advisable for the athlete to limit weight-bearing activities for one to two days, after which rehabilitation may become more aggressive. An elastic wrap might provide comfortable pressure when weight bearing begins. Early functional rehabilitation of the ankle should include range-of-motion exercises and isometric and isotonic strength-training exercises. In the intermediate stage of rehabilitation, a progression of proprioception-training exercises should be incorporated, followed by focusing on sport-specific activities to prepare the athlete for return to competition.[48] When the athlete returns to weight bearing, application of tape may provide an extra measure of protection.[71] Usually an athlete can return to activity in seven to ten days.

Grade 2 inversion ankle sprain A grade 2 ankle sprain has a high incidence among sports participants and causes a great deal of disability with many days of lost time.[67]

Etiology Moderate force on the ankle while it is in a position of inversion, plantar flexion, and adduction can cause a grade 2 sprain.

Symptoms and signs The athlete usually complains of feeling a pop or snap on the lateral side of the ankle. There is moderate pain and disability, weight bearing is difficult, and there is tenderness and edema with blood in the joint. Ecchymosis may occur, as well as a positive talar tilt test. There is also a positive anterior drawer sign between 4 and 14 mm (.16–.55 inch).[6] A grade 2 ankle sprain may be a complete tear of the anterior talofibular ligament and a stretch and tear of the calcaneofibular ligament. The anterior drawer test will elicit slight to moderate abnormal motion. This injury degree can produce a persistently unstable ankle that recurrently becomes sprained and later develops traumatic arthritis.[67]

Management RICE should be used intermittently for at least seventy-two hours. X-ray examination should be routine for this grade of injury. The athlete should use crutches for five to ten days, gradually progressing to full weight bearing during that period. The athlete will need to wear some type of protective immobilization device for one to two weeks.[6] Plantar and dorsiflexion exercises in a pain-free range should begin forty-eight hours after the injury occurs. Early movement helps maintain range of motion and normal proprioception. Proprioceptive neuromuscular facilitation (PNF) exercise improves strength, range of motion, and proprioception. Exercise should include isometrics while the ankle is immobilized, followed by range-of-motion exercises, progressive resistance exercise (PRE), and balance activities lasting up to four weeks.[57] It has been suggested that protection of healing structures may lead to a more optimal long-term outcome.[15]

Taping in a closed basket weave technique may protect the ankle during the early stages of walking (see Figure 8-26). The athlete must be instructed to avoid walking or running on uneven surfaces for two to three weeks after weight bearing has begun. NOTE: The long-term effects of a grade 2 sprain are likely to include chronic instability with a recurrence of injury. Over a period of time, this instability can lead to joint degeneration and osteoarthritis. Once a grade 2 sprain has occurred, the athlete must continue to engage in rehabilitative activities to minimize recurrence of injury.[75]

Grade 3 inversion ankle sprain The grade 3 inversion ankle sprain is relatively uncommon in sports. When it does happen, it is extremely disabling. Often the force causes the ankle to subluxate and then spontaneously reduce.

Etiology The grade 3 sprain is caused by a significant inversion force to the ankle, usually combined with plantar flexion, and adduction. This injury involves varying grades of damage to the anterior talofibular, calcaneofibular, and posterior talofibular ligaments as well as the joint capsule.

Symptoms and signs The athlete complains of severe pain in the region of the lateral malleolus. Weight bearing is not possible because of the great amount of swelling, with or without pain. Hemarthrosis, discoloration, a positive talar tilt, and a positive anterior drawer test are present.[70]

Management Normally RICE is used intermittently for at least three days. It is not uncommon for the physician to apply a dorsiflexion cast or weight-bearing brace for three to six weeks, followed by taping for three to six weeks.[33] Crutches are usually given to the athlete when the cast is removed. Isometric exercise is carried out while the cast is on, followed by range-of-motion, PRE, and balance exercises. In some cases surgery is warranted to stabilize the athlete's ankle. NOTE: A grade 3 ankle sprain creates significant joint laxity and instability. Because of this laxity, the ankle joint is prone to degenerative processes. However, chronic ankle instability does not necessarily have a negative effect on functional performance.[14]

Eversion Ankle Sprains

Etiology Eversion ankle sprains represent only about 5 percent to 10 percent of all ankle sprains. The eversion ankle sprain is less common than the inversion ankle sprain largely because of the bony and ligamentous anatomy (Figure 19-21). As mentioned previously, the fibular malleolus extends further inferiorly than does the tibial malleolus. This protection, combined with the strength of the thick deltoid ligament, prevents excessive eversion. More often, eversion injuries involve an avulsion fracture of the tibia before the deltoid ligament tears.[32] The deltoid ligament may also be contused in inversion sprains due to impingement between the fibular malleolus and the calcaneus. Despite the fact that eversion sprains are less common, they are more severe and may take longer to heal than inversion sprains.

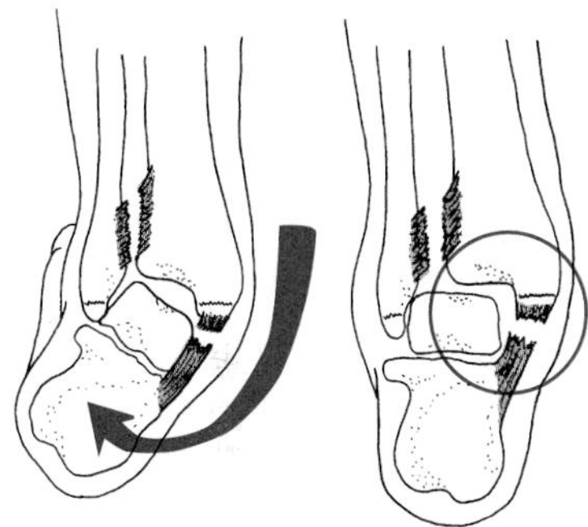

Figure 19-21

An eversion ankle sprain that creates a space between the medial malleolus and the talus.

A foot that is pronated, hypermobile, or has a depressed medial longitudinal arch is more predisposed to eversion ankle injuries (Figure 19-22).[6]

Symptoms and signs Depending on the grade of injury, the athlete complains of pain, sometimes severe, that occurs over the foot and lower leg. Usually the athlete is unable to bear weight on the foot. Both abduction and adduction cause pain, but pressing directly upward against the bottom of the foot will not produce pain.

Management X rays are often necessary to rule out fracture. Initially, RICE and no weight bearing are recommended, and a posterior splint tape is applied. NSAIDs and analgesics are given as needed. Management of eversion sprain will follow the same course described for inversion sprains. The athlete engages in a PRE program for the posteromedial ankle muscles, engages in balance activities, and is fitted with an inner heel wedge shoe insert. NOTE: An eversion sprain with a severity of grade 2 or more can produce significant joint instability. Because the deltoid ligament helps support the medial longitudinal arch, a sprain can cause weakness in this area, leading to excessive pronation or a fallen arch.

19-1

Critical Thinking Exercise

Following a grade 1 ankle sprain, a football player is rehabilitating his injury.

? What would be an appropriate progression for him to use to get from non–weight bearing to sprinting?

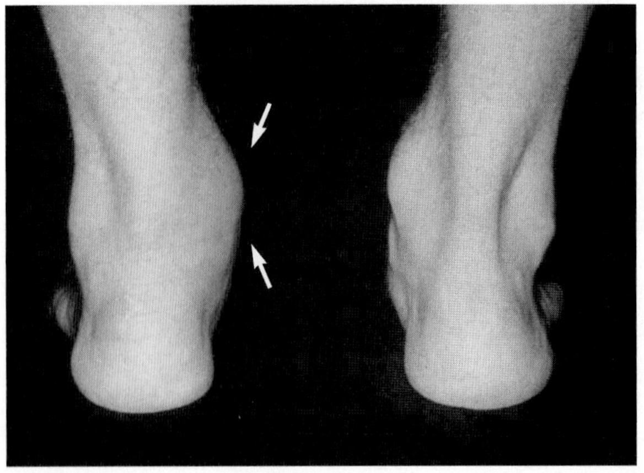

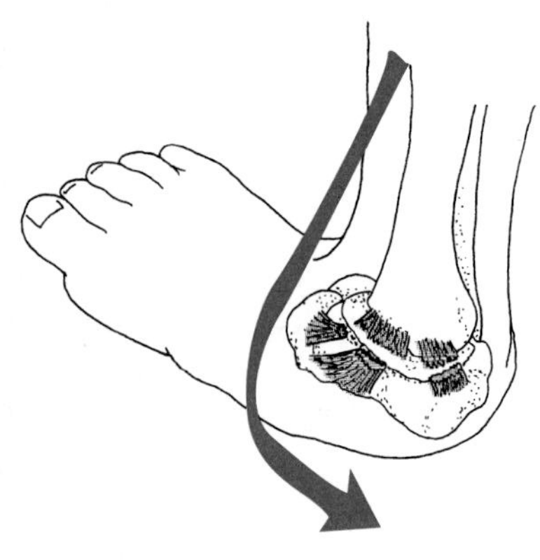

Figure 19-22

A pronated foot can lead to an eversion ankle sprain, with a characteristic swelling pattern.

19-2 Critical Thinking Exercise

A male soccer player cuts for the ball and injures his right ankle. He describes a hyperdorsiflexion mechanism of injury. X rays were negative for this injury.

? What is this athlete's injury? What are special considerations with this injury?

19-3 Critical Thinking Exercise

A basketball player has a history of numerous lateral ankle sprains.

? How may this player reduce the incidence of these ankle sprains?

19-4 Critical Thinking Exercise

A collegiate field hockey player has a history of repeated ankle sprains. She complains of constant pain and aching and says the ankle feels like it catches when she runs. There also appears to be some mild effusion.

? What might the athletic trainer suspect is wrong, and how should this injury be managed?

Syndesmotic Sprain (High Ankle Sprain)

Etiology Isolated injuries to the distal tibiofemoral joint are referred to as syndesmotic sprains,[46,58] or high ankle sprains.[65] The anterior and posterior tibiofibular ligaments are found between the distal tibia and fibula and extend up the lower leg as the interosseous ligament, or syndesmotic ligament. Sprains of the ligaments are more common than has been realized in the past.[18] These ligaments are torn with increased external rotational or forced dorsiflexion and are often injured in conjunction with a severe sprain of the medial and lateral ligament complexes (see Figure 19-19, page 575).[54, 68] Initial rupture of the ligaments occurs distally at the tibiofibular ligament above the ankle mortise. As the force of disruption is increased, the interosseous ligament is torn more proximally.

Symptoms and signs The athlete complains of severe pain and loss of function in the ankle region. When the ankle is passively externally rotated or dorsiflexed, there is a major pain in the lower leg indicating a syndesmotic sprain or possibly a lateral malleolar fracture. Pain normally occurs along the anterolateral leg.

Management Sprains of the syndesmotic ligaments are extremely hard to treat and often take months to heal.[68] Treatments for this problem are essentially the same as for medial or lateral sprains, with the difference being an extended period of immobilization. Functional activities and return to sport may be delayed for a longer period of time than for inversion or eversion sprains.[55]

Ankle Fracture/Dislocation

Etiology There are a number of mechanisms through which an ankle can be fractured or dislocated.[21, 47] A foot that is forcibly abducted can produce a transverse fracture of the distal tibia and fibula. In contrast, a foot that is planted in combination with a forced internal rotation of the leg can produce a fracture to the distal and posterior tibia (Figure 19-23).

Avulsion fractures, in which a chip of bone is pulled off by resistance of a ligament, are common in grade 2 and 3 degree eversion or inversion sprains.

Symptoms and signs In most cases of fracture, swelling and pain may be extreme. There may be some or no deformity; however, if a fracture is suspected, splinting is essential.

Management RICE is used as soon as possible to control hemorrhage and swelling. Once swelling is reduced, a walking cast or brace may be applied. Immobilization will usually last for at least six to eight weeks.[3]

Osteochondritis Dissecans

Etiology While less common than in the knee, osteochondritis dissecans can occur in the superior medial articular surface of the talar dome. One or several fragments of

Management PLAN

Signs & Symptoms
Management Plan
Therapy
Exercise Rehabilitation

Grade 2 Inversion Ankle Sprain

Injury Situation A male, college senior lacrosse player stepped into a rut on the field, causing a major twist of the left ankle. At the time of injury, the athlete felt a severe pain on the lateral aspect of the ankle before he fell to the ground.

Symptoms and Signs After the injury, the athlete complained of moderate pain on the outside of his left ankle. Initially, it was painful to move the ankle. Walking on the left foot was very difficult. There was moderate tenderness over the lateral aspect of the ankle. Swelling rapidly occurred around the lateral malleoli. The ankle displayed a slight positive talor tilt and a positive anterior drawer test of 4 mm.

Phase 1 *Acute Injury*

GOALS: To control hemorrhage, swelling, pain, and spasm.
ESTIMATED LENGTH OF TIME (ELT): 2–3 days.

■ **Therapy** Ice packs are applied (20 minutes) intermittently 6 to 8 times daily. X-ray examination rules out fracture. The athlete should wear elastic wrap during waking hours and elevate leg. The leg should be elevated during sleep. Nonsteroidal antiinflammatory drugs and analgesics should be given. An air splint should be used during this period for support and compression. No weight bearing is allowed. Crutches are used to avoid weight bearing for at least 3 or 4 days or until the athlete can walk without a limp with lateral support.

■ **Exercise rehabilitation** The athlete should begin exercise by toe gripping and spreading if there is no pain (10 to 15 times) every waking hour starting on the second day of injury. General body maintenance exercises should be conducted 3 times a week as long as they do not aggravate the injury.

Phase 2 *Repair*

GOALS: To decrease swelling, permit secondary healing to occur, restore full muscle contraction without pain, restore 50% pain-free movement.
ELT: 3 weeks.

■ **Therapy** All treatment should be followed immediately by exercise. Ice pack should be used (5 to 15 minutes), ice massage (7 minutes), cold whirlpool (60° F, 10 minutes), or massage above and below injury site (5 minutes). When hemorrhage is completely controlled, use whirlpool (90° to 100° F, 10 to 15 minutes).

■ **Exercise rehabilitation** The athlete should crutch walk with a toe touch if he or she is unable to walk without a limp while wearing an air cast, tape, or both for 3 weeks. For the first 2 weeks, toe gripping and spreading (10 to 15 times) every waking hour. Active PNF ankle patterns 3 or 4 times daily for a pain-free range of motion. Avoid any exercise that produces pain or swelling. Ankle circumduction (10 to 15 times each direction) 2 or 3 times daily. Achilles tendon stretch from the floor (30 seconds) in each foot position (toe in, toe out, straight ahead) 3 or 4 times daily. Toe raises (10 times, 1 to 3 sets) 3 or 4 times daily. Eversion exercise using a towel or rubber tube or tire resistance 3 or 4 times daily. Shifting body weight between injured and noninjured ankle (up to 20 times 2 or 3 times daily). Wobble board exercise (1 to 3 minutes) 2 or 3 times daily. Progress to straight-ahead short-step walking if it can be done without a limp. General body maintenance exercises are conducted 3 times a week as long as they do not aggravate injury.

Phase 3 *Remodeling*

GOALS: To restore symptom-free full range of motion, power, endurance, speed, and agility.
ELT: 3–5 days.

■ **Therapy** Therapeutic modalities such as whirlpool (100° to 105° F) (20 minutes) or ultrasound (0.5 W/cm^2) (5 minutes) should be used symptomatically.

Continued

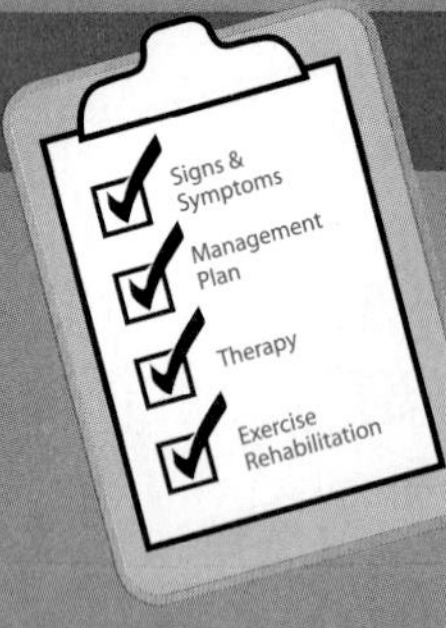

Grade 2 Inversion Ankle Sprain—*continued*

■ **Exercise rehabilitation** Achilles tendon stretch using slant board (30 seconds each foot position) 2 or 3 times daily. Toe raises using slant board and resistance (10 repetitions, 1 to 3 sets) 2 or 3 times daily. Resistance ankle device to strengthen anterior, lateral, and medial muscles (starting with 2 lb and progressing to 10 lb) (1 to 3 sets) 2 or 3 times daily. Wobble board for ankle proprioception (begin at 1 minute in each direction, progress to 5 minutes) 3 times daily. Walk-jog routine as long as athlete is symptom free: begin with alternate walk-jog-run-walk 25 yards straight ahead, jog 25 yards straight ahead; progress to walk 25 yards in lazy S or to perform five figure eights, progress to figure-eight running as fast as possible; progress to run 10 figure eights or Z cuts as fast as possible and to spring up in the air on the injured leg 10 times without pain.

Criteria for Return *to* Competitive Lacrosse

1. The ankle is pain free during motion and no swelling is present.
2. The athlete has full ankle range of motion and strength.
3. The athlete is able to run, jump, and make cutting movements as well as before injury.

articular cartilage and its underlying subchondral bone are either partially detached or completely detached and moving within the joint space. The mechanism of injury may be a single trauma, in which case it may be diagnosed as an osteochondral fracture, or it may be due to repeated episodes of ankle sprain.

Symptoms and signs Initially the athlete may complain of pain and effusion with signs of progressing atrophy. There may also be complaints of catching, locking, or giving way, particularly if the fragment is detached.

Management Diagnosis is usually made by X-ray, although an MRI may also show the articular cartilage overlying the osseous lesion. Incomplete and nondisplaced injuries can be immobilized with early motion and delayed weight bearing until there is evidence of healing. If the fragment is displaced, surgery is recommended to excise the fragment and minimize the risk of nonunion.

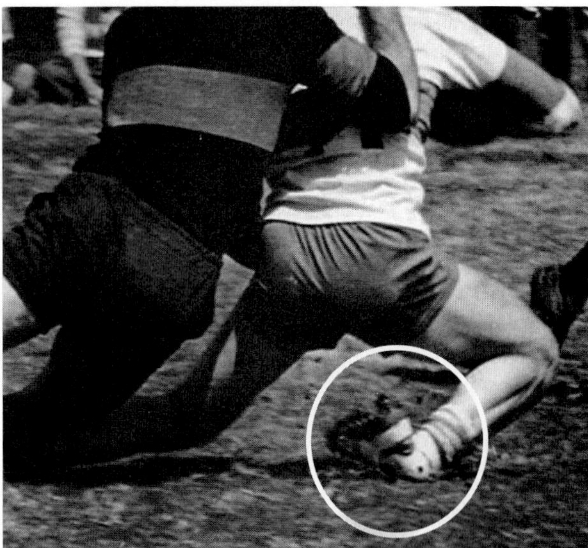

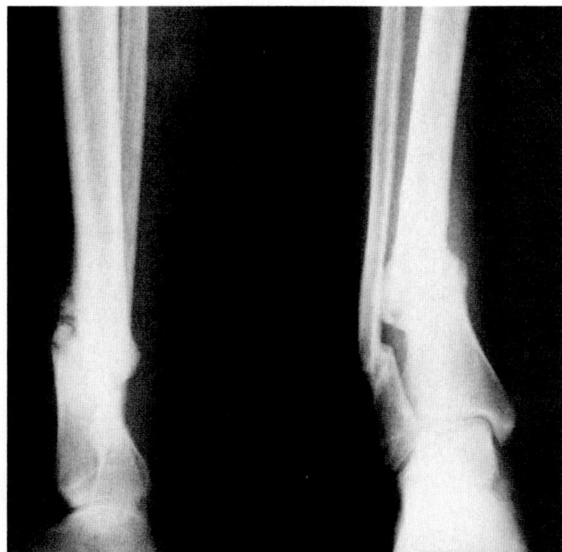

Figure 19-23

Ankle fractures or dislocations can be major sports injuries.

Lower Leg Injuries

Acute Achilles Tendon Strain

Etiology Achilles tendon strains are common in sports and occur most often after ankle sprains or sudden excessive dorsiflexion of the ankle.

Symptoms and signs The resulting injury may be mild to severe. The most severe injury is a partial or complete avulsion or rupturing of the Achilles tendon. While sustaining this injury, the athlete feels acute pain and extreme weakness on plantar flexion.

Management Initially, as with other acute conditions, pressure is first applied with an elastic wrap together with the application of cold. Unless the injury is minor, hemorrhage may be extensive, requiring RICE over an extended period of time. After hemorrhaging has subsided, an elastic wrap should be applied for continued pressure. Because of the tendency for acute Achilles tendon trauma to become a chronic condition, a conservative approach to therapy is required. The athlete should begin stretching and strengthening the heel cord complex as soon as possible. A lift should be placed in the heel of each shoe to decrease stretching of the tendon and thus relieve some stress that contributes to chronic inflammation.

19-5 Critical Thinking Exercise

A tennis player sustains a grade 2 lateral sprain of the left ankle while making a sudden stop.

? Assuming good immediate care was carried out, how should this condition be managed ten days after injury?

Achilles Tendinitis

Etiology Achilles tendinitis is an inflammatory condition that involves the Achilles tendon and/or its tendon sheath, the paratenon. Often, the tendon is overloaded because of excessive tensile stress placed on it during movements of a repetitive nature, such as running or jumping. Achilles tendinitis will often present with a gradual onset over a period of time. The condition worsens with repetitive weight-bearing activities such as running or early season conditioning in which the duration and intensity are increased too quickly with insufficient recovery time. Decreased gastrocnemius and soleus complex flexibility can also increase symptoms.[2]

Symptoms and signs The athlete often complains of generalized pain and stiffness about the Achilles tendon region that, when localized, is usually just proximal to the calcaneal insertion. Uphill running or hill workouts will usually aggravate the condition. There may be reduced gastrocnemius and soleus muscle flexibility in general that may worsen as the condition progresses. Muscle testing may show a deficit when the athlete performs toe raises. Initially, the athlete may ignore symptoms that present at the beginning of activity and resolve as the activity progresses. Symptoms may progress to morning stiffness and discomfort with walking after periods of prolonged sitting. The tendon may be warm and painful to palpation as well as thickened, which may indicate the chronicity of the condition. Crepitus may be palpated with active plantar flexion and dorsiflexion, and pain will be elicited with passive stretching. Chronic inflammation of the Achilles tendon may lead to thickening when compared with the uninvolved side (Figure 19-24).[28]

Management Achilles tendinitis may be resistant to a quick resolution because of the slower healing response of tendinous tissue. It is important to create a proper healing environment by reducing stress on the tendon. Proper shoeware and foot orthotics should be worn to address structural faults that may be causing the irritation, and flexibility exercises should be performed for the heel cord complex. Modalities such as ice can help reduce pain and inflammation early on, and ultrasound can facilitate an increased blood flow to the tendon in the later stages of rehabilitation. Cross friction massage may be used to break down adhesions that may have formed during the healing response and to further improve the gliding ability of the paratenon. Strengthening of the gastrocnemius-soleus musculature must be progressed carefully so as not to cause a recurrence of the symptoms.[28]

19-6 Critical Thinking Exercise

A football player, while lying on the field, has his ankle forced into external rotation by another player.

? What type of injury is sustained by this mechanism? What is a characteristic sign of this injury?

Achilles Tendon Rupture

A rupture of the Achilles tendon (Figure 19-25) is possible in sports that require stop-and-go action. Although most common in athletes who are thirty years of age or

19-7 Critical Thinking Exercise

A thirty-five-year-old racquetball player, while moving backward, experiences a sudden snap and pain in the left Achilles tendon.

? What type of injury does this mechanism describe, and how should it be examined?

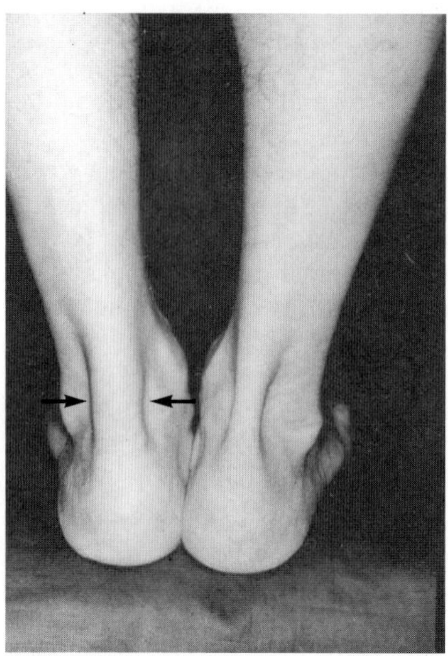

Figure 19-24

A thickened Achilles tendon caused by tendinitis.

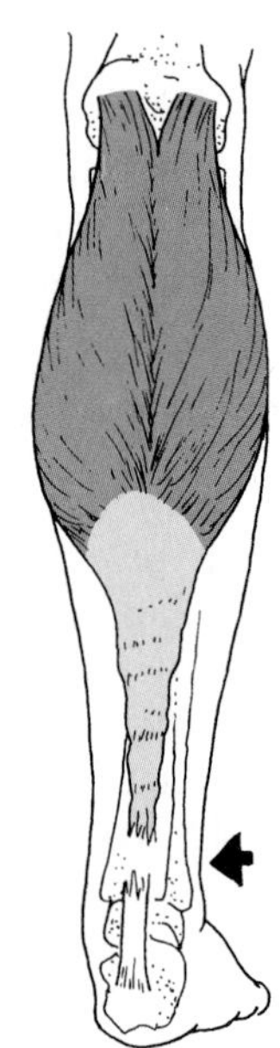

Figure 19-25

Achilles tendon rupture.

older, rupture of the Achilles tendon can occur in athletes of any age.[40] It usually occurs in an athlete with a history of chronic inflammation and gradual degeneration caused by microtears.[2]

A ruptured Achilles tendon may occur because of chronic inflammation.

Etiology The initial insult normally is the result of sudden pushing-off action of the forefoot with the knee being forced into complete extension.

Symptoms and signs When the rupture occurs, the athlete complains of a sudden snap that felt like something kicked him or her in the lower leg. Pain is immediate but rapidly subsides. Point tenderness, swelling, and discoloration are usually associated with the trauma. Toe raising is impossible in an Achilles tendon rupture. The major problem in Achilles tendon rupture is accurate diagnosis, especially in a partial rupture. Any acute injury to the Achilles tendon should be suspected of a rupture. Signs indicative of a rupture are obvious indentation at the tendon site and a positive Thompson test (see Figure 19-10). An Achilles tendon rupture usually occurs 2 to 6 cm (.78 to 2.34 inches) proximal to its insertion onto the calcaneus.

Management Usual management of a complete Achilles tendon rupture is surgical repair.[14] Nonoperative treatment consists of RICE, NSAIDs, and analgesics with a non–weight bearing cast for six weeks followed by a short-leg walking cast for two weeks. With this approach, there is 75 percent to 80 percent return of normal function.[6] Surgery is usually the choice for serious injuries, providing 75 percent to 90 percent return of function. Exercise rehabilitation lasts for about six months and consists of range-of-motion exercises, PRE, and the wearing of a 2 cm heel lift in both shoes.[6]

19-8

***Critical Thinking* Exercise**

A volleyball player with a history of repeated ankle sprains complains of a snapping sensation in the right ankle.

? What procedures should be followed when managing a subluxated peroneal tendon?

Peroneal Tendon Subluxation/Dislocation

The peroneus longus and brevis tendons pass through a common groove located behind the lateral malleolus. The tendons are held in place by the peroneal retinaculum.

Etiology This injury most often occurs in sports that apply dynamic forces to the foot and ankle (e.g., turning and sharply cutting). Wrestling, football, ice skating, skiing, basketball, and soccer have the highest incidence. Another mechanism is a direct blow to the posterior lateral malleolus. A moderate to severe inversion sprain or forceful dorsiflexion of the ankle can tear the peroneal retinaculum, allowing the peroneal tendon to dislocate out of its groove. As discussed previously, one of the major functions of the peroneus longus muscle is to pull the first metatarsal into plantar flexion.

Symptoms and signs The athlete complains that in running or jumping the tendons snap out of the groove and then back in when stress is released. Eversion against manual resistance will often replicate the subluxation. The athlete experiences recurrent pain, snapping, and ankle instability. The lateral aspect of the ankle may show ecchymoses, edema, tenderness, and crepitus over the peroneal tendon.

Management A conservative approach should be used first and should include compression with a felt pad cut in a horseshoe-shaped pattern that surrounds the lateral malleolus. This compression can be reinforced with a rigid plastic or plaster splint until acute signs have subsided, and RICE, NSAIDs, and analgesics are given as needed. The time period for this conservative care is five to six weeks, followed by a gradual exercise rehabilitation program that includes range-of-motion exercises, PRE, and balance training. If a conservative approach fails, surgery is required.

Anterior Tibialis Tendinitis

Etiology Anterior tibialis tendinitis is a common condition of athletes and joggers who run downhill for an extended period of time.

Symptoms and signs There is point tenderness over the anterior tibialis tendon (Figure 19-26).

Management The athlete should be advised to rest (or at least decrease running time and distance) and to avoid hills. In more serious cases, ice packs, coupled with stretching before and after running, should help reduce the symptoms. A daily strengthening program also should be conducted. Oral antiinflammatory medications may be required.[45]

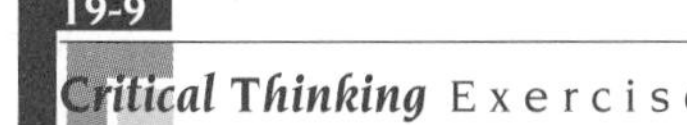

A jogger, after running downhill for an extended period of time, experiences pain in the anterior medial aspect of the left foot. The condition is diagnosed as anterior tibialis tendinitis.

? How should this condition be managed?

Posterior Tibialis Tendinitis

Etiology Posterior tibialis tendinitis is a common overuse condition among runners with hypermobility or pronated feet. It is a repetitive microtrauma occurring during pronation in movements such as jumping, running, or cutting.[20]

Symptoms and signs The athlete complains of pain and swelling in the area of the medial malleolus (see Figure 19-26). Inspection reveals edema and point tenderness directly behind the medial malleolus. In serious cases, the pain becomes more intense during resistive inversion and plantar flexion.[20]

Management Initially, RICE, NSAIDs, and analgesics are given as needed. A non–weight bearing short-leg cast with the foot in inversion may be used. Management consists of correcting the problem of pronation with LowDye taping or an orthotic device.

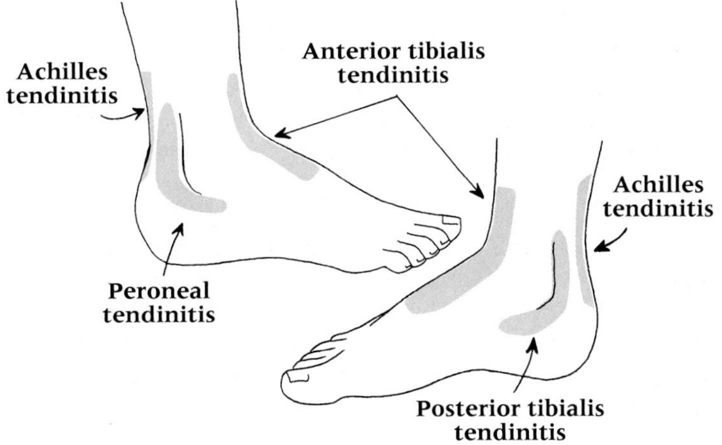

Figure 19-26

Common tendinitis of the foot and ankle region.

Peroneal Tendinitis

Etiology Although not particularly common, peroneal tendinitis can be a problem in athletes with pes cavus. In pes cavus, the foot tends to excessively supinate, which causes weight bearing on the outside of the foot and thus places stress on the peroneal tendon.

Symptoms and signs The athlete complains of pain behind the lateral malleolus when rising on the ball of the foot during jogging, running, cutting, or turning activities. Tenderness is noted over the tendon located at the lateral aspect of the calcaneus distally to beneath the cuboid bone (see Figure 19-26).[43]

Management Initially, management consists of RICE and NSAIDs as required, taping with elastic tape, and appropriate warm-up and flexibility exercises. LowDye taping (see Figure 8-19) or an orthosis to help support the foot and prevent excessive pronation may help.

Shin Contusion

A forceful blow to an unprotected shin can lead to a severe contusion.

Etiology The anterior aspect of the lower leg is often referred to as the shin. The tibia, lying just under the skin, is exceedingly vulnerable and sensitive to blows or bumps. Because of the absence of muscular or adipose padding, the periosteum receives the full force of any impact delivered to the shin. The periosteum is a membrane that surrounds all bony surfaces except articulating surfaces, which are covered by hyaline cartilage. The periosteum is composed of two fibrous layers that adhere closely to the bone and act as a bed for nerves, blood vessels, and bone-forming osteoblasts.

Symptoms and signs The athlete complains of intense pain when the shin is contused. A hematoma forms rapidly and tends to exhibit a jellylike consistency.[15] There could also be an associated compartment syndrome, particularly in the anterior compartment, as well as a potential tibial fracture.

Management RICE, NSAIDs, and analgesics are administered as needed. Maintaining compression in the area of the hematoma is critical. In some cases, the hematoma may need to be aspirated. The athlete, within pain limitations, should perform range-of-motion and PRE exercises. The athlete should be fitted with a doughnut padding under an orthoplast shell for protection.[20]

An inappropriately managed injury to the periosteum may develop into osteomyelitis, a serious condition that results in the destruction and deterioration of bone (Figure 19-27).

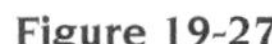

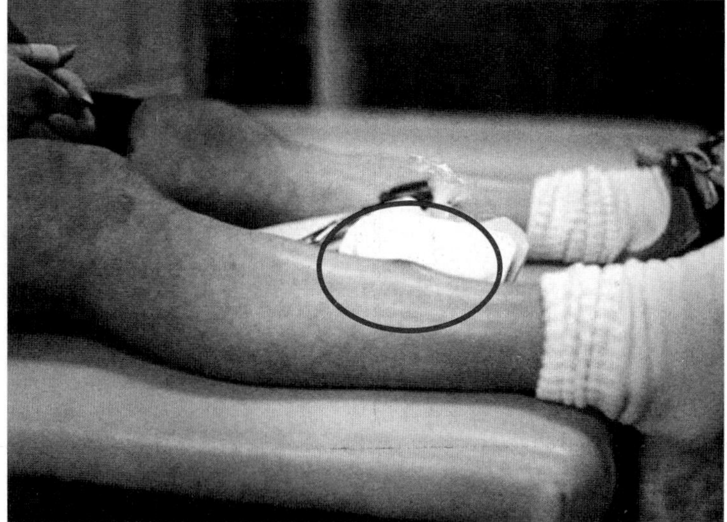

Figure 19-27

A poorly cared-for shin bruise can lead to osteomyelitis.

In sports such as football and soccer in which the shin is particularly vulnerable, adequate protective padding should be used. All injuries in this area are potentially serious; therefore even minor shin bruises should never be permitted to go untended.

Muscle Contusions

Etiology Contusions of the leg, particularly in the area of the gastrocnemius muscle, are common in sports. Most often, contusions occur from being kicked in the back of the leg.

Symptoms and signs A bruise in this area can produce an extremely handicapping injury for the athlete. A bruising blow to the leg will cause pain, weakness, and partial loss of the use of the limb. Palpation may reveal a hard, rigid, and somewhat inflexible area because of internal hemorrhage and muscle guarding.

Management When this condition occurs, it is advisable to stretch the muscles in the region immediately to prevent spasm and then to apply a compression wrap and ice to control internal hemorrhaging.

If cold therapy or other superficial therapy such as massage and whirlpool do not return the athlete to normal activity within two to three days, the use of ultrasound may be warranted. An elastic wrap or tape support will stabilize the part and permit the athlete to participate without aggravating the injury.

Leg Cramps and Spasms

Spasms are sudden, violent, involuntary contractions of one or several muscles and may be either clonic or tonic. A *clonic* spasm is identified by intermittent contraction and relaxation. A *tonic* spasm is identified by constant muscle contraction without an intervening period of relaxation. The clonic spasm has a neurological basis and is seen less often in sports.

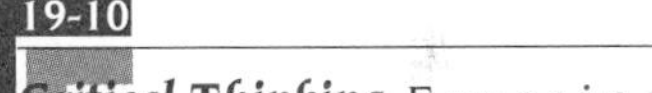

19-10 ***Critical Thinking*** Exercise

A football running back receives a hard, low tackle. He hears a loud pop and feels a sharp pain in his right lower leg. Weight bearing is impossible.

? In this situation, what type of injury is suspected?

Etiology The specific cause of a muscle cramp is often difficult to determine. Fatigue, excess loss of fluid through sweating, and inadequate reciprocal muscle coordination are some of the factors that may predispose an individual to tonic muscle spasm. The gastrocnemius muscle is particularly prone to this condition.

Symptoms and signs The athlete has considerable muscle cramping and pain with the tonic contraction of the calf muscle.

Management Management in such cases includes trying to help the athlete relax to relieve the muscle cramp. A firm grasp of the contracted muscle, together with mild, gradual stretching, relieves most acute spasms. An ice pack or gentle ice massage may also be helpful in reducing spasm. In cases of recurrent spasm, the athletic trainer should make certain that fatigue or abnormal water or electrolyte loss is not a factor.

Gastrocnemius Strain

Etiology The medial head of the gastrocnemius is particularly susceptible to muscle strain near its musculotendinous attachment. Sports that require quick starts and stops or occasional jumping can cause this gastrocnemius strain. Usually the athlete makes a quick stop with the foot planted flat and suddenly extends the knee, placing stress on the medial head of the gastrocnemius (Figure 19-28).

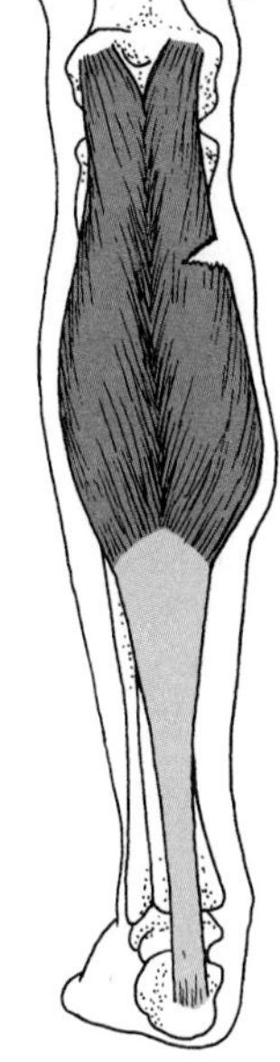

Figure 19-28

Calf strain.

Symptoms and signs Depending on the grade of injury, there is a variable amount of pain, swelling, and muscle disability. The athlete may complain of a sensation of having been "hit in the calf with a stick." Examination reveals edema, point tenderness, and a functional strength loss.[8]

Management Initially, RICE, NSAIDs, and analgesics are given as needed. A grade 1 calf strain should be given a gentle, gradual stretch after muscle cooling. Weight bearing can take place as tolerated. A heel wedge may help reduce stretching of the calf muscle during walking. Appropriate elastic wrap may serve to support the muscle while active. A gradual program of range-of-motion exercises and PRE should be instituted.

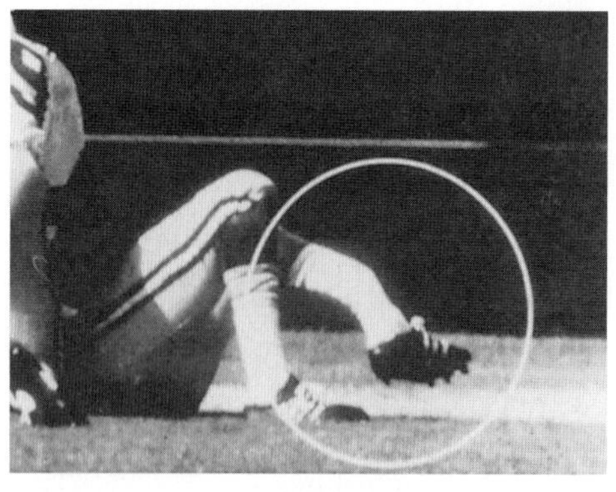

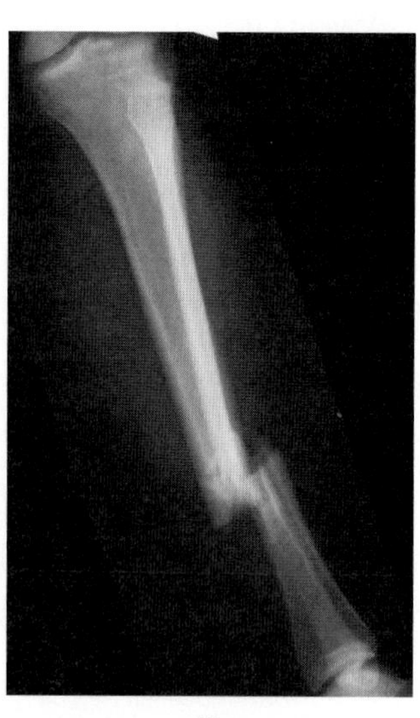

Figure 19-29

A, Fracture of the tibia.
B, X-ray view.

Acute Leg Fractures

Etiology Of all leg fractures, the fibular fracture has the highest incidence. It occurs principally in the middle third, while fractures of the tibia occur predominantly in the lower third. Fractures of the shaft of both the tibia and fibula result from either direct or indirect trauma (Figure 19-29). There may be bony displacement with deformity that results in overriding of the bone ends, particularly if the athlete attempts to move or to stand on the limb after the injury. Crepitus and a temporary loss of limb function are usually present.

Symptoms and signs This injury causes soft-tissue insult and hemorrhaging. The athlete complains of severe pain and disability. The leg appears hard and swollen, which may indicate the beginning of Volkmann's contracture. Volkmann's contracture is the result of internal tension caused by hemorrhage and swelling within closed fascial compartments, which inhibits the blood supply and results in necrosis of muscles and contractures.

Management In most cases, fracture reduction and cast immobilization are applied up to six weeks, depending on the extent of the injury and any complications.

19-11 Critical Thinking Exercise

A gymnast complains of pain in the medial aspect of her right tibia. There is pain before, during, and after activity. Assessment rules out a stress fracture, and the injury is determined to be a grade 3 medial tibial stress syndrome (MTSS).

? What could be the cause of this condition?

Medial Tibial Stress Syndrome

Etiology Medial tibial stress syndrome (MTSS) has in the past been referred to as shinsplints, which is a catchall term that indicates pain in the anterior part of the shin (Figure 19-30). Conditions such as stress fractures, muscle strains, and chronic anterior compartment syndromes have all been termed shinsplints. MTSS accounts for approximately 10 percent to 15 percent of all running injuries and up to 60 percent of all conditions that cause pain in athletes' legs.[38] MTSS is caused by a repetitive microtrauma. It is seen commonly in basketball, running, and gymnastics. Factors that can contribute to MTSS include weakness of leg muscles, shoes that provide little support or cushioning, and training errors such as running on hard surfaces or overtraining.[38] Malalignment problems such as varus foot, a tight heel cord, a hypermobile pronated foot, or a forefoot supination can also lead to MTSS.[38]

MTSS may involve one of two syndromes: a tibial stress fracture or an overuse syndrome that can progress to an irreversible, exertional compartment syndrome.

Symptoms and signs Four grades of pain can be attributed to medial tibial stress syndrome: grade 1 pain occurring after athletic activity; grade 2 pain occurring before and after activity but not affecting performance; grade 3 pain occurring before, during, and after athletic activity and affecting performance; and grade 4 pain, so severe that performance is impossible.

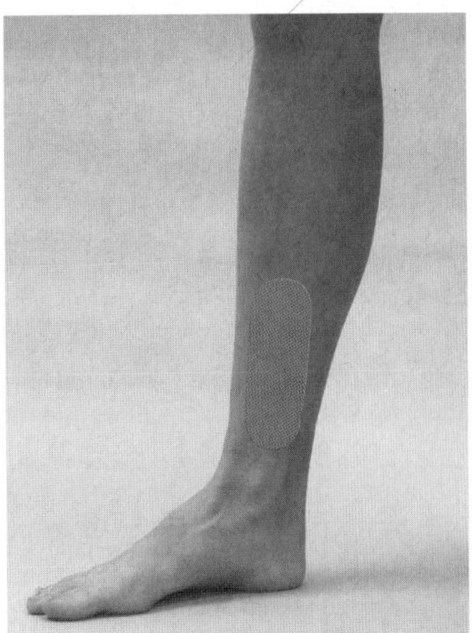

Figure 19-30

In medial tibial stress syndrome, the pain is usually located on the medial aspect of the lower leg just posterior to the tibia (shaded area). Pain is most often associated with the posterior tibialis muscle.

Management Management of this condition should include physician referral to rule out the possibility of stress fracture via the use of bone scans and X rays. Activity modification along with measures to maintain cardiovascular fitness should be set in place immediately. Correction of abnormal pronation during walking and running must also be addressed with shoes and if needed, custom foot orthotics. Ice massage to the area may be helpful in the reduction of localized pain and inflammation. A flexibility program for the gastrocnemius-soleus musculature should be initiated. Arch taping and circumferential tape applied around the area of pain may also be used.

Compartment Syndromes

As discussed earlier in this chapter, the leg is composed of four compartments. Each compartment is bound by fascial sheaths or by fascial sheaths and bone (see Figure 19-6, page 565). Compartment syndromes may be classified as either acute traumatic or chronic exertional.

Etiology The rare acute traumatic syndrome occurs either after being kicked in the lower leg or after excessive exercise in an untrained individual. Excessive swelling within the confines of a fascial compartment compress muscles, blood vessels, and nerves. With the increase in fluid pressure, muscle ischemia that could lead to permanent disability occurs, creating a medical emergency that requires immediate decompression to prevent permanent damage.

A chronic exertional compartment syndrome occurs most frequently among runners and athletes in sports that involve extensive running, such as soccer. Normally internal pressures within the lower leg compartments rise slowly during exercise and subside after exercise is stopped.[7] Chronic exertional compartment syndrome occurs when the tissue fluid pressure increases too much and/or remains elevated after exercise stops, producing ischemia and pain, but neurological involvement is rare.[7] Chronic exertional compartment syndrome is often confused with shinsplints by the athletic trainer. It may also be confused with a stress fracture.

Chronic exertional compartment syndromes occur most commonly in runners, while acute compartment syndromes occur in soccer players.

The compartments most often affected are the anterior and deep posterior, with the anterior having by far the highest incidence.[7,11] On occasion, the lateral compartment may be involved.

Symptoms and signs The more common chronic exertional compartment syndrome symptoms are usually bilateral. The incidence of bilaterality in chronic exertional compartment syndrome is 50 percent to 60 percent.[11] The athlete complains of

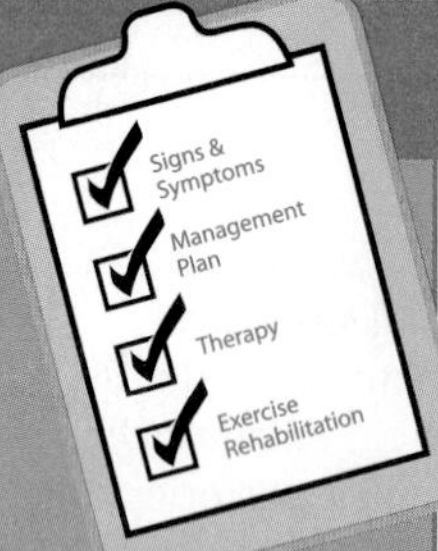

Management PLAN

Medial Tibial Stress Syndrome

Injury Situation A female college field hockey player at the end of the competitive season began to feel severe discomfort in the medial aspect of the right shin.

Symptoms and Signs The athlete complained that her shin seemed to ache all the time but the pain became more intense after practice or a game. During palpation there was severe point tenderness approximately 2 inches (5 cm) in length, beginning 4½ inches (11.25 cm) from the tip of the medial malleolus. The pain was most severe along the medial posterior edge of the tibia. Further evaluation showed that the athlete had pronated feet. X-ray examination showed no indication of stress fracture.

Management Plan The injury was considered to be a medial tibial stress syndrome (shinsplints) involving the long flexor muscle, the great toe, and the posterior tibial muscle.

Phase 1 *Acute Injury*

GOALS: To reduce inflammation, pain, and point tenderness.
ESTIMATED LENGTH OF TIME (ELT): 1–2 weeks.

■ **Therapy** Initially RICE, NSAIDs, and analgesics should be given as needed. The athlete should be instructed to rest and avoid weight bearing as much as possible. Ice massage (7 minutes) should be performed, followed by gentle static stretching to the anterior and posterior muscles 2 to 3 times daily. A LowDye taping or orthotic device should be applied to the arch to correct pronation during weight bearing.

■ **Exercise rehabilitation** Static stretch of Achilles tendon and anterior part of low leg; stretch is held 30 seconds (2 or 3 times); set should be repeated 3 or 4 times daily. General body maintenance exercises should be conducted 3 times weekly if they do not aggravate injury.

Phase 2 *Repair*

GOALS: To heal injury, help athlete become symptom free, return athlete to walking, jogging, and finally, running.
ELT: 2–3 weeks.

■ **Therapy** Cold application (5 to 15 minutes) to shin area before and after walking 1 time daily. Activity should be stopped if there is shin pain. Ultrasound (0.5 to 0.075 W/cm^2) (5 to 10 minutes) 1 to 2 times daily. Transverse friction massage should be given to prevent adhesions. The athlete should wear LowDye taping or orthoses when weight bearing. A counterforce bracing with tape also should be worn 2 to 4 inches (5 to 10 cm) proximal to the malleoli.

■ **Exercise rehabilitation** Ankle range-of-motion exercises plus PRE with rubber tubing to the anterior and posterior leg muscles. Static stretch of lower leg followed by arch and plantar flexion exercises. Towel gathering exercise (10 repetitions, 1 to 3 sets); progress from no resistance to 10 lb of resistance, 3 times daily. Towel scoop exercise (10 repetitions, 1 to 3 sets); progress to 10 lb, 3 times daily. Marble pickup, 3 times daily. General body maintenance exercises should be conducted 3 times weekly if they do not aggravate injury. Athlete should engage in a program of progressive weight bearing and locomotion within pain-free limits starting with slow heel-toe walking, fast walking, jogging, and finally, running. As pain decreases, activity can increase.

Phase 3 *Remodeling*

GOALS: To return to full-field hockey activity.
ELT: 3–6 weeks.

■ **Therapy** The athlete should carry out cryokinetics before and after practice. The athlete should continue to wear counterforce brace and LowDye taping or orthoses for foot pronation.

■ **Exercise rehabilitation** The athlete should continue a daily program of lower leg static stretch after ice application before and after activity. The athlete should carry out a program of ankle range-of-motion exercises and lower leg PRE 3 days a week.

Criteria for Return to Competitive Field Hockey

1. Leg is symptom free after prolonged activity.
2. The lower leg and ankle have full strength and range of motion.
3. Hyperpronation is controlled to prevent reoccurrence.

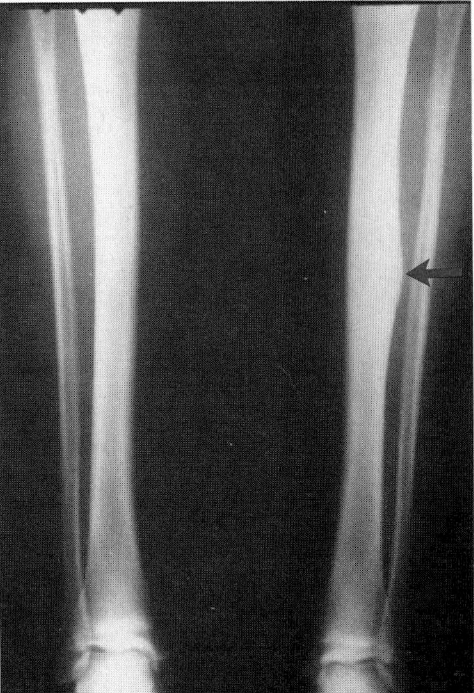

Figure 19-31

Tibial stress fracture.

pain during exercise in the anterolateral region of the leg. Gradually, over time the pain will occur in a predictable manner after running a specific distance or length of time. The athlete commonly complains of an ache or sharp pain and pressure in the region of the anterior compartment when performing a particular activity. The symptoms subside or go away completely when resting. When major symptoms are present, weakness in foot and toe extension and numbness in the dorsal region may occur.

Management Often initial symptoms are aided by the application of RICE, NSAIDs, and analgesia as needed. However, recurrent conditions may require surgical release of the associated fascia. Once surgery is performed, the athlete is allowed to begin a light program of exercise in ten days.

19-12

Critical Thinking Exercise

A soccer player complains of recurrent pain in the anterolateral region of the leg during practice and competition. The pain is described as an ache and a feeling of pressure.

? This condition is determined to be an exertional compartment syndrome. How should it be managed?

Stress Fracture of the Tibia or Fibula

Etiology Stress fractures to the tibia or fibula are a common overuse stress condition, especially among distance runners (Figure 19-31). Stress fractures of the lower leg, like many other overuse syndromes, are more likely to occur in athletes who have structural deformities of the foot. Athletes who have hypermobile pronated feet are more susceptible to fibular stress fracture, whereas those with rigid pes cavus are more prone to tibial stress fractures. The wider the tibia, the lower the incidence of stress fractures. Runners frequently develop a stress fracture in the lower third of the leg; ballet dancers more commonly acquire one in the middle third. Stress fractures often occur to inexperienced and nonconditioned individuals.[13] Training errors are often the cause.[13] Other causes may include amenorrhea and nutritional deficiencies.

Symptoms and signs The athlete complains of pain in the leg that is more intense after than during the activity. There is usually point tenderness, but it may be difficult to discern the difference between bone pain and soft-tissue pain. One technique for distinguishing bone pain from soft-tissue pain is bone percussion. The fibula or tibia is tapped firmly above the level of tenderness. Vibration travels along the bone to the fracture, which may respond with pain. Another percussive technique is to hit the heel upward from below, which causes pain to occur at the fracture site.

19-13

Critical Thinking Exercise

A novice and poorly conditioned recreational runner with a pes cavus experiences pain and discomfort in the lower third of the lower left leg after three weeks of running. The pain and discomfort become more intense immediately after running.

? An X ray shows the beginning of a stress fracture. How should it be managed?

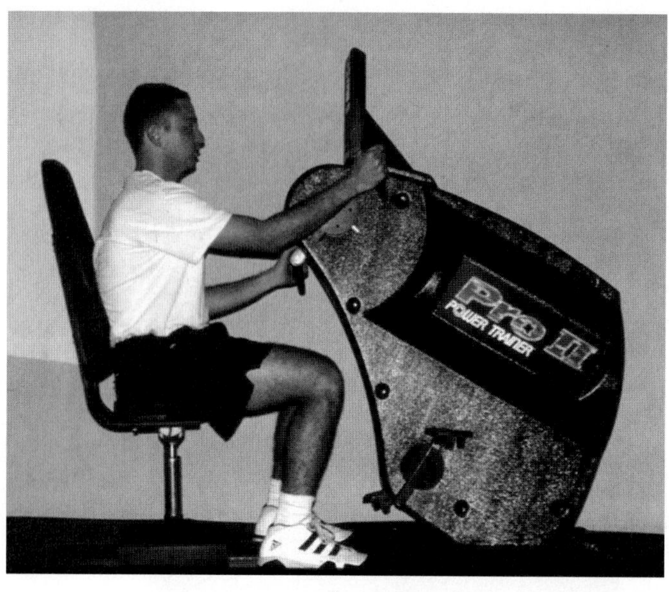

A

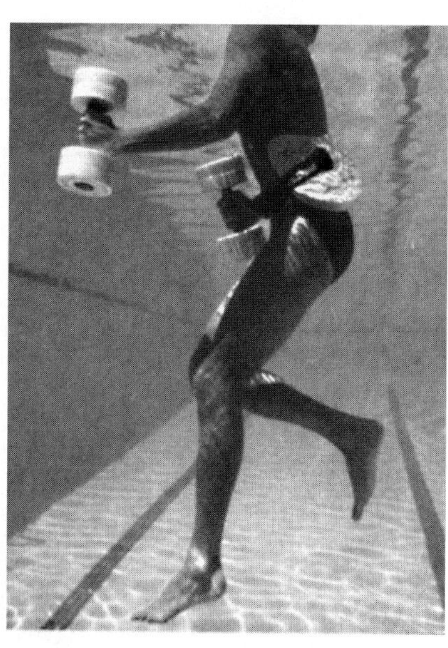

B

Figure 19-32

Non–weight-bearing exercises to maintain cardiorespiratory endurance can be done **A,** on an upper extremity ergometer or **B,** in an exercise pool.

Diagnosis of a stress fracture may be extremely difficult. X-ray examination may or may not detect the problem. A bone scan will more accurately assess the presence of a stress fracture but does not clearly distinguish between a stress fracture and periostitis.

Management The following regimen may be used for a stress fracture of the tibia or fibula:

- The athlete should discontinue running and other stressful locomotor activities for at least fourteen days.
- When pain is severe, the athlete should use a crutch for walking or wear a cast.
- The athlete may resume weight bearing as pain subsides.
- The athlete may bicycle before returning to running.
- After a pain-free period of at least two weeks, the athlete can gradually begin running again.[16]
- Biomechanical foot corrections should be made.

REHABILITATION TECHNIQUES FOR THE LOWER LEG AND ANKLE

General Body Conditioning

The athlete should maintain cardiorespiratory conditioning during the entire rehabilitation process. Pedaling a stationary bike or using an upper extremity ergometer with the hands provides the athlete with excellent cardiovascular exercise without placing stress on the lower leg or ankle (Figure 19-32). Pool running with a float vest and swimming are also good cardiovascular exercises.

Weight Bearing

During the period of maximum protection immediately following injury, the athlete should be either non–weight bearing or perhaps partial weight bearing on crutches. Early limited stress following the initial period of inflammation may promote faster and stronger healing.[32] Partial weight bearing with crutches helps control several complications to healing, including muscle atrophy, proprioceptive loss, circulatory stasis, and tendinitis. For these reasons, early ambulation, even if only touch down weight bearing, is essential.[45] Protected motion facilitates proper collagen reorientation and thus increases the strength of the healing ligament.

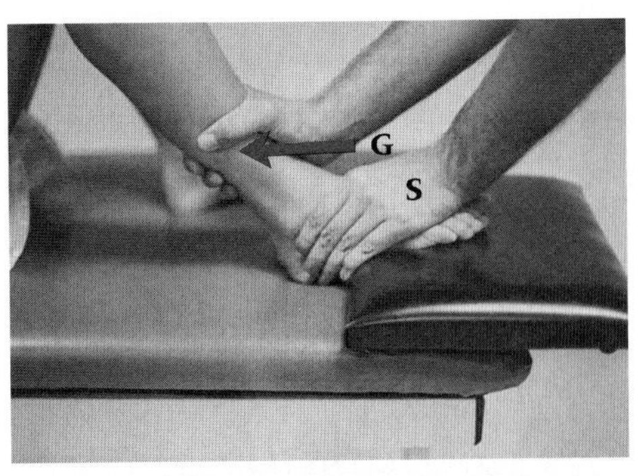

A

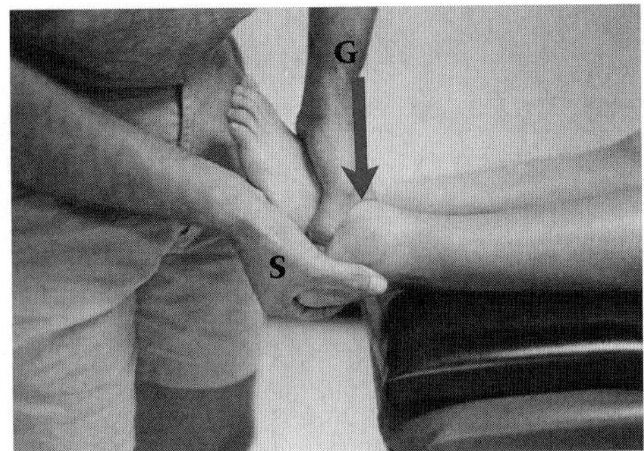

B

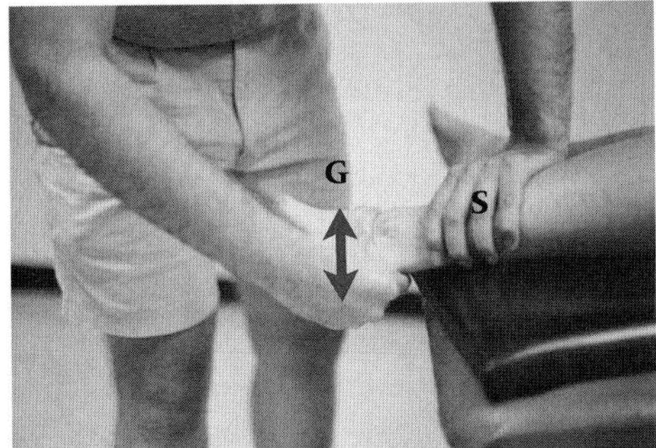

C

Figure 19-33

Ankle joint mobilization techniques. **A,** Posterior tibial glides. **B,** Posterior talar glides. **C,** Subtalar joint medial and lateral glides.

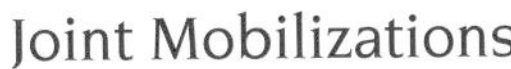

Joint Mobilizations

Movement of an injured joint can be improved by manual joint mobilization techniques (Figure 19-33). Joint mobilizations that concentrate on increasing dorsiflexion and plantar flexion should be started first.[43] Posterior tibial glides and anterior talar glides can be used to improve plantar flexion. Anterior tibial glides and posterior talar glides will increase dorsiflexion. Subtalar joint medial and lateral glides can be used to increase inversion and eversion.

Flexibility

In the early stages of rehabilitation, inversion and eversion should be minimized. Exercises such as towel stretching for the plantar flexors and standing or kneeling stretches for the dorsiflexors can improve range of motion. Athletes are encouraged to do these exercises slowly and without pain and to use high repetitions (two sets of 40). Vigorous heel cord stretching should be initiated as soon as possible[74] (Figure 19-34).

As tenderness decreases, inversion-eversion exercises may be initiated.[74] Such exercises include pulling a towel from one side to the other by alternately inverting and everting the foot, and drawing the alphabet while the foot is in an ice bath. The alphabet should be done in capital letters to ensure that full range is used.

Exercises performed on a BAPS board, wedge board, or KAT system may be beneficial for range of motion and for regaining neuromuscular control.[4] The athlete begins these exercises seated and progresses to standing (Figure 19-35). Initially, the athlete should start in the seated position and move a wedge board in the plantar flexion–dorsiflexion direction. As pain decreases and healing progresses, the board may be turned in the inversion-eversion direction. When seated exercises are performed with ease, standing balance exercises should be initiated. They may be started with the athlete on one leg, standing, without a board. The athlete then supports weight with the hands and maintains balance on a wedge board in either plantar flexion–dorsiflexion or inversion-eversion directions. Next, hand support may be eliminated while the athlete balances on the wedge board. The same sequence is then used on the BAPS board. The BAPS board is initially used with assistance from the hands. Then balance is practiced on the BAPS board unassisted.

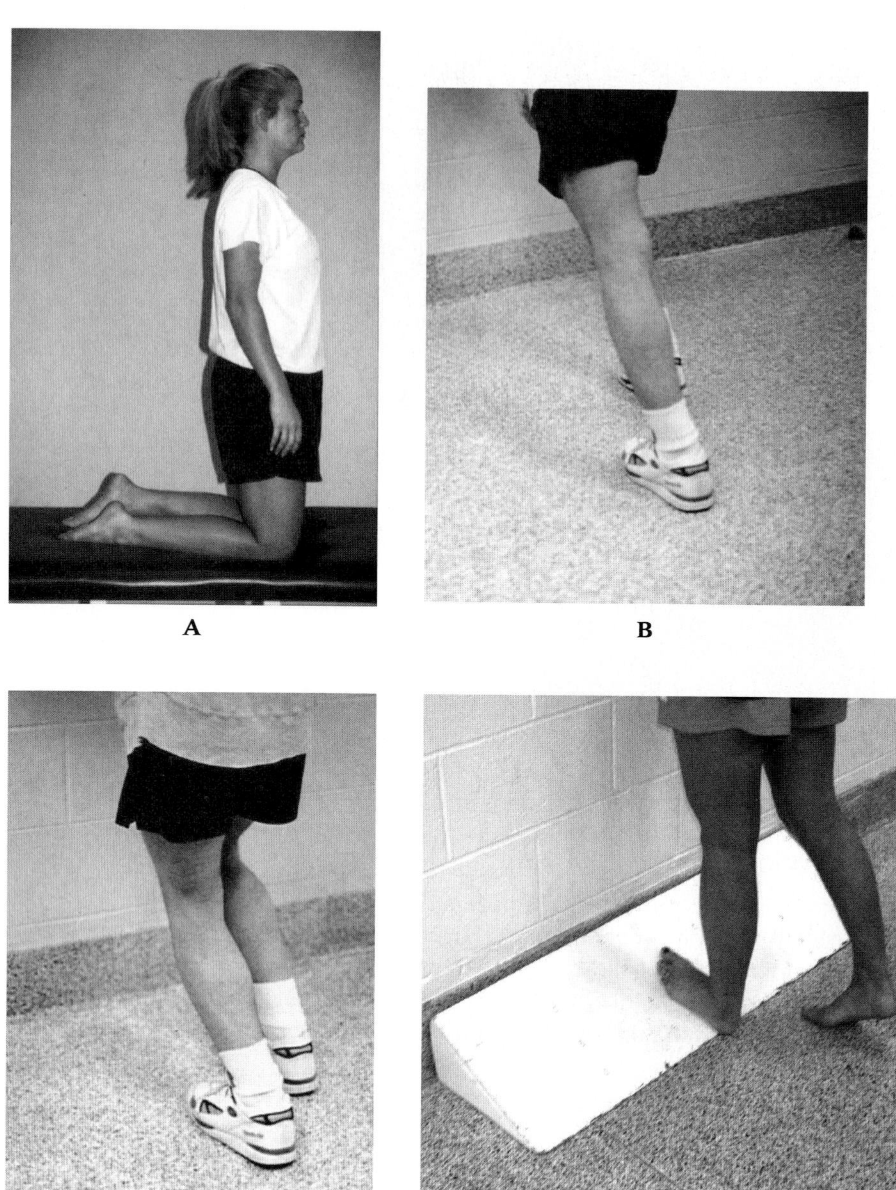

Figure 19-34

Flexibility exercises. **A,** Kneeling stretch for dorsiflexors. **B,** Gastrocnemius stretch with knee straight. **C,** Soleus stretch with knee bent. **D,** Stretches for the heel cord may also be done on an incline board.

Proprioception and Neuromuscular Control

Early weight bearing has previously been mentioned as a method of reducing proprioceptive loss. It has been shown that deficits in ankle proprioception can predispose an athlete to ankle injury.[56,73] Changes in joint position sense and kinesthesia of a magnitude found in subjects with chronically unstable ankles can lead to an increased risk of lateral ankle sprains. Results from a small number of studies suggest that balance and coordination training can restore the increased uncertainty of joint positioning to normal.[37] During the rehabilitation phase, an athlete can recoup proprioception by standing on both feet with eyes closed and progressing to standing on one leg.[28] This exercise may be followed by standing and balancing on a BAPS board, Bosu Balance Trainer, Rocker board, Tremor box, minitramp, or Dynadisc which should be done initially with support from the hands (Figure 19-36). As a final exercise, the athlete can progress to free standing. Regaining control of balance is a key in ankle rehabilitation.[61,62] Postural control is significantly impaired with ankle sprain and may require two to four weeks to return to normal.[25]

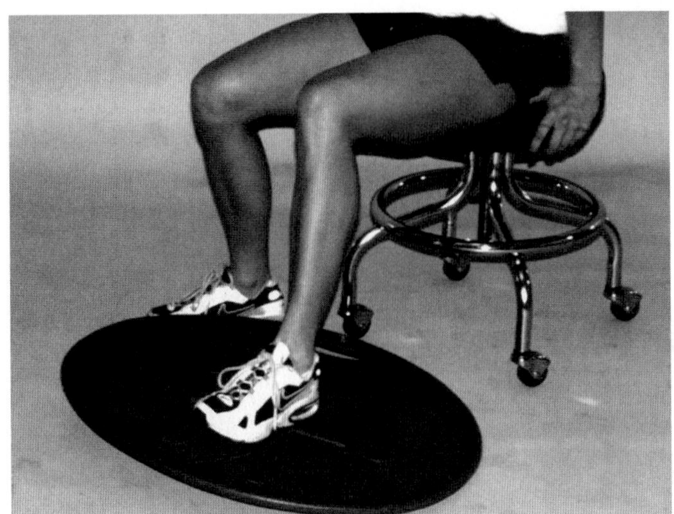

Figure 19-35

BAPS board exercises are used for reestablishing neuromuscular control.

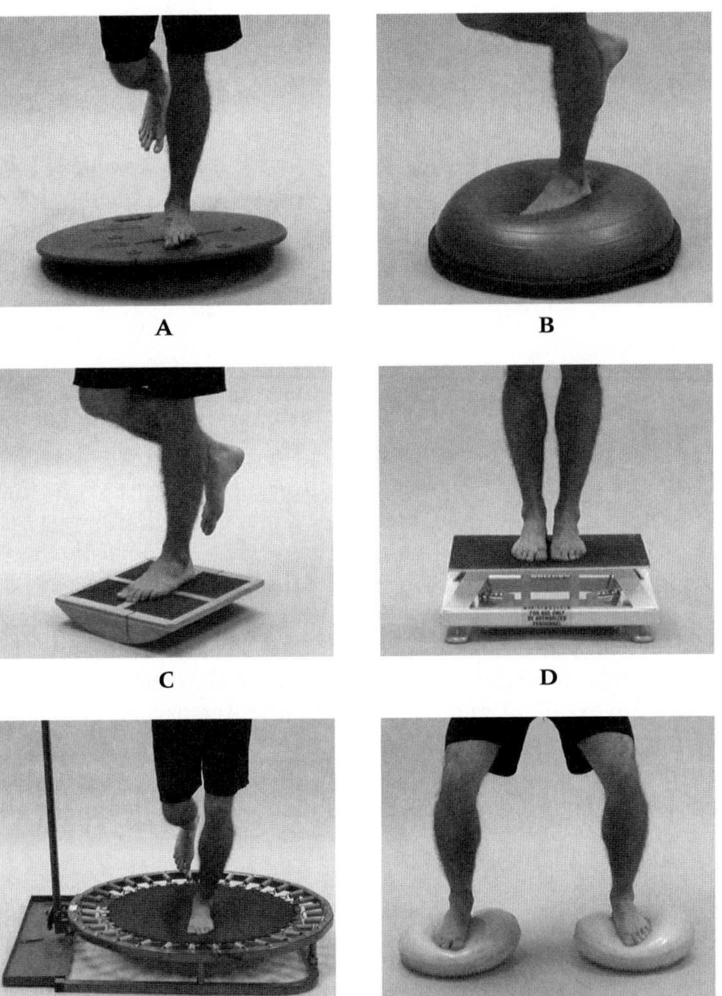

Figure 19-36

Activities to enhance both strength and neuromuscular control. **A,** BAPS board. **B,** Bosu Balance Trainer. **C,** Rocker board. **D,** Tremor box. **E,** Minitramp. **F,** Dynadisc.

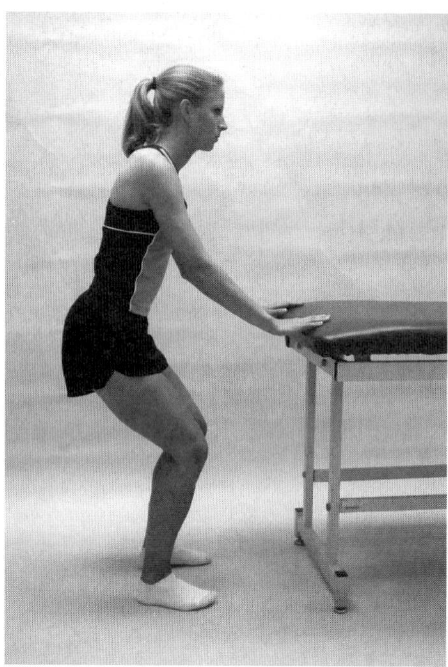

Figure 19-37

Minisquats are helpful both in regaining range of motion and in strengthening.

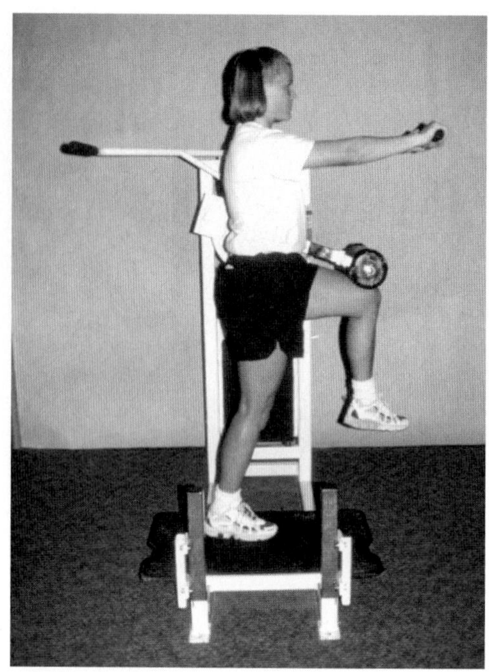

Figure 19-38

Single leg standing kicks on an exercise machine.

Other closed kinetic chain exercises may be beneficial. Leg presses and minisquats (Figure 19-37) on the involved leg will encourage weight bearing and increase proprioceptive return.[17] Single leg standing kicks using abduction, adduction, extension, and flexion of the uninvolved side while weight bearing on the affected side will increase both strength and proprioception. These kicks may be performed with the athlete either standing free or on a machine (Figure 19-38).

Strengthening

Strengthening techniques should concentrate on achieving a balance in muscle groups surrounding the ankle.[34] Isometric strengthening exercises may be done in the four major ankle motion planes. They may be accompanied early in the rehabilitative phase by plantar flexion and dorsiflexion isotonic exercises. As healing progresses and range of motion increases, the athlete may begin strengthening exercises in all planes of motion (Figure 19-39).[49] Care must be taken when exercising in inversion and eversion to avoid tibial rotation as a substitute movement. Pain should be the basic guideline for deciding when to start inversion-eversion isotonic exercises.[35] Light resistance with high repetitions has fewer detrimental effects on the ligaments (two to four sets of 10 repetitions). Resistive tubing exercises, ankle weights around the foot, or a balance board are excellent methods of strengthening inversion and eversion. Tubing has advantages because it may be used both eccentrically and concentrically. Isokinetics have advantages because the athlete may obtain more functional speeds. PNF strengthening exercises that isolate the desired motions at the talocrural joint can also be used.

Taping and Bracing

It is most desirable to have the athlete return to sport without the aid of ankle support. However, it is common practice for some type of ankle support to be worn initially.[22,36] Ankle taping does appear to have a stabilizing effect on unstable ankles without interfering with motor performance.[66] Taping also may help to protect the injured ligaments from excessive loading.[71] The athletic trainer can tape the ankle and

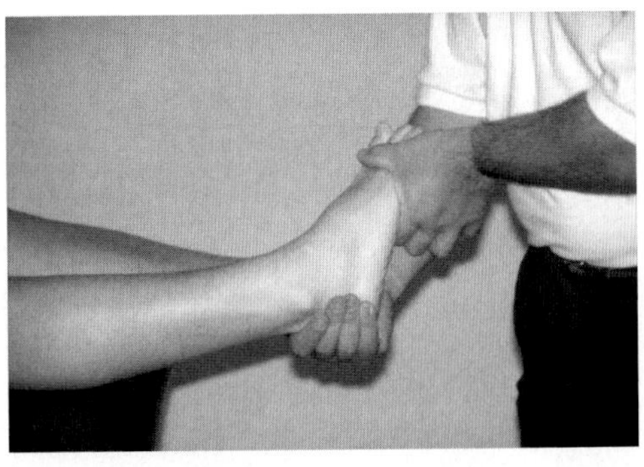

A

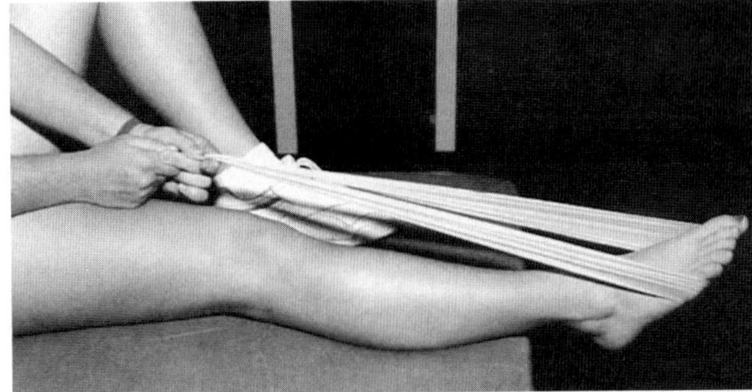

B

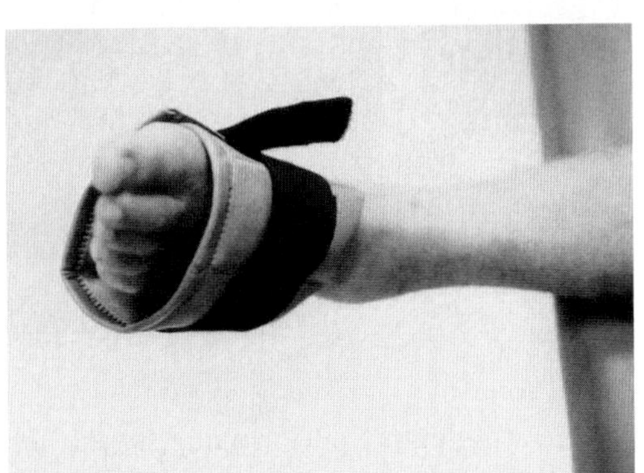

C

Figure 19-39

Ankle strengthening exercises. **A,** Manually resisted strengthening exercises can be done in all four directions. **B,** Resisted tubing exercises. **C,** Ankle weights.

can also tape the shoe onto the foot to make the shoe and ankle function as one unit. High-topped footwear may further stabilize the ankle.[41] If cleated shoes are worn, cleats should be outset along the periphery of the shoe to provide stability. An Aircast or some other supportive ankle brace also can be worn as a substitute for taping (Figure 19-40).[12,23,42,53,64] Bracing may help the athlete detect movement in the ankle and thus may help reduce injury.[16,31]

Functional Progressions

Functional progressions may be as complex or simple as needed. More severe injuries need a more detailed functional progression (see *Focus Box:* "Return to running following ankle injury functional progression.") The typical progression begins early in the rehabilitation process as the athlete becomes partially weight bearing. Full weight bearing should be started when ambulation is performed without a limp.[1]

Running may begin as soon as ambulation is pain free. Pain-free hopping on the affected side may also be a guideline to determine when running is appropriate. Exercising in a pool allows for early running. The athlete is placed in the pool in a swim vest that supports the body in water. The athlete then runs in place without touching the bottom of the pool. Proper running form should be stressed. Eventually the athlete is moved into shallow water so that more weight is placed on the ankle. The athlete then progresses to running on a smooth, flat surface, ideally a track. Initially the athlete should jog the straights and walk the curves and then progress to jogging the entire track. Speed may be increased to a sprint in a straight line. The cutting sequence should begin with circles of diminishing diameter. Cones may be set up for the athlete to run figure-eights as the next cutting progression. The crossover or sidestep is next.[32] The athlete sprints to a predesignated spot and cuts or sidesteps abruptly. When this progression is accomplished, the cut should be done without warning on the command of another person. Jumping and hopping exercises should be started on both legs simultaneously and gradually reduced to only the injured side.[27,32]

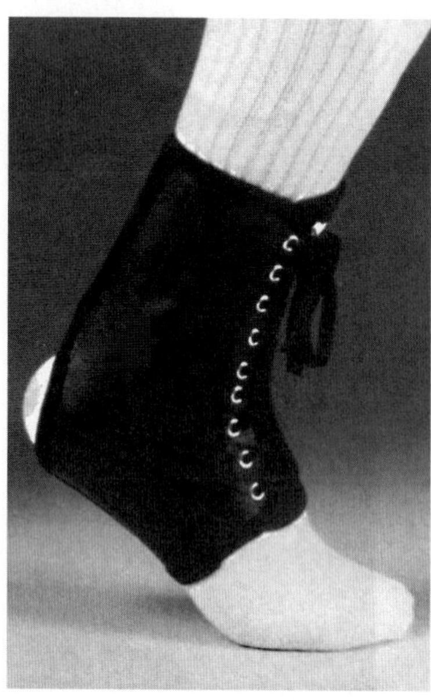

A

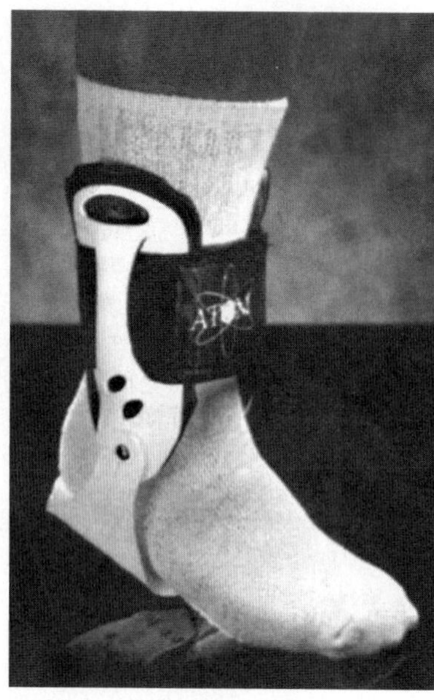

B

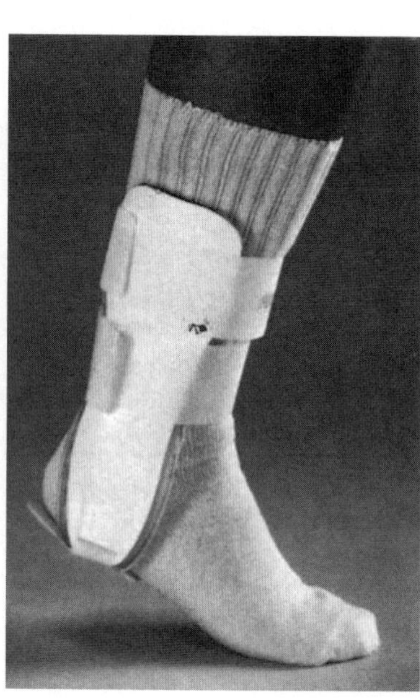

C

Figure 19-40

A number of ankle support devices are available.

The athlete may perform at different levels for each of these functional sequences. One functional sequence may be done at half speed while another is done at full speed. For example, an athlete may run full speed on straights of the track but do figure-eights at only half speed. Once the upper levels of all the sequences are reached, the athlete may return to limited practice, which may include early teaching and fundamental drills.[52]

Return to Activity

The athlete should have complete range of motion and at least 80 percent to 90 percent of preinjury strength before considering a return to the sport.[32] Finally, if full practice is tolerated without insult to the injured part, the athlete may return to competition. Returning to full activity must include a gradual progression of functional activities that slowly increase the stress on the injured structure. The specific demands of each sport dictate the individual drills of this progression.

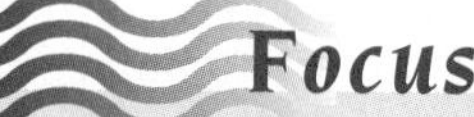

Return to running following ankle injury functional progression

- Walking
- Jogging on track with walking of curves
- Jogging full track
- Running on track with jogging of curves
- Running full track
- Running for fitness—two to three miles three times per week
- Lunges—90 degree, pivot, 180 degree
- Sprints—"W," triangle, 6 second, 20 yd, 40 yd, 120 yd
- Acceleration/deceleration runs
- Shuffle slides progressing to shuffle run
- Carioca

SUMMARY

- The portion of the lower extremity that lies between the knee and the ankle is called the lower leg and contains two bones, the tibia and the fibula. The bones that form the ankle joint, or talocrural joint, are the distal portion of the tibia, the distal portion of the fibula, and the talus. The calcaneus also plays a critical role in the function of the ankle joint.
- The ligamentous support of the ankle consists of the tibiofibular ligaments, three lateral ligaments, and the medial, or deltoid, ligament.
- The musculature of the lower leg is contained within four distinct compartments: muscles of the anterior compartment dorsiflex the ankle; muscles of the lateral compartment evert the ankle; muscles of the superficial posterior compartment plantar flex the ankle; and muscles of the deep posterior compartment invert the ankle.
- Athletes can prevent many lower leg and ankle conditions, especially sprains, by stretching the Achilles tendon, strengthening key muscles, engaging in neuromuscular and proprioceptive training, wearing proper footwear, and using taping and ankle support devices appropriately.
- Ankle sprains are the single most common injury in the athletic population. Ankle sprains are classified as inversion, eversion, or syndesmotic injuries. Occasionally, ankle fractures occur along with ankle sprains.
- The Achilles tendon, or heel cord complex, is subject to acute strain that may lead to a chronic tendinitis. A rupture of the Achilles tendon is common in the older athlete.
- Tendinitis of the anterior tibialis, posterior tibialis, and peroneal tendons are all common around the ankle joint.
- Shin contusions, muscle contusions, muscle cramps, gastrocnemius strains, and fractures of the tibia or fibula are all traumatic injuries that can occur in the lower leg.
- Chronic overuse conditions of the lower leg include medial tibial stress syndrome (shinsplints), exertional compartment syndrome, and stress fractures of the tibia and fibula.
- Perhaps the most important consideration in the rehabilitation of injuries to the lower leg and ankle is to use a gradual progression, beginning with non–weight bearing and subsequently incorporating the appropriate strengthening, range-of-motion, neuromuscular control, and joint mobilization techniques to facilitate the athlete's return to full activity.

Websites

Cramer First Aider:
http://www.cramersportsmed.com/first_aider.jsp

The University of Texas Anatomy of The Human Body:
http://www.bartleby.com/107

American Orthopaedic Foot and Ankle Society:
http://www.aofas.org

World Ortho: http://www.worldortho.com

Readers can use the search engine in this site to locate relevant information on the ankle and lower leg.

American Podiatric Medical Association: http://www.apma.org

Provides a variety of information on foot and ankle injuries from the APMA.

AAOS Online Serivce: Foot and Ankle:
http://orthoinfo.aaos.org/category.cfm?topcategory=foot

Provides answers to a wide range of questions on foot and ankle injuries from the American Academy of Orthopedic Surgeons.

Solutions to Critical Thinking EXERCISES

19-1 The typical progression begins when the athlete becomes partially weight bearing. Full weight bearing should be started when ambulation is performed without a limp. Walking may begin as soon as ambulation is pain free. The athlete then progresses to running on a smooth, flat surface, ideally a track. Initially the athlete should jog the straights and walk the curves and then progress to jogging the entire track. The cutting sequence should begin with circles of diminishing diameter, figure eights, and crossover or side steps. Jumping and hopping exercises should be started on both legs simultaneously and gradually reduced to only the injured side.

19-2 The soccer player most likely has a syndesmotic sprain or sprain of the distal tibiofibular ligaments. This is commonly referred to as a high ankle sprain. This injury may take longer to heal compared with an inversion or eversion ankle sprain.

19-3 The athletic trainer should take a multifaceted approach to reducing ankle sprains. The athlete should stretch his Achilles tendon to allow at least 10 degrees of dorsiflexion and should perform strength training on the peroneals, plantar flexors, and dorsiflexors. The athlete should also perform proprioceptive training on a balance board. The athlete should wear high-top shoes. Ankle taping with an orthosis can also be employed.

19-4 Based on these symptoms it is likely that the athlete has either an osteochondral fracture or osteochondritis dissecans. The athlete should be referred to a physician for X rays to confirm this opinion. It is likely that the physician will recommend an arthroscopic procedure to remove these fragments.

19-5 The athlete should continue to wear a stirrup brace for one to three more weeks. Taping at 90 degrees will be conducted for two to four weeks. The athlete should engage in pain-free plantar flexion and dorsiflexion exercises and proprioceptive exercises on a balance board.

19-6 The mechanism describes a syndesmotic ankle sprain. The athlete experiences severe pain in the anterolateral leg region when the ankle is externally rotated.

19-7 This injury is a possible partial or complete rupture of the Achilles tendon. The athletic trainer should look for pain that eventually subsides, an inability to perform a toe raise, point tenderness, swelling, discoloration, an obvious indentation at the tendon site, and a positive Thompson test.

19-8 The athletic trainer should apply compression with a horseshoe-shaped felt pad around the lateral malleoleus. This pad should be reinforced by a rigid splint. RICE, NSAIDs, and analgesics should be given as needed. The athlete should follow an exercise program to strengthen, stretch, and enhance balance training.

19-9 The athletic trainer should instruct the athlete to rest or reduce the stress of running. The athlete should apply ice packs followed by stretching before and after activity. The athlete should follow a strengthening program along with treatment by oral antiinflammatory medications as needed.

19-10 The athlete has sustained a lower leg fracture. The most common site is in the middle third of the fibula.

19-11 In gymnastics, athletes often run on hard surfaces wearing shoes with little cushioning. This, combined with overtraining and fatigue, could lead to MTSS. Other reasons are a varus or pronated hypermobile foot.

19-12 The conservative approach is to apply RICE and NSAIDs and rest. With weakness in toe extension and numbness in the dorsal region, surgery may be warranted.

19-13 The runner should avoid stressful locomotor activities for at least fourteen days. He or she can engage in bicycling and swimming if pain free. Running can be resumed after a pain-free period of two weeks.

REVIEW QUESTIONS AND CLASS ACTIVITIES

1. Identify and describe the anatomy of the ankle and lower leg.
2. How can ankle injuries be prevented?
3. Demonstrate the steps that should be taken when assessing ankle and lower leg injuries.
4. Describe the three different types of ankle sprains.
5. Contrast the management of grade 1, 2, and 3 ankle sprains.
6. What is the usual mechanism for fractures of the ankle?
7. Describe the various injuries that can occur to the Achilles tendon. Indicate their etiology and symptoms and signs.
8. What tendons are most likely to develop tendinitis around the ankle?
9. Discuss the etiology, symptoms and signs, and management of the various acute or traumatic injuries that can occur in the lower leg.
10. What are the possible causes of medial tibial stress syndrome?
11. Contrast the acute anterior compartment syndrome with the chronic type.
12. Describe the various chronic overuse problems that can occur in the lower leg.
13. Describe the appropriate progression of treatment that should be used in the rehabilitation of ankle and lower leg injuries.

REFERENCES

1. Albensi RJ, Nyland J, Caborn DNM: The relationship of body weight and clinical foot and ankle measurements to the heel forces of forward and backward walking, *J Ath Train* 34(4):328, 1999.
2. Alfredson H, Lorentzon R: Chronic Achilles tendinosis: recommendations for treatment and prevention, *Sports Med* 29(2):135, 2000.
3. Baxter D: *The foot and ankle in sport,* St Louis, 1995, Mosby.
4. Bernier JN, Perrin DH, Rijke A: Effect of unilateral functional instability of the ankle on postural sway and inversion and eversion strength, *J Ath Train* 32(3):226, 1997.
5. Beynnon B, Murphy D, Alosa D: Predictive factors for lateral ankle sprains: a literature review, *J Ath Train* 37(4):376, 2002.
6. Birrer RB: Ankle injuries. In Birrer RB, editor: *Sports medicine for the primary care physician,* ed 2, Boca Raton FL CRC Press, 1995, Mosby.
7. Blackman PG: A review of chronic exertional compartment syndrome in the lower leg, *Med Sci Sports Exerc* 32(3 Suppl):S4, 2000.
8. Booher JM, Thibodeau GA: *Athletic injury assessment,* ed 4, St Louis, 1999, McGraw-Hill.
9. Bot SDM, van Mechelen W: The effect of ankle bracing on athletic performance, *Sports Med* 27(3):171, 1999.
10. Brosky T et al: The ankle ligaments: considerations of syndesmotic injury and implications for rehabilitation, *J Orthop Sports Phys Ther* 21(1):197, 1995.
11. Brown DE: Exertional leg pain. In Brown DE, Neuman RD, editors: *Orthopedic secrets,* Philadelphia, 1995, Hanley & Belfus.
12. Cordova M, Ingersoll C, Palmieri R: Efficacy of prophylactic ankle support: an experimental perspective, *J Ath Train* 37(4):246, 2002.
13. Couture CJ: Tibial stress injuries: decisive diagnosis and treatment of "shin splint," *Physician Sportsmed* 30(6):29, 2002.
14. Demeritt K, Shultz S, Docherty C: Chronic ankle instability does not affect lower extremity functional performance, *J Ath Train* 37(4):507, 2002.

15. Denegar C, Miller S: Can chronic ankle instability be prevented? Rethinking management of lateral ankle sprains, *J Ath Train* 37(4):430, 2002.
16. DesRochers DM: Proprioceptive benefit derived from ankle support. *Athletic Therapy Today* 7(6):44, 2002.
17. Docherty CL, Moore JH, Arnold BL: Effects of strength training on strength development and joint position sense in functionally unstable ankles, *J Ath Train* 33(4):310, 2000.
18. Doughtie M: Syndesmotic ankle sprain in football: a survey of National Football League athletic trainers, *J Ath Train* 34(1):15, 1999.
19. Dugan D, Hobler C: Progressive management of open surgical repair of Achilles tendon rupture, *J Ath Train* 29(4):349, 1994.
20. Geidman WM, Johnson JE: Posterior tibial tendon dysfunction, *J Orthop Sports Phys Ther* 30(2):68, 2000.
21. Glick J, Sampson T: Ankle and foot fractures in athletics. In Nicholas J, Hershman E: *The lower extremity and spine in sports medicine*, St Louis, 1996, Mosby.
22. Guskiewicz KM, Riemann BL, Onate JA: Comparison of 3 methods of external support for management of acute lateral ankle sprains, *J Ath Train* 34(1):5, 1999.
23. Heit E, Lephart S, Rozzi S: The effects of ankle bracing and taping on joint position sense in the stable ankle, *J Sport Rehabil* 5(3):206, 1996.
24. Hertel J: Functional anatomy, pathomechanics, and pathophysiology of lateral ankle instability. *J Ath Train* 37(4):364, 2002.
25. Hertel J: Serial testing of postural control after acute lateral ankle sprain. *J Ath Train* 36(4):363, 2001.
26. Hertel J, Denegar C, Monroe M: Talocrural and subtalar joint instability after lateral ankle sprain, *Med Sci Sports Exerc* 31(11):1501, 1999.
27. Hess DM: Effect of a 4-week agility-training program on postural sway in the functionally unstable ankle. *J Sport Rehabil* 10(1):24, 2001.
28. Hirth C: Rehabilitation of lower leg injuries. In Prentice WE, editor: *Rehabilitation techniques in sports medicine and athletic training*, ed 4, St Louis, 2004, McGraw-Hill.
29. Hockenbury RT, Sammarco GJ: Evaluation and treatment of ankle sprains: clinical recommendations for a positive outcome, *Physician Sportsmed* 29(2):57, 2001.
30. Hubbard TJ: Reliability of intratester and intertester measurements derived from an instrumented ankle arthrometer, *J Sport Rehabil* 12(3):208, 2003.
31. Hubbard T, Kaminski T: Kinesthesia is not affected by functional ankle instability status, *J Ath Train* 37(4):481, 2002.
32. Hunter S, Prentice W: Rehabilitation of ankle injuries. In Prentice WE, editor: *Rehabilitation techniques in sports medicine and athletic training*, ed 4, St Louis, 2004, McGraw-Hill.
33. Jepson KK: The use of orthoses for athletes. In Birrer RB, editor: *Sports medicine for the primary care physician*, ed 2, Boca Raton, Fla, 1994, CRC Press.
34. Kaminski T, Hartsell H: Factors contributing to chronic ankle instability: A strength perspective, *J Ath Train* 37(4):394, 2002.
35. Kaminski TW, Perrin DH, Gansneder BM: Eversion strength analysis of uninjured and functionally unstable ankles, *J Ath Train* 34(3):239, 1999.
36. Kinzey SJ, Ingersoll CD, Knight KL: The effects of selected ankle appliances on postural control, *J Ath Train* 32(4):300, 1997.
37. Konradsen L: Factors contributing to chronic ankle instability: kinesthesia and joint position sense, *J Ath Train* 37(4):381, 2002.
38. Kortebein PM, Kaufman KR, Basford JR, Stuart MJ: Medial tibial stress syndrome, *Med Sci Sports Exerc* 32(3 Suppl):S27, 2000.
39. Kovaleski JE: Instrumented ankle arthrometry. *Athletic Therapy Today* 8(1):44, 2003.
40. Leppilahti I, Orava S: Total Achilles tendon rupture: a review, *Sports Med* 25(2):79, 1998.
41. Lindley T: Taping and semirigid bracing may not affect ankle functional range of motion, *J Ath Train* 30(2):109, 1995.
42. Locke A et al: Long-term use of a softshell prophylactic ankle stabilizer on speed, agility, and vertical jump performance, *J Sport Rehabil* 6(3):235, 1997.
43. Loudin J, Bell S: The foot and ankle: an overview of arthrokinematics and selected joint techniques, *J Ath Train* 31(2):173, 1996.
44. Lynch S: Assessment of the injured ankle in the athlete, *J Ath Train* 37(4):406, 2002.
45. Madras D: Rehabilitation for functional ankle instability, *J Sport Rehabil* 12(2):133, 2003.
46. Mangus B, Hoffman M, Parry S: Management of tibiofibular syndesmosis injuries, *Athletic Therapy Today* 4(5):47, 1999.
47. Mattacola CG: Management of talus fractures. *Athletic Therapy Today* 7(1):32, 2002.
48. Mattacola C, Dwyer M: Rehabilitation of the ankle after acute or chronic injury, *J Ath Train* 37(4):413, 2002.
49. McKnight C, Armstrong C: The role of ankle strength in functional ankle instability. *J Sport Rehabil* 6(1):21, 1997.
50. McPoil Jr TG, Brocoto RS: The foot and ankle: biomechanical evaluation and treatment. In Gould III JA, editor: *Orthopaedic and sports physical therapy*, ed 2, St Louis, 1990, Mosby.
51. Muir IW, Chesworth BM, Vandervoort AA: Effect of a static calf-stretching exercise on the resistive torque during passive ankle dorsiflexion in healthy subjects, *J Orthop Sports Phys Ther* 29(2):106, 1999.
52. Munn J: Do functional-performance tests detect impairment in subjects with ankle instability? *J Sport Rehabil* 11(1):40, 2002.
53. Nishikawa T, Grabiner MD: Peroneal motoneuron excitability increases immediately following application of a semirigid ankle brace, *J Orthop Sports Phys Ther* 29(3):168, 1999.
54. Norkus SA, Floyd RT: The anatomy and mechanisms of syndesmotic ankle sprains, *J Ath Train* 36(1):68, 2001.
55. Norwig J: Recognizing and rehabilitating the high ankle sprain, *Athletic Therapy Today* 3(4):12, 1998.
56. Payne KA, Berg K, Latin RW: Ankle injuries and ankle strength, flexibility, and proprioception in college basketball players, *J Ath Train* 32(3):221, 1997.
57. Pugia ML, Middel CJ, Seward SW: Comparison of acute swelling and function in subjects with lateral ankle injury, *J Orthop Sports Phys Ther* 31(7):384, 2001.
58. Ransone J: Syndesmotic ankle sprains. *Athletic Therapy Today* 6(5):48, 2001.
59. Ricard MD et al: Effects of taping and exercise on dynamic ankle inversion, *J Ath Train* 35(1):31, 2000.
60. Ricard MD, Schulties SS, Saret JJ: Effects of high-top and low-top shoes on ankle inversion, *J Ath Train* 35(1):38, 2000.
61. Riemann B: Is there a link between chronic ankle instability and postural instability, *J Ath Train* 37(4):386, 2002.
62. Rozzi SL et al: Balance training for persons with functionally unstable ankles, *J Orthop Sports Phys Ther* 29(8):478, 1999.
63. Sammarco GJ: Injuries to the tibialis anterior, peroneal tendons, and long flexors and extensions of the toes. In Baxter DE, editor: *The foot and ankle in sport*, St Louis, 1995, Mosby.
64. Sharpe SR, Knapik J, Jones B: Ankle braces effectively reduce recurrence of ankle sprains in female soccer players, *J Ath Train* 32(1):21, 1997.
65. Silvestri PG: Management of syndesmotic ankle sprains. *Athletic Therapy Today* 7(5):48, 2002.
66. Simoneau GG, Degner RM, Kramper CA et al: Changes in ankle joint proprioception resulting from strips of athletic tape applied over the skin, *J Ath Train* 32(2):141, 1997.
67. Stanish WD: Lower leg, foot, and ankle injuries in young athletes. In Micheli LJ, editor: *The young athlete. Clinics in sports medicine*, vol 14, no 3, Philadelphia, 1995, Saunders.

68. Taunton J, Smith C, Magee D: Leg, foot, and ankle injuries. In Zachazewski J, Magee D, Quillen W: *Athletic injuries and rehabilitation,* Philadelphia, 1996, WB Saunders.
69. Thacker SB, Stroup DF, Branche CM: The prevention of ankle sprains in sports: a systematic review of the literature, *Am J Sports Med* 27(6):753, 1999.
70. Vegso JJ: Ankle sprain: nonoperative management injuries to lower extremity. In Torg JS, Shephard RJ, editors: *Current therapy in sports medicine,* ed 3, St Louis, 1995, Mosby.
71. Wilkerson G: Biomechanical and neuromuscular effects of ankle taping and bracing, *J Ath Train* 37(4):236, 2002.
72. Wilkerson GB: Treatment of the inversion ankle sprain through synchronous application of focal compression and cold, *J Ath Train* 26(3):220, 1991.
73. Willems T, Witvrouw E, Verstuyft J: Proprioception and muscle strength in subjects with a history of ankle sprains and chronic instability, *J Ath Train* 37(4):487, 2002.
74. Wright IC, Neptune RR, Van Den Bogert AJ, Nigg BM: The effects of ankle compliance and flexibility on ankle sprains, *Med Sci Sports Exerc* 32(2):260, 2000.
75. Zecher SB, Leach RE: Lower leg and foot injuries in tennis and other racquet sports. In Lehman RC, editor: *Racquet sports. Clinic in sports medicine,* vol 14, no 1, Philadelphia, 1995, Saunders.

ANNOTATED BIBLIOGRAPHY

Baxter D: *The foot and ankle in sport,* St Louis, 1995, Mosby.

This comprehensive text is edited by an orthopedist who specializes in foot and ankle injuries.

Brown DE, Neumann RD, editors: *Orthopedic secrets,* Philadelphia, 1995, Hanley & Belfus.

This text presents an overview of orthopedics in a question-and-answer format. The ankle and lower leg are well presented.

Sammarco GJ: *Rehabilitation of the foot and ankle,* St Louis, 1995, Mosby.

This text specifically addresses the aspects of rehabilitation directed at both the foot and ankle.

Pfeffer R: *Athletic injuries to the foot and ankle,* Park Ridge, Ill, 2000, American Academy of Orthopedic Surgeons.

This book goes into great detail on a wide variety of injuries that occur in the ankle joint.

Prentice WE, editor: *Rehabilitation techniques in sports medicine and athletic training,* ed 4, St Louis, 2004, McGraw-Hill.

Chapters 24 and 25 of this text are dedicated to a discussion of rehabilitation techniques for injuries to the lower leg and ankle. The text first covers the pathomechanics and mechanisms of various injuries and then presents rehabilitation concerns and progressions in specific detail.

Nyska M, Mann G, (editors): *The unstable ankle,* Champaign, Ill, 2002, Human Kinetics.

This book covers the basic concepts and practical applications in the diagnosis, treatment, and prevention of acute ankle ligament injury and acute and chronic ankle instability.

Journal of Athletic Training, 37:4, 2002.

The entire journal contains articles that discuss various aspects of ankle injury.

The Knee and Related Structures

Chapter 20

When you finish this chapter you should be able to

- Recognize the normal structural and functional knee anatomy.
- Demonstrate the various ligamentous and meniscal stability tests discussed in this chapter.
- Explain how knee injuries can be prevented.
- Compare and contrast male/female differences relative to anterior cruciate ligament (ACL) injuries.
- Discuss etiological factors, symptoms and signs, and management procedures for the injuries to the ligaments and menisci.
- Identify the various etiological factors, symptoms and signs, and management procedures for injuries that occur in the patellofemoral joint and in the extensor mechanism.
- Design appropriate rehabilitation protocols for the injured knee.

Because so many sports place extreme stress on the knee, it is one of the most traumatized joints in the physically active population. The knee is commonly considered a hinge joint because its two principal movements are flexion and extension. However, because rotation of the tibia is an essential component of knee movement, the knee is not a true hinge joint. The stability of the knee joint depends primarily on the ligaments, the joint capsule, and the muscles that surround the joint. The knee is designed primarily to provide stability in weight bearing and mobility in locomotion; however, it is especially unstable laterally and medially.

Muscles and ligaments provide the main source of stability in the knee.

ANATOMY OF THE KNEE

Bones

The knee joint complex consists of the femur, the tibia, the fibula, and the patella (Figure 20-1). The distal end of the femur expands and forms the convex lateral and medial condyles, which are designed to articulate with the tibia and the patella. The articular surface of the medial condyle is longer from front to back than is the surface of the lateral condyle. Anteriorly, the two condyles form a hollowed groove to receive the patella. The proximal end of the tibia, the tibial plateau, articulates with the condyles of the femur. On this flat tibial plateau are two shallow concavities that articulate with their respective femoral condyles and are divided by the popliteal notch. Separating these concavities, or articular facets, is a roughened area where the cruciate ligaments attach and from which a process commonly known as the tibial spine arises.

Patella

The patella is the largest sesamoid bone in the human body. It is located in the tendon of the quadriceps femoris muscle and is divided into three medial facets and a lateral facet that articulate with the femur (Figure 20-1). The lateral aspect of the patella is wider than the medial aspect. The patella articulates between the concavity provided by the femoral condyles. Tracking within this groove depends on the pull of the

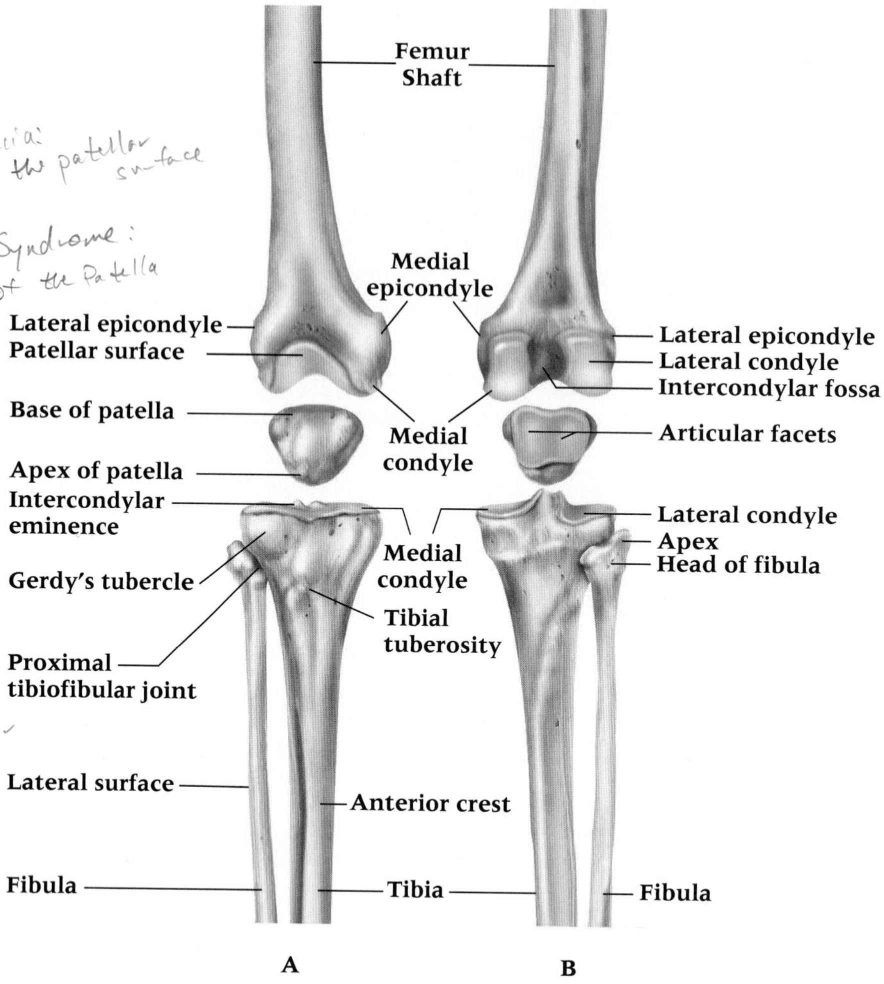

Figure 20-1

The bones of the knee joint. **A,** Anterior view. **B,** Posterior view.

quadriceps muscle and patellar tendon, the depth of the femoral condyles, and the shape of the patella.

Articulations

The knee joint complex consists of several articulations between the femur and the tibia, the femur and the patella, the femur and the fibula, and the tibia and fibula.

Menisci

The menisci (Figure 20-2) are two oval (semilunar) fibrocartilages that deepen the articular facets of the tibia, cushion any stresses placed on the knee joint, and maintain spacing between the femoral condyles and tibial plateau. The consistency of the menisci is much like that of the intervertebral disks. They are located medially and laterally on the tibial tuberosity. The menisci transmit one-half of the contact force in the medial compartment and an even higher percentage of the contact load in the lateral compartment. The menisci help stabilize the knee, especially the medial meniscus, when the knee is flexed at 90 degrees.

Medial Meniscus

The medial meniscus is a **C**-shaped fibrocartilage, the circumference of which is attached firmly to the medial articular facet of the tibia and to the joint capsule by the coronary ligaments. Posteriorly, it is also attached to fibers of the semimembranous muscle.

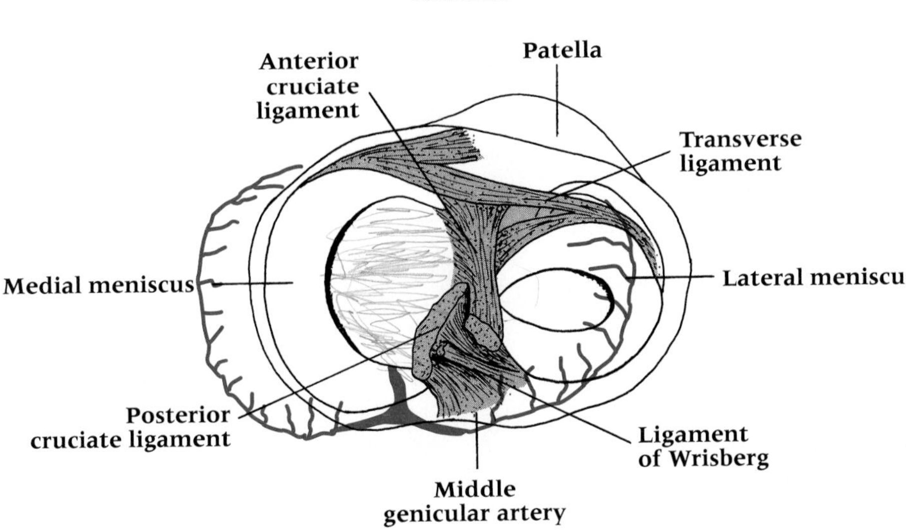

Figure 20-2

Menisci and blood supply of the knee.

Lateral Meniscus

The lateral meniscus is more **O**-shaped and is attached to the lateral articular facet on the superior aspect of the tibia. The lateral meniscus also attaches loosely to the lateral articular capsule and to the popliteal tendon. The ligament of Wrisberg is the part of the lateral meniscus that projects upward, close to the attachment of the posterior cruciate ligament. The transverse ligament joins the anterior portions of the lateral and medial menisci.

Meniscal Blood Supply

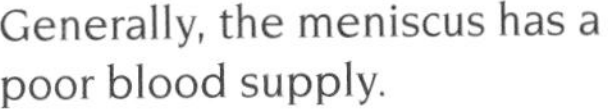

Generally, the meniscus has a poor blood supply.

Blood is supplied to each meniscus by the medial genicular artery. Each meniscus can be divided into three circumferential zones: the red-red zone is the outer, or peripheral, one-third and has a good vascular supply; the red-white zone is the middle one-third and has minimal blood supply; and the white-white zone on the inner one-third is **avascular** (Figure 20-3).[23]

avascular
Devoid of blood circulation.

Stabilizing Ligaments

The major stabilizing ligaments of the knee include the cruciate ligaments, the collateral ligaments, and the capsular ligaments (Figure 20-4).

Cruciate Ligaments

The cruciate ligaments account for a considerable amount of knee stability. They are two ligamentous bands that cross one another within the joint cavity of the knee. The anterior cruciate ligament (ACL) attaches below and in front of the tibia; then, passing backward, it attaches laterally to the inner surface of the lateral condyle. The posterior

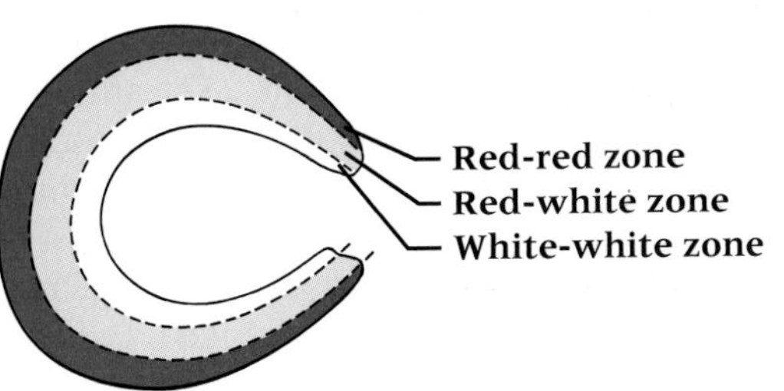

Figure 20-3

The meniscus has three vascular zones.

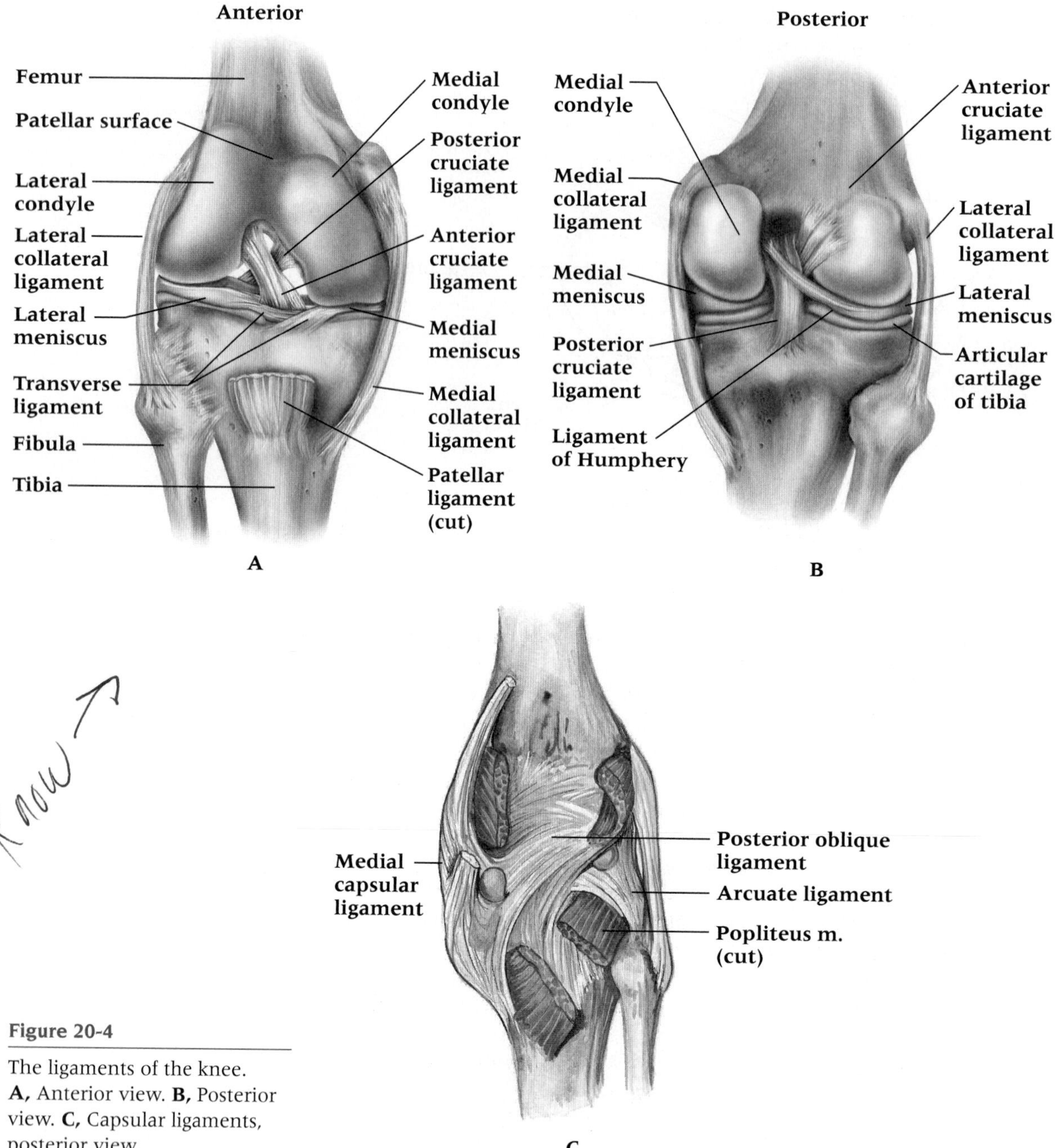

Figure 20-4

The ligaments of the knee. **A,** Anterior view. **B,** Posterior view. **C,** Capsular ligaments, posterior view.

cruciate ligament (PCL), the stronger of the two, crosses from the back of the tibia in an upward, forward, and medial direction and attaches to the anterior portion of the lateral surface of the medial condyle of the femur.

Anterior cruciate ligament The anterior cruciate ligament comprises three twisted bands: the anteromedial, intermediate, and posterolateral bands. In general, the anterior cruciate ligament prevents the femur from moving posteriorly during weight bearing. It also stabilizes the tibia against excessive internal rotation and serves as a secondary restraint for valgus or varus stress with collateral ligament damage.

When the knee is fully extended, the posterolateral section of the cruciate ligament is tight. In flexion the posterolateral fibers loosen and the anteromedial fibers tighten.[61] The anterior cruciate ligament works in conjunction with the thigh muscles, especially the hamstring muscle group, to stabilize the knee joint.

Posterior cruciate ligament Some portion of the posterior cruciate ligament is taut throughout the full range of motion. It acts as a drag during the gliding phase of motion and resists internal rotation of the tibia. In general, the posterior cruciate ligament prevents hyperextension of the knee and femur, sliding forward during weight bearing.

Capsular and Collateral Ligaments

Additional stabilization of the knee is provided by the capsular and collateral ligaments. Besides providing stability, they also direct movement in a correct path. Although they move in synchrony, they are divided into the medial and lateral complexes.

Medial collateral ligament The superficial position of the medial (tibial) collateral ligament (MCL) is separate from the deeper capsular ligament at the joint line. It attaches above the joint line on the medial epicondyle of the femur and below on the tibia, just beneath the attachment of the pes anserinus. The posterior aspect of the ligament blends into the deep posterior capsular ligament and semimembranous muscle. Fibers of the semimembranous muscle go through the capsule and attach to the posterior aspect of the medial meniscus, pulling it backward during knee flexion. Some of its fibers are taut through flexion and extension. Its major purpose is to prevent the knee from valgus and external rotating forces. The medial collateral ligament was thought to be the principal stabilizer of the knee in a valgus position when combined with rotation. It is now known that other structures, such as the anterior cruciate ligament, play an equal or greater part in this function.[69]

Deep medial capsular ligaments The deep medial capsular ligament is divided into three parts: the anterior, medial, and posterior capsular ligaments. The anterior capsular ligament connects with the extensor mechanism and the medial meniscus through the coronary ligaments. It relaxes during knee extension and tightens during knee flexion. The primary purposes of the medial capsular ligaments are to attach the medial meniscus to the femur and to allow the tibia to move on the meniscus inferiorly. The posterior capsular ligament is sometimes called the posterior oblique ligament and attaches to the posterior medial aspect of the meniscus and intersperses with the semimembranous muscle.[4]

Lateral collateral ligament and related structures The lateral (fibular) collateral ligament (LCL) is a round, fibrous cord that is shaped like a pencil. It is attached to the lateral epicondyle of the femur and to the head of the fibula. The lateral collateral ligament is taut during knee extension but relaxed during flexion.

Another stabilizing ligament of importance is the arcuate ligament. It is formed by a thickening of the posterior articular capsule. Its posterior aspect attaches to the fascia of the popliteal muscle and the posterior horn of the lateral meniscus.

Other structures that stabilize the knee laterally are the iliotibial band, popliteus muscle, and biceps femoris. The iliotibial band, a tendon of the tensor fascia latae and gluteus medius, attaches to the lateral epicondyle of the femur and lateral tibial tubercle (Gerdy's tubercle). It becomes tense during both extension and flexion. The popliteus muscle stabilizes the knee during flexion and, when contracting, protects the lateral meniscus by pulling it posteriorly.

The biceps femoris muscle also stabilizes the knee laterally by inserting into the fibular head, iliotibial band, and capsule.

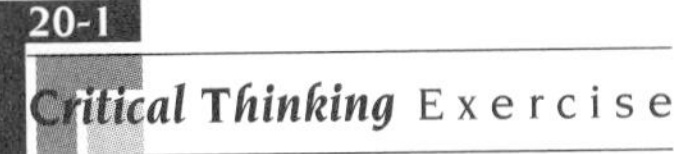

A tennis player injures her knee during a match. As she hits a forehand stroke, her knee is in full extension and she feels pain in it as she rotates on the follow-through. She feels some diffuse pain around her knee joint and is concerned that she has sprained a ligament.

? In a position of full extension, which of the supporting ligaments are taut? Which ligaments are most likely to be injured in this position?

Joint Capsule

The articular surfaces of the knee joint are completely enveloped by the largest joint capsule in the body (Figure 20-5). Anteriorly, the joint capsule extends upward underneath the patella to form the suprapatellar pouch. The inferior portion contains the infrapatellar fat pad and the infrapatellar bursa. Medially, a thickened section of the

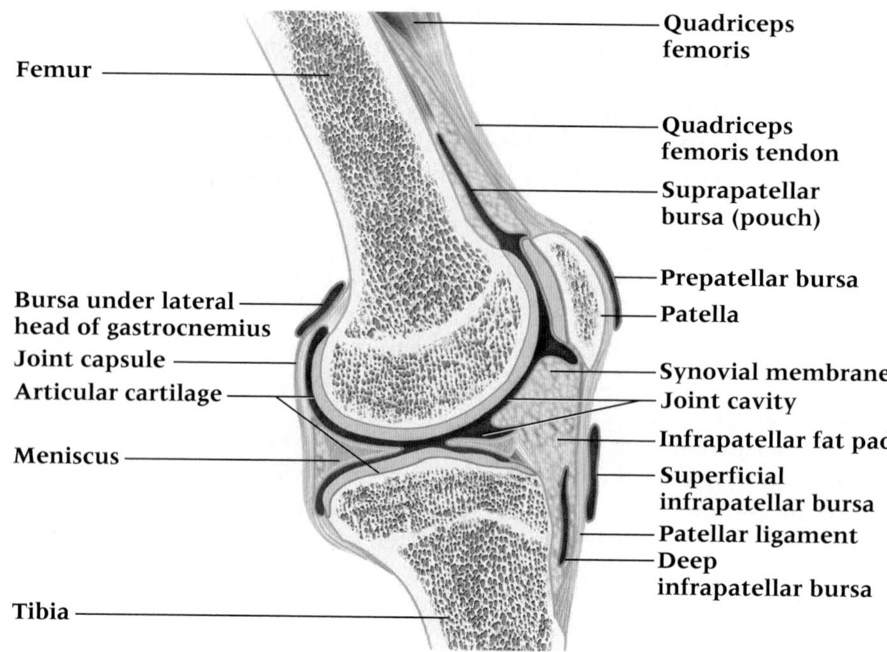

Figure 20-5

Sagittal cross section of the knee showing location of bursae and synovial membranes.

capsule forms the deep portion of the medial collateral ligament. Posteriorly, the capsule forms two pouches that cover the femoral condyles and the tibial plateau. The capsule thickens medially to form the posterior oblique ligament and laterally to form the arcuate ligament (Figure 20-4C).

The joint capsule is divided into four regions: the posterolateral, posteromedial, anterolateral, and anteromedial. Each of these four "corners" of the capsule is reinforced by other anatomical structures. The posterolateral corner is reinforced by the iliotibial band, the popliteus, the biceps femoris, the LCL, and the arcuate ligament. The MCL, the pes anserinus tendons, the semimembranosus, and the posterior oblique ligament reinforce the posteromedial corner. The anterolateral corner is reinforced by the iliotibial band, the patellar tendon, and the lateral patellar retinaculum. The superficial MCL and the medial patellar retinaculum reinforce the anteromedial corner.

Synovial membrane lines the inner surface of the joint capsule, except posteriorly where it passes in front of the cruciates, making them extrasynovial (Figure 20-5).

Knee Musculature

For the knee to function properly, a number of muscles must work together in a highly complex fashion. The following is a list of knee actions and the muscles that initiate them (Figure 20-6):

- Knee flexion is executed by the biceps femoris, semitendinosus, semimembranosus, gracilis, sartorius, gastrocnemius, popliteus, and plantaris muscles.
- Knee extension is executed by the quadriceps muscle of the thigh, consisting of three vasti—the vastus medialis, vastus lateralis, and vastus intermedius—and by the rectus femoris.
- External rotation of the tibia is controlled by the biceps femoris. The bony anatomy also produces external tibial rotation as the knee moves into extension.
- Internal rotation is accomplished by the popliteal, semitendinosus, semimembranosus, sartorius, and gracilis muscles. Rotation of the tibia is limited and can occur only when the knee is in a flexed position.
- The iliotibial band on the lateral side primarily functions as a dynamic lateral stabilizer.

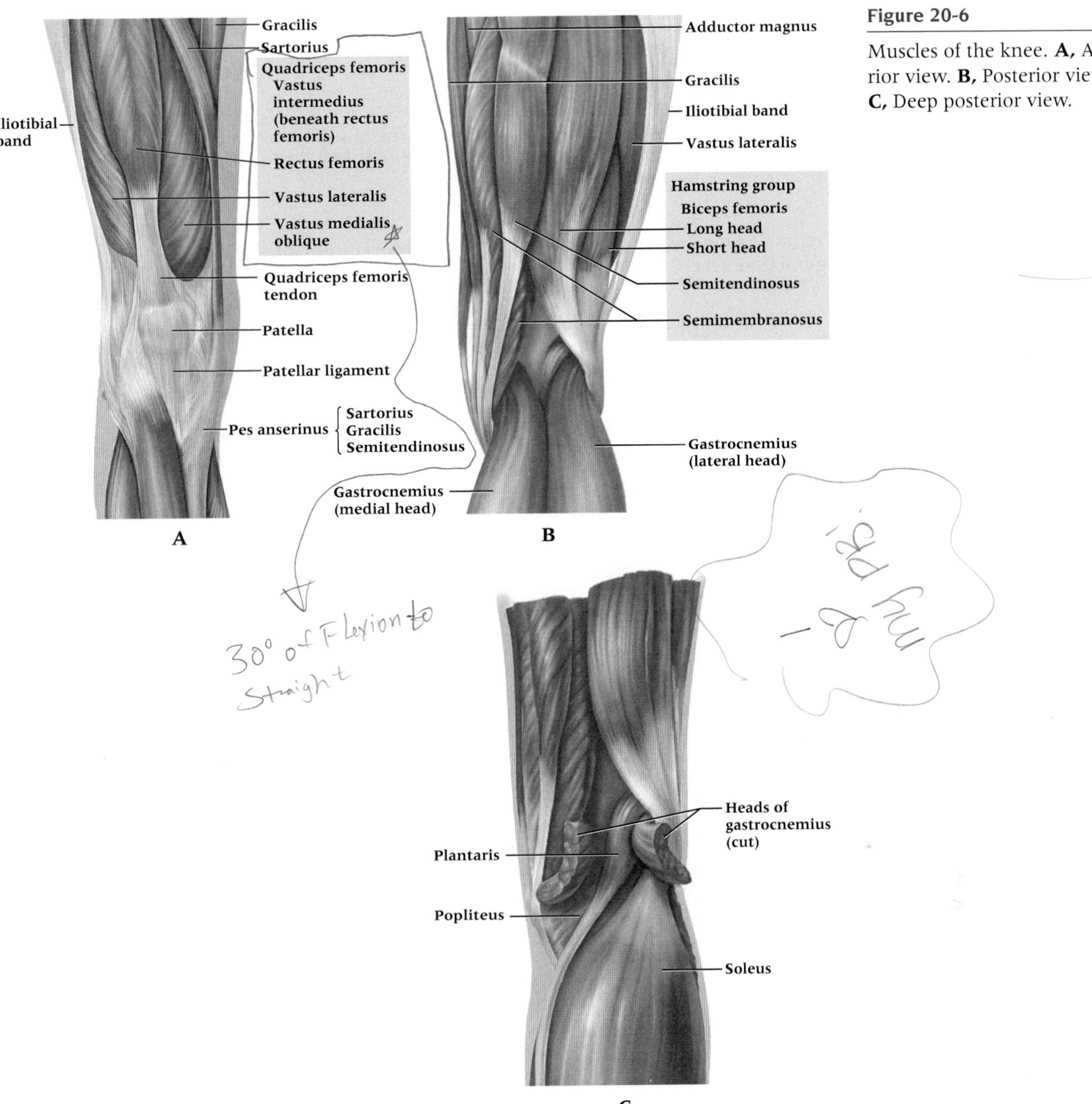

Figure 20-6

Muscles of the knee. **A,** Anterior view. **B,** Posterior view. **C,** Deep posterior view.

Bursae

A bursa is a flattened sac or enclosed cleft composed of synovial tissue that is separated by a thin film of fluid. The function of a bursa is to reduce the friction between anatomical structures. Bursae are found between muscle and bone, tendon and bone, tendon and ligament, and so forth. As many as two dozen bursae have been identified around the knee joint. The suprapatellar, prepatellar, infrapatellar, pretibial, and gastrocnemius bursae are perhaps the most commonly injured about the knee joint.

Fat Pads

There are several fat pads around the knee. The infrapatellar fat pad is the largest. It serves as a cushion to the front of the knee and separates the patellar tendon from the joint capsule. Other major fat pads in the knee include the anterior and posterior

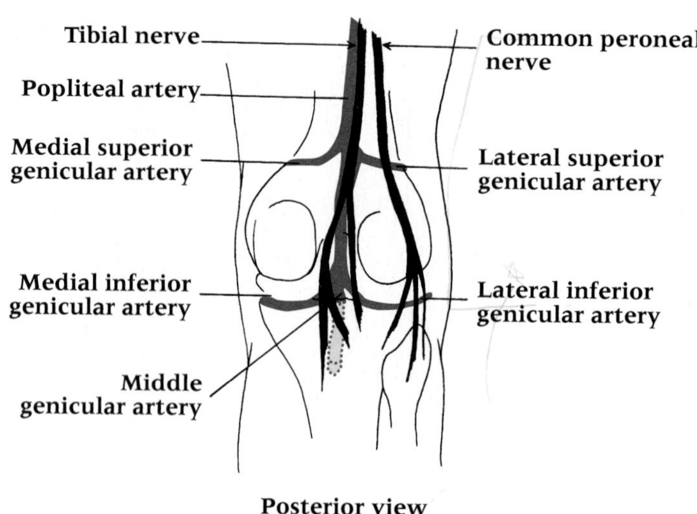

Figure 20-7

Blood and nerve supply to the knee.

suprapatellar and the popliteal. Some fat pads occupy space within the synovial capsule.

Nerve Supply

The tibial nerve innervates most of the hamstrings and the gastrocnemius. The common peroneal nerve innervates the short head of the biceps femoris and then courses through the popliteal fossa and wraps around the proximal head of the fibula. Because the peroneal nerve is exposed at the head of the fibula, contusion of the nerve can cause distal sensory and motor deficits. The femoral nerve innervates the quadriceps and the sartorius muscles (Figure 20-7).

Blood Supply

The main blood supply to the knee comes from the popliteal artery, which stems from the femoral artery. From the popliteal artery, five branches supply the knee: the medial and lateral superior genicular, middle genicular, and medial and lateral inferior genicular arteries (see Figure 20-7).

FUNCTIONAL ANATOMY

Major actions of the knee:

- Flexion
- Extension
- Gliding
- Rolling
- Rotation

Movement between the tibia and the femur involves the physiological motions of flexion, extension, and rotation as well as arthrokinematic motions, including rolling and gliding. As the tibia extends on the femur, the tibia glides and rolls anteriorly. If the femur is extending on the tibia, gliding occurs in an anterior direction, whereas rolling occurs posteriorly.

Axial rotation of the tibia relative to the femur is an important component of knee motion. In the "screw home" mechanism of the knee, as the knee extends, the tibia externally rotates. Rotation occurs because the medial femoral condyle is larger than the lateral condyle. Thus, when weight bearing, the tibia must rotate externally to achieve full extension. The rotational component gives a great deal of stability to the knee in full extension. When weight bearing, the popliteus muscle must contract and externally rotate the femur to "unlock" the knee so that flexion can occur.

The capsular ligaments are taut during full extension and to some extent relaxed during flexion. This is particularly true of the lateral collateral ligament; however, portions of the medial collateral ligament relax as flexion occurs. Relaxation of the more superficial collateral ligaments allows rotation to occur. In contrast, the deeper capsular ligament tightens to prevent excessive rotation of the tibia.

During the last 15 degrees of extension, the tibia externally rotates and the anterior cruciate ligament unwinds.[47] In full extension the anterior cruciate ligament is taut, and

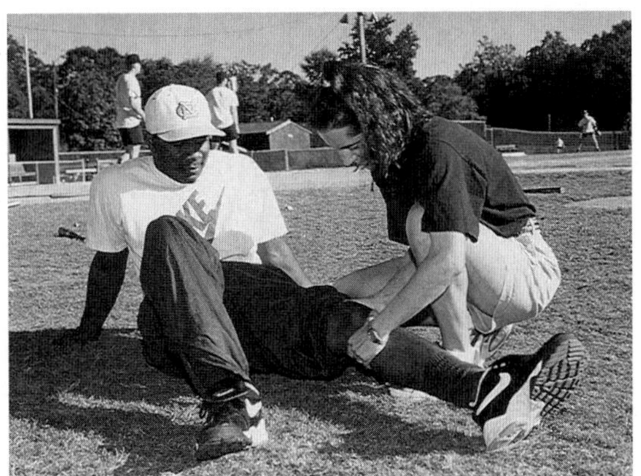

Figure 20-8

It is extremely important that the sequence and mechanism of a knee injury be known before the pathological process can be understood.

it loosens during flexion. As the femur glides on the tibia, the posterior cruciate ligament becomes taut and prevents further gliding. In general, the anterior cruciate ligament stops excessive internal rotation, stabilizes the knee in full extension, and prevents hyperextension. The posterior cruciate ligament prevents excessive internal rotation, guides the knee in flexion, and acts as a drag during the initial glide phase of flexion.[28]

In complete flexion, approximately 140 degrees, the range of the knee movement is limited by the extremely shortened position of the hamstring muscles, the extensibility of the quadriceps muscles, and the bulk of the hamstring muscles. In this position, the femoral condyles rest on their corresponding menisci at a point that permits a small degree of inward rotation.

The patella aids the knee during extension by lengthening the lever arm of the quadriceps muscle.[25] It distributes the compressive stresses on the femur by increasing the contact area between the patellar tendon and the femur.[63] It also protects the patellar tendon against friction. During full extension, the patella lies slightly lateral and proximal to the trochlea. At 20 degrees of knee flexion, there is tibial rotation, and the patella moves into the trochlea. At 30 degrees, the patella is most prominent. At 30 degrees and more, the patella moves deeper into the trochlea. At 90 degrees, the patella again becomes positioned laterally. When knee flexion is 135 degrees, the patella has moved laterally beyond the trochlea.[63]

The Knee in the Kinetic Chain

The knee is part of the kinetic chain that was discussed in Chapter 16. It is directly affected by motions and forces occurring to and being transmitted from the foot, ankle, and lower leg. In turn, the knee must transmit forces to the thigh, hip, pelvis, and spine. Abnormal forces that cannot be distributed must be absorbed by the tissues. When the foot is in contact with the ground, a closed kinetic chain exists. In a closed kinetic chain, forces must either be transmitted to proximal segments or be absorbed in a more distal joint. The inability of this closed system to dissipate these forces typically leads to a breakdown in some part of the system. As part of the kinetic chain, the knee joint is susceptible to injury resulting from the absorption of these forces.[93]

ASSESSING THE KNEE JOINT

It is the responsibility of the team physician to diagnose the severity and exact nature of a knee injury. Although the physician is charged with the final evaluation, the athletic trainer is usually the first person to observe the injury; therefore he or she is charged with initial evaluation and immediate care. The most important aspect of understanding what pathological process has taken place is to become familiar with the traumatic sequence and mechanisms of injury, either through having seen the injury occur or through learning its history (Figure 20-8). Often the team physician is not present when the injury occurs, and the athletic trainer must relate the pertinent information.[69]

History

To determine the history and major complaints involved in a knee injury, the athletic trainer should ask the following questions.

Current Injury

- What were you doing when the knee was hurt?
- What position was your body in?
- Did the knee collapse?
- Did you hear a noise or feel any sensation at the time of injury, such as a pop or crunch? (A pop could indicate an anterior cruciate tear, a crunch could be a sign of a torn meniscus, and a tearing sensation might indicate a capsular tear.)
- Could you move the knee immediately after the injury? If not, was it locked in a bent or extended position? (Locking could mean a meniscal tear.) After being locked, how did it become unlocked?
- Did swelling occur? If yes, was it immediate, or did it occur later? (Immediate swelling could indicate a cruciate or tibial fracture, whereas later swelling could indicate a capsular, synovial, or meniscal tear.)
- Where was the pain? Was it local, all over, or did it move from one side of the knee to the other?
- Have you hurt the knee before?

When first studying the injury, the athletic trainer should observe whether the athlete is able to support body weight flat-footed on the injured leg or whether the athlete needs to stand and walk on the toes. Toe walking is an indication that the athlete is holding the knee in a splinted position to avoid pain or that the knee is being held in a flexed position by a wedge of dislocated meniscus. In first-time acute knee sprains, fluid and blood effusion is not usually apparent until after a twenty-four-hour period. However, in an anterior cruciate ligament sprain, a hemarthrosis may occur during the first hour after injury. Swelling and ecchymosis will occur unless the effusion is arrested through the use of compression, elevation, and cold packs.

Recurrent or Chronic Injury

- What is your major complaint?
- When did you first notice the condition?
- Is there recurrent swelling?
- Does the knee ever lock or catch? (If yes, it may be a torn meniscus or a loose body in the knee joint.)
- Is there severe pain? Is it constant, or does it come and go?
- Do you feel any grinding or grating sensations? (If yes, it could indicate chondromalacia or traumatic arthritis.)
- Does your knee ever feel like it is going to give way, or has it actually done so? (If yes and often, it may be a capsular, cruciate, or meniscal tear, a loose body, or a subluxating patella.)
- What does it feel like to go up and down stairs? (Pain may indicate a patellar irritation or meniscal tear.)
- What past treatment (past surgery, physical therapy, etc.) if any, have you received for this condition?

Observation

If possible, the athlete with an injured knee should be observed in the following actions:

- Walking
- Half squatting
- Going up and down stairs

A visual examination should be performed after the major complaints have been determined. The athlete should be observed in a number of situations: walking, half squatting, and going up and down stairs. The leg also should be observed for alignment and symmetry or asymmetry.

Walking

- Does the athlete walk with a limp, or is the walk free and easy? Is the athlete able to fully extend the knee during heel strike?

- Can the athlete fully bear weight on the affected leg?
- Can the athlete perform a half-squat to extension?
- Can the athlete go up and down stairs with ease? (If stairs are unavailable, stepping up on a box or stool will suffice.)

Leg Alignment

The athlete should be observed for leg alignment. Anteriorly, the athlete should be evaluated for genu valgum, genu varum, and the position of the patella. Next, the athlete should be observed from the side to ascertain conditions such as the hyperflexed or hyperextended knee.

Deviations in normal leg alignment may or may not be a factor in knee injury but should always be considered as a possible cause. Like alignment in any other body segment, leg alignment differs from person to person; however, obvious discrepancies could predispose the athlete to an acute or chronic injury.

Anteriorly, with the knees extended as much as possible, the following points should be noted:

- Are the patellas level with each other (patella alta or baja)?
- Are the patellas facing inward (squinting patella)?
- Can the athlete touch the medial femoral condyles and medial malleoli?

Looking at the athlete's knees from the side:

- Are the knees fully extended with only slight hyperextension?
- Are both knees equally extended?

Leg alignment deviations that may predispose to injury Four major leg deviations could adversely affect the knee and patellofemoral joints: patellar malalignment, genu valgum (knock-knees), genu varum (bowlegs), and genu recurvatum (hyperextended knees).

Patellar malalignment In *patella alta,* the patella sets in a more superior position than normal when the athlete is standing. The ratio of patellar tendon length to the height of the patella is greater than the normal 1:1 ratio. In patella alta, the length of the patellar tendon is 20 percent greater than the height of the patella. In *patella baja,* the patella sets in a more inferior position than normal and the ratio of patellar tendon length to the height of the patella is less than the normal 1:1 ratio.

A patella that is rotated inward or outward from the center may be caused by a complex set of circumstances. For example, a combination of genu recurvatum, genu varum, and internal rotation, or anteversion, of the hip and internal rotation of the tibia could cause the patella to face inward. Internal rotation of the hip also may be associated with knock-knees, along with external rotation of the tibia, or tibial torsion. Athletes who toe-out when they walk may have an externally rotated hip, or retroversion. The normal angulation of the femoral neck after eight years of age is 15 degrees; an increase of this angle is considered anteversion, and a decrease is considered retroversion. If an abnormal angulation seems to be a factor with the patella, malalignment or tibial torsion angles should be measured.

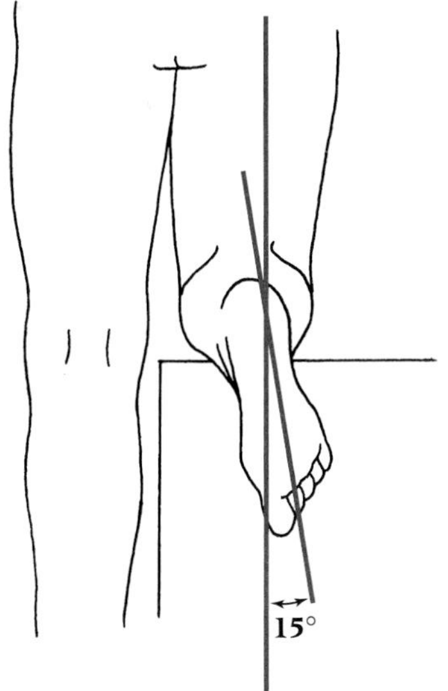

Figure 20-9
Measuring for tibial torsion.

MEASURING FOR TIBIAL TORSION, FEMORAL ANTEVERSION, AND FEMORAL RETROVERSION Tibial torsion is determined by having the athlete kneel on a stool with the foot relaxed. An imaginary line is drawn along the center of the thigh and lower leg, bisecting the middle of the heel and the bottom of the foot. Another line starts at the center of the middle toe and crosses the center of the heel. The angle formed by the two lines is measured (Figure 20-9); an angle measuring more or less than 15 degrees is a sign of tibial torsion.

Femoral anteversion or retroversion can be determined by the number of degrees the thigh rotates in each direction. As a rule, external rotation and internal rotation added together equal close to 100 degrees. If internal rotation exceeds 70 degrees, there may be anteversion of the hip.[80]

Hyperextension of the knee may result in internal rotation of the femur and external rotation of the tibia. Internal rotation at the hip is caused by weak external rotator muscles or foot pronation.

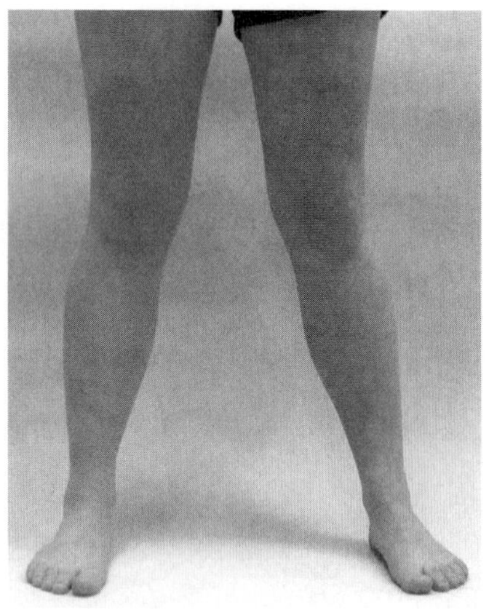
A

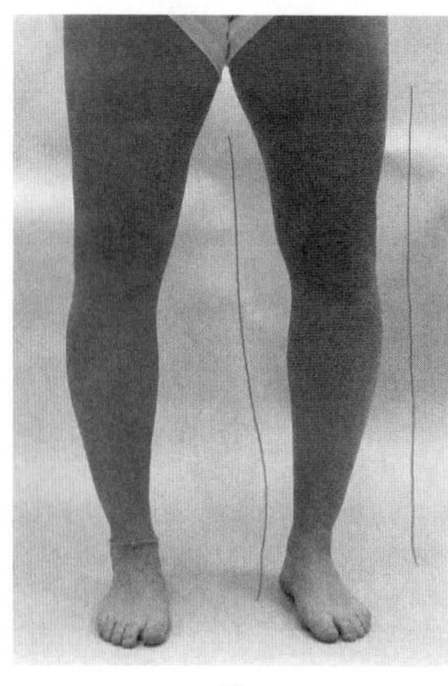
B

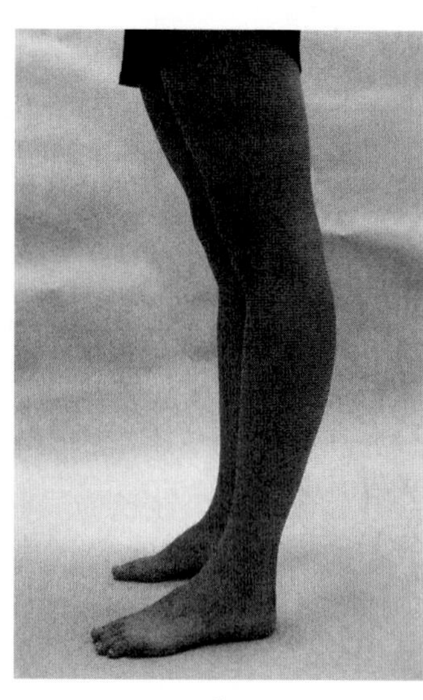
C

Figure 20-10

Leg alignment. **A,** Genu valgum. **B,** Genu varum. **C,** Genu recurvatum.

Patellar orientation *Patellar orientation* refers to the positioning of the patella relative to the tibia.[69] Assessment should be done with the athlete in supine position. Four components should be assessed when looking at patellar orientation: the glide component, the tilt component, the rotation component, and the anteroposterior tilt component. The *glide* component assesses whether the patella is deviated either lateral or medial to the center of the trochlear groove of the femur. Glide should be assessed both statically and dynamically. Patellar *tilt* is determined by comparing the height of the medial patellar border with the lateral patellar border. If the medial border is more anterior than the lateral border, a positive lateral tilt exists. Patellar *rotation* is identified by assessing the deviation of the longitudinal axis (line drawn from superior pole to inferior pole) of the patella relative to the femur. The point of reference is the inferior pole. Thus if the inferior pole is more lateral than the superior pole, a positive external rotation exists. The *anteroposterior tilt* component must be assessed laterally to determine if a line drawn from the inferior patellar pole to the superior patellar pole is parallel to the long axis of the femur. If the inferior pole is posterior to the superior pole, the athlete has a positive anteroposterior tilt component.[69]

Genu valgum The causes of genu valgum, or knock-knees, can be multiple (Figure 20-10A). Normally, toddlers and very young children display knock-knees. When the legs have strengthened and the feet have become positioned more in line with the pelvis, the condition is usually corrected. Commonly associated with knock-knees are pronated feet. Genu valgum places chronic tension on the ligamentous structures of the medial part of the knee, abnormal compression of the lateral aspect of the knee surface, and abnormal tightness of the iliotibial band. One or both legs may be affected, and the hip's external rotator muscles may be weak.

Genu varum The two types of genu varum, or bowlegs, are structural and functional (Figure 20-10B). The structural type, which is seldom seen in athletes, reflects a deviation of the femur and tibia. The more common functional, or postural, type usually is associated with knees that are hyperextended and femurs that are internally rotated. Often when genu recurvatum is corrected, so is genu varum.

Genu recurvatum Genu recurvatum, or hyperextended knees, commonly occurs as a compensation for lordosis, or swayback (Figure 20-10C).[45] There is notable weakness and stretching of the hamstring muscles. Chronic hyperextension can produce undue anterior pressure on the knee joint and posterior ligaments and tendons.

Knee Symmetry or Asymmetry

The athletic trainer must establish whether both of the athlete's knees look the same:

- Do the knees appear symmetrical?
- Is one knee obviously swollen?
- Is muscle atrophy apparent?

Leg-Length Discrepancy

Discrepancies in leg length can occur as a result of many causes, either anatomical or functional. True anatomical leg length can be measured from the anterior superior iliac spine (ASIS) to the lateral malleolus. Functional leg length can be measured from the umbilicus to the medial malleolus.

Anatomical differences in leg length can potentially cause problems in all weight-bearing joints. Functional differences can be caused by rotations of the pelvis or malalignments of the spine.

Palpation

Bony Palpation

The bony structures of the knee are palpated for pain and deformities that might indicate a fracture or dislocation. The athlete sits on the edge of the training table or a bench. With the athlete's knee flexed to 90 degrees, the athletic trainer palpates the following bony structures:

Medial Aspect

- Medial tibial plateau
- Medial femoral condyle
- Adductor tubercle
- Gerdy's tubercle

Lateral Aspect

- Lateral tibial plateau
- Lateral femoral condyle
- Lateral epicondyle
- Head of the fibula

Anterior Aspect

- Tibial tuberosity

Patella

- Superior patellar border (base)
- Inferior patellar border (apex)
- Around periphery with the knee relaxed
- Around periphery with the knee in full extension

Soft-Tissue Palpation

The following soft-tissue structures should be palpated:

Anterior

- Vastus medialis
- Vastus lateralis
- Vastus intermedialis
- Rectus femoris
- Quadriceps tendon
- Sartorius
- Medial patellar plica
- Patellar tendon
- Anterior joint capsule

Medial

- Medial collateral ligament, superficial portion
- Medial collateral ligament—capsular portion

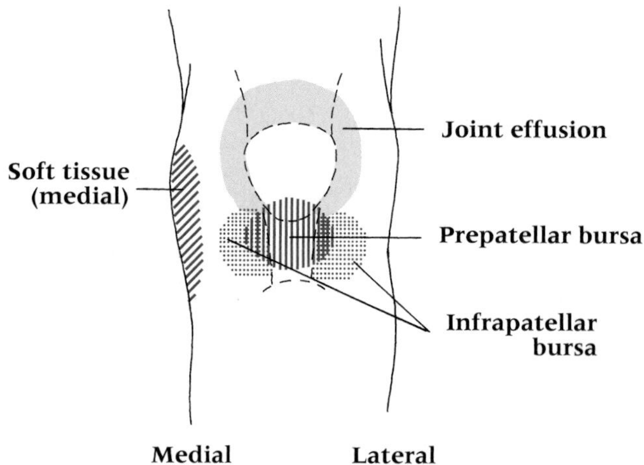

Figure 20-11

Typical swelling sites around the knee.

- Pes anserinus insertion (sartorius, gracilis, semitendinosus)
- Medial joint capsule

Posterior
- Semitendinosus
- Popliteus
- Medial and laterals heads of the gastrocnemius
- Biceps femoris
- Posterior oblique ligament

Lateral
- Lateral collateral ligament
- Iliotibial band
- Lateral joint capsule
- Arcuate complex

Palpation of Swelling Patterns

hemarthrosis (hem **are** throsis)
Blood in a joint cavity.

Of major importance to knee inspection and evaluation is palpating for joint effusion (Figure 20-11). Swelling may be *intracapsular* (inside the joint capsule) or *extracapsular* (outside the joint capsule). Intracapsular swelling may also be referred to as a *joint effusion.* A moderate amount of swelling that occurs immediately following injury and that is caused by synovial fluid and by blood in the joint is called a **hemarthrosis.** A hemarthrosis can only be identified by having the team physician aspirate the joint with a needle. With intracapsular joint effusion, the fluid in the joint can be moved manually from one side of the joint to the other. In a *sweep maneuver,* pressure applied from superior to the patella downward moves fluid into the center of the joint capsule; then pressure from the medial side of the joint line will cause a bulging laterally. Joint effusion can also cause what has been referred to as a *ballotable patella.* With the knee in full extension and the quadriceps relaxed, a release of downward pressure on the patella sitting on top of the joint capsule causes the patella to bounce back to its normal position.

Extracapsular swelling from bursitis, tendinitis, or injury to one of the collateral ligaments tends to localize over the injured structure and then gradually migrate downward toward the foot and ankle because of the effects of gravity.

Special Tests for Assessment of Knee Joint Instability

Both acute and chronic injury to the knee can produce ligamentous instability.[92] It is advisable that the injured knee's stability be evaluated as soon after injury as possible. However, tests of this type should be performed only by well-trained professionals. The injured knee and uninjured knee are tested and contrasted to determine any differences in their stability.

TABLE 20-1 Knee Stability Tests

Test	If Positive
Valgus stress test at 08	Torn MCL and possibly ACL, PCL, PMC
Valgus stress test at 208/308	Torn MCL (if grade 3 check ACL, PCL, PMC)
Varus stress test at 08	Torn LCL and possibly ACL, PCL, PLC
Varus stress test at 208/308	Torn LCL (if grade 3 check ACL, PCL, PLC)
Lachman drawer test (208/308 flexion)	Torn ACL, PCL (positive more often than anterior drawer because hamstrings are relaxed and medial meniscus/collateral ligaments do not block anterior displacement at 208)
Anterior drawer test (neutral)	Torn ACL
Anterior drawer test (158 ER)	Torn PMC, ACL, and possibly MCL
Anterior drawer test (308 IR)	Torn PLC, ACL
Pivot-shift tests (Galaway and McIntosh)	Torn ACL, ALC
Extension/IR/valgus (tibia subluxated) → flexion (tibia reduces at 208)	
Slocum's test	Torn ACL, ALC
Sidelying extension/IR/valgus (tibia subluxated) → flexion (tibia reduces at 208)	
Jerk test (Hughston)	Torn ACL, ALC
Flexion/IR/valgus (tibia reduced) → extension (tibia subluxates at 208)	
Losee test	Torn ACL, ALC
458 flexion/ER/valgus (tibia subluxated anteriorly) → extension (tibia reduces at 208)	
Flexion-rotation drawer test	Torn ACL
458 flex (tibia subluxated anteriorly/femur ER) → flexion (tibia reduces posteriorly/femur IR)	
Posterior drawer test 908	Torn PCL
External rotation recurvatum test (tibia ER)	Torn PCL, PLC
Posterior sag test 908	Torn PCL
Reverse pivot-shift test (Jakob)	Torn PCL
Extension (tibia reduced) ® flexion (tibia subluxated posteriorly with ER)	
McMurray's test	
(IR)	Torn LM
(ER)	Torn MM
Apley's grinding test	Torn MM

ACL 5 anterior cruciate ligament; ALC 5 anterior lateral corner; ER 5 external rotation; IR 5 internal rotation; LCL 5 lateral collateral ligament; LM 5 lateral meniscus; MCL 5 medial collateral ligament; MM 5 medial meniscus; PCL 5 posterior cruciate ligament; PLC 5 posterior lateral corner; PMC 5 posterior medial corner.

Determination of the degree of instability is made by feeling the endpoint during stability testing. As stress is applied to a joint, there will be some motion, which is limited by an intact ligament. In a normal joint, the endpoint will be abrupt with little or no give and no reported pain. With a grade 1 sprain, the endpoint will still be firm with little or no instability, and some pain will be indicated. With a grade 2 sprain, the endpoint will be soft with some instability present and a moderate amount of pain. In a grade 3 complete rupture, the endpoint will be very soft with marked instability, and pain will be severe initially, then mild.[44]

The use of magnetic resonance imaging (MRI) as a diagnostic tool has aided tremendously in the classification of ligamentous sprains. Despite its expense, MRI is being widely used by physicians to detect ligament injuries.

Table 20-1 provides a summary of the various tests and what a positive test indicates in terms of the injured structures.

Classification of Knee Joint Instabilities

A good deal of controversy exists over the most appropriate terminology for classifying instabilities in the knee joint.[52] For years the American Orthopedic Society for Sports Medicine has classified knee laxity as either a straight or a rotatory instability.

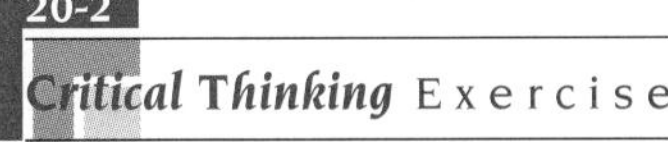

20-2 Critical Thinking Exercise

A cross-country runner is complaining of nonspecific anterior knee pain. She indicates that not only do her knees hurt during her training sessions, but they also bother her when ascending or descending stairs, when she squats and then tries to stand, and when she sits for long periods of time.

? What anatomical and biomechanical factors that might be contributing to the athlete's anterior knee pain should the athletic trainer assess?

TABLE 20-2 Classification of Instabilities

Straight Instabilities	Rotary Instabilities
Medial	Anterolateral
Lateral	Anteromedial
Anterior	Posterolateral
Posterior	

A straight instability implies laxity in a single direction, either medial, lateral, anterior, or posterior. Rotatory instabilities refer to excessive rotation of the tibial plateau relative to the femoral condyles and are identified as anterolateral, anteromedial, posterolateral, or rarely, posteromedial. It is not unusual to see combined instabilities, depending on the structures that have been injured. This classification system is still the most widely used and accepted by athletic trainers (Table 20-2).

translation
Refers to anterior gliding of tibial plateau.

Recently, the concept of tibial translation has been proposed.[57] **Translation** refers to the amount of gliding of the medial tibial plateau as compared with the lateral tibial plateau relative to the femoral condyles. For example, in anterolateral rotatory instability, the anterior translation of the lateral tibial plateau would be much greater than the more stable medial tibial plateau. The amount of anterior translation is determined by the integrity of the anatomical restraints that normally restrict excessive translation. More ligamentous, tendinous, and capsular structures will be damaged as the severity of the injury increases. Classification of knee injury relative to tibial translation is likely to gain popularity among sports medicine professionals.

20-3 *Critical Thinking* Exercise

A football running back is hit on the lateral surface of his knee by an opponent making a tackle. He has significant pain and some immediate swelling on the medial surface of his knee. The athletic trainer suspects that the athlete has sustained a sprain of the MCL.

? What are the most appropriate tests that the athletic trainer should do to determine the exact nature and extent of the injury?

Valgus and Varus Stress Tests

Valgus and varus stress tests are intended to reveal laxity of the medial and lateral stabilizing complexes, especially the collateral ligaments. The athlete lies supine with the leg extended. To test the medial side, the athletic trainer holds the ankle firmly with one hand while placing the other hand over the head of the fibula. The athletic trainer then places a force inward in an attempt to open the side of the knee. This valgus stress is applied with the knee fully extended, or at 0 degrees, and at 30 degrees of flexion (Figure 20-12A). The examination in full extension tests the MCL, posteromedial capsule, and the cruciates. At 30 degrees flexion, the MCL is isolated. The athletic trainer reverses hand positions and tests the lateral side with a varus force on the fully extended knee and then with 30 degrees of flexion (Figure 20-12B). With the knee extended, the LCL and posterolateral capsule are examined. At 30 degrees of flexion, the LCL is isolated.[44] NOTE: The lower limb should be in a neutral position with no internal or external rotation.

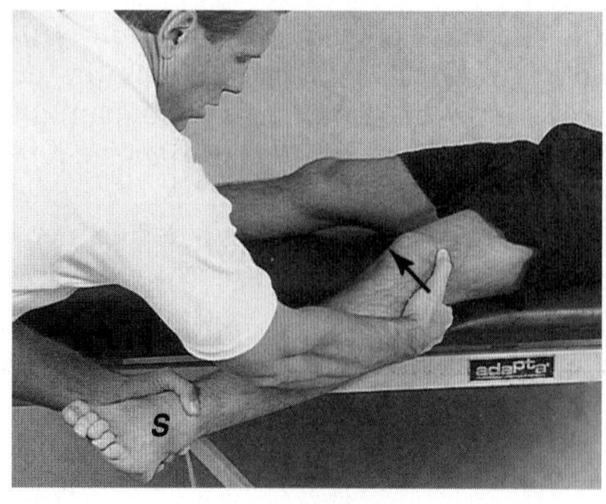

A

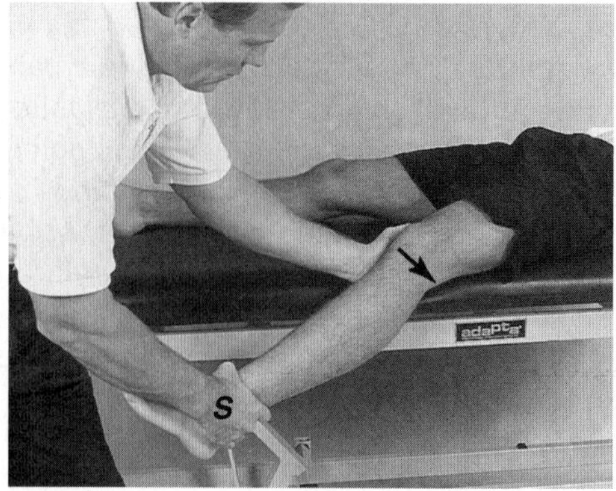

B

Figure 20-12

Valgus and varus knee stress tests. **A,** Valgus. **B,** Varus. (S = Stabilize)

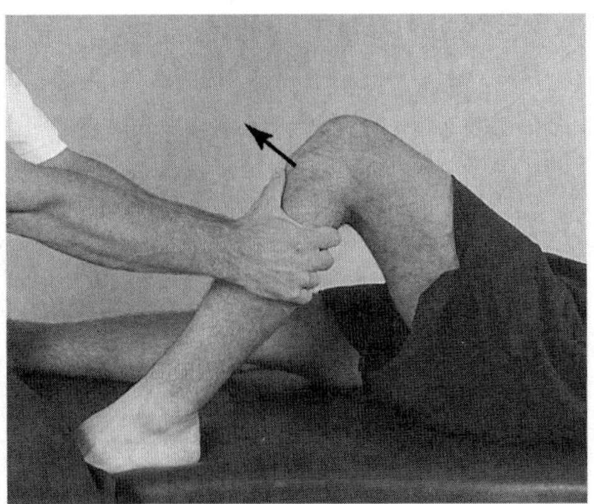

A

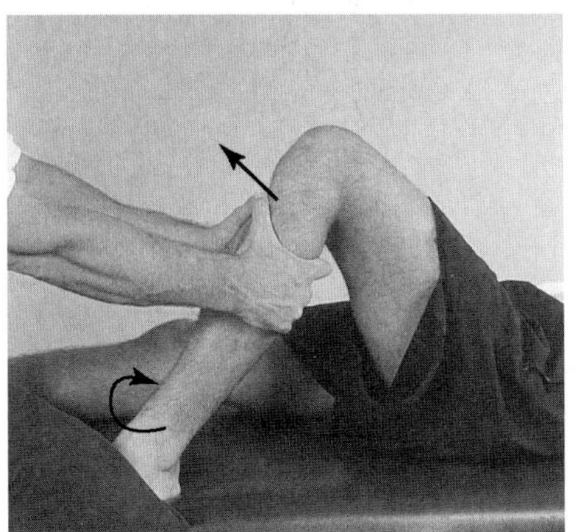

B

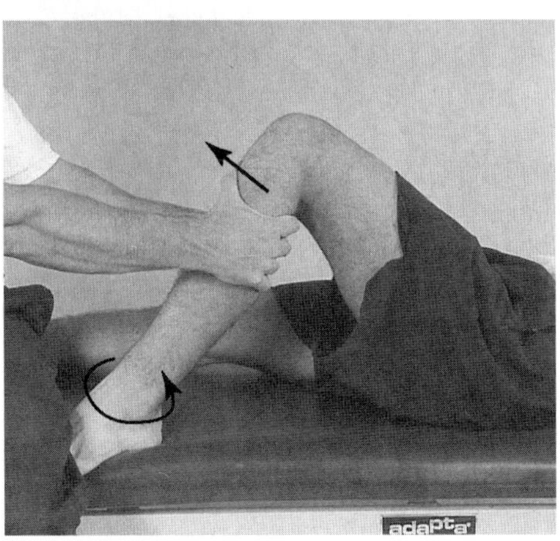

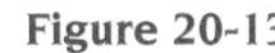

C

Figure 20-13

Drawer test for cruciate laxity. **A,** Knee at 90 degrees, with the foot pointing straight. **B,** Slocum's test with the knee at 90 degrees and the leg internally rotated. **C,** Slocum's test with the knee, at 90 degrees and the leg externally rotated.

Anterior Cruciate Ligament Tests

A number of tests are currently being used to establish the integrity of the cruciate ligaments.[52] They are the drawer test at 90 degrees of flexion, the Lachman drawer test, the pivot-shift test, the jerk test, and the flexion-rotation drawer test.

Drawer test at 90 degrees of flexion The athlete lies on the treatment table with the injured leg flexed. The athletic trainer stands facing the anterior aspect of the athlete's leg, with both hands encircling the upper portion of the leg, immediately below the knee joint. The athletic trainer positions his or her fingers in the popliteal space of the affected leg, with the thumbs on the medial and lateral joint lines (Figure 20-13A). The athletic trainer places his or her index fingers on the hamstring tendon to ensure that it is relaxed before the test is administered. The tibia's sliding forward from under the femur is considered a positive anterior drawer sign.[47] Slocum's test should be performed with the athlete's leg rotated internally 30 degrees and externally 15 degrees (Figure 20-13B and C). A sliding forward of the tibia when the leg is externally rotated is an indication that the posteromedial aspect of the joint capsule, the anterior cruciate ligament, or possibly the medial collateral ligament could be torn. Movement when the leg is internally rotated indicates that the anterior cruciate ligament and posterolateral capsule may be torn. A normal anterior shear is 2 inches (5 mm). Shears of ½ inch, ½ to ¾ inch, and ¾ inch or more (1.25 cm, 1.25 to 1.9 cm, and 1.9 cm or more) correspond to grades 1, 2, and 3, respectively.[52]

Lachman drawer test The Lachman drawer test is considered to be a better test than the drawer test at 90 degrees of flexion (Figure 20-14).[86, 92] This preference is especially true for examinations immediately after injury. One reason for using it

Figure 20-14

Lachman drawer test for anterior cruciate laxity.
A, Standard Lachman drawer test. **B,** Alternative technique one. **C,** Alternative technique two. **D,** Prone Lachman drawer test.

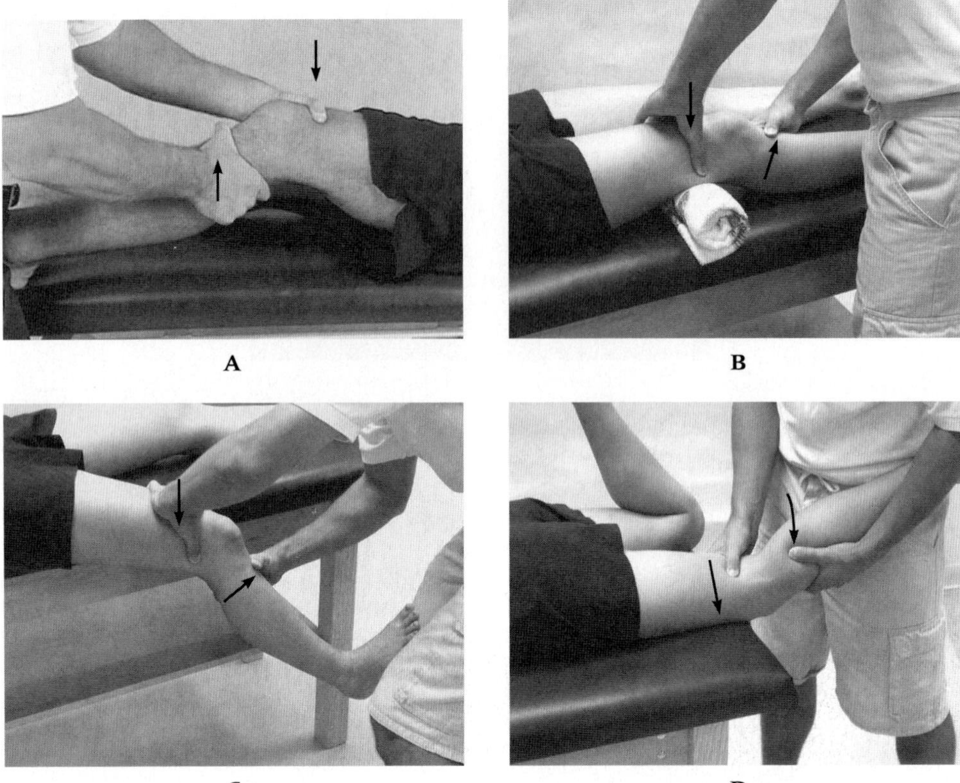

immediately after an injury is that it does not force the knee into the painful 90-degree position but tests it at a more comfortable 20 to 30 degrees. Another reason for its increased popularity is that it reduces the contraction of the hamstring muscles.[56] That contraction causes a secondary knee-stabilizing force that tends to mask the real extent of injury. The Lachman drawer test is administered by positioning the knee in approximately 30 degrees of flexion. The athletic trainer uses one hand to stabilize the leg by grasping the distal end of the thigh, and the other hand to grasp the proximal aspect of the tibia and attempts to move it anteriorly. One problem that exists with the Lachman test is that if the athlete is very large, or if the athletic trainer has small hands, it is difficult to perform this test efficiently.[33] Several alternative methods may be used. First, a tightly rolled towel or other support can be placed under the femur and the athletic trainer can use one hand to stabilize the femur and the other to anteriorly translate the tibia (Figure 20-14B). A second alternative is to slide the lower leg off the edge of the examining table with the knee and femur supported by the edge of the table. Again, one hand should be used to stabilize the femur and the other to anteriorly translate the tibia (Figure 20-14C). Finally, the athlete may be placed prone with the knee and lower leg just off of the edge of the table. This position minimizes any posterior sag of the tibia which can potentially mask a positive test.[56] Using the table to stabilize the femur, the athletic trainer can anteriorly translate the tibia (Figure 20-14D). A positive Lachman test indicates damage to the anterior cruciate.

20-4

Critical Thinking Exercise

A lacrosse player carrying the ball attempts to avoid a defender by planting his right foot firmly on the ground and cutting hard to his left. His knee immediately gives way, and he hears a loud pop. He has intense pain immediately, but after a few minutes he feels as if he can get up and walk.

? What ligament has most likely been injured? What stability tests should the athletic trainer do to determine the extent of the injury to this ligament?

Pivot-shift test The pivot-shift test is designed to determine anterolateral rotary instability (Figure 20-15). It is most often used in chronic conditions and is a sensitive test when the anterior cruciate ligament has been torn. The athlete lies supine. The athletic trainer uses one hand to press against the head of the fibula and the other to grasp the athlete's ankle. To start, the lower leg is internally rotated and the knee is fully extended. The thigh is then flexed 30 degrees at the hip while the knee is also flexed, and the athletic trainer applies a simultaneous valgus force and axial load with

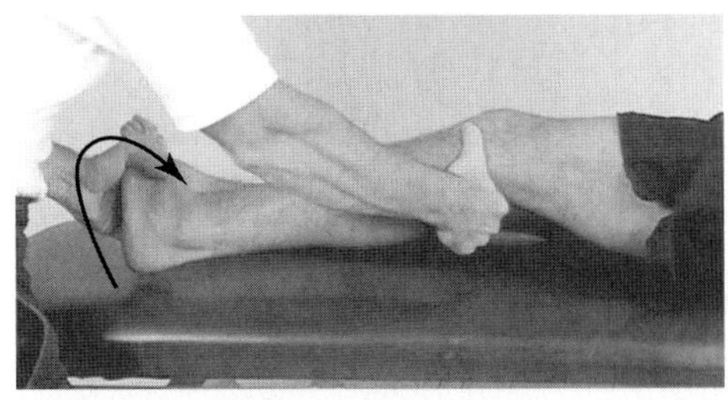

A

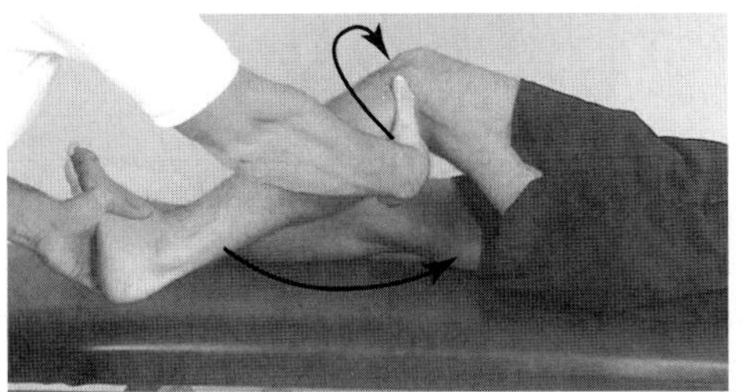

B

Figure 20-15

Pivot-shift test for anterolateral rotary instability. **A,** The tibia is subluxated in extension. **B,** It reduces at 20 degrees of flexion.

his or her upper hand. If the anterior cruciate ligament is damaged, the lateral tibial plateau will be subluxated in the fully extended position. As the knee is flexed to between 20 and 40 degrees, the lateral tibial plateau will reduce itself, producing a palpable shift or clunk.[87] A variation of the pivot-shift test is Slocum's test, which is done in a side-lying position.[87]

Jerk test The jerk test reverses the direction of the pivot-shift test.[44] The position of the knee is identical to that for the pivot-shift test except that the knee is moved from a position of flexion into extension with the lateral tibial plateau in a reduced position. If there is anterior cruciate insufficiency, as the knee moves into extension the tibia will subluxate at about 20 degrees of flexion, once again producing a palpable shift or clunk (Figure 20-16).

Flexion-rotation drawer test With this test, the lower leg is cradled with the knee flexed between 15 and 30 degrees. At 15 degrees, the tibia is subluxated anteriorly with the femur externally rotated. As the knee is flexed to 30 degrees, the tibia reduces posteriorly and the femur rotates internally (Figure 20-17).[87]

Posterior Cruciate Ligament Tests

Tests for posterior cruciate ligament instability include the posterior drawer test, the external rotation recurvatum test, and the posterior sag test.

Posterior drawer test The posterior drawer test is performed with the knee flexed at 90 degrees and the foot in neutral. Force is exerted in a posterior direction at the proximal tibial plateau. A positive posterior drawer test indicates damage to the posterior cruciate ligament (Figure 20-18).

External rotation recurvatum test The athletic trainer grasps the great toe and lifts the leg off the table. If the tibia externally rotates and slides posteriorly, there may be injury to the posterior cruciate ligament and posterolateral corner of the joint capsule, creating posterolateral instability (Figure 20-19).[87]

Posterior sag test (Godfrey's test) With the athlete supine, both knees are flexed to 90 degrees. Observing laterally on the injured side, the tibia will appear to sag posteriorly when compared with the opposite extremity if the posterior cruciate ligament is damaged (Figure 20-20).[87]

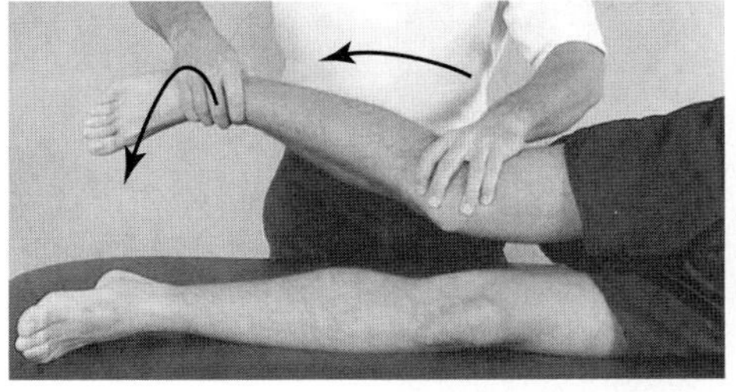

A

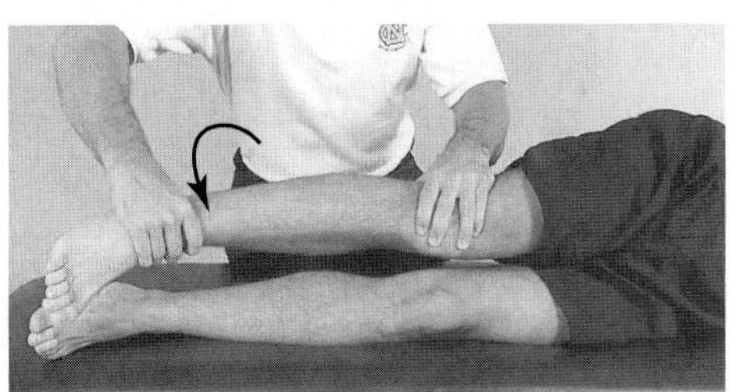

B

Figure 20-16

Jerk test for anterolateral rotary instability. **A,** The tibia is reduced in flexion. **B,** It subluxates at 20 degrees of extension.

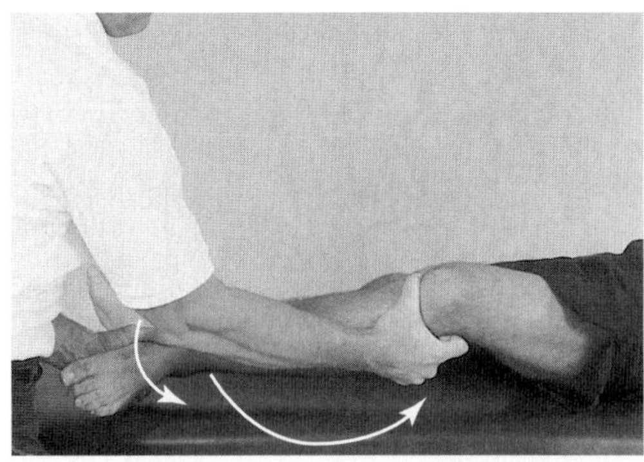

Figure 20-17

Flexion-rotation drawer test.

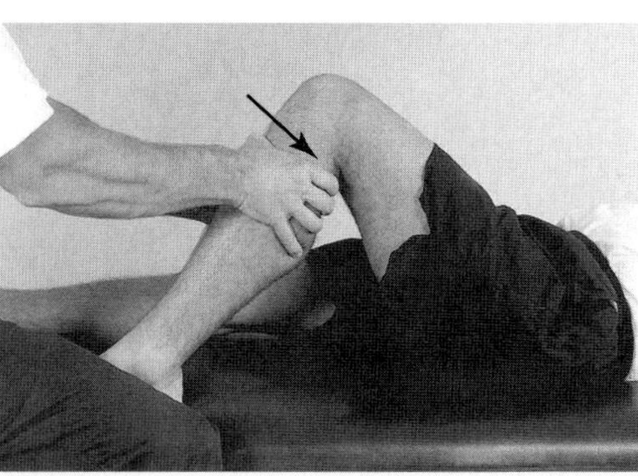

Figure 20-18

Posterior drawer test.

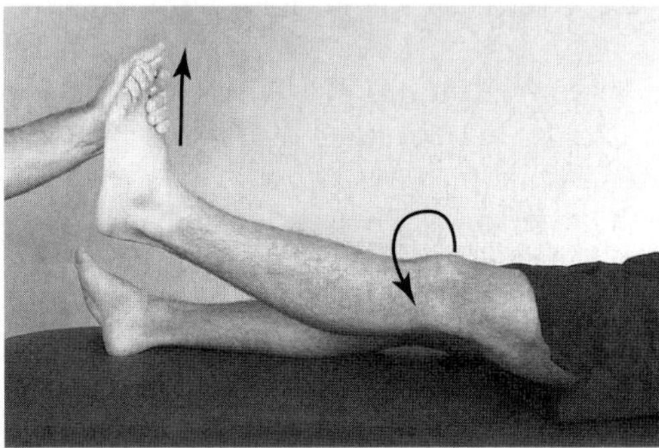

Figure 20-19

External rotation recurvatum test.

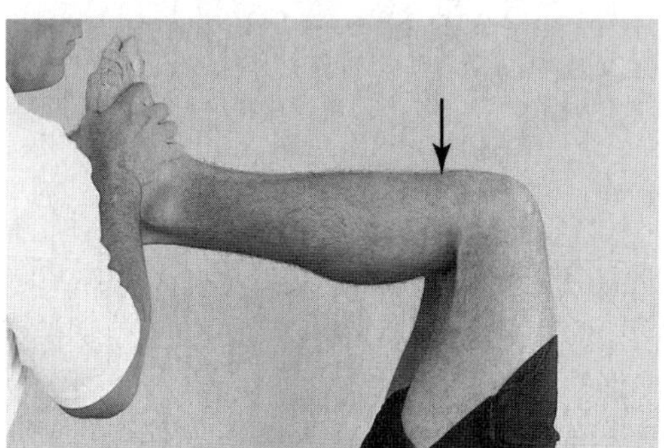

Figure 20-20

Posterior sag test (Godfrey's test).

Instrument Assessment of Cruciate Laxity

Several ligament-testing devices are currently available that objectively quantify the anterior or posterior displacement of the knee joint, thus reducing much of the subjectivity associated with the previously described tests.[93] The KT-2000 knee arthrometer, the Stryker knee laxity tester, and the Genucom are three such testing devices (Figure 20-21).

Measurements taken postoperatively and at periodic intervals throughout the rehabilitation process provide an objective indication to the athletic trainer about the effectiveness of the treatment program in maintaining or reducing anterior or posterior translation.[92]

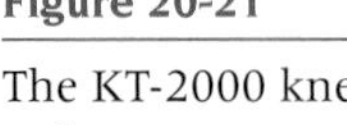

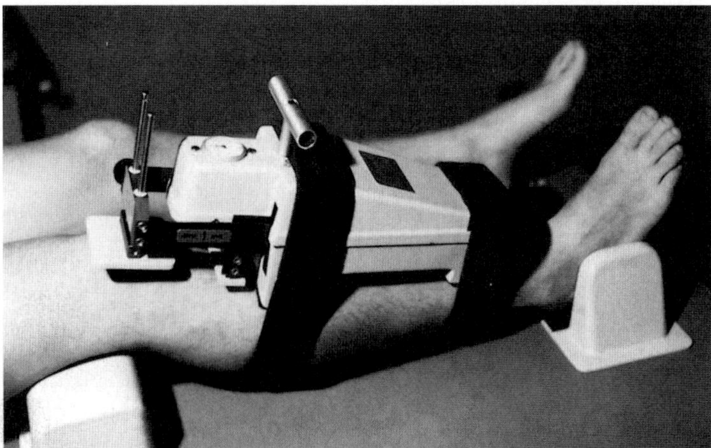

Figure 20-21

The KT-2000 knee arthrometer.

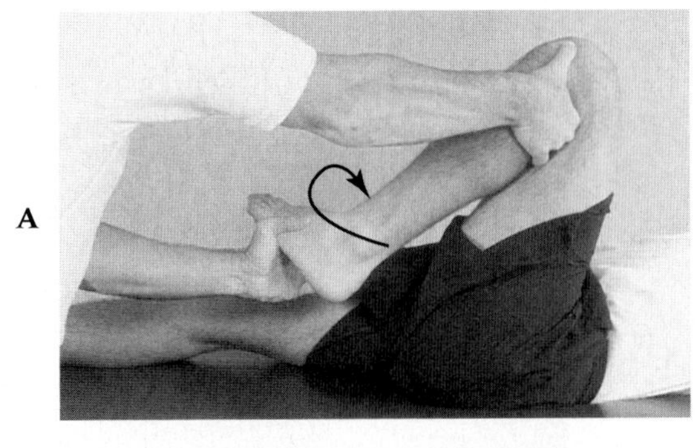

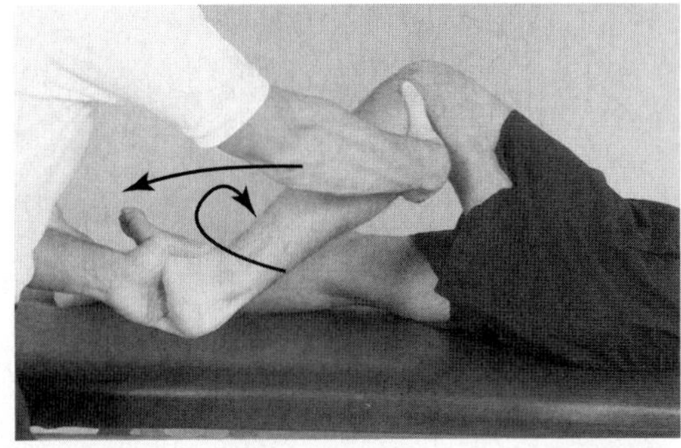

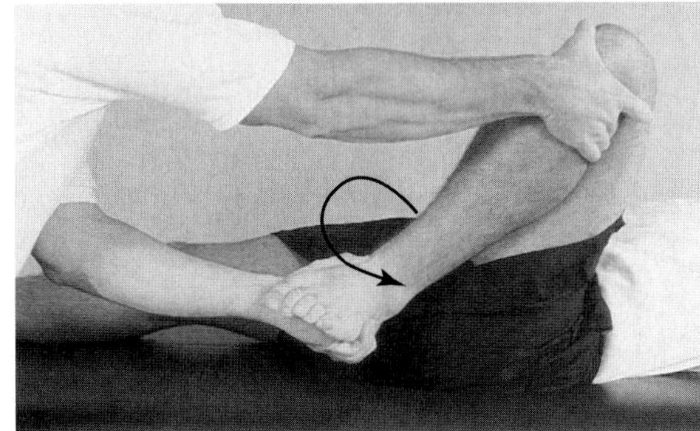

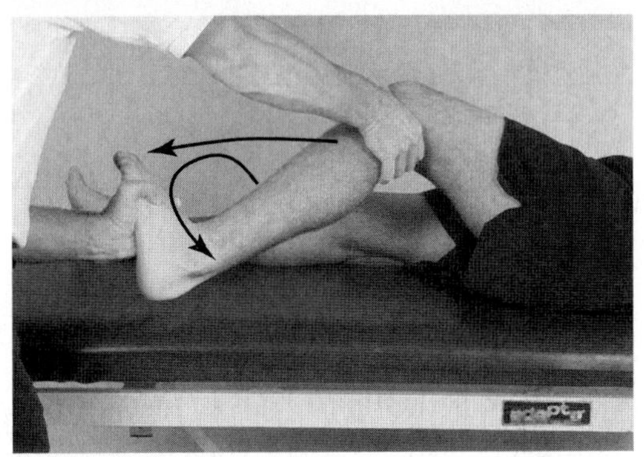

Figure 20-22

The McMurray's meniscal test. **A & B,** Internal rotation of the lower leg into knee extension. **C & D,** External rotation of the lower leg into knee extension.

Meniscal Tests

Determining a torn meniscus often can be difficult. The three most commonly used tests are McMurray's test, the Apley compression test, and the Apley distraction test.

McMurray's meniscal test McMurray's test (Figure 20-22) is used to determine the presence of a displaceable meniscal tear within the knee. The athlete is positioned face up on the table with the injured leg fully flexed. The athletic trainer places one hand on the foot and one hand over the top of the knee, fingers touching the medial joint line. The ankle hand scribes a small circle and pulls the leg into extension. As this occurs, the hand on the knee feels for a clicking response. Medial meniscal tears can be detected when the lower leg is externally rotated, and internal rotation allows detection of lateral tears.

Apley compression test The Apley compression test (Figure 20-23) is performed with the athlete lying face down and the affected leg flexed to 90 degrees. While stabilizing the thigh, the athletic trainer applies a hard downward pressure to the leg and rotates the leg back and forth. If pain results, a meniscal injury has occurred. A medial meniscal tear is noted by external rotation, and a lateral meniscal tear is noted by internal rotation of the lower leg.

Apley distraction test With the athlete in the same position as for the Apley compression test, the athletic trainer applies traction to the leg while moving it back and forth (Figure 20-24). This maneuver distinguishes collateral ligamentous tears from capsular and meniscal tears. If the capsule or ligaments are affected, pain will occur; if the meniscus is torn, no pain will occur from the traction and rotation.[44]

Girth Measurement

A knee injury is almost always accompanied by an eventual decrease in the girth of the thigh musculature. The muscles most affected by disuse are the quadriceps group, which are antigravity muscles and assist humans in maintaining an erect, straight-leg position. They are in constant use in effecting movement. Atrophy results when a lower limb is favored and is not used to its potential. Measurement of the circumference of both thighs can often detect former leg injuries or determine the extent of exercise rehabilitation. Five sites have been suggested for girth measurement: the joint

Because the musculature of the knee atrophies so readily after an injury, girth measurements must be routinely taken.

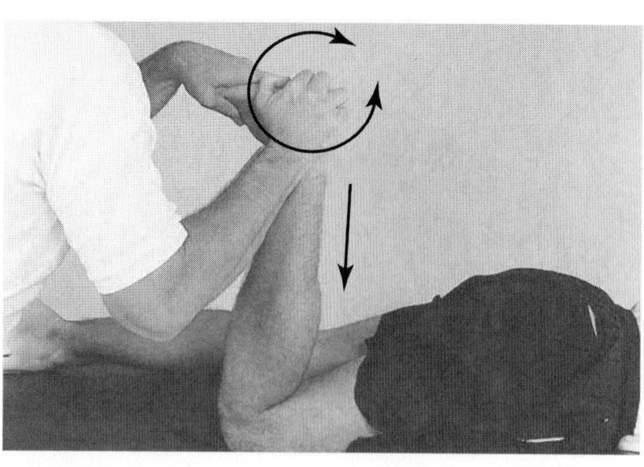

Figure 20-23

The Apley compression test.

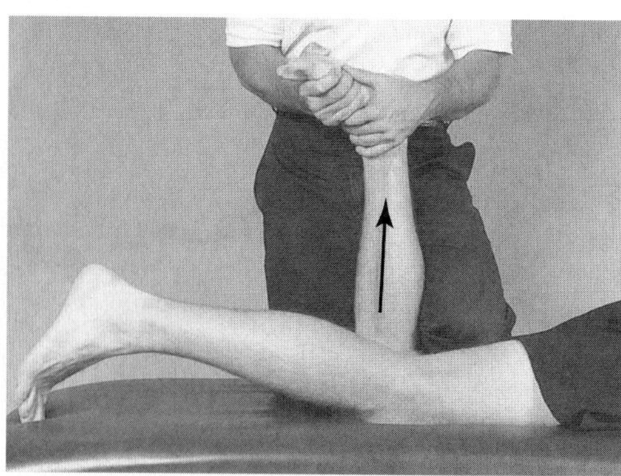

Figure 20-24

The Apley distraction test.

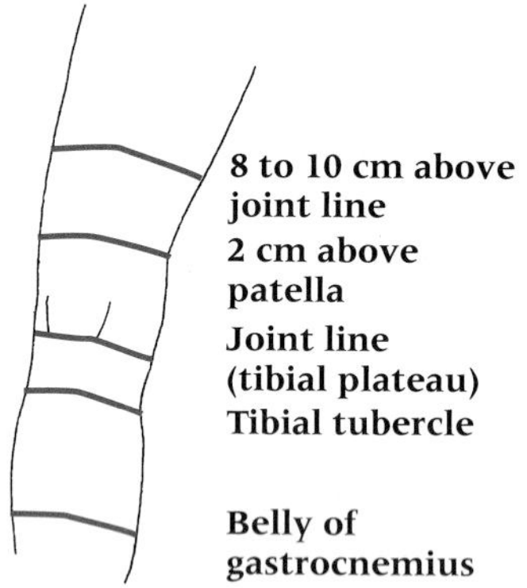

Figure 20-25

The five sites for girth measurement.

line (tibial plateau), 8 to 10 cm above the tibial plateau; the level of the tibial tubercle; the belly of the gastrocnemius muscle measured in centimeters from the tibial tubercle; and 2 cm above the superior border of the patella recorded in centimeters above the tibial tubercle (Figure 20-25).[84]

Subjective Rating Scales

On occasion, subjective rating scales such as the Lysholm Knee Scoring Scale, the Cincinnati Knee Scale, the International Knee Documentation Committee (IKDC) Scale, and the Knee Outcome Survey have been used to determine the patient's perception of how well the injured knee is doing relative to pain, stability, and functional performance. The information obtained from these rating scales can be combined with findings from stability testing to help with an initial diagnosis or evaluation of progress in rehabilitation (*Focus Box:* "Lysholm knee scoring scale").

Functional Examination

It is important that the athlete's knee also be tested for function. The athlete should be observed walking and, if possible, running, turning, performing figure-eights, backing up, and stopping. The co-contraction test, vertical jump, and single-leg hop test are also useful functional tests. If the athlete can do a deep knee bend or duck walk without discomfort, it is doubtful that there is a meniscal tear. The resistive strength of the hamstring and quadriceps muscles should be compared with the strength of the uninjured knee (Figure 20-26).

Patellar Examinations

Any knee evaluation should include inspection of the patella. Numerous evaluation procedures are associated with the patella and its surroundings. The following evaluation procedures can provide valuable information about possible reasons for knee discomfort and problems in functioning.[86]

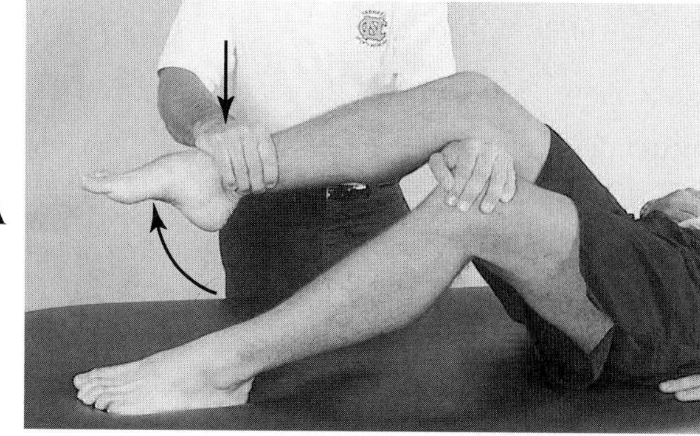

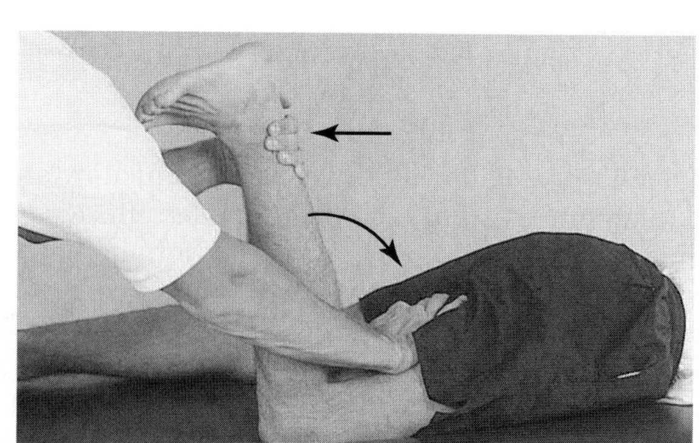

Figure 20-26

A, Testing quadriceps strength.
B, Testing hamstring strength.

Focus

Lysholm knee scoring scale[84]

1. Please check the statement that best describes the way you walk.
   ____ I never walk with a limp.
   ____ I rarely walk with a limp or I walk with a slight limp.
   ____ I walk with a constant and severe limp.
2. Which of the following do you presently use as a support while you walk?
   ____ I can walk without crutches or a cane.
   ____ I can put some weight on my leg, but I need at least one crutch or a cane to walk.
   ____ I cannot put any weight on my leg when walking.
3. Do you experience LOCKING of your knee?
   ____ No, never.
   ____ My knee catches, but does not lock.
   ____ Yes, my knee locks occasionally.
   ____ Yes, my knee locks frequently.
   ____ Yes, my knee is locked all the time.
4. Do you experience slipping or giving way of your knee?
   ____ No, never.
   ____ Yes, rarely during sporting activities or other severe exertion.
   ____ Yes, frequently during sporting activities or other severe exertion.
   ____ Yes, occasionally during daily activities.
   ____ Yes, frequently during daily activities.
   ____ Yes, on every step.
5. Which of the following best describes your level of pain?
   ____ I have no pain in my knee.
   ____ I have occasional pain, which is slight and present only after severe exertion.
   ____ I have marked pain during severe exertion.
   ____ I have marked pain after walking more than 2 miles.
   ____ I have marked pain after walking less than 2 miles.
   ____ I have constant pain.
6. Which of the following best describes swelling in your knee?
   ____ I have no swelling.
   ____ I have swelling only after severe exertion.
   ____ I have swelling after ordinary exertion.
   ____ I have constant swelling.
7. Which of the following best describes your ability to climb stairs?
   ____ I have no problems on stairs.
   ____ I am only slightly impaired on stairs.
   ____ I can negotiate stairs, but only one at a time.
   ____ I cannot go up or down stairs.
8. Can you get into a full squat position?
   ____ Yes, no problems.
   ____ No, but I am only slightly impaired.
   ____ No, I cannot squat with my knee past 90 degrees.
   ____ No, I cannot squat at all.

THANK YOU FOR TAKING TIME TO COMPLETE THIS QUESTIONNAIRE.

From Tegner Y, Lysholm J: Rating systems in the evaluation of knee ligament injuries, *Clin Orthop* 198:43, 1985.

The Q Angle

The Q angle is created when lines are drawn from the middle of the patella to the anterosuperior spine of the ilium and from the tubercle of the tibia through the center of the patella (Figure 20-27). It should be measured with the knee fully extended and with the knee flexed at 30 degrees. The normal Q angle is 10 degrees for males and

A Q angle greater than 20 degrees could predispose the athlete to patellar femoral pathology.

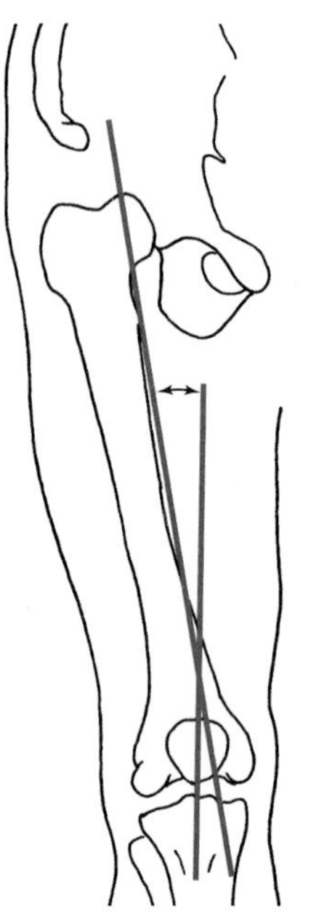

Figure 20-27

Measuring the Q angle of the knee.

15 degrees for females. Q angles that exceed 20 degrees are considered excessive and could lead to a pathological condition associated with improper patellar tracking in the femoral groove.[41] The Q angle can be decreased with isometric quadriceps contraction.

The A Angle

The A angle measures the patellar orientation to the tibial tubercle. It is created by the intersection of a line that bisects the patella longitudinally and a line from the tibial tubercle to the apex of the inferior pole of the patella (Figure 20-28).[3] An A angle of 35 degrees or greater has been correlated with patellofemoral pathomechanics that seem to result in constant patellofemoral pain. The A angle serves as a quantitative measure of patellar realignment after rehabilitative intervention.

Palpation of the Patella

With the athlete's quadriceps muscle fully relaxed, the examiner palpates the patella for pain sites around its periphery and under its sides (Figure 20-29).

Patellar Compression, Patellar Grinding, and Apprehension Tests

With the knee held to create approximately 20 degrees of flexion, the patella is compressed downward into the femoral groove; it is then moved forward and backward (Figure 20-30). If the athlete feels pain or if a grinding sound is heard during the patellar grind test, a pathological condition is probably present. With the knee still flexed, the patella is forced forward and is held in this position as the athlete extends the knee (Figure 20-31). A positive Clark's sign is present when the athlete experiences pain and grinding. Another test that indicates whether the patella can easily be subluxated or dislocated is known as the patellar apprehension test (Figure 20-32). With the knee and patella in a relaxed position, the examiner pushes the patella laterally. The athlete will express sudden apprehension at the point at which the patella begins to dislocate.[67]

PREVENTION OF KNEE INJURIES

Preventing knee injuries in sports is a complex problem. Of major importance are effective physical conditioning, rehabilitation and skill development, and shoe type. The routine use of protective bracing may be a questionable practice.

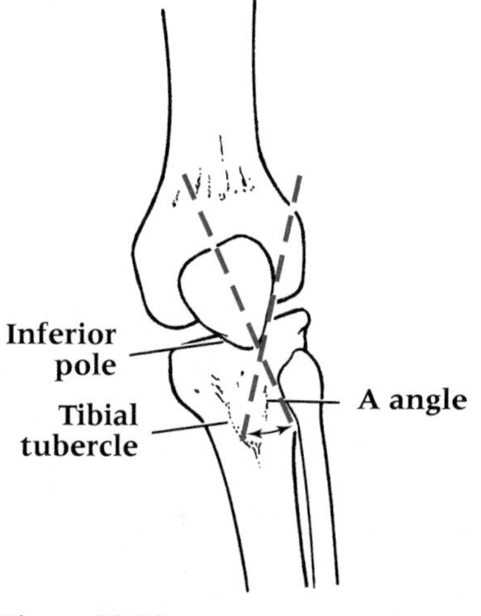

Figure 20-28

Determining the A angle.

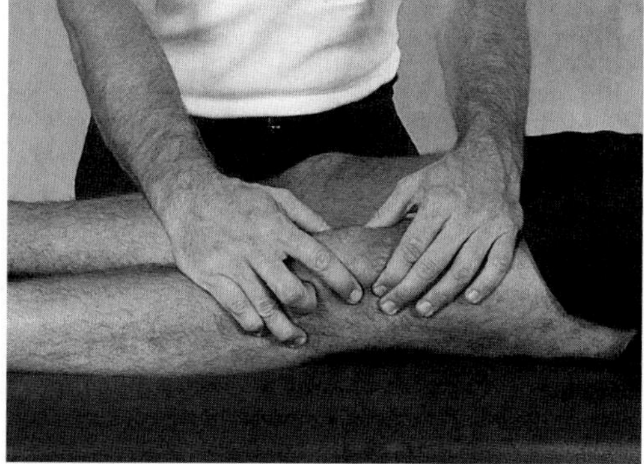

Figure 20-29

Palpating the periphery of the patella while the quadriceps muscle is fully relaxed.

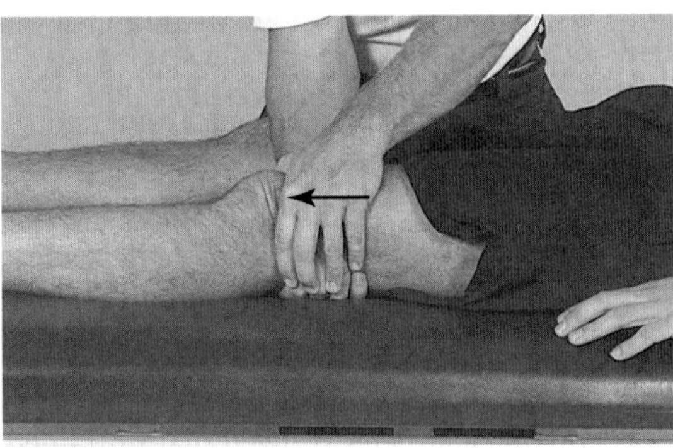

Figure 20-30

Patellar compression test. The patella is pressed downward in the femoral groove and moved forward and backward to elicit pain or crepitus.

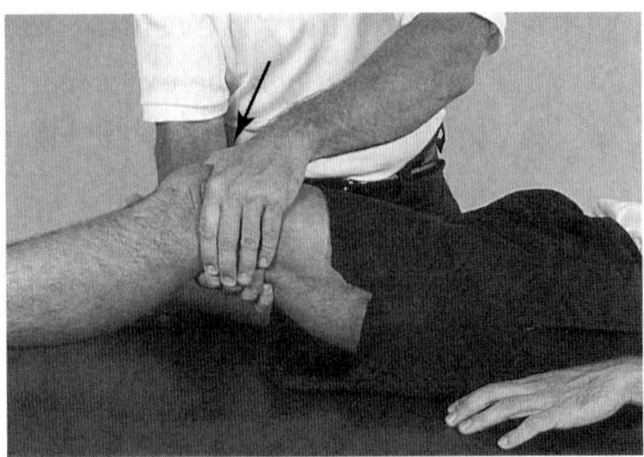

Figure 20-31

Patellar grind test. While the knee is flexed, the patella is forced forward; the athlete then actively contracts the quadriceps. The test reveals a positive Clark's sign if the athlete feels pain or grinding.

Physical Conditioning and Rehabilitation

To avoid knee injuries, the athlete must be as highly conditioned as possible, which means total body conditioning that includes strength, neuromuscular control, flexibility, cardiovascular and muscle endurance, agility, speed, and balance.[69] Specifically, the muscles surrounding the knee joint must be strong and flexible. The joints and soft tissue that make up the kinetic chain of which the knee is a part must also be considered sources of knee injury and therefore must be specifically conditioned for strength and flexibility.[77] Athletes participating in a particular sport should acquire a strength ratio between the quadriceps and hamstring muscle groups. For example, the hamstring muscles of football players should have 60 percent to 70 percent of the strength of the quadriceps muscles.[69] The gastrocnemius muscle should also be strengthened to help stabilize the knee. Although maximizing muscle strength may prevent some injuries, it fails to prevent rotary-type injuries.

Avoiding abnormal contraction of the muscles through flexibility exercises is a necessary protection for the knee. Gradual stretching of the knee musculature helps the muscle fibers become more extensible and elastic.[69] Of special concern in preventing knee injuries is the extensibility of the hamstrings, erector spinae, groin, quadriceps, and gastrocnemius muscles.

Knees that have been injured must be properly rehabilitated. Repeated minor injuries to a knee make it susceptible to a major injury. (See the section on knee joint rehabilitation later in this chapter.)

20-5

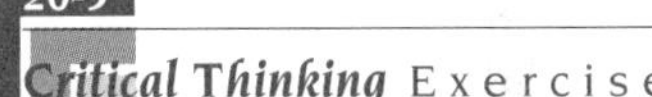

Critical Thinking Exercise

A baseball player is six months post-ACL reconstruction. He has been cleared by the team physician to return to activity. However, he still has a concern about his knee being reinjured. He wants to know whether he should be wearing a functional knee brace.

? What should the athletic trainer recommend to this athlete?

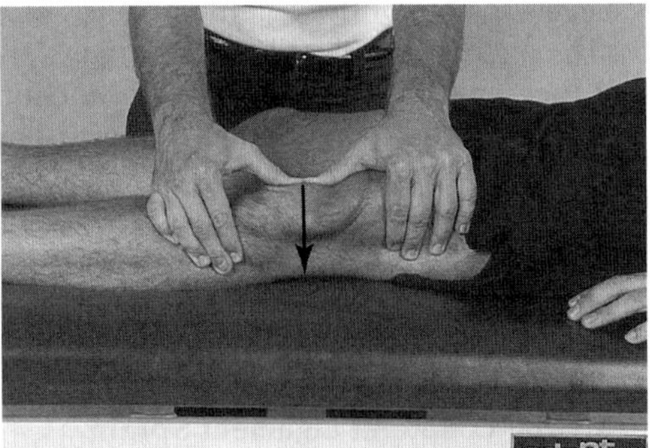

Figure 20-32

Patellar apprehension test for the easily subluxated or dislocated patella.

area is a minimized.[4] Tears that occur within the midsubstance of the meniscus often fail to heal because of lack of adequate blood supply.[4]

Symptoms and signs An absolute diagnosis of meniscal injury is difficult. To determine the possibility of such an injury, the athletic trainer should obtain a complete history which consists of information about past knee injuries and an understanding of how the present injury occurred. Diagnosis of meniscal injuries should be made immediately after the injury has occurred and before muscle spasm and swelling obscure the normal shape of the knee.

A meniscal tear may or may not result in the following:

- Effusion developing gradually over forty-eight to seventy-two hours.
- Joint-line pain and loss of motion.
- Intermittent locking and giving way of the knee.
- Pain when the athlete squats.

Once a meniscal tear occurs, the ruptured edges harden and may eventually atrophy. On occasion, portions of the meniscus may become detached and wedge themselves between the articulating surfaces of the tibia and femur, thus imposing a locking, catching, or giving way of the joint. Chronic meniscal lesions may also display recurrent swelling and obvious muscle atrophy around the knee. The athlete may complain of a sense of the knee collapsing, of a popping sensation, or of an inability to perform a full squat or to change direction quickly without pain when running. Such symptoms and signs usually warrant surgical intervention. NOTE: Symptomatic meniscal tears can eventually lead to serious articular degeneration with major impairment and disability.

Management If the knee is not locked but shows indications of a tear, the physician might initially obtain an MRI. A diagnostic arthroscopic examination may also be performed.

The knee that is locked by a displaced meniscus may require unlocking with the athlete under anesthesia so that a detailed examination can be conducted. If discomfort, disability, and locking of the knee continue, arthroscopic surgery may be required to remove a portion of the meniscus.

Surgical management of meniscal tears should make every effort to minimize loss of any portion of the meniscus.[14] The menisci are critical in preventing degenerative joint disease. Healing of the torn meniscus depends on where the tear has occurred. Tears in the red-red or red-white zones may heal well after surgical repair because they have a good vascular supply. Tears in the inner white-white zone will have to be resected because they are unlikely to heal, even with surgical repair, due to avascularity (see Figure 20-3). Resection, or a partial menisectomy, involves removing as little as possible of the meniscus through an arthroscope. Partial menisectomy of a torn meniscus is much more common than meniscal repair is.

Postsurgical management for a partial menisectomy does not require bracing and allows partial to full weight bearing on crutches as quickly as can be tolerated for about two weeks. It is not uncommon for an athlete to return to full activity in as little as six to fourteen days.

A repaired meniscus requires immobilization in a rehabilitative brace for five to six weeks. The athlete should be on crutches, progressing from partial to full weight bearing at six weeks. During immobilization, the athlete can perform active ROM exercises between 0 and 90 degrees. At six weeks, full ROM resistive exercises can begin. Rehabilitation should concentrate on endurance.[14]

20-7 Critical Thinking Exercise

A wrestler is diagnosed by the team physician as having a torn medial meniscus. On evaluation, McMurray's test was positive, and a subsequent MRI revealed a longitudinal bucket-handle tear in the posterior horn of the medial meniscus.

? What are the typical mechanisms of injury that can result in a tear of a meniscus?

20-8 Critical Thinking Exercise

A gymnast with no history of knee injury comes to the athletic trainer complaining of knee pain. She complains of pain while ascending or descending stairs and when squatting. Her major complaint is recurring episodes of painful pseudo-locking of the knee when she sits for a period of time. There is little or no swelling and no ligamentous laxity. A palpable tenderness begins on the medial wall of the knee joint and extends downward into the infrapatellar fat pad. As the knee passes 15 to 20 degrees of flexion, a snap may be felt or heard.

? Based on the findings of the evaluation, what might be causing these symptoms and signs?

Joint Injuries

Knee Plica

The fetus has three synovial knee cavities whose internal walls, at four months, are gradually absorbed to form one chamber; however, in 20 percent of all individuals, the knee fails to fully absorb these cavities.[66] In adult life, these septa form synovial folds known as plicae.

Etiology The most common synovial fold is the infrapatellar plica, which originates from the infrapatellar fat pad and extends superiorly in a fanlike manner. The

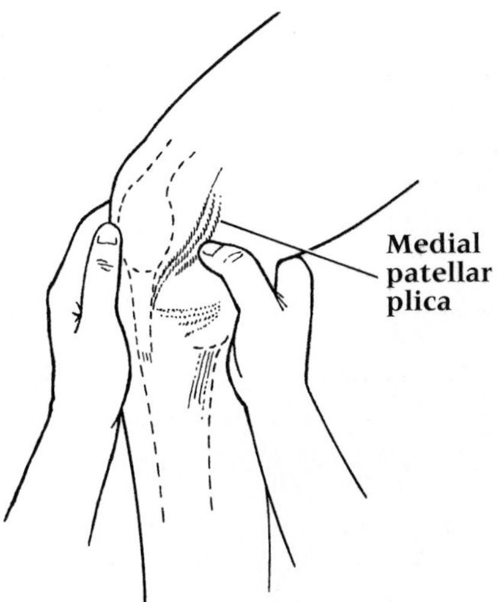

Figure 20-44

Knee plica.

second most common synovial fold is the suprapatellar plica, located in the suprapatellar pouch. The least common, but most subject to injury, is the mediopatellar plica, which is bandlike and begins on the medial wall of the knee joint and extends downward to insert into the synovial tissue that covers the infrapatellar fat pad.[66] Because most synovial plicae are pliable, most are asymptomatic; however, the mediopatellar plica may be thick, nonyielding, and fibrotic, causing a number of symptoms. The mediopatellar plica is associated with chondromalacia of the medial femoral condyle and patella (Figure 20-44).[66]

Symptoms and signs The athlete may or may not have a history of knee injury. If symptoms are preceded by trauma, it is usually from blunt force, such as a fall on the knee, or from a twist with the foot planted. A major complaint is recurrent episodes of painful pseudolocking of the knee when the athlete has been sitting for a period of time. As the knee passes 15 to 20 degrees of flexion, a snap may be felt or heard. Such characteristics of locking and snapping could be misinterpreted as a torn meniscus. The athlete complains of pain while ascending or descending stairs or when squatting. Unlike meniscal injuries, there is little or no swelling and no ligamentous laxity.

Management A knee plica that becomes inflamed as a result of trauma is usually treated conservatively with rest, antiinflammatory agents, and local heat. If the condition recurs, causing a chondromalacia of the femoral condyle or patella, the plica will require surgical excision.

Knee plicae that have become thick and hard are often mistaken for meniscal injuries.

Osteochondral Knee Fractures

Etiology Occasionally the same mechanisms that produce collateral ligamentous, cruciate ligamentous, or meniscal tears can shear off either a piece of bone attached to the anterior cartilage or cartilage alone (Figure 20-45). Twisting, sudden cutting, or being struck directly in the knee are typical causes of this condition.

Symptoms and signs The athlete commonly hears a snap and feels the knee give way. Swelling is immediate and extensive because of hemarthrosis, and there is considerable pain.

Management The diagnosis is usually confirmed by arthroscopic examination. Surgery is performed to replace the fragment as soon as possible to avoid joint degeneration and arthritis. The femoral condyles and the patella are affected.

Osteochondritis Dissecans

Etiology Osteochondritis dissecans is a painful condition involving partial or complete separation of a piece of articular cartilage and subchondral bone.[62] Both teenagers and adults can have this condition. The vast majority of fragments, more

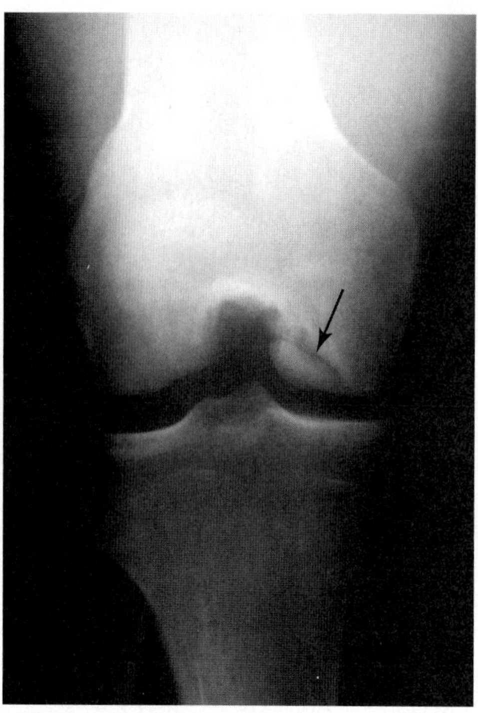

Figure 20-45

Osteochondral fracture with osteochondritis dissecans.

than 85 percent, occur in the lateral portion of the medial femoral condyle.[69] Clinically, osteochondral detachments are seen wherever there is osteochondritis dissecans. Typically, the lesion results in normal articular cartilage with dead subchondral bone underneath separated by a layer of fibrous tissue.

The exact cause of osteochondritis dissecans is unknown. It usually has a very slow onset. Possible etiological factors include the following:

- Direct or indirect trauma.
- Association with certain familial skeletal or endocrine abnormalities.
- A prominent tibial spine impinging on the medial femoral condyle.
- A facet of the patella impinging on the medial femoral condyle.

Symptoms and signs The athlete with osteochondritis dissecans complains of a knee that aches, swells recurrently, and on occasion, may catch or lock. There may be atrophy of the quadriceps muscle and point tenderness.

Management For children, rest and immobilization using a cylinder cast are usually prescribed. This management affords proper resolution of the injured cartilage and normal ossification of the underlying bone. Like many other osteochondroses, osteochondritis dissecans may take as long as one year to resolve. This condition in the teenager and adult may warrant surgery such as multiple drilling in the area to stimulate healing, pinning loose fragments, or bone grafting.

Loose Bodies Within the Knee

A knee that locks and unlocks during activity may indicate a torn meniscus.

Etiology Because of repeated trauma to the knee during sports activities, osteochondral fragments, or loose bodies ("joint mice"), can develop within the joint cavity. Loose bodies can stem from osteochondritis dissecans, fragments from the menisci, pieces of torn synovial tissue, or a torn cruciate ligament.

Symptoms and signs The loose body may move in the joint space and become lodged, causing locking and popping. The athlete will complain of pain and a feeling of instability, and the knee may give way.

Management When the loose body becomes wedged between articulating surfaces, irritation can occur. If not surgically removed, the loose body can create conditions that lead to joint degeneration.

Joint Contusions

Etiology A blow struck against the muscles crossing the knee joint can result in a handicapping condition. One of the muscles frequently involved is the vastus medialis of the quadriceps group, which is primarily involved in locking the knee in a position of full extension.

Symptoms and signs Bruises of the vastus medialis produce all the appearances of a knee sprain, including severe pain, loss of movement, and signs of acute inflammation. Such bruising is often manifested by swelling and discoloration caused by the tearing of muscle tissue and blood vessels. If adequate first aid is given immediately, the knee will usually return to functional use twenty-four to forty-eight hours after the trauma.

Bruising of the capsular tissue that surrounds the knee joint is often associated with muscle contusions and deep bone bruises. A traumatic force delivered to capsular tissue may cause capillary bleeding, irritate the synovial membrane, and result in profuse fluid effusion into the joint cavity and surrounding spaces, thereby producing intraarticular swelling. Effusion often takes place slowly and almost imperceptibly. The athlete should not engage in further activity for at least twenty-four hours after he or she receives a capsular bruise. Activity causes an increase in circulation and may cause extensive swelling and hematoma at the knee joint. Scar tissue develops wherever internal bleeding with clot organization is present. If this condition is repeated time after time, chronic synovitis or an arthritic sequela may develop.

Because the knee joint and patella are poorly padded, they are prone to bruising.

Management Care of a bruised knee depends on many factors. However, management principally depends on the location and severity of the contusion. The following procedures are suggested:

- Apply compression bandages and cold until resolution has occurred.
- Prescribe inactivity and rest for twenty-four hours.
- If swelling occurs, continue cold application for seventy-two hours. If swelling and pain are intense, refer the athlete to the physician.
- Once the acute stage has ended and there is little or no swelling, conduct cold application with active ROM exercises within a pain-free range. If a gradual use of heat is elected, great caution should be taken to prevent swelling.
- Allow the athlete to return to normal activity, with protective padding, when pain and the initial irritation have subsided.
- If swelling is not resolved within a week, it is possible that a chronic condition of either synovitis or bursitis may exist, indicating the need for rest and medical attention.

Peroneal Nerve Contusion

Etiology Compression of the peroneal nerve as it crosses directly behind the underlying neck of the fibula most commonly occurs from a kick or direct blow.

Symptoms and signs Immediately following the impact the athlete experiences local pain from the contusion and pain (likened to an electric shock) radiating down the anterior leg into the dorsum of the foot. Numbness and paresthesia in the cutaneous distribution of the nerve may also be present. Locally, there may be skin abrasions or ecchymosis with tenderness of the underlying peroneal nerve. Local pressure may exacerbate the tingling. Usually this neuropraxia lasts only a few seconds or minutes, but if the injury is severe, the hypesthesia and weakness of the peroneals and dorsiflexors persist, and it is possible that the athlete could develop a drop foot. However, most of the time the contusion of the nerve is minor, and usually the athlete recovers within one or two days following injury.

Management Initially the injury is managed with RICE. The athlete may return to play as soon as the symptoms abate and there is no weakness of the peroneals or dorsiflexors. Protective padding over the fibular head area should be used to protect the nerve for a few weeks. An orthosis for a drop foot is rarely necessary.

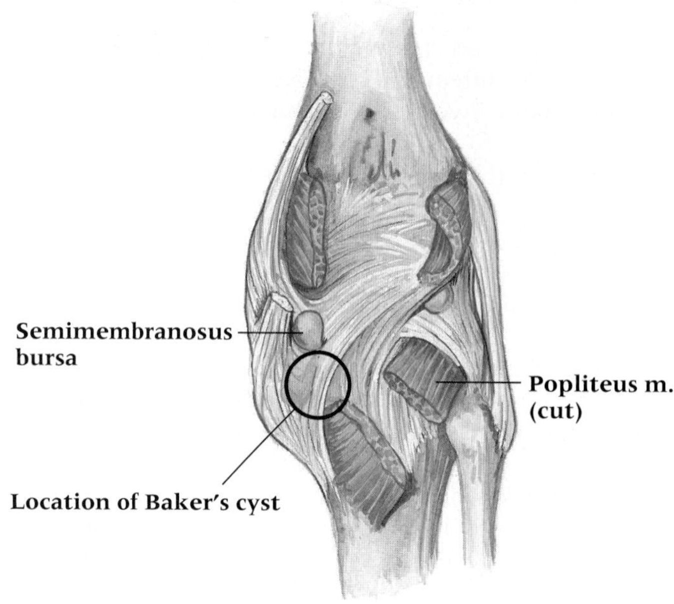

Figure 20-46

Location of a Baker's cyst in the popliteal fossa.

Bursitis

The knee has many bursae; the prepatellar, deep infrapatellar, and suprapatellar bursae are most often irritated.

Bursitis in the knee can be acute, chronic, or recurrent. Although any one of the numerous knee bursae can become inflamed, anteriorly the prepatellar, deep infrapatellar, and suprapatellar bursae have the highest incidence of irritation in sports (see Figure 20-5).

Etiology The prepatellar bursa often becomes inflamed from continued kneeling, and the deep infrapatellar bursa becomes irritated from overuse of the patellar tendon.

Symptoms and signs Prepatellar bursitis results in localized swelling above the knee that is ballotable. Swelling is not intraarticular, and there may be some redness and increased temperature. Swelling in the popliteal fossa does not necessarily indicate bursitis but could instead be a sign of a Baker's cyst (Figure 20-46). A Baker's cyst is associated with the semimembranosus bursa and occurs under the medial head of the gastrocnemius muscle. It is connected directly to the joint, and it swells because of a problem in the joint and not because of bursitis. A Baker's cyst is commonly painless, causing no discomfort or disability. Some inflamed bursae may be painful and disabling because of the swelling and should be treated accordingly.

20-9 *Critical Thinking* Exercise

An ice hockey player comes to the athletic training room with significant knee swelling after falling straight down on his knee. The swelling is found to be extracapsular and some redness is also present on the knee.

? What is most likely this athlete's injury? What tests can be used to evaluate the swelling?

Management Management usually follows a pattern of eliminating the cause, prescribing rest, and reducing inflammation. Perhaps the two most important techniques for controlling bursitis are the use of elastic compression wraps and antiinflammatory medication. When the bursitis is chronic or recurrent and the synovium has thickened, the use of aspiration and a steroid injection may be warranted.

Patellar Conditions

Patellofemoral disorders are likely the single most common knee pathology encountered by the athletic trainer.[35,85] In fact they may be among the most common musculoskeletal conditions seen by the athletic trainer.[95] Traditionally there has been difficulty in classifying specific patellofemoral disorders because of the similarity in the reported symptoms.[32]

Patellar Fracture

Etiology Fractures of the patella can be caused by either direct or indirect trauma (Figure 20-47). Most patellar fractures are the result of indirect trauma in which a severe pull of the patellar tendon occurs against the femur when the knee is semiflexed.

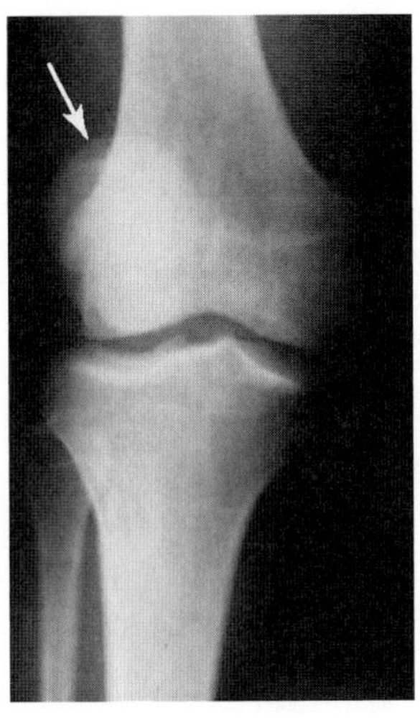

A

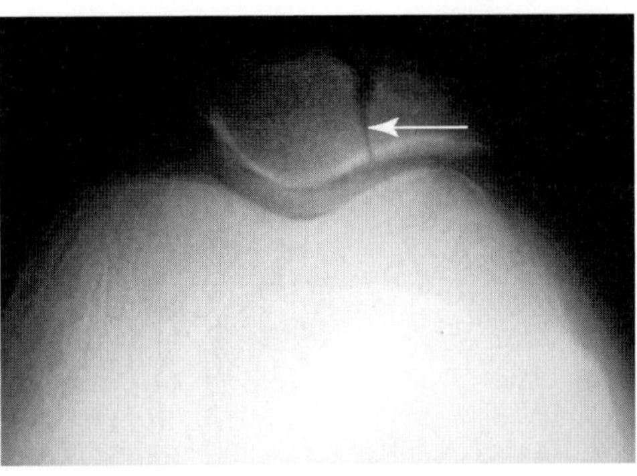

B

Figure 20-47

A, Patellar dislocation.
B, Patellar fracture (sunrise view).

This position subjects the patella to maximum stress from the quadriceps tendon and the patellar ligament. Forcible muscle contraction may then fracture the patella at its lower half. Direct injury most often produces fragmentation with little displacement. Falling, jumping, or running may result in a fracture of the patella. NOTE: Approximately 3 percent of the population has a bipartite patella, meaning there are two portions of the patella. This condition can be misdiagnosed as a patellar fracture.

Symptoms and signs The fracture causes hemorrhage and joint effusion, resulting in generalized swelling. Indirect fracture causes capsular tearing, separation of bone fragments, and possible tearing of the quadriceps tendon. Direct fracture involves little bone separation.

Management Diagnosis is accomplished through use of the history, palpation of separated fragments, and an X-ray confirmation. As soon as the examiner suspects a patellar fracture, a cold wrap should be applied, followed by an elastic compression wrap and splinting. The athletic trainer should then refer the athlete to the team physician. The athlete will normally be immobilized for two to three months.

Acute Patellar Subluxation or Dislocation

Etiology When an athlete plants his or her foot, decelerates, and simultaneously cuts in an opposite direction from the weight-bearing foot, the thigh rotates internally while the lower-leg rotates externally, causing a forced knee valgus. The quadriceps muscle attempts to pull in a straight line and as a result pulls the patella laterally—a force that may dislocate the patella. As a rule, displacement takes place outwardly, with the patella resting on the lateral condyle (Figure 20-47).

Knees that give way or catch have a number of possible pathological conditions, including:

- Subluxating patella
- Meniscal tear
- Anterior cruciate ligamentous tear
- Hemarthrosis

With this mechanism, the patella is forced to slide laterally into a partial or full dislocation. Some athletes are more predisposed to this condition than others because of the following anatomical structures:[17,69]

- A wide pelvis with anteverted hips
- Genu valgum, which increases the Q angle
- Shallow femoral grooves
- Flat lateral femoral condyles
- High-riding and flat patellas
- Vastus medialis and ligamentous laxity with genu recurvatum and externally rotated tibias
- Pronated feet
- Externally pointing patellas

A patella that subluxates repeatedly places abnormal stress on the patellofemoral joint and the medial restraints. The knee may be swollen and painful. Pain is a result

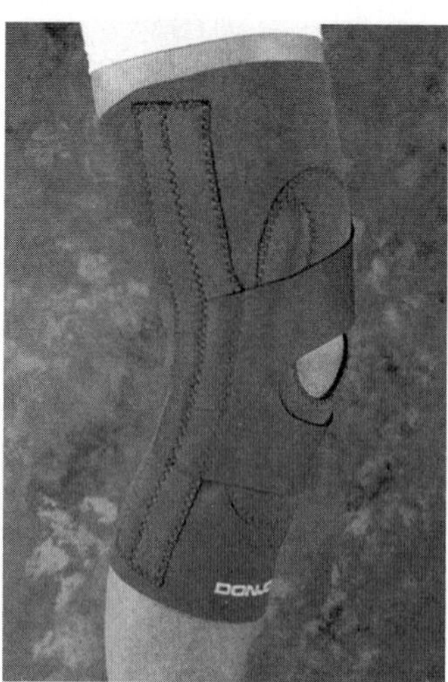

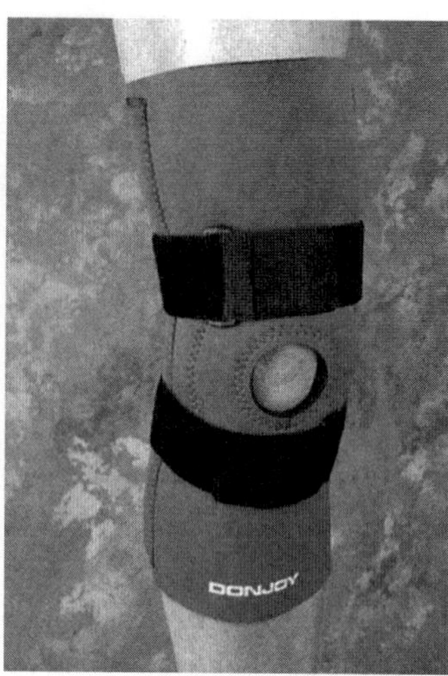

Figure 20-48

Special pads for the dislocated patella.

of swelling but also results because the medial capsular tissue has been stretched and torn. Because of the associated swelling, the knee is restricted in flexion and extension. There may also be a palpable tenderness over the adductor tubercle where the medial retinaculum (patellar femoral ligament) attaches.

An acute patellar dislocation is often associated with sudden twisting of the body while the foot or feet are planted and is associated with a painful giving way episode, creating injury to the ACL, PCL, or P/ACL.[49]

Symptoms and signs The athlete experiences pain, swelling, and a complete loss of knee function, and the patella rests in an abnormal position. The physician immediately reduces the dislocation by applying mild pressure on the patella with the knee extended as much as possible. If a period of time has elapsed before reduction, a general anesthetic may have to be used. After aspiration of the joint hematoma, ice is applied, and the joint is splinted. A first-time patellar dislocation is sometimes associated with a chondral or osteochondral fracture. X-ray evaluation is performed before and after reduction.

Management To reduce a dislocation, the hip is flexed, and the patella is gently moved medially as the knee is slowly extended. After reduction, the knee is immobilized in extension for four weeks or longer, and the athlete is instructed to use crutches when walking. During immobilization, the athlete should perform isometric exercises at the knee joint. After immobilization, the athlete should wear a horseshoe-shaped felt pad that is held in place around the patella by an elastic wrap or sewn into an elastic sleeve that is worn while the athlete runs or performs in sports. Commercial braces are also available (Figure 20-48).

Muscle rehabilitation should focus on all the musculature of the knee, thigh, and hip. Knee exercise should be confined to straight-leg raises.

If surgery is performed, it is usually to release constrictive ligaments or to reconstruct the patellofemoral joint. It is important to strengthen and to balance the strength of all musculature associated with the knee joint. Postural malalignments must be corrected as much as possible. Shoe orthotic devices may be used to reduce foot pronation, tibial internal rotation, and subsequently, stress to the patellofemoral joint.

Injury to the Infrapatellar Fat Pad

The two most important fat pads of the knee are the infrapatellar fat pad and the suprapatellar fat pad. The infrapatellar fat pad lies between the synovial membrane on the anterior aspect of the joint and the patellar tendon, and the suprapatellar fat pad lies between the anterior surface of the femur and the suprapatellar bursa. Of the two pads, the infrapatellar is more often injured in sports, principally as a result of its large size and particular vulnerability during activity.

Etiology The infrapatellar fat pad may become wedged between the tibia and the patella, irritated by chronic kneeling pressures, or traumatized by direct blows.

Symptoms and signs Repeated injury to the fat pad produces capillary hemorrhaging and swelling of the fatty tissue; if the irritation continues, scarring and calcification may develop. The athlete may complain of pain below the patellar ligament, especially during knee extension, and the knee may display weakness, mild swelling, and stiffness during movement.

Management Care of acute fat pad injuries involves rest from irritating activities until inflammation has subsided, heel elevation of ½ to 1 inch (1.25 to 2.5 cm), and the therapeutic use of cold. Heel elevation prevents added irritation during full extension; the application of hyperextension taping may also be necessary to prevent the occurrence of full extension.

Patellofemoral Arthralgia (Patellofemoral Pain Syndrome)

The patella, in relation to the femoral groove, can be subject to direct trauma or disease that leads to chronic pain and disability.[83] Of primary concern among athletes are those conditions that stem from abnormal patellar tracking within the femoral groove, of which the two most common are chondromalacia patella and patellofemoral stress syndrome.[6,96] Patellofemoral pain syndrome is a catchall term that is used to refer to any type of pain that occurs in or around the patellofemoral joint.[11]

Chondromalacia patella

Etiology Chondromalacia patella is a softening and deterioration of the articular cartilage on the back of the patella (Figure 20-49). Chondromalacia undergoes three stages:

- Stage 1—swelling and softening of the articular cartilage
- Stage 2—fissuring of the softened articular cartilage
- Stage 3—deformation of the surface of the articular cartilage caused by fragmentation

The exact cause of chondromalacia is unknown. As indicated previously, abnormal patellar tracking could be a major etiological factor; however, individuals with normal tracking have acquired chondromalacia, and some individuals with abnormal tracking are free of it.[6] Abnormal patellofemoral tracking can be produced by genu valgum,

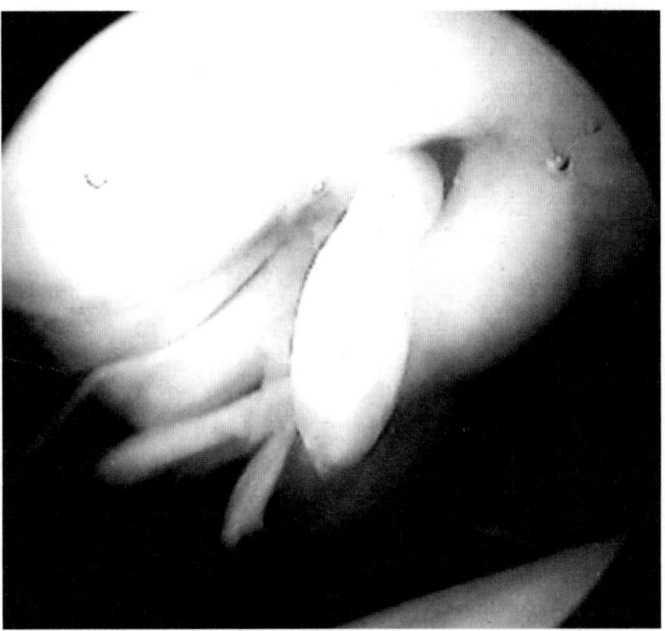

Figure 20-49

Chrondromalacia with chipping away of the articular surface of the patella.

external tibial torsion, foot pronation, femoral anteversion, a quadriceps Q angle greater than 15 to 20 degrees, patella alta, a shallow femoral groove, a shallow articular angle of the patella, an abnormal articular contour of the patella, or laxity of the quadriceps tendon.

Symptoms and signs The athlete may experience pain in the anterior aspect of the knee while walking, running, ascending and descending stairs, or squatting. There may be recurrent swelling around the kneecap and a grating sensation when flexing and extending the knee.

The patella displays crepitation during the patellar grind test. During palpation, there may be pain on the inferior border of the patella or when the patella is compressed within the femoral groove while the knee is passively flexed and extended. The athlete has one or more lower-limb alignment deviations.

Degenerative arthritis occurs on the medial facet of the patella, which makes contact with the femur when the athlete performs a full squat.[6] Degeneration first occurs in the deeper portions of the articular cartilage, followed by blistering and fissuring that stems from the subchondral bone and appears on the surface of the patella.[6,12]

Management In some cases, patellofemoral arthralgia is initially treated conservatively as follows:

- Avoidance of irritating activities such as stair climbing and squatting
- Isometric exercises that are pain free to strengthen the quadriceps and hamstring muscles
- Oral antiinflammatory agents and small doses of aspirin
- A neoprene knee sleeve
- An orthotic device to correct pronation and reduce tibial torsion

If conservative measures fail to help, surgery may be the only alternative. Some of the following surgical measures may be indicated:[6]

- Moving the insertion of the vastus medialis muscle forward through realignment procedures such as lateral release of the retinaculum
- Shaving and smoothing the irregular surfaces of the patella, femoral condyle, or both
- In cases of degenerative arthritis, removing the blister through drilling
- Elevating the tibial tubercle
- As a last resort, completely removing the patella

20-10 Critical Thinking Exercise

A triathlete has been complaining of knee pain for several months. She has never had an acute injury to the knee, but her training regimen is intense, involving three hours of training each day. She has been diagnosed by a physician as having chondromalacia patella.

? She has been referred to the athletic trainer for evaluation and rehabilitation. What can the athletic trainer do to help reduce the athlete's symptoms and signs?

Patellofemoral stress syndrome

Etiology Patellofemoral stress syndrome results from some lateral deviation of the patella as it tracks in the femoral groove. This tendency toward lateral tracking may be the result of several factors:[69]

- Tightness of the hamstrings and gastrocnemius
- Tightness of the lateral retinaculum, which compresses the lateral facet of the patella against the lateral femoral condyle
- Increased Q angle
- Tightness of the iliotibial band
- Pronation of the foot
- Patella alta (the patellar tendon is longer than the patella)
- Vastus medialis oblique (VMO) insufficiency caused by imbalance with the strength of the vastus lateralis (VL) or by inhibition resulting from the presence of 20 to 30 milliliters of effusion in the knee[6]
- Weak hip adductors to which the VMO is attached

Symptoms and signs There will be tenderness of the lateral facet of the patella and some swelling associated with irritation of the synovium as well as reports of a dull ache in the center of the knee. Patellar compression will elicit pain and crepitus. The athlete will be apprehensive when the patella is forced laterally.

Management The causes underlying patellofemoral pain as identified during the evaluation process should provide the basis for treatment.[65] The athlete must engage in

20-11 Critical Thinking Exercise

A track athlete complains of pain in the anterior aspect of the knee while walking, running, ascending and descending stairs, or squatting. There is a grating sensation when flexing and extending the knee.

? What condition should the athletic trainer suspect and what treatment should he or she recommend?

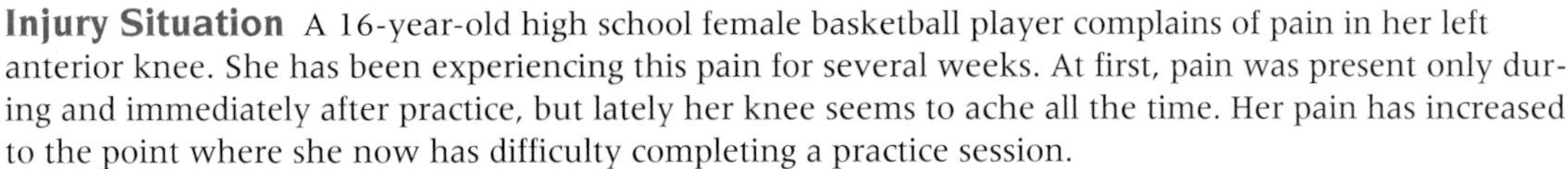

Management PLAN

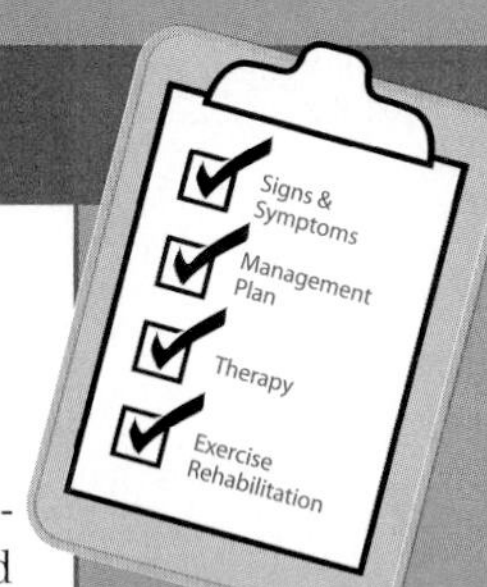

Patellofemoral Pain

Injury Situation A 16-year-old high school female basketball player complains of pain in her left anterior knee. She has been experiencing this pain for several weeks. At first, pain was present only during and immediately after practice, but lately her knee seems to ache all the time. Her pain has increased to the point where she now has difficulty completing a practice session.

Symptoms and Signs The athlete complains of pain in the anterior aspect of the knee while walking, running, ascending and descending stairs, or squatting. Pain is increased during the patellar grind test. During palpation, there may be pain on the inferior border of the patella or when the patella is compressed within the femoral groove while the knee is passively flexed and extended. She has tightness of the hamstrings, an increased Q angle, excessive pronation in her left foot, and weakness in her vastus medialis obliques (VMO).

Management Plan The goal is to reduce pain initially and then to identify and correct faulty biomechanics that may collectively contribute to her anterior knee pain.

Phase 1 *Acute Injury*

GOALS: To modulate pain and begin appropriate strengthening exercises.
ESTIMATED LENGTH OF TIME (ELT): 1 to 4 days.

- **Therapy** Use ice and electrical stimulation to decrease pain. If there appears to be inflammation, anti-inflammatory medications may be helpful. McConnell taping should be used to try and correct any patellar malalignment. The athlete may need to sit out of practice for a couple of days to remove the source of irritation.
- **Exercise rehabilitation** An orthotic insert should be constructed to correct the excessive pronation that occurs during gait. Quadriceps strengthening begins with isometric exercises, specifically, quad sets. Isometric contractions may be done at several positions throughout the range from 90 degrees of flexion to full extension.

Phase 2 *Repair*

GOALS: Increase VMO strength and improve hamstring flexibility.
ELT: 5 days to 2 weeks.

- **Therapy** Ice and electrical stimulation may be continued. McConnell taping technique should also be continued, with day-to-day reassessment of its effectiveness. The use of biofeedback may help the athlete to learn to contract the VMO.
- **Exercise rehabilitation** The effectiveness of the orthotic should be reassessed with appropriate correction adjustments. Aggressive hamstring stretching exercises should be used. Quadriceps strengthening exercises should concentrate on the VMO and should progress from isometrics to full-range isotonics as soon as full range-of-motion resisted exercise no longer causes pain. Closed kinetic chain exercises, particularly minisquats and lateral step-ups, should be recommended. The athlete may resume practice; however, those activities that seem to increase pain should be modified or replaced with alternative activities. Fitness levels must be maintained by either stationary cycling or aquatic exercise.

Phase 3 *Remodeling*

GOALS: To completely eliminate pain and fully return to activity.
ELT: 2 weeks to full return.

- **Therapy** The athlete gradually can be weaned from McConnell taping. She may find it helpful to wear a neoprene sleeve during activity.

Continued

Patellofemoral Pain—*continued*

■ **Exercise rehabilitation** The athlete must continue quadriceps strengthening and hamstring stretching exercises. The athlete should now be accustomed to the orthotic insert. It may be necessary to continue to use alternative fitness activities indefinitely.

Criteria for Return to Competitive Basketball

1. Pain is eliminated in squatting and in ascending or descending stairs.
2. The athlete has good hamstring flexibility.
3. Quadriceps strength, particularly VMO strength, is good.

a strengthening program for the adductor muscles and for correcting the imbalance between the VMO and the VL through the use of biofeedback techniques.[39,51] Stretching exercises for the hamstrings, gastrocnemius, and iliotibial band are also necessary.[66] Orthotics can be used to correct pronation and other malalignments.[22] The McConnell taping technique (see Chapter 8) has been demonstrated to be extremely effective in regaining proper patellar alignment and thus a more symmetrical loading on the lower extremity.[15,22] Taping is designed to correct the orientation of the patella.[66]

If conservative treatment measures fail, lateral retinacular release has been advocated by some physicians.

Extensor Mechanism Injuries

Many extensor mechanism problems can occur in the physically active individual. They can occur in the immature adolescent's knee or as a result of jumping and running.

Osgood-Schlatter Disease and Larsen-Johansson Disease

Conditions that may be mistaken for one another:
- Osgood-Schlatter disease
- Larsen-Johansson disease
- Jumper's or kicker's knee

Etiology Two conditions common to the immature adolescent's knee are Osgood-Schlatter disease and Larsen-Johansson disease. Osgood-Schlatter disease is an apophysitis characterized by pain at the attachment of the patellar tendon to the tibial tubercle. This condition most often represents an avulsion fracture of the tibial tubercle. This fragment is cartilaginous initially, but with growth, a bony callus forms and the tuberosity enlarges. This condition usually resolves when the athlete reaches the age of eighteen or twenty. The only remnant is an enlarged tibial tubercle.

The most commonly accepted cause of Osgood-Schlatter disease is repeated avulsion of the patellar tendon at the apophysis of the tibial tubercle. Complete avulsion of the patellar tendon is a major complication of Osgood-Schlatter disease.

Larsen-Johansson disease is similar to Osgood-Schlatter disease, but it occurs at the inferior pole of the patella (Figure 20-50). Like the cause of Osgood-Schlatter disease, the cause of Larsen-Johansson disease is believed to be excessive repeated strain on the patellar tendon. Swelling, pain, and point tenderness characterize Larsen-Johansson disease. Later, degeneration can be noted during X-ray examination.

Symptoms and signs Repeated irritation causes swelling, hemorrhage, and gradual degeneration of the apophysis as a result of impaired circulation. The athlete complains of severe pain when kneeling, jumping, and running. There is point tenderness over the anterior proximal tibial tubercle (see Figure 20-50).

Management Management is usually conservative and includes the following:[8]

- Stressful activities are decreased until the epiphyseal union occurs, within six months to one year.
- Severe cases may require a cylindrical cast.
- Ice is applied to the knee before and after activities.
- Isometric strengthening of quadriceps and hamstring muscles is performed.

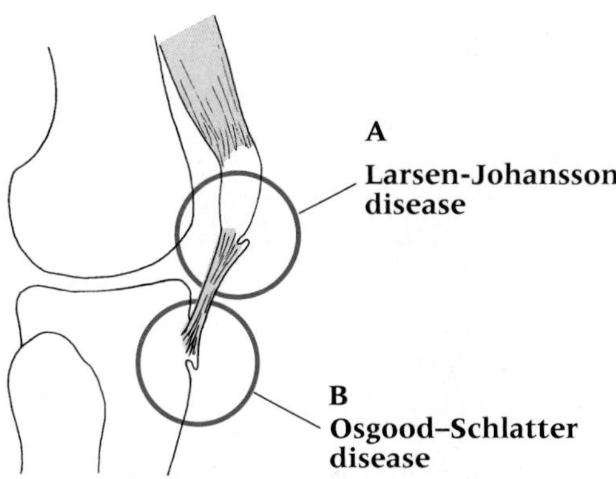

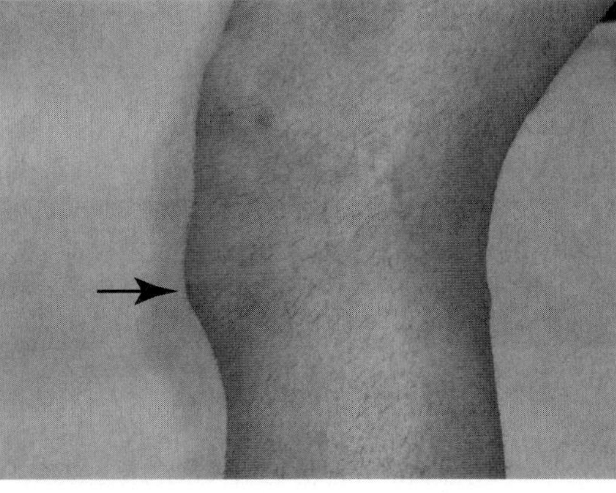

Figure 20-50

Two conditions of the immature extensor mechanism. **A,** Larsen-Johansson disease. **B,** Osgood-Schlatter disease. **C,** An enlarged tibial turbercle.

Patellar Tendinitis (Jumper's and Kicker's Knee)

Etiology Jumping, as well as kicking or running, may place extreme tension on the knee extensor muscle complex. As a result of one or more commonly repetitive injuries, tendinitis occurs in the patellar or quadriceps tendon.[7] On rare occasions, a patellar tendon may completely fail and rupture. Sudden or repetitive forceful extension of the knee may begin an inflammatory process that will eventually lead to tendon degeneration.

Symptoms and signs The athlete will report pain and tenderness at the inferior pole of the patella on the posterior aspect. Patellar tendinitis has three stages of pain:

- Stage 1—pain after sports activity
- Stage 2—pain during and after activity (the athlete is able to perform at the appropriate level)
- Stage 3—pain during activity and prolonged after activity (athletic performance is hampered); may progress to constant pain and complete rupture

Management Any pain in the patellar tendon must preclude sudden explosive movement such as that characterized by heavy plyometric-type exercising. Many approaches to treating athletes with inflammation associated with jumper's knee have been reported, including the use of ice, phonophoresis, iontophoresis, ultrasound, and various forms of superficial heat modalities, such as whirlpool, together with a program of exercise.[97] A patellar tendon tenodesis brace or strap may also be used (Figure 20-51).

Deep transverse friction massage has been used successfully for treating jumper's knee.[60] Friction is created by firm massage of the patellar tendon at the inferior patellar pole perpendicular to the direction of the fibers. Friction massage is used to increase the process of inflammation so that healing may progress to the fibroblastic phase. Thus, when transverse friction massage is used, other techniques for reducing inflammation should not be used.

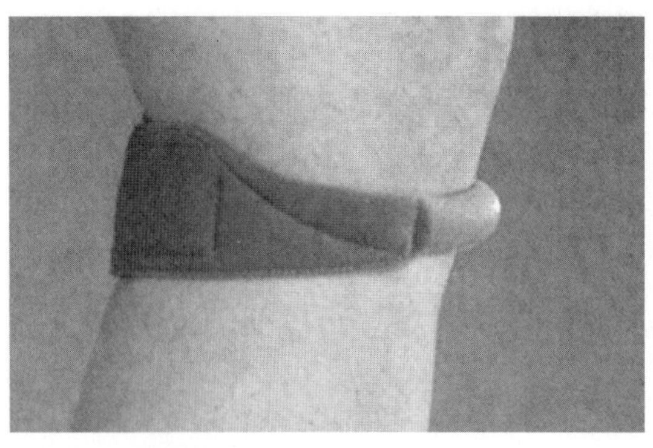

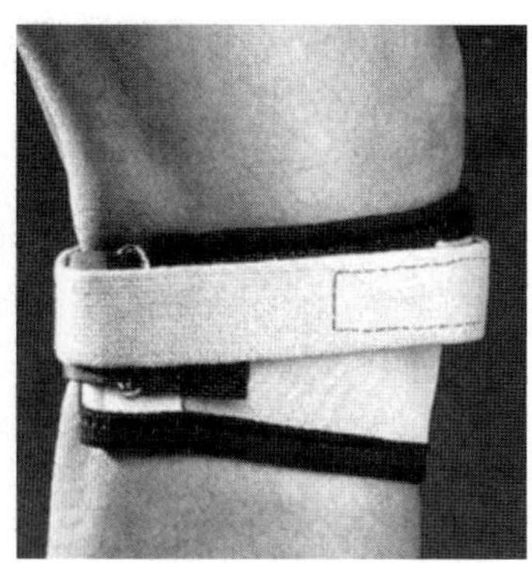

A B

Figure 20-51

Patellar tendon tenodesis braces or straps for patellofemoral pain.

20-12 Critical Thinking Exercise

A high jumper has been diagnosed as having patellar tendinitis, or jumper's knee. In three weeks, he has two important track meets and wants to know what he can do to get rid of the problem as soon as possible.

? What options does the athletic trainer have in treating the athlete with patellar tendinitis?

Patellar Tendon Rupture

Etiology A sudden powerful contraction of the quadriceps muscle with the weight of the body applied to the affected leg can cause a rupture.[95] The rupture may occur to the quadriceps tendon or to the patellar tendon. Usually rupture does not occur unless there has been an inflammatory condition over a period of time in the region of the knee extensor mechanism, causing tissue degeneration. A rupture seldom occurs in the middle of the tendon; usually it is torn from its attachment. The quadriceps tendon ruptures from the superior pole of the patella, whereas the patellar tendon ruptures from the inferior pole of the patella.

Symptoms and signs The patella moves upward toward the thigh and the defect can be palpated. The athlete cannot extend the knee. There is considerable swelling with significant pain initially, followed by a feeling that the injury may not be all that serious.

Management A rupture of the patellar tendon usually requires surgical repair. Proper conservative care of jumper's knee can minimize the chances of patellar tendon rupture. Athletes who use antiinflammatory drugs such as steroids must avoid intense exercise involving the knee. Steroids injected directly into these tendons weaken collagen fibers and mask pain.[95]

Runner's Knee (Cyclist's Knee)

Etiology Runner's knee is a general expression for many repetitive and overuse conditions. Many runner's knee problems can be attributed to malalignment and structural asymmetries of the foot and lower leg, including leg-length discrepancy. Common are patellar tendinitis and patellofemoral problems that may lead to chondromalacia. Two conditions that are prevalent among joggers, distance runners, and cyclists are iliotibial band friction syndrome and pes anserinus tendinitis or bursitis.

iliotibial band friction syndrome (ill ee **oh** tibial) Runner's knee.

ILIOTIBIAL BAND FRICTION SYNDROME **Iliotibial band friction syndrome** is an overuse condition commonly occurring in runners and cyclists who have genu varum and pronated feet.[71] Irritation develops at the band's insertion and, where friction is created, over the lateral femoral condyle. Ober's test (see Chapter 21) will cause pain at the point of irritation. Treatment includes stretching the iliotibial band and reducing inflammation.[71]

PES ANSERINUS TENDINITIS OR BURSITIS The pes anserinus is where the sartorius, gracilis, and semitendinosus muscles join to the tibia (see Figure 20-6). Associated with pes anserinus tendinitis is pes anserinus bursitis. Inflammation results from excessive genu valgum and weakness of the vastus medialis muscle. This condition is commonly produced by running on a slope with one leg higher than the other.

Management Management of runner's or cyclist's knee involves correction of foot and leg alignment problems. Therapy includes cold packs or ice massage before and after activity, proper warm-up and stretching, and avoidance of activities, such as running on inclines, that aggravate the problem. Other management procedures may include antiinflammatory medications and orthotic shoe devices to reduce leg conditions such as genu varum.

The Collapsing Knee

Knee collapse can occur for a variety of reasons. The most common causes of frequent knee collapse include a weak quadriceps muscle; chronic instability of the medial collateral ligament, anterior cruciate ligament, or posterior capsule; a torn meniscus; loose bodies within the knee; a subluxating patella; chondromalacia; and meniscal tears. Frequently, the knee will give way in response to pain produced by one of these conditions.

KNEE JOINT REHABILITATION

Rehabilitation of the injured knee joint in an athlete presents a challenge to the athletic trainer who is overseeing the rehabilitation process.[54] The goal of every rehabilitation program is to achieve return to normal activity. For the athlete, "normal" activity involves psychological and physiological stresses that are at a considerably higher level than those experienced by the average person in the population. The athletic trainer must assume the responsibility for rehabilitating the whole athlete and not just the injured knee.

Every athlete who is injured must be treated individually. The athletic trainer who attempts to use a cookbook approach to rehabilitation protocols will become frustrated because a rehabilitation program needs the flexibility to be altered based on the specific needs of the individual athlete.[69]

It is difficult for anyone supervising rehabilitation programs to stay abreast of the newest techniques and philosophies, which are constantly being updated or altered. This difficulty is perhaps more true for injuries involving the knee joint than any other body part. Rapid advances in technology and surgical techniques, along with an ever-increasing understanding of the physiological, biomechanical, and neural components of knee function, have drastically and repeatedly changed the approach to knee rehabilitation in recent years.

General Body Conditioning

The athlete must work hard to maintain levels of cardiorespiratory endurance. Full return to activity will be delayed if endurance levels must be improved after the injured knee is rehabilitated. The athlete can engage in non–weight bearing activities such as using an upper-extremity ergometer, aquatic exercise, and if range of motion permits, riding a stationary bicycle (see Figure 4-21). It is essential for the athlete to concentrate on maintaining existing levels of strength, flexibility, and proprioception in all other areas of the body throughout the rehabilitation process.

Weight Bearing

Generally, it is best for the athlete to go non–weight bearing on crutches for at least one to two days after acute injury to the knee. This precaution will allow the healing process to progress well into the inflammatory stage before the athlete does anything that may interfere with healing. Frequently the athlete will be allowed to progress gradually to weight bearing while continuing to wear a rehabilitative brace. The athlete should then progress to touch down weight bearing, to three-point gait, to four-point gait, and finally, to full weight bearing as soon as the healing constraints of the particular injury allow. Injured structures in the knee joint will not heal fully until they are subjected to normal tensile forces and strains.

Knee Joint Mobilization

Mobilization techniques should be incorporated as early as possible to reduce the arthrofibrosis that normally occurs with immobilization.[69] After surgery, patellar mobility is generally considered to be the key to regaining normal knee motion. Patellar mobilizations that include medial, lateral, superior, and inferior glides should be used along

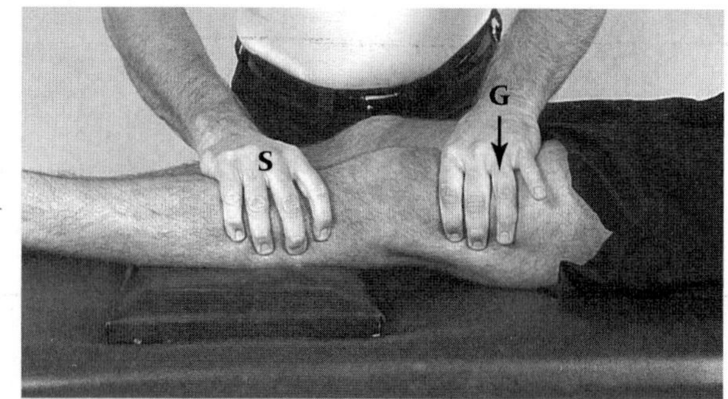

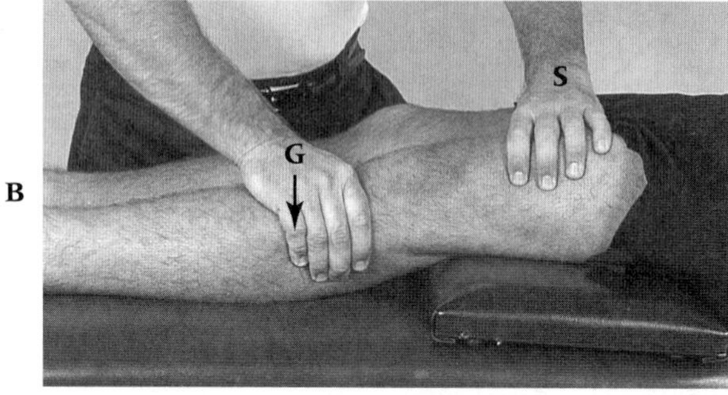

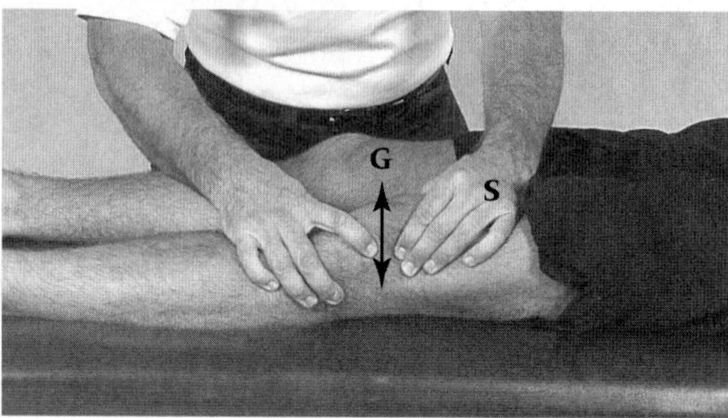

Figure 20-52

Knee mobilization techniques.
A, Posterior femoral glides.
B, Posterior tibial glides.
C, Patellar glides.
(S = Stabilize, G = Glide)

with anterior and posterior tibial glides to ensure the return of normal joint arthrokinematics (Figure 20-52). Constant passive motion (CPM) machines are commonly used to maintain motion in a pain-free arc immediately after surgery (Figure 20-53).

Flexibility

Regaining full range of motion after knee injury is one of the most critical aspects of a knee rehabilitation program. Regardless of whether an injury is treated conservatively or surgically, efforts toward achieving full range of movement are begun on the first day. The athletic trainer should emphasize active ROM exercises throughout the rehabilitation program. Once normal movement of the knee joint has been achieved, efforts should be directed toward maintaining or improving flexibility of each of the muscle groups surrounding the knee joint through stretching. PNF stretching techniques are most effective.[68]

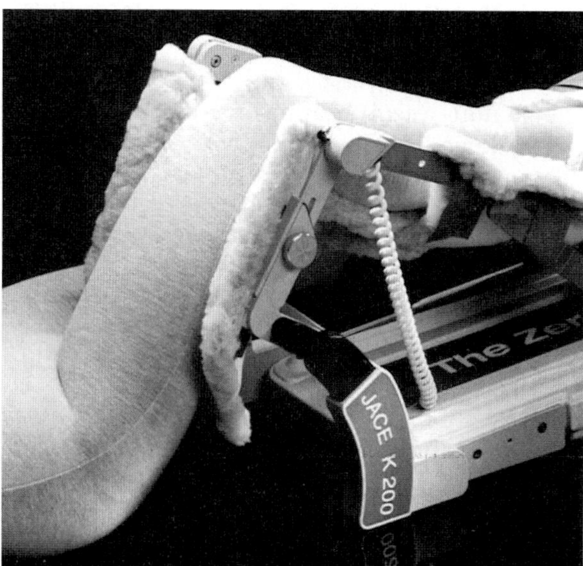

Figure 20-53

Constant passive motion for the knee.

Muscular Strength

Strengthening generally follows a progression from isometric exercise (i.e., straight-leg raises, quad setting) (Figure 20-54), to isotonic exercise stressing both concentric and eccentric components, to isokinetic exercise, to plyometric exercise. It is essential to concentrate on strengthening all the muscle groups that have some function at the knee joint, including the quadriceps, hamstrings, abductors, adductors, and gastrocnemius.[69]

Eccentric muscle contraction should be routinely incorporated into strengthening programs through both isotonic and isokinetic exercise. Eccentric contraction of the quadriceps is necessary for deceleration of the lower leg during running. Conversely, the hamstrings must decelerate the lower leg in a kicking motion.[94] Plyometric exercises used during the later phases of rehabilitation use a quick, eccentric muscle contraction to facilitate a concentric contraction.

Traditionally, rehabilitation has tended to make use of the open kinetic chain strengthening exercises that use ankle band weights, free weights, machines, and so on. It is important to emphasize closed kinetic chain exercises, in which the foot is in contact with the ground.[19] Closed chain activities are more functional and eliminate many of the stress and shearing forces associated with an open-lever system. Thus, they are safer than open chain exercises. Minisquats, step-ups onto a box,[43] leg presses on a machine, and the use of stationary bicycles, stair climbing machines, and exercise tubing are examples of closed chain activities (Figure 20-55).[94] These exercises also emphasize and facilitate cocontraction of antagonistic muscle groups (e.g., quadriceps and hamstrings). This cocontraction aids in providing appropriate neuromuscular control of opposing muscle groups and thus promotes stability about the joint.[69] Strengthening exercises should also incorporate balance and postural control activities.[50]

20-13

***Critical Thinking* Exercise**

A field hockey player is three days postop after reconstruction of her knee using a patellar tendon graft. It is essential that she begin active range-of-motion and strengthening exercises as soon as possible.

? What type of strengthening exercises should the athletic trainer recommend?

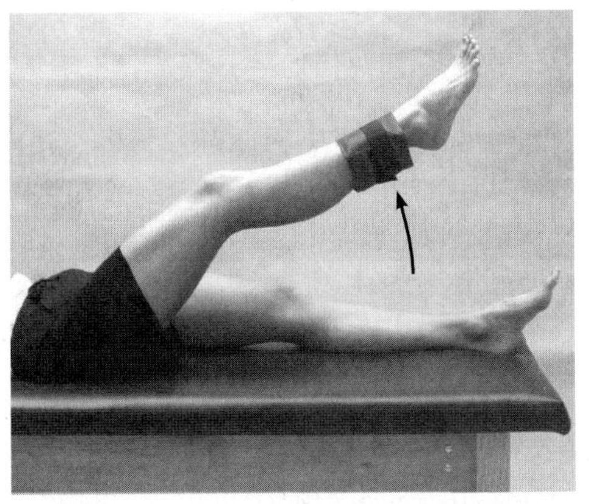

A

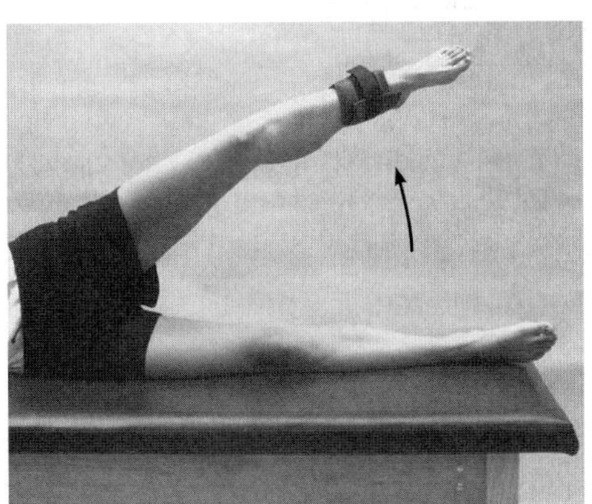

B

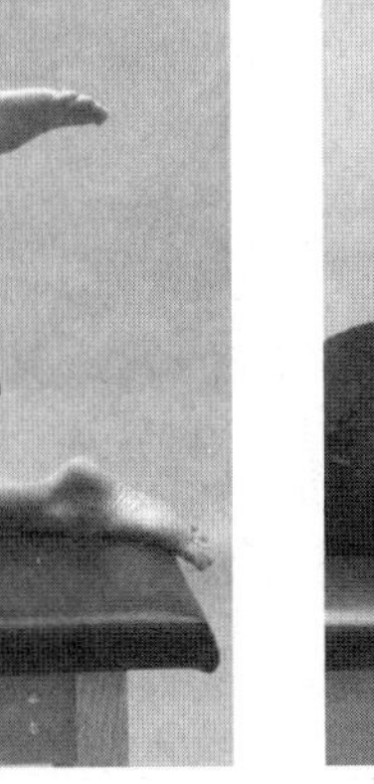

C

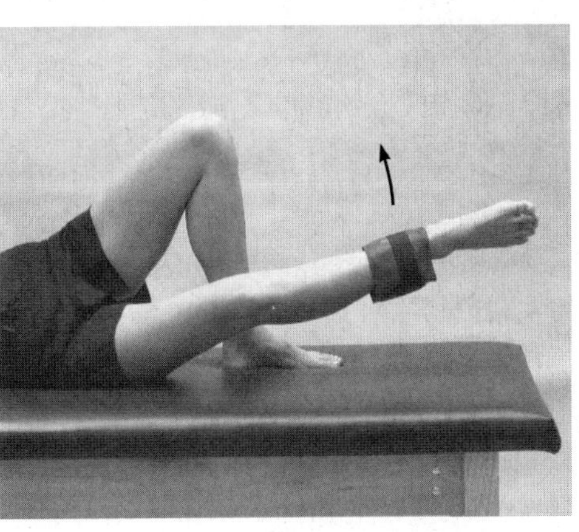

D

Figure 20-54

Straight leg raising with knee slightly flexed. **A,** Hip flexion. **B,** Hip abduction. **C,** Hip extension. **D,** Hip adduction.

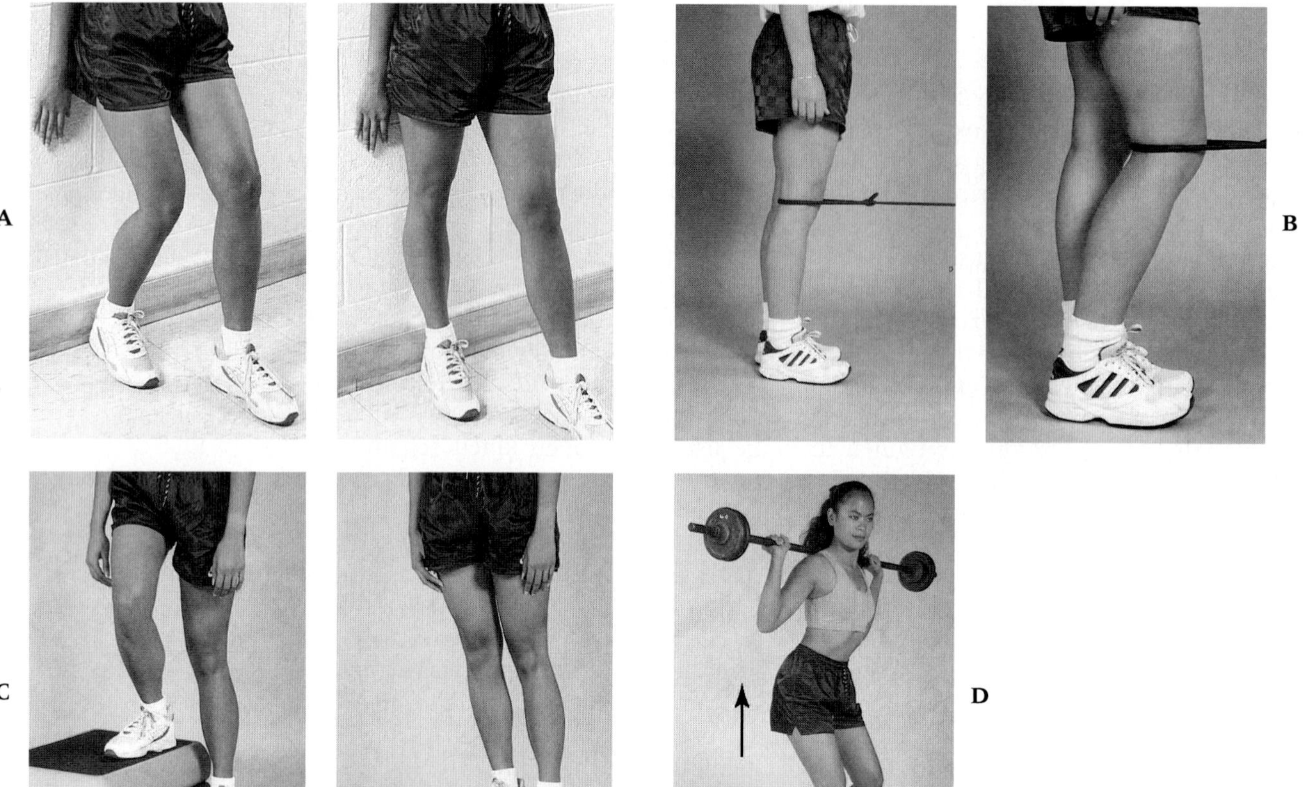

Figure 20-55

Terminal knee extension—closed kinetic chain. **A,** Wall standing—starting position; stopping position. **B,** Using rubber tubing—starting position; stopping position. **C,** Lateral step-ups—starting position; stopping position. **D,** Minisquats.

PNF strengthening techniques using D1 and D2 lower-extremity patterns allow the athletic trainer to work on coordinated movement patterns and, in particular, emphasize the tibial rotation component of knee motion (see Figure 16-12A to 16-12H).[69]

Neuromuscular Control

Regaining neuromuscular control of joint motion after injury is also important. The athlete quickly "forgets" how to contract a muscle after injury. Loss of neuromuscular control usually occurs because of pain inhibition or swelling. Efforts directed toward proprioceptive control are begun immediately after injury to the knee with weight-shifting exercises on crutches, straight-leg lifts, and quad sets. Strengthening and flexibility exercises mentioned previously will help facilitate the return of proprioception. The BAPS board, Bosu Balance trainer rocker board, tremor box, minitramp, and Dynadisc (see Figures 19-36A through F), can all be used to improve proprioception and balance, as can the balance shoes (see Figure 18-42).

Bracing

Rehabilitative knee braces have been designed to allow protected motion of either operative or nonoperative knees.[67] Braces enclose the thigh and calf with fabric fasteners, are lightweight, and are hinged so that motion can be limited within a specific degree range (see Figure 20-56A). Depending on the specific injury or the surgical technique used, the knee must be protected in limited ranges for some period of time. The braces are removed during rehabilitation sessions to allow the athlete to work in the greatest range of motion possible. Rehabilitative braces are typically worn for three to six weeks after surgery.

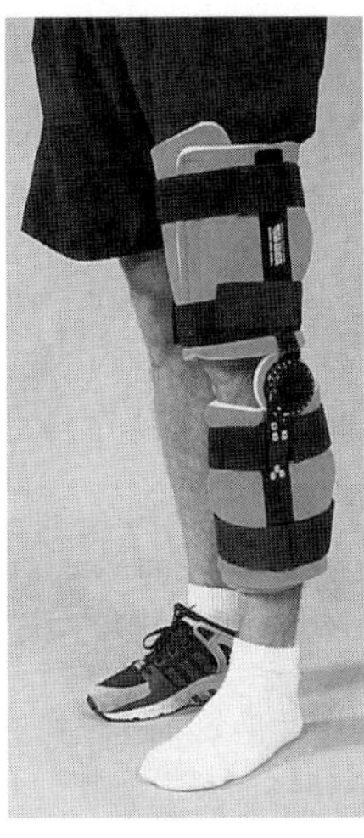
A

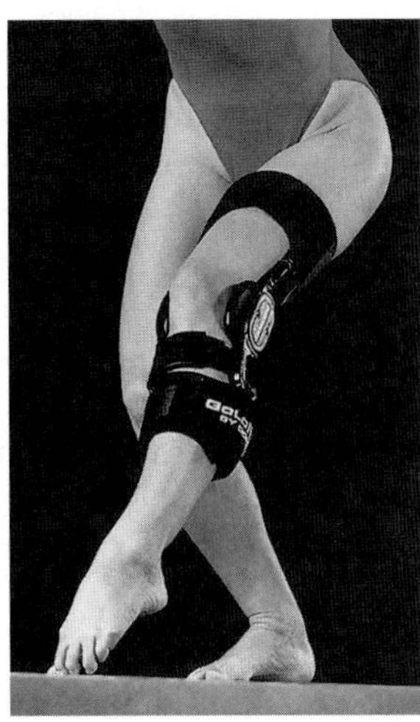
B

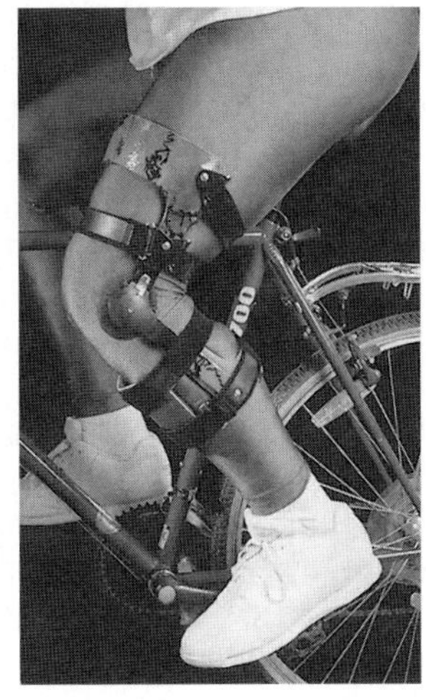
C

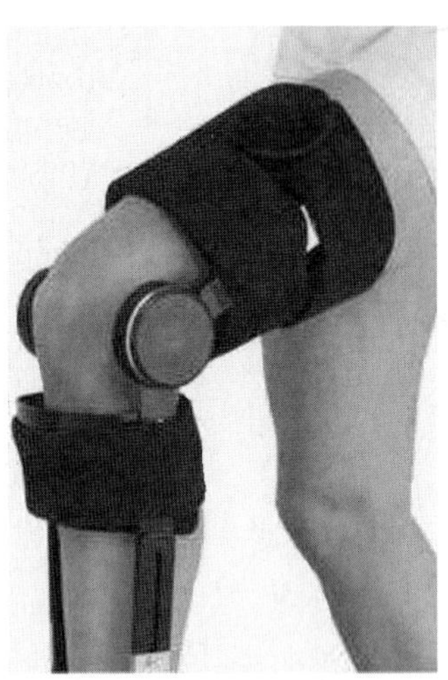
D

Figure 20-56

A, Rehabilitative knee brace.
B & C, Functional knee braces.
D, Functional resistance brace.

Functional knee braces are worn to provide support to the unstable knee on return to activity.[67] All functional braces are custom fitted to some degree and use hinges and posts for support. Some braces use custom-molded thigh and calf enclosures to hold the brace in place, whereas others rely on straps for suspension (Figure 20-56B and C). Braces are designed to improve the stability of the ACL-deficient knee by preventing full extension. Some braces attempt to control rotation or varus force. Functional knee braces alone do not seem to be able to control pathological laxity associated with ACL deficiency. However, if combined with an appropriate rehabilitation program, these braces have been shown to restrict anterior-posterior translation of the tibia at low loads.

Functional resistance braces have been designed for use in individuals who have patellofemoral pain syndrome (Figure 20-56D). This brace provides variable resistance to knee flexion that can be adjusted to provide progressive increasing resistance. The brace is worn both during rehabilitative exercise and during activities of daily living.[18]

Functional Progression

Sport-specific skills should be broken down into component parts, and the athlete should be gradually reintroduced to them and should progress through their individual components. For the athlete with an injured knee, a gradual return to running is essential. The athlete should begin with walking (forward, backward, straight line, curve) and progress to jogging (straight, curve, uphill, downhill), running (forward, backward), and then sprinting (straight, curve, large figure-eight, small figure-eight, zigzag, carioca).[45]

Return to Activity

The decision to permit the athlete to return to full activity should be based on a number of criteria.[13] It is perhaps most important to make sure that the healing process has been given a sufficient chance to repair the injured structure. Objective criteria for return include isokinetic evaluation (torque values of at least 90 percent of the uninjured extremity), arthrometer measurement, and functional performance tests (figure-eights at speed, carioca, hop test, etc.).[90]

SUMMARY

- The knee is a hinge joint that also glides and has some rotation, it is also one of the most traumatized joints in sports. Three types of structures are most often injured: the medial and lateral collateral capsules and ligaments, the menisci, and the cruciate ligaments.

- Knee injuries may be avoided if athletes maximize muscle strength and wear appropriate shoes. The use of protective knee bracing is questionable.
- Ligamentous and capsular sprains occur frequently to the medial aspect of the knee and less often to the lateral aspect. The most common ligamentous injury occurs to the anterior cruciate ligament.
- A meniscus can be injured in a variety of ways, including a rotary force to the knee with the foot planted, a sudden valgus or varus force, or sudden flexion or extension of the knee. There may be severe pain and loss of motion, locking of the knee, and pain in the area of the tear.
- The patella and its surrounding area can develop a variety of injuries from sports activities. Some of these injuries are fracture, dislocation, and chronic articular degeneration such as chondromalacia. Other conditions in the region include Osgood-Schlatter disease and jumper's knee.
- The goal of the knee rehabilitation program is to restore the athlete's muscular strength, power, endurance, flexibility, neuromuscular control, and functional capability. The program varies according to the sport and condition.

Websites

Knee 1.com: http://www.knee1.com

This is a complete, free knee resource. Find healing technology/rehabilitation for knee pain, ACL injuries, osteoarthritis, other diseases, and knee replacements. Talk online to surgeons and patients.

Iliotibial Band Syndrome: http://www. itbs.info

ITBS is a common running and cycling injury around the knee. This site lists causes, therapies, treatments, and personal experiences with this problem.

What is Chondromalacia? http://healthlink.mcw.edu/article/926052680.html

This article discusses the causes and treatment of the knee disorder chondromalacia patellae.

World Ortho: http://www.worldortho.com

Wheeless' Textbook of Orthopaedics: http://www.wheelessonline.com

Anatomy of the Knee Tutorial: http://scoi.com/kneeanat.htm

Knee Surgery Information: http://www.arthroscopy.com

MEDLINEplus: Knee Injuries and Disorders www.nlm.nih.gov/medlineplus/kneeinjuriesanddisorders.html

A site from the National Institute of Health for research on knee injuries and disorders.

Solutions to Critical Thinking EXERCISES

20-1 When the athlete is weight bearing with the knee in full extension, the femur is internally rotated relative to the tibia and is "locked" in this position. The collateral, the cruciates, and the capsular ligaments are tightest in full extension and tend to become more relaxed when moving into flexion. It is possible to injure any of the ligaments in full extension. The posterior cruciate has the least chance of being injured when the knee is fully extended.

20-2 During the evaluation, the athletic trainer should look for tightness of the hamstrings or gastrocnemius, tightness of the lateral retinaculum, increased Q angle, tightness of the iliotibial band, pronation of the foot, patella alta, vastus medialis oblique (VMO) insufficiency, inhibition resulting from the presence of effusion in the knee, or weak hip adductors to which the VMO is attached.

20-3 A valgus stress test should be used to test the MCL. The examination in full extension tests the MCL, posteromedial capsule, and the cruciates. At 30 degrees of flexion, the MCL is isolated. If some instability is present with the knee in full extension, the athletic trainer should closely evaluate the integrity of the cruciate ligaments.

20-4 This mechanism is typical for a sprain of the anterior cruciate ligament, although other ligamentous, capsular, and meniscal structures may be injured as well. Appropriate stability tests for the ACL include the anterior drawer test done in neutral, internal, and external rotation; the Lachman test; the pivot-shift test; the jerk test; and the flexion-rotation drawer test.

20-5 If the baseball player still is concerned about his knee not being ready to return to full activity, then he is not ready, regardless of whether he is wearing a knee brace. The athletic trainer should design a series of functional progression activities that will help the athlete gain confidence in his abilities while continuing to work on strengthening and neuromuscular control exercises. If the athlete feels strongly about wearing a brace, the athletic trainer should make every effort to provide him with one despite the fact that the literature supporting the use of functional knee braces is unclear.

20-6 It is important to understand that once a ligament has been sprained, the inherent stability provided to the joint by that ligament has been lost and will never be totally regained. Thus, the athlete must rely on the other structures that surround the joint—the muscles and their tendons—to help provide stability. It is essential for the athlete to work hard at strengthening all the muscle groups that play a role in the function of the knee joint.

20-7 The most common mechanism is weight bearing combined with a rotary force while the knee is extended or flexed. A large number of medial meniscus lesions are the outcome of a sudden, strong internal rotation of the femur with a partially flexed knee while the foot is firmly planted. Another way a longitudinal tear occurs is by forceful extension of the knee from a flexed position while the femur is internally rotated. During extension, the medial meniscus is suddenly pulled back, causing the tear.

20-8 It is likely that the athlete has an inflamed or irritated mediopatellar plica. The mediopatellar plica may be thick, nonyielding, and fibrotic, which can cause a number of symptoms. The presence of an inflamed mediopatellar plica is sometimes associated with chondromalacia of the medial femoral condyle and patella.

20-9 The injury is most likely prepatellar bursitis due to the extracapsular swelling pattern, redness, and the mechanism of injury. A possible fracture should be ruled out as well. Ballotable patella or a sweep maneuver can be used to evaluate the swelling pattern to determine whether the swelling is intracapsular or extracapsular.

20-10 The athletic trainer should recommend that the athlete reduce the length of her training sessions, in particular, limiting the running phase of training. Pain-free isometric exercises to strengthen the quadriceps and hamstring muscles can be used initially, and the athlete can progress to closed kinetic chain strengthening exercises. Oral antiinflammatory agents and small doses of aspirin may also be helpful. A neoprene knee sleeve may also help modulate pain. Use of an orthotic device to correct pronation and reduce tibial torsion can sometimes help eliminate pain.

20-11 It is likely that this athlete has chondromalacia patella. The athletic trainer should recommend avoiding irritating activities such as stair climbing and squatting. The athletic trainer should recommend isometric exercises that are pain free to strengthen the quadriceps and hamstring muscles and wearing a neoprene knee sleeve. If conservative measures fail to help, surgery may be the only alternative.

20-12 A conservative approach would be to use the normal techniques to reduce inflammation, such as rest, ice, ultrasound, and antiinflammatory medications. An alternative and more aggressive technique would be to use a deep transverse friction massage technique to increase the inflammatory response, which will ultimately facilitate healing. If successful, the more aggressive treatment may allow a quicker return to full activity.

20-13 Closed kinetic chain strengthening exercises such as mini-squats, lateral or forward step-ups onto a box, leg presses on a machine, terminal knee extensions using exercise tubing, and use of stationary bicycles, stair climbing machines, and stepping machines are all appropriate exercises that can be used safely and effectively almost immediately after surgery. Limited range of motion secondary to pain and swelling may restrict the athlete's ability to perform these strengthening exercises.

REVIEW QUESTIONS AND CLASS ACTIVITIES

1. Describe the major structural and functional anatomical features of the knee.
2. Explain how a knee injury can best be prevented. What injuries are most difficult to prevent?
3. Demonstrate the steps that should be taken when assessing a knee injury.
4. Describe the symptoms, signs, and management of knee contusions and bursitis.
5. Distinguish collateral ligament sprains from cruciate sprains.
6. What is the difference between a meniscal lesion and a knee plica?
7. Explain how different fractures (e.g., patellar and epiphyseal fractures) may occur in the knee.
8. Describe the relationship of loose bodies within the knee to osteochondritis dissecans.
9. How do the patella fracture and the patellar dislocation occur?
10. Compare the causes of patellofemoral arthralgia.
11. What types of injuries can occur to the extensor mechanism in a physically immature athlete?
12. Describe and compare the iliotibial band friction syndrome and pes anserinus tendinitis or bursitis.
13. What causes the knee to collapse?
14. Describe knee rehabilitation after conservative treatment of a second-degree medial collateral sprain and after surgical repair of a torn anterior cruciate ligament.

REFERENCES

1. Arangio G, Cohen E: Incidence of associated knee lesions with torn anterior cruciate ligament: retrospective cohort assessment, *J Sport Rehabil* 7(1):1, 1998.
2. Arendt EA, Agel J, Dick R: Anterior cruciate ligament injury patterns among collegiate men and women, *J Ath Train* 34(2):86, 1999.
3. Arno S: The A angle: a quantitive measurement of patella alignment and realignment, *J Orthop Sports Phys Ther* 12(6):237, 1990.
4. Arnoczky SP, Warren RF: Microvasculature of the human meniscus, *Am J Sports Med* 10:90, 1982.
5. Arnosky P: Physiologic principles of ligament injuries and healing. In Scott N, editor: *Ligament and extensor mechanism injuries of the knee: diagnosis and treatment,* St Louis, 1991, Mosby.
6. Baker MM, Juhn MS: Patellofemoral pain syndrome in the female athlete, *Clin Sports Med* 19(2):315, 2000.
7. Bazluki J: Surgical intervention and rehabilitation of chronic patellar tendinitis, *J Ath Train* 31(1):65, 1996.
8. Bedigrew S: Inexpensive Osgood-Schlatter management. *Athletic Therapy Today* 8(3):54, 2003.
9. Bernstein J: Meniscal tears of the knee: diagnosis and individualized treatment, *Physician Sportsmed* 28(3):83, 2000.
10. Birmingham TB, Kramer JF, Kirkley A: Knee bracing after ACL reconstruction: effects on postural control and proprioception, *Med Sci Sports Exerc* 33(8):1253, 2001.
11. Boden BP, Griffin LY, Garrett WE: Etiology and prevention of noncontact ACL injury, *Physician Sportsmed* 28(4):53, 2000.
12. Bonci C: Assessment and evaluation of predisposing factors to anterior cruciate ligament injury, *J Ath Train* 34(2):155, 1999.
13. Borsa PA, Lephart SM, Irrgang JJ: Sport-specificity of knee scoring systems to assess disability in anterior cruciate ligament-deficient athletes, *J Sport Rehabil* 7(1):44, 1998.
14. Brindle T, Nyland J, Johnson DL: The meniscus: review of basic principles with application to surgery and rehabilitation, *J Ath Train* 36(2):160, 2001.
15. Callaghan MJ: The effects of patellar taping on knee joint proprioception. *J Ath Train* 37(1):19–24, 2002.
16. Caraffa A, et al: Prevention of anterior cruciate ligament injuries in soccer: a prospective controlled study of proprioceptive training, *Knee Surgery, Sport Traumatology, Arthroscopy* 4(1):19, 1996.
17. Cosgerea AJ: Evaluation and management of the unstable patella, *Physician Sportsmed* 30(10):33, 2002.
18. Earl J, Piazza S, Hertel J: The Protonics brace unloads the quadriceps muscle in healthy subjects, *J Ath Train* 39(1):44, 2004.
19. Escamilla RF, Fleisig GS, Zheng N: Biomechanics of the knee during closed kinetic chain and open kinetic chain exercises, *Med Sci Sports Exerc* 30(4):556, 1998.
20. Fagenbaum R: Jump landing strategies in male and female college athletes and the implications of such strategies for anterior crucial ligament injuries, *Am J SportsMed* 31(2):233, 2003.

21. Gastel J et al: Surgical management for the athlete with a PCL-deficient knee, *J Sport Rehabil* 8(4):289, 1999.
22. Gilleard W, McConnell J, Parsons D: The effect of patellar taping on the onset of vastus medialis obliquus and vastus lateralis muscle activity in persons with patellofemoral pain, *Phys Ther* 78(1):25, 1998.
23. Gray JC: Neural and vascular anatomy of the menisci of the human knee, *J Orthop Sports Phys Ther* 29(1):23, 1999.
24. Greene DL, Hamson KR, Bay RC, Bryce CD: Effects of protective knee bracing on speed and agility, *Am J Sports Med* 28(4):453, 2000.
25. Grelsamer RP, Klein JR: The biomechanics of the patellofemoral joint, *J Orthop Sports Phys Ther* 28(5):286, 1998.
26. Griffin LY, Agel J, Albohm MJ: Noncontact anterior cruciate ligament injuries: risk factors and prevention strategies, *Journal American Academy Orthopaedic Surgeon* 8(3):141, 2000.
27. Griffis ND, Vequist SW, Yearout KM, Henning CE, Lynch MA: Injury prevention of the anterior cruciate ligament. Presented at American Orthopaedic Society for Sports Medicine, Traverse City, Mich, June 1999.
28. Harner C, Vogrin T, Woo S: Anatomical and biomechanical considerations of the PCL, *J Sport Rehabil* 8(4):260, 1999.
29. Heitz NA et al: Hormonal changes throughout the menstrual cycle and increased anterior cruciate ligament laxity in females, *J Ath Train* 34(2):144, 1999.
30. Hewett TE, Stroupe AL, Nance TA, Noyes FR: Plyometric training in female athletes: decreased impact forces and increased hamstring torques, *Am J Sports Med* 24(6):765, 1996.
31. Hewett TE: Neuromuscular and hormonal factors associated with knee injuries in female athletes: strategies for intervention, *Sports Med* 29(5):313, 2000.
32. Holmes SW, Clancy WG: Clinical classification of patellofemoral pain and dysfunction, *J Orthop Sports Phys Ther* 28(5):299, 1998.
33. Hurley WL: Influences of clinician technique on performance and interpretation of the Lachman test. *J Ath Train* 38(1):34, 2003.
34. Indelicato P: Isolated MCL tear: nonoperative management. In Torg J, Shephard R, editors: *Current therapy in sports medicine,* St Louis, 1995, Mosby.
35. Ingersoll CD: Assessment of patellofemoral pain, *Athletic Therapy Today* 3(2):45, 1998.
36. Ireland ML: Anterior cruciate ligament injury in female athletes: epidemiology, *J Ath Train* 34(2):150, 1999.
37. Irrgang J, Harner C: Recent advances in ACL rehabilitation: clinical factors that influence the program, *J Sport Rehabil* 6(2):111, 1997.
38. Janousek AT, Jones DG, Clatworthy M, Higgins LD, Fu FH: Posterior cruciate ligament injuries of the knee joint, *Sports Med* 28(6):429, 1999.
39. Laprade J, Culham E, Brouwer B: Comparison of five isometric exercises in the recruitment of the vastus medialis oblique in persons with and without patellofemoral pain syndrome, *J Orthop Sports Phys Ther* 27(3):197, 1998.
40. Lathinghouse LH, Trimble MH: Effects of isometric quadriceps activation on the Q-angle in women before and after quadriceps exercise, *J Orthop Sports Phys Ther* 30(4):211, 2000.
41. Livingston L: The quadriceps angle: a review of the literature, *J Orthop Sports Phys Ther* 28(2):105, 1998.
42. Loudon JK, Goist HL, Loudon KL: Genu recurvatum syndrome, *J Orthop Sports Phys Ther* 27(5):361, 1998.
43. Loudon J, Wiesner D, Goist-Foley H: Intrarater reliability of functional performance tests for individuals with patellofemoral pain syndrome, *J Ath Train* 37(3):256, 2002.
44. Lynch M, Henning C: Physical examination of the knee. In Nicholas J, Hershman E, editors: *The lower extremity and spine in sports medicine,* St Louis, 1995, Mosby.
45. MacLean CL: Functional rehabilitation for the PCL-deficient knee. *Athletic Therapy Today* 6(6):32, 2001.
46. Mangine R, Kremchek T: Evaluation-based protocol of the anterior cruciate ligament, *J Sport Rehabil* 6(2):157, 1997.
47. Martin D, Guskiewicz K, Perrin D: Tibial rotation affects anterior displacement of the knee, *J Sport Rehab* 3(4):275, 1994.
48. Martin M: Problematic external wound healing after ACL-reconstructive surgery. *Athletic Therapy Today* 7(3):36, 2002.
49. Matheny M: Acute, traumatic rupture of the PCL, ACL, and MCL with patellar dislocation. *Athletic Therapy Today* 6(3):52, 2001.
50. Mattacola C, Perriin D, Gansneder B: Strength, Functional outcome, and postural stability after anterior cruciate ligament reconstruction, *J Ath Train* 37(3):262, 2002.
51. Miller JP, Sedory D, Croce RV: Vastus medialis obliquus and vastus lateralis activity in patients with and without patellofemoral pain syndrome, *J Sport Rehabil* 6(1):1, 1997.
52. Mont M, Scott N: Classification of ligament injuries. In Scott N, editor: *Ligament and extensor mechanism injuries of the knee: diagnosis and treatment,* St Louis, 1991, Mosby.
53. Moul JL: Differences in selected predictors of anterior cruciate ligament tears between male and female NCAA Division I collegiate basketball players, *J Ath Train* 33(2):118, 1998.
54. Mullin MJ: Functional rehabilitation of the knee, *Athletic Therapy Today* 5(2):28, 2000.
55. Nichols C, Johnson R: Cruciate ligament injuries: nonoperative treatment. In Scott N, editor: *Ligament and extensor mechanism injuries of the knee: diagnosis and treatment,* St Louis, 1991, Mosby.
56. Norkus SA: Advantages of the prone Lachman Test. *Athletic Therapy Today* 7(2):52, 2002.
57. Noyes F, Grood E: Classification of ligament injuries: why an anterolateral or anteromedial laxity is not a diagnostic entity. In Griffin P, editor: *Instructional course lectures,* Park Ridge, Ill, 1987, American Academy of Orthopaedic Surgeons.
58. Onate JA, Guskiewicz KM, Sullivan RJ: Augmented feedback reduces jump-landing forces, *J Orthop Sports Phys Ther* 31(9):511, 2001.
59. Onate JA: Non-contact knee injury prevention plan (NC-LEIPP). Workshop presented at National Athletic Trainers' Association 52d Annual Meeting, Los Angeles, Calif, June 2001.
60. Pellecchia G, Hame H, Behnke P: Treatment of infrapatellar tendinitis: a combination of modalities and transverse friction massage, *J Sport Rehab* 3(2):125, 1994.
61. Pepe MD: Assessment and surgical decision making for PCL injuries in athletes. *Athletic Therapy Today* 6(6):9, 2001.
62. Peters TA, McLean ID: Osteochondritis dissecans of the patellofemoral joint, *Am J Sports Med* 28(1):63, 2000.
63. Pitman M, Frankel V: Biomechanics of the knee in athletics. In Nicholas J, Hershman E, editors: *The lower extremity and spine in sports medicine,* St Louis, 1995, Mosby.
64. Pizzari T, McBurney H, Taylor N: Adherence to anterior cruciate ligament rehabilitation: a qualitative analysis. *J Sport Rehabil* 11(2):90, 2002.
65. Post WR: Patellofemoral pain: let the physical exam define treatment, *Physician Sportsmed* 26(1):68, 1998.
66. Powers CM: Rehabilitation of patellofemoral joint disorders: a critical review, *J Orthop Sports Phys Ther* 28(5):345, 1998.
67. Powers CM, Shellock FG, Beering TV, Garrido DE, Goldbach RM, Molnar T: Effect of bracing on patellar kinematics in patients with patellofemoral joint pain, *Med Sci Sports Exerc* 31(12):1714, 1999.
68. Prentice WE: Techniques of manual therapy in the injured knee, *J Sport Rehabil* 1(3):249, 1992.
69. Prentice W, Onate J: Rehabilitation of the knee. In Prentice W, editor: *Rehabilitation techniques in sports medicine and athletic training,* St Louis, 2004, McGraw-Hill.
70. Prentice W, Toriscelli T: The effects of lateral knee stabilizing braces on running speed and agility, *Ath Train* 21(2):112, 1986.
71. Racioppi EA, Gulick DT: Iliotibial band friction syndrome, *Athletic Therapy Today* 4(5):9, 1999.

72. Reinold MM: Rehabilitation after PCL reconstruction. *Athletic Therapy Today* 6(6):23, 2001.
73. Rettig A: Medial and lateral ligament injuries. In Scott N, editor: *Ligament and extensor mechanism injuries of the knee: diagnosis and treatment,* St Louis, 1991, Mosby.
74. Risberg MA et al: Prospective study of changes in impairments and disabilities after anterior cruciate ligament reconstruction, *J Orthop Sports Phys Ther* 29(7):400, 1999.
75. Roberts D et al: Proprioception in people with anterior cruciate ligament–deficient knees: comparison of symptomatic and asymptomatic patients, *J Orthop Sports Phys Ther* 29(10):587, 2000.
76. Rosene JM, Fogarty TD: Anterior tibial translation in collegiate athletes with normal anterior cruciate ligament integrity, *J Ath Train* 34(2):93, 1999.
77. Ryder S, et al: Prevention of ACL injuries, *J Sport Rehabil* 6(2):80, 1997.
78. Safran M et al: Effects of injury and reconstruction of the posterior cruciate ligament on proprioception and neuromuscular control, *J Sport Rehabil* 8(4):304, 1999.
79. Shelbourne D, Gray T: Natural history study of athletes with PCL-deficient knees, *J Sport Rehabil* 8(4):279, 1999.
80. Shelbourne D, Klootwyk T, De Carlo M: Ligamentous injuries. In Griffin L, editor: *Rehabilitation of the injured knee,* St Louis, 1995, Mosby.
81. Shelbourne D, Trumper R: Accelerated rehabilitation after ACL reconstruction. In Torg J, Shephard R, editors: *Current therapy in sports medicine,* St Louis, 1995, Mosby.
82. Slauterbeck J, Fuzie S, Smith M: The menstrual cycle, sex, hormones, and anterior cruciate ligament injury. *J Ath Train* 37(3):275, 2002.
83. Somes S, Worrell TW, Corey B, Ingersol CD: Effects of patellar taping on patellar position in the open and closed kinetic chain: a preliminary study, *J Sport Rehabil* 6(4):299, 1997.
84. Tegner Y, Lysholm J: Rating systems in the evaluation of knee ligament injuries, *Clin Orthop* 198:43, 1985.
85. Thomee R, Augustsson J, Karlsson J: Patellofemoral pain syndrome: a review of current issues, *Sports Med* 28(4):245, 1999.
86. Toy B et al: Anatomy of the ACL: influence on anterior drawer and Lachman test, *Athletic Therapy Today* 4(2):54, 1999.
87. Tria A, Hosea T: Clinical diagnosis of knee ligament injuries. In Scott N, editor: *Ligament and extensor mechanism injuries of the knee: diagnosis and treatment,* St Louis, 1991, Mosby.
88. Trulock S: Modifying postsurgical ACL rehabilitation for associated pathology. *Athletic Therapy Today* 7(4):34, 2002.
89. Udry E, Shelbourne D, Gray T: Psychological readiness for anterior cruciate ligament surgery: describing and comparing the adolescent and adult experiences, *J Ath Train* 38(2):176, 2003.
90. Urabe Y, Ochi M, Onari K: Changes in isokinetic muscle strength of the lower extremity in recreational athletes with anterior cruciate ligament reconstruction, *J Sport Rehabil* 11(4):252, 2002.
91. Van Lunen B, Roberts J, Branch D: Association of menstrual-cycle hormone changes with anterior cruciate laxity measurements, *J Ath Train* 38(4):298, 2003.
92. Weiss J et al: A functional assessment of anterior cruciate ligament deficiency in an acute and clinical setting, *J Orthop Sports Phys Ther* 11(8):372, 1990.
93. Wilk K, et al: Kinetic chain exercise: implications for the anterior cruciate ligament patient, *J Sport Rehabil* 6(2):125, 1997.
94. Wilk KE, Arrigo C, Andrews J: Rehabilitation after anterior cruciate ligament reconstruction in the female athlete, *J Ath Train* 34(2):177, 1999.
95. Wilk KE: Patellofemoral disorders: a classification system and clinical guidelines for nonoperative rehabilitation, *J Orthop Sports Phys Ther* 28(5):307, 1998.
96. Wilkerson GB: Quadriceps strength and knee osteoarthritis, *Athletic Therapy Today* 8(1):25, 2003.
97. Wilson JK, Sevier TL, Helfst R: A comparison of rehabilitation methods in the treatment of patellar tendinitis, *J Sport Rehabil* 9(4):304, 2000.
98. Wu GKH, Ng GYF, Mak AFT: Effects of knee bracing on the functional performance of patients with anterior cruciate ligament reconstruction, *Arch Phys Med Rehabil* 82(2):282, 2001.
99. Yasuda K, Yohyama H, Inoue M: The effect of PCL injury on muscle performance, *J Sport Rehabil* 8(4):322, 1999.

ANNOTATED BIBLIOGRAPHY

Ellenbecker T: *Knee ligament rehabilitation,* Philadelphia, 2000, Churchill-Livingston.

This book provides data to diagnose and rehabilitate knee ligament injuries. Includes protocols for nonoperative and postoperative rehabilitation.

Fanelli, G: *The multiple ligament injured knee,* New York, 2004, Springer-Verlag.

This text presents a review of the most recent and advanced knowledge needed to successfully diagnose and treat knee ligament injuries.

Fulkerson J, Buuck D, Post W: *Disorders of the patellofemoral joint,* Baltimore, 2004, Lippincott, Williams & Wilkins.

This text explains such aspects of patellofemoral joint conditions as the normal anatomy, biomechanics, nonarthritic anterior knee pain, dysplasias, patellar dislocation, nonoperative and surgical treatments, and chronic pain.

Grelsamer R, McConnell J: *The patella: a team approach,* Austin, TX, 2004, PRO-ED, Inc.

This text provides a comprehensive discussion that concentrates specifically on the patella from both a physician's and a physical therapist's perspective.

Griffin L: *Rehabilitation of the knee,* St Louis, 1995, Mosby.

This text incorporates new advances in rehabilitation techniques and equipment and emphasizes to sport-specific functional rehabilitation programs.

Nicholas J, Hershman E: *The lower extremity and spine in sports medicine,* St Louis, 1995, Mosby.

This two-volume set looks at the entire lower extremity and spine; it is an excellent comprehensive reference for all joints.

Prentice W: *Rehabilitation techniques in sports medicine and athletic training,* St Louis, 2004, McGraw-Hill.

This is a comprehensive, well-illustrated text on rehabilitation techniques used in sports medicine. Chapter 23 deals specifically with rehabilitation of the knee and provides up-to-date recommendations for a rehabilitation program.

Scott N: *Ligament and extensor mechanism injuries of the knee,* St Louis, 1991, Mosby.

This comprehensive text looks at all aspects of the knee joint, including anatomy, biomechanics, ligamentous stability testing, injuries, surgical procedures, bracing, and rehabilitation; it provides an outstanding review of the existing literature on all topics.

Special Issue: Anterior cruciate ligament injury in the female athlete, *Journal of Athletic Training* 34(2), 1999.

The articles in this entire issue are devoted to a discussion of various aspects of ACL injury in female athletes.

Special Issue: Concepts and clinical considerations for the patellofemoral joint, *Journal of Orthopedic and Sports Physical Therapy* 28(5), 1998.

This issue contains a series of articles that are related to the function and rehabilitation of the patellofemoral joint.

Darrow M, Brazina G: *The knee source book,* New York, 2001, McGraw-Hill.

This straightforward guide discusses causes, symptoms, and treatments for common injuries and chronic conditions of the knee and explains what to do immediately after an injury to avoid more harm. It also discusses the benefits of rehab versus surgery.

Chapter 21 The Thigh, Hip, Groin, and Pelvis

When you finish this chapter you should be able to

- Recognize the normal structural anatomy of the thigh.
- Conduct an assessment of the injured thigh.
- Correctly recognize the various injuries that can occur to the different anatomical structures in the thigh.
- Review the anatomy of the pelvis, hip, and groin region.
- Be able to accurately evaluate injuries that occur in or around the groin, hip, and pelvis.
- Outline the etiological factors, symptoms and signs, and management procedures for the injuries that occur in the pelvis, hip, and groin.
- Develop a generalized rehabilitation plan for dealing with injuries to the thigh, hip, pelvis, and groin.

Although the thigh, hip, and pelvis have relatively lower incidences of injury than the knee and ankle, they are subject to considerable trauma from a variety of sports activities. Of major concern are thigh strains and contusions and chronic and overuse stresses affecting the thigh and hip.

ANATOMY OF THE THIGH

The thigh is generally considered that part of the leg between the hip and the knee. Several important anatomical units must be considered in terms of their relationship to sports injuries: the shaft of the femur, musculature, nerves and blood vessels, and the fascia that envelops the thigh.

Bones

The femur (Figure 21-1) is the longest and strongest bone in the body and is designed to permit maximum mobility and support during locomotion. The cylindrical shaft is bowed forward and outward to accommodate the stresses placed on it during bending of the hip and knee and during weight bearing. The proximal head of the femur articulates with the pelvis to form the hip joint, and the distal femoral condyles articulate with the tibia at the knee joint.

Thigh Musculature

The muscles of the thigh may be categorized according to their location: anterior, posterior, and medial (Table 21-1).

Anterior Thigh Muscles

The anterior thigh muscles consist of the sartorius and the quadriceps femoris group. The sartorius muscle (Figure 21-2) consists of a narrow band that is superficial throughout its whole length. It stems from the anterosuperior iliac spine and crosses obliquely downward and medially across the anterior aspect of the thigh where it attaches to the anteromedial aspect of the tibial head. It helps flex the thigh at the hip joint, abducts and outwardly rotates the thigh at the hip joint, and inwardly rotates the flexed knee. When the legs are stabilized, the sartorius acts to flex the pelvis on the thigh. When the sartorius muscle contracts, the pelvis is rotated.

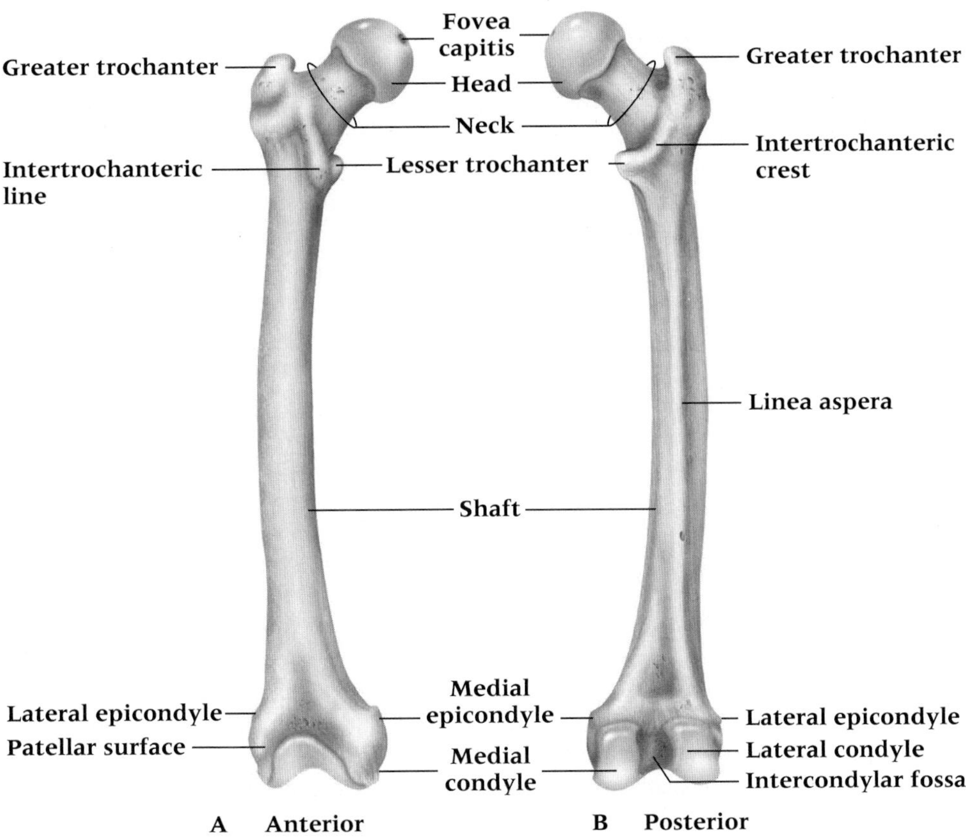

Figure 21-1

The femur. **A,** Anterior view. **B,** Posterior view.

The quadriceps femoris muscle group (Figure 21-2) consists of four muscles: rectus femoris, vastus medialis, vastus lateralis, and vastus intermedius. These four muscles form a common tendon that attaches distally at the superior border of the patella and indirectly into the patellar ligament, which attaches to the tibial tuberosity. The rectus femoris muscle is attached superiorly to the anterior inferior iliac spine and the ilium above the acetabulum and inferiorly to the patella and patellar ligament. The vastus medialis and vastus lateralis muscles originate from the lateral and medial linea aspera of the femur. The vastus intermedius muscle originates mainly from the anterior and lateral portion of the femur. Inferiorly, the three vastus muscles are attached to the rectus femoris muscle and to the lateral and proximal aspects of the patella. Of particular importance is the vastus medialis muscle, which serves as a major stabilizer for patellar tracking.

Posterior Thigh Muscles

The posterior thigh muscles include the popliteus and the hamstring muscles. The function of the popliteus muscle was discussed in Chapter 20. It externally rotates the femur in weight bearing to unlock the knee so that flexion can occur (see Figure 20-6C). Located posteriorly, the hamstring muscle group (Figure 21-2) consists of three muscles: the biceps femoris, semimembranosus, and semitendinosus muscles.

The biceps femoris muscle, as its name implies, has two heads. Its long head originates with the semitendinosus at the medial aspect of the ischial tuberosity. Its short head is attached to the linea aspera below the gluteus maximus attachment on the femur and medial to the attachment of the vastus lateralis. Both muscle heads attach with a common tendon to the head of the fibula.

The semitendinosus muscle originates at the medial aspect of the ischial tuberosity along with the biceps femoris muscle. Together with the semimembranosus muscle, the semitendinosus muscle attaches to the medial aspect of the proximal tibia. This

TABLE 21-1 Muscles of the Thigh

Muscle	Origin	Insertion	Muscle Action	Innervation
Anterior Compartment				
Sartorius	Anterior superior iliac spine	Proximal medial surface of the tibia, below the tuberosity	Flexes the thigh and the leg and laterally rotates the thigh	Femoral
Quadriceps femoris:				
Rectus femoris	Anterior inferior iliac spine and just above the acetabulum of the os coxae	Tibial tuberosity, via the patella and the patellar ligament	Extends the leg; the rectus femoris also flexes the thigh	Femoral
Vastus lateralis	Greater trochanter and lateral lip of the linea aspera of the femur			
Vastus medialis	Medial lip of the linea aspera of the femur			
Vastus intermedias	Anterior surface of the shaft of the femur			
Posterior Compartment				
Hamstrings:				
Biceps femoris	*Long head:* ischial tuberosity *Short head:* lateral lip of the linea aspera	Lateral surface of the head of the fibula, and the lateral condyle of the tibia	Flexes the leg; the long head extends the thigh	Sciatic
Semitendinosus	Ischial tuberosity	Medial surface of the proximal end of the tibia	Flexes the leg and extends the thigh	Tibial
Semimembranosus	Ischial tuberosity	Medial surface of the proximal end of the tibia	Flexes the leg and extends the thigh	Tibial
Medial Compartment				
Adductor magnus **Adductor longus** **Adductor brevis** **Pectineus**	These muscles act only on the femur		Adducts and laterally rotates the thigh	Obturator
Gracilis	Symphysis pubis and the pubic arch	Medial surface of the tibia just below the condyle	Adducts the thigh: flex the leg	Obturator

attachment is just behind those of the sartorius and gracilis muscles, which all together form the pes anserinus tendon. The tibial branch of the sciatic nerve supplies this muscle.

The semimembranosus muscle originates from the lateral aspect of the upper half of the ischeal tuberosity. Moving downward, it attaches into the medial femoral condyle. It also attaches to the medial side of the tibia, the popliteus muscle fascia, and the posterior capsule of the knee joint. The tibial branch of the sciatic nerve supplies this muscle.

Medial Thigh Muscles

The medial thigh muscles include the gracilis, sartorius, pectineus, and three adductor muscles. All act as adductors and lateral rotators of the thigh at the hip joint (Figure 21-2). These muscles collectively make up a part of the anatomic region on the inner thigh referred to as the *groin.*

The gracilis muscle is attached superiorly to the body of the inferior ramus of the pubis and inferiorly to the medial aspect of the proximal tibia. It is a relatively narrow-appearing muscle that adducts the thigh at the hip and flexes and medially rotates the leg at the knee joint. The anterior branch of the obturator nerve serves this muscle.

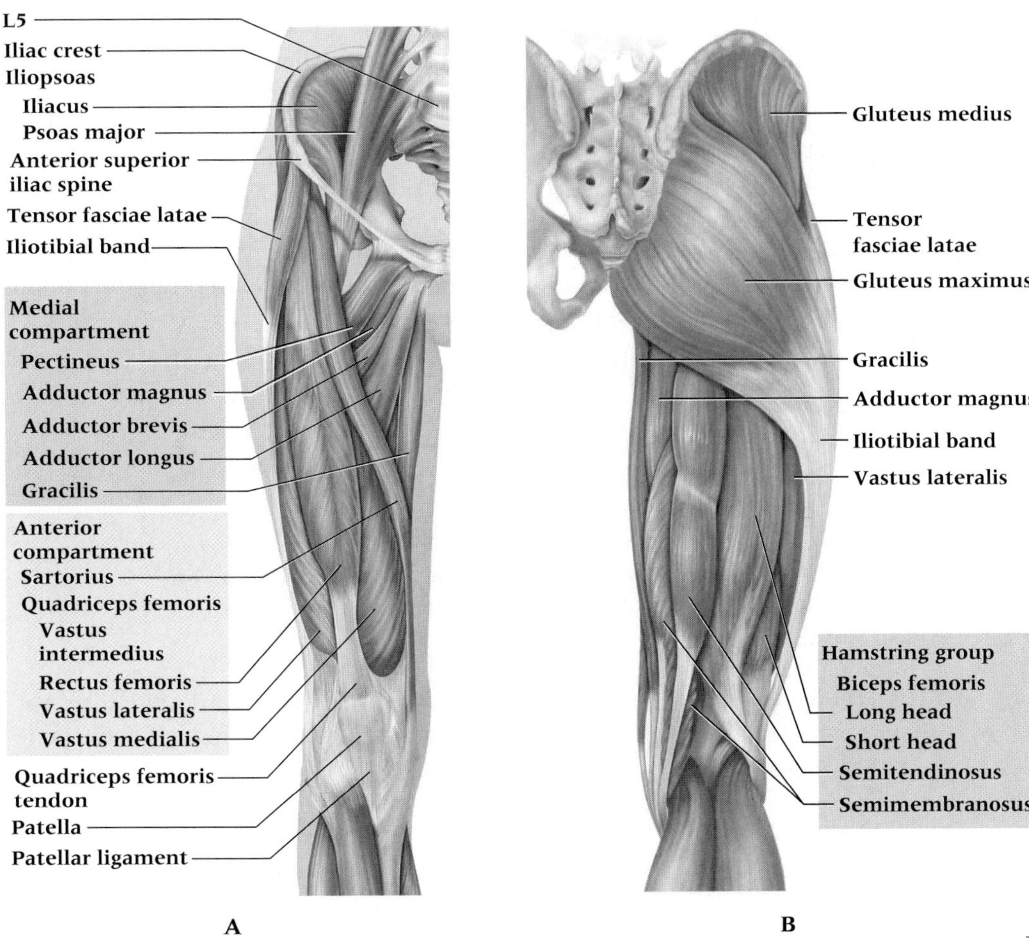

ure 21-2

Muscles of the hip and thigh. **A,** Anterior view. **B,** Posterior view.

The pectineus muscle arises from the pectineal crest of the pubis and attaches distally on the pectineal line of the femur. As one of the adductors, it also flexes and outwardly rotates the thigh.

The adductor longus, brevis, and magnus muscles originate at the ramus of the pubis and attach inferiorly on the linea aspera of the femur. The muscles adduct the thigh at the hip and outwardly rotate the thigh. All these muscles assist in the flexion of the thigh.

Nerve Supply

Among nerves that emerge from the sacral plexus are the tibial and common peroneal nerves, which in the thigh form the largest nerve in the body, the greater sciatic nerve. The sciatic nerve supplies the muscles of the thigh and lower leg (see Figure 21-14, page 673).

Blood Supply

The main arteries that supply the thigh are the medial circumflex femoral, deep femoral, and femoral artery. The two main veins are the superficial great saphenous and the femoral vein (see Figure 21-14).

Fascia

The fascia lata femoris is that part of the deep fascia that invests the thigh musculature. It is relatively thick anteriorly, laterally, and posteriorly but thin on the medial side where it covers the adductors. On its most lateral part, the iliotibial track, an attachment is provided for the tensor fascia lateral and greater aspect of the gluteus maximus.

FUNCTIONAL ANATOMY OF THE THIGH

The quadriceps inserts by a common tendon to the proximal patella. The rectus femoris is the only quadriceps muscle that crosses the hip joint. It not only extends the knee but also flexes the hip. This is very important in differentiating hip flexor strains (i.e. iliopsoas versus rectus femoris) and the ensuing treatment and rehabilitation programs.[17]

The hamstrings all cross the knee joint posteriorly, and all except the short head of the biceps cross the hip joint. These biarticular muscles produce forces that depend upon the position of both the knee joint and the hip joint. The position of the hip and knee during movement and the injury mechanism provide important information for rehabilitating and preventing hamstring injuries.[17]

ASSESSMENT OF THE THIGH

History

The athletic trainer should ask the following questions:

- Was the onset sudden or slow?
- Has this injury occurred before?
- How was the thigh injured?
- Can the athlete describe the intensity or duration of the pain?
- Is the pain constant? If not, when does it occur?
- Can the athlete specify exactly where the pain is?
- Is the pain related to risk?
- What type of pain is there? Muscle pain is dull, achy, and hard to localize. Vascular pain is sharp, bright, and sometimes burning. Bone pain feels deep, penetrating, and highly localized.

Observation

The athletic trainer should compare the thighs:

- Are they symmetrical?
- Are both the same size? Is there swelling?
- Are the skin color and texture normal?
- Is the athlete in obvious pain?
- Is the athlete willing to move the thigh?

Palpation

Both thighs should be palpated for comparison while the athlete is as relaxed as possible.

Bony Palpation

The following bony landmarks should be palpated:

- Medial femoral condyle
- Lateral femoral condyle
- Greater trochanter
- Lesser trochanter
- Anterior superior iliac spine

Soft Tissue Palpation

The following soft tissue structures should be palpated:

Anterior

- Sartorious
- Rectus femoris
- Vastus lateralis
- Vastus medialis
- Vastus intermedialis

Posterior
- Semimembranosis
- Semitendinosis
- Biceps femoris

Medial
- Adductor brevis
- Adductor longus
- Adductor magnus
- Gracilis
- Pectineus

Lateral
- Iliotibial band
- Gluteus medius
- Tensor fasciae latae

Special Tests

NOTE: If a fracture is suspected, the following tests should not be performed.

- Beginning in extension, the knee is passively flexed. A normal muscle will elicit full range of motion that is pain free. A muscle that has swelling or spasm will have restricted passive motion.
- Active movement from flexion to extension that is strong and painful may indicate muscle strain. A movement that is weak and pain free may indicate a third-degree or partial muscle rupture.[32]
- Muscle weakness against an isometric resistance may indicate a nerve injury.[2]

PREVENTION OF THIGH INJURIES

Like all other muscles in sports, the thigh must have maximum strength, endurance, and extensibility to withstand strain. In collision sports such as football, thigh guards are mandatory.

RECOGNITION AND MANAGEMENT OF THIGH INJURIES

Injuries to the thigh muscles are among the most common in sports. Contusions and strains occur most often, with the former having the higher incidence.[11]

Quadriceps Contusions

Etiology The quadriceps group is continually exposed to traumatic blunt blows in a variety of vigorous sports. Contusions usually develop as the result of a severe impact to the relaxed thigh that compresses the muscle against the hard surface of the femur. The extent of the force and the degree of thigh relaxation determine the depth of the injury and the amount of structural and functional disruption that take place.[8]

Symptoms and signs Contusions of the quadriceps display all the classic symptoms of most muscle bruises. Pain, a transitory loss of function, and immediate capillary effusion usually occur at the instant of trauma. The athlete usually describes having been hit by a sharp blow to the thigh, which produces intense pain and weakness. Early detection and avoidance of profuse internal hemorrhage are vital, both in effecting a fast recovery by the athlete and in preventing widespread scarring. Palpation may reveal a circumscribed swollen area that is painful to the touch.

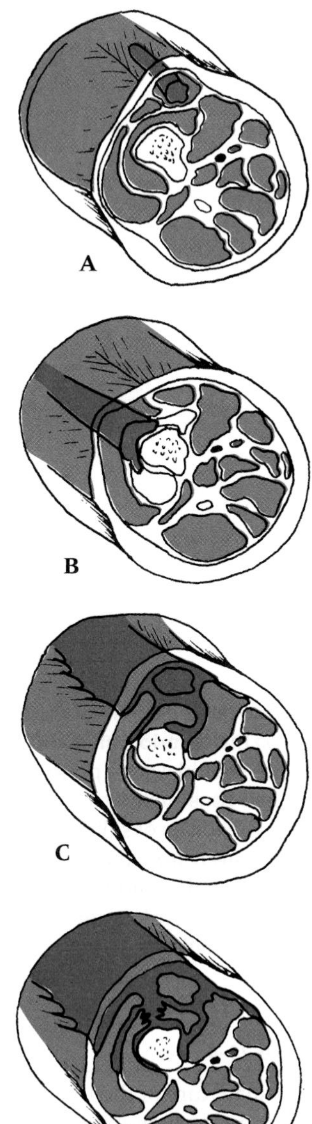

Figure 21-3

Quadriceps contusion. **A,** Grade 1 mild hemorrhage. **B,** Grade 2 mild pain and point tenderness. **C,** Grade 3 moderate pain and swelling. **D,** Grade 4 deep intramuscular hematoma.

The grade 1 quadriceps contusion is a superficial intramuscular bruise that produces mild hemorrhage, little pain, no swelling, and mild point tenderness at the site of the trauma. There is no restriction of the range of motion (Figure 21-3A; Table 21-2). The grade 2 contusion is deeper than grade 1 and produces mild pain, mild swelling, and point tenderness, with the athlete unable to flex the knee more than 90 degrees (Figure 21-3B). The grade 3 quadriceps contusion is of moderate intensity, causing pain, swelling, and a range of knee flexion that is 90 to 45 degrees and an

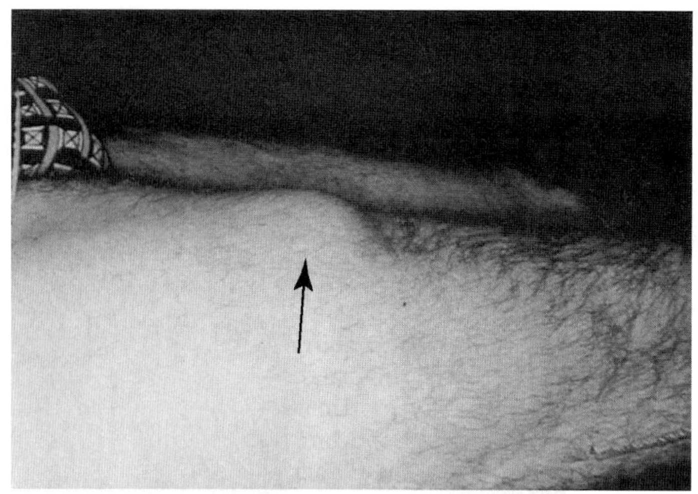

Figure 21-6

Rupture of the rectus femoris.

Quadriceps Muscle Strain

Quadriceps tendon strain is discussed in the section on jumper's knee in Chapter 20.

Etiology On occasion, the rectus femoris muscle will be strained by a sudden stretch, such as when an athlete falls on a bent knee, or a sudden contraction, such as when an athlete jumps in volleyball or kicks in soccer. Usually the strain is associated with a muscle that is weakened or one that is overly constricted.

A tear in the region of the rectus femoris muscle may cause partial or complete disruption of muscle fibers (Figure 21-6). The incomplete tear may be located centrally within the muscle or more peripheral to the muscle.

Symptoms and signs A peripheral quadriceps femoris muscle tear causes fewer symptoms than the deeper tear. In general, there is less point tenderness and a smaller hematoma. A more centrally located partial muscle tear causes the athlete more pain and discomfort than the peripheral tear does. With the deep tear there is a great deal of pain, point tenderness, spasm, and loss of function but little discoloration from internal bleeding. In contrast, complete muscle tear of the rectus femoris muscle may leave the athlete with little disability and discomfort but with some deformity of the anterior thigh.

Management Initially, RICE, NSAIDs, and analgesics are given as needed. The extent of the tear should be ascertained as soon as possible before swelling. Swelling can mask the grade of injury. Crutches may be warranted for the first, second, and third days. After the acute inflammatory phase has progressed to resolution and healing has begun, a regimen of isometric muscle contraction, within pain-free limits, can be initiated along with cryotherapy. Other therapy approaches such as cold whirlpool and ultrasound may also be used. Gentle stretching should not be started until the thigh is pain free. A neoprene or elastic sleeve may be worn for support (Figure 21-7).

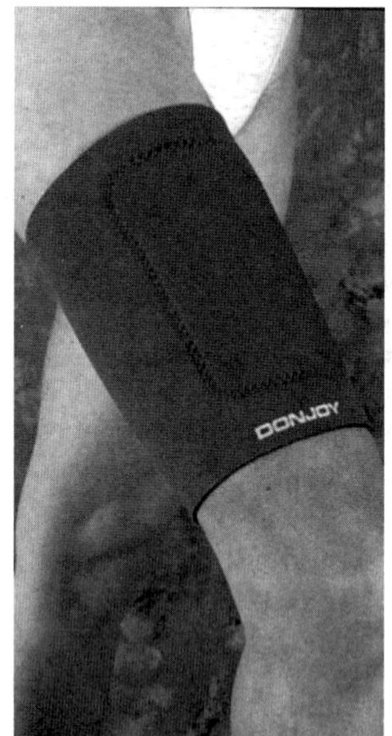

Figure 21-7

A neoprene sleeve may be worn for soft-tissue support.

In order of incidence of sports injury to the thigh, quadriceps contusions rank first and hamstring strains rank second.

Hamstring Muscle Strains

Hamstring strains are among the most common injuries to the thigh. Athletes suffer more strains to the hamstrings than to any other thigh muscle.

Etiology The exact cause of hamstring strain is not known. One theory is that the short head of the biceps femoris muscle is subject to the highest incidence of hamstring strain because, as a result of an idiosyncracy of innervation, it contracts at the same time that the quadriceps muscle does. Another speculation is that a quick change of the hamstring muscle from the role of knee stabilization to that of extending the hip when running could be a major cause of strain (Figure 21-8). What leads to this muscle failure and deficiency in the complementary action of opposing muscles is not clearly understood.[34] Possible reasons include muscle fatigue, faulty posture, leg-length discrepancy,

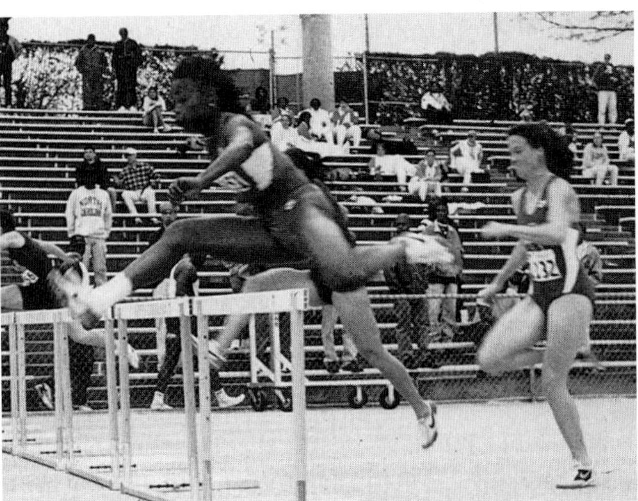

Figure 21-8

There is a high incidence of hamstring strain in hurdling and sprinting.

tight hamstrings, improper form, adverse neural tension,[45] or an imbalance of strength between hamstring muscle groups. NOTE: Hamstring muscles function as decelerators of leg swing and commonly become injured when an athlete suddenly changes direction or starts too slow. In most athletes, the hamstring muscle group should have a strength 60 percent to 70 percent of that of the quadriceps group.[8,40]

Symptoms and signs Hamstring strain can involve the muscle belly or bony attachment. The extent of injury can vary from the pulling apart of a few muscle fibers to a complete rupture or an avulsion fracture (Figure 21-9).[34]

Capillary hemorrhage, pain, and immediate loss of function vary according to the degree of trauma. Discoloration may occur a day or two after injury.

Grade 1 hamstring strain usually is evidenced by muscle soreness during movement, accompanied by point tenderness. These strains are often difficult to detect when they first occur. Irritation and stiffness do not become apparent until the athlete has cooled down after activity. The soreness of the mild hamstring strain in most instances can be attributed to muscle spasm rather than to the tearing of tissue. Fewer than 20 percent of fibers are torn in a grade 1 hamstring strain.

A grade 2 hamstring strain represents a partial tearing of muscle fibers, identified by a sudden snap or tear of the muscle accompanied by severe pain and a loss of function during knee flexion. Fewer than 70 percent of fibers are torn in a grade 2 hamstring tear.

A grade 3 hamstring strain constitutes the rupturing of tendinous or muscular tissue and involves major hemorrhage and disability. With more than 70 percent of fibers torn, there is severe edema, tenderness, loss of function, ecchymosis, and a palpable mass or palpable gap in the muscle.[30]

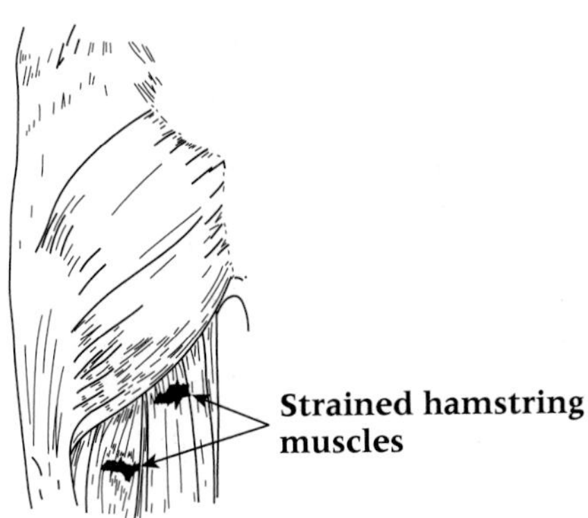

Figure 21-9

A hamstring strain results in separation or tearing of muscle fibers.

21-2

***Critical Thinking* Exercise**

A sprinter competing in a 100-yard dash experiences a sudden snap, severe pain, and weakness in the left hamstring muscle. Examination reveals a grade 2 strain.

? In terms of exercise, how should this injury be managed?

Management Initially, RICE, NSAIDs, and analgesics are given as needed. Activity should be reduced until soreness has been completely alleviated. An athlete with a grade 1 hamstring strain, as with the other grades of strain, should not be allowed to resume full sports participation until complete function of the injured part is restored.

Grade 2 and 3 strains should be treated extremely conservatively. For grade 2 strains, RICE should be used for twenty-four to forty-eight hours, and for grade 3 strains, for forty-eight to seventy-two hours. After the early inflammatory phase of injury has stabilized, a treatment regimen of isometric exercise, cryotherapy, and ultrasound may be of benefit. In later stages of healing, gentle stretching within pain limits, jogging, stationary cycling, and isokinetic exercise at high speeds may be used. After the elimination of soreness, the athlete may begin isotonic knee curls. Full recovery may take from one month to a full season.

Strains are always a problem to the athlete because they tend to recur as a result of the inelastic, fibrous scar tissue that sometimes forms during the healing process. The higher the incidence of strains at a particular muscle site, the greater the amount of scar tissue and the greater the likelihood of further injury will be. The fear of another pulled muscle becomes, to some individuals, almost a neurotic obsession, which is often more handicapping than the injury itself.

Muscle rehabilitation after injury should emphasize eccentric exercise (Table 21-3).

Acute Femoral Fractures

Femoral stress fractures are becoming more prevalent because of the increased popularity of repetitive, sustained activities such as distance running.

Etiology Femoral fractures are rare in the adolescent athlete, occur more often in middle-age athletes, and are relatively common in elderly individuals with osteoporosis.[44] A significant trauma is necessary to cause a hip fracture in the young athletic population. Even though femoral fractures are relatively rare in young athletes, the potential complications of this injury are significant.[35] Due to a limited blood supply in the region of the femoral head, there is a high incidence of avascular necrosis,

TABLE 21-3 Management of Muscle-Tendon Injuries of the Hip, Groin, and Pelvis

	Stage of Healing		
Management	Phase I Acute Inflammation (1 to 72 hrs)	Phase II Healing and Repair	Phase III Maturation and Remodeling
Ice	X		
Compression	X		
Elevation	X		
Rest	X		
Nonsteroidal antiinflammatory medication	X		
Contrast baths		X	
Whirlpool hydrotherapy		X	
Active range of motion		X	X
Ultrasound	X	X	X
Muscle stimulation	X	X	X
Isometric exercise		X	X
Isokinetic/isotonic exercise			X
Stretching			X
Aerobic exercise			X
Proprioceptive activities			X
Agility training			X
Sport-specific activities			X
Jogging			X
Straight-ahead sprint			X
Return to sport			X
Strength and flexibility maintenance			X

which is an important consideration until the athlete becomes skeletally mature and collateral blood supply has been well established. The prognosis of the fracture is dependent on the specific location of the injury and the degree to which the blood supply is compromised. Those fractures that occur across the epiphysis have the highest likelihood of developing avascular necrosis.[1]

Symptoms and signs After injury, the athlete complains of significant pain and generally cannot stand or walk. The athlete is muscle guarding and resists any attempts to move. The hip is usually externally rotated and slightly adducted. Shortening of the limb may also be evident.

Management The athlete must be immediately immobilized and transported for medical care. The physician will perform either an open or closed reduction with some type of rigid internal fixation using multiple pins or plates.[27] Following surgery the athlete must be immobilized with a hinged brace. Rehabilitation requires a slow progression over approximately a 4-month period.

Femoral Stress Fractures

Etiology Stress fractures of the femoral neck are fairly uncommon and femoral shaft stress fractures rarely occur. They occur most often in endurance athletes (i.e., triathalon, marathon) and thus the primary mechanism of injury is attributed to overuse.[18] These injuries are more likely in females than males.

Symptoms and signs Onset of symptoms may occur several weeks after increasing the intensity of a training program. The athlete with a stress fracture complains of pain in the groin or anterior thigh which increases during activity and may persist after activity. Pain may be referred to the knee. Pain is relieved with longer periods of rest. Eventually pain becomes constant even with no activity. The athlete walks with an antalgic gait using an abduction lurch-type movement. There is also a positive Trendelenburg's sign. Early X rays may not show any clear signs.

Management Initial treatment requires complete rest with no running. The prognosis varies according to the location of the stress fracture. Stress fractures on the medial side of the femoral neck tend to heal well with conservative management. Stress fractures on the lateral side of the femoral neck are more likely to eventually displace and cause additional complications. Stress fractures of the femoral shaft usually heal with conservative management but in rare cases can progress to failure of cortical bone. If a fracture does occur, surgery may be indicated, and the time required for fracture healing and remodeling can be as long as 12 months.

ANATOMY OF THE HIP, GROIN, AND PELVIC REGION

Normal function of the hip and pelvis is necessary for sports performance. Normal body movement is highly important for sports that predominantly use the lower extremities or the upper extremities. The hip and pelvis are part of the kinetic chain that transmits a load from the foot to the spine and vice versa in all three planes of movement.[41]

Bones

The pelvis, or pelvic girdle, is a bony ring formed by the two innominate bones, the sacrum and the coccyx (Figure 21-10). Each innominate bone is composed of an ilium, ischium, and pubis (Figure 21-11). The functions of the pelvis are to support the spine and trunk and to transfer their weight to the lower limbs. In addition to providing skeletal support, the pelvis serves as a place of attachment for the trunk and thigh muscles and as protection for the pelvic viscera. The basin formed by the pelvis is separated into a false and a true pelvis. The false pelvis is composed of the wings of the ilium. The true pelvis is composed of the coccyx, the ischium, and the pubis.

The innominate bones are three bones that ossify and fuse early in life. They include the ilium, which is positioned superiorly and posteriorly; the pubis, which forms the anterior part; and the ischium, which is located inferiorly. Lodged between the innominate bones is the wedge-shaped sacrum, composed of five fused vertebrae.

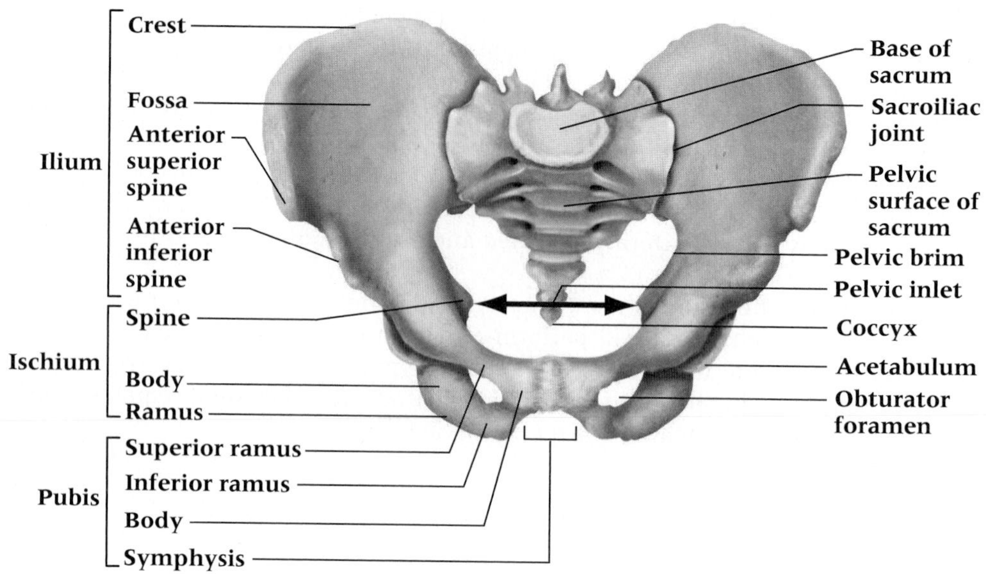

Figure 21-10

The pelvic girdle.

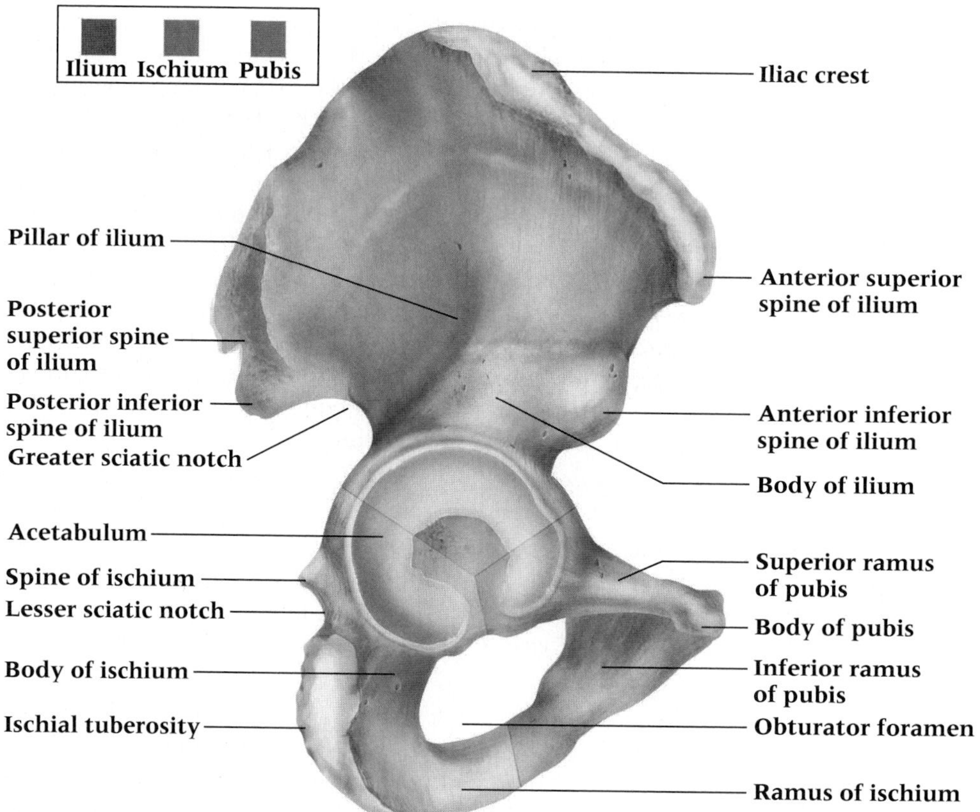

Figure 21-11

The innominate bone consists of the ilium, ischium, and pubic bones.

Articulations

Sacroiliac Joint and Coccyx

The sacrum is joined to other parts of the pelvis by strong ligaments, forming the sacroiliac joint. A small backward-forward movement is present at the sacroiliac junction. The coccyx is composed of four or five small fused vertebral bodies that articulate with the sacrum. The sacroiliac joint is discussed in detail in Chapter 25.

Hip Joint

The hip joint is formed by articulation of the femur with the innominate, or hip, bone. The articulating, spherical head of the femur fits into a deep socket in the innominate bone called the acetabulum, which is padded at its center by a mass of fatty tissue, ligaments, and capsule. The acetabulum forms an incomplete bony ring that is interrupted by a notch on the lower aspect of the socket. The ring is completed by the transverse ligament that crosses the notch. The socket faces forward, downward, and laterally. The femoral head is a sphere that fits into the acetabulum in a medial, upward, and slightly forward direction.

Ligaments, Joint Capsule, and Synovial Membrane

Surrounding its rim is a fibrocartilage known as the glenoid labrum. A loose sleeve of articular tissue is attached to the circumference of the acetabulum above and to the neck of the femur below. The capsule is lined by an extensive synovial membrane, and the iliofemoral, pubocapsular, and ischiocapsular ligaments give it strong reinforcement. Hyaline cartilage completely covers the head of the femur, with the exception of the fovea capitis, a small area in the center to which the ligamentum teres is attached. The ligamentum teres gives little support to the hip joint; its main function is the transport of nutrient vessels to the head of the femur. Because of its bony, ligamentous, and muscular arrangements, this joint is considered by many to be the strongest articulation in the body.

The synovial membrane is a vascular tissue enclosing the hip joint in a tubular sleeve, with the upper portion surrounding the acetabulum. The lower portion is fastened to the circumference of the neck of the femur. Except for the ligamentum teres, which lies outside the synovial cavity, the membrane lines the acetabular socket.

The articular capsule is a fibrous, sleevelike structure covering the synovial membrane; its upper end attaches to the cartilaginous labrum and its lower end to the neck of the femur. The circular fibers that surround the femoral neck serve as a tight collar. This area is called the zona orbicularis, and it holds the femoral head in the acetabulum. Many strong ligaments—the iliofemoral, the pubofemoral, and the ischiofemoral—reinforce the hip joint (Figure 21-12).

The iliofemoral ligament (Y ligament of Bigelow) is the strongest ligament of the body. It prevents hyperextension, controls external rotation and adduction of the thigh, and limits the pelvis during any backward rolling of the femoral head during weight bearing. It reinforces the anterior aspect of the capsule and is attached to the anterior iliac spine and the intertrochanteric line on the anterior aspect of the femur.

The pubofemoral ligament prevents excessive abduction of the thigh and is positioned anterior and inferior to the pelvis and femur.

The ischiofemoral ligament prevents excessive internal rotation and adduction of the thigh and is located posterior and superior to the articular capsule.

Hip Musculature

The muscles of the hip can be divided into anterior and posterior groups (Table 21-4). The anterior group includes the iliacus and psoas muscles (see Figure 21-2A, page 659). The posterior group's muscles include the tensor fasciae latae, gluteus maximus, gluteus medius, gluteus minimus, and the six deep outward rotators—the piriformis, gemellus superior, gemellus inferior, obturator internus, obturator externus, and quadratus femoris (see Figure 21-2B, page 659 and Figure 21-13, page 672).

Anterior Hip Muscles

The iliacus and psoas muscles are the anterior hip muscles. The triangular-shaped iliacus is contained within the iliac fossa within the abdomen. Its tendon merges with the psoas major muscles, forming a common tendon that is called the iliopsoas. The iliopsoas attaches on the iliac fossa and part of the inner surface of the sacrum proximally,

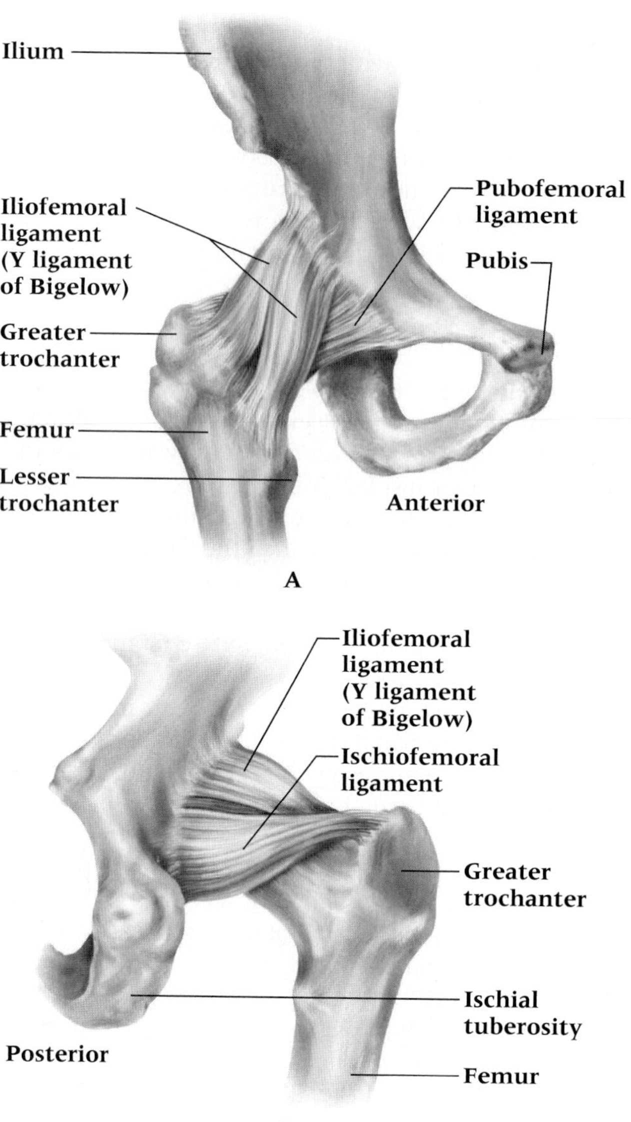

Figure 21-12

Ligaments of the hip. **A,** Anterior view. **B,** Posterior view.

and it attaches distally on the lesser trochanter of the femur. The psoas muscle attaches proximally on the transverse processes and bodies of the lumbar vertebrae. Its distal attachment is on the lesser trochanter. The iliopsoas muscle flexes the thigh at the hip joint and tends to rotate the thigh outwardly and to adduct the thigh when free to move. When fixed, the iliopsoas assists in flexing the trunk and hip.

Posterior Hip Muscles

The posterior muscles of the hip consist of the tensor fasciae latae, the three gluteal muscles, and the six deep outward rotators (see Figure 21-2B, page 659 and Figure 21-13).

The tensor fasciae latae muscle is located on the upper anterior aspect of the lateral thigh. It is attached superiorly to the iliac crest just behind the anterior superior iliac spine and is inserted inferiorly into the iliotibial tract. Its primary action is flexion and medial rotation of the thigh. It is innervated by the superior gluteal nerve.

The gluteus maximus muscle forms the buttocks in the hip region. Lateral to and underneath the gluteus maximus are the gluteus medius and the gluteus minimus muscles (see Figure 21-2B, and Figure 21-13). The gluteus maximus muscle is attached above to

TABLE 21-4 Muscles of the Hip

Muscle	Origin	Insertion	Muscle Action	Innervation
Iliopsoas				
Psoas major and minor	Transverse processes and bodies of the last thoracic and all of the lumbar vertebrae	Lesser trochanter of the femur	Flexes the thigh and the trunk on the femur	Femoral and first lumbar
Iliacus	Iliac crest and fossa			
Tensor fasciae latae	Anterior portion of the iliac crest and the anterior superior iliac spine	Iliotibial band of the fasciae latae	Tenses the fascia lata and assists in flexion, abduction, and medial rotation of the thigh	Superior gluteal
Gluteus maximus	Posterior gluteal line of the ilium and the posterior surface of the sacrum and the coccyx	Gluteal tuberosity of the femur; iliotibial band	Extends and laterally rotates the thigh	Inferior gluteal
Gluteus medius	Outer surface of the ilium between the posterior and the anterior gluteal lines	Lateral surface of the greater trochanter of the femur	Abducts and medially rotates the thigh	Superior gluteal
Gluteus minimus	Outer surface of the ilium between the anterior and the inferior gluteal lines	Anterior surface of the greater trochanter of the femur	Abducts and medially rotates the thigh	Superior gluteal
Piriformis	Anterior surface of the sacrum	Superior border of the greater trochanter of the femur	Rotates the thigh laterally and assists in extending and abducting the thigh	Second sacral
Superior gemellus	Ischial spine	Greater trochanter of the femur	Rotates the thigh laterally	Fifth lumbar and first and second sacral
Inferior gemellus	Ischial tuberosity	Greater trochanter of the femur	Rotates the thigh laterally	Fourth and fifth lumbar and first sacral
Obturator internus	Inner surface of the obturator membrane and the bony margins of the obturator foramen	Greater trochanter of the femur	Rotates the thigh laterally	Fifth lumbar and first and second sacral
Obturator externus	Outer surface of the obturator membrane and the bony margins of the obturator foramen	Trochanteric fossa of the femur	Rotates the thigh laterally	Obturator
Quadratus femoris	Ischial tuberosity	Shaft of the femur just below the greater trochanter	Rotates the thigh laterally	Fourth and fifth lumbar

the posterior aspect of the iliac crest, the sacrum, and the coccyx as well as to the fascia in the area. Inferiorly, this muscle attaches to the iliotibial tract and into the gluteal tuberosity of the femur between the linea aspera and greater trochanter. The gluteus maximus muscle acts as a lateral rotator of the thigh at the hip joint and allows the body to rise from a sitting to a standing position. Through its attachment to the iliotibial tract, the muscle helps extend the flexed knee. The inferior gluteal nerve supplies this muscle. The gluteus medius muscle is located lateral to the hip. It is attached superiorly to the lateral aspect of the ilium and inferiorly to the lateral aspect of the trochanter. The gluteus maximus muscle covers this muscle posteriorly, and it is covered anteriorly by the

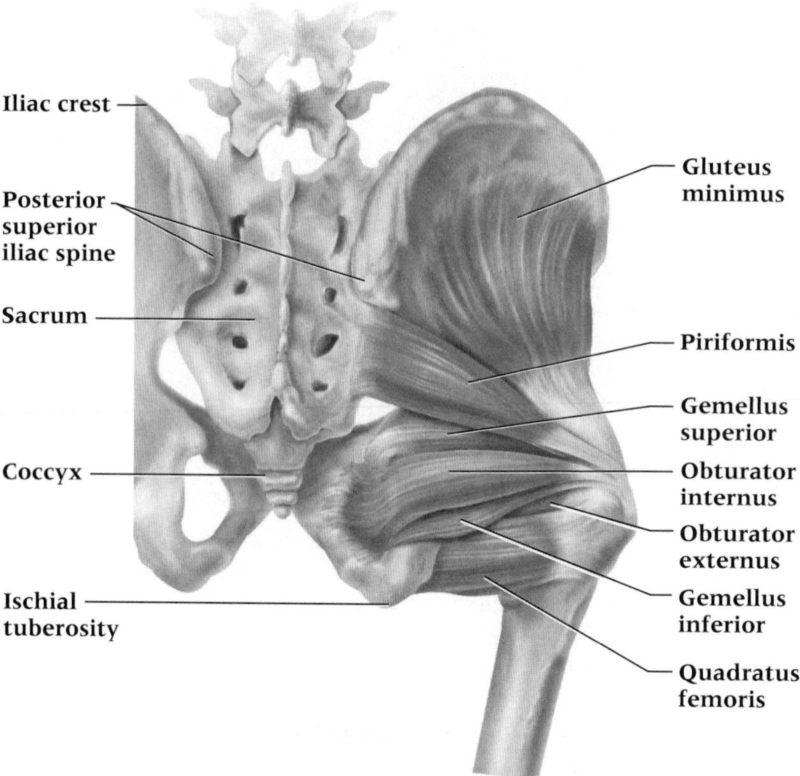

Figure 21-13

The six deep muscles of the hip.

tensor fasciae latae. The gluteus medius muscle acts primarily as a thigh abductor at the hip, with some flexion and medial rotation occurring from its anterior aspect and some extension and lateral rotation occurring from its posterior aspect. It is innervated by the superior gluteal nerve. The gluteus minimus muscle originates above the lateral aspect of the ilium and attaches inferiorly to the anterior aspect of the greater trochanter of the femur. Its main action is to cause medial rotation at the hip joint; its secondary action is abduction of the thigh at the hip joint. It is innervated by the superior gluteus nerve.

Underneath these larger muscles are much smaller muscles that, along with the gluteus maximus, laterally rotate the hip: the piriformis, the quadratus femoris, the obturator internus and externus, and the gemellus superior and inferior (Figure 21-13). Collectively, they stabilize the head of the femur in the acetabulum.

Bursae

The hip joint has many bursae. Clinically, the most important of them are the iliopsoas bursa and the deep trochanteric bursa. The iliopsoas bursa is located between the articular capsule and the iliopsoas muscle on the anterior aspect of the joint. The deep trochanteric bursa lies between the greater trochanter and the deep fibers of the gluteus maximus muscle.

Nerve Supply

The lumbar plexus is created by the intertwining of the fibers stemming from the first four lumbar nerves (see Chapter 25). The femoral nerve, a major nerve emerging from this plexus, later divides into many branches to supply the thigh and lower leg. Nerve fibers from the fourth and fifth lumbar nerves and the first, second, and third sacral nerves form the sacral plexus within the pelvic cavity, anterior to the piriformis muscle (see Chapter 25.) Along with other nerves, the tibial and common peroneal nerves emerge from the sacral plexus and form the large sciatic nerve in the thigh (Figure 21-14).

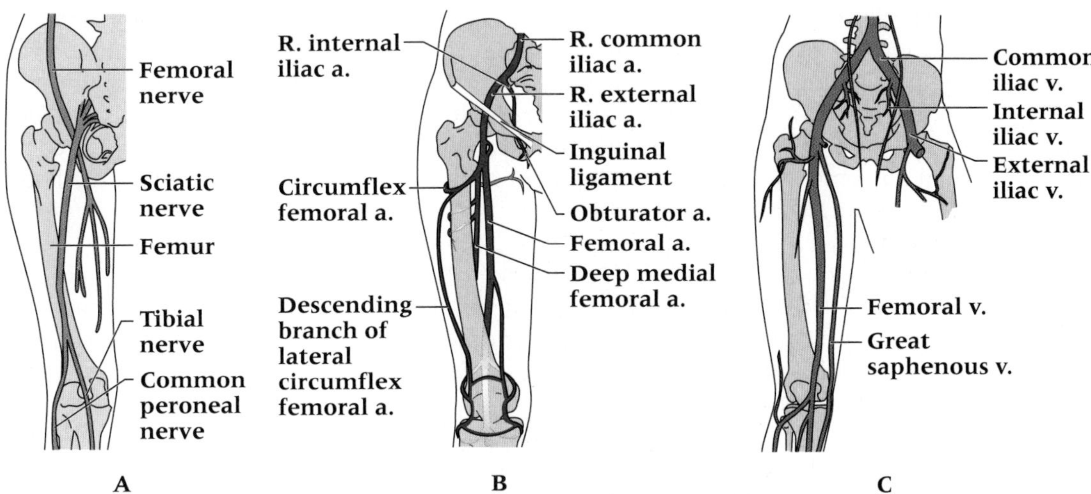

Figure 21-14

Blood and nerve supply to the hip region. **A,** Nerves of the pelvis and thigh. **B,** Arterial blood supply. **C,** Veins of the pelvis, hip, and thigh.

Blood Supply

Arteries

Opposite the fourth lumbar vertebra, the aorta divides to become the two common iliac arteries (see Figure 21-14). They in turn pass downward to divide, opposite the sacroiliac joint, into the internal and external iliac arteries. Most of the branches of the internal iliac artery supply blood to the pelvic viscera. The external iliac artery is the primary artery to the lower limb.

Veins

Three major veins are found in the region of hips, groin, and pelvis. The first is the common iliac vein, which stems from the inferior vena cava on both sides draining the lower body. The second is the internal iliac vein, which ascends behind its iliac artery to the brim of the true pelvis, where it joins the external vein to form the common iliac vein. Its tributaries drain the pelvis and adjoining area. Third is the external iliac vein, which passes upward from the femoral vein behind the inguinal ligament and follows the brim of the true pelvis, where it joins the internal iliac vein.

FUNCTIONAL ANATOMY OF THE HIP, GROIN, AND PELVIC REGION

The pelvis and hip are made up of the pelvic girdle and the articulation of the femoral head to the bony socket of the pelvic girdle, the acetabulum, forming a ball-in-socket joint. This joint connects the lower extremity to the pelvic girdle. The pelvis itself moves in three directions, anteroposterior tilting, lateral tilting, and rotation. The iliopsoas muscle and other hip flexors, as well as extensors of the lumbar spine, perform anterior tilting in the sagittal plane and facilitate lumbar lordosis. The gluteus maximus and hamstrings, along with the rectus abdominus and the obliques, posteriorly tilt the pelvis and cause a decrease in lumbar lordosis. During lateral tilting in the frontal plane, the hip joint acts as the center of rotation. Hip abduction or adduction is a result of pelvic lateral tilting. The hip abductors control lateral tilting by contracting isometrically or eccentrically. Pelvic rotation occurs in the transverse plane, again using the hip joint as the axis of rotation. The gluteal muscles, external rotators, adductors, pectineus, and iliopsoas all act together to perform this movement in the transverse plane. These movements of the pelvis play an important role in gait analysis, injury evaluation, and teaching correct gait.[17]

The hip joint is a true ball-in-socket joint and has intrinsic stability not found in other joints. This intrinsic stability does not prevent the hip joint from retaining great mobility. During normal gait, the hip joint moves in all three planes, sagittal, frontal, and transverse. To participate in athletic activities a greater range of motion is needed. With its great range of motion, the hip is capable of performing a wide range of combined movements. Forces at the hip joint have been increased to five times the body weight during running. These forces can also contribute to injuries, both muscular and bony.[32]

The most frequently injured structures of the groin, hip, pelvis, and thigh are the muscles and tendons that perform the movements.[47] The majority of these muscles originate on the pelvis or the proximal femur. The iliac crest serves as the attachment site for the abdominal muscles, the ilium serves as the attachment for the gluteals, and the gluteals insert to the proximal femur. The pubis serves as the attachment for the adductors, and the iliopsoas inserts distally to the lesser trochanter of the proximal femur. Due to all the attachments in a small area, injury to these structures can be very disabling and difficult to distinguish.[17]

ASSESSMENT OF THE HIP, GROIN, AND PELVIS

The hip, groin, and pelvis form the body's core. The body's center of gravity is located just in front of the upper part of the sacrum. Injuries to the hip, groin, or pelvis cause the athlete major disability in the lower limb, trunk, or both.[3,11]

Because of the close proximity of the hip and pelvis to the low back region, many evaluative procedures overlap (see Chapter 25).

History

The athletic trainer should determine following information:

- What are the athlete's symptoms (e.g., weakness, disability, pain)?
- When did the athlete first notice a problem with the hip or pelvis?
- Describe types of pain (hip pain is felt mainly in the groin and medial or frontal side of thigh; hip pain may also be referred to the knee).
- Describe the sacroiliac pain. Does it radiate in the posterior thigh, iliac fossa, or buttock on the affected side?
- When does the pain occur (e.g., during activity, while turning in bed)?
- Note the age and gender of the athlete (e.g., boys three to twelve years old can have Legg-Calvé-Perthes disease; distance-running amenorrheic girls may develop a hip stress fracture).

Observation

The athlete with an external pelvic pain must be observed for postural asymmetry.

The athlete should be observed for postural asymmetry and while standing on one leg and during ambulation.

Postural Asymmetry

From the front view, do the hips look even? A laterally tilted hip could mean a leg-length discrepancy or abnormal muscle contraction on one side of the hip or low back region.

- From the side view, is the pelvis abnormally tilted anteriorly or posteriorly? This tilting may indicate lordosis or flat back, respectively.
- In lower-limb alignment, is there indication of genu valgum, genu varum, foot pronation, or genu recurvatum? The patella should also be noted for relative position and alignment.
- The posterior superior iliac spines, represented by the skin depressions above the buttocks, should be horizontal to one another. Uneven depressions could indicate that the pelvis is laterally tilted.

Standing on One Leg

Standing on one leg may produce pain in the hip, abnormal movement of the symphysis pubis, or a fall of the pelvis on the opposite side as a result of abductor weakness.

Ambulation

The athlete should be observed during walking and sitting. Pain in the hip and pelvic region will normally be reflected in movement distortions.

Palpation

The following bony landmarks should be palpated:

Bony Palpation

- Iliac crest
- Anterior superior iliac spine
- Anterior inferior iliac spine
- Greater trochanter
- Femoral neck
- Lesser trochanter
- Pubic symphysis
- Ischial tuberosity
- Posterior inferior iliac spine
- Posterior superior iliac spine

Soft-Tissue Palpation

The soft-tissue sites of major concern are in the regions of the groin, femoral triangle, sciatic nerve, and major muscles. Groin pain could result from swollen lymph glands, indicating an infection, or from an adductor muscle strain.

The following soft tissue structures should be palpated:

Anterior

- Rectus femoris
- Sartorius
- Iliopsoas
- Inguinal ligament

Medial

- Gracilis
- Adductor magnus
- Adductor longus
- Adductor brevis
- Pectineus

Posterior

- Gluteus maximus
- Piriformis
- Hamstrings

Lateral

- Gluteus medius
- Gluteus minimus
- Tensor fasciae latae
- Iliotibial band

Special Tests

Functional Evaluation

The athlete is led through all possible hip movements, both passive and active, to evaluate range of motion and active and resistive strength. These movements are as follows:

hip abduction, hip adduction, hip flexion, hip extension, and internal and external hip rotation.

Tests for Hip Flexor Tightness

Contractures of the hip flexors are major causes of lordosis and susceptibility to groin pain and discomfort. Two tests can be used: the Kendall test and the Thomas test.

Kendall test The athlete lies supine on a table with one knee flexed on the chest and the back completely flat (Figure 21-15). The other knee is flexed over the table's end. Normal extensibility of the hip flexors allows the thigh to touch the table with the knee flexed approximately 70 degrees. Tight hip flexors are revealed by the inability of the thigh to lie flat on the table. If only the rectus femoris muscle is tight, the thigh will touch the table, but the knee will extend more than 70 degrees (Figure 21-16).

Thomas test The Thomas test indicates whether hip contractures are present (Figure 21-17). The athlete lies supine on a table, arms across the chest, legs together and fully extended. The athletic trainer places one hand under the athlete's lumbar curve; one thigh is brought to the chest, flattening the spine. In this position, the extended thigh should be flat on the table. If not, there is a hip contracture. When the athlete fully extends the leg again, the curve in the low back returns.

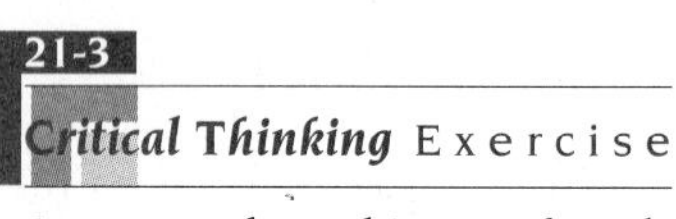

21-3 Critical Thinking Exercise

A gymnast has a history of moderate groin pain. She is susceptible to strains in that region. The athlete also appears to have an exaggerated lumbar lordotic curve.

? What tests should be given to evaluate the tightness of the groin region?

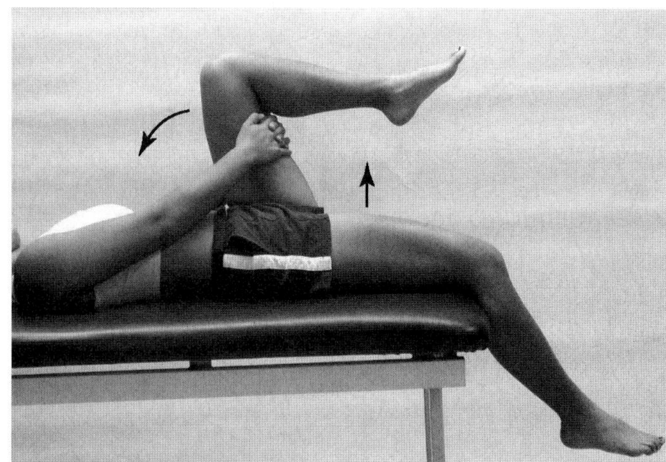

Figure 21-15

Kendall test for hip flexor tightness.

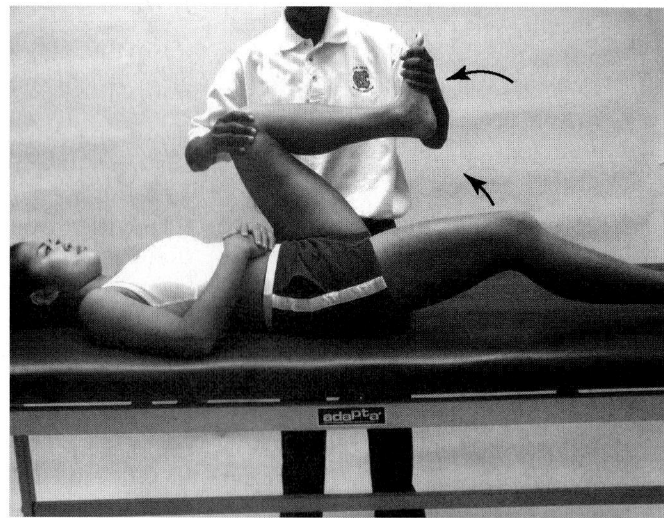

Figure 21-16

Demonstrating tight hip flexors.

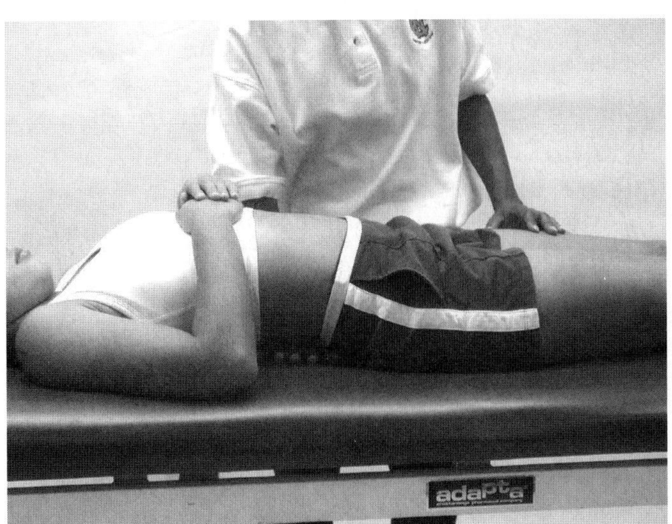
A

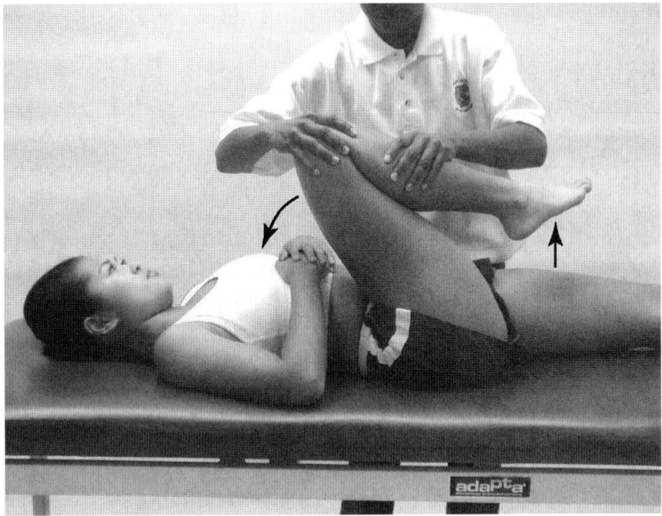
B

Figure 21-17

Thomas test for hip contractures. **A,** Starting positon. **B,** Test position.

Femoral Anteversion and Retroversion

The athlete with a painful hip problem may also have a discrepancy in the relationship between the neck of the femur and the shaft of the femur. The normal angle of the femoral neck is 15 degrees anterior to the long axis of the shaft of the femur and femoral condyles. Athletes who walk in a toe-in manner may be reflecting a hip deformity in which the femoral neck is directed anteriorly (femoral anteversion). In contrast, athletes who walk in a pronounced toe-out manner may be displaying a condition in which the femoral neck is directed posteriorly (femoral retroversion) (Figure 21-18). Internal hip rotation in excess of 35 degrees is characteristic of femoral anteversion, and hip rotation in excess of the normal 45 degrees of external rotation is characteristic of femoral retroversion.

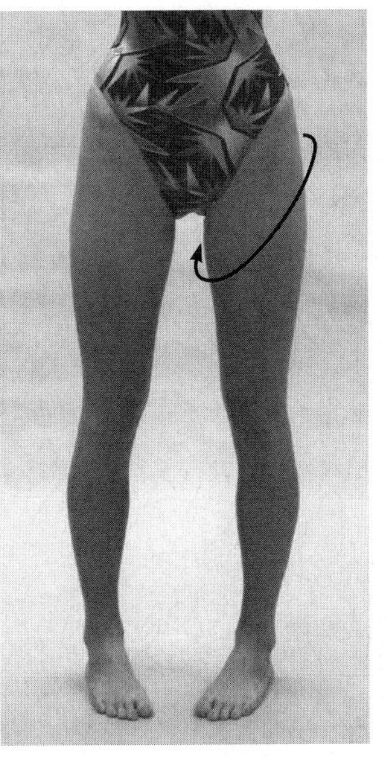
A

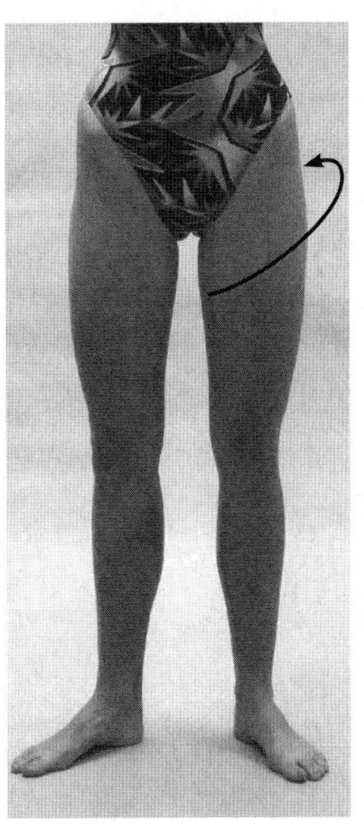
B

Figure 21-18

A, Anteversion of the femoral neck. When the knee is directed anteriorly, the femoral neck is directed anteriorly to some degree. **B,** Retroversion of the femoral neck. When the knee is directed posteriorly, the femoral neck is directed posteriorly to some degree.

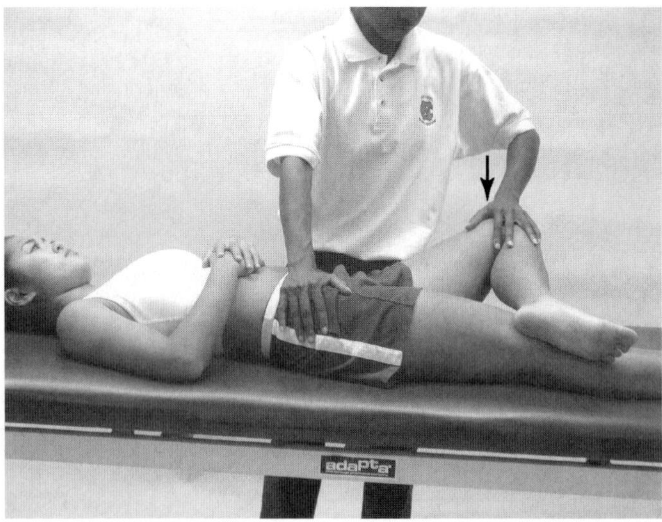

Figure 21-19

The Patrick test for a pathological condition of the hip and sacroiliac joint.

Test for the Hip and Sacroiliac Joint

Patrick test (FABER) The Patrick test, or FABER test (flexion, abduction, external rotation of the hip), detects pathological conditions of the hip and sacroiliac joint (Figure 21-19). The athlete lies supine on the examining table. The foot on the side of the painful sacroiliac is placed on the opposite extended knee. Pressure is then applied downward on the bent knee. Pain may be felt in the hip or sacroiliac joint.

Gaenslen's test In a supine position, with the affected side on the edge of the table, the unaffected thigh is flexed toward the abdomen. Pressure is applied to the knee on the affected side, moving the sacroiliac joint into extension. The test is positive if hyperextension on the affected side increases pain (Figure 21-20).

Testing the Tensor Fasciae Latae and Iliotibial Band

Three tests that can be used to discern iliotibial band tightness and inflammation of the bursa overlying the lateral femoral epicondyle or direct irritation of the iliotibial band and periosteum are Renne's test, Nobel's test, and Ober's test.[2]

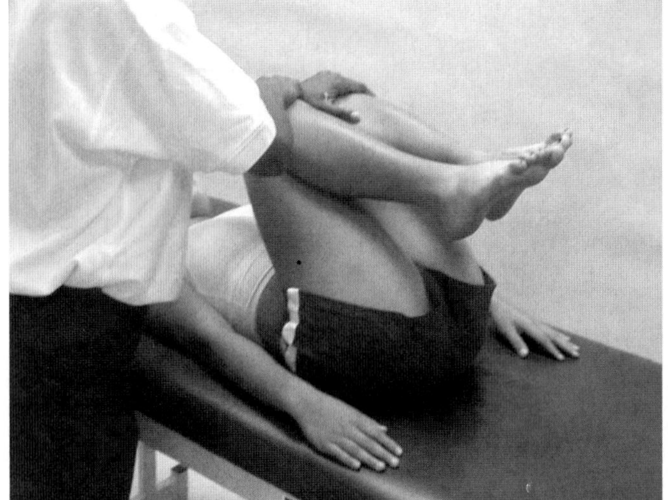

A

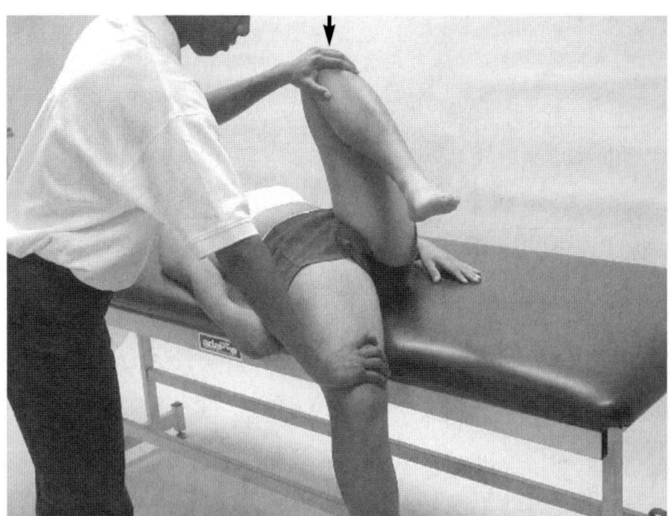

B

Figure 21-20

Gaenslen's test. **A,** Starting position. **B,** Test position.

Renne's test The athlete stands and supports his or her full weight on the affected leg with the knee bent at 30 degrees to 40 degrees. A positive response of fasciae latae tightness occurs when pain is felt at the lateral femoral condyle[28] (Figure 21-21).

Nobel's test Lying supine, the athlete's knee is flexed to 90 degrees, and pressure is applied to the lateral femoral epicondyle while the knee is gradually extended. A positive response occurs when severe pain is felt at the lateral femoral epicondyle with the knee at 30 degrees of flexion (Figure 21-22).[38]

Ober's test The athlete lies on the unaffected side. With the knee flexed at 90 degrees, the affected thigh is abducted as far as possible. With the pelvis stabilized, the abducted thigh is then relaxed and allowed to drop into adduction. A contracted tensor fasciae latae or iliotibial band will keep the thigh in an abducted position, not allowing it to fall into adduction (Figure 21-23).

Trendelenburg's Test While the athlete stands, the foot on the unaffected side is lifted so that the hip flexes. Normally in this position, the iliac crest on the unaffected side will be higher than on the affected side. If the iliac crest on the affected side is higher than on the unaffected side, the test is positive, indicating weakness in the hip abductors, particularly the gluteus medius (Figure 21-24).

Piriformis Test The athlete lies on the unaffected side with the affected leg in 60 degrees of hip flexion and the knee relaxed. The pelvis is stabilized and pressure is applied downward on the knee, rotating the hip internally. Tightness or pain is indicative of piriformis tightness (Figure 21-25).

Ely's Test While the athlete lies in a prone position, the pelvis is stabilized and the knee on the affected side is flexed. If the hip on that side extends as the knee is flexed, there is tightness of the rectus femoris (Figure 21-26).

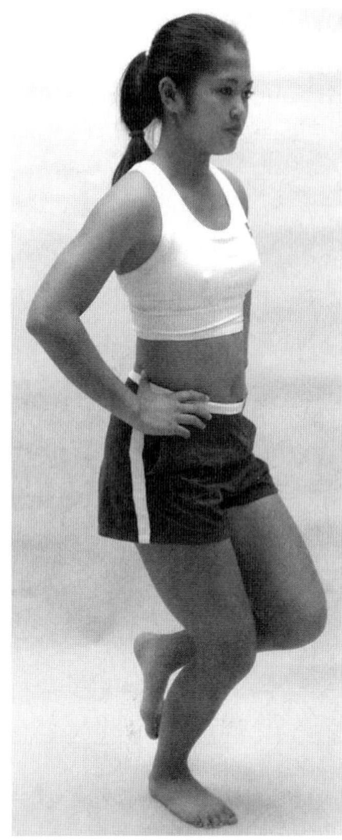

Figure 21-21

Renne's test for iliotibial band tightness.

Measuring Leg-Length Discrepancy

In individuals who are not physically active, leg-length discrepancies of more than one inch may produce symptoms; however, shortening of as little as ⅛ inch (3 mm) may cause symptoms in highly active athletes. Such discrepancies can cause cumulative stresses to the lower limbs, hip, and pelvis, or low back.[9]

There are two types of leg-length discrepancy: (1) true, or anatomical, shortening and (2) apparent, or functional, shortening. X-ray examination is the most valid

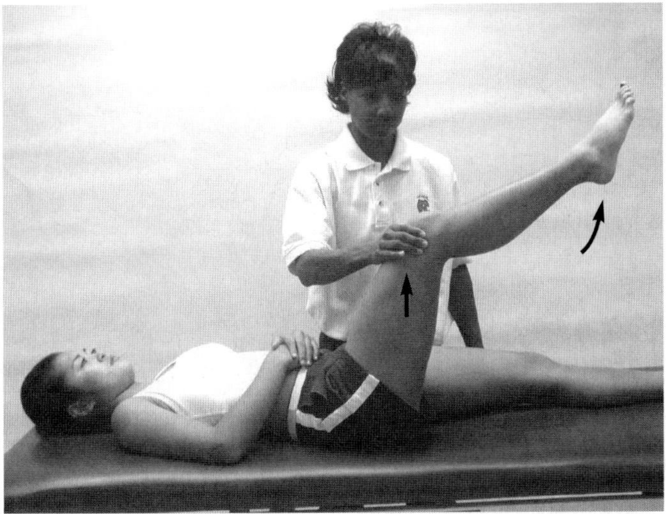

Figure 21-22

Nobel's test for iliotibial band tightness.

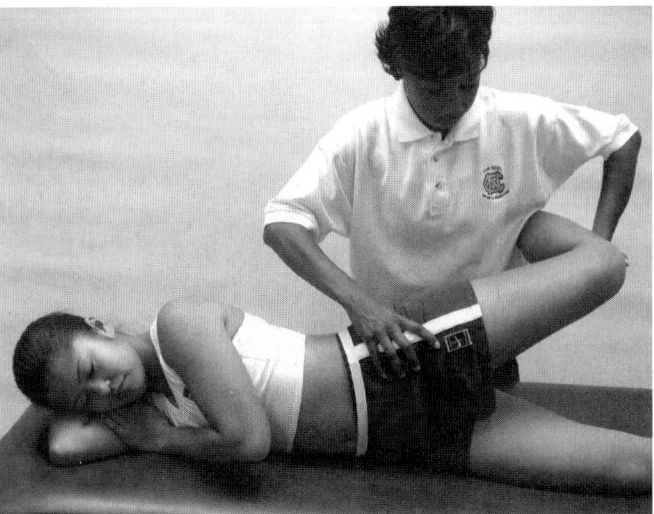

Figure 21-23

Ober's test for iliotibial band tightness.

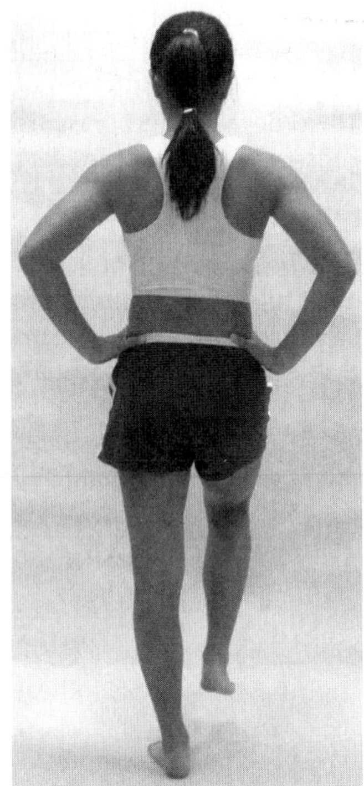

A

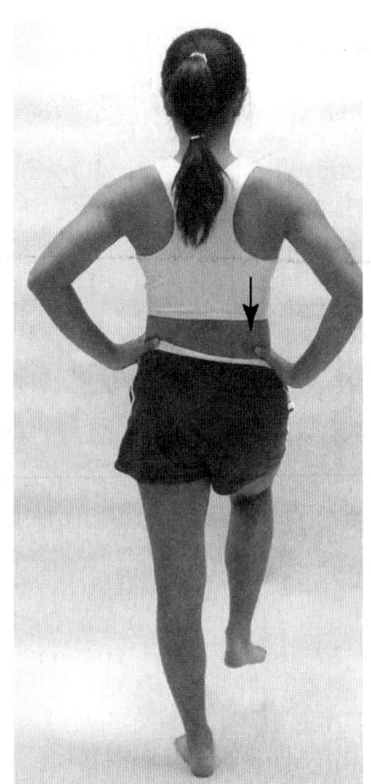

B

Figure 21-24

Trendelenburg's test.
A, Normal. **B,** Positive.

21-4
***Critical Thinking* Exercise**

During a gait evaluation, an athletic trainer notices one of the basketball players walks with a swinging hip where one side of the pelvis drops to the side during single leg stance.

? What could be a cause of this movement?

means of measurement. It is difficult to be completely accurate because of mobility of the soft tissue over bony landmarks (Figure 21-27A).[36]

Anatomical discrepancy In an anatomical discrepancy, shortening may be equal throughout the lower limb or localized within the femur or lower leg. The athlete lies supine and fully extended on the table. Measurement is taken between the medial malleoli and the anterior superior iliac spine of each leg (Figure 21-27B).

Functional discrepancy Functional leg shortening can occur as the result of lateral pelvic tilt (obliquely) or from a flexion or adduction deformity. Measurement is taken from the umbilicus to the medial malleoli of each ankle (Figure 21-27C).

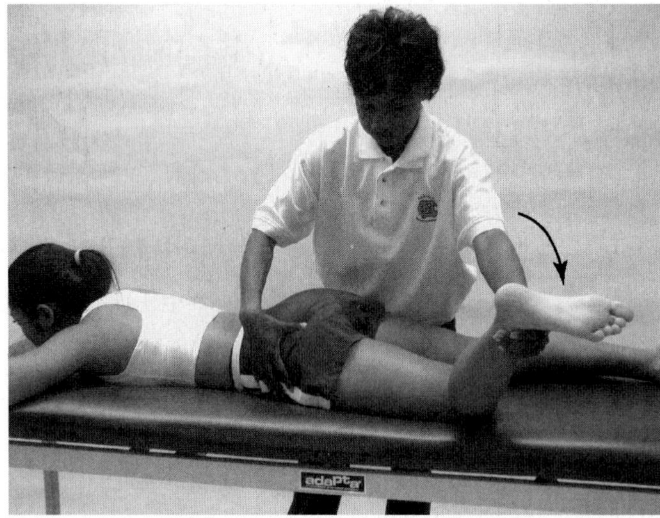

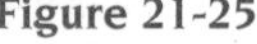

Figure 21-25

Piriformis tightness test.

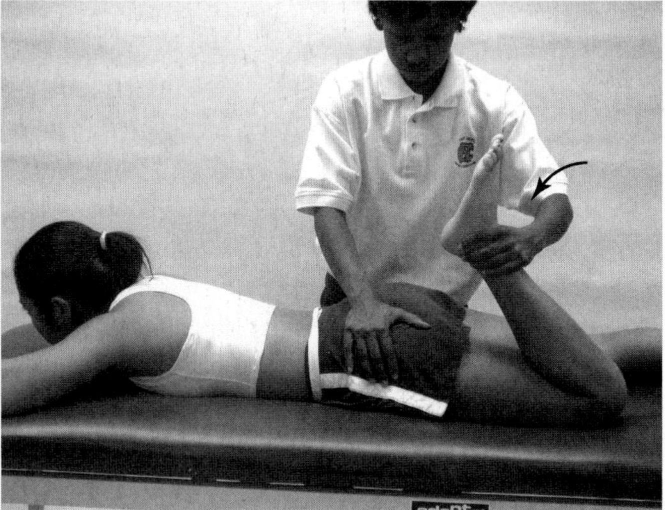

Figure 21-26

Ely's test.

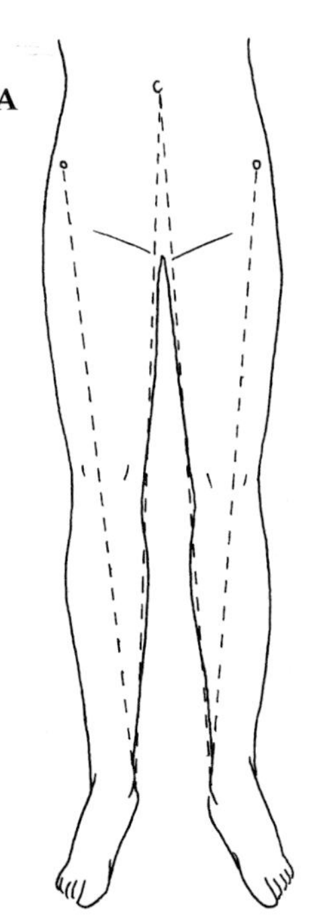

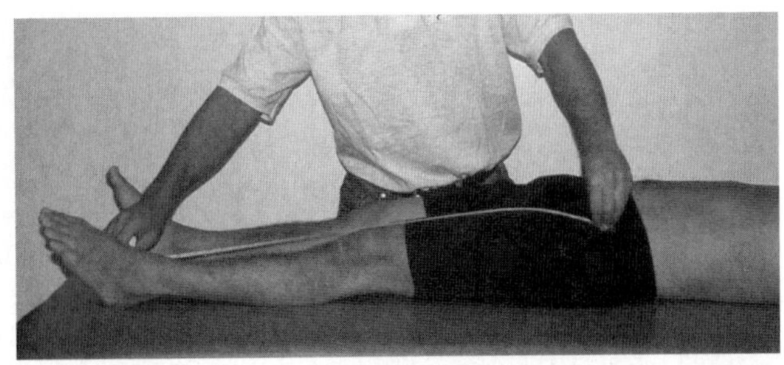

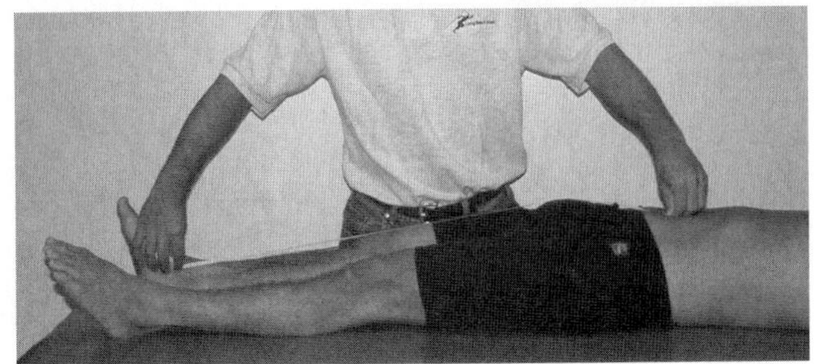

Figure 21-27

A, Measuring for leg-length discrepancy. **B,** Anatomical discrepancy. **C,** Functional discrepancy.

RECOGNITION AND MANAGEMENT OF SPECIFIC HIP, GROIN, AND PELVIC INJURIES

Hip Joint

Groin Strain

Etiology The groin is the region that lies on the medial and anterior aspect of the upper thigh. The musculature of this area includes the iliopsoas, the rectus femoris, and the adductor group (the gracilis, pectineus, adductor brevis, adductor longus, and adductor magnus). Groin pain is one of the more difficult problems to diagnose, especially if it is chronic.[2]

Leg-length discrepancy in an athlete can lead to stress-related physical injuries.

Any one of the muscles in the region of the groin can be injured during sports activity and elicit what is commonly considered a groin strain (Figure 21-28). The adductor

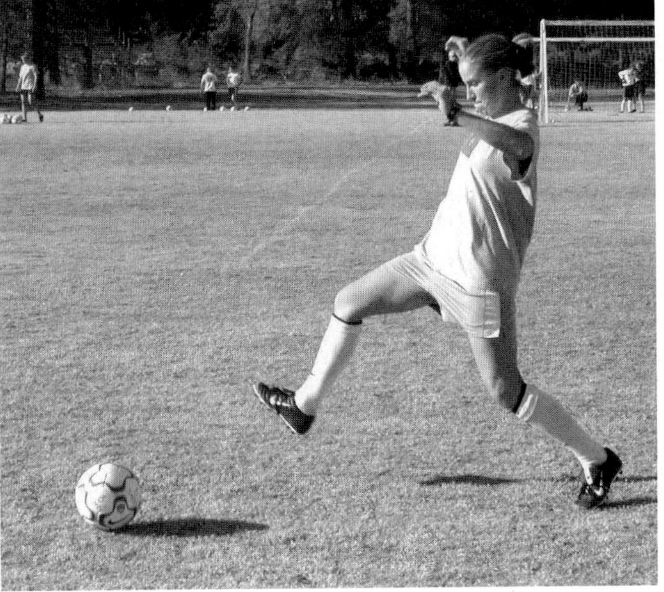

Figure 21-28

Many sports that require stretch of the hip region can cause a groin strain.

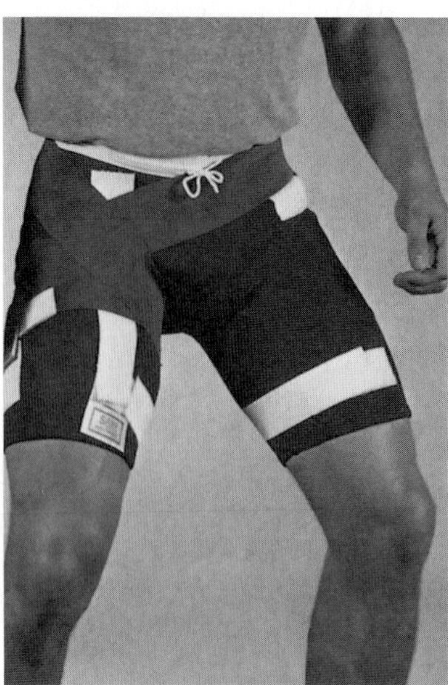
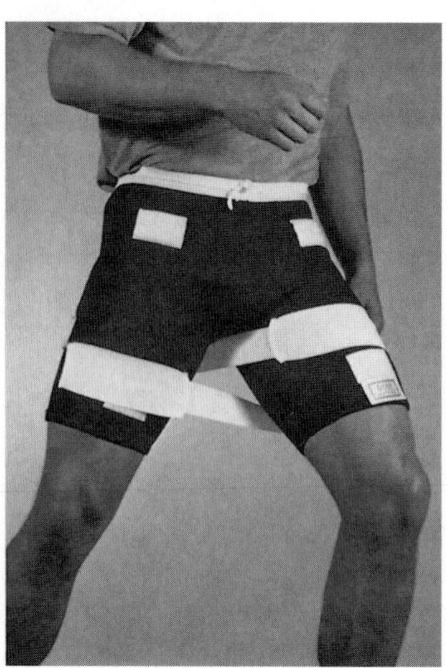

Figure 21-29

Commercial restraints such as the Sawa groin and thigh braces are increasingly being used by athletic trainers.

longus muscle is most often strained.[26] Running, jumping, or twisting with external rotation can produce such injuries.

Symptoms and signs The groin strain is one of the most difficult injuries to care for in sports.[12] The strain can be felt as a sudden twinge or feeling of tearing during an active movement, or the athlete may not notice it until after the termination of activity.[13] Like most tears, the groin strain produces pain, weakness, and internal hemorrhage.

Management If it is detected immediately after it occurs, the strain should be treated by RICE, NSAIDs, and analgesics as needed for forty-eight to seventy-two hours. Passive, active, and resistive muscle tests should be given to ascertain the exact muscle or muscles that are involved.

The athletic trainer frequently encounters difficulty when attempting to care for a groin strain. Rest has been the best treatment. Daily whirlpool therapy or cryotherapy are palliative; ultrasound offers a more definite approach. Exercise should be delayed until the groin is pain free. Exercise rehabilitation should emphasize gradual stretching and restoration of the normal range of motion. Until normal flexibility and strength are developed, a protective spica bandage or a commercial brace should be applied (Figure 21-29).

Trochanteric Bursitis

Etiology Trochanteric bursitis is a relatively common condition of the greater trochanter of the femur (Figure 21-30). Although commonly called bursitis, the condition also could be an inflammation at the site where the gluteus medius muscle inserts or the iliotibial band passes over the trochanter.

Symptoms and signs The athlete complains of pain in the lateral hip. Pain may radiate down to the knee, causing a limp. Palpation reveals tenderness over the lateral aspect of the greater trochanter. The athletic trainer should perform tests for tensor fasciae latae and iliotibial tightness.

An increased Q angle or leg-length discrepancy can lead to trochanteric bursitis in women runners.

Management Therapy initially includes RICE, NSAIDs, and analgesics as needed. ROM exercises and PRE directed toward hip abductors and external rotators should follow. Phonophoresis may be added if the athlete does not respond in three to four days. The athlete's return to running should be cautious; the athlete should avoid running on inclined surfaces. Faulty running form, leg-length discrepancy, and faulty foot

Signs & Symptoms
Management Plan
Therapy
Exercise Rehabilitation

Acute Groin Strain

Injury Situation A female varsity basketball player had a history of tightness in her groin. During a game she suddenly rotated her trunk while also stretching to the right side. The athlete experienced a sudden, sharp pain and a sense of "giving way" in the left side of the groin that caused her to immediately stop play and limp to the sidelines.

Symptoms and Signs As the athlete described it to the athletic trainer, there was severe pain when rotating her trunk to the right and flexing her left hip. Inspection revealed the following:

1. There was major point tenderness in the groin, especially in the region of the adductor magnus muscle.
2. There was no pain during passive movement of the hip, but severe pain did occur during both active and resistive motion.
3. When the groin and hip were tested for injury, the hip joint, illiopsoas, and rectus femoris muscles were ruled out as having been injured; however, when the athlete adducted the hip from a stretch position, it caused her extreme discomfort.

Management Plan Based on the athletic trainer's inspection, with findings confirmed by the physician, it was determined that the athlete had sustained a grade 2 strain of the groin, particularly to the adductor magnus muscle.

Phase 1 *Acute Injury*

GOALS: To stop hemorrhage, reduce pain, and stop muscle spasms.
ESTIMATED LENGTH OF TIME (ELT): 2 to 3 days.

■ **Therapy** Careful physical examination plus MRI to rule out conditions other than a strain. IMMEDIATE CARE: RICE (20 min) intermittently, 6 to 8 times daily. When weight bearing, the athlete should wear a 6-inch elastic hip spica.

■ **Exercise rehabilitation** No exercise—as much complete rest as possible.

Phase 2 *Repair*

GOALS: To reduce pain, control spasm, and restore full ability to contract and stretch the adductor longus muscle. To maintain cardiorespiratory fitness.
ELT: 2 to 3 weeks.

■ **Therapy** Ice massage (1 min) 3 to 4 times daily followed by hip ROM movements. Muscle electrical stimulation using the surge current at 7 or 8, depending on athlete's tolerance, together with ultrasound, set at 1 W/cm^2 (7 min), once daily. Cold therapy in the form of ice massage (7 min) or ice packs (10–15 min) followed by exercise, 2 to 3 times daily.

■ **Exercise rehabilitation** Proprioceptive neuromuscular facilitation hip patterns 2 to 3 times daily after cold application, progressing to PRE using pulley, isokinetic, or free weights (10 repetitions, 3 sets) once daily. Jogging in chest-level water (10 to 20 min) 1 or 2 times daily for first exercise rehabilitation week followed by flutter kick swimming (pain free) once daily during subsequent weeks. General body maintenance exercises should be conducted 3 times a week as long as they do not aggravate the injury.

Phase 3 *Remodeling*

GOALS: To restore full power, endurance, and muscle extensibility. The athlete gradually returns to precompetition exercise and finally competition, wearing a groin restraint.
ELT: 3 to 6 weeks.

Continued

Acute Groin Strain—*continued*

■ **Therapy** If symptom free, precede exercise with ice massage (7 min) or ice pack (5 to 15 min).

■ **Exercise rehabilitation** Engage in ROM exercise and PRE. Begin a program of jogging on flat course, slowly progressing to a 3-mile run once daily and then progressing to figure eights, starting with obstacles 10 feet apart and gradually shortening distance to 5 feet, from one-half speed to full speed.

Criteria for Return to Competitive Basketball

1. As measured by an isokinetic dynamometer, the athlete's injured hip should have strength equal to that of the uninjured hip.
2. Hip has full range of motion.
3. The athlete is able to run figure eights around obstacles set 5 feet apart at full speed.

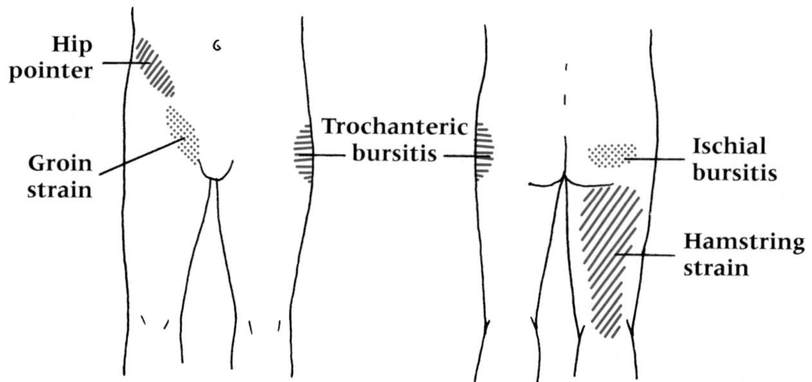

Figure 21-30

Tenderness sites in the region of the hip and pelvis.

biomechanics must be taken into consideration. The condition is most common among women runners who have an increased Q angle or a leg-length discrepancy.

21-5 Critical Thinking Exercise

A gymnast performs a dismount from the rings. Landing off balance, he violently twists his right hip.

? From the information provided, what type of injury could he have sustained?

Sprains of the Hip Joint

Etiology The hip joint, the strongest and best-protected joint in the human body, is seldom seriously injured during sports activities.[21] The hip joint is substantially supported by the ligamentous tissues and muscles that surround it, so any unusual movement that exceeds the normal range of motion may result in tearing of tissue. Such an injury may occur as the result of a violent twist, produced either via an impact force delivered by another participant, via forceful contact with another object, or via a situation in which the foot is firmly planted and the trunk is forced in an opposing direction.[1]

Symptoms and signs A hip sprain displays all the signs of an acute injury but is best revealed through the athlete's inability to circumduct the thigh. Symptoms are similar to a stress fracture. There is significant pain in the hip region. Hip rotation increases pain.

Management X rays or MRIs should be done to rule out fracture; RICE, NSAIDs, and analgesics should be given as needed. Depending on the grade of sprain, weight bearing should be restricted. Crutch walking is used for grade 2 and 3 sprains. ROM exercises and PRE should be delayed until the hip is pain free.

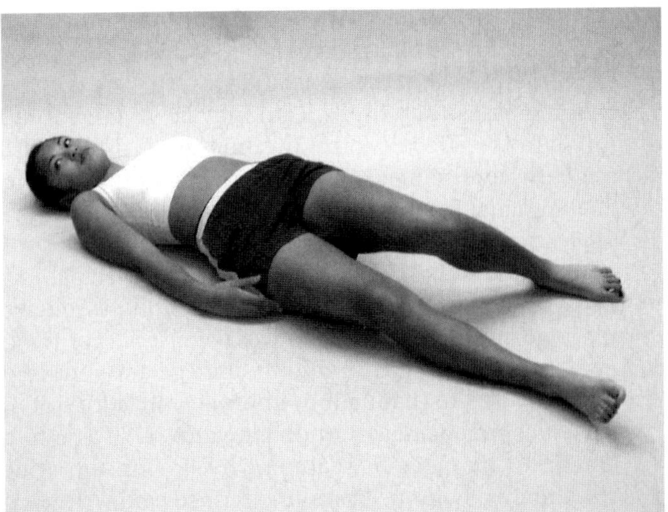

Figure 21-31

Typical position for a hip dislocation: slightly flexed, adducted and internally rotated.

Dislocated Hip Joint

Etiology Dislocation of the hip joint rarely occurs in sports and then usually only as the end result of traumatic force directed along the long axis of the femur. Such dislocations are produced when the knee is bent. The most common displacement is one posterior to the acetabulum, with the femoral shaft adducted and flexed.

Symptoms and signs The injury presents a picture of a flexed, adducted, and internally rotated thigh (Figure 21-31). Palpation will reveal that the head of the femur has moved to a position posterior to the acetabulum. A hip dislocation causes serious pathology by tearing capsular and ligamentous tissue. A fracture is often associated with this injury, accompanied by possible damage to the sciatic nerve.

Management Medical attention must be secured immediately after displacement, or muscle contractures may complicate the reduction. Immobilization usually consists of two weeks of bed rest and the use of a crutch for walking for a month or longer.

Complications Complication of the posterior hip dislocation is likely, with such possibilities as a palsy of the sciatic nerve and later the development of osteoarthritis. Hip dislocation also can lead to disruption of the blood supply to the head of the femur, which eventually leads to the degenerative condition known as avascular necrosis.[16]

21-6

Critical Thinking **Exercise**

A field hockey player has been determined to have a Q angle of 22 degrees. Her left leg is ¾ inch shorter than her right leg. She complains of pain at the point just over the left greater trochanter when she runs.

? Based on the information provided, what could the condition be?

Avascular Necrosis

Etiology Avascular necrosis is a condition that results from the temporary or permanent loss of the blood supply to the proximal femur. Without blood, the bone tissue dies and causes a collapse of the joint surface. Avascular necrosis has several causes. Loss of blood supply to the bone can be caused by an injury such as a hip dislocation (trauma-related avascular necrosis) in which the blood vessels may be damaged, thus interfering with the blood circulation to the bone. In a hip dislocation, the lateral circumflex artery, which supplies most of the blood to the femoral head, can be compromised thus interfering with circulation. If this condition is not rectified quickly the chances of developing avascular necrosis are markedly increased. Certain other risk factors (nontraumatic avascular necrosis), such as the use of some medications (steroids), blood coagulation disorders, or excessive alcohol use, create increased pressure within the bone, causing the blood vessels to narrow and making it hard for the vessels to deliver enough blood to the bone cells.

Symptoms and signs In the early stages of avascular necrosis, the athlete may not have any symptoms. As the disease progresses, however, most individuals experience

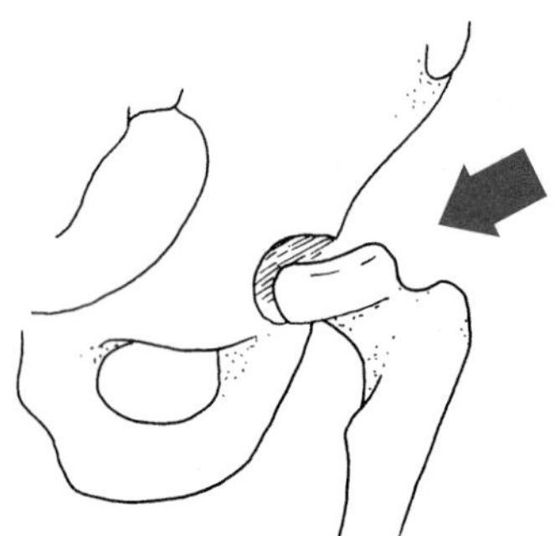

Figure 21-32

Legg-Calvé-Perthes disease (coxa plana). Arrow indicates avascular necrosis of the femoral head.

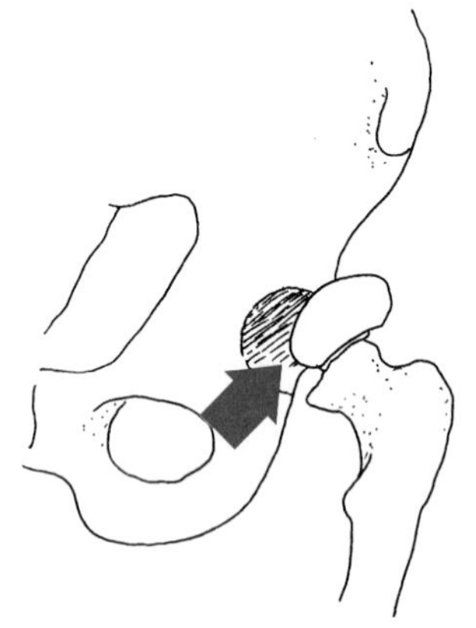

Figure 21-33

Slipped capital femoral epiphysis (arrow).

A young athlete complaining of pain in the groin, abdomen, or knee and walking with a limp may display signs of Legg-Calvé-Perthes disease or a slipped capital femoral epiphysis.

joint pain—at first, only when weight bearing on the affected joint, and then even when resting. Pain usually develops gradually and may be mild or severe. If avascular necrosis progresses and the bone and surrounding joint surface collapse, pain may develop or increase dramatically. Pain may be severe enough to limit the athlete's range of motion in the affected joint. In some cases, osteoarthritis may develop. The period of time between the first symptoms and loss of joint function is different for each individual, ranging from several months to more than a year.

Management In cases of suspected avascular necrosis, the athlete should be referred to a physician for an MRI, X ray, or CT scan. The goal in treating avascular necrosis is to improve the athlete's use of the affected joint, stop further damage to the bone, and ensure bone and joint survival. Several conservative treatments are available that can help prevent further bone and joint damage and reduce pain. Range-of-motion exercises may be used to maintain or improve joint range of motion. Electrical stimulation has been recommended to induce bone growth. If avascular necrosis is diagnosed early, the physician may begin treatment by having the athlete be non–weight bearing. When combined with medication to reduce pain, reduced weight bearing can be an effective way to avoid or delay surgery. The use of medications to reduce fatty substances (lipids) that increase with corticosteroid treatment or to reduce blood clotting in the presence of clotting disorders is also recommended. In most cases the athlete will eventually require surgery to repair the joint permanently.

Hip Joint Problems in the Young Athlete

The athletic trainer working with a child or adolescent should understand three major problems. They are Legg-Calvé-Perthes disease, slipped capital femoral epiphysis, and the snapping hip.

Legg-Calvé-Perthes Disease (Coxa Plana)

Etiology Legg-Calvé-Perthes disease is avascular necrosis of the femoral head (Figure 21-32). It occurs in children ages four to ten and in boys more often than in girls. For the most part this condition is not clearly understood. Trauma accounts for 25 percent of the cases seen.[5] It is listed under the broad heading of osteochondrosis. Because of a disruption of circulation at the head of the femur, articular cartilage becomes necrotic and flattens.[20]

Symptoms and signs The young athlete commonly complains of pain in the groin that sometimes is referred to the abdomen or knee. Limping is also typical. The condition can have a rapid onset, but more often it comes on slowly over a number of months. Examination may show limited hip movement and pain.

Management Care of this condition could mean complete bed rest to alleviate synovitis. The athlete may have to wear a special brace to avoid direct weight bearing on the hip. If treated in time, the head of the femur will revascularize and reossify.

Complications If the condition is not treated early enough, the head of the femur will become ill shaped, creating problems of osteoarthritis in later life.

Slipped Capital Femoral Epiphysis

Etiology The problem of a slipped capital femoral epiphysis (Figure 21-33) is found mostly in boys between the ages of ten and seventeen who are characteristically tall and thin or obese. Although idiopathic, it may be related to the effects of a growth hormone. One-quarter of the cases seen have the condition in both hips. Trauma accounts for 25 percent of the cases seen.[5] X-ray examination may show femoral head slippage posteriorly and inferiorly.

Symptoms and signs Like Legg-Calvé-Perthes disease, a slipped capital femoral epiphysis causes the athlete pain in the groin that comes on suddenly as a result of trauma or over weeks or months as a result of prolonged stress. In the early stages of this condition, signs may be minimal. In its most advanced stage, however, there is hip and knee pain during passive and active motion; limitations of abduction, flexion, and medial rotation; and a limp.[25]

Management In minor slippage, rest and non–weight bearing may prevent further slipping. Major displacement usually requires corrective surgery.

Complications If the slippage goes undetected or if surgery fails to properly restore normal hip mechanics, severe hip problems may occur in later life.

The Snapping Hip Phenomenon

Etiology The snapping hip phenomenon is common to young female dancers, gymnasts, and hurdlers, who make similar use of their hips. The problem stems from habitual movements that predispose muscles around the hip to become imbalanced.[27] This condition commonly occurs when the individual laterally rotates and flexes the hip joint as part of the exercise or dance routine. This condition is related to a structurally narrow pelvic width, greater range of motion of hip abduction, and less range of motion in lateral rotation. As hip stability lessens, the hip joint capsule and ligaments and adductor muscles become less stable.

Symptoms and signs The athlete complains that snapping occurs, especially when balancing on one leg. Such a problem should not go unattended, especially if pain and inflammation are associated with the snapping.

Management Management should focus on cryotherapy and ultrasound to stretch tight musculature and strengthen weak musculature in the hip region.

21-7 Critical Thinking Exercise

A fifteen-year-old male football player complains of pain in his hip off and on during the season. There is increasing hip and knee pain during movement. The athlete has a restriction of hip abduction, flexion, and medial rotation. He is beginning to walk with a limp.

? What should the athletic trainer be concerned about in this fifteen-year-old, and what steps should be taken?

Pelvic Conditions

Athletes who perform activities that involve jumping, running, and violent collisions can sustain serious acute and overuse injuries to the pelvic region.[4] When an athlete runs, the pelvis rotates along a longitudinal axis proportionate to the amount of arm swing. It also tilts up and down as the leg engages in support and nonsupport. This combination of motion causes shearing at the sacroiliac joint and symphysis pubis. Tilting of the pelvis also produces both a decrease and an increase in lumbar lordosis, depending on the slant of the running surface. Running downhill increases lumbar lordosis, and running uphill decreases it.[10]

Contusion (Hip Pointer)

Etiology Iliac crest contusion and contusion of the abdominal musculature, commonly known as a hip pointer, occurs most often in contact sports (Figure 21-34). The hip pointer results from a blow to an inadequately protected iliac crest. The hip pointer is considered one of the most handicapping injuries in sports and one that is difficult to manage. A direct force to the unprotected iliac crest causes severe pinching action to the soft tissue of that region.

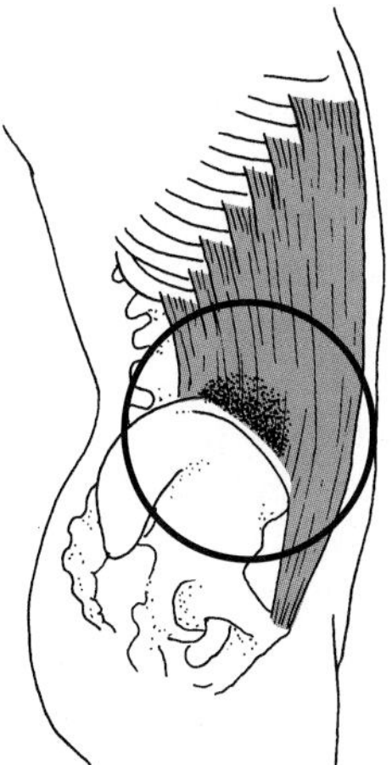

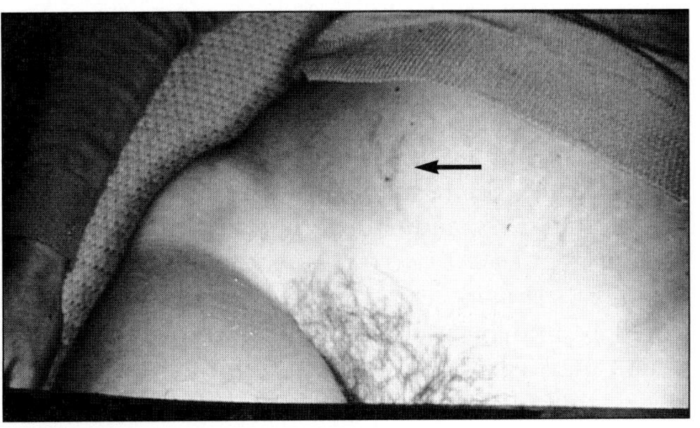

'Figure 21-34

A blow to the pelvic rim can cause a bruise and hematoma known as a hip pointer.

21-8 Critical Thinking Exercise

A young female gymnast complains to the athletic trainer that her hip snaps when she stands on one leg.

? What is the possible cause of this snapping hip phenomenon?

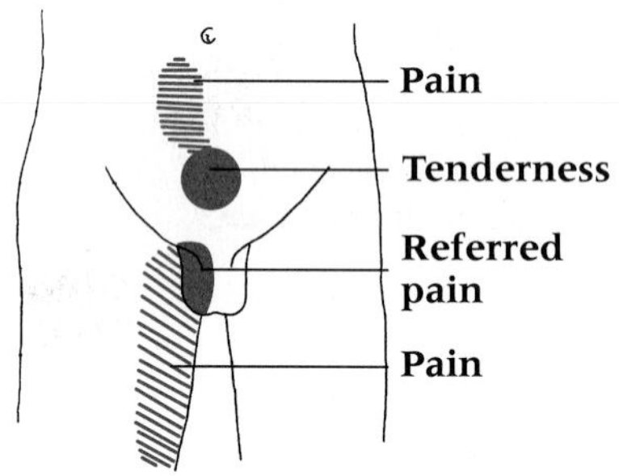

Figure 21-35

Osteitis pubis and other pain sites in the region of the pelvis and groin.

Symptoms and signs A hip pointer produces immediate pain, spasms, and transitory paralysis of the soft structures. As a result, the athlete is unable to rotate the trunk or to flex the thigh without pain.

Management RICE should be applied immediately after injury and should be maintained intermittently for at least forty-eight hours. In severe cases, bed rest for one to two days will speed recovery. The mechanisms for the hip pointer are the same as those for an iliac crest fracture or epiphyseal separation.

The athlete must be referred to a physician, and an X-ray examination must be performed. A variety of treatment procedures can be used for this injury. Ice massage and ultrasound have been found to be beneficial. Initially the injury may be injected with a steroid. Later, oral antiinflammatory agents may be used. Recovery time usually ranges from one to three weeks.

Osteitis Pubis

Etiology Because the popularity of distance running has increased, a condition known as osteitis pubis has become more prevalent. It is also caused by the sports of soccer, football, and wrestling. Repetitive stress on the pubic symphysis and adjacent bony structures caused by the pull of muscles in the area creates a chronic inflammatory condition (Figure 21-35).

Symptoms and signs The athlete has pain in the groin region and in the area of the symphysis pubis. There is point tenderness on the pubic tubercle, and the athlete experiences pain while running, doing sit-ups, and doing squats. Acute osteitis pubis may occur as a result of pressure from a bicycle seat.

Management Follow-up care usually consists of rest, an oral antiinflammatory agent, and a gradual return to activity.

Athletic Pubalgia

Etiology The term *pubalgia* is a catchall term that generally refers to chronic pubic region or inguinal pain. It may be caused by repetitive stress to the pubic symphysis from kicking and twisting or cutting at high speeds, such as occurs in soccer or ice hockey[39]. Forceful hip adduction from a hyperextended position creates shear forces that are transmitted through the pubic symphysis to the common insertion of the rectus abdominus, the hip adductors, and the conjoined tendon at the pubic tubercle. These forces may result in microtears of the transversalis abdominis fascia or the aponeurosis of the internal and external obliques, or a defect or weakness at the conjoint tendon. These factors collectively can create a weakness in the anterior wall of the inguinal canal, although there is no direct or indirect hernia present.[19]

Symptoms and signs Chronic pain often occurring only during exertion may persist for several months. Sharp, burning pain localizes to the lower abdominal and inguinal region initially and later radiates to the adductors and testicles. There is point tenderness at the pubic tubercle. Pain is increased with resisted hip flexion, internal rotation, and abdominal muscle contraction. Pain also occurs with resisted hip adduction, although the adductors are not tender, which differentiates this condition from an adductor strain.

Management Conservative treatment is rarely effective and pain often returns with activity. Nevertheless, conservative treatment should be attempted, beginning initially with deep tissue massage of the affected structures. After a week, stretching of the hip flexors, adductors and rotators, the hamstrings, and low back muscles can be incorporated. At two weeks, strengthening of the abdominals and hip adductors and flexors should begin. At three to four weeks running can begin, followed as tolerated by jumping and kicking. If conservative treatment is not effective, cortisone injection may be used cautiously. Surgical intervention to tighten the pelvic floor may be necessary if more conservative measures fail.

21-9 Critical Thinking Exercise

A soccer player complains of a sharp, burning pain in his groin and his testicles whenever he kicks the ball. He has palpable tenderness over his pubic tubercle and indicates there is also pain on resisted adduction. The athlete is concerned that he has a hernia.

? What might the athletic trainer suspect is wrong with this athlete?

Stress Fractures

Etiology Stress fractures in the pelvic area are seen mostly in distance runners. Repetitive cyclical forces created by ground reaction forces can produce stress fractures in the pelvis and the proximal femur. They constitute approximately 16 percent of all stress fractures and are more common in women than in men. The most common sites are the inferior pubic ramus and the femoral neck and subtrochanteric area of the femur.

Symptoms and signs Commonly, the athlete complains of groin pain along with an aching sensation in the thigh that increases with activity and decreases with rest. Standing on one leg may be impossible for the athlete. Deep palpation will cause severe point tenderness. Pelvic stress fracture has a tendency to occur during intensive interval training or competitive racing. For the ischium and the pubis, crutch walking is recommended.[5]

Management Rest is usually the treatment of choice for two to five months. Normally a bone scan will pick up osteoclastic activity early.[5] Freestyle swimming can be performed for aerobic exercise. The breast stroke must be avoided.

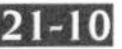

21-10
Critical Thinking Exercise

A football player who was not wearing hip pads receives a hard, compressive hit to his left iliac crest region.

? What injury has this athlete sustained? What are the expected symptoms and signs?

Avulsion Fractures and Apophysitis

Etiology The pelvis has a number of apophyses where major muscles make their attachments. An apophysis, or traction epiphysis, is a bony outgrowth and is contrasted to pressure epiphyses, which are the growth plates for long bones. The three most common sites for avulsion fractures and apophysitis in the pelvic region are the ischial tuberosity and the hamstring attachment, the anterior inferior iliac spine and the rectus femoris muscle attachment, and the anterior superior iliac spine where the sartorius muscle makes its attachment (Figure 21-36). Sports that have sudden acceleration or deceleration, such as football, soccer, and basketball, can cause a convulsion, a fracture, or an apophysitis.[7]

Symptoms and signs The athlete complains of a sudden localized pain with limited movement. There is swelling and point tenderness. Muscle testing increases pain.

Management X-ray examination is routinely given with apophysical pain. Uncomplicated conditions can be treated with RICE and crutches, with toe-touch weight bearing for one to two months.[4] After the control of pain and inflammation (two to three weeks), a gradual stretch program should begin. When 80 degrees of range of motion have been returned, a PRE program should be instituted.[2] When full range of motion and strength have been regained, the athlete can return to competition.

21-11
Critical Thinking Exercise

A cross-country runner complains of pain in her groin and in the area of her symphysis pubis. She says she experienced pain when running and when doing sit-up exercises.

? What conditions might be indicated by this athlete's complaints?

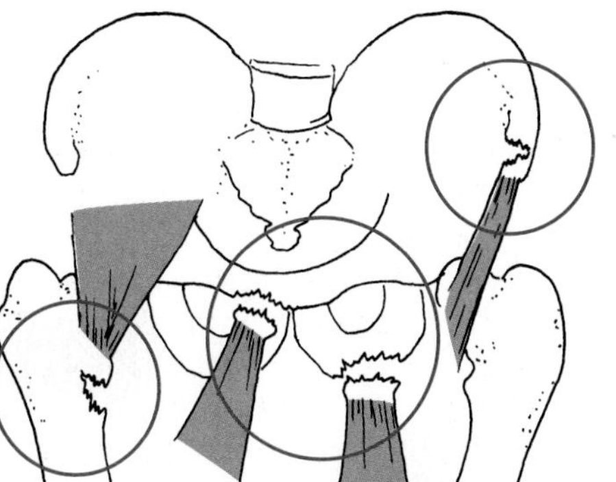

Figure 21-36

Potential avulsion fractures to the pelvic apophyses.

THIGH AND HIP REHABILITATION TECHNIQUES

General Body Conditioning

As with other sports injuries, the athlete must maintain cardiorespiratory fitness, muscle endurance, and strength of the total body. If weight bearing is painful or if the athlete is not capable of performing functional activities while fully weight bearing, fitness can be maintained by engaging in aquatic exercise, riding a stationary bike, or using an upper body ergometer.

Flexibility

In the rehabilitation of injuries in the hip and thigh region, regaining pain-free range of motion is a primary concern.[22] Muscle injuries, particularly of the quadriceps, hamstrings, and groin muscles, can significantly restrict motion, thus limiting function. Likewise, injuries to the strong ligamentous and capsular structures of the hip can limit motion. Stretching exercises usually progress from gentle passive stretching to static stretching to proprioceptive neuromuscular facilitation stretching, all within pain-free limits.[43] A complete rehabilitation program must include stretching exercises for those muscles that produce internal and external rotation, adduction, abduction, extension, flexion, and circumduction (Figure 21-37).

Mobilization

If limitations in motion are caused by injury and subsequent tightness in the ligaments and capsule surrounding the hip, joint mobilization techniques should be incorporated to regain normal arthrokinematic movements at the hip. The basic joint mobilization techniques may include but are not limited to the following techniques. Inferior femoral glides at 90 degrees of hip flexion are used to increase abduction and flexion. With the athlete supine, a posterior femoral glide can be done by stabilizing underneath the pelvis and using the body weight applied through the femur to glide posteriorly. Posterior glides are used to increase hip flexion. Anterior femoral glides increase extension and are accomplished by using some support to stabilize under the pelvis and applying an anterior glide posteriorly on the femur. Medial femoral rotations may be used for increasing medial rotation and are done by stabilizing the opposite innominate while internally rotating the hip through the flexed knee (Figure 21-38).

Figure 21-37

Stretching exercises for the thigh and hip. **A,** Hamstrings. **B,** Gluteals.

Continued

A

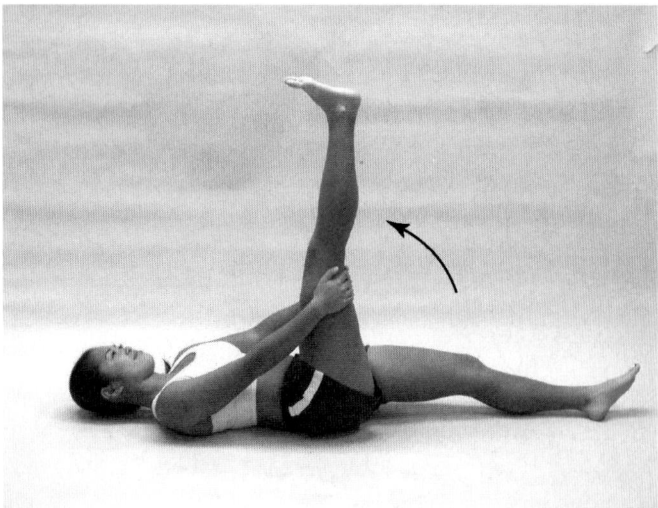

B

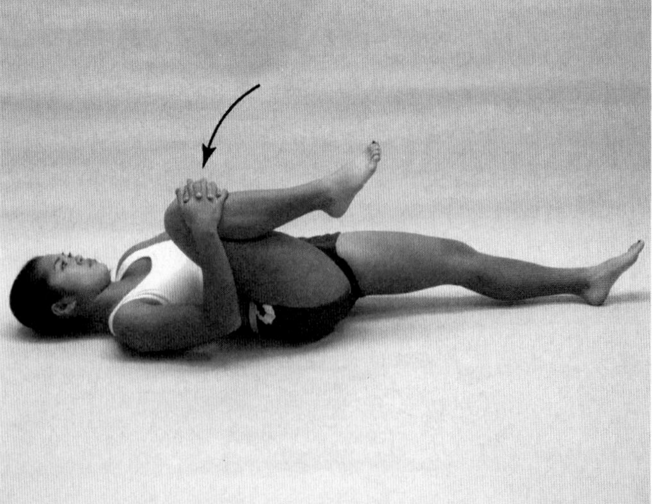

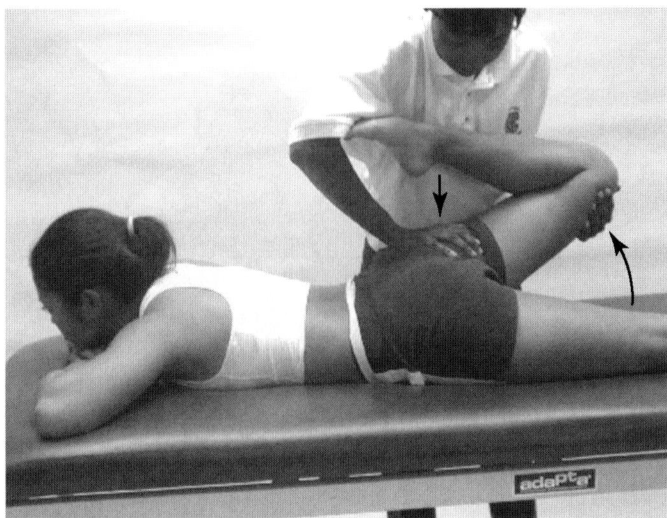

C

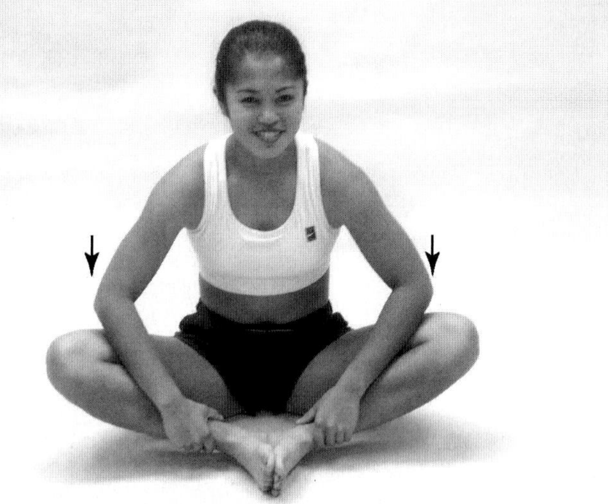

D

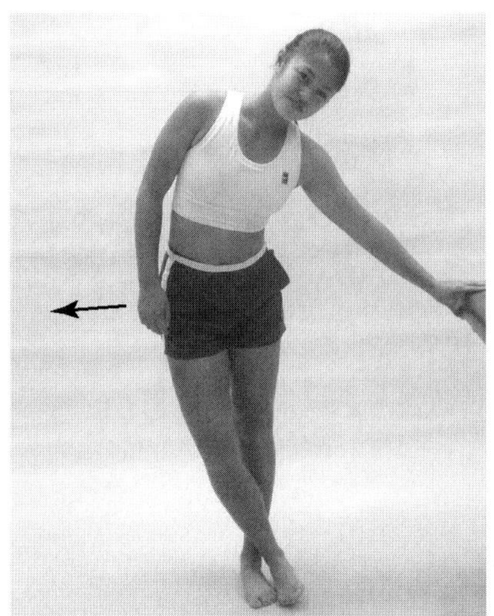

E

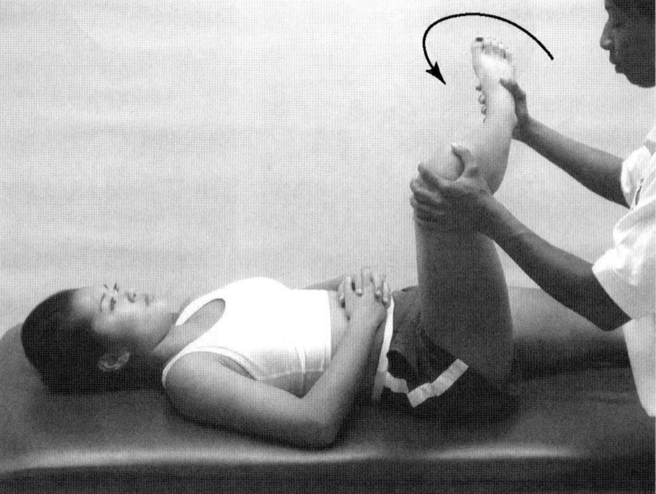

F

Figure 21-37—continued

C, Quadriceps iliopsoas. **D,** Groin (adductors). **E,** Iliotibial band. **F,** Internal rotators. **G,** External rotators. **H,** Piriformis.

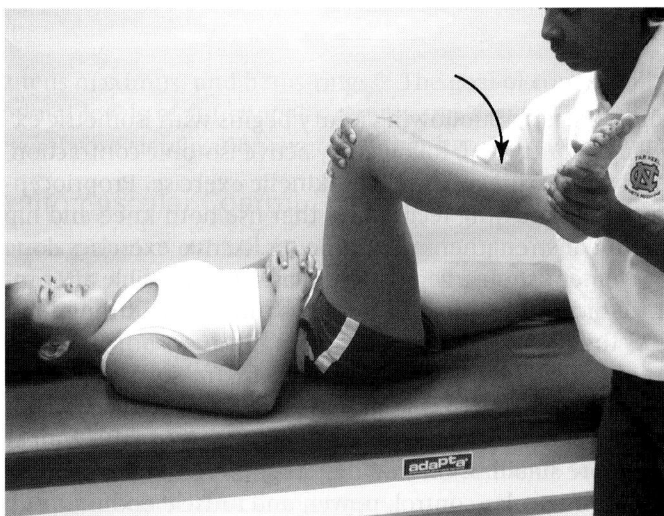

G

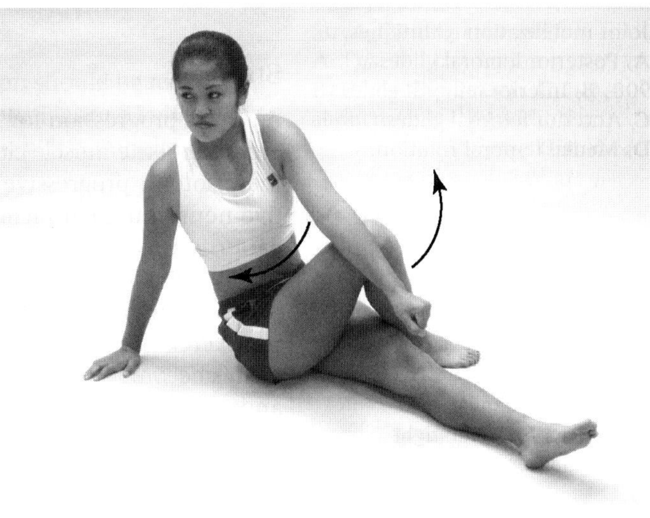

H

34. Panariello RA: CKC exercises for rehabilitating hamstring injuries, *Athletic Therapy Today* 4(4):11, 1999.
35. Parr K: Fractured femur in a middle-distance sprinter. *Athletic Therapy Today* 6(1):50, 2001.
36. Petrone M, Guinn J, Reddin A: The accuracy of the palpation meter (PALM) for measuring pelvic crest height difference and leg length discrepancy. *J Orthop Sports Phys Ther* 33(6):319, 2003.
37. Prentice WE: Mobilization and traction techniques in rehabilitation. In Prentice WE, editor: *Rehabilitation techniques in sports medicine and athletic training,* ed 4, St Louis, 2004, McGraw-Hill.
38. Reese N, Bandy W: Use of an inclinometer to measure flexibility of the iliotibial band using the ober test and the modified ober test: differences in magnitude and reliability of measurements. *J Orthop Sports Phys Ther* 33(6):226, 2003.
39. Rodriguez C, Miguel A, Lima H: Osteitis pubis syndrome in the professional soccer athlete: a case report, *J Ath Train* 36(4):437, 2001.
40. Rosene J, Fogarty T, Mahaffey B: Isokinetic hamstrings: quadriceps ratios in intercollegiate athletics. *J Ath Train* 36(4):378, 2001.
41. Ruane J, Rossi TA: When groin pain is more than just a strain, *Physician Sportsmed* 26(4):78, 1996.
42. Schmitz R, Riemann B, Thompson T: Gluteus medius activity during isometric closed-chain hip rotation, *J Sport Rehabil* 11(3):179, 2002.
43. Spernoga S, Uhl T, Arnold B: Duration of maintained hamstring flexibility after a 1-time modified hold-relax stretching protocol, *J Ath Train* 36(1):44, 2001.
44. Trudelle-Jackson E, Emerson R, Smith S: Outcomes of total hip arthroplasty: study of patients one year postsurgery, *J Orthop Sports Phys Ther* 32(6):260, 2002.
45. Turl SE, George KP: Adverse neural tension: a factor in repetitive hamstring strain? *J Orthop Sports Phys Ther* 27(1):16, 1998.
46. Wissen W: An aggressive approach to managing quadriceps contusions, *Athletic Therapy Today* 5(1):36, 2000.
47. Woolf JM: Pathoanatomy of the painful hip. In *Proceedings, National Athletic Trainers' Association 51st Annual Meeting and Clinical Symposia,* Champaign, Ill, 2000, Human Kinetics: National Athletic Trainers' Association.

ANNOTATED BIBLIOGRAPHY

Fagerson T: *The hip handbook,* Burlington, Ma 1998, Butterworth-Heinemann.

This book provides a clinical resource for physical therapists involved in hip rehabilitation.

Journal of Science and Medicine in Sport 2(1 Supplement), March, 1999.

This issue of this journal contains a number of concise abstracted articles that deal with a variety of injuries to the hip, thigh, pelvis, and groin region.

Koval K, Zuckerman J: Hip fractures: A practical guide to management, New York, 1999, Springer-Verlag.

This book addresses the issues, complications and treatments that face the hip specialist and the general orthopaedic surgeon in both the surgical and non-surgical treatment and management of hip fractures.

Tile M, Helfet D, Kellam J: *Fractures of the pelvis and acetabulum,* Philadelphia, 2003, Lippincott, Williams & Wilkins.

This text discusses anatomy, biomechanics, pathoanatomy, and aspects of trauma and examines the various diagnosis, treatment, and management options.

Torg JS, Shephard RJ, editors: *Current therapy in sports medicine,* ed 3, St. Louis, 1995, Mosby.

This detailed sports medicine text contains extensive coverage of thigh, hip, and pelvic injuries.

The Shoulder Complex

Chapter 22

When you finish this chapter you should be able to

- Point out the critical anatomical features of the four articulations in the shoulder complex.
- Perform an in-depth evaluation of the shoulder complex.
- Recognize those steps that can be taken to minimize the chances of injury to the shoulder complex.
- Explain how shoulder stability is maintained by the joint capsule, ligaments, and muscles.
- Summarize the anatomical and functional relationship between shoulder stability and shoulder impingement.
- Identify the etiology and recognize the symptoms and signs of specific injuries that occur around the shoulder joint, and discuss plans for management.
- Formulate a general plan that may be effectively incorporated into a rehabilitation program for treating a variety of injuries in the shoulder complex.

The shoulder complex, as the name implies, is an extremely complicated region of the body. Because of its anatomical structure, the shoulder complex has a great degree of mobility. This mobility requires some compromise in stability, and thus the shoulder is highly susceptible to injury. Many sport activities, in particular those that involve repetitive overhead movements such as throwing, swimming, or serving in tennis or volleyball, place a great deal of stress on the supporting structures (Figure 22-1). Consequently, injuries related to overuse in the shoulder are commonplace in the athlete. Some understanding of the anatomy and mechanics of this joint is essential for the athletic trainer.

ANATOMY OF THE SHOULDER

Bones

The bones that make up the shoulder complex and shoulder joint are the clavicle, scapula, and humerus (Figure 22-2).

Clavicle

The clavicle is a slender, S-shaped bone approximately 6 inches (15 cm) long. It supports the anterior portion of the shoulder, keeping it free from the thoracic cage. It extends from the sternum to the tip of the shoulder, where it joins the acromion process of the scapula. The shape of the medial two-thirds of the clavicle is primarily circular, and its lateral third assumes a flattened appearance. The medial two-thirds bend convexly forward, and the lateral third is concave. The point at which the clavicle changes shape and contour presents a structural weakness, and the largest number of fractures to the bone occur at this point. Lying superficially with no muscle or fat protection makes the clavicle subject to direct blows.

Scapula

The scapula is a flat, triangular-shaped bone that serves mainly as an articulating surface for the head of the humerus. It is located on the dorsal aspect of the thorax and

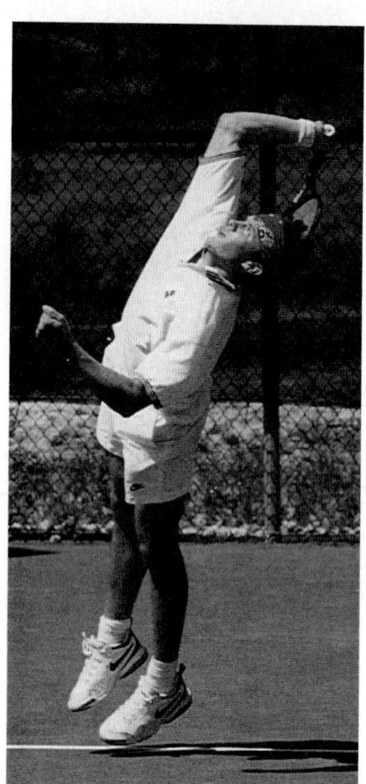

Figure 22-1

Vigorous overhead activities can produce a number of shoulder problems.

has three prominent projections: the spine, the acromion, and the coracoid process. The spine divides the posterior aspect unequally. The superior dorsal aspect is a deep depression called the supraspinous fossa, and the area below, a more shallow depression, is called the infraspinous fossa. The acromion is a process at the lateral tip of the spine. A hooklike projection called the coracoid process arises anteriorly from the scapula. It curves upward, forward, and outward in front of the glenoid fossa, which is the articulating cavity for the reception of the humeral head. The glenoid cavity is situated laterally on the scapula below the acromion and is relatively shallow. However, the presence of the fibrocartilaginous glenoid labrum increases the depth of articulation. The scapula serves as a site of attachment for many muscles that act to move the shoulder complex.

Humerus

The head of the humerus is spherical, with a shallow, constricted neck; it faces upward, inward, and backward, articulating with the scapula's shallow glenoid fossa. Circumscribing the humeral head is a slight groove called the anatomical neck, which is the attachment for the articular capsule of the glenohumeral joint. The greater and lesser tubercles are located adjacent and immediately inferior to the head. The lesser tubercle is positioned anteriorly and medially, with the greater tubercle placed somewhat higher and laterally. Lying between the two tubercles is a deep groove called the bicipital groove, which retains the long tendon of the biceps brachii muscle.

Articulations

There are four major articulations associated with the shoulder complex: the sternoclavicular joint, the acromioclavicular joint, the glenohumeral joint, and the scapulothoracic joint (Figure 22-2).

Sternoclavicular Joint

The clavicle articulates with the manubrium of the sternum to form the sternoclavicular (SC) joint, the only direct connection between the upper extremity and the trunk. The sternal articulating surface is larger than the sternum, causing the clavicle to rise much higher than the sternum. A fibrocartilaginous disk is interposed between the two articulating surfaces. It functions as a shock absorber against the medial forces and also helps prevent any displacement upward. The articular disk is placed so that the clavicle moves on the disk and the disk in turn moves separately on the sternum. The clavicle is permitted to move up and down, forward and backward, in combination, and in rotation.

Acromioclavicular Joint

Shoulder complex articulations:

- Sternoclavicular
- Acromioclavicular
- Glenohumeral
- Scapulothoracic

The acromioclavicular (AC) joint is a gliding articulation of the lateral end of the clavicle with the acromion process. It is a rather weak junction. A fibrocartilaginous disk separates the two articulating surfaces. A thin, fibrous capsule surrounds the joint.

Glenohumeral Joint

The glenohumeral joint (shoulder joint) is an enarthrodial, or ball-and-socket, joint in which the round head of the humerus articulates with the shallow glenoid cavity of the scapula. The cavity is deepened slightly by a fibrocartilaginous rim called the glenoid labrum. The glenohumeral joint is maintained by both a passive and an active mechanism; the passive mechanism relates to the glenoid labrum and capsular ligaments, and the active mechanism relates to the deltoid and rotator cuff muscles.

Scapulothoracic Joint

The scapulothoracic joint is not a true joint; however, the movement of the scapula on the wall of the thoracic cage is critical to shoulder joint motion. Contraction of the scapular muscles, which attach the scapula to the axial skeleton, is critical in sta-

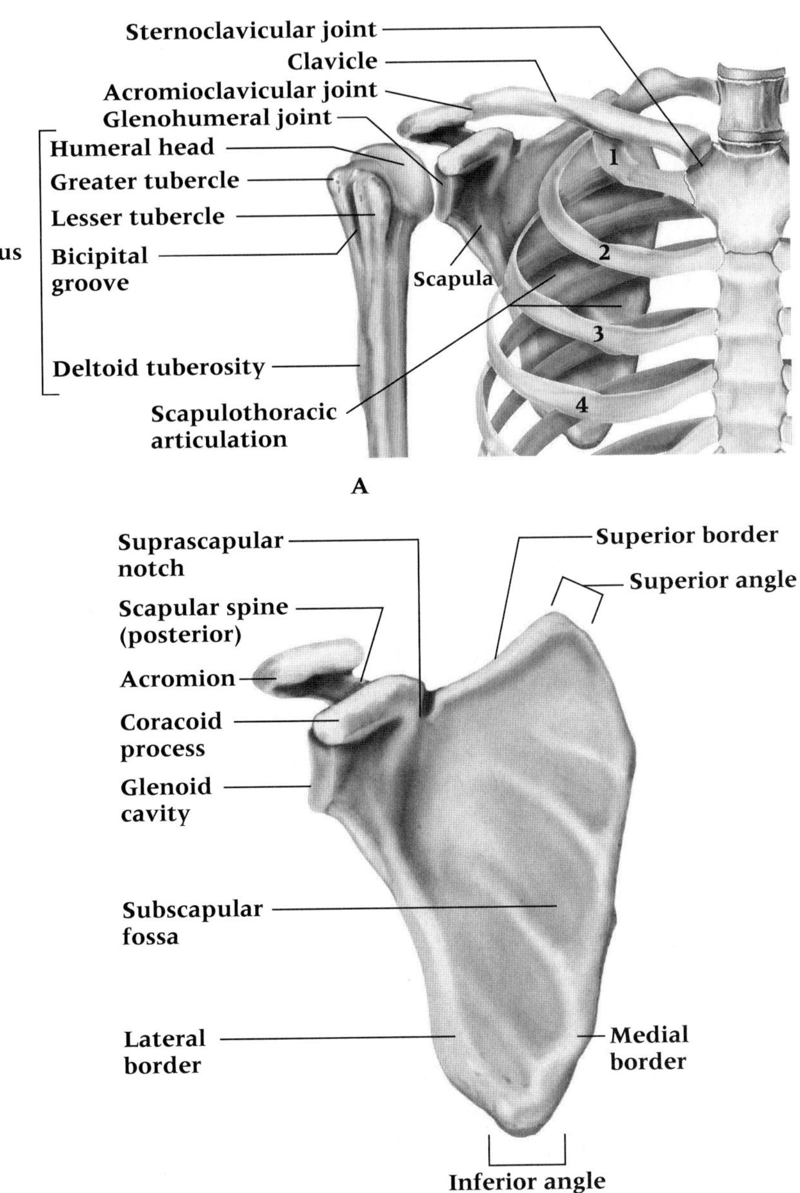

Figure 22-2

A, Skeletal anatomy of the shoulder complex. **B,** Anatomy of the scapula.

bilizing the scapula and thus in providing a base on which a highly mobile joint can function.

Ligaments

Figure 22-3 shows the ligamentous arrangement of the shoulder complex.

Sternoclavicular Joint Ligaments

The sternoclavicular joint is extremely weak because of its bony arrangement, but it is held securely by strong ligaments that tend to pull the sternal end of the clavicle downward and toward the sternum, in effect, anchoring it. The main ligaments are the anterior sternoclavicular, which prevents upward displacement of the clavicle; the posterior sternoclavicular, which also prevents upward displacement of the clavicle; the interclavicular, which prevents lateral displacement of the clavicle; and the costoclavicular, which prevents lateral and upward displacement of the clavicle.[3]

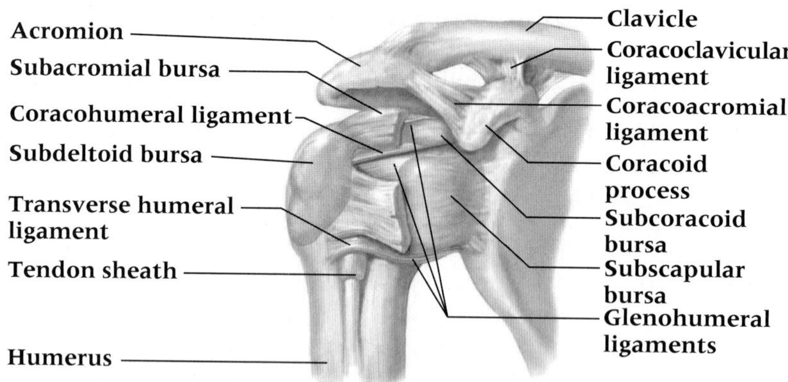

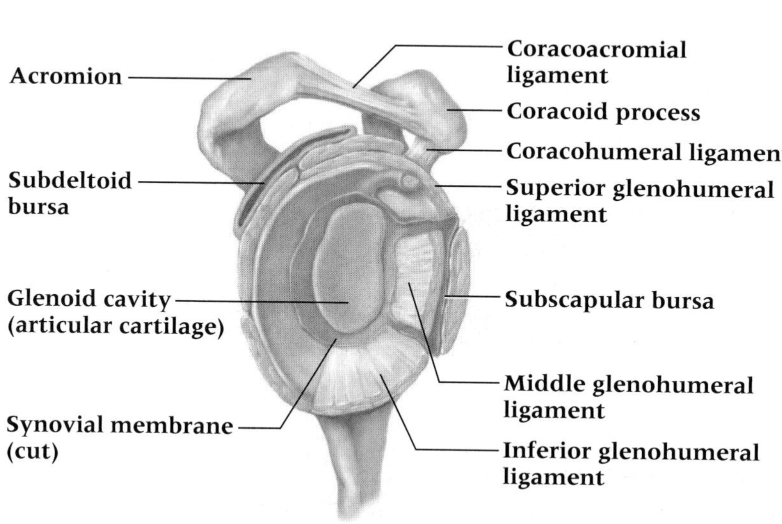

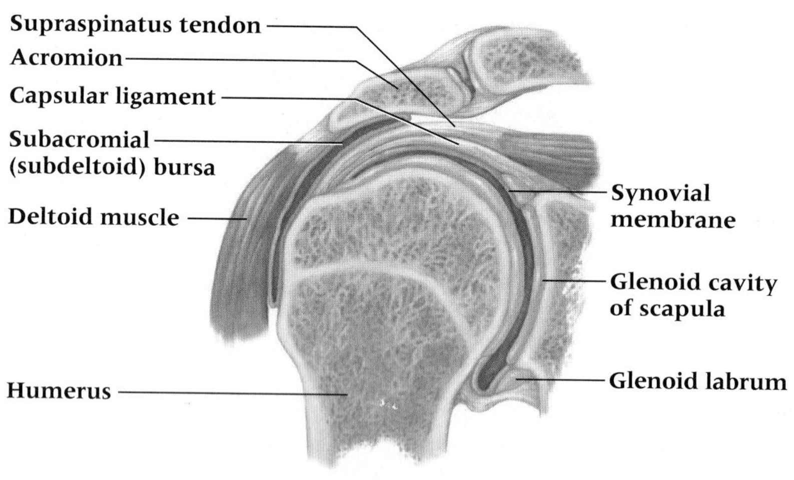

Figure 22-3

Shoulder complex articulations, ligaments and bursae. **A,** Anterior view. **B,** Lateral view. **C,** Frontal section.

Acromioclavicular Joint Ligaments

The acromioclavicular ligament consists of anterior, posterior, superior, and inferior portions. In addition to the acromioclavicular ligament, the coracoclavicular ligament joins the coracoid process and the clavicle and helps maintain the position of the clavicle relative to the acromion. The coracoclavicular ligament is further divided into the conoid and trapezoid ligaments. The coracoclavicular ligament, because of the rotation of the clavicle on its long axis, develops some slack, which permits movement of the scapula at the acromioclavicular joint to take place. The coracoacromial ligament connects the coracoid to the acromion. This ligament along with the acromion forms the coracoacromial arch.

Glenohumeral Joint Ligaments

Surrounding the glenohumeral articulation is a loose, articular capsule. This capsule is strongly reinforced by the superior, middle, and inferior glenohumeral ligaments and by the tough coracohumeral ligament, which attaches to the coracoid process and to the greater tuberosity of the humerus.[53] The glenohumeral ligaments appear to produce a major restraint in shoulder flexion, extension, and rotation. The anterior glenohumeral ligament is tense when the shoulder is in extension, abduction, or external rotation. The posterior glenohumeral ligament's greatest tension is in extension with external rotation. The middle glenohumeral ligament is in greatest tension when in flexion and external rotation. The inferior glenohumeral ligament is most tense when the shoulder is abducted, extended, or externally rotated. The posterior capsule is tense when the shoulder is in flexion, abduction, internal rotation, or any combination of these. The superior and middle segment of the posterior capsule has the greatest tension while the shoulder is internally rotated. The inferior glenohumeral ligament is primarily a check against both anterior and posterior dislocation of the humeral head. The long tendon of the biceps brachii muscle passes across the head of the humerus and then through the bicipital groove. In the anatomical position, the long head of the biceps moves in close relationship with the humerus. The transverse ligament retains the long biceps tendon within the bicipital groove by passing over it from the lesser and the greater tuberosities, converting the bicipital groove into a canal.

22-1
Critical Thinking **Exercise**

A football quarterback has a multidirectional instability of the glenohumeral joint resulting from a series of two anterior dislocations. He is just beginning preseason practice and wants to know what he can do to strengthen his shoulder so that it does not dislocate again.

? What muscles are important in providing dynamic stability specifically to the glenohumeral joint, and will strengthening these muscles prevent a subsequent dislocation?

Shoulder Musculature

Muscles Acting on the Glenohumeral Joint

The muscles that cross the glenohumeral joint produce dynamic motion and establish stability to compensate for a bony and ligamentous arrangement that allows for a great deal of mobility (Figure 22-4). Movements at the glenohumeral joint include flexion, extension, abduction, adduction, horizontal adduction/abduction, internal/external rotation, and circumduction. The muscles acting on the glenohumeral joint may be separated into two groups. The first group consists of muscles that originate on the axial skeleton and attach to the humerus and includes the latissimus dorsi and the pectoralis major. The second group originates on the scapula and attaches to the humerus and includes the deltoid, the teres major, and the coracobrachialis. Additionally, the subscapularis, the supraspinatus, the infraspinatus, and the teres minor muscles constitute the short rotator muscles, commonly called the rotator cuff, whose tendons adhere to the articular capsule and serve as reinforcing structures (Figure 22-5). The biceps and triceps muscles attach on the glenoid and effect elbow motion (Table 22-1).

Glenohumeral joint movements:

- Flexion
- Extension
- Abduction
- Adduction
- External rotation
- Internal rotation
- Horizontal abduction
- Horizontal adduction
- Circumduction

Rotator cuff muscles:

- Subscapularis
- Supraspinatus
- Infraspinatus
- Teres minor

Scapular Muscles

A third group of muscles attaches the axial skeleton to the scapula and includes the levator scapulae, the trapezius, the rhomboids, and the serratus anterior and posterior. The scapular muscles are important in providing dynamic stability to the shoulder complex (see Table 22-1).

Bursae

Several bursae are located around the shoulder joint, the most important of which is the subacromial bursa (see Figure 22-3), located between the coracoacromial arch and the glenohumeral capsule and reinforced by the supraspinous tendon. The subacromial bursa is easily subjected to trauma when the humerus is in the overhead position because it becomes compressed under the coracoacromial arch.

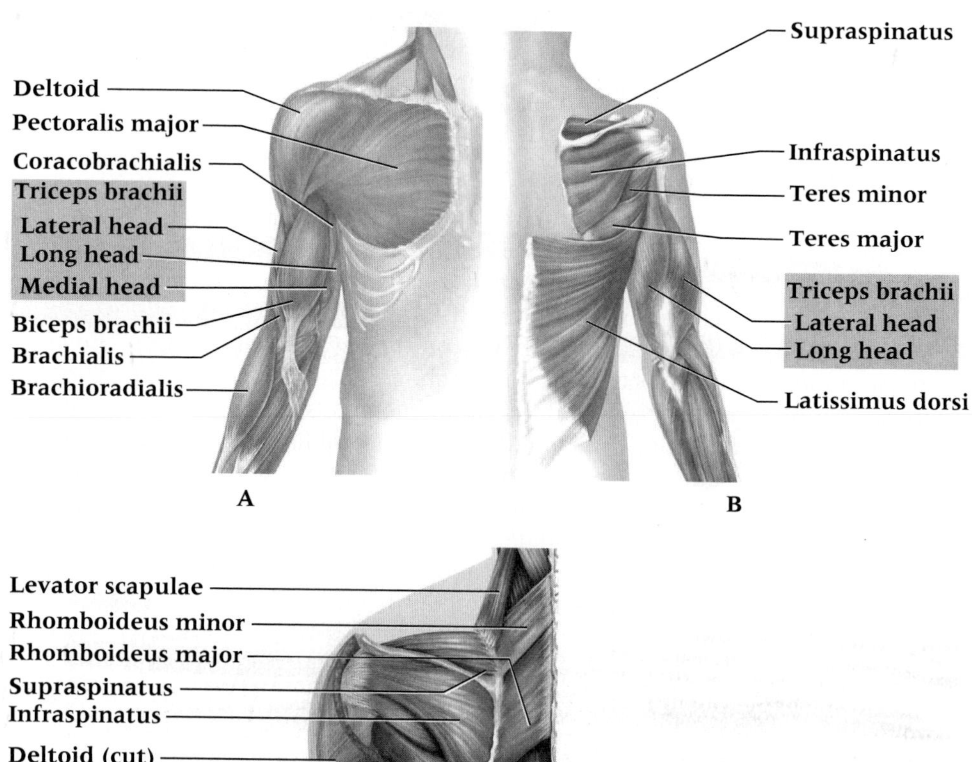

Figure 22-4

Shoulder musculature.
A, Anterior muscles.
B, Posterior muscles.
C, Scapular muscles.

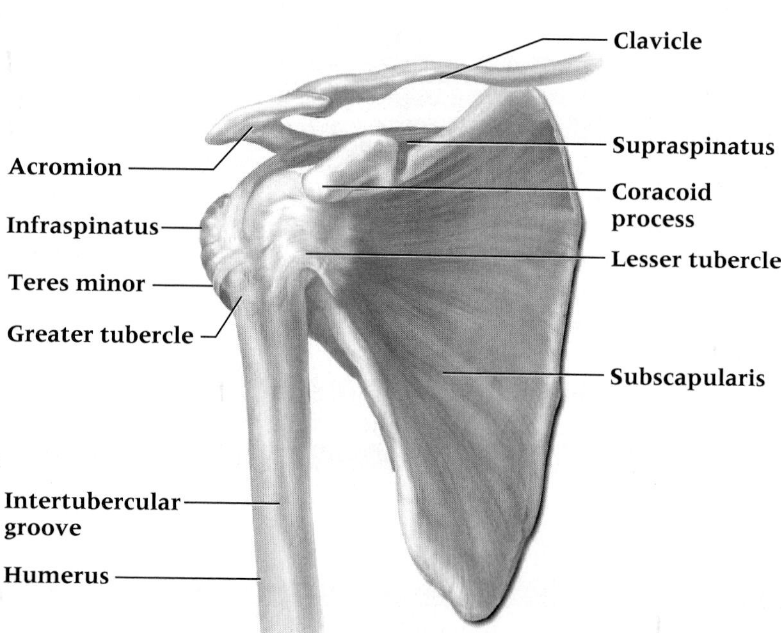

Figure 22-5

Rotator cuff muscles.

TABLE 22-1 Muscles of the Shoulder Girdle

Muscle	Origin	Insertion	Muscle Action	Innervation
Muscles Acting on Humerus				
Pectoralis major	Medial half of the clavicle, the sternum, the costal cartilages of the upper six ribs, and the aponeurosis of the external oblique muscle	Greater turbercle of the humerus	Flexes, adducts, and medially rotates the arm	Medial and lateral pectoral
Latissimus dorsi	Spinous processes of the lower six thoracic and the lumbar vertebrae, the sacrum, the posterior iliac crest—all via the lumbodorsal fascia	Medial margin of the intertubercular groove of the humerus	Extends, adducts, and medially rotates the arm; pulls shoulder downward	Thoracodorsal
Deltoid	Lateral third of the clavicle, the acromion process, and the spine of the scapula	Deltoid tuberosity of the humerus	Abducts arm; anterior fibers flex and medially rotate the arm; posterior fibers extend and laterally rotate the arm	Axillary
Supraspinatus	Supraspinatus fossa of the scapula	Greater tubercle of the humerus	Abducts the arm; slight lateral rotation	Suprascapular
Infraspinatus	Infraspinatus fossa of the scapula	Greater tubercle of the humerus (posterior to the supraspinatus)	Rotates the arm laterally; slight adduction	Suprascapular
Subscapularis	Subscapular fossa of the scapula	Lesser tubercle of the humerus	Rotates the arm medially	Subscapular
Teres major	Dorsal surface of the interior angle of the scapula	Lesser tubercle of the humerus	Adducts, extends, and medially rotates the arm	Subscapular
Teres minor	Axillary border of the scapula	Greater tubercle of the humerus (posterior to the infraspinatus)	Rotates the arm laterally	Axillary
Coracobrachialis	Coracoid process of the scapula	Middle of the humerus, medial surface	Flexes and adducts the arm	Musculocutaneous
Muscles Acting on Scapula				
Trapezius	Occipital bone, the ligamentum nuchae, and the spinous processes of the seventh cervical and all of the thoracic vertebrae	Lateral third of the clavicle, the acromion process, and the spine of the scapula	Elevates (upper portion) or depresses (lower portion), rotates, adducts, and stabilizes the scapula	Spinal accessory (cranial nerve XI)
Rhomboideus major	Spinous processes of the seventh cervical and first thoracic vertebrae	Vertebral border of the scapula, below the spine of the scapula	Adduct, stabilize, and rotate the scapula, lowering its lateral angle	Dorsal scapular (fifth cervical)
Rhomboideus minor	Spinous processes of the second through the fifth thoracic vertebrae	Vertebral border of the scapula, at the base of the spine of the scapula		
Levator scapulae	Transverse processes of the upper four cervical vertebrae	Vertebral border of the scapula, above the spine of the scapula	Elevates scapula and bends the neck laterally when the scapula is fixed	Dorsal scapular
Pectoralis minor	Anterior surface of the third through the fifth ribs	Coracoid process of the scapula	Draws the scapula anteriorly and downward	Medial pectoral (eight cervical and first thoracic)
Serratus anterior	Outer surface of the first nine ribs	Entire length of the ventral surface of the vertebral border of the scapula	Stabilizes, abducts, and rotates the scapula	Long thoracic (fifth through seventh cervical)

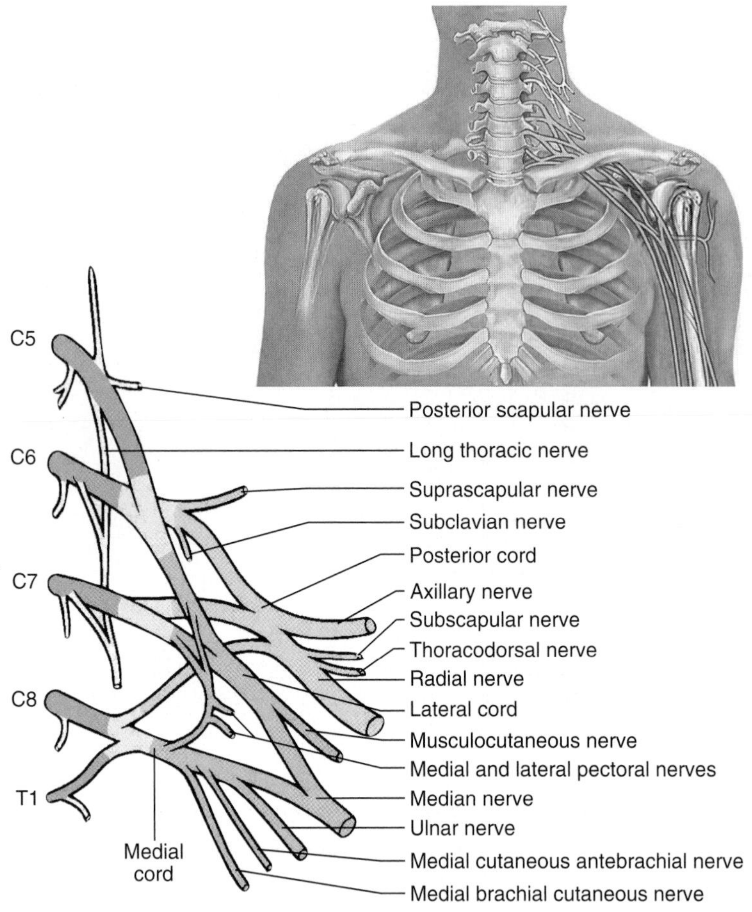

Figure 22-6

The brachial plexus and nerve supply of the shoulder.

Nerve Supply

The spinal nerve roots from the fifth cervical vertebra through the first thoracic vertebra to create the complex nerve network called the brachial plexus, which is discussed in Chapter 25 (Figure 22-6). Stemming from this plexus are the peripheral nerves that innervate muscles of the upper extremity, including the axillary (C5–6), the musculocutaneous (C5–7), the subscapular (C5–6), the suprascapular (C5–6), the dorsal scapular (C5), the pectoral (C5–T1), and the radial (C5–T1) nerves.[2]

Blood Supply

The subclavian artery, which lies distal to the sternoclavicular joint, arches upward and outward, passes the anterior scalene muscle, and then moves downward laterally behind the clavicle and in front of the first ribs (see Figure 22-7). The subclavian artery continues on to become the axillary artery at the outer border of the first rib and to become the brachial artery in the region of the teres major muscle in the upper arm.

FUNCTIONAL ANATOMY

The anatomy of the shoulder complex allows for a great degree of mobility.[75] To achieve this mobility, stability of the complex is sometimes compromised. Instability of the shoulder frequently leads to injury, particularly in those sports that involve overhead activity. In the glenohumeral joint, the rounded humeral head articulates with a relatively flat glenoid on the scapula. Thus, in movement of the shoulder joint, it is critical to maintain the positioning of the humeral head relative to the glenoid. The muscles of the rotator cuff—the subscapularis, infraspinatus, supraspinatus, and teres minor—along with the long head of the biceps function to provide dynamic stability, to control the po-

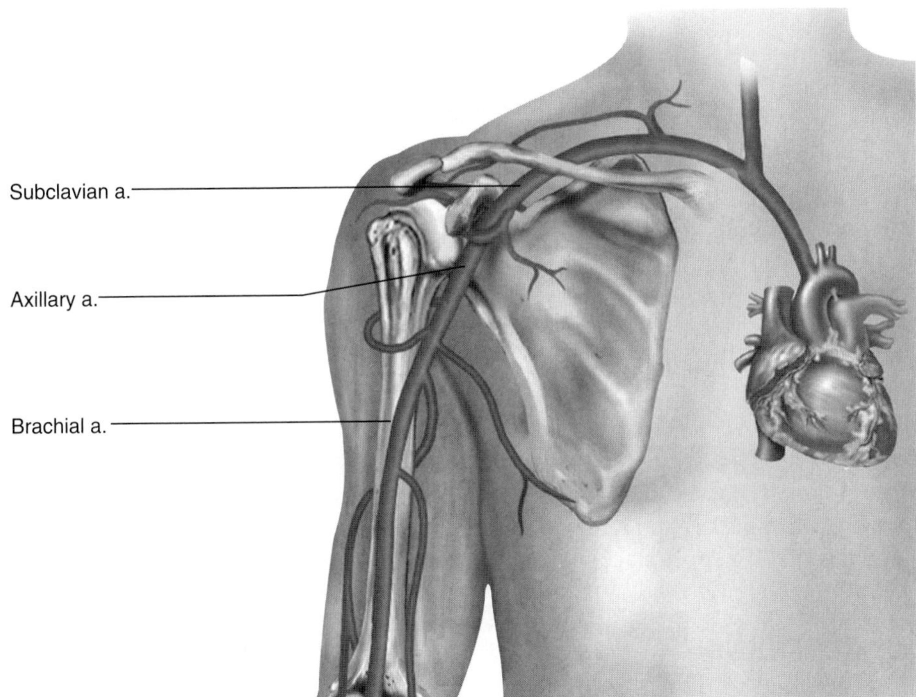

Figure 22-7

Blood supply of the shoulder complex.

sition, and to prevent excessive displacement of the humeral head relative to the position of the glenoid.[32] The supraspinatus compresses the humeral head into the glenoid while cocontraction of the infraspinatus, teres minor, and subscapularis depresses the humeral head during overhead movements.[25,53]

The glenohumeral joint capsule also helps control humeral head movement. The tendons of the rotator cuff blend into the glenohumeral joint capsule. As the muscles contract, they dynamically tighten the joint capsule, which helps center the humeral head relative to the glenoid.[69]

Dynamic movement, as well as stabilization of the shoulder complex, requires integrated functioning of not only the glenohumeral joint, but also of the scapulothoracic, acromioclavicular, and sternoclavicular joints.[75] The muscles that produce movement of the scapula on the thorax help maintain the position of the glenoid relative to the moving humerus and include the levator scapula and upper trapezius, which elevate the scapula; the middle trapezius and rhomboids, which adduct the scapula; the lower trapezius, which adducts and depresses the scapula; and the serratus anterior, which abducts and upwardly rotates the scapula.[34,55,72]

Scapulohumeral Rhythm

Scapulohumeral rhythm describes the movement of the scapula relative to the movement of the humerus throughout a full range of abduction (Figure 22-8). As the humerus elevates to 30 degrees, there is no movement of the scapula. This phase is referred to as the setting phase, during which a stable base is being established on the thoracic wall. From 30 to 90 degrees, the scapula abducts and upwardly rotates 1 degree for every 2 degrees of humeral elevation. From 90 degrees to full abduction, the scapula abducts and upwardly rotates 1 degree for each 1 degree of humeral elevation.[13]

For the scapula to abduct and upwardly rotate throughout 180 degrees of humeral abduction, clavicular movement must occur at both the sternoclavicular and acromioclavicular joints. The clavicle must elevate approximately 40 degrees and must rotate in a posterosuperior direction at least 10 degrees.[3]

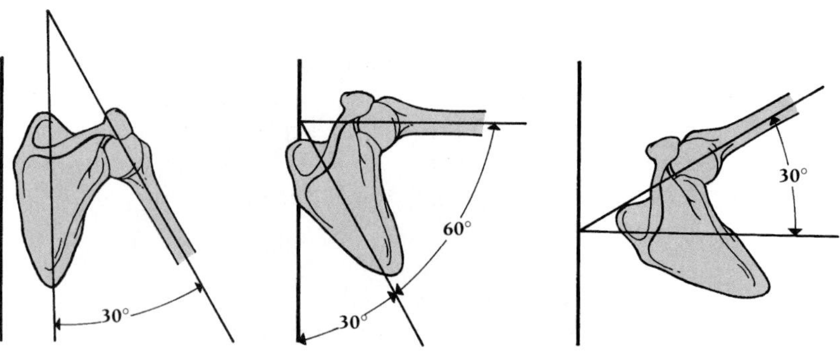

Figure 22-8
Scapulohumeral rhythm.

22-2 Critical Thinking Exercise

A tennis player has a history of chronic shoulder pain. During an injury evaluation, the athletic trainer notes that as the arm elevates above 90 degrees, the athlete seems to be leaning the body toward the side opposite the injured shoulder in an effort to achieve full overhead range of motion. On closer inspection, it seems that the scapula is not moving freely above 90 degrees. The athletic trainer suspects that for some reason the athlete is not exhibiting a normal scapulohumeral rhythm as the arm moves from adduction to a full overhead position.

? What is a normal scapulohumeral rhythm?

PREVENTION OF SHOULDER INJURIES

Proper physical conditioning is of major importance in preventing many shoulder injuries. Like all preventive conditioning programs, the shoulder program should be directed toward general body development and development of specific body areas for a given sport. If a sport places extreme, sustained demands on the arms and shoulders or if the shoulder is at risk for sudden traumatic injury, an athlete should extensively condition that area. Strengthening through a full range of motion of all the muscles involved in movement of the shoulder complex is essential.

An athlete should perform a proper warm-up gradually before attempting explosive arm movements. This warm-up includes a general increase in body temperature, followed by sport-specific stretching of selected muscles.

All athletes in collision and contact sports should be instructed and drilled on how to fall properly. They must be taught not to try to catch themselves with an outstretched arm. Performing a shoulder roll is a safer way to absorb the shock of the fall. Specialized protective equipment such as shoulder pads must be properly fitted to help prevent shoulder injuries in tackle football.

To avoid overuse shoulder injuries, it is essential that athletes be correctly taught the appropriate techniques of throwing, spiking, overhead smashing, overhand serving, tackling and blocking, and the proper swimming strokes.

ASSESSMENT OF THE SHOULDER COMPLEX

The shoulder complex is one of the most difficult regions of the body to evaluate.[37] One reason for this difficulty is that the biomechanical demands placed on these structures during overhand accelerations and decelerations are not yet clearly understood.[52]

History

It is essential that the athletic trainer understand the athlete's major complaints and the possible mechanism of the injury. It is also necessary to know whether the condition was produced by a sudden trauma or was of slow onset. If the injury was sudden, the athletic trainer must determine whether the precipitating cause was external and direct trauma or some resistive force.[8] The following questions can help the athletic trainer determine the nature of the injury:

- What happened to cause this pain?
- Has the athlete ever had this problem before?
- What are the duration and intensity of the pain?
- Where is the pain located?
- Is there crepitus during movement, numbness, or distortion in temperature such as a cold or warm feeling?
- Is there a feeling of weakness or a sense of fatigue?
- What shoulder movements or positions seem to aggravate or relieve the pain?
- If therapy has been given before, what, if anything, offered pain relief (e.g., cold, heat, massage, or analgesic medication)?

Observation

The athlete should be generally observed while walking and standing. Observation during walking can reveal an asymmetrical arm swing or a lean toward the painful shoulder. Next, the athlete should be observed from the front, side, and back while in a standing position. The athletic trainer should look for any postural asymmetries, bony or joint deformities, or muscle spasm or guarding patterns.

Anterior Observation

- Are both shoulder tips even with one another, or is one depressed?
- Is one shoulder held higher because of muscle spasm or guarding?
- Is the lateral end of the clavicle prominent (indicating a step deformity caused by acromioclavicular sprain or dislocation)?
- Is one lateral acromion process more prominent than the other (indicating a possible glenohumeral dislocation)?
- Does the clavicular shaft appear deformed (indicating possible fracture)? Is there loss of the normal lateral deltoid muscle contour (indicating glenohumeral dislocation)?
- Is there an indentation in the upper biceps region (indicating rupture of biceps tendon)?
- Are the deltoid muscles symmetrical?

Lateral Observation

- Is there thoracic kyphosis, or shoulders slumped forward (indicating weakness of the erector muscles of the spine and tightness in the pectoral region)?
- Is the position of the head normal or is it forward?
- Is there forward or backward arm hang (indicating possible scoliosis)?

Posterior Observation

- Is there asymmetry such as a low shoulder, and are the scapulae even? (One scapula being unusually high may indicate Sprengel's deformity, which is a congenital deformity in which the scapula does not descend.)
- Is the scapula protracted because of constricted pectoral muscles?
- Is there a distracted or winged scapula on one or both sides? (A winged scapula on both sides could indicate a general weakness of the serratus anterior muscles; if only one side is winged, the long thoracic nerve may be injured. Winging of one scapular and not the other may indicate scoliosis.)
- Are the muscles symmetrical on both sides?
- Is there normal scapulohumeral rhythm?

Palpation

Bony Palpation

Palpation of the bony structures should be done with the athletic trainer standing in front of and then behind the athlete. The athletic trainer should palpate both shoulders at the same time for pain sites and deformities.

Anterior structures

- Sternoclavicular joint
- Clavicular shaft
- Acromioclavicular joint
- Coracoid process
- Acromion process
- Humeral head
- Greater tuberosity of the humerus
- Lesser tuberosity of the humerus
- Bicipital groove

Posterior structures

- Scapular spine
- Scapular vertebral border
- Scapular lateral border
- Scapular superior angle
- Scapular inferior angle

Soft-Tissue Palpation

Palpation of the soft tissue of the shoulder detects pain sites, abnormal swelling or lumps, muscle spasm or guarding, and trigger points. Trigger points are commonly found in the following muscles: levator scapulae, lesser rhomboid, supraspinous, infraspinous, scalene, deltoid, subscapular, teres major, trapezius, serratus anterior, and pectoralis major and minor. The shoulder is again palpated anteriorly and posteriorly.

Anterior palpation

- Sternoclavicular ligament
- Acromioclavicular ligament
- Coracoclavicular ligament
- Anterior and middle deltoid muscle
- Rotator cuff tendons
- Subacromial bursa
- Pectoralis major muscle
- Sternocleidomastoid muscle
- Biceps muscle and tendon
- Coracoacromial ligament
- Glenohumeral joint capsule

Posterior palpation

- Posterior deltoid
- Rhomboids
- Latissimus dorsi
- Serratus anterior
- Levator scapulae
- Trapezius
- Supraspinatus
- Infraspinatus
- Teres major and minor

Special Tests

A number of special tests can help determine the nature of an injury to the shoulder complex.

Active and Passive Range of Motion

The shoulder's active and passive range of motion should be noted and compared with the opposite side. The following are normal ranges for shoulder motion:

- Flexion 5 180 degrees
- Extension 5 50 degrees
- Abduction 5 180 degrees
- Adduction 5 40 degrees
- Internal rotation 5 90 degrees
- External rotation 5 90 degrees

Muscle Testing

The strength of the shoulder musculature should be assessed by manual muscle testing. Both the muscles that act on the glenohumeral joint and the muscles that act on the scapula should be tested. Muscle actions were described in the section on anatomy.

Test for Sternoclavicular Joint Instability

With the athlete sitting, pressure is applied anteriorly, then superiorly, and then inferiorly to the proximal clavicle to determine any instability or increased pain associated with a sprain (Figure 22-9A). Pressure applied to the tip of the shoulder in a medial direction may also increase pain.

Test for Acromioclavicular Joint Instability

The acromioclavicular joint is first palpated to determine if there is any displacement of the acromion process and the distal head of the clavicle. Next, pressure is applied to the distal clavicle in all four directions to determine stability and any associated increase in pain (Figure 22-9B). Pressure is applied to the tip of the shoulder, which compresses the acromioclavicular joint and may also increase pain.[53]

Tests for glenohumeral instability:

- Load and shift test
- Anterior drawer test
- Posterior drawer test
- Sulcus test
- Clunk test
- O'Brien's test
- Apprehension test
- Relocation test

Tests for Glenohumeral Instability

Glenohumeral translation (load and shift test) This test may be done with the athlete either sitting or supine. First, the athletic trainer places one hand over the shoulder to stabilize the scapula (Figure 22-10). With the other hand he or she grasps the humeral head between the thumb and index finger. A stress load is applied and translation of the humerus is assessed in both an anterior and a posterior direction.

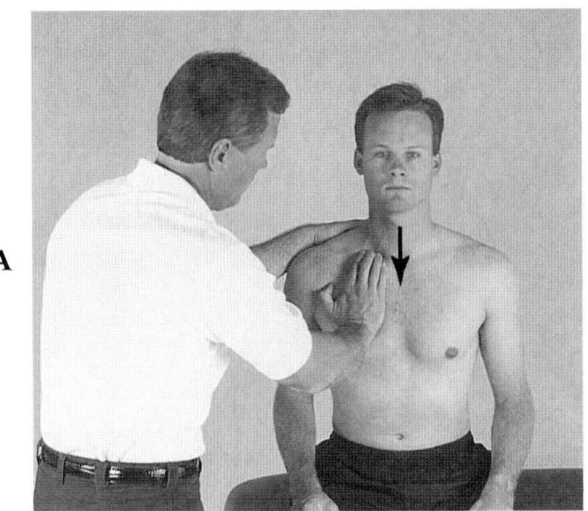

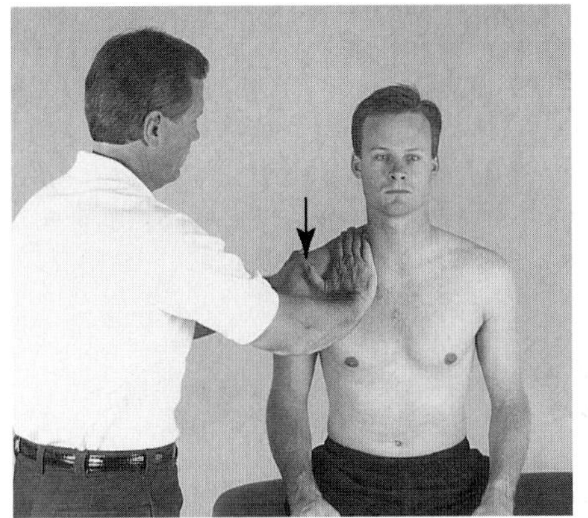

Figure 22-9

A, Assessing sternoclavicular joint stability. **B,** Assessing acromioclavicular joint stability.

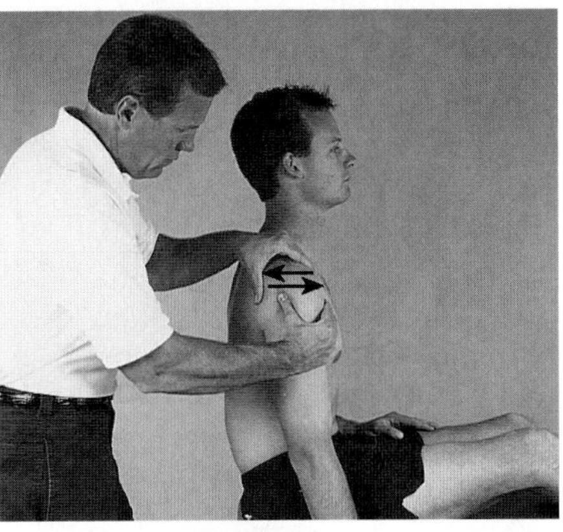

Figure 22-10

Test for anterior-posterior translation.

Anterior and posterior drawer tests The anterior drawer test checks for anterior glenohumeral instability. The athlete lies supine with the arm abducted 80 degrees, horizontally adducted 10 degrees, and externally rotated 10 degrees. The scapula is stabilized, and the humeral head is glided anteriorly while slight distraction is applied to the glenohumeral joint (Figure 22-11A).

The posterior drawer test checks for posterior glenohumeral instability. The athlete lies supine with the arm abducted 90 degrees and horizontally adducted 20 degrees, and the elbow flexed at 90 degrees. The scapula is stabilized, and the humerus is internally rotated as the humeral head is glided posteriorly (Figure 22-11B).

Sulcus test The the athletic trainer grasps the elbow and applies traction in an inferior direction. With excessive inferior translation, a depression occurs just below the acromion. The appearance of this sulcus is a positive sign (Figure 22-12).[49]

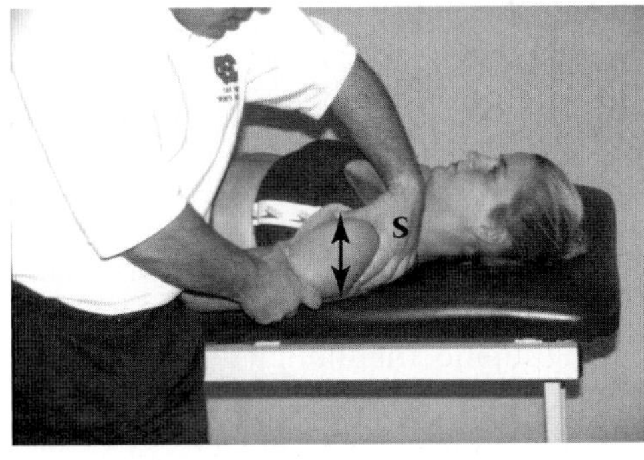

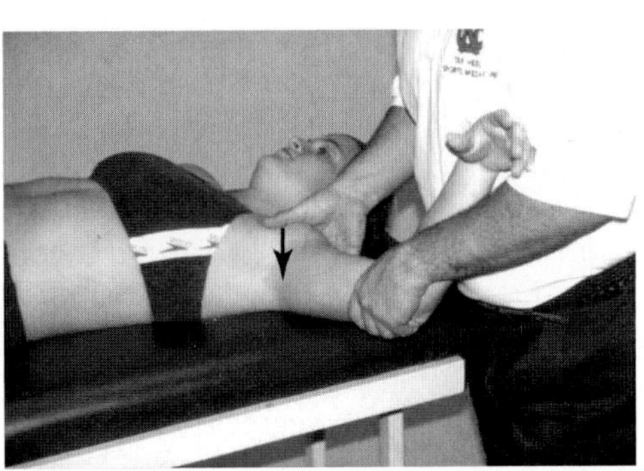

Figure 22-11

A, Anterior drawer test. **B,** Posterior drawer test.

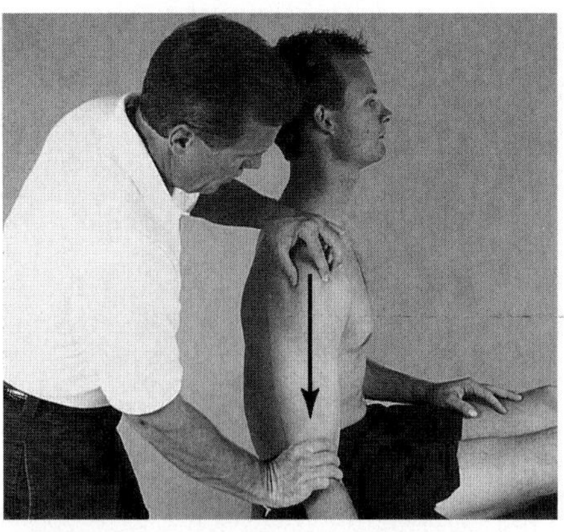

Figure 22-12

Sulcus test.

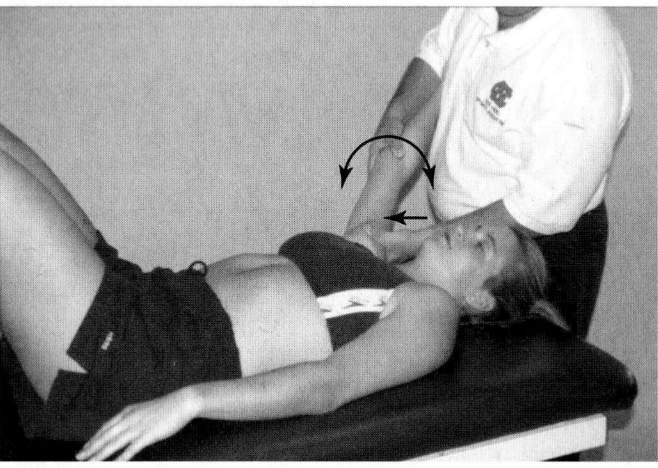

Figure 22-13

Clunk test.

Clunk test While the athlete lies supine, the athletic trainer grasps the elbow with one hand and places the other hand on the posterior humerus. The arm is passively abducted and externally rotated with an anterior force applied to the humeral head. The arm is then circumducted while the athletic trainer feels for a clunking sensation. A positive test may indicate the presence of a tear in the glenoid labrum (Figure 22-13).[3]

O'Brien's Test (Active Compression Test) With the athlete sitting, the glenohumeral joint is flexed to 90 degrees and horizontally adducted 15 degrees from the sagittal plane. The humerus is fully internally rotated with the forearm pronated (Figure 22-14). The athletic trainer applies downward pressure over the distal forearm. The test is repeated with the humerus externally rotated and the forearm supinated. If pain is present when the humerus is internally rotated but decreases in external rotation, and if there is clicking within the glenohumeral joint, this may indicate an anteroposterior tear in the superior glenoid labrum, which is called a SLAP lesion. Pain in the acromioclavicular joint with this test may indicate AC joint pathology.

Apprehension test (crank test) and relocation test With the arm abducted 90 degrees, the shoulder is slowly and gently externally rotated as far as the athlete will allow. The athlete with a history of anterior glenohumeral instability will show great apprehension that is reflected by a facial grimace before an endpoint can be reached. At no time should the athletic trainer force this movement (Figure 22-15A).

Posterior instability also can be determined through an apprehension maneuver. With the athlete in a supine position, the shoulder is flexed to 90 degrees and internally rotated while a force is applied through the long axis of the humerus (Figure 22-15B).

The relocation test is done with the athlete lying supine, the shoulder at 90 degrees, and the elbow at 90 degrees. As the shoulder is externally rotated, pressure is applied anteriorly to stabilize the humeral head, which allows for a greater degree of external rotation than does the apprehension test (Figure 22-15C).[3]

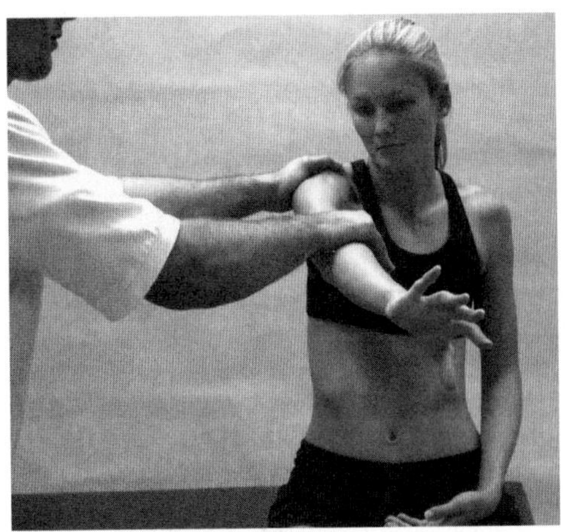

A

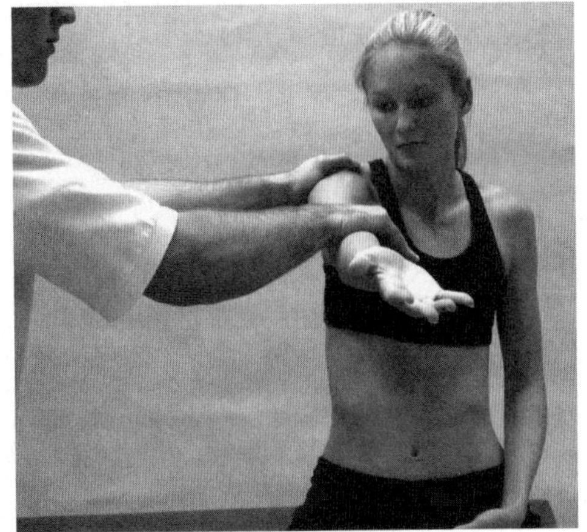

B

Figure 22-14

O'Brien's test. **A,** Pronated position. **B,** Supinated position.

A

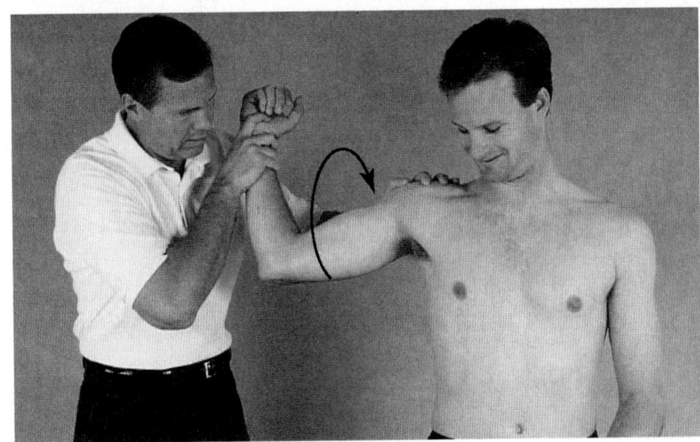

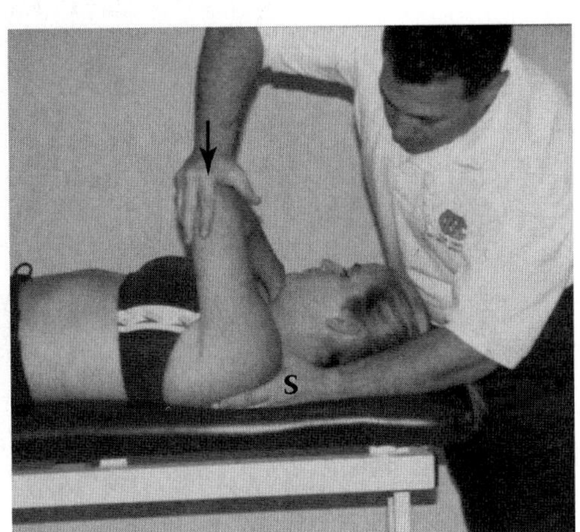

B

C

Figure 22-15

A, Shoulder apprehension test. **B,** Posterior apprehension test. **C,** Relocation test.

Tests for Shoulder Impingement

Neer's Test In Neer's test, forced flexion of the humerus in the overhead position may cause impingement of soft-tissue structures between the humeral head and the coracoacromial arch (Figure 22-16A).

Hawkins-Kennedy Test The Hawkins-Kennedy impingement test involves horizontal adduction with forced internal rotation of the humerus, which also produces impingement (Figure 22-16B). A positive sign is indicated if the athlete feels pain and reacts with a grimace.[31]

Tests for Supraspinatus Muscle Weakness

Drop arm test The drop arm test is designed to determine tears of the rotator cuff, primarily of the supraspinatus muscle. The athlete abducts the arm as far as possible and then slowly lowers it to 90 degrees. From this position the athlete with a torn

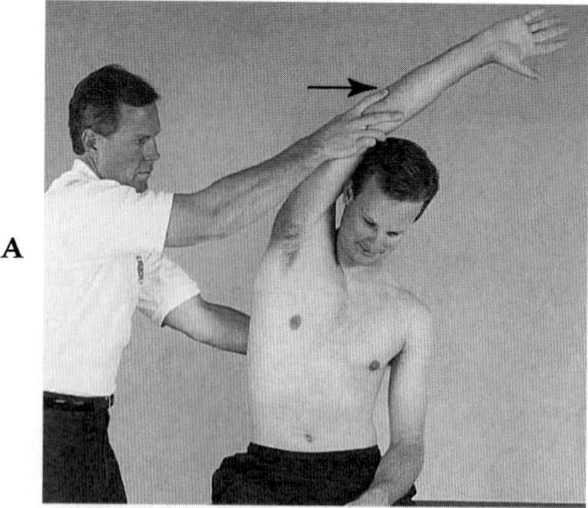
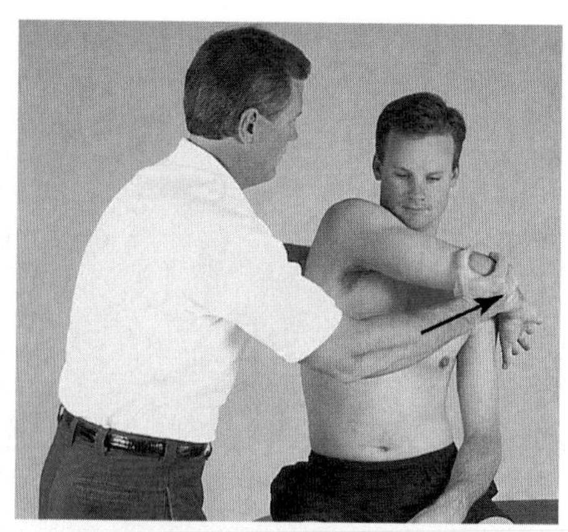

Figure 22-16

Shoulder impingement test. **A,** Full elevation. **B,** Horizontal adduction with internal rotation.

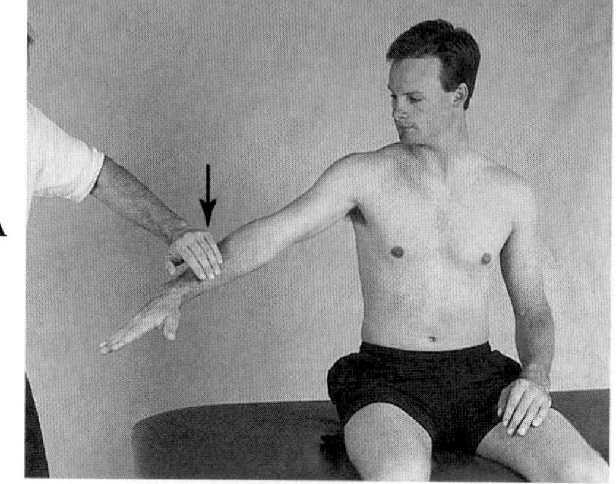
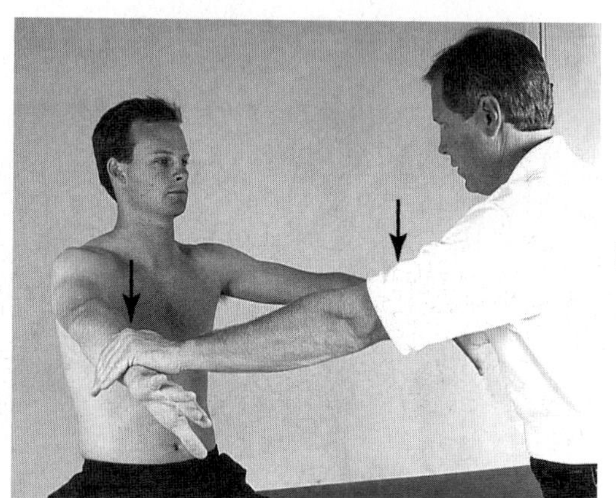

Figure 22-17

Supraspinatus tests. **A,** Drop arm test. **B,** Empty can test.

Tests for supraspinatus weakness:
- Drop arm test
- Empty can test

supraspinatus muscle will be unable to lower the arm further with control (Figure 22-17A). If the athlete can hold the arm in a 90-degree position, pressure on the wrist will cause the arm to fall.

Empty can test The empty can test for supraspinatus muscle strength has the athlete bring both arms into 90 degrees of forward flexion and 30 degrees of horizontal abduction (Figure 22-17B). In this position, the arms are internally rotated as far as possible, thumbs pointing downward. The athletic trainer then applies a downward pressure. Weakness and pain can be detected as well as comparative strength between the two arms.

Test for Serratus Anterior Muscle Weakness

The athlete performs a push-up movement against a wall. Winging of the scapula indicates weakness of the serratus anterior muscle. Winging of only one scapula could indicate an injury to the long thoracic nerve (Figure 22-18).[24]

Tests for Biceps Tendon Irritation

Tests for biceps tendon irritation
- Yergason's test
- Speed's test
- Ludington's test

Yergason's test involves keeping the elbow at 90 degrees with the forearm pronated while the athlete attempts to actively supinate against the resistance of the athletic trainer as the humerus is also being pulled downward (Figure 22-19A). *Speed's test* is performed with the elbow extended, the forearm supinated, and resistance applied as the humerus elevates to 60 degrees (Figure 22-19B). Both tests are positive if the athletic trainer feels pain in the region of the bicipital groove. If there is instability, the tendon may subluxate out of its groove. *Ludington's test* is performed with the athlete in a seated position with hands clasped behind the head. The biceps muscles are alternately contracted and relaxed. The athletic trainer palpates the biceps muscles, and if no contraction is felt on one side, there is likely a rupture (Figure 22-19C).

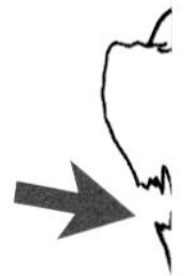

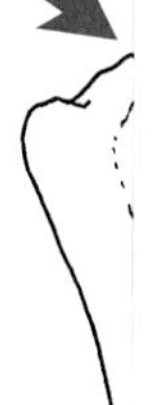

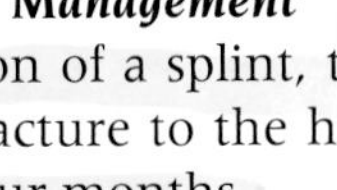

Management tion of a splint, t fracture to the h four months.

A suspected fr sling and swathe to six months.

Initial treatme referral to a phys approximately tl damage to the ep

Sternoclavicul

Etiology A st rence in sports, l mas affecting the an indirect force lence such as a b

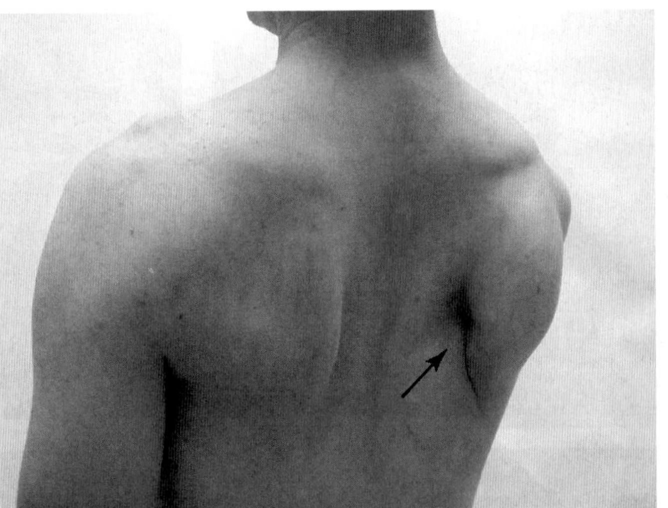

Figure 22-18

Winged scapula.

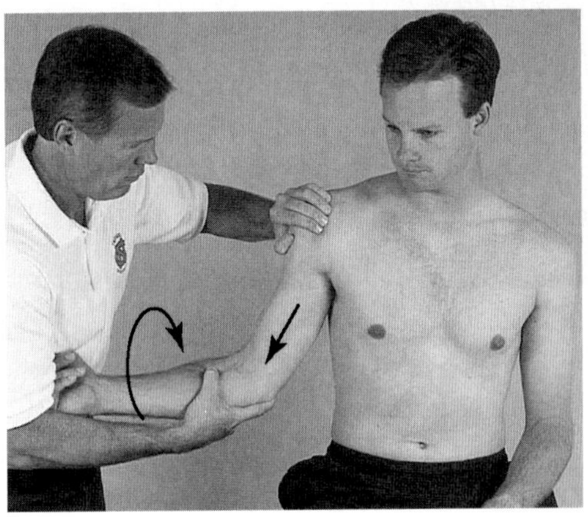

A

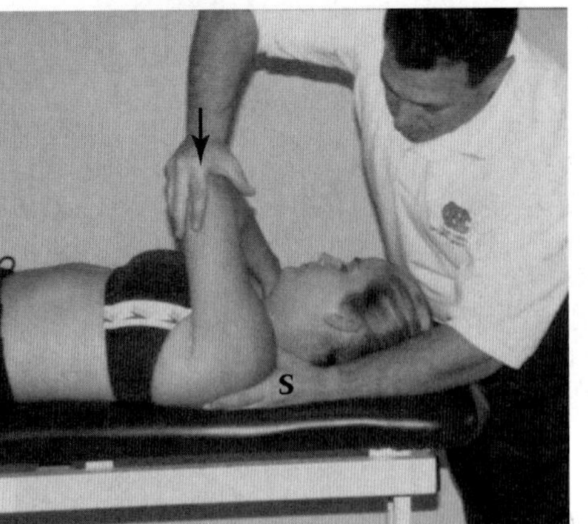

B

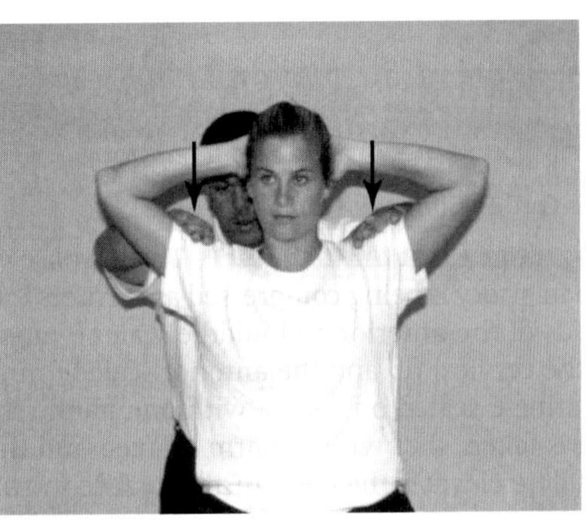

C

Figure 22-19

Bicipital tendinitis and subluxation tests.
A, Yergason's test. **B,** Speed's test. **C,** Ludington's test.

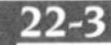

22-3

Critical Thinking Exercise

A wrestler comes into the training room complaining of paresthesia and pain extending down the arm, of a sensation of cold, impaired circulation in the fingers, and of muscle weakness. During the evaluation it also becomes apparent that the wrestler has some muscle atrophy in the affected extremity. The athletic trainer suspects that the wrestler may have thoracic outlet compression syndrome.

? What specific tests should the athletic trainer do to determine whether thoracic outlet compression syndrome is present, and what do those tests indicate?

Circulatory Assessment

It is essential that athletes with shoulder complaints be evaluated for impaired circulation. Pulse rates are routinely obtained over the axillary, brachial, and radial arteries. The axillary artery is found in the axilla against the shaft of the humerus. The brachial artery is a continuation of the axillary artery and follows the medial border of the biceps brachii muscle toward the elbow. The radial pulse is found at the anterior lateral aspect of the wrist over the radius. Taking the radial pulse provides an indication of the total circulation of the shoulder and arm.

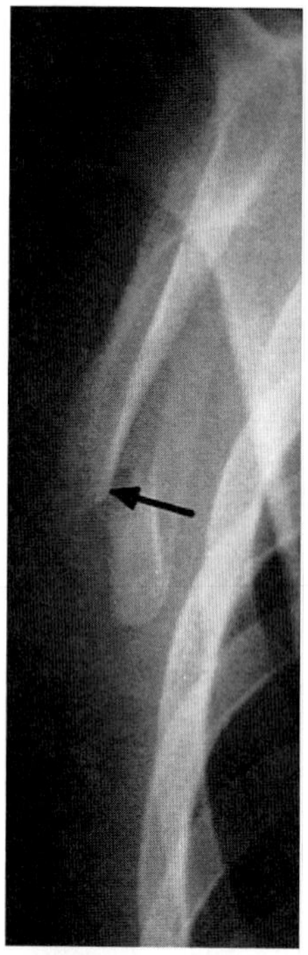

Figure 22-22

Fractures of the scap
infrequent in sports.

CONTUSION TO THE DISTAL END OF THE CLAVICLE Contusions of this type are often called shoulder pointers and cause a bone bruise and subsequent irritation to the periosteum. During initial inspection, this injury may be mistaken for a grade 1 acromioclavicular sprain. In most cases, these conditions are self-limiting. When the athlete is able to move the shoulder freely, he or she can return to sports activities.

Symptoms and signs The grade 1 acromioclavicular sprain reflects point tenderness and discomfort during movement at the junction between the acromion process and the outer end of the clavicle. There is no disruption of the acromioclavicular joint, indicating only mild stretching of the acromioclavicular and coracoclavicular ligaments (see Figure 22-26A).

A grade 2 sprain indicates tearing or rupture of acromioclavicular ligaments with associated stretching of the coracoclavicular ligament. There is partial displacement and prominence of the lateral end of the clavicle when compared with the unaffected side, especially when the acromioclavicular stress test is initiated (Figure 22-27). In this moderate sprain, there is point tenderness during palpation of the injury site, and the athlete is unable to fully abduct through a full range of motion or to bring the arm completely across the chest (see Figure 22-26B).

Although it occurs less frequently, the grade 3 sprain involves complete rupture of the acromioclavicular and coracoclavicular ligaments (see Figure 22-26C).

A grade 4 sprain exhibits posterior dislocation of the clavicle with complete disruption of the acromioclavicular ligament (see Figure 22-26D). In some grade 4 sprains, the coracoclavicular ligaments may remain intact.

In a grade 5 sprain, there is complete loss of both the acromioclavicular and coracoclavicular ligaments in addition to tearing of the trapezius and deltoid attachment to the clavicle and acromion. Such an injury reflects gross deformity and prominence of the distal clavicle, severe pain, loss of movement, and instability of the shoulder complex (see Figure 22-26E).

A grade 6 injury is very rare in the athletic setting and involves the clavicle being displaced inferior to the coracoid behind the coracobrachialis tendon (see Figure 22-26F).

Management Immediate care of the acromioclavicular sprain involves three basic procedures: (1) application of cold and pressure to control local hemorrhage, (2) stabilization of the joint by a sling and swathe bandage, and (3) referral to a physician for definitive diagnosis and treatment.

A grade 1 sprain requires use of a sling for three or four days. A grade 2 sprain requires ten to fourteen days of protection in a sling. The current recommended management for a grade 3 sprain is nonoperative with approximately two weeks of protection in a sling. Grades 4 through 6 require surgical intervention using open reduction with internal fixation.[48] If there is posterior displacement of the clavicle, surgical reduction and fixation will be necessary. With all grades, an aggressive rehabilitation program involving joint mobilization, flexibility exercises, and strengthening exercises should begin immediately after the recommended period of protection. Progression should be as rapid as the athlete can tolerate without increased pain or swelling. The joint should also be protected with appropriate padding until a pain-free, full range of motion returns (Figure 22-27C).[5]

Glenohumeral Joint Sprain

Etiology The mechanism of this injury is similar to that which produces dislocations and strains. Anterior capsular sprains occur when the arm is forced into abduction (e.g., when making an arm tackle in football). Sprains can also occur from external rotation of the arm. A direct blow to the shoulder could also result in a sprain. The pathological process of a sprain to the glenohumeral joint often involves the rotator cuff muscles.

The infraspinatus–teres minor muscle group is the most effective in controlling external rotation of the humerus and in reducing ligamentous injury.[46] The posterior capsule can be sprained by a forceful movement of the humerus posteriorly when the arm is flexed.

22-5

Critical Thinking Exercise

A football player has suffered an anterior dislocation of the glenohumeral joint while making a tackle. He is really concerned about missing the remainder of the season and is the type of athlete who wants to know everything there is to know about the injury. He asks the athletic trainer to explain to him exactly what has happened and what other problems might exist along with this injury.

? What should the athletic trainer tell this player about the possible ramifications of this injury?

A
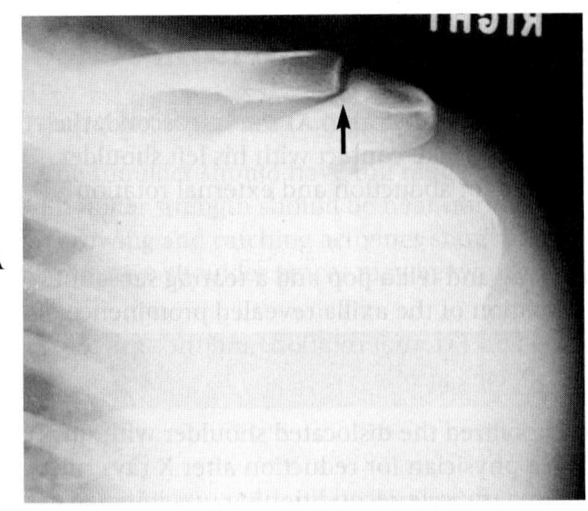

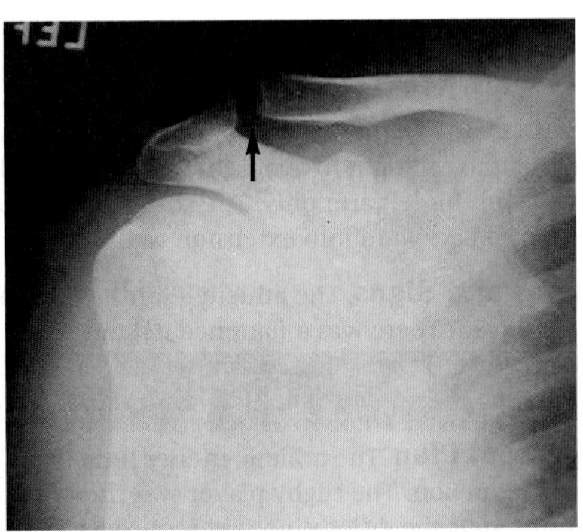

B

C
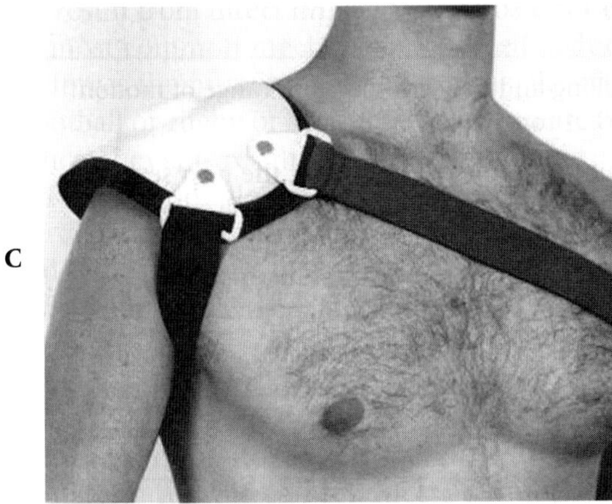

Figure 22-27

Comparison of **A,** a normal shoulder with **B,** a grade 2 acromioclavicular sprain. **C,** Domed pad protection for sprain of the AC joint.

Symptoms and signs The athlete complains of pain during arm movement, especially when the sprain mechanism is reproduced. There may be decreased range of motion and pain during palpation.

Management Care after acute trauma to the shoulder joint requires the use of a cold pack for twenty-four to forty-eight hours, elastic or adhesive compression, rest, and immobilization by a sling. After hemorrhage has subsided, a program of cryotherapy or ultrasound and massage may be added, and mild passive and active exercise is advocated for regaining full range of motion. Once the athlete can execute full shoulder range of movement without signs of pain, a resistance exercise program should be initiated. Any traumatic injury to the shoulder joint can lead to a subacute and chronic condition of either synovitis or bursitis, which, in the absence of shoulder movement, will allow muscle contractures, adhesions, and atrophy to develop, resulting in an ankylosed shoulder joint.

Acute Subluxations and Dislocations

Shoulder dislocations account for up to 50 percent of all dislocations. The extreme range of mobility in the normal shoulder creates an inherent instability in the joint, which is thus susceptible to dislocation. The most common kind of displacement is that occurring anteriorly. Posterior dislocations account for 1 percent to 4.3 percent of all shoulder dislocations. Inferior dislocations are extremely rare. Of dislocations caused by direct trauma, 85 percent to 90 percent recur.[65]

Etiology

SUBLUXATIONS With glenohumeral subluxations, there is excessive translation of the humeral head without complete separation of the joint surfaces. Subluxation is a brief, transient occurrence in which the humeral head quickly returns to its normal position relative to the glenoid. Subluxation can occur anteriorly, posteriorly, or inferiorly.

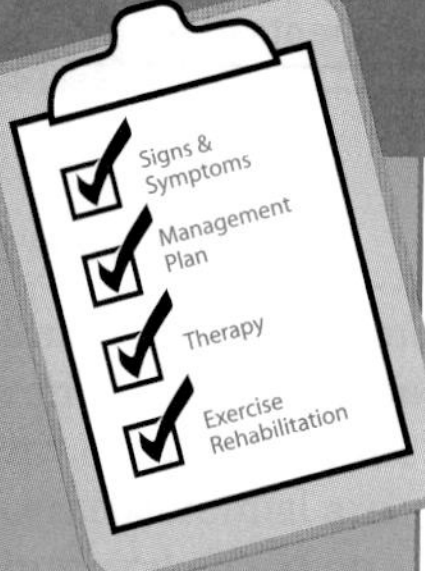

Management PLAN

Shoulder Impingement

Injury Situation An eighteen-year-old female middle distance swimmer is in the third week of her preseason training program. She has significantly increased the distance she has been swimming during the last three weeks. Her workouts have increased to twice a day and she has been swimming all freestyle. She is complaining of an aching pain in her left shoulder.

Symptoms and Signs The swimmer complains of diffuse pain around the acromion with point tenderness over the supraspinatus or biceps tendons. Palpation of the subacromial space increases the pain. Overhead activities also increase the pain. There is an achy feeling when she finishes her workout. The external rotators are generally weaker than the internal rotators. There is tightness in the posterior and inferior joint capsule. There is a positive impingement sign, and both the empty can test and the drop arm test increase pain.[62]

Management Plan Management involves restoring normal biomechanics to the shoulder joint in an effort to maintain space under the coracoacromial arch during her swimming workout.

Phase 1 Acute Injury

GOALS: To control pain and inflammation.
ESTIMATED LENGTH OF TIME (ELT): 1 to 6 days.

▪ **Therapy** RICE and electrical stimulating currents can be used to modulate pain initially. Ultrasound and antiinflammatory medications should be used to reduce inflammation.

▪ **Exercise rehabilitation** Her aggressive swimming workout, which caused the problem in the first place, should be modified so that there is some initial control over the frequency and the duration of the workout with a gradual and progressive increase in distance. It may be necessary to keep her out of the pool during phase 1 to allow the inflammation to subside. To maintain her level of fitness, she should substitute running or exercising on a stationary bike for her swimming workout. She may continue her strengthening program, but she must discontinue any strengthening exercise using her sore shoulder.

Phase 2 Repair

GOALS: To alter joint biomechanics to reduce the likelihood of impingement.
ELT: 1 to 2 weeks.

▪ **Therapy** Continue using electrical stimulation and ice to modulate pain. Ultrasound is also helpful in reducing inflammation. Continue antiinflammatory medication.

▪ **Exercise rehabilitation** She may now get back into the pool and begin with a short workout initially and then gradually increase the duration and intensity, using increased pain or stiffness as a guide for progression. Exercises should concentrate on strengthening the rotator cuff and the muscles that abduct, elevate, and upwardly rotate the scapula. The external rotators should also be strengthened. It may be necessary to limit strengthening exercises in flexion or abduction. Any exercise that places the shoulder in impingement should be avoided. Posterior and inferior glenohumeral joint mobilizations should be done to reduce tightness in the posterior and inferior joint capsule.

Phase 3 Remodeling

GOALS: To return to unrestricted activity.
ELT: 2 weeks to full return.

▪ **Therapy** Use ultrasound before the workout and ice after completing the workout. Continue antiinflammatory medication.

▪ **Exercise rehabilitation** Strengthening exercises should progress to full-range overhead activities. PNF D1 AND D2 strengthening patterns may be used with either manual or surgical tubing resistance. She must continue to work on strengthening the appropriate scapular muscles as she did in phase 2. Exercises designed to stretch the inferior and posterior capsule should also be continued.

Continued

A

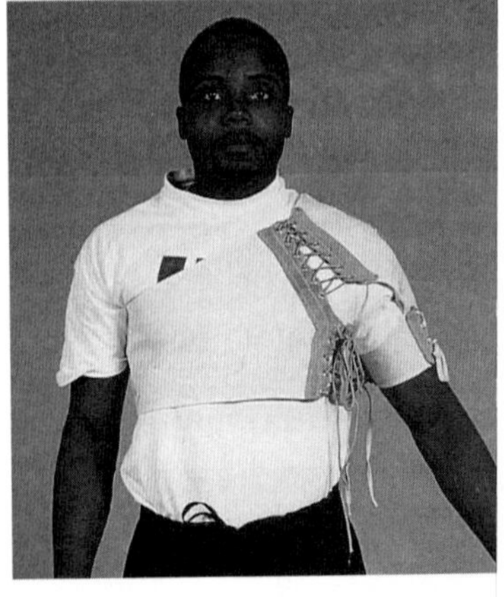

movement and consequently sacr
ity.[29] Achieving the necessary b
performance athlete.

In recent years, the shoulder jo
tention within the sports medici
treatment, management, and reh
athletic trainers to use cookbook a
to allow for essential alteration o
the individual athlete. The athlet
der rehabilitation programs. Ther
not necessary to use a lot of expe

Immobilization after Injury

Rehabilitation programs should
gressive approach should be used
mobilization period will vary dep
injury, and whether the injury is
Regardless of the injury, the inju
while wearing an immobilization
be unnecessary to wear a sling o
be worn twenty-four hours a da
tain injuries may require that a s
ing, that a motion-limiting brace
that no sling or brace be worn a
an angle of 90 degrees be limited
of motion and strengthening tec
the physiological process of heal
swelling associated with increase

General Body Conditioning

It is essential for the athlete to r
throughout the rehabilitation p
running, speed walking, or ridin
piratory endurance. Because ma
in such training for a shoulder in
the rehabilitation of an ankle sp
extremity endurance, such as sw
activities as soon as the activities
may be modified so that the ath
neuromuscular control through
rehabilitation. Even though wei
the upper extremity, aquatic ex

Shoulder Impingement—*continued*

Criteria for Return to Competitive Swimming

1. The gradual program that has been used to increase the duration and intensity of the workout has allowed her to complete a workout without pain.
2. She exhibits improved strength in the rotator cuff and the scapular muscles.
3. She no longer has a positive impingement sign, drop arm test, or empty can test.
4. She can discontinue the use of antiinflammatory medications without a return of pain.

Frozen Shoulder (Adhesive Capsulitis)

Adhesive capsulitis is also called a frozen shoulder.

Etiology Adhesive capsulitis, or frozen shoulder, is a condition more characteristic of an older person, but occasionally it occurs in the younger athlete. The exact cause of adhesive capsulitis is unclear. However, it involves a contracted and thickened joint capsule that is tight around the humeral head with little synovial fluid. There is also chronic inflammation with some fibrosis. The rotator cuff muscles are also contracted and inelastic. Constant, generalized inflammation causes pain on both active and passive motion. Thus the individual will progressively resist moving the joint because of pain. The result is a stiff or frozen shoulder.

Symptoms and signs Pain is reported in all directions of movement about the shoulder with restriction or limitation of both active and passive movement.

Management The objectives are to relieve discomfort and restore motion. Treatment usually involves aggressive joint mobilizations and stretching tight muscles. Electrical stimulating currents may be used to reduce pain. Ultrasound is useful in providing penetrating heat to the area.

Thoracic Outlet Compression Syndrome

Etiology Thoracic outlet compression syndromes involve compression of the brachial plexus, subclavian artery, and subclavian vein (neurovascular bundle) in the neck and shoulder.[57] Neurovascular compression can occur as a result of the following conditions:

- Compression of the neurovascular bundle in the narrowed space between the first rib and clavicle (costoclavicular syndrome)
- Compression between the anterior and middle scalene muscles
- Compression by the pectoralis minor muscle as the neurovascular bundle passes beneath the coracoid process or between the clavicle and first rib
- The presence of a cervical rib (an abnormal rib originating from a cervical vertebra and the thoracic rib)

Symptoms and signs Abnormal pressure on the subclavian artery, subclavian vein, and brachial plexus produces a variety of symptoms, including paresthesia and pain, a sensation of cold, impaired circulation in the fingers, muscle weakness, muscle atrophy, and radial nerve palsy. Three tests described earlier in this chapter can be used to determine thoracic outlet compression syndrome: the anterior scalene test, the costoclavicular test, and the hyperabduction test.

Management A conservative approach should be taken with early and mild cases of thoracic outlet compression syndromes. Conservative treatment is favorable in 50 percent to 80 percent of cases.[57] It involves correcting the anatomical condition that is responsible for this syndrome with a series of stretching and strengthening exercises. Exercises should be done to strengthen the trapezius, rhomboids, serratus anterior, and erector muscles of the spine. Stretching exercises for the pectoralis minor and the scalene muscles should also be used.

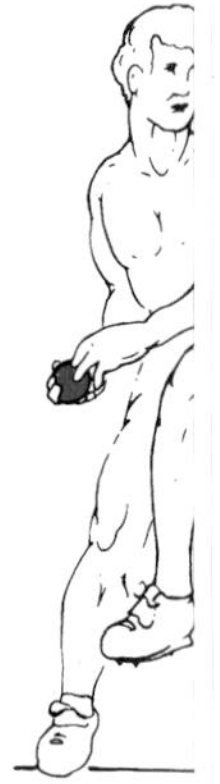

Figure 22-31

Phases of throwing from left to right: windup, early cocking, late cocking, acceleration, follow-through, and deceleration.

22-11

Critical Thinking **Exercise**

A baseball pitcher is throwing a fastball. To effectively execute this motion, the pitcher must develop significant velocity in glenohumeral internal rotation during the acceleration phase. During the follow-through phase, this high-velocity internal rotation must quickly decelerate.

? What muscles function to actively internally rotate the glenohumeral joint during the acceleration phase, and what muscles decelerate internal rotation during follow-through?

and position the scapula. In movement of the shoulder joint, it is critical to maintain the positioning of the humeral head relative to the glenoid.

- The athletic trainer, when evaluating injuries to the shoulder complex, must take into consideration all four joints. A number of special tests can provide insight into the nature of a particular injury.
- Fractures may occur to the clavicle, scapula, or humerus. Sprains may occur at the sternoclavicular, acromioclavicular, or glenohumeral joints.
- Shoulder dislocations and subluxations are relatively common, with an anterior dislocation and posterior subluxation being the most likely to occur. After a dislocation has been reduced and immobilized, muscle reconditioning should be initiated as soon as possible.
- Chronic or recurrent shoulder instability can occur after acute subluxation or dislocation. Recurrent instabilities may be either anterior, posterior, inferior, or multidirectional. The causes of shoulder instabilities may be traumatic (macrotraumatic), atraumatic, microtraumatic (repetitive use), congenital, or neuromuscular.
- Shoulder impingement is closely related to shoulder instability. Athletes involved with overhead activities often exhibit hypermobility and significant capsular laxity. Shoulder impingement involves a mechanical compression of the supraspinatus tendon, the subacromial bursa, and the long head of the biceps tendon under the coracoacromial arch.
- A number of injuries, including subacromial bursitis, contusions, bicipital tenosynovitis, adhesive capsulitis, peripheral nerve injuries, and thoracic outlet compression syndromes, are common injuries of the shoulder complex in athletes.
- Rehabilitation after injury to the shoulder joint may require a brief period of immobilization. Joint mobilization, flexibility, and strengthening exercises should be initiated as soon as possible after injury. Progression in range of motion and strengthening techniques should be dictated by a lack of pain and swelling associated with increased activity. Activities that stress closed kinetic chain function emphasize co-contraction of antagonistic muscle groups, and thus provide neuromuscular control of opposing muscle groups and promote stability about the shoulder joint. For the athlete with an injured shoulder joint, functional progressions usually incorporate some sport-specific skill that involves overhead motions.

Websites

Anatomy of the Shoulder Tutorial:
http://www.innerbody.com/tutorial3/tutorial.html

Cramer First Aider:
http://www.cramersportsmed.com/first_aider.jsp

World Ortho: http://www.worldortho.com

Wheeless' Textbook of Orthopaedics:
http://www.wheelessonline.com

American Orthopaedic Society for Sports Medicine:
http://www.sportsmed.org

MedFacts Sports Doc: http://www.medfacts.com

Readers can click on the medical library for information about common injuries.

OrthoNet: http://www.orthonet.on.ca

Solutions to Critical Thinking EXERCISES

22-1 The athletic trainer should point out to the athlete that regardless of the strengthening exercises, there is still a high probability that a recurrent dislocation will occur. The dynamic stabilizers of the glenohumeral joint include the subscapularis, infraspinatus, teres minor, and supraspinatus. It is perhaps just as important to strengthen the scapular muscles.

22-2 Normal scapulohumeral rhythm exhibits no movement of the scapula as the humerus elevates to 30 degrees. As the humerus elevates from 30 degrees to 90 degrees, the scapula should abduct and upwardly rotate 1 degree for every 2 degrees of humeral elevation. From 90 degrees to full abduction of the humerus, the scapula should abduct and rotate upward 1 degree for each 1 degree of humeral elevation.

22-3 Thoracic outlet compression syndromes involve compression of the brachial plexus, subclavian artery, and subclavian vein. The anterior scalene syndrome test, or Adson's test, tests for compression by the heads of the anterior and middle scalene muscles or between the cervical rib and the anterior scalene muscle. The costoclavicular syndrome test (Roo's test or the military brace position test) tests for compression between the first rib and the clavicle. The hyperabduction syndrome test, or Allen test, tests for compression behind the pectoral muscle and beneath the coracoid process.

22-4 Falling on the tip of the shoulder is a typical mechanism of injury for a sprain of both the acromioclavicular and sternoclavicular joints. It is also possible that a clavicular fracture has occurred.

22-5 In an anterior glenohumeral dislocation, the head of the humerus is forced out of its articular capsule in an anterior direction past the glenoid labrum and then downward to rest under the coracoid process. Torn capsular and ligamentous tissue, a possible tendinous avulsion of the rotator cuff muscles or long head of the biceps, a possible tear or detachment of the glenoid labrum, a possible injury to the brachial plexus, and profuse hemorrhage are all potential problems.

22-6 A dislocation can cause a variety of injuries within the glenohumeral joint, including a Bankart lesion, a Hill-Sachs lesion, and a SLAP lesion. A Bankart lesion is a defect of the anterior labrum while a Hill-Sachs lesion is a defect on the posterior lateral aspect of the humeral head. A SLAP lesion involves a tear of the superior labrum that may also involve the biceps tendon.

22-7 It is most likely that the pitcher has some anterior instability that is allowing for excessive translation of the humeral head on the glenoid. During throwing this can create a repetitive compression of the rotation cuff, consequently causing impingement of soft tissues under the coracoacromial arch.

22-8 If the dynamic stabilizers (rotator cuff) and the static stabilizers (joint capsule) of the glenohumeral joint cannot maintain the position of the humeral head relative to the glenoid, there will be excessive translation of the humeral head. Excessive translation of the humerus in the overhead position can result in mechanical impingement of those structures under the coracoacromial arch. If the scapular muscles do not maintain the position of the glenoid relative to the humerus, impingement can result.

22-9 Her pain is probably due to mechanical impingement or compression of the supraspinatus tendon, the subacromial bursa, or the long head of the biceps under the coracoacromial arch as the arm moves into a fully abducted or flexed position. The space under the arch becomes even more compressed as the humerus is internally rotated, as would occur during the follow-through.

22-10 Restoring normal biomechanics to the shoulder joint in an effort to maintain space under the coracoacromial arch during overhead activities is critical. The athletic trainer should use techniques that strengthen the rotator cuff muscles, which act to both compress and depress the humeral head relative to the glenoid, and strengthen the scapular muscles, which abduct, elevate, and upwardly rotate the scapula. The athletic trainer should also incorporate posterior and inferior glenohumeral joint mobilizations to reduce tightness in the posterior and inferior joint capsule.

22-11 The subscapularis, pectoralis major, latissimus dorsi, teres major, and anterior deltoid must all contract concentrically to produce internal rotation during the acceleration phase. The infraspinatus, teres minor, and posterior deltoid must contract eccentrically during the follow-through to decelerate internal rotation.

22-12 Efforts toward regaining neuromuscular control should begin immediately in the rehabilitation program. Closed kinetic chain exercises emphasize cocontraction of antagonistic muscle groups, which provides neuromuscular control of opposing muscle groups and promotes stability about the shoulder joint. Activities that stress closed kinetic chain function include weight shifting on the hands or on a ball and push-ups. Biofeedback techniques can help the athlete regain control of specific muscle actions.

22-13 Because the athlete is having difficulty regaining active range of motion, the athletic trainer might try using diagonal 1 and 2 upper-extremity PNF patterns with rhythmic initiation. This technique involves a progression from passive to active assisted to active contraction throughout a functional range. The trainer should also use joint mobilization techniques for not only the acromioclavicular joint but also the sternoclavicular, glenohumeral, and scapulothoracic joints if needed.

REVIEW QUESTIONS AND CLASS ACTIVITIES

1. Explain why a full range of motion of the shoulder joint requires motion at all four joints in the shoulder complex.
2. Explain how the positioning of the humeral head is maintained relative to the glenoid in overhead throwing motions.
3. What is the relationship between shoulder instability and shoulder impingement?
4. What are the mechanisms of an anterior dislocation and a posterior dislocation?
5. How do recurrent instabilities develop?
6. What can be done to minimize the chances of a baseball pitcher developing shoulder impingement?
7. What is myositis ossificans and how can its development be prevented?
8. How may an athlete acquire bicipital tenosynovitis? How does this condition lead to a ruptured biceps tendon?
9. Describe the various tests for thoracic outlet compression syndrome.
10. Discuss the mechanics involved in throwing a baseball.
11. Explain why closed kinetic chain exercises are useful in rehabilitation of shoulder injuries.
12. Develop an exercise rehabilitation program for a rotator cuff injury, a glenohumeral dislocation, and an acromioclavicular sprain.

REFERENCES

1. Allegrucci M, Whitney S, Lephart S: Shoulder kinesthesia in healthy unilateral athletes participating in upper extremity sports, *J Orthop Sports Phys Ther* 22(4):220, 1995.
2. Allen J: Recognizing, managing, and treating an axillary-nerve dysfunction, *Athletic Therapy Today* 7(2):28, 2002.
3. Andrews J, Wilk K: *The athlete's shoulder,* New York, 1994, Churchill Livingstone.
4. Aronen JG, Chronister RD: Anterior shoulder dislocations: easing reduction by using linear traction techniques, *Physician Sportsmed* 23(10):65, 1995.
5. Axe MJ: Acromioclavicular joint injuries in the athlete, *Sports Med Arthroscopy Review* 8(2):182, 2000.
6. Axe M, Windley W, Synder-Mackler L: Data-based interval throwing programs for collegiate softball players, *J Ath Train* 37(2):194, 2002.
7. Axe M, Windley W, Synder-Mackler L: Data-based interval throwing programs for baseball position players from age 13 to college level, *J Sport Rehabil* 10(4):267, 2001.
8. Baker CL, Merkley MS: Clinical evaluation of the athlete's shoulder, *J Ath Train* 35(3):256, 2000.
9. Beim GM: Acromioclavicular joint injuries, *J Ath Train* 35(3):261, 2000.

10. Blackburn TA, Guido JA: Rehabilitation after ligamentous and labral surgery of the shoulder: guiding concepts, *J Ath Train* 35(3):373, 2000.
11. Blackburn T, McLeod W: EMG analysis of posterior rotator cuff exercises, *Ath Train* 25(1):40, 1990.
12. Borsa P, Timmons M, Sauer E: Scapular positioning patterns during humeral elevation in nonimpaired shoulders, *J Ath Train* 38(1):12, 2003.
13. Borsa P, Lephart S, Kocher M: Functional assessment and rehabilitation of shoulder proprioception for glenohumeral instability, *J Sport Rehabil* 3(1):84, 1994.
14. Butters K: The scapula. In Rockwood C, Masten F, editors: *The shoulder*, Philadelphia, 2004, Elsevier Science.
15. Cavallo RJ, Speer KP: Shoulder instability and impingement in throwing athletes, *Med Sci Sports Exerc* 30(4 suppl.):S18, 1998.
16. Chu J, Kane E, Arnold B: The effect of a neoprene shoulder stabilizer on active joint-reposition sense in subjects with stable and unstable shoulders, *J Ath Train* 37(2):141, 2002.
17. Conroy DE, Hayes KW: The effect of joint mobilization as a component of comprehensive treatment for primary shoulder impingement syndrome, *J Orthop Sports Phys Ther* 28(1):3, 1998.
18. Cordasco F: Understanding multidirectional instability of the shoulder, *J Ath Train* 35(3):278, 2000.
19. Cordasco FA, Wolfe IN, Wootten ME, Bigliani LU: An electromyographic analysis of the shoulder during a medicine ball rehabilitation program, *Am J Sports Med* 24(5):386, 1996.
20. Craig E: Fractures of the clavicle. In Rockwood C, Masten F, editors: *The shoulder*, Philadelphia, 1998, Saunders.
21. D'Alessandro DF, Fleischli JE, Connor PM: Superior labral lesions: diagnosis and management, *J Ath Train* 35(3):286, 2000.
22. DeCarlo M, Malone K, Gerig B, Hunker M: Evaluation of shoulder instability braces, *J Sport Rehabil* 5(2):143, 1996.
23. Dover G, Powers M: Reliability of joint position sense and force production measures during internal and external rotation of the shoulder, *J Ath Train* 38(4):304, 2003.
24. Duralde XA: Neurologic injuries in the athlete's shoulder, *J Ath Train* 35(3):316, 2000.
25. Durall C, Davies G, Kernozek T: The effects of training the humeral rotators on arm elevation in the scapular plane, *J Sport Rehabil* 10(2):79, 2001.
26. Ellenbecker TS, Davies GJ: The application of isokinetics in testing and rehabilitation of the shoulder complex, *J Ath Train* 35(3):338, 2000.
27. Ellenbecker TS, Mattalino AJ: Glenohumeral joint range of motion and rotator cuff strength following arthroscopic anterior stabilization with thermal capsulorraphy, *J Orthop Sport Phys Ther* 29(3):160, 1999.
28. Floyd R, Behrhorst K, Walters S: Innovative tools for shoulder rehabilitation, *Athletic Therapy Today* 4(4):47, 1999.
29. Greenfield B, Catlin P, Coats P: Posture in patients with shoulder overuse injuries and healthy individuals, *J Orthop Sports Phys Ther* 22(5):287, 1995.
30. Hayes K, Callanan M, Walton J: Shoulder instability: management and rehabilitation, *J Orthop Sports Phys Ther* 32(10):497, 2002.
31. Hillman S: Principles and techniques of open kinetic chain rehabilitation: the upper extremity, *J Sport Rehabil* 3(4):319, 1994.
32. Henry T, Lephart S, Giraldo J: The effect of muscle fatigue on muscle force-couple activation of the shoulder, *J Sport Rehabil* 10(42):24, 2001.
33. Irrgang J, Whitney S, Harner C: Nonoperative treatment of rotator cuff injuries in throwing athletes, *J Sport Rehabil* 1(3):197, 1992.
34. Janwantanakul P, Jones M, Magarey M: Characteristics of shoulder-position sense: effects of mode of movement, scapular support, and arm orientation, *J Sport Rehabil* 11(3):157, 2002.
35. Jobe CM, Coen MJ: Evaluation of impingement syndromes in the overhead-throwing athlete, *J Ath Train* 35(3):293, 2000.
36. Karas S: Thoracic outlet syndrome. In Hershman E, editor: *Clinics in sports medicine*, Philadelphia, 1990, Saunders.
37. Keskula D, Lott J: Defining and measuring functional limitations and disability in the athletic shoulder, *J Sport Rehabil* 10(3):221, 2001.
38. Kibler WB: The role of the scapula in athletic shoulder function, *Am J Sports Med* 26(2):325, 1998.
39. Kibler WB: Shoulder rehabilitation: principles and practice, *Med Sci Sports Exerc* 30(4 suppl):S40, 1998.
40. Li et al: Shoulder function in patients with unoperated anterior shoulder instability, *Am J Sports Med* 19(5):469, 1992.
41. Line L, Murret L: Labral tears: diagnosis, treatment and rehabilitation, *Athletic Therapy Today* 4(4):18, 1999.
42. Ludewig P, Cook T: Translations of the humerus in persons with shoulder impingement symptoms, *J Orthop Sports Phys Ther* 32(6): 248, 2002.
43. Manske R, Davies: G: Postrehabilitation outcomes of muscle power (torque-acceleration energy) in patients with selected shoulder dysfunctions, *J Sport Rehabil* 12(3):181, 2003.
44. Masten F, Arntz C: Subacromial impingement. In Rockwood C, Masten F, editors: *The shoulder*, Philadelphia, 2004, Elsevier Science.
45. Masten F, Thomas S, Rockwood C: Glenohumeral instability. In Rockwood C, Masten F, editors: *The shoulder*, Philadelphia, 2004, Elsevier Science.
46. McCluskey GM, Getz BA: Pathophysiology of anterior shoulder instability, *J Ath Train* 35(3):268, 2000.
47. McLoda T, Murphy K, Davison S: Functional effects of inertial training of the upper extremity, *J Sport Rehabil* 12(3):229, 2003.
48. Mendoza F, Main K: Peripheral nerve injuries of the shoulder in the athlete. In Hershman EB, editor: *Neurovascular injuries. Clinics in sports medicine*, vol 9, no 2, Philadelphia, 1995, Saunders.
49. Mendoza F et al: Principles of shoulder rehabilitation in the athlete. In Nicholas JA, Hershman EB, editors: *The upper extremity in sports medicine*, St Louis, 1995, Mosby.
50. Meyers JB, Lephart SM: The role of the sensorimotor system in the athletic shoulder, *J Ath Train* 35(3):351, 2000.
51. Myers J: Conservative management of shoulder impingement syndrome in the athletic population, *J Sport Rehabil* 8(3):230, 1999.
52. Norris T: History and physical examination of the shoulder. In Nicholas JA, Hershman EB, editors: *The upper extremity in sports medicine*, St Louis, 1995, Mosby.
53. O'Brien S et al: The anatomy and histology of the inferior glenohumeral ligament complex of the shoulder, *Am J Sports Med* 18(5): 449, 1990.
54. Perkins S, Massie J: Patient satisfaction after thermal shrinkage of the glenohumeral-joint capsule, *J Sport Rehabil* 10(3):157, 2001.
55. Plafcan DM, Turczany PJ, Guenin BA, Kegerreis S, Worrell TW: An objective measurement technique for posterior scapular displacement, *J Orthop Sports Phys Ther* 25(5):336, 1997.
56. Ragol IM, Ernst G, Perrin DH: Open and closed kinetic chain exercises improve shoulder joint reposition sense equally in healthy subjects, *J Ath Train* 33(4):315, 1998.
57. Richardson AB: Thoracic outlet syndrome in aquatic athletes, *Clin Sports Med* 18(2):361, 1999.
58. Rockwood CA, Williams GR, Young DC: Injuries to the acromioclavicular joint. In Rockwood CA, Green DP, Bucholz RW: *Rockwood and Green's fractures in adults*, Philadelphia, 2001, JB Lippincott.
59. Rofii M et al: Computed tomography (CT) arthrography of shoulder instabilities in athletes, *Am J Sports Med* 16(4):353, 1988.
60. Roskin D, Speer K, Gallagher A: Accelerated post-operative management of shoulder injuries, *Athletic Therapy Today* 4(4):27, 1999.
61. Satterwhite YE: Evaluation and management of recurrent anterior shoulder instability, *J Ath Train* 35(3):273, 2000.

62. Sawa T: An alternate conservative management of shoulder dislocations and subluxations, *J Ath Train* 27(4):366, 1992.
63. Schneider R, Prentice W: Rehabilitation of shoulder injuries. In Prentice W: *Rehabilitation techniques in sports medicine and athletic training,* St Louis, 2004, McGraw-Hill.
64. Scovazzo ML et al: The painful shoulder during freestyle swimming, *Am J Sports Med* 19(6):577, 1991.
65. Skyhar M, Warren R, Altcheck D: Instability of the shoulder. In Nicholas JA, Hershman EB, editors: *The upper extremity in sports medicine,* St Louis, 1995, Mosby.
66. Stone J, Lueken J, Partin N: Closed kinetic chain rehabilitation for the glenohumeral joint, *J Ath Train* 28(1):34, 1993.
67. Taylor M, Fruth S, Kegerreis S: The glenoid labrum: basic science and clinical correlation, *J Sport Rehabil* 4(1):42, 1995.
68. Terry G et al: The function of passive shoulder restraints, *Am J Sports Med* 19(1):26, 1991.
69. Terry GC, Chopp TM: Functional anatomy of the shoulder, *J Ath Train* 35(3):248, 2000.
70. Thein JM, Brody LT: Aquatic-based rehabilitation and training for the shoulder, *J Ath Train* 35(3):382, 2000.
71. Uhl T, Carver T, Mattacola C: Shoulder musculature activation during upper extremity weight-bearing exercise, *J Orthop Sports Phys Ther* 33(3):109, 2003.
72. Voight ML, Thomson BC: The role of the scapula in the rehabilitation of shoulder injuries, *J Ath Train* 35(3):364, 2000.
73. Watson K: Impingement and rotator cuff lesions. In Nicholas JA, Hershman EB, editors: *The upper extremity in sports medicine,* St Louis, 1995, Mosby.
74. Weise K, Sitler M, Tierney R: Effectiveness of glenohumeral joint stability braces in limiting active and passive shoulder range of motion in collegiate football players, *J Ath Train* 39(2):151, 2004.
75. Weldon EJ III, Richardson AB: Upper extremity overuse injuries in swimming: a discussion of swimmer's shoulder, *Clin Sports Med* 20(3):423, 2001.
76. Wilk KE, Arrigo CA, Andrews JR: Current concepts: the stabilizing structures of the glenohumeral joint, *J Orthop Sports Phys Ther* 25(6): 364, 1997.
77. Wilk K, Reinold M, Dugas J: Rehabilitation following thermal-assisted capsular shrinkage of the glenohumeral joint: current concepts, *J Orthop Sports Phys Ther* 32(6):268, 2002.
78. Williams GR, Kelley M: Management of rotator cuff and impingement injuries in the athlete, *J Ath Train* 35(3):300, 2000.
79. Wolin PM, Tarbet JA: Rotator cuff injury: addressing overhead overuse, *Physician Sportsmed* 25(6):54, 1997.
80. Yanai T, Hay JG, Miller GF: Shoulder impingement in front-crawl swimming: I. a method to identify impingement, *Med Sci Sports Exerc* 32(1):21, 2000.
81. Zheng N, Fleisig G, Andrews J: Biomechanics and injuries of the shoulder during throwing, *Athletic Therapy Today* 4(4):6, 1999.

ANNOTATED BIBLIOGRAPHY

Andrews J, Wilk K: *The athlete's shoulder,* New York, 1994, Churchill Livingstone.

This text concentrates on both conservative and surgical treatment of shoulder injuries that occur specifically in the athletic population.

Cailliet R: *Shoulder pain,* ed 3, Philadelphia, 1991, Davis.

This text provides excellent coverage of the fundamental principles for assessing and treating shoulder pain syndromes.

Hartley A: *Practical joint assessment: a sports medicine manual,* St Louis, 1991, Mosby.

This concise manual of joint assessment includes detailed shoulder evaluation.

Hawkins RJ, editor: *Basic science and clinical application in the athlete's shoulder. Clinics in sports medicine,* vol 10, no 4, Philadelphia, 1991, Saunders.

This detailed monograph is dedicated to all aspects of the shoulder in sports.

Iannotti JP, Williams GR: *Disorders of the shoulder: diagnosis and management,* Baltimore, 1999, Lippincott, Williams & Wilkins.

This text presents the basic concepts of diagnosis and management of the common shoulder disorders.

Kirshnan S, Hawkins R: *The shoulder and the overhead athlete,* Philadelphia 2004, Lippincott, Williams & Wilkins.

Written by a multidisciplinary team of expert shoulder surgeons, athletic trainers, and physical therapists, this reference delivers comprehensive and up-to-date information on the evaluation, treatment, rehabilitation, and prevention of shoulder injuries in athletes who throw and use other overhead movements.

Nicholas JA, Hershman EB, editors: *The upper extremity in sports medicine,* St Louis, 1995, Mosby.

This text has a great deal of information on the recognition, evaluation, and management of shoulder injuries in addition to injuries of the elbow, wrist, and hand.

Rockwood C, Masten F: *The shoulder,* Philadelphia, 2004, Elsevier Science.

This complete, two-volume set covers every subject relative to the shoulder complex.

Special Issue: Evaluation and management of shoulder injuries in the athlete, *Journal of Athletic Training,* 35(3), 2000.

An entire issue of this quarterly journal is dedicated to research articles dealing with injuries to the shoulder joint.

Chapter 23

The Elbow

When you finish this chapter you should be able to

- Recall the structural and functional anatomy of the elbow and relate it to sports injuries.
- Explain the process for assessing the injured elbow.
- Demonstrate proper immediate and follow-up management of elbow injuries.
- Devise appropriate rehabilitation techniques that can be used following injury to the elbow.
- Design a functional progression for the throwing athlete to return to activity.

ANATOMY OF THE ELBOW JOINT

Bones

The elbow joint is composed of three bones: the humerus, the radius, and the ulna (Figure 23-1). The distal end of the humerus forms two articulating condyles. The lateral condyle is the capitulum, and the medial condyle is the trochlea. The convex capitulum articulates with the concave head of the radius. The trochlea, which is spool shaped, fits into an articulating groove, the semilunar notch, which is provided by the ulna between the olecranon and coronoid processes. Above each condyle is a projection called the epicondyle. The structural design of the elbow joint permits flexion and extension through the articulation of the trochlea with the semilunar notch of the ulna. Forearm pronation and supination are made possible because the head of the radius rotates against the capitulum freely without any bone limitations.[22]

Articulations

The elbow complex consists of three separate joints: the humeroulnar joint, the humeroradial joint, and the proximal radioulnar joint (Figure 23-2). The humeroulnar joint is the articulation between the distal humerus medially and the proximal ulna. When the elbow is in flexion, the ulna slides forward until the coronoid process of the ulna stops in the floor of the coronoid fossa of the humerus. In extension, the ulna will slide backwards until the olecranon process of the ulna makes contact with the olecranon fossa of the humerus posteriorly. The humeroradial joint is the articulation of the lateral distal humerus and the proximal radius. In flexion, the radius is in contact with the radial fossa of the distal humerus, whereas in extension, the radius and the humerus are not in contact. The proximal radioulnar joint is the articulation between the radial notch of the proximal lateral aspect of the ulna, the radial head, and the capitulum of the distal humerus. The proximal and distal radioulnar joints are important in supination and pronation. The proximal and distal aspects of this joint cannot function without each other.

Ligaments and Capsule

The capsule of the elbow, both anteriorly and posteriorly, is relatively thin and is covered by the brachialis muscle in front and the triceps brachii behind. The capsule is

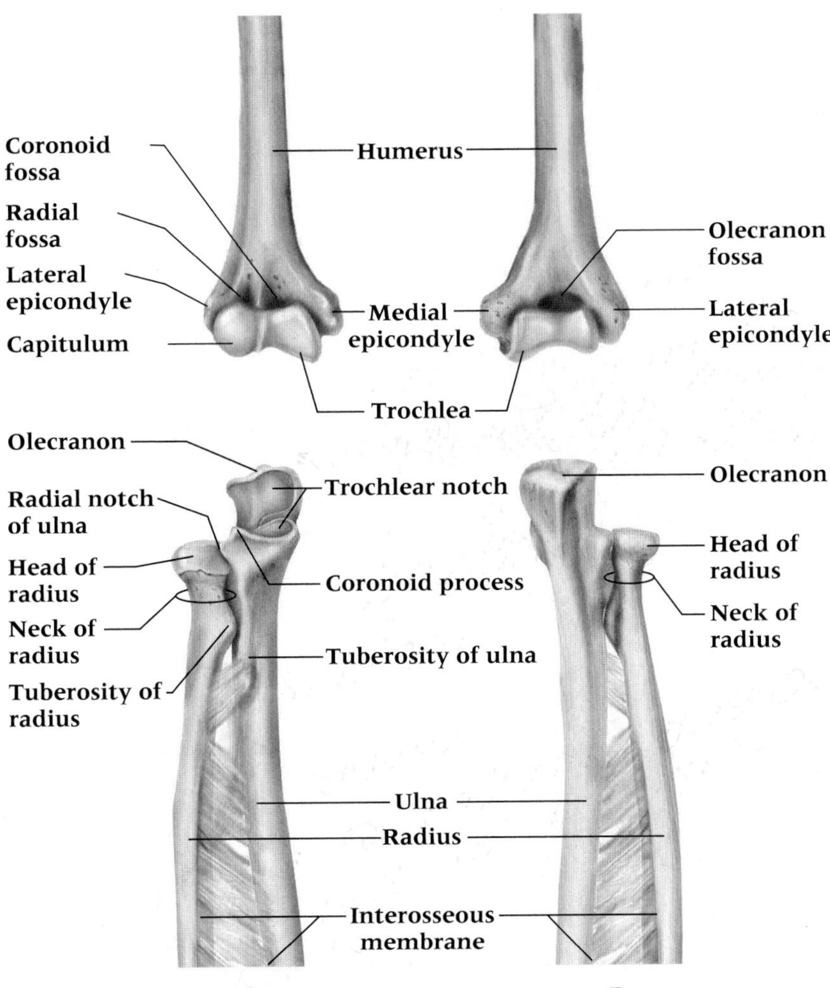

Figure 23-1

Bones of the elbow joint. **A,** Anterior view. **B,** Posterior view.

reinforced by the ulnar and radial collateral ligaments (Figure 23-2). The ulnar collateral ligament is composed of a strong anterior band with weaker transverse and middle sheets. The radial collateral ligament does not attach to the radius, which is free to rotate. The radius rotates in the radial notch of the ulna and is stabilized by a strong annular ligament. The annular ligament is attached to the anterior and posterior margins of the radial notch and encircles the head and neck of the radius.

Valgus elbow stability depends mainly on the integrity of the medial collateral ligament. Lateral elbow stability depends on two factors: the integrity of the lateral collateral ligament and stabilization by the annular ligament, which maintains the relationship of the radial head to the proximal radioulnar joints. The medial collateral ligament is of major importance in activities that produce forceful flexion-supination movements. Varus elbow joint forces are uncommon. The main stability of the elbow is contingent on the integrity of radiocapitular articulation, the trochlear-ulnar joint with its coronoid process, and intact medial and lateral ligaments. Additional elbow support is provided by the muscle tendons.

Synovium and Bursae

A common synovial membrane invests the elbow and the superior radioulnar articulations, lubricating the deeper structures of the two joints; a sleevelike capsule surrounds the entire elbow joint. The most important bursae in the area of the elbow are the bicipital and olecranon bursae. The bicipital bursa lies in the anterior aspect of the

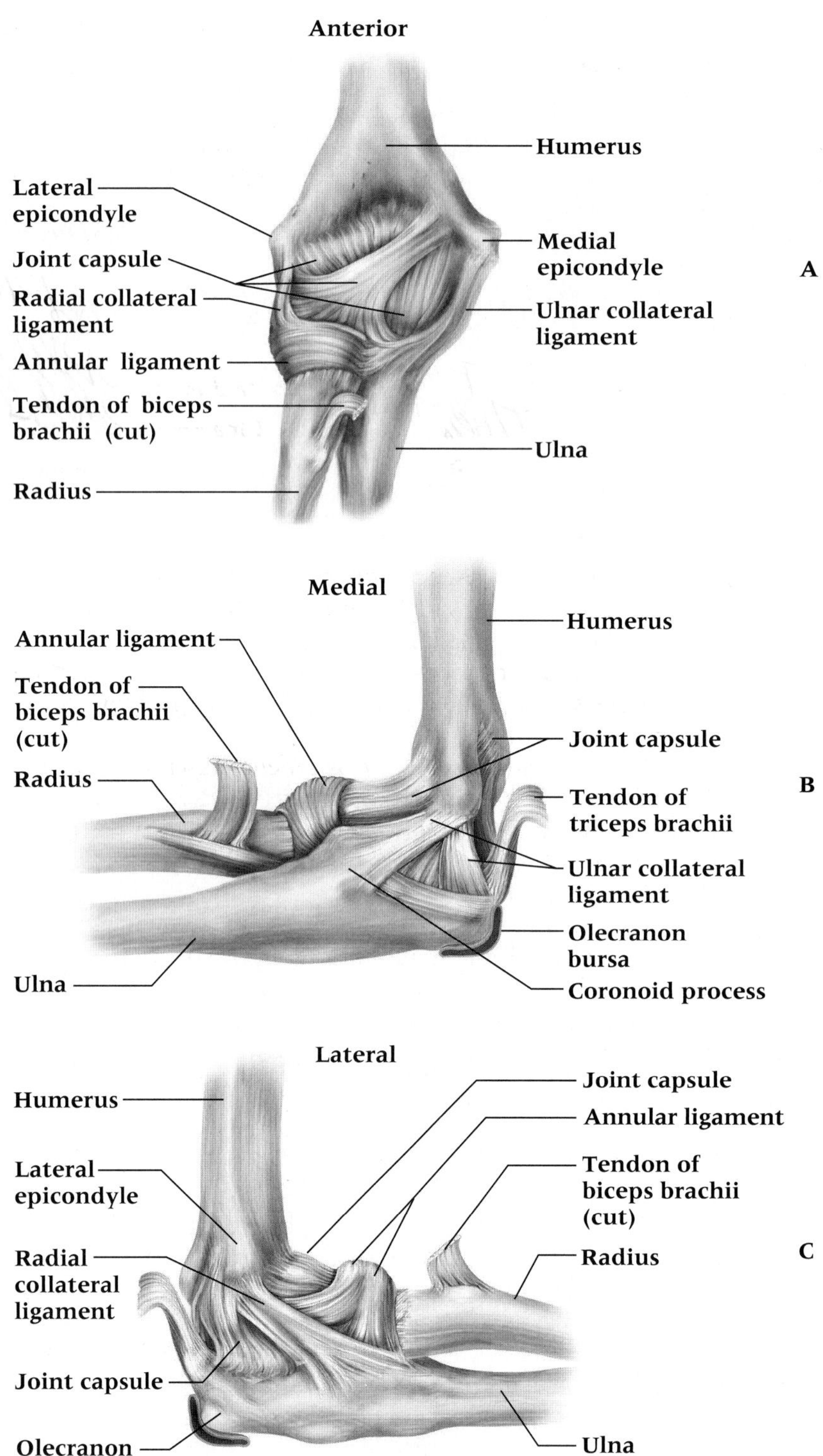

Figure 23-2

Joint capsule and ligaments of the elbow. **A,** Anterior. **B,** Mechanical. **C,** Lateral.

bicipital tuberosity and cushions the tendon when the forearm is pronated. The olecranon bursa lies between the olecranon process and the skin (Figure 23-2B).

Elbow Musculature

The elbow flexors are the biceps brachii, brachialis, and brachioradialis muscles (Figure 23-3). The biceps brachii originates via two heads proximally at the shoulder; the long head from the supraglenoid tuberosity of the scapula and the short head from the coracoid process of the scapula. The insertion is from a common tendon at the radial

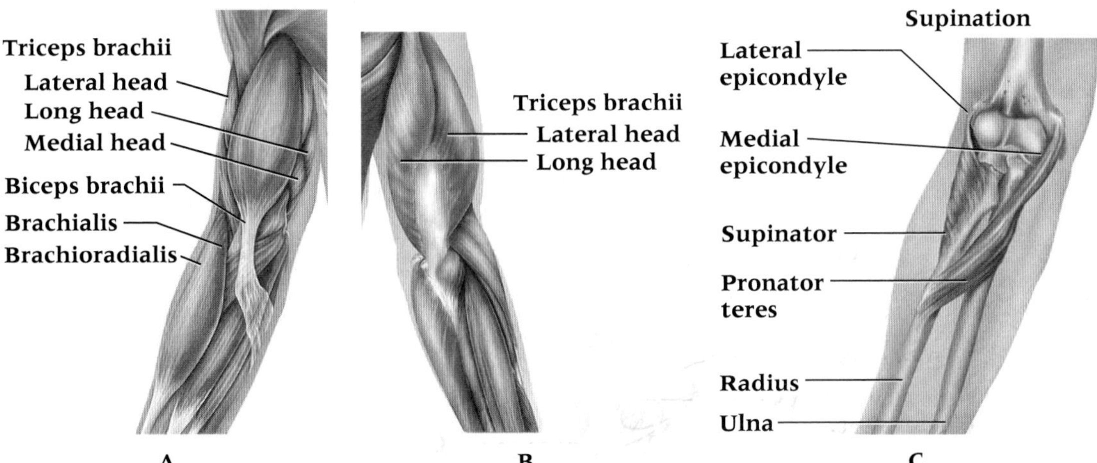

Figure 23-3

Muscles of the elbow joint. **A,** Anterior view. **B,** Posterior view. **C,** Deep pronator teres and supinator muscles.

tuberosity. The biceps brachii flexes the elbow and supinates the forearm. The brachialis originates from the lower two-thirds of the anterior humerus and inserts on the coronoid process and the tuberosity of the ulna. It flexes the elbow. The brachioradialis, which originates from the lower two-thirds of the lateral humerus and attaches to the lateral styloid process of the distal radius, functions as an elbow flexor, pronator, and semisupinator.

The elbow extensors are the triceps brachii and the anconeus muscles. The triceps brachii consists of long, medial, and lateral heads. The long head originates at the infraglenoid tuberosity of the scapula. The lateral and medial heads originate at the posterior aspect of the humerus. The insertion is via the common tendon posteriorly at the olecranon process. The triceps and the anconeus muscle cause extension of the elbow complex.

The pronator teres at the elbow joint and pronator quadtratus at the distal aspect of the wrist cause pronation of the forearm. Supination is caused by a combined action of the biceps brachii and the supinator muscle. With both supination and pronation, the radius will move on the ulna.

Nerve Supply

Nerves stemming from brachial plexus (C4–T2) innervate the muscles that control movement around the elbow joint (see Figure 22-6). In the cubital fossa, these nerves become the musculocutaneous, radial, ulnar, and median nerves (Table 23-1).

Blood Supply

Superficial and close to the skin in front of the elbow lie the veins that return the blood of the forearm to the heart. Deep within the antecubital fossa lie the brachial and medial arteries that supply the area with oxygenated blood (Figure 23-4).

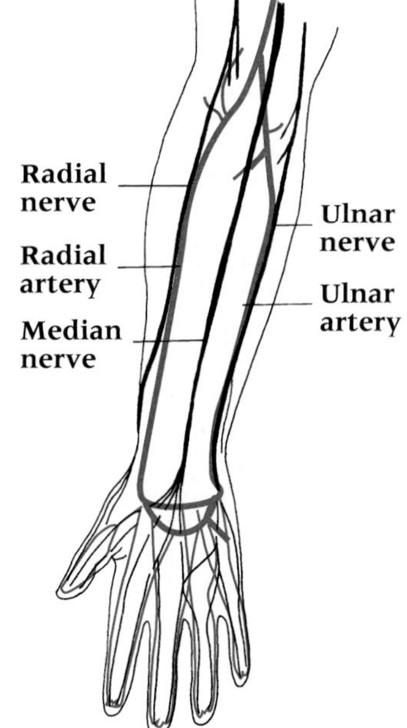

Figure 23-4

Arteries and nerves supplying the elbow joint, wrist, and hand.

FUNCTIONAL ANATOMY

The anatomic arrangement of the elbow complex allows for flexion, extension, pronation, and supination. The elbow has approximately 145 degrees of flexion and 90 degrees of both supination and pronation. The bony limitations, ligamentous support, and muscular stability at the elbow help to protect it from overuse and traumatic injury. Because of the more distal projection of the humerus medially, the elbow complex will demonstrate a carrying angle that is an abducted position of the elbow in the anatomical position[22] (Figure 23-5). The normal carrying angle in females is 10 to 15 degrees and in males 5 to 10 degrees. In the athletic environment, the elbow complex can be subjected to forces ranging from overhead throwing activities to blunt trauma that can cause various injuries.

TABLE 23-1 Muscles Acting on the Elbow Joint

Muscle	Origin	Insertion	Muscle Action	Innervation
Biceps brachii	*Long head:* Supraglenoid tuberosity of the scapula *Short head:* Coracoid process of the scapula	Tuberosity of the radius	Flexes the elbow and the arm; supinates the forearm	Musculocutaneous
Brachialis	Anterior surface of the distal half of the humerus	Coronoid process of the ulna	Flexes the elbow	Musculocutaneous and radial
Brachioradialis	Lateral supracondular ridge of the humerus	Styloid process of the radius	Flexes the elbow	Radial
Triceps brachii	*Long head:* Infraglenoid tuberosity of the scapula *Lateral head:* Posterior surface of the humerus above the radial groove *Medial head:* Posterior surface of the humerus below the radial groove	Olecranon process of the ulna	Extends the elbow and the arm	Radial
Supinator	Lateral epicondule of the humerus	Proximal end of the lateral surface of the shaft of the radius	Supinates the elbow	Radial
Pronator teres	Medial epicondyle of the humerus and the coronoid process of the ulna	Middle of the lateral surface of the shaft of the radius	Pronates the elbow	Median
Anconeus	Lateral epicondyle of the humerus	Lateral surface of the olecranon process of the ulna	Extends the elbow	Radial

The elbow is a critical link in the kinetic chain of the upper extremity. Functionally, the hand and the shoulder need the elbow for normal function. The connection between multijoint muscles that affect the elbow will work both proximally and distally in the upper extremity as a whole.

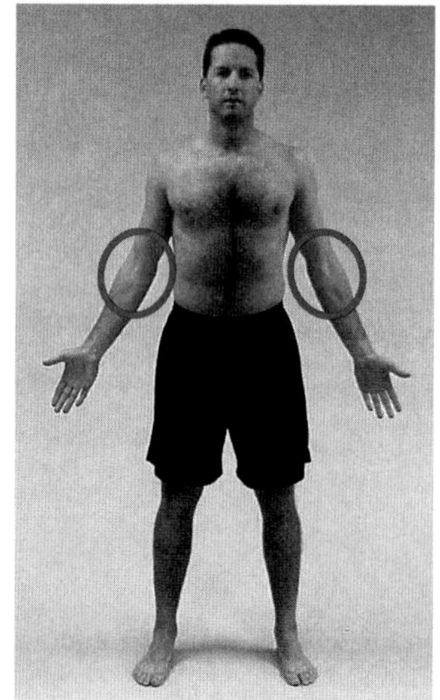

Figure 23-5

Observing for elbow carrying angle and the extent of cubitus valgus and cubitus varus.

ASSESSMENT OF THE ELBOW

History

Like all sports injuries, an elbow injury requires the athletic trainer to first understand the possible mechanism of injury. The athletic trainer should ask the following questions when evaluating the elbow:

- Is the pain or discomfort caused by a direct trauma such as falling on an outstretched arm or landing on the tip of a bent elbow (the most common mechanism for a variety of elbow injuries)?[31]
- Can the problem be attributed to sudden overextension of the elbow or to repeated overuse of a throwing motion?[12]
- What are the location and duration of the pain? Like shoulder pain, elbow pain or discomfort could be from internal organ dysfunction or referred from a nerve root irritation or nerve impingement.
- Are there movements or positions of the arm that increase or decrease the pain?
- Has a previous elbow injury been diagnosed or treated?
- Is there a feeling of locking or crepitation during movement?

Observation

The athlete's elbow should be observed for obvious deformities and swelling. The carrying angle, flexion, and extensibility of the elbow should be observed.[12] If the carrying

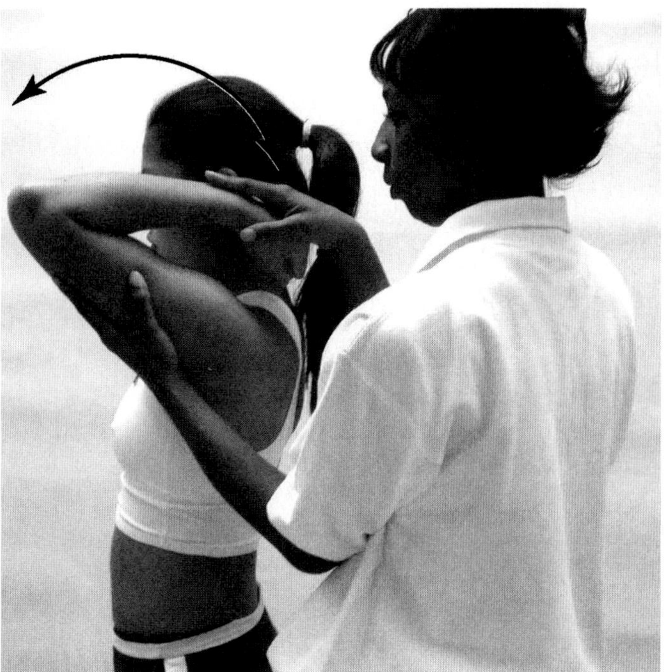

Figure 23-6

Testing for elbow flexion and extension.

angle is abnormally increased, a cubitus valgus is present; if it is abnormally decreased, a cubitus varus is present (Figure 23-5). Over the long term, overhead throwing activities can increase this angle. The athlete is next observed for the extent of elbow flexion and extension. Both elbows are compared (Figure 23-6). A decrease in normal flexion, an inability to extend fully, or extending beyond normal extension (cubitus recurvatus) could be precipitating reasons for joint problems (Figure 23-7). Next, the elbow is bent to a 45-degree angle and observed from the rear to determine whether the two epicondyles and olecranon process form an isosceles triangle (Figure 23-8).

Palpation

Bony Palpation

The following bony landmarks should be palpated:

- Medial epicondyle
- Lateral epicondyle
- Olecranon process
- Radial head
- Radius
- Ulna

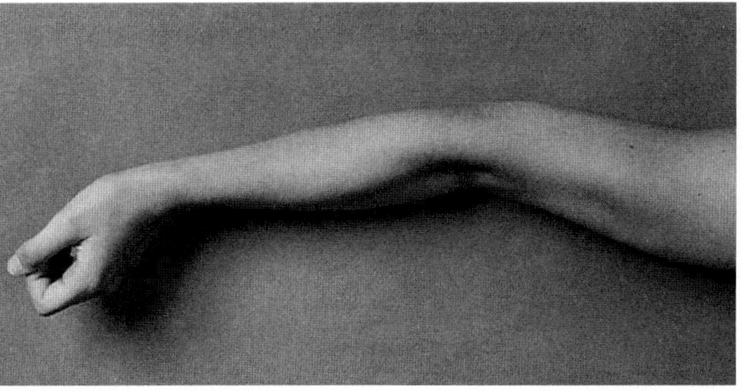

Figure 23-7

Testing for cubitus recurvatus (elbow hyperextension).

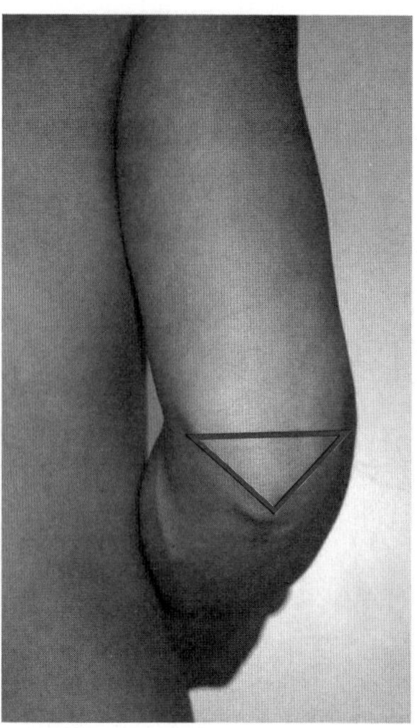

Figure 23-8

Determining whether the lateral and medial epicondyles, along with the olecranon process, form an isosceles triangle.

Soft Tissue Palpation

The following soft tissue structures should be palpated:

Anterior

- Biceps brachii
- Brachialis
- Brachioradialis
- Pronator teres

Posterior

- Triceps
- Supinator

Medial

- Ulnar collateral ligament
- Wrist flexor muscles

Lateral

- Radial collateral ligament
- Annular ligament
- Wrist extensor muscles

Special Tests

Circulatory and Neurological Evaluation

With an elbow injury, a pulse should routinely be taken at the brachial artery and at the radial artery at the wrist. Alteration of skin sensation also should be noted, which could indicate nerve root compression or irritation in the cervical or shoulder region or in the elbow itself. Additional nerve evaluation is made through active and resisted muscle tests (see Table 23-1).

Tinel's sign Tinel's test is designed to determine ulnar nerve compromise. The subject is seated with the elbow in slight flexion. The athletic trainer stands and grasps the athlete's wrist and, with the other hand, taps the ulnar notch between the olecranon process and medial epicondyle with the reflex hammer or the index finger. A positive Tinel's sign is when the athlete complains of a tingling sensation along the forearm, hand, and fingers (Figure 23-9).[19]

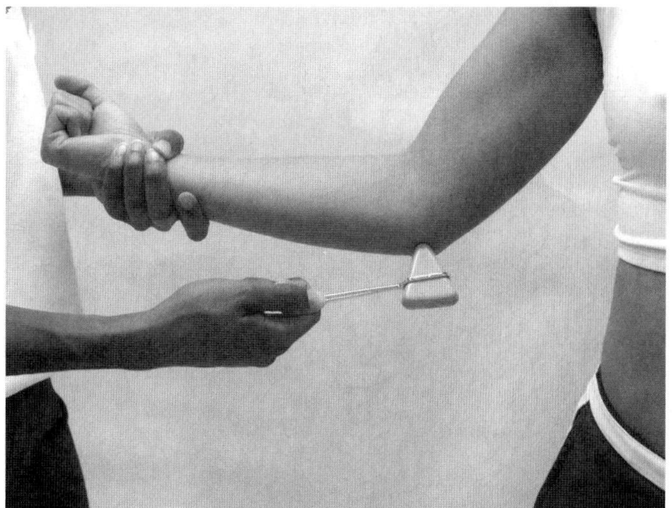

Figure 23-9

Tinel's sign.

Tests for Capsular Injury

To test for capsular pain after hyperextension of the elbow, the elbow is flexed in a 45-degree position. The wrist is flexed as far as possible and then extended as far as possible (Figure 23-10). If joint pain is severe during this test, a moderate to severe capsular sprain or fracture should be suspected. However, a chronic injury may also produce capsular pain.

Valgus/Varus Stress Test

A valgus stress test checks for sprain of the medial collateral ligament. A varus stress test checks for sprain or instability of the lateral collateral ligament. The athletic trainer grasps the athlete's wrist and extends the arm in an anatomical position and places the other hand over either the lateral or medial epicondyle. While the hand that is over the epicondyle acts as a fulcrum, the hand holding the athlete's wrist attempts to move the forearm. In applying the stress, the athletic trainer should notice whether there is gapping of the lateral or medial collateral ligament (Figure 23-11).

The athlete complains of severe pain on the medial aspect of the elbow that becomes relieved by flexing the elbow. There is point tenderness on the medial epicondyle, distal aspect of the ulna, or lateral collateral ligament.

23-1

Critical Thinking Exercise

An athlete sustains a serious sprain to the left elbow.

? What tests and basic examination procedures should be performed to determine the nature of this injury?

Medial and Lateral Epicondylitis Tests

The elbow is flexed to 45 degrees and wrist extension is resisted, which increases pain at the lateral epicondyle (Figure 23-12). When wrist flexion is resisted, pain increases at the medial epicondyle.

A

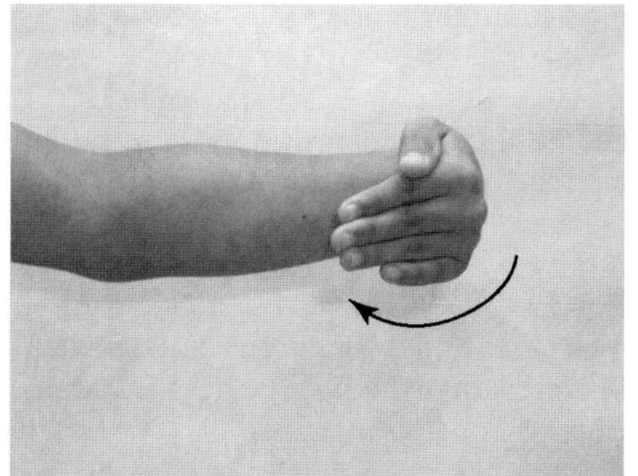

B

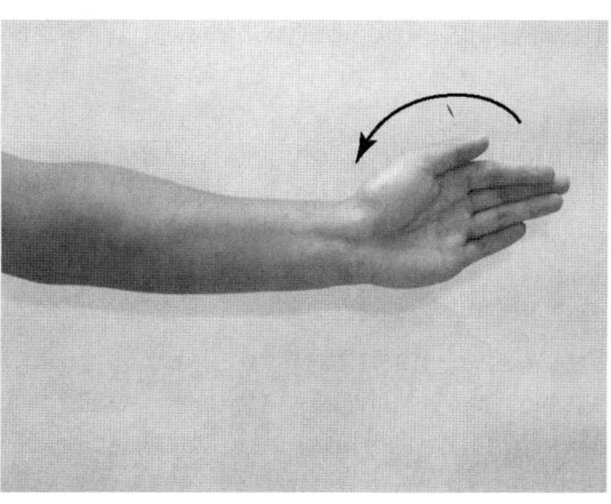

Figure 23-10

Testing for capsular pain after hyperextension of the elbow. **A,** Wrist flexion. **B,** Wrist extension.

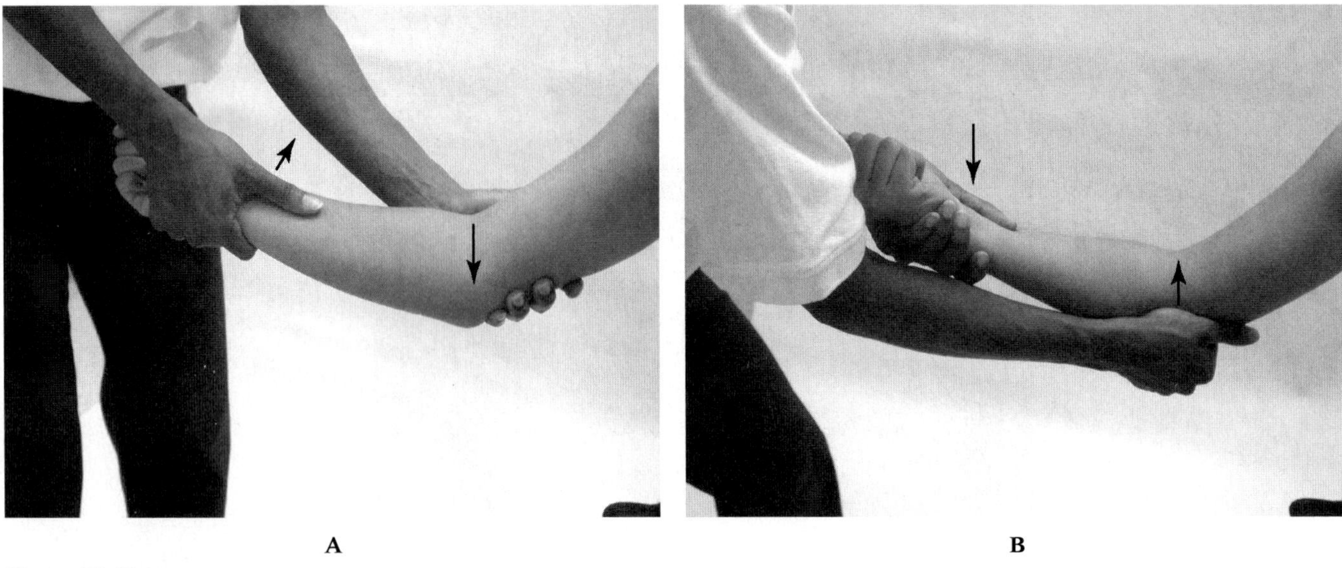

A B

Figure 23-11

Collateral ligament test of the elbow. **A,** Medial collateral ligament. **B,** Lateral collateral ligament.

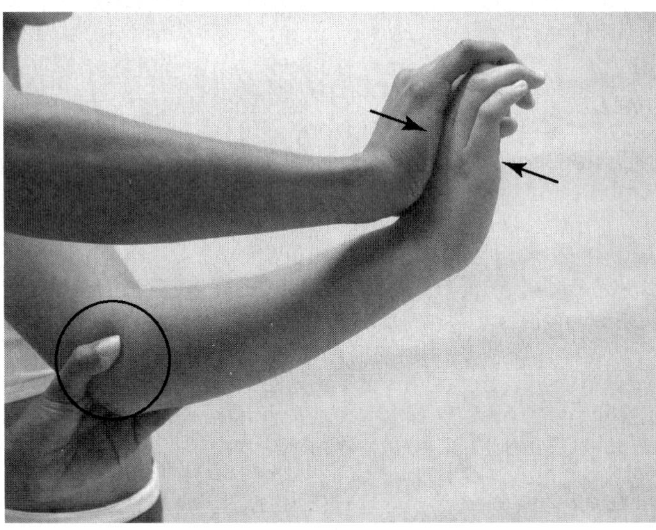

Figure 23-12

Tennis elbow test.

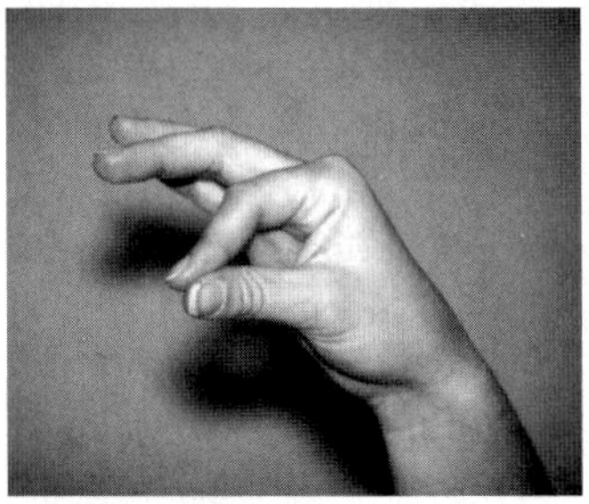

Figure 23-13

Pinch grip test

Pinch Grip Test

The athlete is instructed to pinch the tips of the thumb and index finger together. An inability to touch the thumb and index finger indicates entrapment of the anterior interrosseous nerve between the two heads of the pronator muscle (Figure 23-13).

Pronator Teres Syndrome Test

While the athlete is in a seated position, the athletic trainer resists forearm pronation. Increased pain proximally over the pronator teres would indicate a positive test (Figure 23-14).

Functional Evaluation

The joint and the muscles are evaluated for pain sites and weakness through passive, active, and resistive motions consisting of elbow flexion and extension (Figure 23-15) and forearm pronation and supination (Figure 23-16). Range of motion is particularly noted in passive and active pronation and supination.

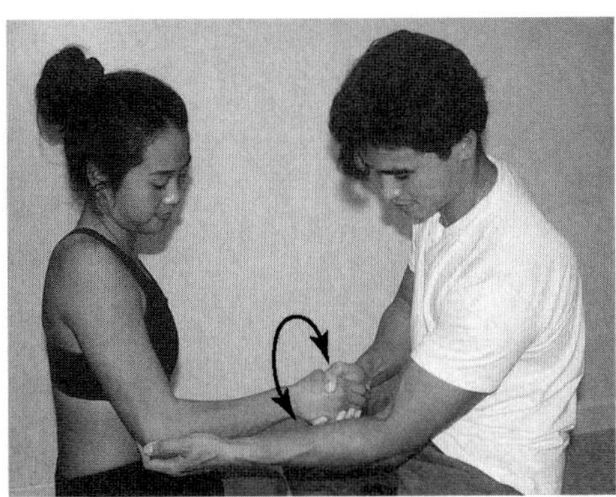

Figure 23-14

Elbow evaluation includes performing passive, active, and resistive forearm pronation and supination.

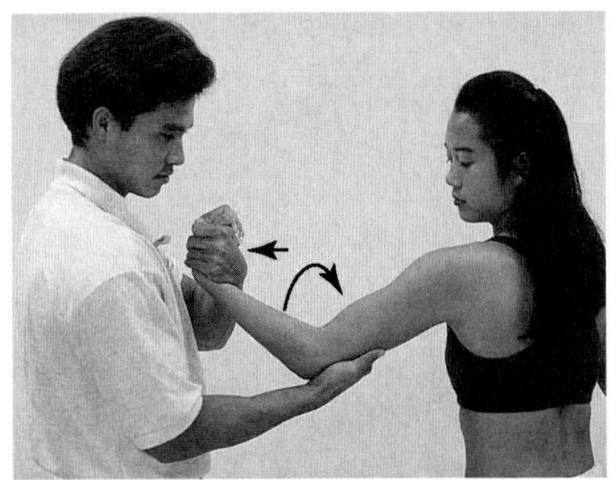

Figure 23-15

Functional evaluation includes performing passive resistance flexion and extension to determine joint restrictions and pain sites.

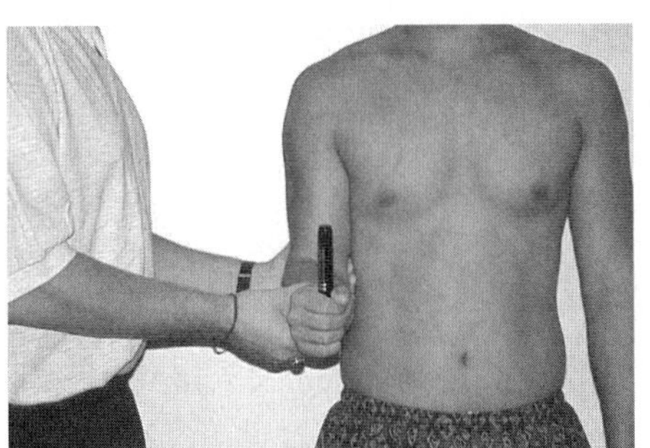

Neutral

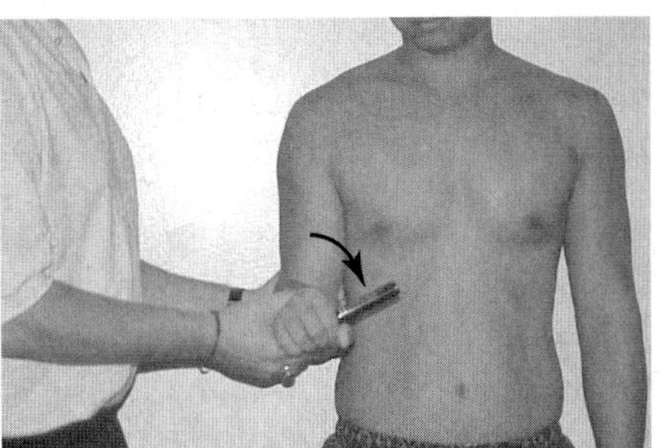

Pronation

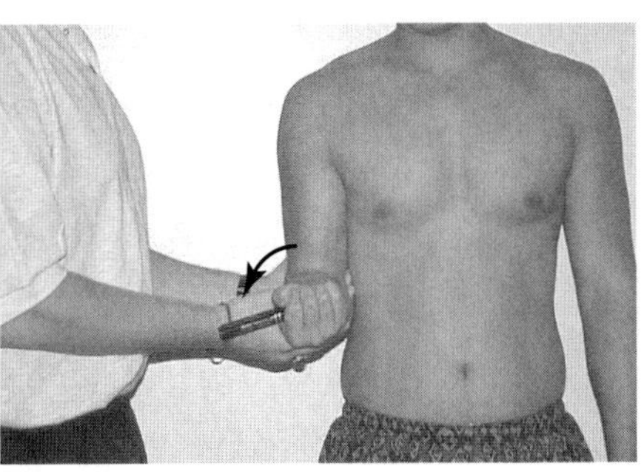

Supination

Figure 23-16

The range of motion of forearm pronation and supination is routinely tested in athletes with elbow conditions.

RECOGNITION AND MANAGEMENT OF INJURIES TO THE ELBOW

The elbow is subject to injury in sports because of its broad range of motion, weak lateral bone arrangement, and relative exposure to soft-tissue damage.[49] Many sports place excessive stress on the elbow joint. Locking of the elbow in gymnastics or using implements such as racquets, golf clubs, and javelins can cause injuries. The throwing mechanism in baseball pitching can injure the elbow during both the acceleration and follow-through phases.[23]

The two most common mechanisms of elbow injury:
- Throwing
- Falling on the outstretched hand

Contusions

Etiology Because of its lack of padding and its general vulnerability, the elbow often becomes contused during contact sports. Bone bruises arise from a deep penetration or a succession of blows to the sharp projections of the elbow.

Symptoms and signs A contusion of the elbow may swell rapidly after an irritation of the olecranon bursa or the synovial membrane.

Management The contused elbow should be treated immediately with cold and pressure for at least twenty-four hours. If injury is severe, the athlete should be referred to a physician for X-ray examination to determine whether a fracture exists.

Olecranon Bursitis

Etiology The olecranon bursa, lying between the end of the olecranon process and the skin, is the most frequently injured bursa in the elbow (Figure 23-17).[28] Its superficial location makes it prone to acute or chronic injury, particularly as the result of direct blows.[7]

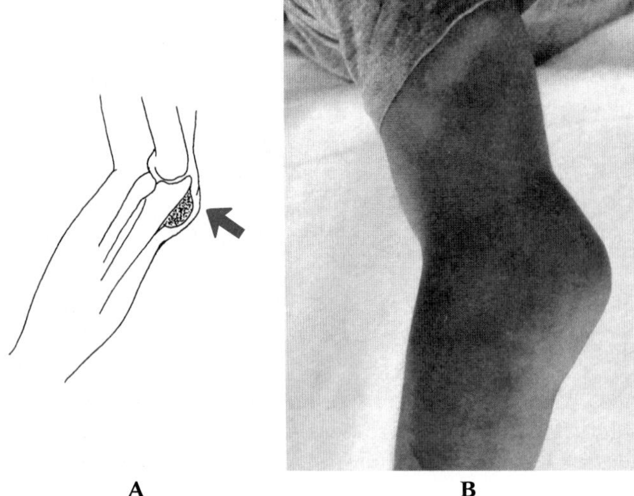

Figure 23-17

Olecranon bursitis.

23-2

Critical Thinking Exercise

A wrestler, not wearing elbow pads, complains of irritation and a mild pain at the tip of the right elbow.

? What is a possible condition?

Symptoms and signs The inflamed bursa produces pain, severe swelling, and point tenderness. Occasionally, swelling will appear almost spontaneously and without the usual pain and heat.

Management If the condition is acute, a cold compress should be applied for at least one hour. Chronic olecranon bursitis requires a program of superficial therapy primarily involving compression. If swelling fails to resolve, in some cases aspiration will hasten healing. Although seldom serious, olecranon bursitis can be annoying and should be well protected by padding while the athlete is engaged in competition.

Strains

Etiology The acute mechanisms of muscle strain associated with the elbow joint are usually excessive resistive motions such as a fall on the outstretched hand with the elbow in extension, which forces the joint into hyperextension. Repeated microtears that cause chronic injury are discussed in the section on epicondylitis.[34]

The biceps, brachialis, and triceps muscles should be tested through active and resistive movement. The muscles of pronation and supination are also tested. Rupture of the distal biceps brachii at its radial attachment is the most common muscle rupture in the upper extremity.[44]

Symptoms and signs During active or resistive movement, the athlete complains of pain. There is usually point tenderness in the muscle, tendon, or lower part of the muscle belly.

Management Immediate care includes RICE as well as sling support for the most severe cases. Follow-up management may include cryotherapy, ultrasound, and rehabilitative exercises. Conditions that cause moderate to severe loss of elbow function should routinely be referred for X-ray examination. It is important to rule out the possibility of an avulsion or epiphyseal fracture.

23-3

Critical Thinking Exercise

A minor league baseball pitcher is complaining of pain on the medial side of his elbow and some tingling and numbness in the ring and little fingers of his throwing arm. On examination the athletic trainer can palpate an area of tenderness over the medial collateral ligament and determines that there is minimal laxity with valgus stress.

? What is most likely to be this athlete's problem, and what should the athletic trainer recommend in terms of management?

Ulnar Collateral Ligament Injuries

Etiology The ulnar collateral ligament provides the primary resistance to valgus stresses that occur during the late cocking and early acceleration phases of throwing,[39] during a forehand stroke in tennis, or in the trailing arm during an improper golf swing. In athletes, the ulnar collateral ligament is most often injured as a result of a valgus force from repetitive trauma.[14] Stress of the medial complex can also result in ulnar nerve inflammation or impairment or wrist flexor tendinitis.[10] Stresses are applied to the medial elbow joint, frequently resulting in ligament failure, tendinitis, or osseous changes.[18] Injuries can vary in degree from an overuse flexor/pronator muscular strain to sprains of the ulnar collateral ligament. These injuries can result in elbow flexion contractures or can increase the instability of the elbow in adolescents.

Symptoms and signs On examination the athlete typically complains of pain along the medial aspect of the elbow. There is tenderness over the medial collateral ligament, usually at the distal insertion and occasionally in a more diffuse distribution. In some cases the athlete may describe associated paresthesias in the distribution of the ulnar nerve with a positive Tinel's sign.[16] When valgus stress is applied to the elbow at 20 to 30 degrees of flexion, local pain, tenderness, and endpoint laxity are assessed. On standard X-ray, hypertrophy of the humeral condyle and posteromedial aspect of the olecranon, marginal osteophytes of the ulnohumeral or radiocapitellar joints, calcification within the medial collateral ligament, and/or loose bodies in the posterior compartment may be present.

Management Conservative treatment of athletes with chronic ulnar collateral ligament injury should begin with rest and NSAID medication. With resolution of symptoms, rehabilitation should be instituted with an emphasis on strengthening. The athletic trainer along with the coach should analyze the athlete's throwing mechanics, which may include video assessment, to correct any existing faulty mechanics. If periods of rest and rehabilitation fail to resolve symptoms, surgical intervention may be necessary.

Operative management consists of repair or reconstruction, which is fairly common, particularly among higher-level baseball players.[19] In the case of an acute rupture, surgical repair can be considered; however, the indications are extremely limited.[4] In baseball players, surgical repair of the ulnar collateral ligament has been referred to as a "Tommy John" procedure. Generally the throwing athlete can return to competitive levels at about twenty-two to twenty-six weeks after surgery.[42]

23-4

Critical Thinking **Exercise**

A tennis player complains of an aching pain around the lateral epicondyle. She indicates that the pain seems to be worse when she tries to hit a backhand shot.

? What is likely the cause of her pain, and how should the athletic trainer choose to treat this problem?

Lateral Epicondylitis

Epicondylitis is a chronic condition that may affect athletes who execute repeated forearm flexion and extension movements such as are performed in tennis, pitching, golf, javelin throwing, and fencing. The elbow is particularly predisposed to mechanical trauma in the activities of throwing and striking.[38]

Etiology Lateral epicondylitis is one of the most common problems of the elbow occurring in sports. It is most often seen in tennis players and is also seen in baseball, swimming, gymnastics, fencing, golfing, and hammer throwing.[26] The cause of lateral epicondylitis is repetitive microtrauma with overuse of the extensor muscles. It usually involves the exterior carpi radialis brevis and extensor digitorum communis laterally and occasionally the pronator teres and flexor carpi radialis medially and the triceps posteriorly, and it can cause tendinopathy at the lateral epicondyle.[6] Microtrauma or overuse can be caused by an activity that involves repetitive wrist extension, supination, or repetitive heavy lifting. Whether there is inflammation is debatable. However it is likely that there is *tendinosis* in which there is a degeneration of the tendon without inflammation.[33] Tennis elbow is another name for lateral epicondylitis that stems from a backhand stroke involving wrist overextension.[38]

Lateral epicondylitis:
- Tennis elbow

Symptoms and signs The athlete complains of an aching pain in the region of the lateral epicondyle during and after activity. The pain gradually becomes worse, and weakness develops in the hand and wrist. Inspection reveals tenderness at the lateral epicondyle and pain on resisted dorsiflexion of the wrist and full extension of the elbow. The elbow has decreased range of motion.[36]

Management Treatment includes the immediate use of RICE, NSAIDs, and analgesics as needed. Rehabilitation includes ROM exercises, PRE, deep friction massage, hand grasping while in supination, and avoiding pronation movements.[43] Mobilization and stretching may be used within pain-free limits. The athlete may wear a counterforce or neoprene elbow sleeve for one to three months.[32] The athlete must be taught proper skill techniques and the proper use of equipment to avoid recurrence of the injury.[26]

23-5

Critical Thinking **Exercise**

A gymnast sustains a serious injury to his right elbow following a fall from the parallel bars.

? The athletic trainer, after ruling out fracture, should provide what immediate and follow-up care to this injury?

Medial Epicondylitis

Etiology Irritation and inflammation of the medial epicondyle may result from a number of different sport activities that require repeated forceful flexions of the wrist

Medial epicondylitis:
- Pitcher's elbow
- Racquetball elbow
- Golfer's elbow
- Javelin-thrower's elbow

Websites

World Ortho: http://www.worldortho.com

Wheeless' Textbook of Orthopaedics: http://www.wheelessonline.com

American Orthopaedic Society for Sports Medicine: http://www.sportsmed.org

MedFacts Sports Doc: http://www.medfacts.com

OrthoNet: http://www.orthonet.on.ca

Tennis Elbow Central: http://www.tennis-elbow.net/

The Physician and Sportsmedicine: Elbow Injuries: http://www.physsportsmed.com/issues/may_96/nirschl.htm

Braces and Supports for Tennis Elbow and Elbow Pain: http://orthobionics.com/elbow/index.htm

MEDLINEplus: Elbow Injuries and Disorders: http://medlineplus.nlm.nih.gov/medlineplus/elbowinjuriesanddisorders.html

Solutions to Critical Thinking EXERCISES

23-1 The athletic trainer should perform tests for ligamentous and capsular stability. Pulses should be taken at the wrist and antecubital fossa. Changes of skin sensation and the athlete's pain reaction to passive, active, and resistive exercise should be noted.

23-2 Swelling in the region of the olecranon process following irritation may indicate olecranon bursitis. This condition is best treated with a compression wrap and antiinflammatory medications.

23-3 It is most likely that this pitcher has a sprain of the ulnar collateral ligament due to valgus forces created during throwing. He should be referred to a physician for X rays and then treated conservatively with NSAIDs and activity modification. It is likely that he will ultimately require surgical reconstruction if he is to continue to perform at a high level.

23-4 It is likely that this tennis player has an inflammation of the lateral epicondyle, which is typically called tennis elbow. Tennis elbow occurs from repeated and forceful hyperextension of the wrist. It is best treated using rest, ice, compression, and antiinflammatory medications.

23-5 Immediate care consists of RICE and NSAIDs. More definitive management can include ROM exercises, PRE, friction massage, and hand grasping exercises while the elbow is in supination. Pronation movements should be avoided. Mobilization and stretching can also be employed within pain-free limits.

23-6 This injury is most likely an inflammation of the medial epicondyle that is caused by forceful hyperflexion of the wrist. Often called golfer's elbow, this condition almost always occurs in the trailing arm (for a right-handed golfer, the trailing arm would be the right arm). Rest, antiinflammatory medication, and ice should be used to treat this problem.

23-7 The young pitcher's condition indicates the possibility of an elbow osteochondritis dissecans, sometimes called Panner's disease.

23-8 This javelin thrower is showing signs of a cubital tunnel syndrome. Because of a pronounced elbow cubitus valgus, the ulnar recurrently subluxates. Because of ligamentous laxity, there is nerve impingement and compression.

23-9 Immediate treatment is critical for an elbow dislocation because of the tissues involved. Ice should be applied and the elbow should be immobilized until a physician is able to reduce the dislocation. If treatment is delayed, the soft tissue can be seriously damaged and the neurovascular supply can be compromised. Due to their close proximity to the joint, the brachial artery and the radial and median nerves are subject to injury. Fractures and ligamentous ruptures may also be present and need to be evaluated before and after reduction.

23-10 The athletic trainer should be concerned that this injury can cause a Volkmann's ischemic contracture. The brachial and radial pulses must be monitored for the possibility of a decrease in normal circulation.

23-11 This athlete must have regained full ROM in flexion, extension, pronation, and supination and must have regained full strength in these muscles.

23-12 This wrestler should do bicep curls to strengthen the biceps brachii, brachialis, and brachioradial muscles, all of which in some way act in flexion; tricep extensions to strengthen the triceps muscle; supination to strengthen the biceps brachii and supinator muscles; and pronation to strengthen the pronator teres and pronator quadratus.

REVIEW QUESTION AND SUGGESTED ACTIVITIES

1. Describe the procedures for assessing an elbow injury.
2. Describe the mechanism and management of elbow strains and sprains.
3. Describe how and why the elbow becomes chronically strained from throwing mechanisms.
4. Describe a dislocated elbow—its cause, appearance, and care.
5. How does the elbow sustain epicondylitis? Describe its appearance and management.
6. Compare elbow osteochondritis dissecans and knee osteochondritis dissecans. How does each occur?
7. What are the symptoms and signs of the elbow osteochondritis dissecans?
8. What causes a Volkmann's contracture? How may it be detected early?
9. Discuss the many aspects of elbow exercise rehabilitation.

REFERENCES

1. Allman FL, Carlson CA: Rehabilitation of elbow injuries. In Nicholas JA, Hershman EB, editors: *The upper extremity in sports medicine,* St Louis, 1995, Mosby.
2. Andrews JR, Whiteside JA: Common elbow problems in the athlete, *J Orthop Sports Phys Ther* 17(6):289, 1993.
3. Andrish JT: Osteochondritis dissecans in a young pitcher, *Physician Sportsmed* 25(3):85, 1997.
4. Azar FM, Andrews JR, Wilk KE: Operative treatment of ulnar collateral ligament injuries of the elbow in athletes, *Am J Sports Med* 28(1):16, 2000.
5. Barrett J: Reflex sympathetic dystrophy, *Physician Sportsmed* 23(4):51, 1995.
6. Benjamin SJ et al: Normalized forces and active range of motion in unilateral radial epicondylalgia (tennis elbow), *J Orthop Sports Phys Ther* 29(11):668, 1999.
7. Bennett JB: Acute injuries to the elbow. In Nicholas JA, Hershman EB, editors: *The upper extremity in sports medicine,* St Louis, 1995, Mosby.

8. Blackard D, Sampson J: Management of an uncomplicated posterior elbow dislocation, *J Ath Train* 32(1):63, 1997.
9. Boyd Jr DW: Osteochondritis dissecans of the elbow, *Sports Med Digest* 15(7):2, 1993.
10. Brown DE et al: *Orthopedic secrets*, Philadelphia, 1999, Hanley & Belfus.
11. Bruce SL, Wasielewski N, Hawke RL: Cubital tunnel syndrome in a collegiate wrestler: a case report, *J Ath Train* 32(2):151, 1997.
12. Brukner P: Elbow and forearm pain. In Brukner P, editor: *Clinical sports medicine*, ed 2, Sydney, 2002, McGraw-Hill.
13. Buettner C, Leaver-Dunn D: Prevention and treatment of elbow injuries in adolescent pitchers, *Athletic Therapy Today* 5(3):19, 2000.
14. Cain EL: Elbow injuries in throwing athletes: a current concept review, *Am J Sports Med* 31(4):621, 2003.
15. Cordasco F, Parkes J: Overuse injuries of the elbow. In Nicholas JA, Hershman EB, editors: *The upper extremity in sports medicine*, St Louis, 1995, Mosby.
16. David TS: Medial elbow pain in the throwing athlete. *Orthopedics* 26(1):94, 2003.
17. Ellenbecker T, Roetert P: Isokinetic profile of elbow flexion and extension strength in elite junior tennis players, *J Orthop Sports Phys Ther* 33(2), 2003.
18. Ellenbecker TS et al: Medial elbow joint laxity in professional baseball pitchers, *Am J Sports Med* 26(3):420, 1998.
19. Field L, Savoie F: Surgical treatment of ulnar collateral ligament injuries, *Athletic Therapy Today* 5(3):25, 2000.
20. Fincher AL, Trudeau RL: Managing epicondylitis in the golfer, *Athletic Therapy Today* 5(6):38, 2000.
21. Fleisig GS et al: Kinetics of baseball: pitching with implications about injury mechanisms, *Am J Sports Med* 23(2):233, 1995.
22. Fornalski S: Anatomy and biomechanics of the elbow joint. *Sports Med Arthroscopy Review* 11(1):1, 2003.
23. Frostick SP, Mohammad M, Ritchie DA: Sport injuries of the elbow, *British Journal of Sports Medicine* 33(5):301, 1999.
24. Grana W: Medial epicondylitis and cubital tunnel syndrome in the throwing athlete, *Clin Sports Med* 20(3):541, 2001.
25. Hall TL, Galea AM: Osteochondritis dissecans of the elbow: diagnosis, treatment, and prevention, *Physician Sportsmed* 27(2):75, 1999.
26. Halperin BC: Elbow and arm injuries. In Birrer RB, editor: *Sports medicine for the primary care physician*, ed 3, Boca Raton, Fla, 2004, CRC Press.
27. Hannafin JA: How I manage tennis and golfer's elbow, *Physician Sportsmed* 24(2):63, 1996.
28. Hocutt JE: General type injuries. In Birrer RB, editor: *Sports medicine for the primary care physician*, ed 3, Boca Raton, Fla, 2004, CRC Press.
29. Hoffman DF: Elbow dislocations, *Physician Sportsmed* 21(11):57, 1993.
30. Hughes PE: Little Leaguer's elbow, medial epicondyle injury, and osteochondritis dissecans. *Sports Med Arthroscopy Review* 11(1):30, 2003.
31. Kaminski T, Powers M, Buckley B: Differential assessment of elbow injuries, *Athletic Therapy Today* 5(3):6, 2000.
32. Knebel PT, Avery DW, Gebhardt TL: A. Effects of the forearm support band on wrist extensor muscle fatigue. *J Orthop Sports Phys Ther* 29(11):677, 1999.
33. Nirschl RP: Elbow tendinopathy: tennis elbow, *Clin Sports Med* 22(4): 813, 2003.
34. Nirschl RP, Kraushaar BS: Guidelines for elbow injuries, *Physician Sportsmed* 24(5):43, 1996.
35. Nuber GW, Bower MK: Olecranon stress fracture in throwing athletes. In Torg JS, Shephard RJ, editors: *Current therapy in sports medicine*, ed 3, St Louis, 1995, Mosby.
36. Peters T, Baker CL Jr., Lateral epicondylitis, *Clin Sports Med* 20(3): 549, 2001.
37. Prentice WE: Mobilization and traction techniques. In Prentice WE, editor: *Rehabilitation techniques in sports medicine and athletic training*, ed 4, St Louis, 2004, McGraw-Hill.
38. Regan WD: Lateral elbow pain in the athlete: a clinical review, *Clin Sports Med* 1(1):53, 1991.
39. Reinold M et al: Biomechanics and rehabilitation of elbow injuries during throwing, *Athletic Therapy Today* 5(3):12, 2000.
40. Rettig AC et al: Epidemiology of elbow, forearm, and wrist injuries in the athlete. In Plancher KD, editor: *The athletic elbow and wrist. Part I. Clinics in sports medicine*, vol 14, no 2, Philadelphia, 1995, Saunders.
41. Ross G: Acute elbow dislocation: on-site treatment, *Physician Sportsmed* 27(2):121, 1999.
42. Safran MR: Injury to the ulnar collateral ligament: diagnosis and treatment, *Sports Med Arthroscopy Review* 11(1):15, 2003.
43. Sevier TL, Wilson JK: Treating lateral epicondylitis, *Sports Med* 28(5):375, 1999.
44. Thompson KL: Rupture of the distal biceps tendon in a collegiate football player: a case report, *J Ath Train* 33(1):62, 1998.
45. Torg JS: Injuries to the upper extremity—Little League elbow. In Torg JS, Shephard RJ, editors: *Current therapy in sports medicine*, St Louis, 1995, Mosby.
46. Tracy J, Obuchi S, Johnson B: Kinematic and electromyographic analysis of elbow flexion during inertial exercise, *J Ath Train* 30(3): 254, 1995.
47. Uhl T: Uncomplicated elbow dislocation rehabilitation, *Athletic Therapy Today* 5(3):31, 2000.
48. Wells M, Bell G: Concerns on Little League elbow, *J Ath Train* 30(3): 249, 1995.
49. Werner SL: Biomechanics of the elbow during baseball pitching, *J Orthop Sports Phys Ther* 17(6):274, 1993.
50. Zulia P, Prentice W: Rehabilitation of elbow injuries. In Prentice W: *Rehabilitation techniques in sports medicine and athletic training*, ed 4, St Louis, 2004, McGraw-Hill.

ANNOTATED BIBLIOGRAPHY

Altchek D, Andrews J: *The Athlete's Elbow*, Baltimore, 2001, Lippincott, Williams & Wilkins.

This text is based on the work of leading authorities on elbow injuries in athletes and provides information on the biomechanics and anatomy of the elbow, as well as guidelines for the evaluation and treatment of injury to the joint.

Ellenbecker T, Mattalino A: *The elbow in sports*, Champaign, Ill, 1997, Human Kinetics.

Intended for physical therapist, athletic trainers, and sports medicine specialists, this comprehensive guide covers the anatomy, biomechanics, musculoskeletal evaluation, and surgical techniques involved in sport-related elbow injuries.

Morrey B: *The elbow and its disorders*, Philadelphia, 2000, WB Saunders.

This text is primarily for orthopedic surgeons and residents and includes evaluation, diagnosis, children's conditions, adult trauma, sports and overuse injuries, reconstruction, septic and nontraumatic conditions.

Plancher KD, editor: *The athletic elbow and wrist.* Part I. Clinics in sports medicine, vol 14, no 2, Philadelphia, 1995, Saunders.

This in-depth monograph covers the diagnosis and conservative treatment of athletic elbow and wrist injuries.

Plancher KD, editor: *The athletic elbow and wrist.* Part II. Clinics in sports medicine, vol 15, no 2, Philadelphia, 1996, Saunders.

This monograph offers detailed discussions of the most common injuries and of overuse injuries to the elbow and wrist that occur in sports.

Sports medicine and arthroscopy review 11(1), 2003.

This entire journal is dedicated to a discussion of the elbow.

Winkle D et al: *Diagnosis and treatment of the upper extremity*, Amsterdam, 1997, Aspen.

This text is a detailed discussion of the orthopedic examination and treatment based on the Cyriax model.

Chapter 24

The Forearm, Wrist, Hand, and Fingers

When you finish this chapter you should be able to

- Review the structural and functional anatomy of the forearm, wrist, hand, and fingers.
- Outline the process of assessment for injuries to the forearm, wrist, hand, and fingers.
- Incorporate management techniques for dealing with injuries to the forearm, wrist, hand, and fingers.
- Implement the appropriate rehabilitation techniques for dealing with injuries to the forearm, wrist, hand, and fingers.

ANATOMY OF THE FOREARM

Bones

The bones of the forearm are the ulna and the radius (Figure 24-1). The ulna, which may be thought of as a direct extension of the humerus, is long, straight, and larger proximally than distally. The radius, considered an extension of the hand, is thicker distally than proximally.

Articulations

The forearm has three articulations: the superior, middle, and distal radioulnar joints. The superior radioulnar articulation is a pivot joint that moves in a ring formed by the ulna and the annular ligament.

The middle radioulnar joint, which is the junction between the shafts of the ulna and the radius, is held together by an oblique ligamentous cord and the interosseous membrane. The oblique cord is a small band of ligamentous fibers that are attached to the lateral side of the ulna and pass downward and laterally to the radius. The interosseous membrane is a thin sheet of fibrous tissue that runs downward between the radius and the ulna and transmits forces directly through the hand from the radius to the ulna. The middle radioulnar joint provides a surface for muscle attachments, and there are openings for blood vessels at the upper and lower ends.

The distal radioulnar joint is a pivot joint formed by the articulation of the head of the ulna with a small notch on the radius. It is held securely by the anterior and posterior radioulnar ligaments. The inferior ends of the radius and ulna are bound by an articular, triangular disk that allows radial movement of 180 degrees into supination and pronation.

Forearm Musculature

The forearm muscles consist of flexors and pronators that are positioned anteriorly and extensors and supinators that lie posteriorly. The flexors of the wrist and fingers are separated into superficial muscles and deep muscles (Figure 24-2). The deep flexors arise from the ulna, the radius, and the interosseous tissue anteriorly, and the superficial flexors come from the internal humeral condyle. The extensors of the wrist

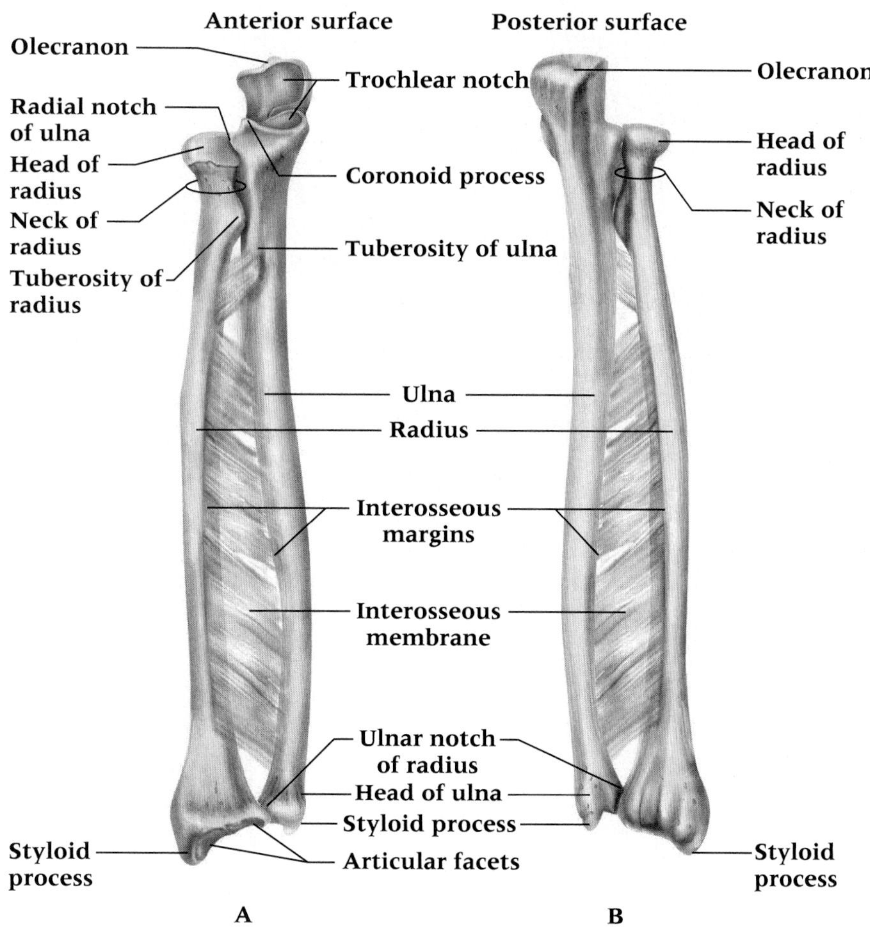

Figure 24-1

Bony anatomy of the forearm. **A,** Anterior view. **B,** Posterior view.

and fingers originate on the posterior aspect and the external condyle of the humerus (Table 24-1).

Nerve and Blood Supply

Except for the flexor carpi ulnaris and half of the flexor digitorum profundus, most of the flexor muscles of the forearm are supplied by the median nerve. The majority of the extensor muscles are controlled by the radial nerve. The major blood supply stems from the brachial artery, which divides into the radial and ulnar arteries in the forearm.

ASSESSMENT OF THE FOREARM

History

The following questions should be asked to determine forearm injuries:

- What caused the injury (e.g., blunt trauma, throwing, or chronic overuse)?
- What were the symptoms at the time of injury? Did symptoms occur later?
- Were symptoms localized or diffused?
- Was there swelling or discoloration?
- Was there immediate loss of function?
- What treatment was given?
- How does the forearm feel now?

Observation

The entire forearm, including the wrist and elbow, is first visually inspected for obvious deformities, swelling, and skin defects. If a deformity is not present, the athlete then is observed pronating and supinating the forearm.

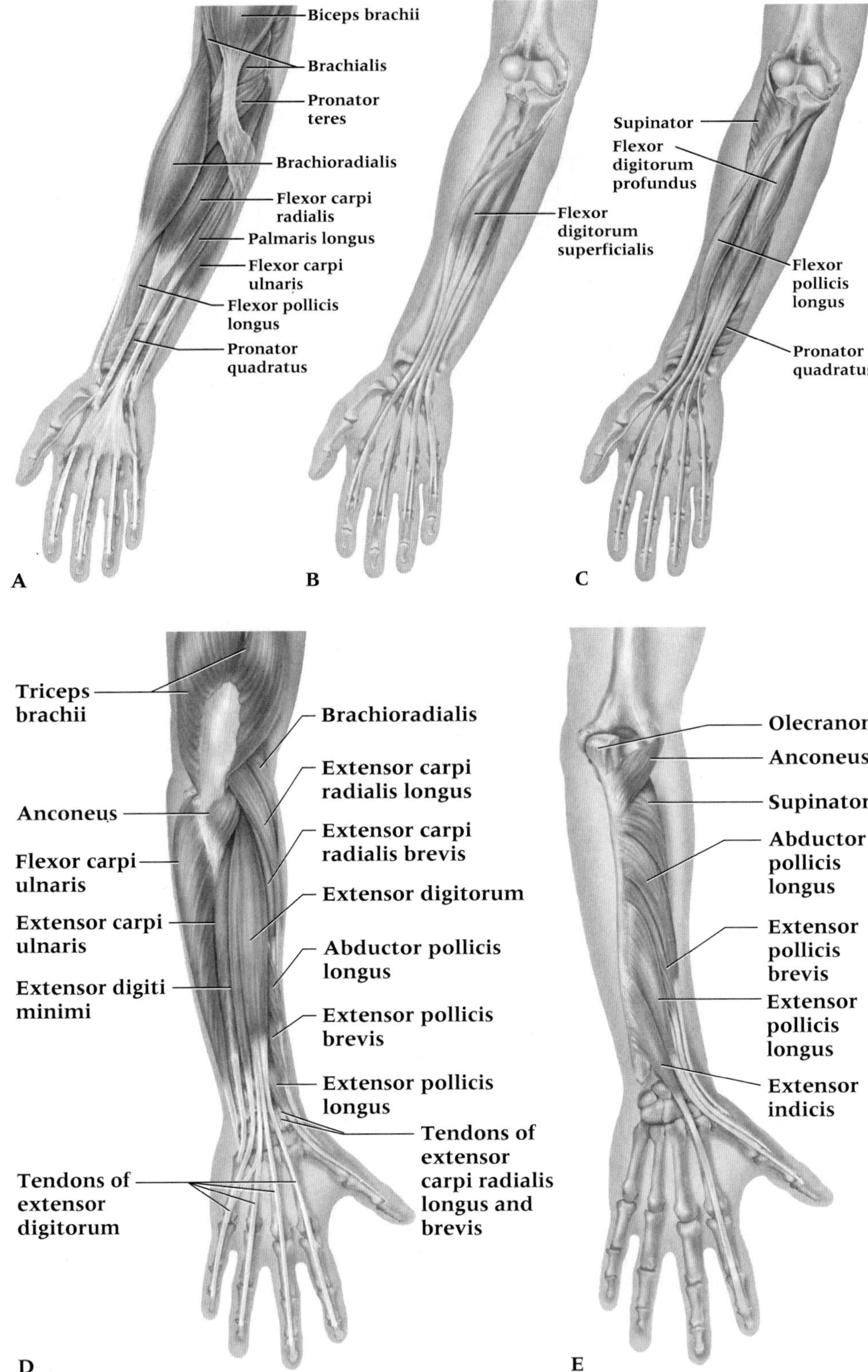

Figure 24-2

Muscles of the forearm. **A,** Superficial flexors. **B,** The flexor digitorum superficialis, deep to the muscles in A but also classified as a superficial flexor. **C,** Deep flexors. **D,** Superficial extensors. **E,** Deep extensors.

TABLE 24-1 Muscles of the Forearm Acting on the Wrist, Hand, and Fingers

Muscle	Origin	Insertion	Action	Innervation
Flexor carpi radialis	Medial epicondyle of the humerus	Ventral surface of the second and third metacarpals	Flexes the wrist and abducts the hand; aids in flexion of the elbow and pronation	Median
Palmaris longus	Medial epicondyle of the humerus	Palmar aponeurosis	Flexes the wrist	Median
Flexor carpi ulnaris	Medial epicondyle of the humerus, olecranon process, and the proximal two-thirds of the posterior surface of the ulna	Pisiform, hamate, and fifth metacarpal	Flexes the wrist and adducts the hand	Ulnar
Flexor digitorum superficialis	Medial epicondyle of the humerus, coronoid process of the ulna, and the anterior of the radius	Ventral surface of the middle phalanges of the second through the fifth fingers	Flexes the wrist and the phalanges	Median
Flexor digitorum profundus	Medial epicondyle and the coronoid process of the humerus, the interosseus membrane, and the ventral surface of the ulna	Ventral surface of the base of the distal phalanges of the second through the fifth fingers	Flexes the wrist and the phalanges	Median and ulnar
Flexor pollicis longus	Ventral surface of the radius and the interosseus membrane	Ventral surface of the base of the distal phalanx of the thumb	Flexes the thumb and aids in flexing the wrist	Median
Pronator quadratus	Distal ventral surface of the ulna	Distal ventral surface of the radius	Pronates the hand	Median
Extensor carpi radialis longus	Lateral supracondylar ridge of the humerus	Dorsal surface of the base of the second metacarpal	Extends the wrist and abducts the hand	Radial
Extensor carpi radialis brevis	Lateral epicondyle of the humerus	Dorsal surface of the base of the third metacarpal	Extends the wrist and abducts the hand	Radial
Extensor digitorum communis	Lateral epicondyle of the humerus	Dorsal surface of the phalanges of the second through the fifth fingers	Extends the fingers and the wrist	Radial
Extensor digiti minimi	Tendon of the extensor digitorum communis	Tendon of the extensor digitorum communis on the dorsum of the little finger	Extends the little finger	Radial
Extensor carpi ulnaris	Lateral epicondyle of the humerus	Base of the fifth metacarpal	Extends the wrist and adducts the hand	Radial
Abductor pollicis longus	Posterior surface of the middle of the radius and ulna and the interosseus membrane	Base of the first metacarpal	Abducts the thumb and the hand	Radial
Extensor pollicis brevis	Posterior surface of the middle of the radius and the interosseus membrane	Base of the first phalanx of the thumb	Extends the wrist and adducts the hand	Radial
Extensor pollicis longus	Posterior surface of the middle of the ulna and the interosseus membrane	Base of the last phalanx of the thumb	Extends the thumb and abducts the hand	Radial
Extensor indicis	Posterior surface of the distal end of the ulna and the interosseus membrane	Tendon of the extensor digitorum communis to the index finger	Extends the index finger	Radial

Palpation

The injured forearm is palpated at distant sites as well as at the point of injury. Palpation can reveal tenderness, edema, fracture deformity, change in skin temperature, a false joint, bone fragments, or a lack of continuity between bones.

Bony Palpation

The following bony landmarks should be palpated:

- Proximal radial head
- Olecranon process
- Radial shaft
- Ulnar shaft
- Distal radius
- Radial styloid process
- Ulnar head
- Ulnar styloid

Soft-Tissue Palpation

The following soft tissue structures should be palpated:

Articulations

- Distal radioulnar joint
- Radiocarpal joint
- Extensor retinaculum (posterior wrist)
- Flexor retinaculum (anterior wrist)

Extensor muscles (posterolateral)

- Extensor carpi radialis longus
- Extensor carpi radialis brevis
- Extensor carpi ulnaris
- Brachioradialis
- Extensor pollicis longus
- Extensor pollicis brevis
- Abductor pollicis longus
- Extensor indicus supinator

Flexor muscles (anteromedial)

- Flexor carpi radialis
- Flexor carpi ulnaris
- Palmaris longus
- Flexor digitorum superficialis
- Flexor digitorum profundus
- Flexor pollicis longus
- Pronator quadratus
- Pronator teres

RECOGNITION AND MANAGEMENT OF INJURIES TO THE FOREARM

The forearm, lying between the elbow joint and the wrist, is indirectly influenced by injuries to these areas; however, direct injuries can also occur.

Contusions

Etiology The forearm is constantly exposed to bruising in contact sports such as football. The ulnar side receives the majority of blows in arm blocks and, consequently, a greater amount of bruising. Bruises to this area may be classified as acute or chronic. The acute contusion can result in a fracture, but this happens only rarely.

Symptoms and signs Most often a muscle or bone develops varying degrees of pain, swelling, and hematoma. The chronic contusion develops from repeated blows to the forearm with attendant multiple irritations. Heavy fibrosis may take the place of the hematoma, and a bony callus has been known to arise out of this condition.

Management Care of the contused forearm requires proper attention in the acute stages through the application of RICE for at least one hour, followed the next day by cryotherapy. Protection of the forearm is important for athletes who are prone to this condition. The best protection consists of a full-length sponge rubber pad for the forearm early in the season.

Forearm Splints

Etiology Forearm strain can occur in a variety of sports; most such injuries come from a severe static contraction. Repeated static contraction can lead to forearm splints. Forearm splints, like the medial tibial stress syndrome (shinsplints), are difficult to manage. They occur most often in gymnasts, particularly those who perform on the side horse, and in wrestlers.[5]

Forearm splints, like shinsplints, commonly occur either early or late in the sports season.

Symptoms and signs The main symptom is a dull ache between the extensor muscles, which cross the back of the forearm. There also may be weakness and extreme pain during muscle contraction. Palpation reveals an irritation of the interosseous membrane and surrounding tissue. The cause of this condition is uncertain; like shinsplints, forearm splints usually appear either early or late in the season, which indicates poor conditioning or fatigue, respectively. The pathological process is believed to result from the constant static muscle contractions of the forearm (e.g., those contractions required to stabilize the side horse participant).[30] Continued isometric contraction causes minute tears in the area of the interosseous membrane.

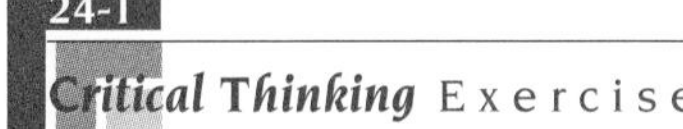
24-1 Critical Thinking Exercise

A rower sustains an overuse injury to the posterior aspect of the right wrist, resulting in pain, swelling, and crepitation.

? What common athletic injury results from repetitive use of the wrist in rowers?

Management Care of forearm splints is symptomatic. If the problem occurs early in the season, the athlete should concentrate on increasing the strength of the forearm through resistance exercises, but if it arises late in the season, emphasis should be on rest and cryotherapy or heat and use of a supportive wrap during activity.

The forearm can also sustain an acute or chronic exertional compartment syndrome, although this condition is much less common than in the lower leg. It can occur in sports such as gymnastics and weight lifting and can result from direct injuries such as muscle avulsion, distal radius fracture, or a crushing injury. The deep forearm compartment containing the flexor digitorum profundus, flexor pollicus longus, and pronator quadratus is most susceptible to changes of muscle and nerve ischemia. Detection and management of this condition are the same as for the lower leg condition.

Forearm Fractures

Etiology Fractures of the forearm (Figure 24-3) are particularly common among active children and youths and occur as the result of a blow or a fall on the outstretched hand.[22] Fractures to the ulna or the radius alone are much rarer than simultaneous fractures to both. A direct blow to the forearm usually results in a fracture to the ulna. The forearm break usually presents all the features of a long-bone fracture: pain,

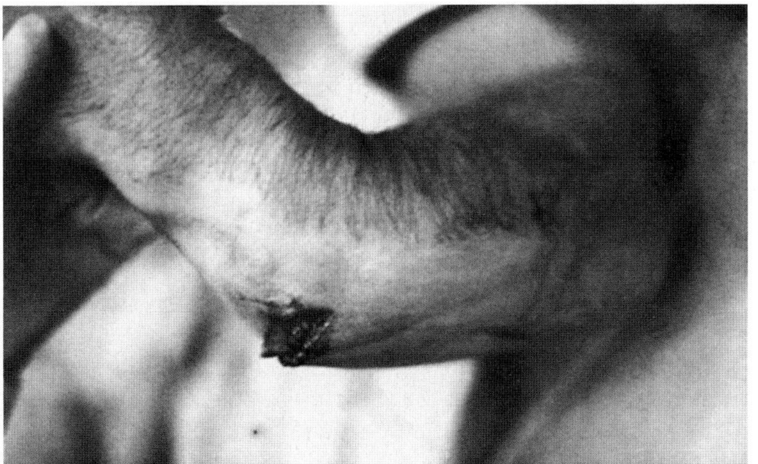

Figure 24-3

An open fracture of the ulna.

swelling, deformity, and a false joint. If the break is in the upper third, the pronator teres muscle has a tendency to pull the forearm into an abduction deformity, whereas fractures of the lower portion of the arm are often in a neutral position. The older the athlete, the greater the danger of extensive damage to soft tissue and the greater the possibility of paralysis from Volkmann's contractures.

Symptoms and signs The athlete experiences an audible pop or crack followed by moderate to severe pain, swelling, and disability. There is localized tenderness, edema, and ecchymosis with possible crepitus.[22]

Management Initially, RICE is applied, followed by splinting until definitive care is available. Definitive care consists of a long-arm plaster or fiberglass cast followed by a program of rehabilitation.

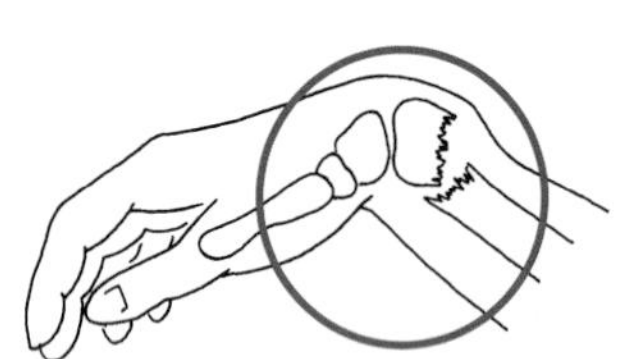

Figure 24-4

Common appearance of the forearm in Colles' fracture.

Colles' Fracture

Etiology Colles' fractures are among the most common types of forearm fractures and involve the lower end of the radius or ulna (Figure 24-4).[14] The mechanism of injury is usually a fall on the outstretched hand, forcing the radius and ulna backward and upward (hyperextension). Much less common is the reverse of Colles' fracture. The mechanism of this fracture is the result of a fall on the back of the hand.[38]

Symptoms and signs In most cases, there is forward displacement of the radius that causes a visible deformity to the wrist, which is commonly called a *silver fork* deformity. Sometimes no deformity is present, and the injury may be passed off as a bad sprain—to the detriment of the athlete. Bleeding is profuse in this area, and the extravasated fluids can cause extensive swelling in the wrist and, if unchecked, in the fingers and forearm. Ligamentous tissue is usually unharmed, but tendons may be torn and avulsed, and there may be median nerve damage.[38]

Management The main responsibility is to apply a cold compress, splint the wrist, put the limb in a sling, and then refer the athlete to a physician for X-ray examination and immobilization. Severe sprains should always be treated as possible fractures. Lacking complications, the Colles' fracture will keep an athlete out of sports for one to two months. What appears to be a Colles' fracture in children and youths is often a lower epiphyseal separation.[44]

24-2

Critical Thinking **Exercise**

A young athlete falls off the parallel bars onto his outstretched left hand, forcing the wrist into hyperextension. There is a visible deformity to the wrist.

? Describe the deformity presented and the actions that the athletic trainer should take.

Madelung Deformity

Etiology Madelung deformity is a developmental abnormality of the wrist. It is characterized by anatomic changes in the radius, ulna, and carpal bones, leading to palmar and ulnar wrist subluxation. It is more common in female athletes, particularly gymnasts, and is usually present bilaterally. The deformity usually becomes evident clinically between the ages of 6 and 13. Epiphyseal plate changes is the distal radius and closure of the plate as of result of loading the wrist and forearm in gymnastics produces a skeletal deformity in which the carpus is wedged between the radius and ulna. There is a concomitant bowing to the radius that is evident on radiograph.[6]

Symptoms and Signs Madelung deformity can result in wrist pain and loss of forearm rotation, leading to decreased function of the wrist and hand. There may be palmar subluxation with prominence of the radial and ulnar styloid processes.

Management The deformity is treated with therapeutic modalities and nonsteroidal anti-inflammatory medication for pain. The wrist should be taped or the athlete should wear a commercially available wrist brace to prevent end-range wrist extension. Although rare, Madelung deformity is typically corrected surgically in athletes with chronic pain and disability.[6]

ANATOMY OF THE WRIST, HAND, AND FINGERS

Bones

The wrist, or carpus, is the region that connects the distal forearm to the hand. It is formed by the distal aspect of the radius and the ulna with a proximal row of four and a distal row of four carpal bones that articulate with five metacarpals. Appearing in order from the radial to the ulnar side in the first, or proximal, row of carpal bones are the scaphoid (navicular), lunate, triquetral, and pisiform bones; the distal row consists

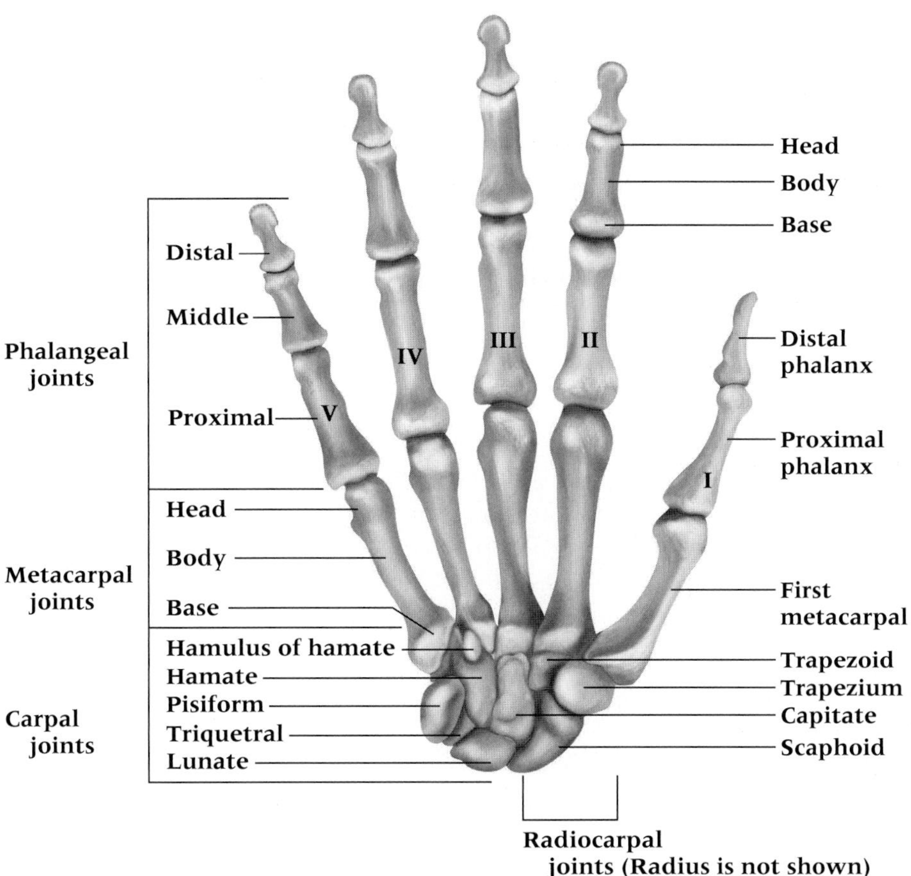

Figure 24-5

Bones of the wrist, hand, and fingers.

of the greater multangular (trapezium), lesser multangular (trapezoid), capitate, and hamate bones (Figure 24-5).

The concave surfaces of the lower ends of the radius and ulna articulate with the convex surfaces of the first row of carpal bones, with the exception of the pisiform, which articulates with the triangular fibrocartilage complex (TFCC) interposed between the head of the ulna and the triquetral bone.

Articulations

Radiocarpal Joints

The radiocarpal joint is a condyloid joint and permits flexion, extension, abduction, and circumduction. Its major strength is drawn from the great number of tendons that cross it rather than from its bone structure or ligamentous arrangement. The articular capsule is a continuous cover formed by the merging of the radial and the ulnar collateral, volar radiocarpal, and dorsal radiocarpal ligaments.

Carpal Joints

The carpal bones articulate with one another in arthrodial, or gliding, joints and combine their movements with those of the radiocarpal joint and the carpometacarpal articulations. They are stabilized by anterior, posterior, and connecting interosseous ligaments.

Metacarpal Joints

The metacarpal bones are five bones that join the carpal bones above and the phalanges below, forming metacarpophalangeal (MCP) articulations of a condyloid type and permitting flexion, extension, abduction, adduction, and circumduction. The thumb varies slightly at its carpometacarpal joint and is classified as a saddle joint that allows rotation on its long axis in addition to the other metacarpophalangeal movements.

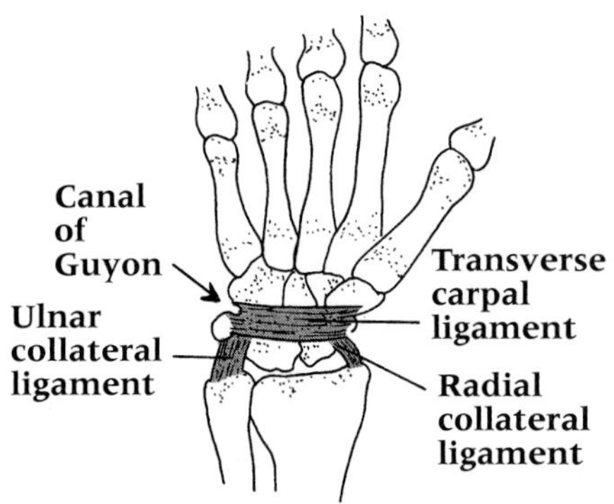

Figure 24-6

Ligaments of the wrist.

Phalangeal Joints

Each phalangeal joint, like the carpal joints, has an articular capsule that is reinforced by collateral and accessory volar ligaments. The interphalangeal articulations are of the hinge type, permitting only flexion and extension. Their ligamentous and capsular support is basically the same as that of the MCP joints.

Ligaments

There are many wrist, hand, and finger ligaments; however, only those most likely to be injured in sports are discussed here.

Ligaments of the Wrist

The wrist is composed of many ligaments that bind the carpal bones to one another, to the ulna and radius, and to the proximal metacarpal bones. Of major interest in wrist injuries are the ulnar collateral ligament, which extends from the tip of the styloid process of the ulna to the pisiform bone, and the triquetral bone and radial collateral ligament that extends from the styloid process to the radius to the navicular bone (scaphoid). Crossing the volar aspect of the carpal bones is the transverse carpal ligament. This ligament serves as the roof of the carpal tunnel, in which the median nerve is often compressed (Figure 24-6).

Ligaments of the Phalanges

The proximal interphalangeal (PIP) joints have the same design as the distal interphalangeal (DIP) joints. They comprise the collateral ligaments, palmar fibrocartilages, and a loose posterior capsule or synovial membrane protected by an extensor expansion (Figure 24-7).

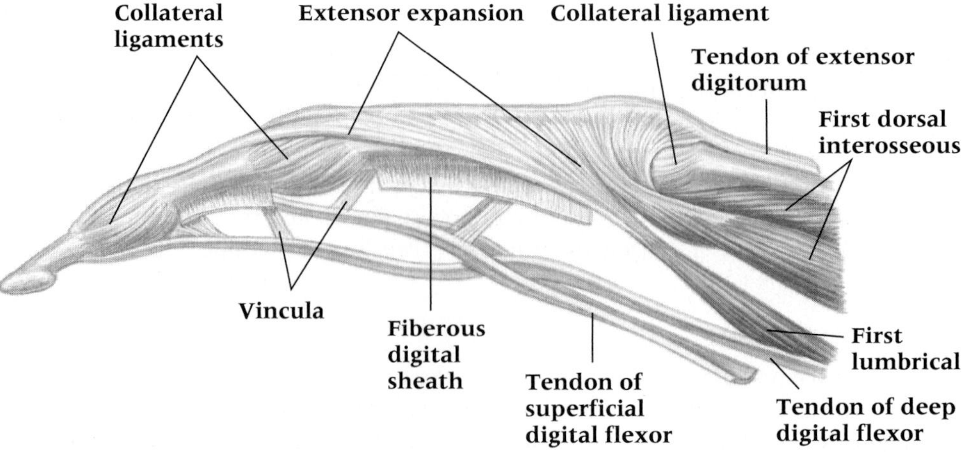

Figure 24-7

Ligamentous and muscular anatomy of the fingers.

TABLE 24-2 Intrinsic Muscles of the Hand

Muscle	Origin	Insertion	Action	Innervation
Palmar Muscles				
Lumbricales	Tendons of the flexor digitorum profundus	Tendons of the extensor digitorum communis	Flexes the metacarpophalangeal joints and extends the interphalangeal joints	Median and ulnar
Dorsal interossei (4)	Adjacent sides of all of the metacarpals	Proximal phalanx of second, third, and fourth fingers	Abducts the fingers from the middle finger	Ulnar
Palmar interossei (3)	Medial side of the second metacarpal and lateral side of the fourth and fifth metacarpals	Proximal phalanx of the same finger	Adducts the fingers toward the middle finger	Ulnar
Thenar Muscles				
Abductor pollicis brevis	Flexor retinaculum, scaphoid, and trapezium	Proximal phalanx of the thumb	Abducts the thumb	Median
Opponens pollicis	Flexor retinaculum and trapezium	Lateral border of the metacarpal of the thumb	Pulls the thumb in front of the palm to meet the little finger	Median
Flexor pollicis brevis	Flexor retinaculum, trapezium, and first metacarpal	Base of the proximal phalanx of the thumb	Flexes and adducts the thumb	Median
Adductor pollicis	Capitate and second and third metacarpals	Proximal phalanx of the thumb	Adducts the thumb	Ulnar
Hypothenar Muscles				
Palmaris brevis	Flexor retinaculum	Skin on the ulnar border of the hand	Pulls the skin toward the middle of the palm	Ulnar
Abductor digiti minimi	Pisiform, and the tendon of the flexor carpi ulnaris	Base of the proximal phalanx of the little finger	Abducts the little finger	Ulnar
Flexor digiti minimi brevis	Flexor retinaculum and hamate	Base of the proximal phalanx of the little finger	Flexes the little finger	Ulnar
Opponens digiti minimi	Flexor retinaculum and hamate	Metacarpal of the little finger	Brings the little finger out to meet the thumb	Ulnar

Musculature

Several muscles of the forearm have long tendons that cross the metacarpophalangeal (MCP) joints and move the fingers. On the flexor surface the flexor digitorum superficialis flexes the proximal interphalangeal (PIP) joint, and the flexor digitorum profundus flexes the distal interphalangeal (DIP) joint. Dorsally as the extensor digitorum longus tendons cross the MCP joints they expand into a tendinous aponeurosis called the extensor expansion that extends the PIP and DIP joints of the fingers (Figure 24-7).

There are a number of muscles that are intrinsic to the hand (Table 24-2). The dorsal and palmar interossei muscles are lateral to the MCP joints and are responsible for abduction and adduction of the MCP joints. The lumbrical muscles are volar to the axis of rotation of the MCP joint, but then they insert into the lateral bands and are dorsal to the PIP and DIP joints. Their function is MCP joint flexion and IP joint extension. The three thenar muscles act on the thumb, and the three hypothenar muscles act on the little finger (Figure 24-8).

Blood and Nerve Supply

Circulation impairment must be noted as soon as possible in any wrist or hand injury.

The three major nerves of the hand are the ulnar, radial, and median nerves. The ulnar nerve comes to the hand by passing between the pisiform bone and the hook of

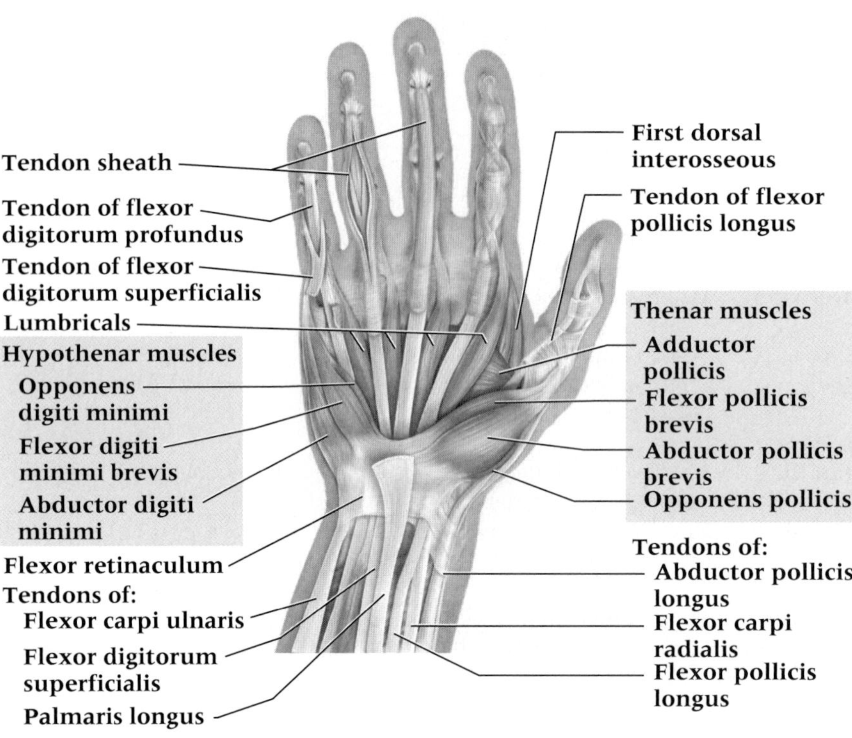

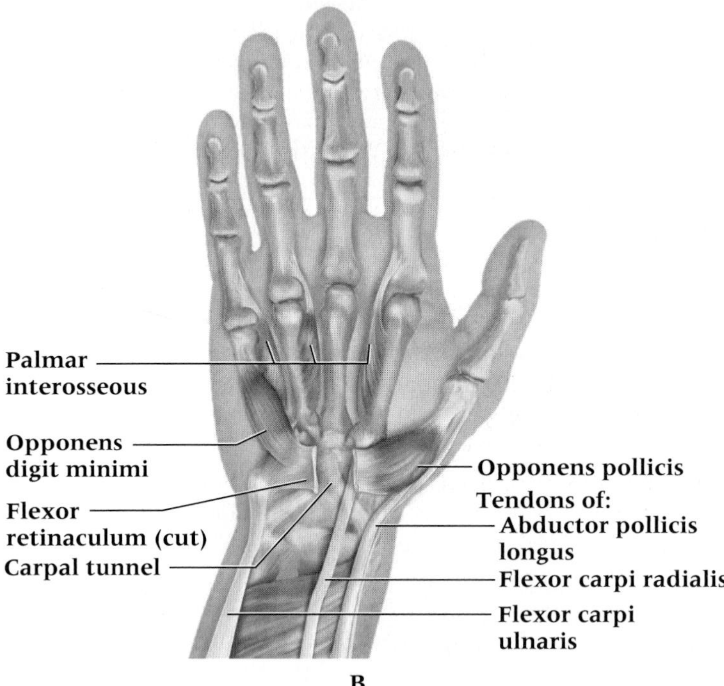

Figure 24-8

Intrinsic muscles of the hand. **A,** Superficial muscles, anterior (palmar) view. **B,** Deep muscles, anterior view.

Continued

the hamate bone. The radial nerve enters the wrist from the back of the forearm between the superficial and deep extensor muscles, where it terminates in the back of the carpus. The median nerve enters the palm of the hand through the carpal tunnel (see Figure 24-9). The sensory pattern of peripheral nerves can be seen in Figure 24-10. The radial nerve may or may not follow this pattern.

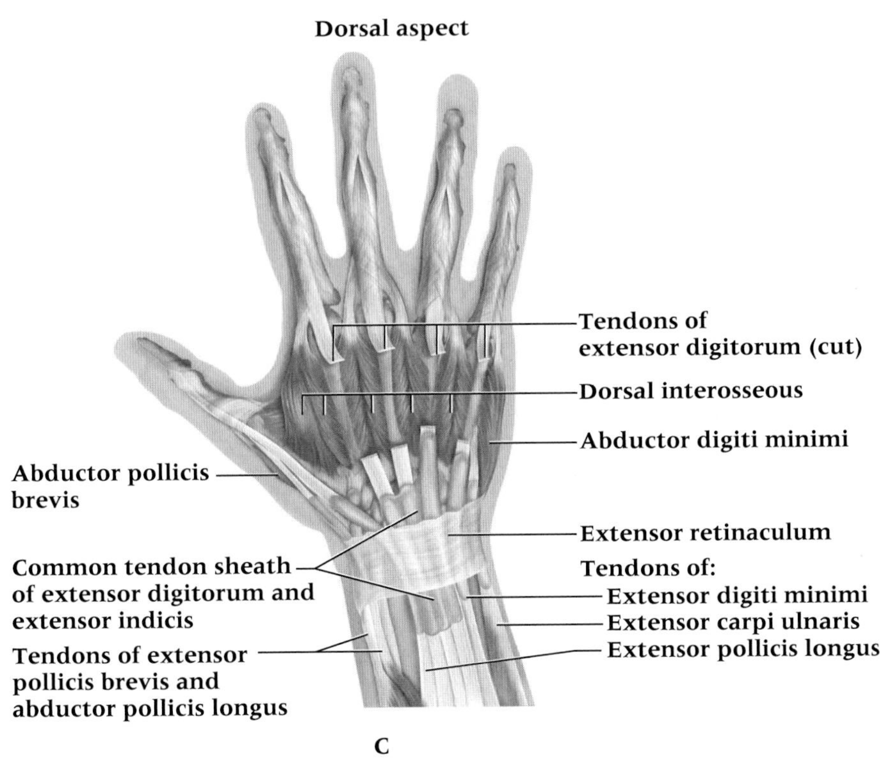

Figure 24-8—continued

C, Superficial muscles, posterior (dorsal) view.

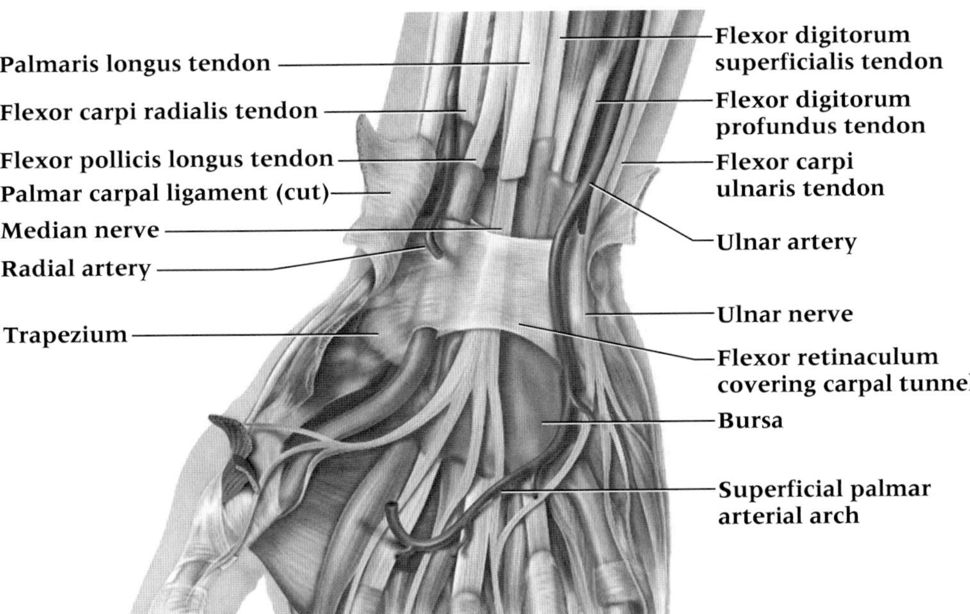

Figure 24-9

Anatomy of the anterior aspect of the wrist and hand.

The arteries that supply the wrist and the hand are the radial and ulnar arteries. They create two arterial arches: the superficial palmar arch, which is the largest and most distal to the hand, and the deep palmar arch.

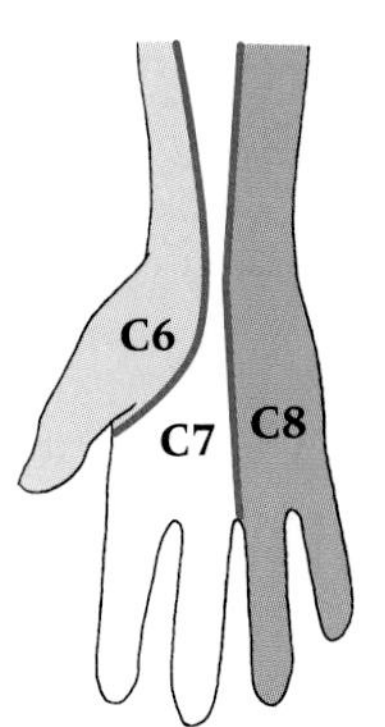

Figure 24-10

Sensory patterns of peripheral nerves in the hand.

ASSESSMENT OF THE WRIST, HAND, AND FINGERS

History

The athletic trainer should ask these questions about the location and type of pain:

- What was the mechanism of injury?
- What increases or decreases the pain?
- Has there been a history of trauma or overuse?
- What therapy if any, has been given in the past?

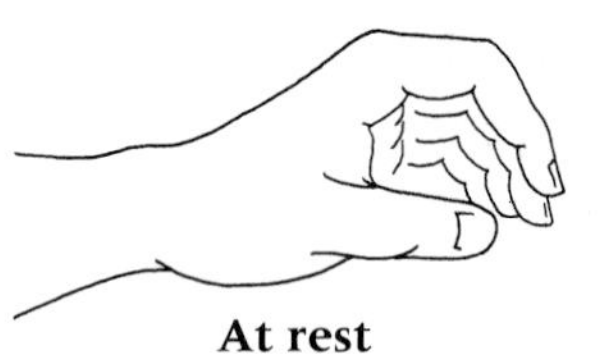

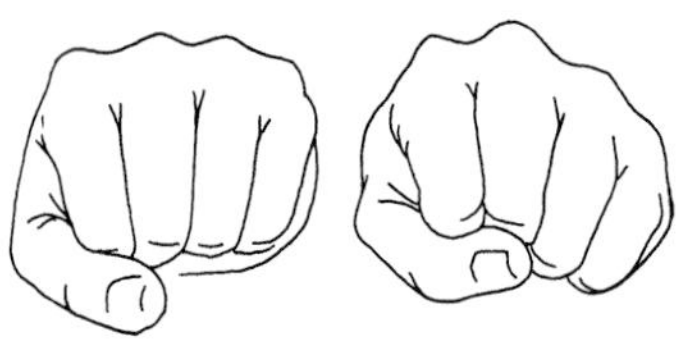

Figure 24-11

General normal attitudes of the hand.

Observation

As the athletic trainer observes athlete, he or she should note arm and hand asymmetries.

- Are there any postural deviations?
- Does the athlete hold the part in a stiff or protected manner?
- Is the wrist or hand swollen?

Hand usage such as writing or unbuttoning a shirt should be noted. The general attitude of the hand should be observed (Figure 24-11). When the athlete is asked to open and close the hand, the athletic trainer should note whether this movement can be performed fully and rhythmically. Another general functional activity is to have the athlete touch the tip of the thumb to each fingertip several times. The last factor to be observed is the color of the fingernails. Nails that are very pale instead of pink may indicate a problem with blood circulation.[22]

Palpation

Bony palpation

The following bony landmarks should be palpated:

- Scaphoid
- Trapezoid
- Trapezium
- Lunate
- Capitate
- Triquetral
- Pisiform
- Hamate (hook of the hamate)
- Metacarpals 1–5
- Proximal, middle, and distal phalanges of the fingers
- Proximal and distal phalanges of the thumb

Soft Tissue Palpation

The following soft tissue structures should be palpated:

General

- Triangular fibrocartilage
- Ligaments of the carpal bones
- Carpometacarpal joints and ligaments
- Metacarpophalangeal joints and collateral ligaments
- Proximal interphalangeal joints and collateral ligaments
- Distal interphalangeal joints and collateral ligaments

Anterior

- Flexor carpi radialis tendon
- Flexor carpi ulnaris tendon
- Lumbricale muscles
- Flexor digitorum superficialis tendons
- Flexor digitorum profundus tendons
- Palmar interossei muscles
- Flexor pollicis brevis
- Flexor pollicis longus tendon
- Abductor pollicis brevis
- Opponens pollicis muscle
- Opponens digiti minimi muscle

Posterior

- Extensor carpi radialis longus tendon
- Extensor carpi radialis brevis tendon
- Extensor carpi ulnaris tendon
- Extensor digitorum tendons
- Extensor indicis tendon

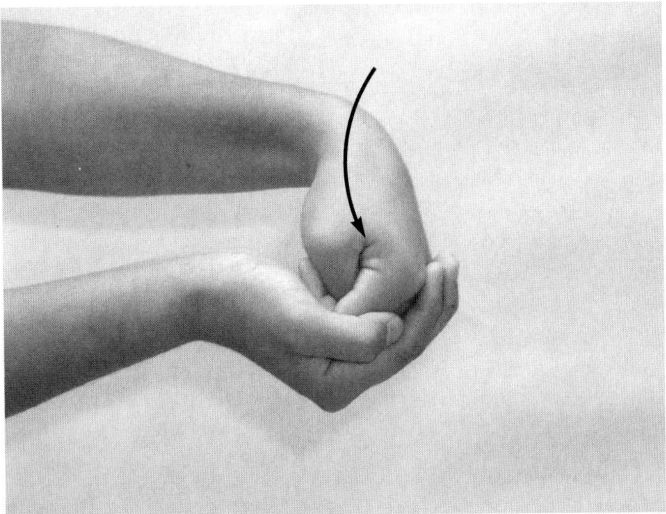

Figure 24-12

Finkelstein's test for deQuervain's syndrome.

- Extensor digiti minimi tendon
- Dorsal interossei muscles
- Extensor pollicis brevis tendon
- Extensor pollicis longus tendon
- Abductor pollicis longus tendon

Special Tests

Finklestein's Test

Finklestein's test is a test for de Quervain's syndrome (Figure 24-12). The athlete makes a fist with the thumb tucked inside. The wrist is then deviated into ulnar flexion. Sharp pain is evidence of stenosing tenosynovitis. Pain over the carpal tunnel could mean a carpal tunnel syndrome affecting the median nerve. On occasion, the flexor tendons also become trapped, making finger flexion difficult. Any symptoms of carpal tunnel syndrome are an indication for testing, using Tinel's sign and Phalen's test.[28]

Tinel's Sign

Tinel's sign is produced by tapping over the transverse carpal ligament of the carpal tunnel, which causes tingling and parasthesia over the thumb, index finger, middle finger, and the lateral half of the ring finger. This sensory distribution of the median nerve indicates the presence of carpal tunnel syndrome (Figure 24-13).

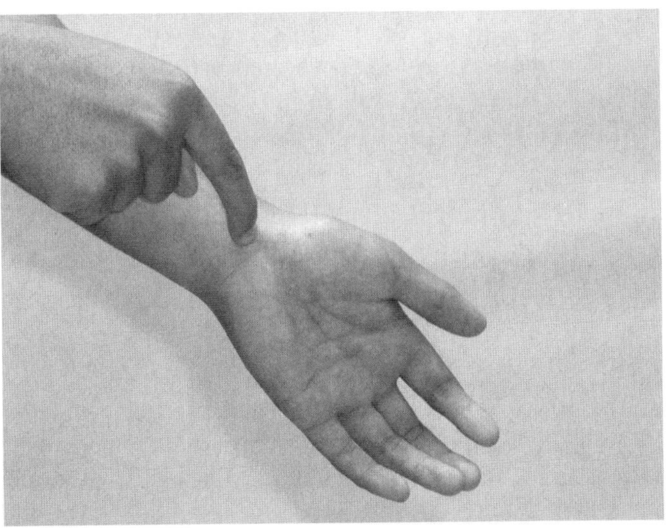

Figure 24-13

Tapping over the transverse carpal ligament to test for carpal tunnel syndrome (Tinel's sign).

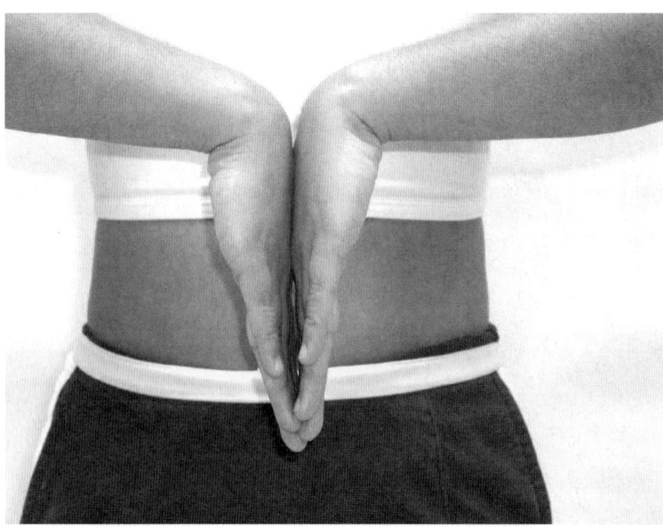

Figure 24-14

Wrist press for carpal tunnel syndrome (Phalen's test).

Phalen's Test

Another common test for carpal tunnel syndrome is Phalen's test. The athlete is instructed to flex both wrists as far as possible and press them together. This position is held for approximately one minute. If this test is positive, pain will be produced in the region of the carpal tunnel (Figure 24-14).[28]

Valgus/Varus and Glide Stress Tests for Wrist, Metacarpophalangeal, and Interphalangeal Joints

A series of tests can be done to stress the ligamentous integrity of the joints in the hand and fingers. Applying valgus and varus stress as well as anterior and posterior glides collectively determines whether a sprain has occurred to one of the many ligaments that connect the carpal bones (Figure 24-15A). Valgus/varus stress to the interphalangeal joints of the fingers stress the collateral ligaments, while anterior/posterior glides stress the joint capsule (Figure 24-15B). Increased pain or instability with any of these tests usually indicates a ligament sprain.[25]

Lunotriquetral Ballotment Test

This test requires the examiner to stabilize the lunate with thumb and index finger while sliding the triquetrum anteriorly and posteriorly to look for laxity, pain, and crepitus. A positive test indicates instability of the lunotriquetral joint that often results in dislocation of the lunate (Figure 24-16).

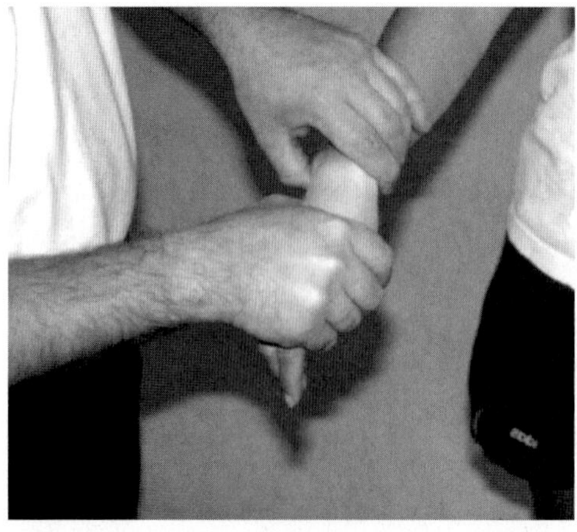

A

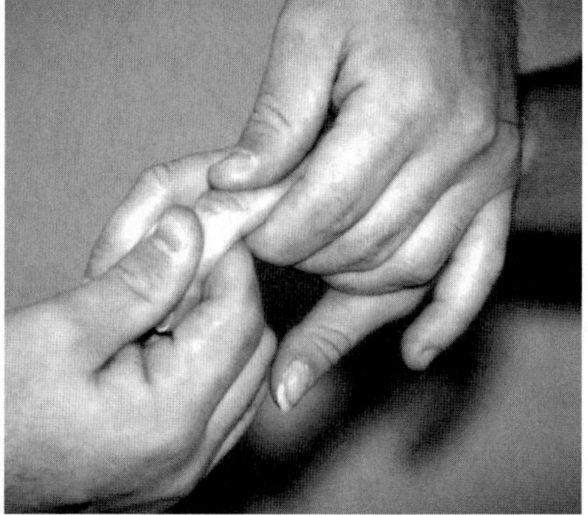

B

Figure 24-15

A, Valgus/varus stress to the wrist. **B,** Anterior/posterior glide to the PIP joint.

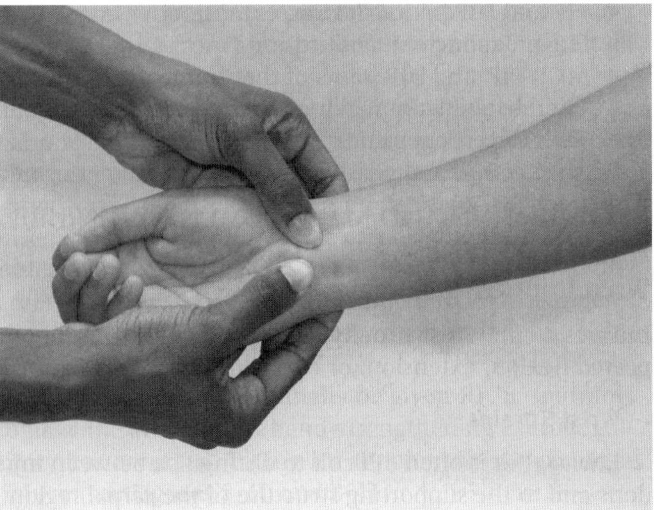

Figure 24-16

Lunotriquetral ballotment test.

Circulatory and Neurological Evaluation

The athletic trainer should inspect the athlete's hands to determine whether circulation is being impeded. The hands should be felt for their temperature. A cold hand or portion of a hand is a sign of decreased circulation. Pinching the fingernails can also help detect circulatory problems. Pinching will blanch the nail, and on release, there should be rapid return of a pink color. Another objective test is the Allen's test.

Allen's test Allen's test is used to determine the function of the radial and ulnar arteries supplying the hand. The athlete is instructed to squeeze the hand tightly into a fist and then open it fully three or four times. While the athlete is holding the last fist, the athletic trainer places firm pressure over each artery. The athlete is then instructed to open the hand. The palm should now be blanched. One of the arteries is then released, and if normal, the hand will instantly become red. The same process is repeated with the other artery (Figure 24-17).

The hand is next evaluated for sensation alterations, especially in cases of suspected tunnel impingements. Nerve involvements will be further evaluated when active and resistive movements are initiated.

24-3 Critical Thinking Exercise

An athlete who sustained a major wrist sprain complains of a decrease in hand circulation.

? How should this injury be evaluated for a circulation problem?

Functional Evaluation

Range of motion is noted in all movements of the wrist and fingers. Active and resistive movements are then compared with those of the uninjured wrist and hand.[25] The following sequence should be conducted:

- Wrist: flexion, extension, radial and ulnar deviation
- MCP joint: flexion, extension

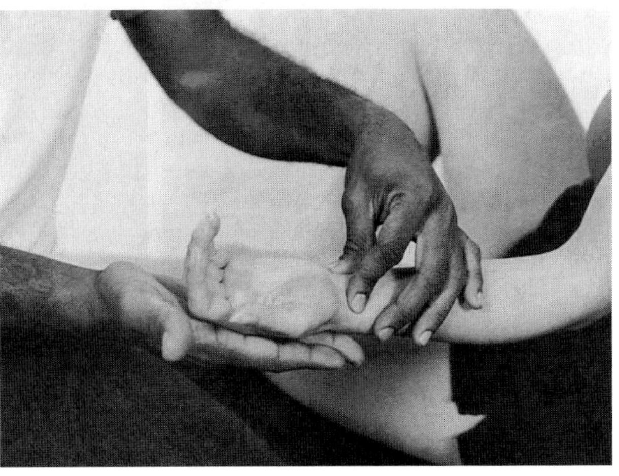

Figure 24-17

Testing the radial and ulmar arteries of the hand (Allen's test).

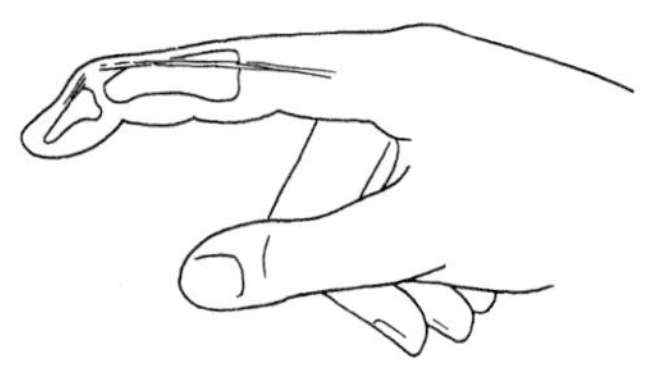

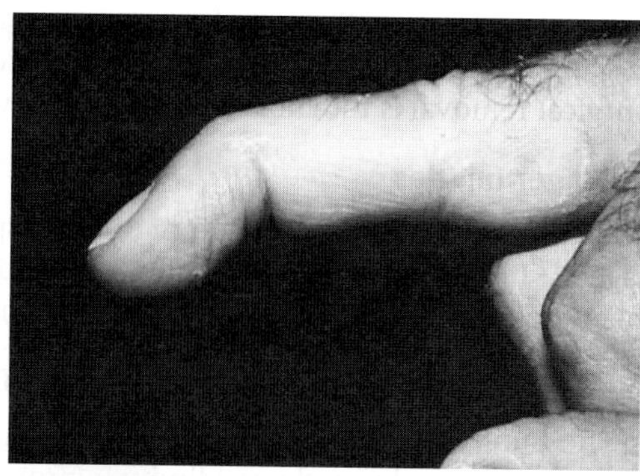

Figure 24-28

Mallet finger occurs from a rupture of the extensor tendon from the distal phalanx.

Symptoms and signs The athlete senses pain, tingling during pressure to the irritated area, and numbness.

Management Early management includes padding of the thumbhole and a decrease in the amount of bowling. If the condition continues, however, surgery may be warranted.

Trigger Finger or Thumb

Etiology Repeated movement can cause the tendons of the wrist and hand to sustain irritation that results in tenosynovitis. An inflammation of the tendon sheath leads to swelling, crepitation, and painful movement. Most commonly affected are the extensor tendons of the wrist: the extensor carpi ulnaris, extensor pollicis longus, extensor pollicis brevis, and abductor pollicis longus.[40]

The trigger finger or thumb is an example of stenosing tenosynovitis. It most commonly occurs in a flexor tendon that runs through a common sheath with other tendons. Thickening of the sheath or tendon can occur, which constricts the sliding tendon. A nodule in the synovium of the sheath adds to the difficulty of gliding.[18] The cause of trigger finger or thumb is nonspecific overuse.

Symptoms and signs The athlete complains that when the finger or thumb is flexed, there is resistance to reextension, producing a snapping that is both palpable and audible. During palpation, tenderness is produced, and a lump can be felt at the base of the flexor tendon sheath.

Management Treatment initially is the same as for de Quervain's disease; however, if treatment is unsuccessful, steroid injections may produce relief. If steroid injections do not provide relief, splinting the tendon sheath is the last option.

Mallet Finger

24-8

***Critical Thinking* Exercise**

A baseball catcher receives a pitch that jams and avulses the extensor tendon of the distal interphalangeal joint of the second finger.

? How should this condition be managed?

Etiology The mallet finger, common in sports, is sometimes called baseball finger or basketball finger. It is caused by a blow from a thrown ball that strikes the tip of the finger, jamming and avulsing the extensor tendon from its insertion along with a piece of bone.

Symptoms and signs The athlete complains of pain at the distal interphalangeal joint. X-ray examination may show a bony avulsion from the dorsal proximal distal phalanx. The athlete is unable to extend the finger, carrying it at approximately a 30-degree angle. There is also point tenderness at the site of the injury, and the avulsed bone often can be palpated (Figure 24-28).

Management RICE is given for the pain and swelling. If there is no fracture, the distal phalanx should immediately be splinted in a position of extension for six to eight weeks (Figure 24-29).

Boutonniere Deformity

Etiology The boutonniere, or buttonhole, deformity is caused by a rupture of the extensor tendon dorsal to the middle phalanx. Trauma occurs to the tip of the finger, which forces the DIP joint into extension and the PIP joint into flexion.[45]

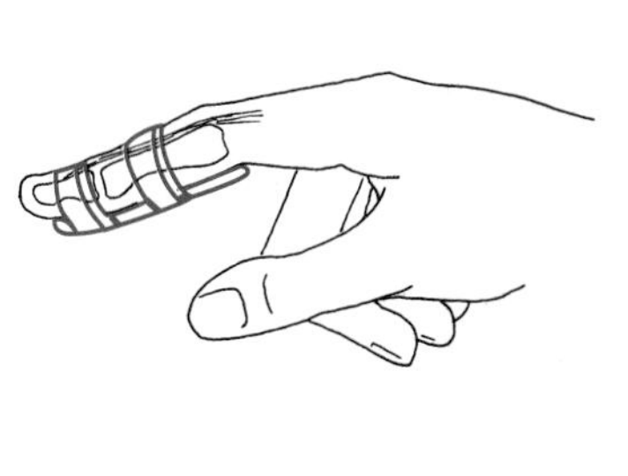
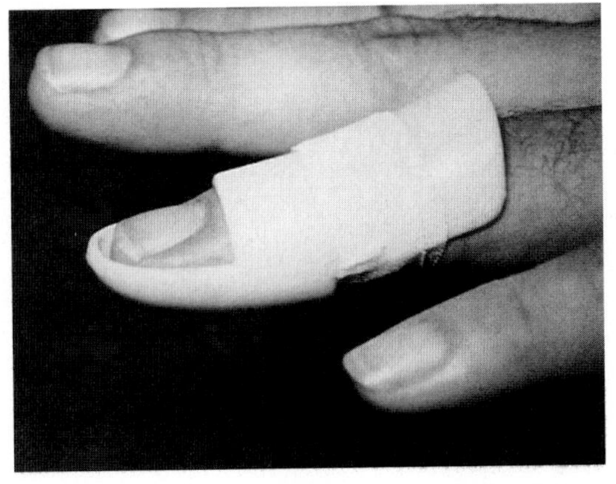

A B

Figure 24-29

A, Splinting of the mallet finger. **B,** Using a Stax splint.

Symptoms and signs The athlete complains of severe pain and inability to extend the DIP joint. There is swelling, point tenderness, and an obvious deformity (Figure 24-30).

Management Management of the boutonniere deformity includes cold application followed by splinting of the PIP joint in extension. NOTE: If this condition is inadequately splinted, the classic boutonniere deformity will develop. Splinting is continued for five to eight weeks. While the finger is splinted, the athlete is encouraged to flex the distal phalanx (Table 24-3).

Jersey Finger

Etiology Jersey finger is a rupture of the flexor digitorum profundus tendon from its insertion on the distal phalanx. This condition most often occurs in the ring finger when the athlete tries to grab the jersey of an opponent and either ruptures the tendon or avulses a small piece of bone.[39]

Symptoms and signs Because the tendon is no longer attached to the distal phalanx, the DIP joint cannot be flexed and the finger is in an extended position (Figure 24-31). There is pain and point tenderness over the distal phalanx.

Management If the tendon is not surgically repaired, the athlete will never be able to flex the DIP joint, causing weakness in grip strength; otherwise, function will be relatively normal. If surgery is done, the course of rehabilitation requires about twelve weeks, and there is often poor gliding of the tendon with the possibility of rerupture.[39]

Dupuytren's Contracture

Etiology The cause of Dupuytren's contracture is unknown. Nodules develop in the palmar aponeurosis that limit finger extension and eventually cause a flexion deformity.

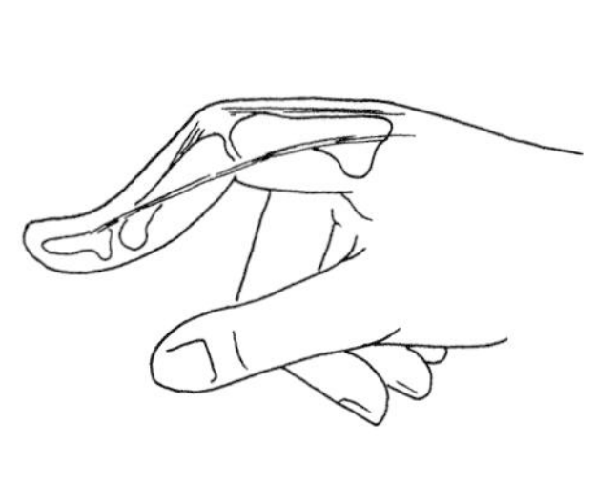
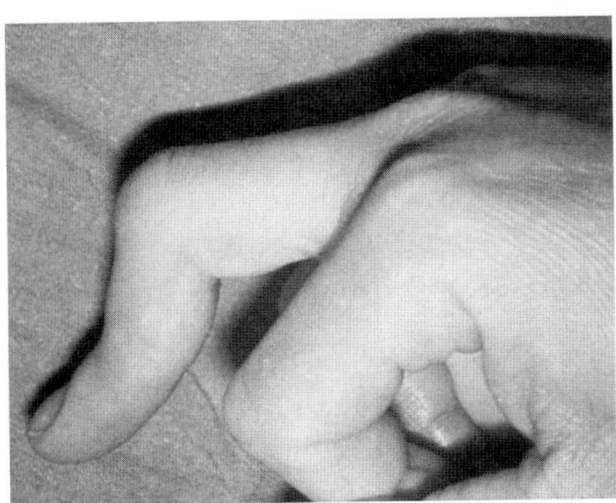
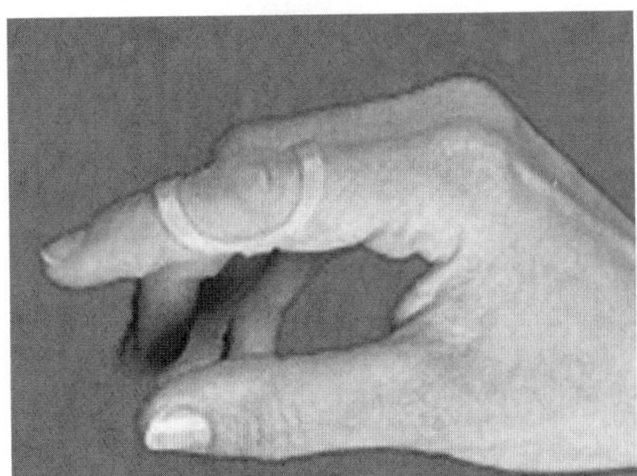

A B C

Figure 24-30

A & B, A Boutonniere deformity occurs from rupture of the tendon dorsal to the PIP joint. **C,** Splinting using an Oval-8 splint.

TABLE 24-3 **Conservative Treatment and Splinting of Finger Injuries**

Injury	Constant Splinting	Begin Motion	Additional Splinting during Competition	Joint Position
Mallet finger	6–8 wk	6–8 wk	6–8 wk	Slight DIP hyperextension
Collateral ligament sprains	3 wk	2 wk	4–6 wk	30-degree flexion
PIP and DIP dislocations	3 wk	3 wk	3 wk	30-degree flexion
Phalangeal fractures	4–6 wk	4–6 wk	3 wk	N/A
PIP and DIP fractures	9–11 wk	3 wk	3 wk	30-degree flexion
Pseudoboutonniere volar plate injuries	5 wk	3 wk	3 wk	20- to 30-degree flexion
Boutonniere deformity	6–8 wk	6–8 wk	6–8 wk	PIP in extension; DIP and MCP not included
MCP fractures	3 wk	3 wk	4–6 wk	30-degree flexion
Flexor digitorum profundus repair	5 wk	3 wk	3 wk	Depends on repair

24-9

Critical Thinking Exercise

A volleyball player attempts to pass a ball and injures her right thumb. She describes a hyperextension with abduction mechanism of injury. The thumb is point tender over the ulnar side of the metacarpophalangeal joint and there is mild swelling.

? What is this injury? What special test can be used to evaluate this injury?

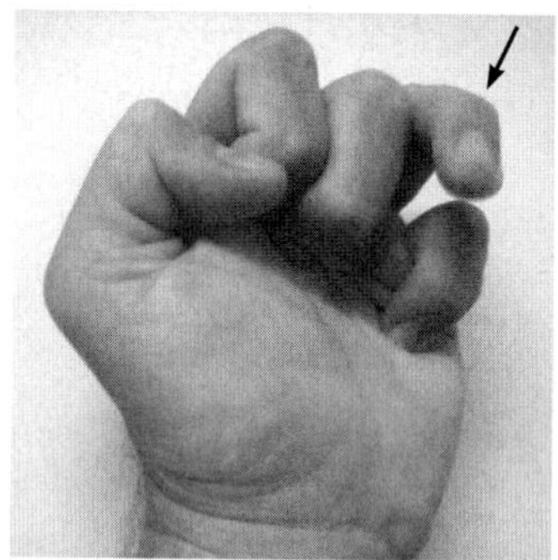

Figure 24-31

A Jersey finger involves ruture of the flexor tendon and loss of ability to flex the finger.

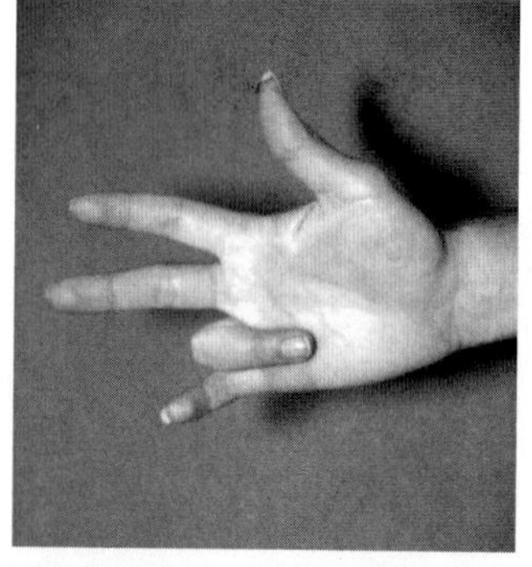

Figure 24-32

Dupuytren's contracture is a flexion deformity of the ring finger

Symptoms and signs A flexion deformity most often develops in which the ring or little finger moves into the palm of the hand and cannot be extended (Figure 24-32).

Management A flexion contracture deformity of this type can significantly interfere with normal hand function. The tissue nodules causing the contracture must be removed surgically.

Sprains, Dislocations, and Fractures of the Phalanges

Etiology The phalanges, particularly of the thumb, are prone to sprains caused by a blow delivered to the tip or by violent twisting (Figure 24-33). The mechanism of injury is similar to that of fractures and dislocations. The sprain, however, mainly affects the capsular, ligamentous, and tendinous tissues.

Symptoms and signs Recognition is accomplished primarily through the history and the sprain symptoms: pain, severe swelling, and hematoma.

Gamekeeper's Thumb

Etiology A sprain of the ulnar collateral ligament of the MCP joint of the thumb is common among athletes, especially skiers and tackle football players.[8]

The mechanism of injury is usually a forceful abduction of the proximal phalanx, which is occasionally combined with hyperextension (Figure 24-34).[19]

Symptoms and signs The athlete complains of pain over the ulnar collateral ligament in addition to a weak and painful pinch. Inspection demonstrates tenderness and swelling over the medial aspect of the thumb.[21]

Management Because the stability of pinching can be severely deterred, proper, immediate, and follow-up care must be performed. If there is instability in the joints, the athlete should be immediately referred to an orthopedist. If the joint is stable, X-ray examination should be performed to rule out fracture. A thumb splint should be applied for protection for three weeks or until the thumb is pain free.[27] The splint, extending from the end of the thumb to above the wrist, is applied with the thumb in a neutral position. After the splint is removed, thumb spica taping should be worn during sports participation (see Figure 8-43).

Sprains of the Interphalangeal Joints of the Fingers

Etiology Interphalangeal finger sprains can include the PIP joint or the DIP joint. Injury can range from minor to complete tears of the collateral ligament, a volar plate

Management Initially, R
tions. Deformity is reduced,
ter which early ROM is carr

Bennett's Fracture

Etiology A Bennett's fra
thumb as the result of an ax
Symptoms and signs Th
the thumb. The thumb's CM
Management This condi
thopedic surgeon.

Distal Phalangeal Fractu

Etiology The primary ca
Symptoms and signs Th
lanx. A subungual hematon
Management Initially, R
as a means for relief of pain

Middle Phalangeal Fract

Etiology A middle phala
Symptoms and signs Th
phalanx. There may be def
Management RICE and
site and if there is no deforn
for sports activity. If there
weeks and a protective splin

Proximal Phalangeal Fra

Etiology Fractures of th
Symptoms and signs Th
spection reveals varying de
Management RICE and
tained by immobilization o
ion, and buddy taping.

PIP Fracture and Disloc

Etiology The cause of t
on a partially flexed finger.
Symptoms and signs Th
PIP joint. There is localized
Management RICE and
fracture. If there is a small f
a splint of 30 to 60 degrees

Fingernail Deformities

Changes in the normal app
different diseases. Some o
causes are listed here:

- Scaling or ridging—p
- Ridging and poor dev
- Clubbing and cyanosi
- Spooning or depressi

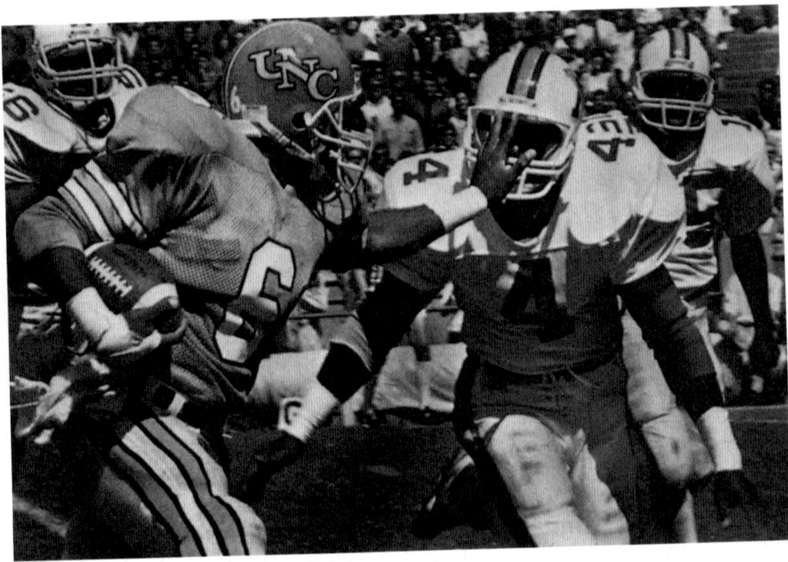

Figure 24-33

Football often places the phalanges at risk of severe injury

tear, or a central extensor slip tear (Table 24-3).[19] A collateral ligament sprain of the interphalangeal joint is common in sports such as basketball, volleyball, and football. A common cause is an axial force that produces a jammed finger. This mechanism places valgus or varus stress on the interphalangeal joint.

Symptoms and signs The athlete complains of pain and swelling at the involved joint. There is severe point tenderness at the joint site, especially in the region of the collateral ligaments. There may be a lateral or medial instability when the joint is in 150 degrees of flexion. Collateral ligamentous injuries may be evaluated by the application of a valgus and varus joint stress test.

Management Management includes RICE for the acute stage, X-ray examinations, and splinting. Splinting of the PIP joint is usually at 30 to 40 degrees of flexion for ten days. If the sprain is to the DIP joint, splinting a few days in full extension assists in the healing process. If the sprains are minor, taping the injured finger to a noninjured one will provide protective support. Later, a protective checkrein can be applied for either thumb or finger protection (see Figure 8-45).

24-10 *Critical Thinking* Exercise

A volleyball player, going up to block a spike, receives an axial force to the middle finger, which causes a valgus force.

? What soft tissue injuries would be expected with such a force?

Swan Neck Deformity and Pseudoboutonniere Deformity

Etiology The volar plate of the PIP joint is most commonly injured in sports from a severe hyperextension force. A distal tear may cause a swan neck deformity, whereas injury to the proximal part of the plate may cause a pseudoboutonniere deformity.

Symptoms and signs There is pain and swelling at the PIP joint, and it displays varying degrees of hyperextension. Tenderness is over the volar aspect of the PIP. A major indication of a tear is that the PIP joint can be passively hyperextended in comparison with other PIP joints.

Management Initially, the athlete is treated with RICE and analgesics as required. Management consists of splinting at 20 to 30 degrees of flexion for three weeks, followed by buddy taping and then PRE.

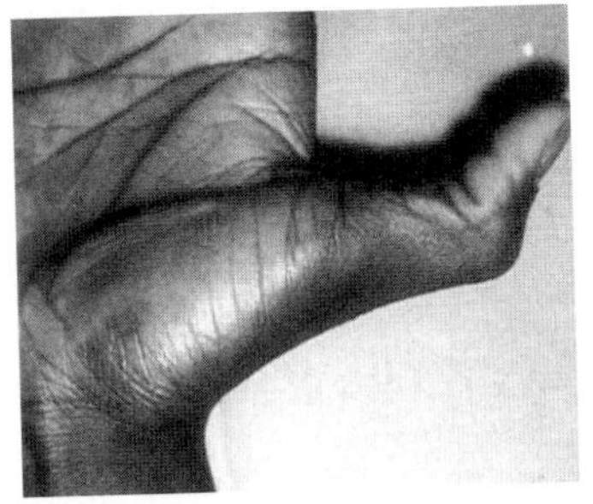

Figure 24-34

A Gamekeeper's thumb is a sprain of the ulnar collateral ligament at the MCP joint of the thumb.

PIP Dorsal Dislocation

Etiology Dislocations of the phalanges have a high rate of occurrence in sports (Figure 24-35).[1] Dislocations can occur at a number of joints, for example, PIP dorsal dislocation, PIP palmar dislocation, and MCP dislocation. Most dislocations are seen in collision or contact sports. The mechanism that produces a PIP dislocation is hyperextension that produces a disruption of the volar plate at the middle phalanx.

Figure 24-35

Open dislocation of the interphalangeal joint of a thumb.

24-11

Critical Thinking Exercise

A football player gets into a fistfight on the field and injures his right hand through an axial force to the fifth metacarpal bone.

? What type of injury should be suspected, and how should it be managed?

capitus and cervicis regions) (Table 25-1). These muscles collectively extend and rotate the spine.

Spinal Cord

The spinal cord is that portion of the central nervous system that is contained within the vertebral canal of the spinal column. It extends from the foramen magnum of the cranium to the filum terminale in the vicinity of the first or second lumbar vertebra. The lumbar roots and the sacral nerves form a horselike tail called the cauda equina (Figure 25-6).

TABLE 25-1 Muscles that Move the Vertebral Column

Muscle	Origin	Insertion	Action	Innervation
Erector Spinae				
Iliocostalis lumborum thoracis cervicis	Crest of the sacrum; spinous processes of the lumbar and lower thoracic vertebrae; iliac crests; angles of the ribs	Angles of the ribs; transverse processes of the cervical vertebrae	Extends the vertebral column and bends it to one side	Branches of the spinal nerves
Longissimus thoracis cervicis capitis	Transverse processes of the lumbar, thoracic, and lower cervical vertebrae	Transverse processes of the vertebra above the vertebra of origin, and the mastoid process of the temporal bone (capitis)	Extends the vertebral column and head; rotates the head toward the same side	Branches of the spinal nerves
Spinalis thoracis cervicis	Spinous process of the upper lumbar, lower thoracic, and seventh cervical vertebrae	Spinous processes of the upper thoracic and the cervical vertebrae	Extends the vertebral column	Branches of the spinal nerves
Multifidus	Posterior surface of the sacrum and the ilium, and the transverse processes of the lumbar, thoracic, and lower cervical vertebrae	Spinous processes of the lumbar, thoracic, and cervical vertebrae	Extends the vertebral column; rotates it toward the opposite side	Branches of the spinal nerves
Rotatores*	Transverse processes of all the vertebrae	Base of the spinous process of the vertebra above the vertebra of origin	Extends the vertebral column; rotates it toward the opposite side	Branches of the spinal nerves
Interspinales*	Superior surface of all the spinous processes	Inferior surface of the spinous process of the vertebra above the vertebra of origin	Extends the vertebral column	Branches of the spinal nerves
Semispinalis thoracis cervicis capitis	Transverse processes of the thoracic and the seventh cervical vertebrae	Spinous processes of the second cervical through the fourth thoracic vertebrae, and the occipital bone	Extends the vertebral column and the head (capitis); rotates them to the opposite side	Branches of the spinal nerves
Splenius capitis cervicis	Spinous processes of the upper thoracic and the seventh cervical vertebrae, and from the ligamentum nuchae	Occipital bone, mastoid process of the temporal bone, and the transverse processes of the upper three cervical vertebrae	Acting together, they extend the head and the neck; acting singly, they abduct and rotate the head toward the same side	Branches of the spinal nerves

*Too small to see on Figure 25-5.

Spinal Nerves and Peripheral Branches

Thirty-one pairs of spinal nerves extend from the sides of the spinal cord: eight cervical, twelve thoracic, five lumbar, five sacral, and one coccygeal (Figure 25-6). Each of these nerves has an anterior root (motor root) and a posterior root (sensory root). The two roots in each case join together and form a single spinal nerve, which passes downward and outward through the intervertebral foramen. As the spinal nerves are conducted through the intervertebral foramina, they pass near the articular facets of

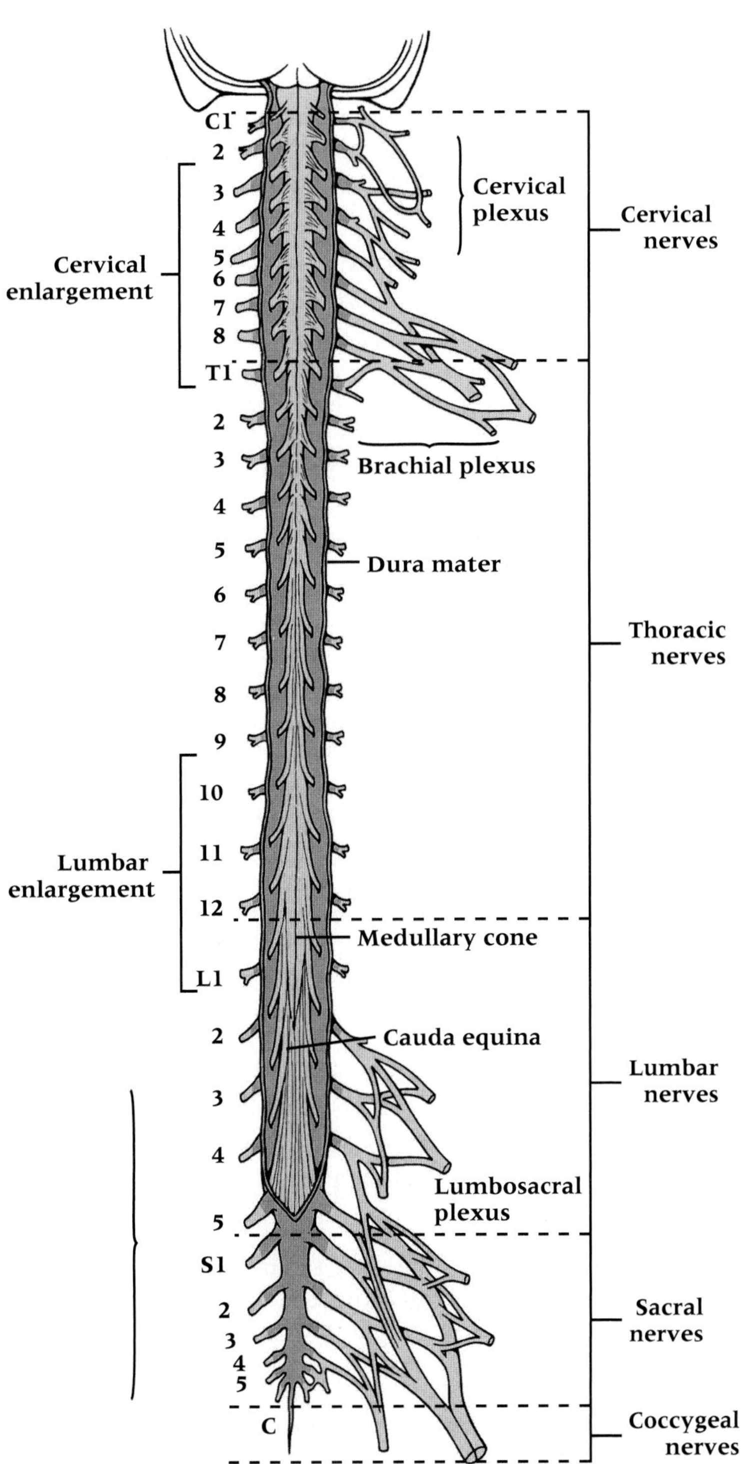

Figure 25-6

Spinal cord and spinal nerves.

the vertebrae. Any abnormal movement of these facets, such as in a dislocation or a fracture, may expose the spinal nerves to injury. Injuries that occur below the third lumbar vertebra usually result in nerve root damage but do not cause spinal cord damage.

Each pair of spinal nerves, with the exception of C1, has a specific area of cutaneous sensory distribution called a *dermatome.* Loss of sensation in a specific dermatome can provide information about the location of nerve damage.

The spinal nerve roots combine to form a network of nerves, or a plexus. There are five nerve plexuses: *cervical, brachial, lumbar, sacral,* and *coccygeal.* The cervical plexus originates from spinal nerves C1 through C4; the brachial plexus, from C5 through T1; the lumbar plexus, from L1 through L4; the sacral plexus, from L4 through S4; and the coccygeal plexus, from S4 through S5 and the coccygeal nerve. Tables 25-2 and 25-3 indicate each nerve; its nerve roots; the muscle it innervates and that muscle's accompanying action; and the cutaneous innervation for the brachial plexus, the lumbar plexus, and the sacral plexus, respectively.

FUNCTIONAL ANATOMY

Movements of the Vertebral Column

Movements of the vertebral column:
- Flexion
- Extension
- Lateral flexion
- Rotation

The movements of the vertebral column are flexion and extension, right and left lateral flexion, or bending, and rotation to the left and right. The degree of movement differs in the various regions of the vertebral column. The cervical and lumbar regions allow extension and flexion. Although the thoracic vertebrae have minimal movement, their combined movement between the first and twelfth thoracic vertebrae can account for 20 to 30 degrees of flexion and extension.

Flexion of the cervical region is produced primarily by the sternocleidomastoid muscles and the scalene muscle group on the anterior aspect of the throat. The scalenes flex the head and stabilize the cervical spine as the sternocleidomastoids flex the neck. The upper trapezius, semispinalis capitis, splenius capitus, and splenius cervicis muscles extend the neck. Lateral flexion of the neck is accomplished by all the muscles on one side of the vertebral column contracting unilaterally. Rotation is produced when the sternocleidomastoid, the scalenes, the semispinalis cervicis, and the upper trapezius on the side opposite the direction of rotation contract in addition to a contraction of the splenius capitus, splenius cervicis, and longissimus capitus on the same side as the direction of rotation.

25-2
***Critical Thinking* Exercise**

A wrestler has normal neck flexion and extension and lateral flexion but is having difficulty rotating his head toward his left shoulder. The athletic trainer suspects a strain of one of the muscles that rotate the head.

? Which muscles rotate the head to the left?

Flexion of the trunk involves the lengthening of the deep and superficial back muscles and the contraction of the abdominal muscles (rectus abdominus, internal oblique, external oblique) and hip flexors (rectus femoris, iliopsoas, tensor fasciae latae, sartorius). Seventy-five percent of flexion occurs at the lumbosacral junction (L5–S1), whereas 15 percent to 20 percent occurs between L4 and L5. The rest of the lumbar vertebrae execute 5 percent to 10 percent of flexion.[9] Extension involves the lengthening of the abdominal muscles and the contraction of the erector spinae and the gluteus maximus, which extends the hip. Trunk rotation is produced by the external obliques and the internal obliques. Lateral flexion is produced by the quadratus lumborum muscle along with the obliques, latissimus dorsi, iliopsoas, and the rectus abdominus on the side of the direction of movement.

PREVENTION OF INJURIES TO THE SPINE

Cervical Spine

Acute traumatic injuries to the spine can be potentially life threatening, particularly if the cervical region of the spinal cord is involved. Thus the athlete must do everything possible to minimize potential injury.

Muscle Strengthening

Strengthening of the musculature of the neck is critical. The neck muscles can protect the cervical spine by resisting excessive hyperflexion, hyperextension, or rotational forces. During participation, the athlete should constantly be in a state of readiness

TABLE 25-2 Brachial Plexus

Nerve	Origin	Function, Muscle Innervated	Cutaneous Innervation
Axillary	Posterior cord, C5–C6	Abducts arm Deltoid Laterally rotates arm Teres minor	Inferior lateral shoulder
Radial	Posterior cord, C5–T1	Extends forearm Triceps brachii Anconeus Flexes forearm Brachialis (part) Brachioradialis Supinates forearm Supinator Extends wrist Extensor carpi radialis longus (also abducts wrist) Extensor carpi radialis brevis (also abducts wrist) Extensor carpi ulnaris (also adducts wrist) Extends fingers Extensor digitorum Extensor digiti minimi Extensor indicis Thumb muscles Abductor pollicis longus Extensor pollicis longus Extensor pollicis brevis	Posterior surface of arm and forearm, lateral two-thirds of dorsum of hand
Musculocutaneous	Lateral cord, C5–C7	Flexes arm Coracobrachialis Flexes forearm Biceps brachii (also supinates) Brachialis (also small amount of innervation from radial)	Lateral surface of forearm
Ulnar	Medial cord, C8–T1	Flexes wrist Flexor carpi ulnaris (also adducts wrist) Flexes fingers Part of flexor digitorum profundus (distal phalanges of little and ring finger) Abducts/adducts fingers Interossei Thumb muscle Adductor pollicis Hypothenar muscles Flexor digiti minimi brevis Abductor digiti minimi Opponens digiti minimi Midpalmar muscles Two medial lumbricals Interossei	Medial one-third of hand, little finger, and medial one-half of ring finger
Median	Medial and lateral cord, C8–T1	Pronates forearm Pronator teres Pronator quadratus Flexes wrist Flexor carpi radialis (also abducts wrist) Palmaris longus Flexes fingers Part of flexor digitorum profundus (distal phalanges of middle and index finger) Flexor digitorum superficialis	Lateral two-thirds of palm of hand, including lateral half of ring finger and tarsal tips of the same finger

Continued

TABLE 25-2 Brachial Plexus—continued

Nerve	Origin	Function, Muscle Innervated	Cutaneous Innervation

		Thumb muscle
		  Flexor pollicis longus
		Thenar muscles
		  Abductor pollicis brevis
		  Opponens pollicis
		  Flexor pollicis brevis
		Midpalmar
		  Two lateral lumbricals	

and, when making contact with an opponent, should "bull" the neck by elevating both shoulders and isometrically cocontracting the muscles surrounding the neck. Protective cervical collars can also help limit movement of the cervical spine. Athletes with long, weak necks are especially at risk. Tackle football players and wrestlers must have highly stable necks. Specific strengthening exercises are essential for the development of this stability. A variety of different exercises that incorporate isotonic, isometric, or isokinetic contractions can be used.[68] One of the best methods is manual resistance by the athlete or by a partner who selectively uses isometric and isokinetic resistance exercises. Manual resistance should not be performed just before an individual engages in a collision sport such as football or ice hockey because of the danger of participating in these activities with fatigued neck muscles.

Range of Motion

In addition to strong muscles, the athlete's neck should have a full range of motion. Ideally, the athlete should be able to place his or her chin on the chest and to extend the head back until the face is parallel with the ceiling. There should be at least 40 to 45 degrees of lateral flexion and enough rotation to allow the chin to reach a level even with the tip of the shoulder. Flexibility is increased through stretching exercises and strength exercises that are in full range of motion. Where flexibility is restricted, manual static stretching can be beneficial.

Using Correct Techniques

Athletes involved in collision sports—in particular, American football and rugby, which involve tackling an opponent—must be taught and required to use techniques that reduce the likelihood of cervical injury. The head, especially one in a helmet, should not be used as a weapon. Football helmets do not protect players against neck injury. In the illegal spearing maneuver, the athlete uses the helmet as a weapon by striking the opponent with its top. Most serious cervical injuries in football result from deliberate axial loading while spearing.[65]

In other sports, such as diving, wrestling, and bouncing on a trampoline, the athlete's neck can be flexed at the time of contact. Energy of the forward-moving body mass cannot be fully absorbed, and fracture or dislocation or both can occur. Diving into shallow water causes many catastrophic neck injuries.[5] Most accidents happen when the diver dives into water that is less than five feet deep and fails to keep the arms extended in front of the face. The head strikes the bottom, which produces a cervical fracture at the C5 or C6 level. Many of the same forces are applied in wrestling. In such trauma, paraplegia, quadriplegia, or death can result. Coaches cannot stress enough to the athlete the importance of using appropriate tackling techniques.

Lumbar Spine

Low back pain is one of the most common and disabling ailments known to humans. In the athlete, however, most cases of low back pain do not involve serious or long-lasting pathology.

TABLE 25-3 Lumbar and Sacral Plexuses

Nerve	Origin	Function, Muscle Innervated	Cutaneous Innervation
Obturator	L2–L4	Adducts thigh Adductor magnus Adductor longus Adductor brevis Gracilis (also flexes thigh) Rotates thigh laterally Obturator externus	Superior medial side of thigh
Femoral	L2–L4	Flexes thigh Iliacus Psoas major Pectineus Sartorius (also flexes leg) Extends leg Rectus femoris (also flexes thigh) Vastus lateralis Vastus medialis Vastus intermedius	Anterior and lateral branches supply the thigh; the saphenous branch supplies the medial leg and foot
Tibial	L4–S3	Extends thigh, flexes leg Biceps femoris (long head) Semitendinosus Semimembranosus Adductor magnus Flexes leg Popliteus Plantar flexes foot Gastrocnemius Soleus Plantaris Tibialis posterior Flexes toes Flexor hallucis longus Flexor digitorum longus	None
Medial and lateral plantar	Tibial	Plantar muscles of foot	Medial and lateral sole of foot
Sural	Tibial	None	Lateral and posterior one-third of leg and lateral side of foot
Common peroneal	L4–S2	Extends thigh, flexes leg Bicep femoris (short head)	Lateral surface of knee
Deep peroneal	Common peroneal	Dorsiflexes foot Tibialis anterior Peroneus tertius Extends toes Extensor hallucis longus Extensor digitorum longus	Skin over great and second toe
Superficial peroneal	Common peroneal	Plantar flexes and everts foot Peroneus longus Peroneus brevis Extends toes Extensor digitorum brevis	Distal anterior third of leg and dorsum of foot

Avoiding Stress

The athlete, like everyone else in the population, can prevent low back pain by avoiding unnecessary stresses and strains that are associated with activities of daily living. The back is subjected to these stresses and strains when standing, sitting, lying, working, or exercising. Care should be taken to avoid postures and positions that can cause injuries (see *Focus Box:* "Recommended postures to prevent low back pain").

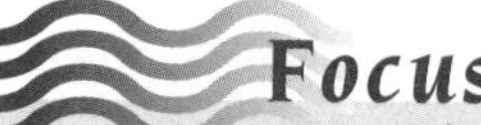

Recommended postures to prevent low back pain

Sitting

1. Do not sit for long periods.
2. Avoid sitting forward on a chair with back arched.
3. Sit on a firm, straight-backed chair.
4. Sit with the low back slightly rounded or positioned firmly against the back of the chair.
5. Sit with the feet flat on the floor and the knees above the level of the hips (if unable to adequately raise the knees, place the feet on a stool).
6. Avoid sitting with legs straight and raised on a stool.

Standing

1. If standing for long periods:
   a. Shift position from one foot to another.
   b. Place one foot on a stool.
2. Stand tall, flatten low back, and relax knees.
3. Avoid arching back.

Lifting and carrying

1. To pick up an object:
   a. Bend at knees and not the waist.
   b. Do not twist to pick up an object—face it squarely.
   c. Tuck in buttocks and tighten abdomen.
2. To carry an object:
   a. Hold object close to body.
   b. Hold object at waist level.
   c. Do not carry object on one side of the body—if it must be carried unbalanced, change from one side to the other.

Sleeping

1. Do not stay in one position too long.
2. Use a bed that is flat and firm yet comfortable.
3. Do not sleep on the abdomen.
4. Do not sleep on the back with legs fully extended.
5. If sleeping on the back, place a pillow under the knees.
6. Ideally, sleep on the side with the knees drawn up.
7. Never extend the arms overhead.
8. Remember that the least strain on the back is in the fully recumbent position with the hips and knees at angles of 90 degrees. In the case of a chronic or a subacute lower back condition, use a firm mattress—it will afford better rest and relaxation of the lower back. Placing ¾-inch plywood underneath the mattress gives a firm, stable surface for the injured back. Sleeping on a water bed will often relieve low back pain, because a water bed supports the body curves equally and decreases abnormal pressures to any one body area.

Correction of Biomechanical Abnormalities

The athletic trainer should be aware of any biomechanical anomalies that the athletes possess. This knowledge helps the athletic trainer establish individual corrective programs. Basic conditioning should include an emphasis on trunk flexibility. Every effort should be made to produce maximum range of motion in rotation and both lateral and forward flexion.[47] Both strength and flexibility should be developed in the spinal extensors (erector spinae). Abdominal strength is essential to ensure proper postural alignment.[31]

Using Correct Lifting Techniques

Weight lifters can minimize their chance of injury to the lumbar spine by using proper lifting techniques.[11] They can help stabilize the spine by incorporating appropriate breathing techniques that involve inhaling and exhaling deeply during lifting. Weight belts can also help stabilize the lumbar spine. Spotters can greatly enhance safety by helping lift and lower the weight.

Core Stabilization

Core stabilization, dynamic abdominal bracing, and maintaining a neutral position are all aspects of a technique that can be used by an athlete to increase the stability of the spine and the lumbo-pelvic-hip complex. This increased stability helps the athlete to maintain the spine and pelvis in a comfortable and acceptable mechanical position that will control the effects of repetitive microtrauma and protect the structures in the back from further damage.[22] Abdominal muscle control also gives the athlete the ability to stabilize the trunk and control posture.[36,85]

ASSESSMENT OF THE SPINE

Assessment of injuries to the spine is somewhat more complex than assessment of injuries to the joints of the extremities because of the number of articulations involved in spinal movement.[33,48] It is also true that injury to the spine, or in particular the spinal cord, may have life-threatening or life-altering implications. Thus, the athletic trainer must perform systematic and detailed evaluations.

History

The most critical part of the evaluation is to rule out the possibility of spinal cord injury. Questions that address this possibility should first establish the mechanism of injury.

- What do you think happened?
- Did you hit someone with, or land directly on, the top of your head?
- Were you knocked out or unconscious? (Anytime an impact is sufficient to cause unconsciousness, the potential for injury to the spine exists.)
- Do you have any pain in your neck?
- Do you have tingling, numbness, or burning in your shoulders, arms, or hands?
- Do you have equal muscle strength in both hands? (Any sensory or motor change bilaterally may indicate a spinal cord injury.)
- Are you unable to move your ankles and toes?

A positive response to any of these questions will necessitate extreme caution when the athlete is moved. The athletic trainer who is handling a suspected cervical spine injury should err only in being overly cautious. *Emergency care of the athlete with suspected cervical spine injury was discussed in detail in Chapter 12.*

Once cervical spine injury has been ruled out, other general questions may provide some indication as to the nature of the problem.

- Where is the pain located?
- What kind of pain do you have?
- What were you doing when the pain began?
- Were you standing, sitting, bending, or twisting?
- Did the pain begin immediately?
- How long have you had this pain?
- Do certain movements or positions cause more pain?
- Can you assume a position that gets rid of the pain?
- Is there any tingling or numbness in the arms or legs?
- Is there any pain in the buttocks or the back of the legs?
- Have you ever had any back pain before?
- What position do you usually sleep in? How do you prefer to sit?

It is important to remember that pain in the back may be caused by many different conditions. The source may be musculoskeletal or visceral, or it may be referred.

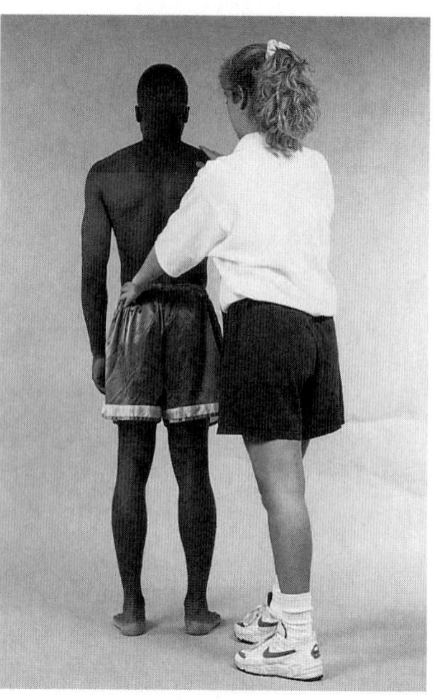

Figure 25-7

Observing spinal alignment.

Observation

Observing the posture and movement capabilities of the athlete during the evaluation can help clarify the nature and extent of the injury.

Posture Evaluation

It is important to observe the athlete's total static posture, paying special attention to the low back, pelvis, and hips.[44] The athletic trainer also should make some decision about somatotype (i.e., ectomorph, mesomorph, or endomorph). When observing the athlete's standing static posture, the athletic trainer must accept the fact that postural alignment varies considerably among individuals; therefore only obvious asymmetries should be considered.[42] The entire body should be observed from all angles—lateral, anterior, and posterior (Figure 25-7). To ensure accuracy of observation, a plumb line or posture screen may be of use (Figure 25-8). A trained observer with a good background in postural observation may not require any special devices. Figure 25-9 shows typical vertical alignment landmarks from a lateral view. In the anterior and posterior assessment, the athletic trainer should look for asymmetries or differences in height between anatomical landmarks on each side (Figure 25-10).[42]

General observations relative to posture include the following:

- Head is tilted to one side.
- Shoulder is lower on one side.
- One shoulder is carried forward.
- One scapula is lower and more prominent than the other.
- Trunk is habitually bent to one side (hips look shifted to one side).
- Space between the body and arm is greater on one side.
- One hip is more prominent than the other.
- Hips are tilted to one side (iliac crests are not same height).
- Ribs are more pronounced on one side.
- One arm hangs longer than the other.
- One arm hangs farther forward than the other.
- One patella is lower than the other (level of popliteal creases is different).
- Trochanters are of unequal height.
- Level of malleoli is different.
- PSIS (posterior superior iliac spine) levels are different.
- ASIS (anterior superior iliac spine) levels are different.

Classic postural deviations include kyphosis, forward head posture, lordosis, flatback posture, swayback posture, and scoliosis.

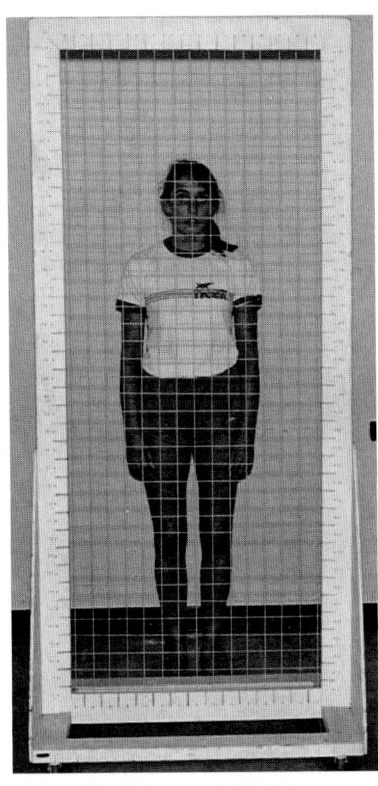

Figure 25-8

Using a grid can produce more accurate results during posture screening.

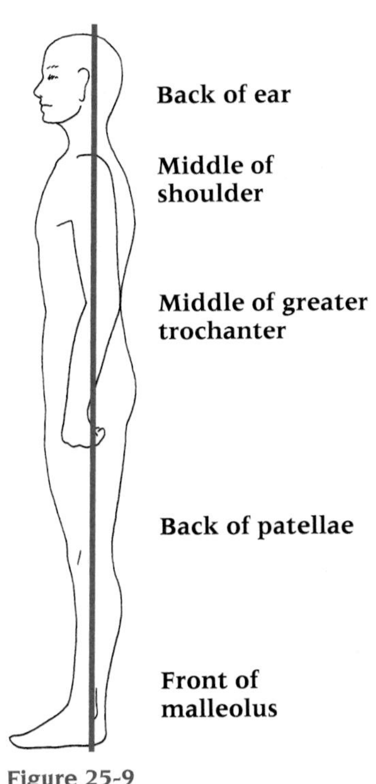

Figure 25-9

Typical vertical alignment landmarks.

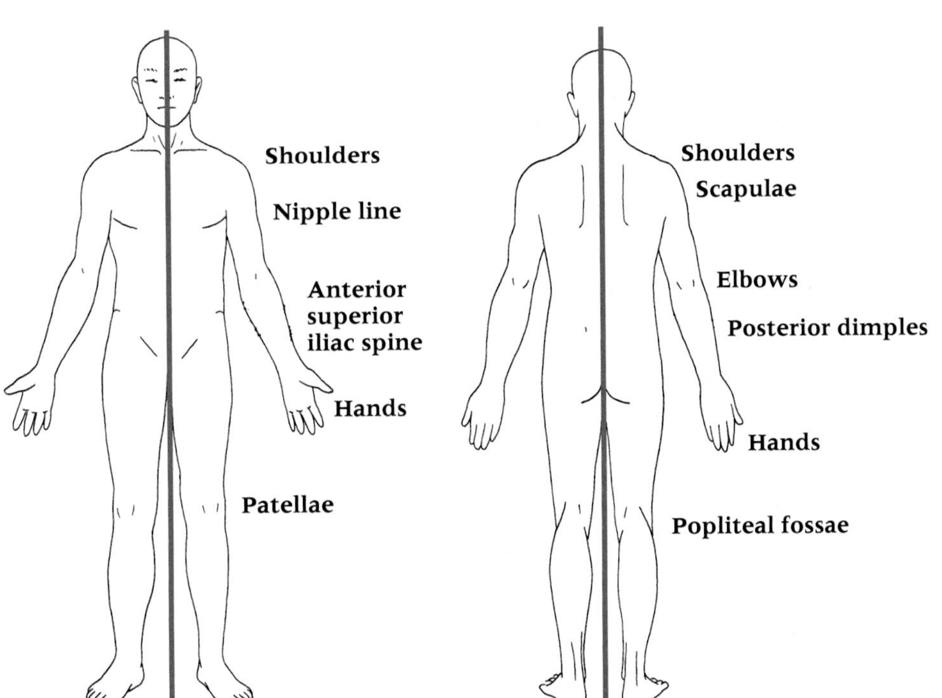

Figure 25-10

Typical horizontal alignment landmarks. (Colored line indicates vertical landmarks.)

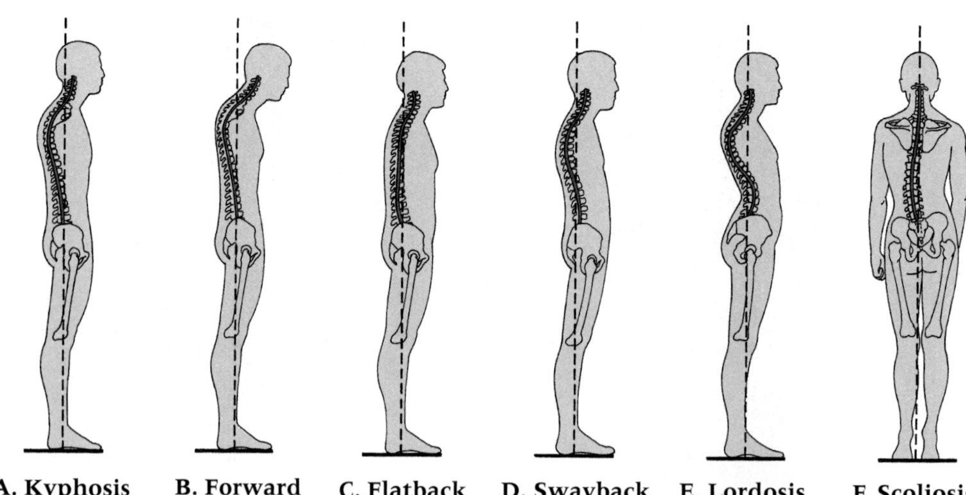

Figure 25-11

Postural malalignments.

Classic postural deviations include kyphosis, forward head posture, flatback posture, swayback posture, lordosis, and scoliosis.

Kyphosis Kyphosis is characterized by an increased thoracic curve and by scapulae that are protracted, which produces a rounded shoulder appearance (Figure 25-11A). Kyphosis is usually associated with a forward head posture.

Scheuermann's disease is a disease of unknown etiology that usually affects adolescent males. This condition is not only painful but also may cause progressive thoracic or lumbar kyphosis.

Forward head posture If the upper back exhibits a kyphotic posture in standing or sitting, there will be a compensatory change in the position of the head and neck. To keep the eyes level in spite of a slumped or rounded shoulder posture, the athlete must extend the cervical spine, which tends to produce short but strong neck extensors and weak, long neck flexors. Thus, the head will be held in a forward position (Figure 25-11B).

Flatback posture Flatback posture is caused by a decreased lumbar curve and an increase in posterior pelvic tilt and in hip flexion (Figure 25-11C).

Swayback posture A swayback posture involves an anterior shifting of the entire pelvis that results in hip extension. The thoracic segment shifts posteriorly, causing flexion of the thorax on the lumbar spine. Thus, there is a decrease in lordosis in the lumbar spine and an increase in kyphosis in the thoracic spine (Figure 25-11D).

Lordosis Lordotic posture is characterized by an increased curve in the lumbar spine and an increase both in anterior tilt of the pelvis and in hip flexion (Figure 25-11E). Lordosis combined with kyphosis and a forward head posture is referred to as a kypho-lordotic posture.

Scoliosis Scoliosis is a lateral curvature of the spine (Figure 25-11F). The athlete with scoliosis exhibits a recognizable abnormal curve in one direction and a compensatory secondary curve in the opposite direction. Scoliosis can be functional or structural. A functional scoliosis can be caused by some nonspinal defect such as unequal leg length, muscle imbalance, or nutritional deficiency. Structural scoliosis is caused by some defect in the bony structure of the spine. When the athlete bends forward, the spine with a functional scoliosis may straighten, whereas the spine with a structural scoliosis remains twisted. With the athlete in this position, one side of the spine may be more prominent than the other.

Cervical Spine Observation

When evaluating a case of cervical injury, the athletic trainer should look at the position of the head and neck. Are the shoulders level and symmetrical? Is the athlete willing to move the head and neck freely? The athletic trainer should check passive,

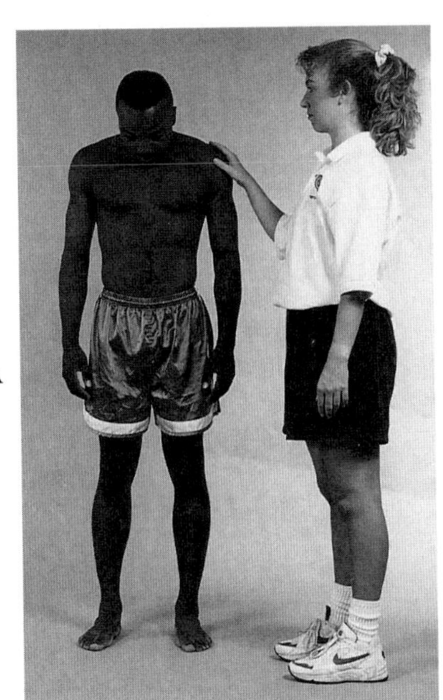
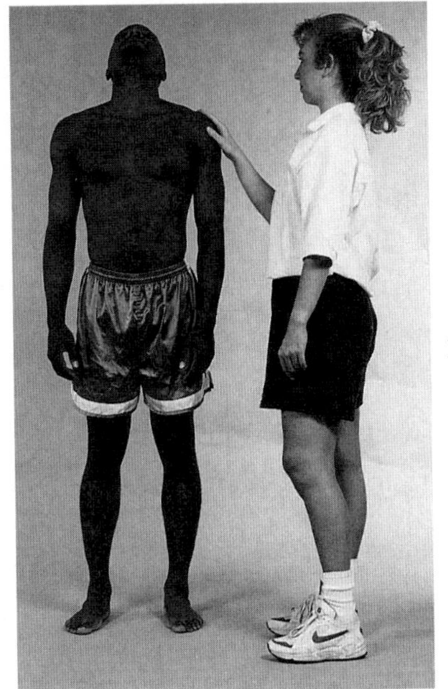
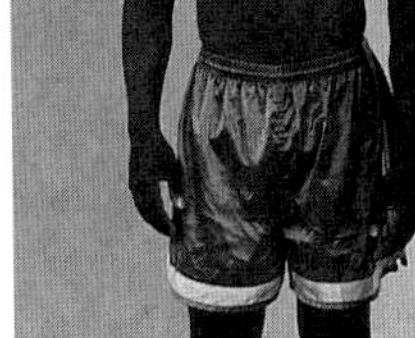
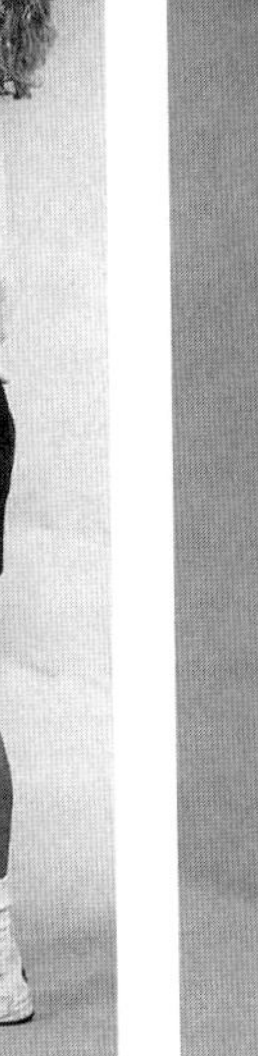
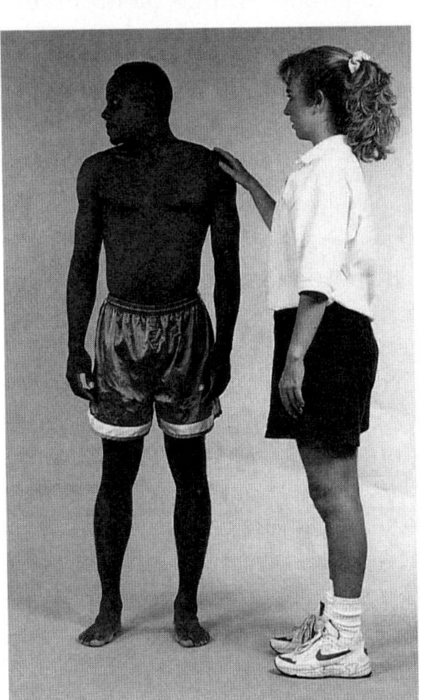

A B C D

Figure 25-12

Checking neck range of motion. **A,** Flexion. **B,** Extension. **C,** Lateral flexion. **D,** Rotation.

active, and resisted range of motion in the neck including flexion, extension, rotation, and lateral bending (Figure 25-12).[51]

Thoracic Spine Observation

The athlete is first asked to flex, extend, laterally flex, and rotate the neck. Pain accompanying the movement in the upper back region could be referred from a lesion of the cervical disk. Additionally, pain in the scapular area could stem from an irritation of a myofascial trigger point or from irritation of the long thoracic or supra-scapular nerves, which requires evaluation of the shoulder complex (see Chapter 22). The athlete should also be asked to flex forward laterally and to extend and rotate the trunk. Pain felt during movement may indicate nerve root irritation to the lower thoracic region.

The most common cause of thoracic pain is dysfunction of one or more joint articulations and usually involves the facet joints. Increased pain upon placing the chin on the chest or upon deep inspiration is often indicative of a facet joint problem.

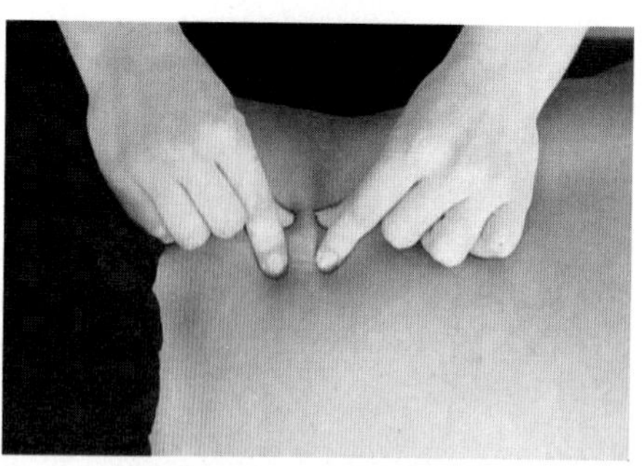

Figure 25-13

Each spinous process should be in a direct line with the one above and below.

Lumbar Spine and Sacroiliac Joint Observation

Normal functional movement in the low back region depends on coordinated motion of the lumbar vertebrae, the sacrum, and the pelvis. The pelvis and shoulders should be level. Both the soft tissue and bony structures on both sides of the midline should be symmetrical. Any unusual curve in the lumbar area that is observed when the athlete is standing or walking could be due to muscular, capsular, or ligamentous injuries, to disk-related problems, or to some idiopathic or structural problem.

The athlete should be observed in standing, sitting, supine, side-lying, and prone positions, and special tests should be done in each of those positions to determine the nature of the problem.[58]

Palpation

Palpation should be performed with the athlete lying prone and the spine as straight as possible. The head and neck should be slightly flexed. In cases of low back pain, a pillow placed under the hips might make the athlete more comfortable. Palpation should progress from proximal to distal as the athletic trainer attempts to identify points of tenderness, muscle spasm or guarding, or defects in bone or soft tissue.

The musculature on each side of the spine should be palpated for tenderness or guarding. Referred pain can produce tender areas. At some point in the evaluation of the lumbar spine, the abdominal musculature should also be palpated; the athlete should perform a partial sit-up to determine symmetry and tone.

The spinous processes are the easiest landmark to locate. Pressure and release should be applied to the spinous process of each vertebra in an anterior direction to determine if pain is increased either centrally or laterally. The gaps between the spinous processes should be palpated. Tenderness may indicate some ligamentous or disk-related problem. Each spinous process should be in a direct line with the one directly above and directly below (Figure 25-13). Misalignment usually occurs in the cervical or lumbar areas, indicating some rotation of an individual vertebral segment. The transverse processes on both sides of each vertebra can also be palpated. Pressure on one side only produces rotation of that segment, which can increase pain. The facet joints and laminae are difficult to palpate because of the paraspinal muscles.

The sacroiliac joints should be palpated bilaterally for tenderness. Posterior pressure on the sacrum may increase pain if the sacroiliac joint is involved.

Special Tests for the Cervical Spine

Special tests for the cervical spine should not be done until trauma to either the vertebrae or the spinal cord has been ruled out.

Brachial plexus test Lateral flexion or bending of the cervical spine by the application of pressure on both the head and the shoulder duplicates the mechanism of injury to the brachial plexus (Figure 25-14). If the cervical spine is flexed to the right and pain radiates to the right shoulder and arm, a compression injury exists. Conversely, if the pain radiates to the left shoulder and arm, a traction or stretch injury has occurred.

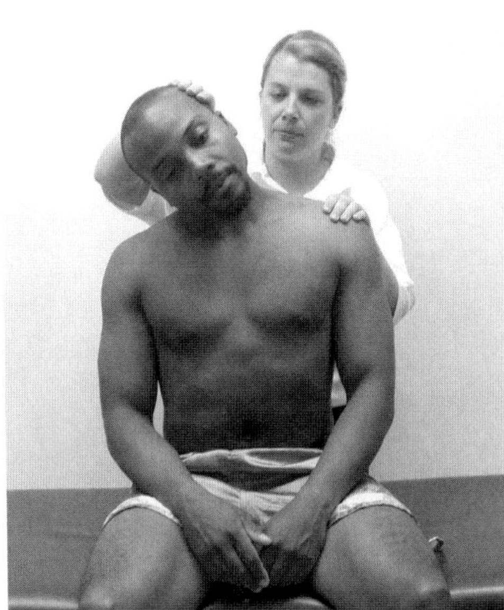

Figure 25-14

Brachial plexus test.

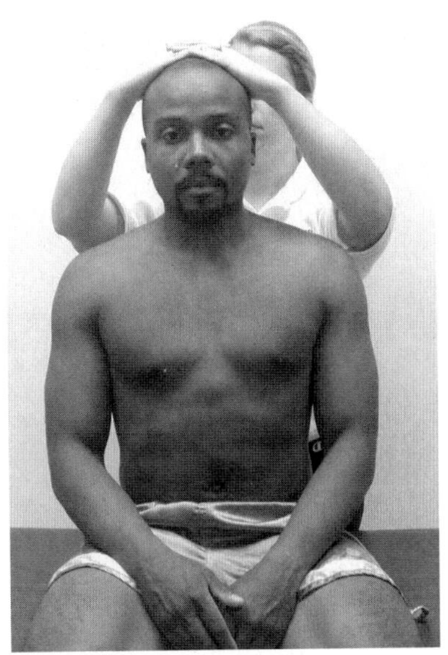

Figure 25-15

Cervical compression test.

Cervical compression and Spurling's tests Axial compression of the cervical spine by the application of a downward force compresses cervical facet joints and the cervical spinal nerve roots (Figure 25-15). The level of the associated pain will determine specifically which nerve root has been injured. Spurling's test also uses cervical compression but with lateral bending and slight extension, which produces pain in the shoulder and arm on the side of flexion (Figure 25-16). Pain is caused by impingement of the nerve root.

Vertebral artery test This test is done with the athlete supine. The athletic trainer extends, then laterally bends and rotates the cervical spine in the same direction (Figure 25-17). Dizziness or abnormal movement of the eyes (nystagmus) indicates that the cervical vertebral artery is being partially occluded because of some abnormal compression. The athlete should be immediately referred to a physician for additional testing and diagnosis.[86]

25-3

Critical Thinking **Exercise**

A cross country runner stepped in a hole while running. He immediately felt pain in his left low back below his waist and had to stop running. He comes to the athletic trainer, who suspects that the mechanism of injury has caused a problem with the sacroiliac joint.

? What signs should the athletic trainer look for during the evaluation that would likely indicate some injury to the sacroiliac joint?

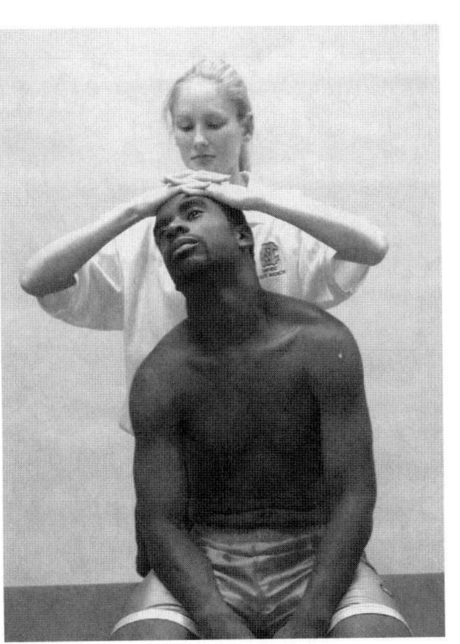

Figure 25-16

Spurling's test.

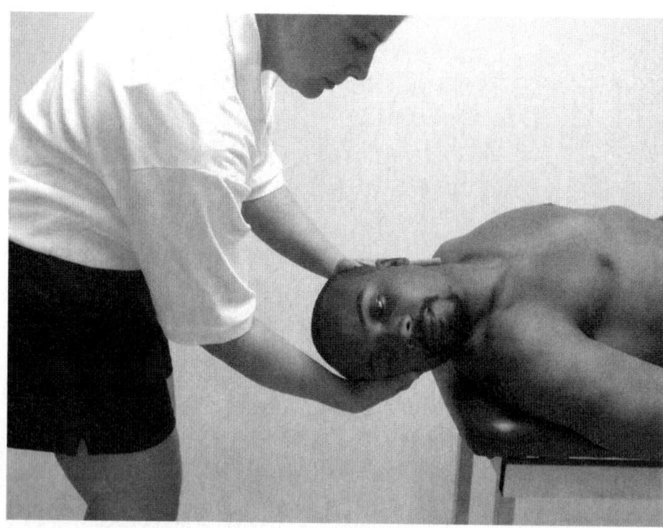

Figure 25-17

Vertebral artery test.

Shoulder abduction test The athlete abducts the shoulder by placing the hand on top of the head (Figure 25-18). A decrease in symptoms may indicate the presence of a nerve root compression, possibly due to a herniated disk.

Special Tests for the Lumbar Spine

Special tests for the lumbar spine should be performed in standing, sitting, supine, side-lying, and prone positions.[21,70]

Tests Done in Standing Position

The athletic trainer should observe the athlete's gait. Is the patient's trunk bent, or are the hips shifted to one side? Is there a limp or any difficulty in walking? The athletic trainer should check the alignment and symmetry of the malleoli, popliteal crease, trochanters, anterior and posterior superior iliac spines (ASIS and PSIS), and iliac crests.

Forward bending Forward bending involves stretching of the posterior spinal ligaments (Figure 25-19A). With forward bending or flexion, the PSISs on each side should move together. If one moves further than the other, a motion restriction is likely present on the side that moves most. If they move at different times, the side that moves first usually has a restriction.

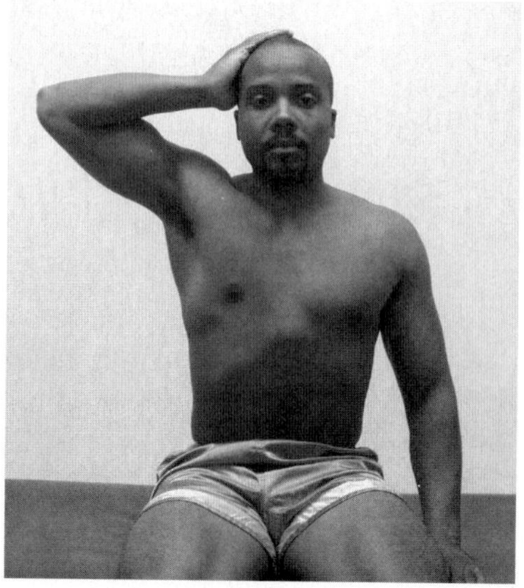

Figure 25-18

Shoulder abduction test.

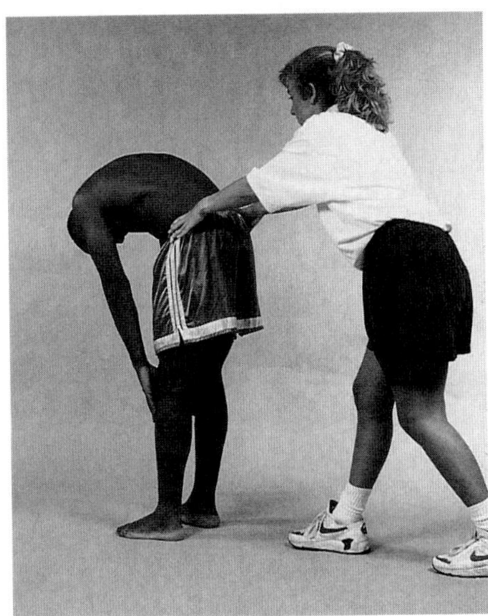

A

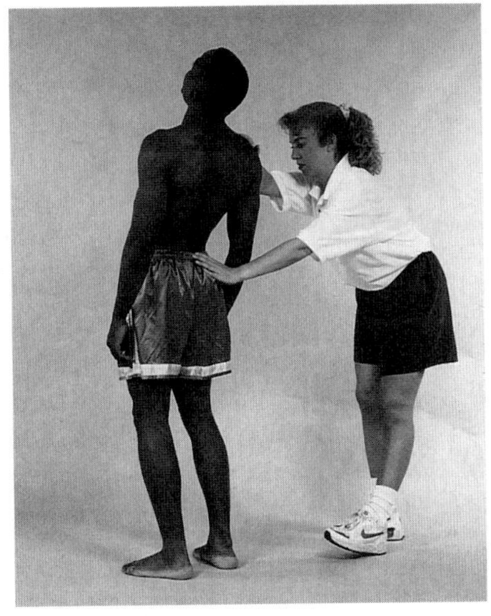

B

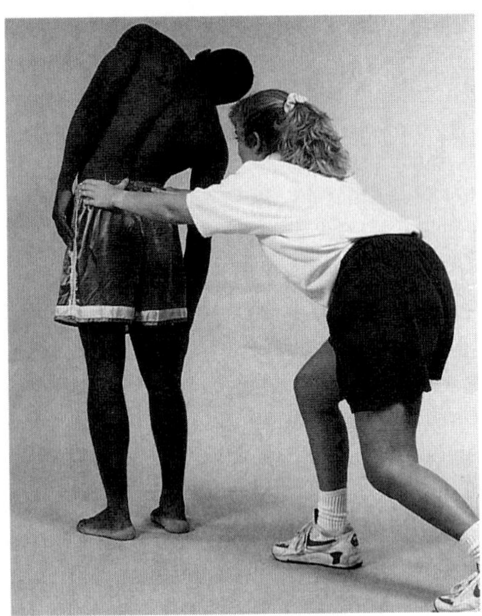

C

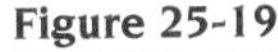

Figure 25-19

Checking lumbar range of motion in standing position. **A,** Forward bending. **B,** Backward bending. **C,** Side bending.

Backward bending Backward bending places the spine in a hyperextended position and stretches the anterior ligaments of the spine (Figure 25-19B). Restrictions or pain present in backward bending are usually associated with a disk problem. However, the pain may also be related to spondylolysis or spondylolisthesis (to be discussed later in this chapter). Extension done in the one-leg standing position (stork position) is a good indicator of a spondylolysis (Figure 25-20).

Side bending For the athlete with a lumbar lesion or with sacroiliac dysfunction, side bending toward the painful side will increase the pain (Figure 25-19C). In the case of a herniated disk, the athlete will usually side bend toward the side of the herniation to relieve the nerve from external compression by the disk.

Rotation While the athlete is standing with his or her arms folded across the chest, the athletic trainer should rotate the trunk to the left, then to the right, checking the

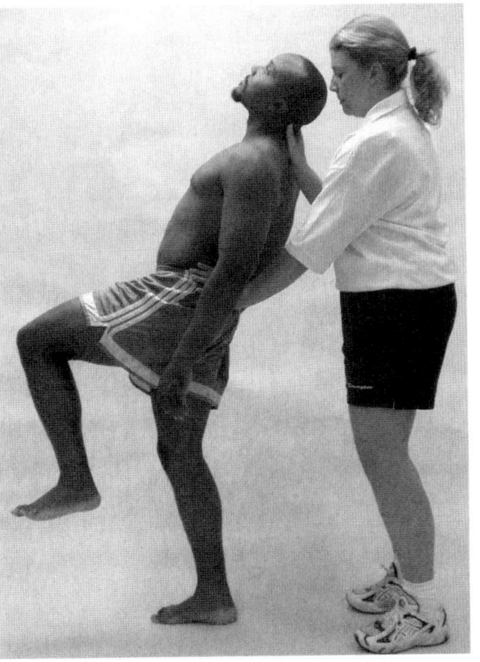

Figure 25-20

Stork test—single leg stance extension.

25-4

***Critical Thinking* Exercise**

A gymnast complains of a centrally located back pain that radiates down her left leg. She describes a sudden onset after a workout that becomes more severe as she tries to rest it. Forward bending and sitting postures increase pain. Backward bending is restricted. Side bending toward the affected side increases pain.

? Based on the athletic trainer's assessment, what would likely be causing this pain?

movement of the lumbar spine for symmetry. The pelvis should not move during the rotation.

Tests Done in Sitting Position

Forward bending In seated forward bending or flexion, like in standing forward bending, the PSISs should move together. If one moves further than the other, a motion restriction is likely present on the side that moves most.

Rotation The athlete sits with arms folded across the chest and rotates the trunk to the left and then to the right while the athletic trainer checks the movement of the lumbar spine for symmetry and provides overpressure to see if pain increases (Figure 25-21A).

Hip rotation With the athlete in the same sitting position, the hip should be rotated internally and externally (Figures 25-21B and C). Internal rotation that produces pain will likely be a piriformis irritation (discussed later in this chapter), and pain is produced as the muscle is stretched.

A "sign of the butt" is a cluster of tests designed to identify a potentially serious hip pathology. The individual tests that make up this sign are usually included in most lumbar and sacroiliac exams, but they are not grouped together in our synthesis of the information. The three component tests are (1) a noncapsular pattern of restriction of the passive range of motion and very definite sharp reproduction of hip pain during

A

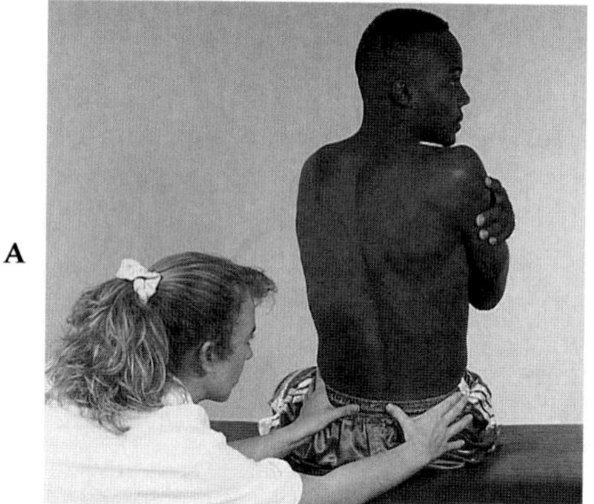

B

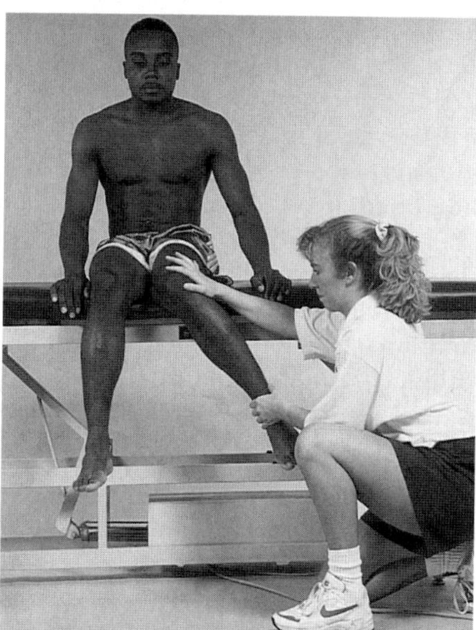

C

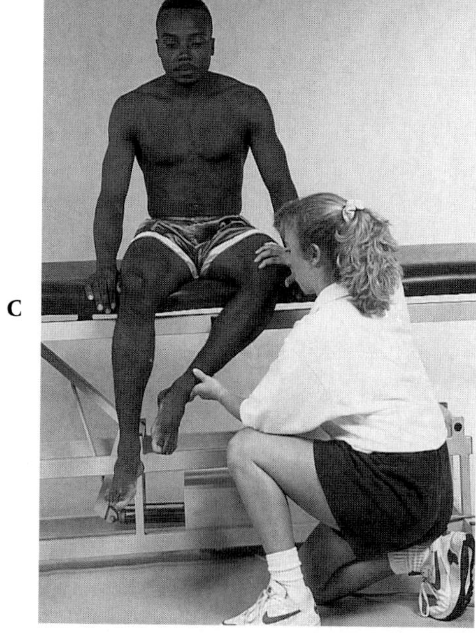

Figure 25-21

Checking lumbar range of motion in sitting position. **A,** Rotation. **B,** Internal hip rotation. **C,** External hip rotation.

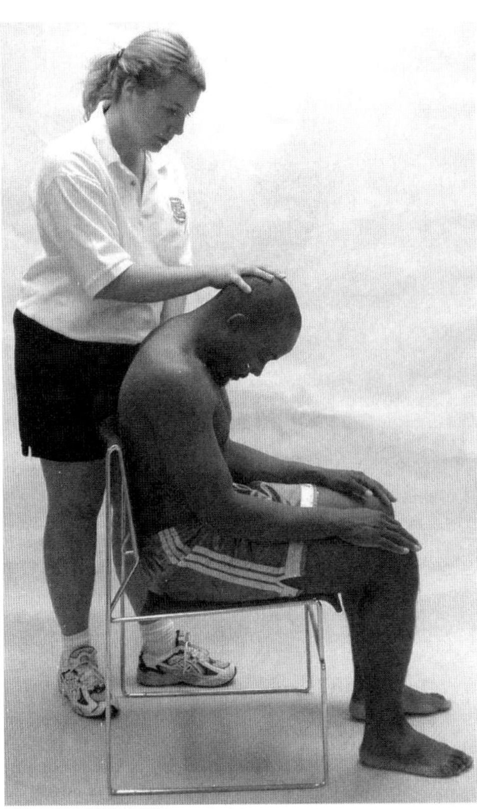

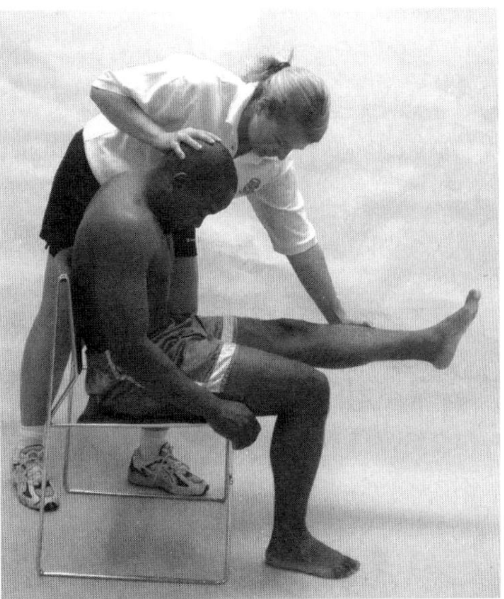

Figure 25-22

Slump test.

passive hip range of motion testing, (2) limited and painful straight leg raise test, and (3) limited and painful hip flexion range of motion with the knee flexed. A capsular pattern of the hip is defined as a gross limitation of hip flexion, abduction, and internal rotation with a slight limitation in hip extension and no limitation of external rotation. An athlete who has gross limitations of all ranges has a noncapsular pattern of limitation. External rotation limitation is the key motion loss in this test.

Slump test The slump test begins with the athlete sitting with knees flexed and feet on the ground (Figure 25-22). The thoracic and lumbar spines are flexed with overpressure. Pain is assessed first in this starting position. From this starting position, the following series of positional changes occurs, with pain being assessed in each position: (1) The cervical spine is flexed, (2) one knee is extended, (3) the ankle is dorsiflexed, (4) neck flexion is released, (5) both legs are extended simultaneously, and (6) steps 1 through 4 are repeated with the other leg. This test is done to detect an increase in nerve root tension that has recently been labeled *neural tension*, which may be caused by lateral disk herniation, nerve root adhesions, or vertebral impingement.[8,26,38]

25-5

Critical Thinking Exercise

A volleyball player comes to the athletic trainer complaining of recurring low back pain. She has been seen by a therapist in her hometown who has told her that she has a positive straight leg raising test, but the athlete still does not understand what is causing her pain.

? How should the athletic trainer explain what having a positive straight leg raising test means?

Tests Done in Supine Position

The athletic trainer should first note the leg position. If there is asymmetrical and exaggerated external rotation on one side, there may be a piriformis contracture on that side. The iliopsoas, adductors, pubic tubercles, and symphysis pubis should be palpated for symmetry and tenderness in the supine position prior to performing the following tests.

Straight leg raises The *straight leg raising* test applies pressure to the sacroiliac joint and may indicate a problem in either the sciatic nerve, the sacroiliac joint, or the lumbar spine (Figure 25-23). Pain at 30 degrees of straight leg raising indicates either a hip problem or an inflamed nerve. Pain from 30 degrees to 60 degrees indicates some sciatic nerve involvement. If dorsiflexing the ankle at maximum straight leg raising increases the pain, the problem is likely due to some nerve root (L3–4, S1–3)

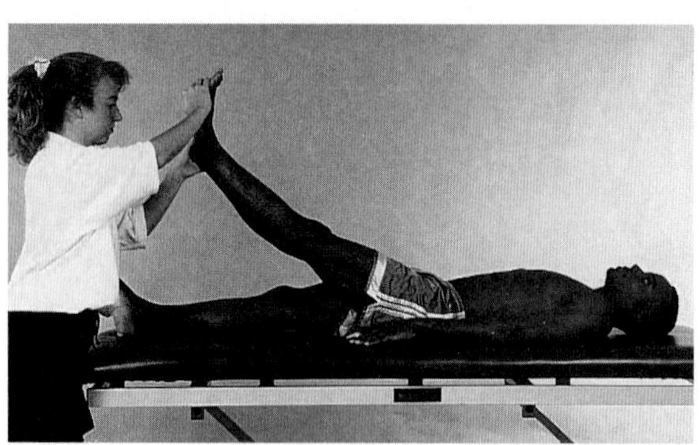

Figure 25-23

Straight leg raising test.

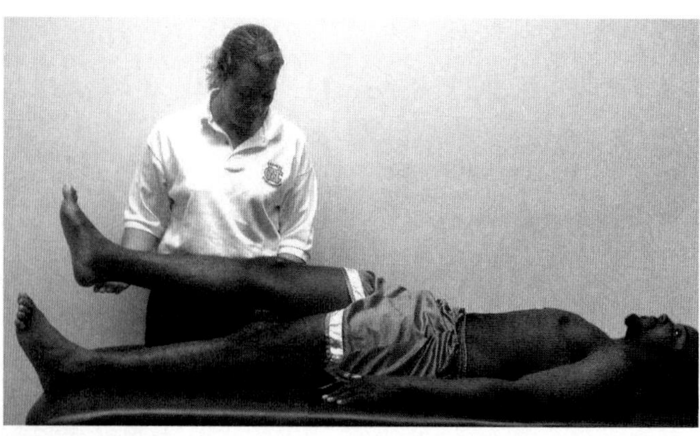

Figure 25-24

Kernig's test.

or sciatic nerve irritation (Laseague's sign). Pain between 70 degrees and 90 degrees is indicative of a sacroiliac joint problem.

Kernig's test In Kernig's test, the athlete performs a unilateral straight leg raise with the knee extended, which creates lumbar pain that possibly radiates into the buttocks. Pain indicates some impingement of the nerve root that is caused by a bulging disk or bony entrapment or by irritation of the meninges (Figure 25-24).

Brudzinski's test Brudzinski's test is a modification of Kernig's test. Pain that increases when the neck is flexed may indicate either a lumbar disk or some nerve root irritation (Figure 25-25).[35]

Well straight leg raising test The well straight leg raising test, done on the unaffected side, may also produce pain in the low back on the affected side as well as radiating along the sciatic nerve. This test provides additional proof of nerve root inflammation (Figure 25-26).

Milgram and Hoover straight leg raising tests An inability to hold both legs off the treatment table for thirty seconds on the Milgram straight leg raising test indicates some problem with the lumbar spine. This test increases intrathecal pressure that causes a disk to put pressure on a lumbar nerve root (Figure 25-27A). The Hoover test is a variation of the Milgram test; it uses a unilateral straight leg raise to check for nerve root problems (Figure 25-27B).

Bowstring test The bowstring test is another way to determine sciatic nerve irritation. The leg on the affected side is lifted until pain is felt. The knee is then flexed until the pain is relieved, at which time pressure is applied to the popliteal fossa. The test result is positive if pain is felt during palpation along the sciatic nerve (Figure 25-28).

Figure 25-25

Brudzinski's test.

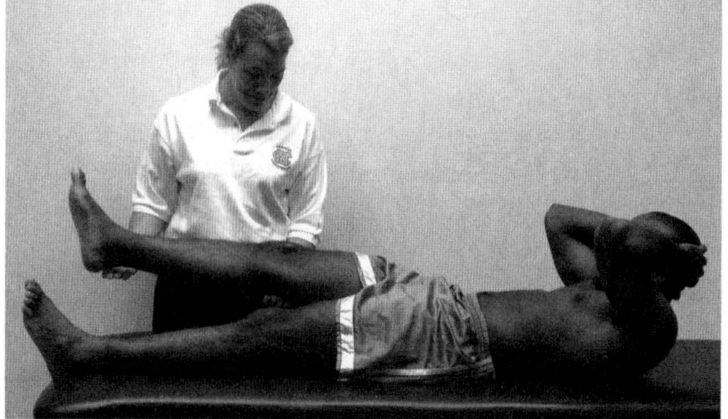

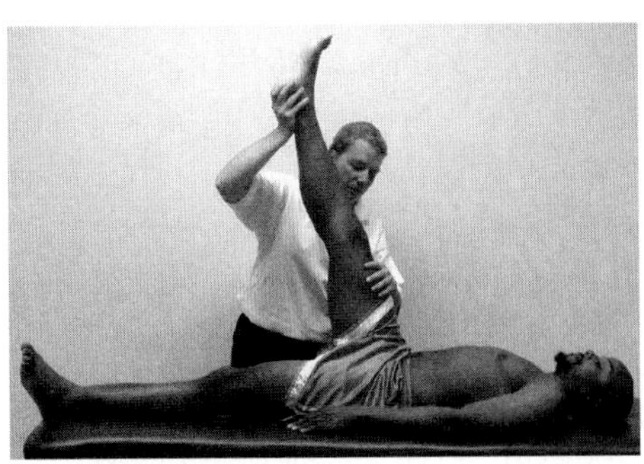
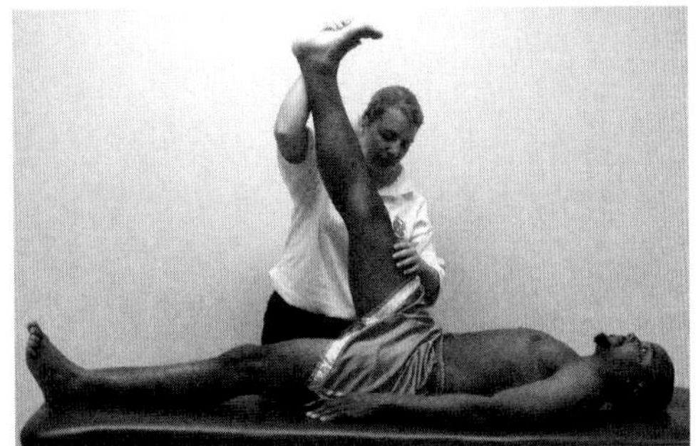

Figure 25-26

Well straight leg raising test.

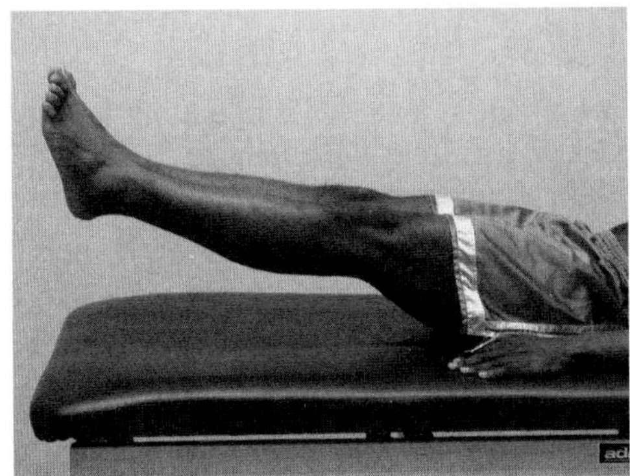
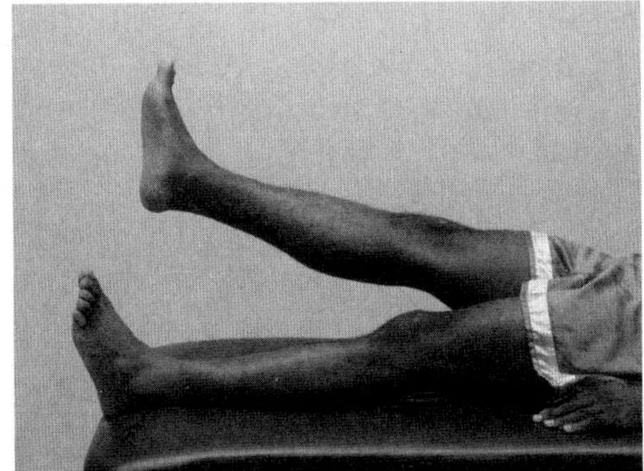
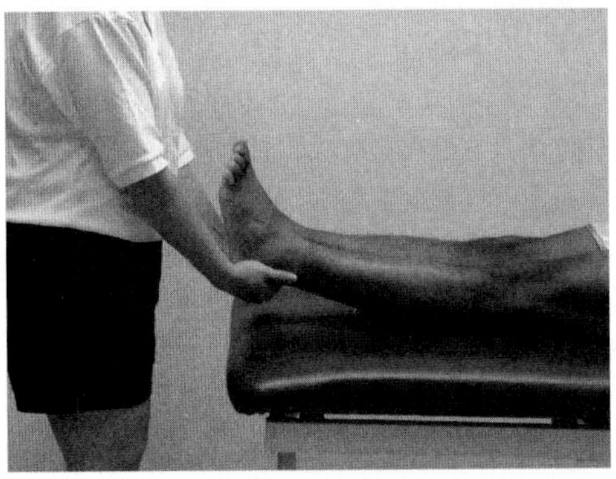
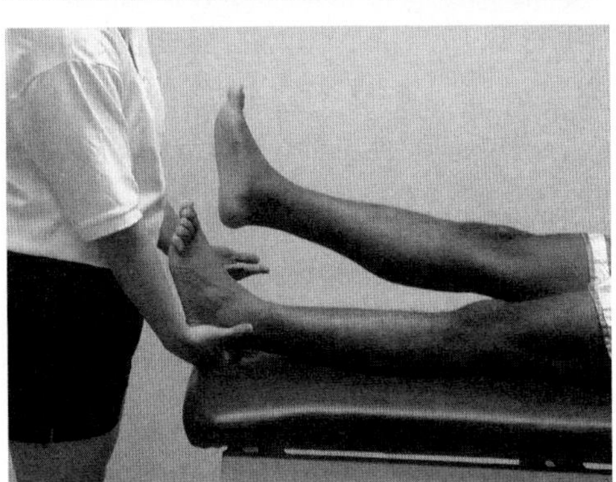

A B

Figure 25-27

A, Milgram straight leg raising test. **B,** Hoover test.

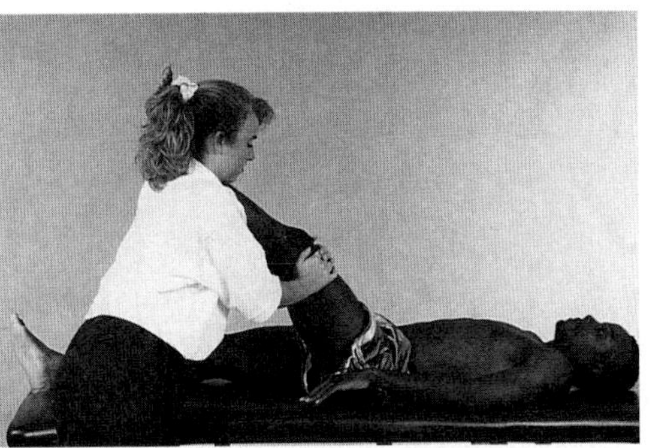

Figure 25-28

Bowstring test for sciatic nerve irritation.

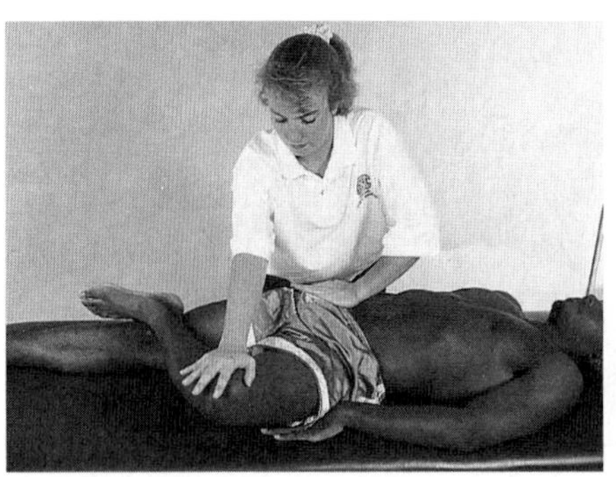

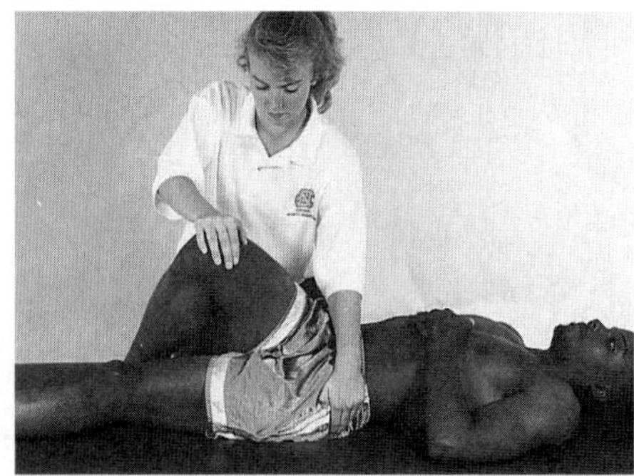

Figure 25-29

A, FABER test (Patrick's test).
B, FADIR test.

To confirm that the pain stems from a nerve root involvement and not from hamstring tightness, the leg is lowered to a point at which pain ceases. In this position, the foot is dorsiflexed and the neck flexed. If pain returns, it is a verification of a pathological condition of the nerve root.

FABER and FADIR tests A FABER (flexion, abduction, external rotation of the hip), or Patrick test, indicates a problem with the hip or sacroiliac joint (Figure 25-29A). A FADIR test (flexion, adduction, internal rotation of the hip) indicates a problem in the lumbar area (Figure 25-29B).

Knees to chest tests Pulling the knees to the chest bilaterally will increase symptoms in the lumbar spine (Figure 25-30A). If pulling a single knee to the chest causes pain in the posterolateral thigh, there may be some irritation to the sacrotuberous ligament (Figure 25-30B). If pain is reported in the area of the PSIS when pulling a single knee to the opposite shoulder, there may be sacroiliac ligament irritation (Figure 25-30C).

SI compression and distraction tests Sacroiliac compression and distraction tests are useful in determining if there is a problem in the sacroiliac joint (Figure 25-31).

Pelvic tilt tests Anterior and posterior pelvic tilts that increase the pain on the side being stressed indicate irritation of the sacroiliac joint (Figure 25-32). Occasionally this test may be done on an athlete in a side-lying position.

Tests Done in a Prone Position

Before performing the following special tests in a prone position, the athletic trainer should palpate a number of structures, feeling for increased tension, attempting to

A

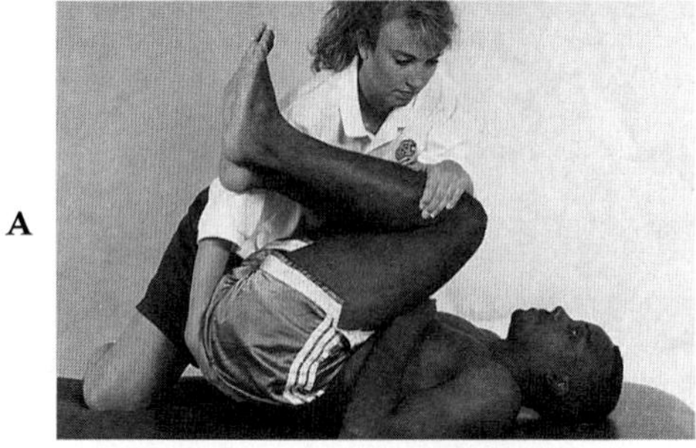

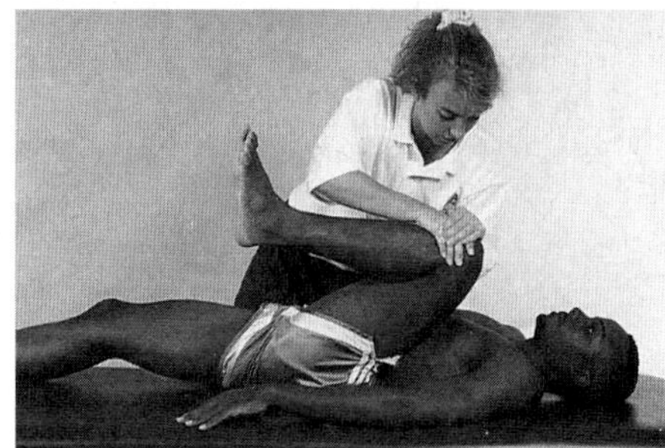

B

C

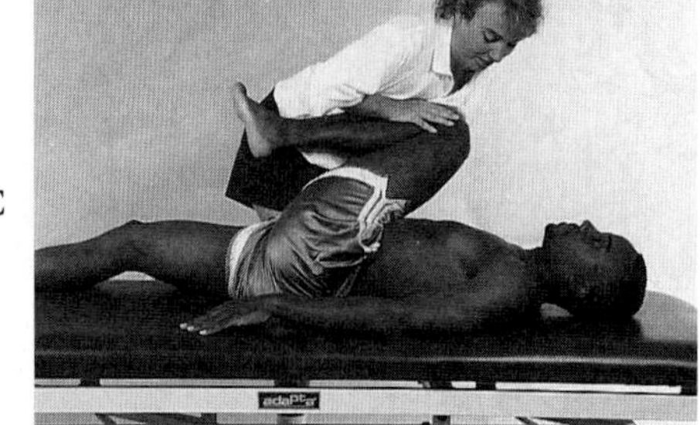

Figure 25-30

A, Bilateral knees to chest.
B, Single knee to chest.
C, Knee to opposite shoulder.

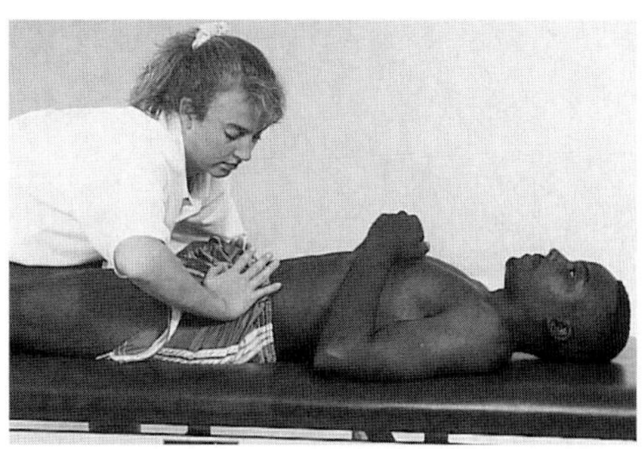
A

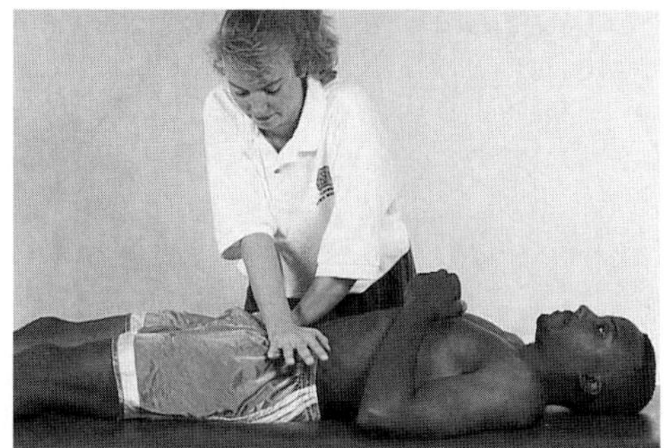
B

Figure 25-31

A, Sacral compression.
B, Sacral distraction.

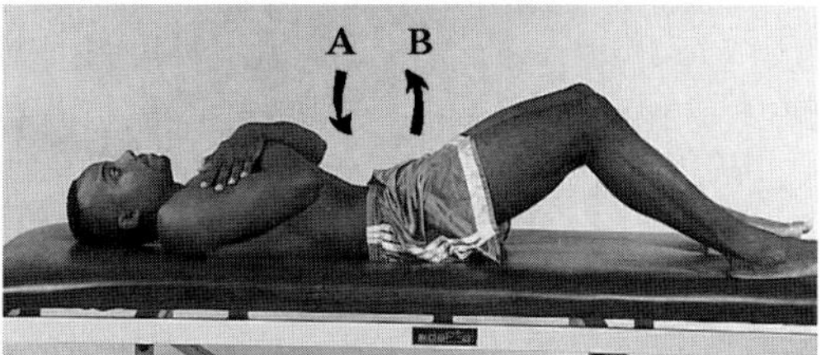

Figure 25-32

A, Anterior pelvic tilt.
B, Posterior pelvic tilt.

provoke a tender pain response, and checking for landmark asymmetries. The structures that are easily palpated in a prone position include the lumbar spinous processes, iliac crests, PSIS, sacrum, trochanters, sacral sulcus, sacrotuberous ligament, sacrospinous ligament, sciatic nerve region, quadratus lumborum, erector spinae, gluteus maximus, gluteus medius, and piriformis.

Press-ups Press-ups, which extend the spine, are done to see if pain radiates into the buttocks or thigh, which may indicate a herniated disk. If pain localizes in this position, conservative care is recommended. If pain is more generalized, surgical care may be required (Figure 25-33).

Reverse straight leg raise test In a reverse straight leg raise, the athlete lies prone and lifts the affected leg. If pain occurs in the low back, an L4 nerve root irritation may be present (Figure 25-34).

Spring test In the spring test, a downward pressure is applied through the spinous process of each vertebra to assess anterior/posterior motion. The spring test can also be done on the transverse process to assess rotational movement. This test can determine either hypermobility or hypomobility of a specific vertebral segment.

Prone knee flexion test A comparison of apparent leg lengths is made with the athlete prone with knees extended and prone with knees flexed to 90 degrees. The leg lengths are compared by inspecting the heels; if there is a short side, that side is indicative of a posterior rotated SI joint. If on flexing the knees, the apparent length of the legs equalizes, this indicates a posteriorly rotated SI joint on that side (Figure 25-35).

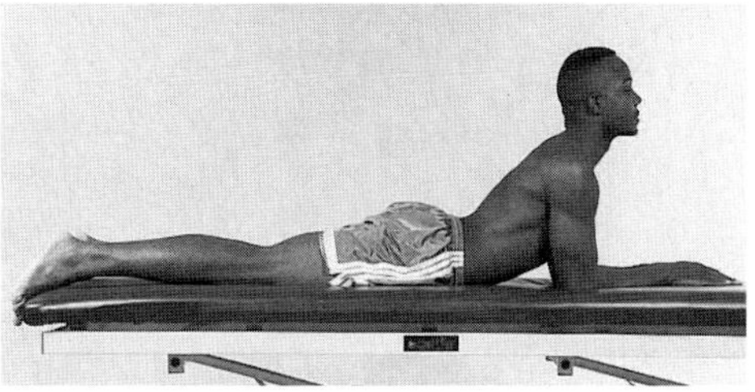

Figure 25-33

Press-ups.

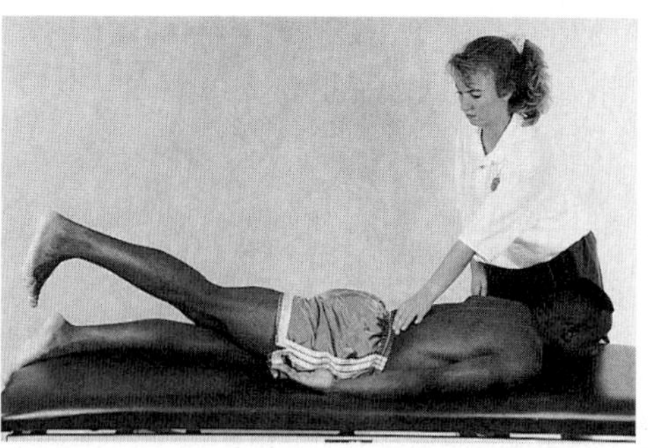

Figure 25-34

Reverse straight leg raise.

Tests Done in a Side-Lying Position

Posterior rotation stress test Pain on movement located near the PSIS indicates irritation in the sacroiliac joint. This does not indicate the direction of the dysfunctional movement, but the pain localizes the problem to a specific side (Figure 25-36).

Iliotibial band stretch test Long-standing SI joint problems sometimes lead to shortness of the iliotibial band and a perpetuation or reoccurrence of the SI problem. This test will often provoke pain in the contralateral PSIS area, indicating an SI problem (Figure 25-37).

Quadratus lumborum stretch test A pillow roll placed under the athlete's waist will side bend the lumbar spine and open the upper quadratus to easy palpation. Dropping the leg off the side of the table while maintaining this position will provide some stretch to the muscle, provoking pain or demonstrating tightness (Figure 25-38).

Piriformis muscle stretch test Flexing both hips to 90 degrees and lifting the top leg places the piriformis muscle in a position of stretch. An increase in pain would indicate tightness or myofascial pain in that muscle (Figure 25-39).

Femoral nerve traction test The femoral nerve traction test is done with the hip extended and the knee flexed to 90 degrees. As the hip is extended, pain occurs in the anterior thigh, which indicates nerve root impingement in the lumbar area. This test may also be done in a prone position (Figure 25-40).

Neurological Exam

The neurological exam was discussed in detail in Chapter 13. In cases in which the spinal cord and associated nerve roots are potentially injured, sensation testing and reflex testing should be a routine aspect of the assessment process.

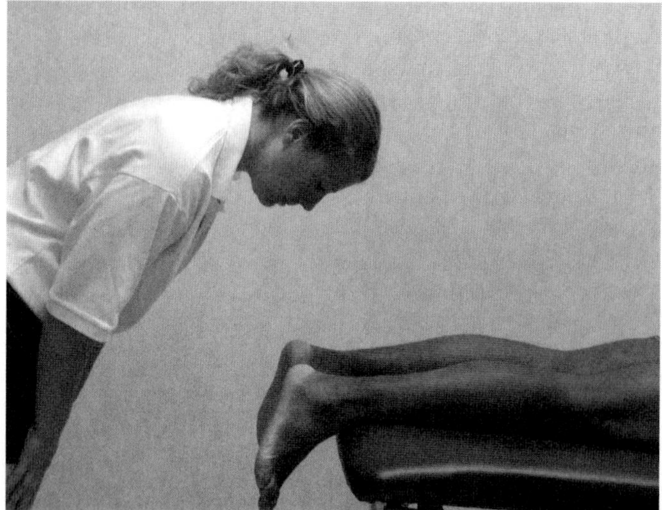

A

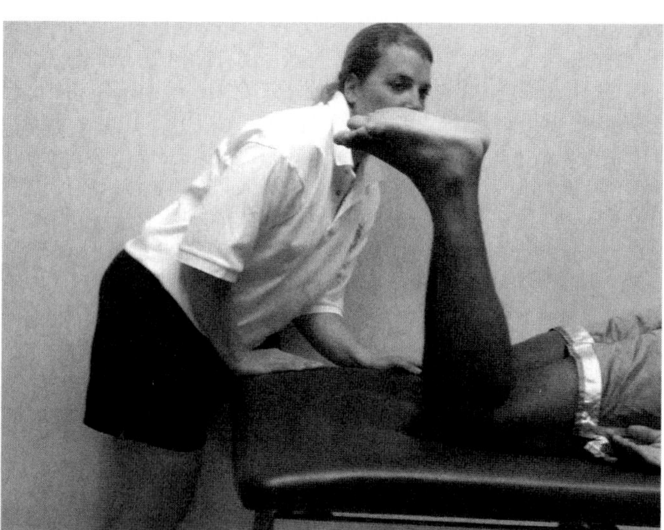

B

Figure 25-35

Prone knee flexion test. **A,** Knees extended. **B,** Knees flexed.

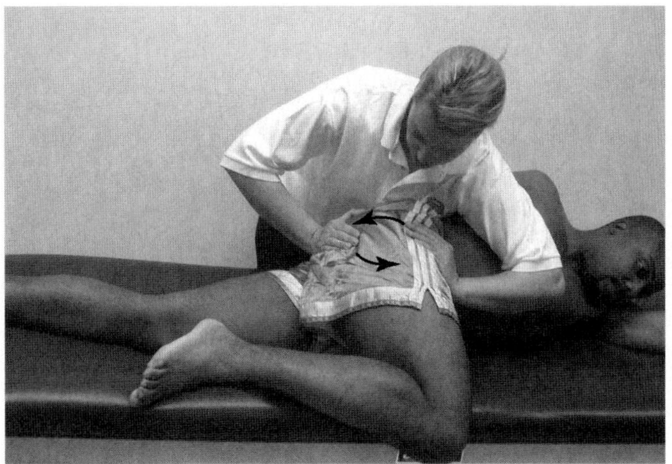

Figure 25-36

Posterior rotation stress test.

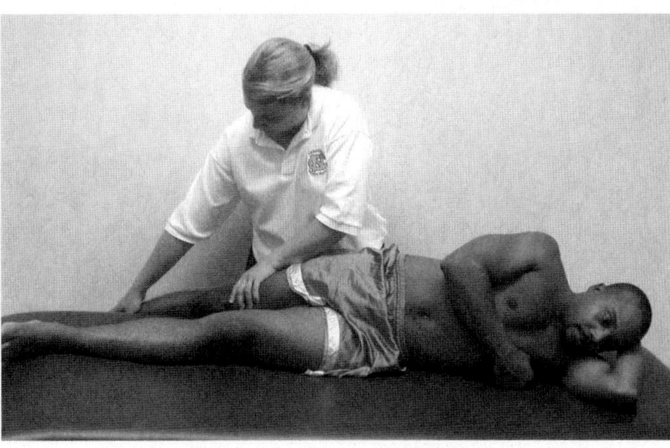

Figure 25-37

Iliotibial band stretch test.

Sensation testing When there is a nerve root involvement, sensation can be partially or completely disrupted in dermatomal patterns. Figures 25-41A and B indicate the locations of general disruption or loss of sensation as a result of cervical and lumbosacral nerve root involvement.

Reflex testing Deep tendon reflexes were discussed in Chapter 13. Three reflexes in the upper extremity are the biceps, brachioradialis, and triceps reflexes. In the biceps reflex, the C5 and C6 nerve roots are being tested. The brachioradialis reflex assesses the C6 nerve root. C7 nerve root dysfunction is indicated by the triceps reflex.

Two reflexes in the lower extremity are the patellar and the Achilles tendon reflexes. A diminished or absent patellar reflex is an indication of an L4 nerve root problem. The Achilles tendon reflex can determine the presence or absence of an S1 nerve root problem.

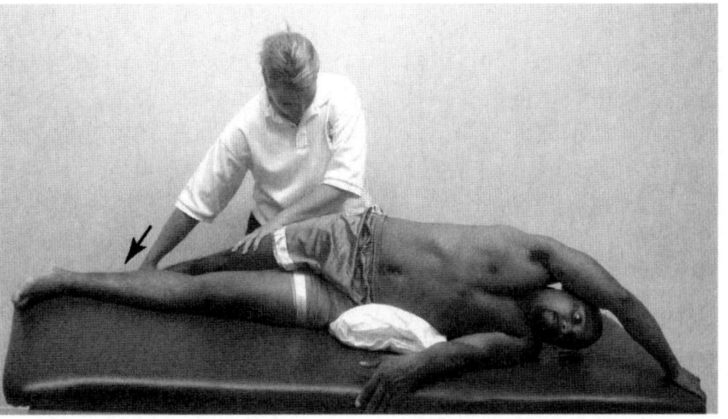

Figure 25-38

Quadratus lumborum stretch test.

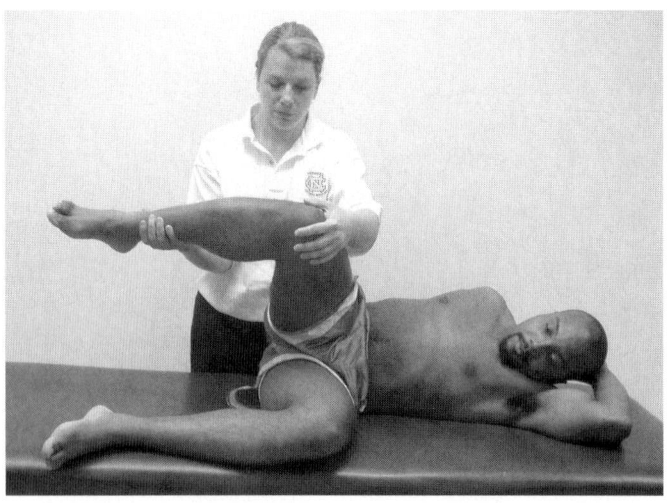

Figure 25-39

Piriformis muscle stretch test.

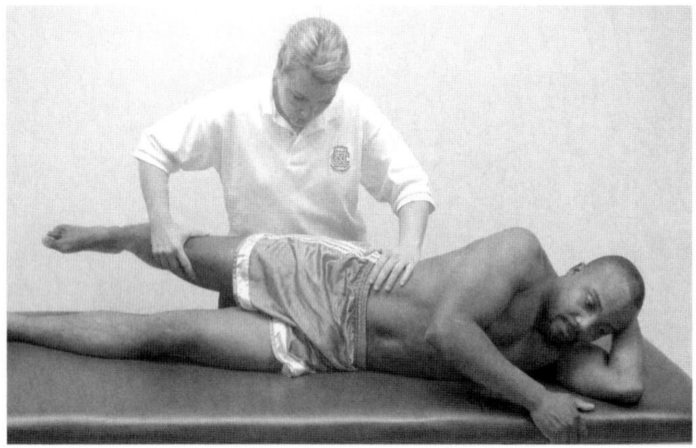

Figure 25-40

Femoral nerve traction test.

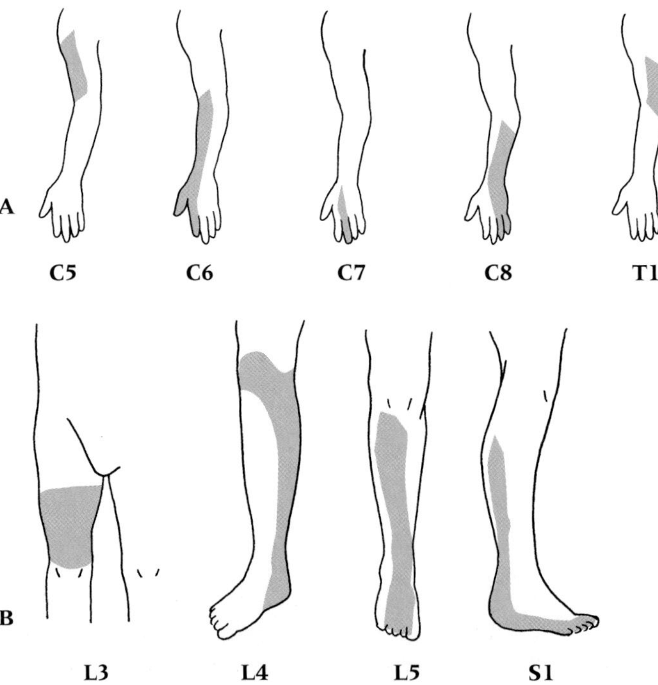

Figure 25-41

Dermatomal patterns of sensation. **A,** Upper extremity. **B,** Lower extremity.

TABLE 25-4 **Special Tests for the Spine**

Test	A Positive Test Indicates
Cervical Spine	
Brachial plexus test	Brachial plexus injury
Cervical compression test	Nerve root impingement
Spurling's test	Nerve root impingement
Vertebral artery test	Occluded cervical vertebral artery
Shoulder abduction test	Nerve root impingement
Lumbar Spine	
Standing Position	
Forward bending	Restriction in PSIS
Backward bending	Disk problem; spondylolysis
Side bending	Herniated disk; SI dysfunction
Stork test	Spondylolysis
Sitting Position	
Forward bending	Restriction in PSIS
Rotation	Asymmetry in lumbar spine
Internal hip rotation	Piriformis injury
Slump test	Increased neural tension
Supine Position	
Straight leg raising 30°	Hip problem; nerve root impingement
Straight leg raising 30–60°	Sciatic nerve; nerve root impingement
Straight leg raising 70–90°	SI joint dysfunction
Kernig's test	Nerve root irritation
Brudzinski's test	Lumbar disk; Nerve root irritation
Well straight leg raising	Nerve root irritation
Milgram straight leg raising	Lumbar disk
Hoover test	Nerve root irritation
Bow string	Sciatic nerve irritation
FABER/Patrick test	SI joint dysfunction
FADIR test	Lumbar strain
Bilateral knees to chest	Lumbar sprain
Single knee to chest	Sacrotuberous ligament sprain
Single knee to opposite shoulder	Sacroiliac ligament sprain
SI joint compression	SI joint dysfunction
SI joint distraction	SI joint dysfunction
Pelvic tilt	SI joint irritation
Prone Position	
Press-ups	Herniated disk
Reverse straight leg raise	L4 nerve root irritation
Spring test	Vertebral hypermobility/hypomobility
Prone knee flexion test	Posteriorly rotated SI joint
Side-Lying Position	
Posterior rotation stress test	SI joint irritation
Iliotibial band stretch test	SI joint irritation
Quadratus lumborum stretch test	Quadratus lumborum tightness
Piriformis muscle stretch test	Piriformis muscle tightness
Femoral nerve traction test	Nerve root irritation

Table 25-4 summarizes the special tests for the spine.

RECOGNITION AND MANAGEMENT OF SPECIFIC INJURIES AND CONDITIONS

Cervical Spine Conditions

Because the neck is so mobile, it is extremely vulnerable to a wide range of sports injuries.[82] Severe sports injury to the neck, although relatively uncommon, can produce catastrophic impairment of the spinal cord (Figure 25-42).[84] The neck can be seriously

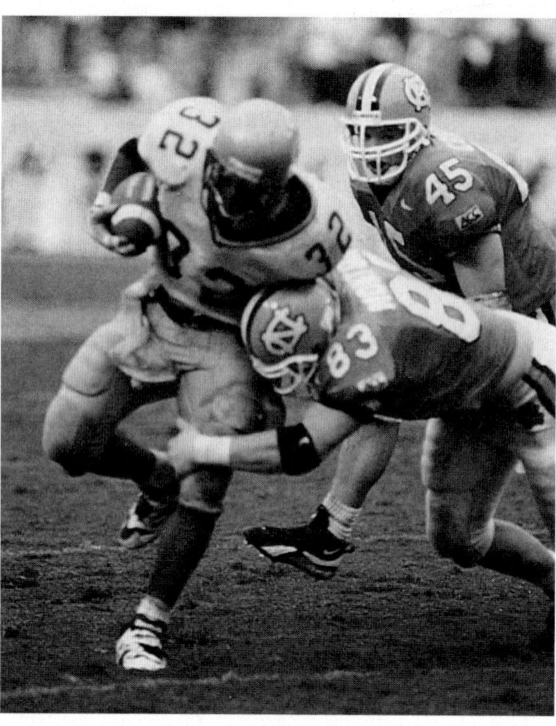

Figure 25-42

The possibility of cervical neck injury, is always present in sports.

injured by the following traumatic events (Figure 25-43): an axial load force to the top of the head, a flexion force, a hyperextension force, a flexion-rotation force, a hyperextension-rotation force, or a lateral flexion force.[74] The neck is also prone to subtle injuries stemming from stress, tension, and postural malalignments.

Cervical Fractures

Etiology Fortunately, the incidence of neck fracture is relatively uncommon in athletics. The spinal cord is well protected by a bony vertebral canal, a connective tissue sheath, fat, and fluid cushioning. Despite this protection, vertebral dislocations and fractures have the potential to result in paralysis. The athletic trainer must con-

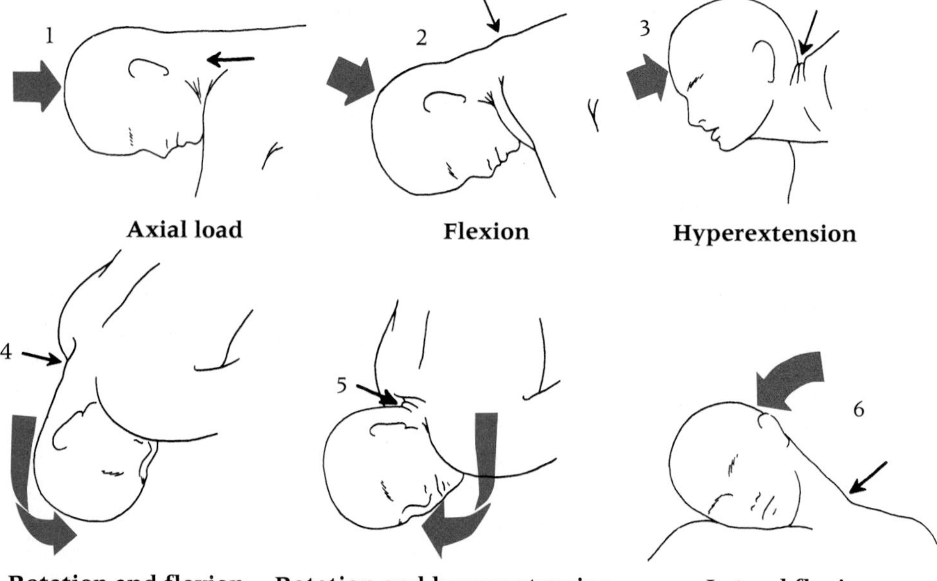

Figure 25-43

Mechanisms of cervical neck injury.

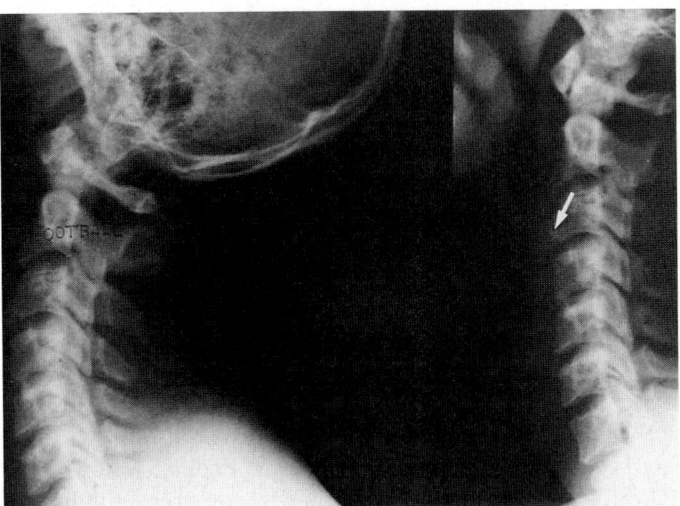

Figure 25-44

Fractures of C3 resulting from a football injury.

stantly be prepared to handle such a situation should it arise. Sports that have the highest incidence of cervical fracture are gymnastics, ice hockey, diving, football, and rugby.[75]

Axial loading of the cervical vertebra from a force to the top of the head combined with flexion of the neck can result in an anterior compression fracture or possibly a dislocation.[73] Fractures are most common in the fourth, fifth, or sixth cervical vertebra. If the head is also rotated when contact is made, a dislocation may occur along with the fracture. Fractures can also occur during a sudden forced hyperextension of the neck (Figure 25-44).

Symptoms and signs The athlete may have one or more of the following signs of cervical fracture: neck point tenderness and restricted movement, cervical muscle spasm, cervical pain and pain in the chest and extremities, numbness in trunk and/or limbs, weakness or paralysis in limbs and/or trunk, loss of bladder and/or bowel control.

Management An unconscious athlete should be treated as if a serious neck injury is present until this possibility is ruled out by the physician.[82] Extreme caution must be used in moving the athlete.[1] The athletic trainer must always be aware that an athlete can sustain a catastrophic spinal injury from improper handling and transportation[19] (see Chapter 12 for *detailed* emergency care of spinal injuries).

Cervical Dislocations

Etiology Cervical dislocations are not common, but they do occur much more frequently in sports than do fractures. Cervical dislocations usually result from violent flexion and rotation of the head. Most injuries of this type happen in pool diving accidents. The mechanism is analogous to the situation that occurs in football when blocks and tackles are poorly executed. The cervical vertebrae are more easily dislocated than are the vertebrae in other spinal regions, principally because of their horizontally arranged articular facets. The superior articular facet moves beyond its normal range of motion and either completely passes the inferior facet (luxation) or catches on its edge (subluxation). The latter is far more common and, as in the case of the complete luxation, most often affects the fourth, fifth, or sixth vertebra.

Symptoms and signs For the most part, a cervical dislocation produces many of the same signs as a fracture. Both can result in considerable pain, numbness, and muscle weakness or paralysis. The most easily discernible difference is the position of the neck in a dislocation: a unilateral dislocation causes the neck to be tilted toward the dislocated side with extreme muscle tightness on the elongated side and a relaxed muscle state on the tilted side.

Management Because a dislocation of a cervical vertebra has a greater likelihood of causing injury to the spinal cord, even greater care must be exercised when moving the patient. Again, the procedures described in Chapter 12 should be applied to cervical dislocations.

Acute Strains of the Neck and Upper Back

Etiology In a strain of the neck or upper back, the athlete has usually turned the head suddenly or has forced flexion, extension, or rotation. Muscles involved are typically the upper trapezius, sternocleidomastoid, the scalenes, and the splenius capitis and cervicis.[43]

Symptoms and signs Localized pain, point tenderness, and restricted motion are present. Muscle guarding resulting from pain is common, and the athlete is reluctant to move the neck in any direction.

Management Care usually includes the use of RICE immediately after the strain occurs and the application of a cervical collar. Follow-up management may include ROM exercises, followed by isometric exercises, and progressing to full-range isotonic strengthening exercises; cryotherapy or superficial heat; and analgesic medications as prescribed by the physician.

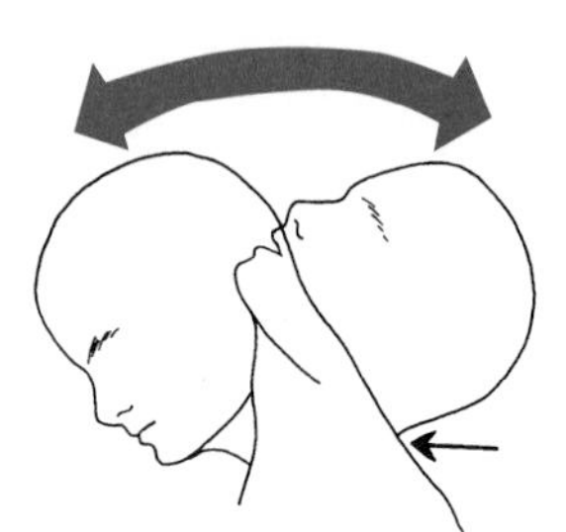

Figure 25-45

Whiplash injury.

Cervical Sprain (Whiplash)

Etiology A cervical sprain can occur from the same mechanism as the strain but usually results from a more violent motion. More commonly, cervical sprain occurs from a sudden snap of the head, such as when the athlete is tackled or blocked while unprepared (Figure 25-45). Frequently, muscle strains occur with ligament sprains. A sprain of the neck produces tears in the major supporting tissue of the anterior or posterior longitudinal ligaments, the interspinous ligament, and the supraspinous ligament.[36]

Symptoms and signs The sprain displays all the signs of the strained neck but the symptoms persist longer. There may also be tenderness over the transverse and spinous processes that serve as sites of attachment for the ligaments.

Pain may not be experienced initially but always appears the day after the trauma. Pain stems from the inflammation of injured tissue and a protective muscle spasm that restricts motion.

Management As soon as possible, the athlete should have a physician evaluation to rule out the possibility of fracture, dislocation, or disk injury.[28] Neurological examination is performed by the physician to ascertain spinal cord or nerve root injury. A soft cervical collar may be applied to reduce muscle spasm. RICE is used for forty-eight to seventy-two hours while the injury is in the acute stage of healing. For an athlete with a severe injury, the physician may prescribe two to three days of bed rest along with analgesics and antiinflammation agents. Therapy might include cryotherapy or heat and massage. Mechanical traction may also be prescribed to relieve pain and muscle spasm.

Acute Torticollis (Wryneck)

Etiology Acute torticollis, a very common condition, is more frequently called wryneck, stiff neck, or occasionally acute cervical joint lock. The athlete usually complains of pain on one side of the neck upon awakening. Wryneck usually occurs when a small piece of synovial membrane lining the joint capsule is impinged or trapped within a facet joint in the cervical vertebra. This problem also can occasionally follow exposure to a cold draft of air or holding of the head in an unusual position over a period of time.

Symptoms and signs During inspection, there is palpable point tenderness and muscle spasm. Head movement is restricted to the side opposite the irritation with marked muscle guarding. X-ray examination will rule out a more serious injury.

Management Various therapeutic modalities may be used to modulate pain in an attempt to break a pain-spasm-pain cycle. Muscle guarding can be reduced through

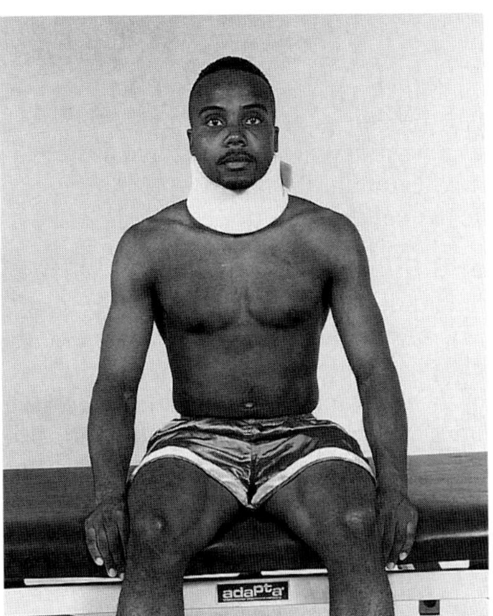

Figure 25-46

A soft collar can make the neck feel more comfortable.

joint mobilizations that involve gentle traction, rotation, and lateral bending, first in the pain-free direction, then in the direction of pain. The athlete may find it helpful to wear a soft cervical collar for comfort (Figure 25-46). This muscle guarding will generally last for two to three days while the athlete progressively regains motion.

Cervical Cord and Nerve Root Injuries

The spinal cord and nerve roots may be injured via four basic mechanisms: laceration by bony fragments, hemorrhage, contusion, and shock.

Etiology The spinal cord and nerve roots may be injured via four basic mechanisms: laceration by bony fragments, hemorrhage (hematomyelia), contusion, and shock. These mechanisms may be combined into a single trauma or may act as separate conditions.

LACERATION Laceration of the cord is usually produced by the combined dislocation and fracture of a cervical vertebra. The jagged edges of the fragmented vertebral body cut and tear nerve roots or the spinal cord and cause varying degrees of paralysis below the point of injury.

HEMORRHAGE Hemorrhage develops from all vertebral fractures and from most dislocations as well as from sprains and strains. It seldom causes harmful effects in the musculature extradurally or even within the arachnoid space, where it dissipates faster than it can accumulate. However, hemorrhage within the cord itself causes irreparable damage.

CONTUSION Contusion in the cord or nerve roots can arise from any force that is applied to the neck violently but does not cause a cervical dislocation or fracture. Such an injury may result from sudden displacement of a vertebra that compresses the cord and then returns to its normal position. This compression causes edematous swelling within the cord, resulting in various degrees of temporary and/or permanent damage.

CERVICAL CORD NEUROPRAXIA Occasionally a situation arises in which an athlete, after receiving a severe twist or snap of the neck, presents all the signs of a spinal cord injury. The athlete is unable to move certain parts of the body and complains of a numbness and a tingling sensation in the arms. After a short while, all these signs leave. The athlete is then able to move the limbs quite freely and has no symptoms other than a sore neck. This condition is considered a cervical cord neuropraxia and is caused by cervical spine stenosis. In such cases, the athlete should be cared for in the same manner used for any severe neck injury.

SPINAL CORD SHOCK Spinal cord shock is usually seen with severe trauma to the spinal cord, most often a cord transaction, in which there is immediate loss of function below the level of the lesion. The limbs are flaccid, in contrast to the later development

Management PLAN

Signs & Symptoms
Management Plan
Therapy
Exercise Rehabilitation

Cervical Sprain (Whiplash)

Injury Situation While at practice, a male ice hockey player was checked hard against the boards. Because he was not properly set for the force, his head was snapped vigorously backward into extension and forward into flexion. In this process the athlete experienced a sudden sharp pain and a tearing sensation at the base of the posterior neck region.

Symptoms and Signs The athlete complained to the athletic trainer that immediately after the injury there was a dull ache, stiffness, and weakness in the neck region. He also complained of headache, dizziness, and nausea approximately 1 hour after the injury.

Palpation revealed severe muscle spasm and point tenderness of the erector spinae muscles and the lateral aspect of the neck and upper shoulder. A neurologic exam did not reveal any changes in motor or sensory abilities. X-ray examination ruled out fracture, dislocation, or spinal cord injury. Gentle passive movement produced some pain. A soft neck collar was applied for immobilization. During further evaluation, there was pain during both gentle active and resistive movement. The condition was considered to be a second-degree neck sprain with muscle involvement produced by a whiplash mechanism.

Management Plan The nature of a neck sprain dictates that management should follow a conservative course. A soft cervical collar was to be worn 24 hours a day for comfort until the athlete was symptom free. Wearing this collar could be followed by wearing the brace just during the waking hours for 1 or 2 additional weeks.

Phase 1 Acute Injury

GOALS: to control initial hemorrhage, swelling, spasm, and pain.
ESTIMATED LENGTH OF TIME (ELT): 2 to 3 days.

- **Therapy** Ice pack (20 min) intermittently 6 to 8 times daily. Transcutaneous electrical nerve stimulation (TENS) was used successfully to reduce spasm and pain in the early stages of injury.
- **Exercise rehabilitation** Athlete should wear soft cervical collar. Athlete should be taught to hold head in good alignment in relation to shoulder and spine; this alignment should be practiced every waking hour. Begin gentle grade 1 and 2 cervical mobilizations as tolerated.

Phase 2 Repair

GOALS: to restore 90% neck range of motion and 50% strength.
ELT: 7 to 11 days.

- **Therapy** Ice pack (5 to 15 min) or ice massage (7 min) 3 or 4 times; precedes active motion.
- **Exercise rehabilitation** Active stretching 2 or 3 times daily, including neck flexion with depressed shoulders, lateral neck flexion, and right and left head rotation; each position should be held 5 to 10 seconds and repeated 5 times or within pain-free limits. Gentle passive static stretching within pain-free limits (2 to 3 times each direction) once daily; each stretch should be held for 20 to 30 seconds. Manual isotonic resistive exercise to the neck should be performed once daily by the athlete or athletic trainer (5 repetitions). Progress to grade 3 and 4 cervical mobilizations as tolerated.

Phase 3 Remodeling

GOALS: to restore full range of motion and full strength. To return to ice hockey competition and full neck muscle bulk.
ELT: 4 to 7 days.

- **Therapy** Ice pack (5 to 15 min) or ice massage (7 min) once daily preceding exercise.
- **Exercise rehabilitation** Continue manual resistive exercise once daily; add resistance devices such as weighted helmet and/or machine neck strengthener (3 sets of 10 repetitions) using DAPRE concept, 3 times a week. Begin practice once daily with a neck roll protective brace during first few weeks of return. Work on maximum neck resistance 3 to 4 times daily.

Continued

Cervical Sprain (Whiplash)—*continued*

Criteria for Return to Competitive Ice Hockey

1. The athlete is completely symptom free.
2. The athlete's head has full range of motion.
3. The athlete's neck has full strength and bulk.

of spasticity. Also there is a total loss of deep tendon reflexes, again in contrast to the later development of hyperreflexia.

Symptoms and signs Each of these situations can result in various types of paralysis that affect the motor and/or sensory systems. The level of the injury obviously will determine the extent of the functional deficits. Spinal cord lesions may be either complete or incomplete. A complete lesion is one in which the spinal cord has been totally severed and there is a complete loss of all motor function and sensation below the level of the injury. Recovery of significant function below the level of the injury is unlikely, although some nerve root function may eventually recover one to two levels below the injury. Complete cord lesions at or above C3 will impair respiration and result in death. Lesions at spinal segment levels below C4 will allow for return of some nerve root function as follows:

- C4–C5—Return of deltoid function
- C5–C6—Return of elbow flexion and wrist extension
- C6–C7—Return of elbow and finger extension and wrist flexion
- C7–T1—Return of grip function

Incomplete lesions can result in central cord syndrome, Brown-Sequard syndrome, anterior cord syndrome, or posterior cord syndrome.[54] Central cord syndrome is caused by hemorrhage or ischemia in the central portion of the cord and results in complete quadriplegia with nonspecific sensory loss and in sexual as well as bowel-bladder dysfunction. Brown-Sequard syndrome is caused by an injury to one side of the spinal cord that results in loss of motor function, touch, vibration, and position sense on one side of the body, and loss of pain and temperature sensation on the other side. Anterior cord syndrome is caused by an injury to the anterior two-thirds of the cord that results in loss of motor function and pain and temperature sensation. However, sexual and bowel-bladder function are present. Posterior cord syndrome, although rare, is caused by injury to the posterior cord. Motor function is completely intact.

Management Like suspected cervical fractures and dislocations, suspected injuries to the spinal cord must be handled with extreme caution. Care must be taken to minimize potential damage to the spinal cord. In cases in which evidence of spinal cord damage accompanied by varying degrees of paralysis exists immediately with injury, management efforts must attempt to minimize additional trauma to the cord.[24] Chapter 12 presents a detailed discussion of the recommended procedures for managing athletes with suspected spinal cord injury.

Cervical Spine Stenosis

Etiology Cervical spine stenosis is a syndrome characterized by a narrowing of the spinal canal in the cervical region that can impinge the spinal cord. This stenosis occurs either as a congenital variation or from some change in the vertebrae, including the development of bone spurs, osteophytes, or disc bulges. There are two methods of determining cervical spinal stenosis: the Torg ratio and the space available for the cord

(SAC).[69] The Torg ratio is determined by dividing the sagittal spinal-canal diameter by the corresponding sagittal vertebral-body diameter. The SAC is determined by subtracting the sagittal spinal-cord diameter from the corresponding sagittal spinal-canal diameter. The Torg ratio and SAC are measured in millimeters. The SAC measure relies more on the spinal canal compared with the Torg ratio and, therefore, may be a more effective indicator of spinal stenosis. This is relevant clinically because neurologic injury related to stenosis is a function of the spinal canal and the spinal cord and not the vertebral body.[69] A ratio of the sagittal canal diameter relative to anteroposterior width of the same vertebrae at its midpoint of less than .80 suggests cervical stenosis.[75]

Symptoms and signs Transient quadriplegia may occur from axial loading, hyperextension, or hyperflexion. Neck pain may be absent initially. The symptoms may be purely sensory with burning or tingling, or the athlete may have some associated motor weakness in either the arms or the legs or all four extremities.[81] Complete recovery normally occurs within ten to fifteen minutes but may be delayed. Following neurologic recovery, full neck ROM is possible.

25-6 Critical Thinking Exercise

A football linebacker is making a tackle and makes initial contact with the ball carrier with his head, forcing the neck into hyperflexion. The athlete immediately has transcient quadriplegia with burning and tingling and associated motor weakness in the arms and legs. Neck pain is absent initially. Within fifteen minutes, the athlete recovers completely and has full range of motion.

? What type of injury should the athletic trainer suspect with this athlete, and how should this condition be managed?

Management Cervical spine stenosis may be present without any symptoms and signs. The presence of transient quadriplegia necessitates extreme caution initially. The athlete must have diagnostic tests, including X rays or MRI to determine the extent of the problem. Athletes, particularly those in contact sports, who have been identified as having some degree of cervical stenosis should be advised of the potential risks of continued participation in that sport. There is a growing consensus among physicians that continued participation should be discouraged.[9]

Brachial Plexus Neurapraxia (Burner)

Etiology Transient neuropraxia, resulting from stretching or compression of the brachial plexus, is the most common of all cervical neurological injuries in the athlete.[54] Neurapraxia involves a disruption in normal function of a peripheral nerve without any degenerative changes.[78] Other terms commonly used to indicate this condition are *stinger, burner,* or *pinched nerve.*[77] The primary mechanism of injury is stretching of the brachial plexus when the neck is forced laterally to the opposite side while the shoulder is depressed, as would occur with a shoulder block in football. A second mechanism compresses the brachial plexus when the neck is extended, compressed, and rotated toward the affected side.

An injury mimicking the stretch palsy is the direct injury to the upper brachial plexus from the edge of the shoulder pads impacting this area. The tip-off here is that there is usually exquisite tenderness over the trapezius and the rhomboid muscles are spared, if there is associated weakness.

Symptoms and signs With the common burner or stinger, the athlete usually comes off the field with pain and numbness, radiating into all fingers of the hand. This implies involvement of, at least, cervical roots 6, 7, and 8. But if there is associated weakness (most of the time there isn't) it is limited to the deltoid and biceps/brachialis muscles (especially the deltoid) implicating the C5 root. Therefore, if there is no weakness of the deltoid on on-field testing, the athlete can return to play when asymptomatic.

25-7 Critical Thinking Exercise

An ice hockey player reports to the athletic trainer for preseason screenings and describes a history of stingers.

? What is a stinger and what are the symptoms associated with this injury?

The player complains of a burning sensation, numbness and tingling, and pain extending from the shoulder down to the hand, with some loss of function of the arm and hand that lasts for several minutes.[32] Rarely, symptoms may persist for several days. Neck range of motion is usually normal. Repeated brachial plexus nerve stretch injuries may result in neuritis, muscular atrophy, and permanent damage.[41]

Management Once the symptoms have completely resolved and there are no associated neurological symptoms, the athlete may return to full activity. Thereafter the athlete should begin strengthening and stretching exercises for the neck musculature.[46] A football player should be fitted with shoulder pads and a cervical neck roll to limit neck range of motion during impact.[79]

Cervical Disk Injuries

Etiology Herniation of a cervical disk is relatively common and can affect athletes in any sport. A herniation usually develops from an extruded posterolateral disk fragment or from degeneration of the disk. The primary mechanism involves sustained repetitive cervical loading during contact sports.

Symptoms and signs The symptoms and signs include neck pain with some restriction in neck motion. There is radicular pain (nerve root) in the upper extremity with associated motor weakness or sensory changes.

Management Initial treatment involves rest and immobilization of the neck to decrease discomfort. Neck mobilizations may help the athlete regain some range of motion. Cervical traction may also help reduce symptoms. If conservative treatment is not helpful or if the neurologic deficits increase, surgery may be necessary.

Thoracic Spine Conditions

Injuries to the thoracic region of the spine have a much lower rate of incidence than do injuries to the cervical or lumbar regions. This lower rate of injury is due to the articulation of the thoracic vertebrae with the ribs, which acts to stabilize and limit motion of the vertebrae and thus minimizes the likelihood of injury to this area. Thoracic fractures, therefore, are relatively rare and occur in high-impact sports such as skiing, tobogganing, skydiving, or automobile racing.

Scheuermann's Disease (Dorsolumbar Kyphosis)

Etiology Scheuermann's disease is characterized by kyphosis that results from wedge fractures of 5 degrees or greater in three or more consecutive vertebral bodies with associated disk space abnormalities and irregularity of the epiphyseal endplates.[57] This degeneration allows the disk's nucleus pulposus to prolapse into a vertebral body. Characteristically, there is an accentuation of the kyphotic curve and backache in the young athlete. Adolescents engaging in sports such as gymnastics and swimming—the butterfly stroke particularly—are prone to this condition. Scheuermann's disease is idiopathic, but the occurrence of multiple minor injuries to the vertebral epiphyses seems to be an etiological factor. These injuries apparently disrupt circulation to the epiphyseal endplate, causing avascular necrosis.

Symptoms and signs In the initial stages, the young athlete will have kyphosis of the thoracic spine and lumbar lordosis without back pain. In later stages, there is point tenderness over the spinous processes, and the young athlete may complain of backache at the end of a very physically active day. Hamstring muscles are characteristically very tight.

Management The major goal of management is to prevent progressive kyphosis. In the early stages of the disease, extension exercises and postural education are beneficial. Bracing, rest, and antiinflammatory medication may also be helpful. The athlete may stay active but should avoid aggravating movements.

Lumbar Spine Conditions

Mechanisms of Low Back Pain

Pain in the low back is second only to foot problems in order of incidence in humans throughout their life span.[50] In sports, back problems are relatively common and are most often the result of either congenital or idiopathic (i.e., mechanical or traumatic) causes.[4] Congenital back disorders are conditions that are present at birth. Many authorities think that the human back is still undergoing structural changes as a result of its upright position and, therefore, humans are prone to slight spinal defects at birth that may cause pain later in life. The usual cause of back pain among athletes is overuse that produces strains and/or sprains of paravertebral muscles and ligaments.

Low back problems are most often either congenital or idiopathic.

Congenital anomalies Anomalies of bony development are the underlying cause of many back problems in sports. Such conditions would have remained undiscovered had it not been for some abnormal stress or injury in the area of the anomaly. The most common causes of these anomalies are excessive length of the transverse process of the fifth lumbar vertebra, incomplete closure of the neural arch (spina bifida occulta), nonconformities of the spinous processes, atypical lumbosacral angles or articular facets, and incomplete closures of the vertebral laminae. All these anomalies may

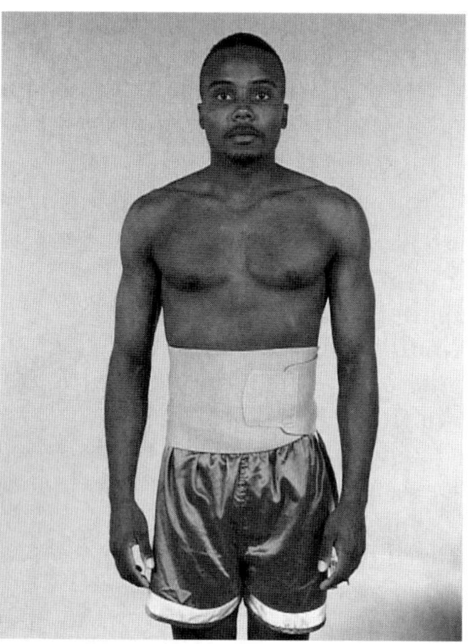

Figure 25-48

An abdominal brace helps support the lumbar area.

Management In the acute phase of this injury, it is essential that cold packs and/or ice massage be used intermittently throughout the day to decrease muscle spasm. An elastic wrap or corset-type brace will help to compress the area. A graduated program of stretching and strengthening begins slowly during the acute stage. Progressive strengthening exercises should concentrate on extension, whereas stretching should focus on both flexion and extension. Injuries of moderate-to-severe intensity may require complete bed rest to help break the pain–muscle spasm cycle. The physician may prescribe oral analgesic medication. Cryotherapy, ultrasound, and an abdominal support (Figure 25-48) are often beneficial following the acute phase. Exercise must not cause pain.

Myofascial Pain Syndrome

Etiology Myofascial pain syndrome is defined as a regional pain with referred pain to a specific area that occurs with pressure or palpation of tender spots or trigger points within a specific muscle.[36] A trigger point is an area of tenderness in a tight band of muscle. Palpation of the trigger point produces pain in a predictable distribution of referred pain.[52] There may also be some restricted range of motion because of pain. Pressure on the trigger point produces a twitch or jump response from the pain. Pain can be increased by passive or active stretching of the involved muscle. In the athlete, painful or active trigger points most often develop because of some mechanical stress to the muscle. This stress could involve either an acute muscle strain or static postural positions that produce constant tension in the muscle.[20] Trigger points occur most typically in the neck, upper back, and lower back. In the lower back, there are two muscles in which trigger points commonly occur: the piriformis and the quadratus lumborum.

The piriformis muscle was discussed in Chapter 21. It is an external rotator of the thigh and is located posterior to the hip joint in the sciatic notch. The piriformis muscle is important because of its proximity to the sciatic nerve. The sciatic nerve either pierces the piriformis or courses directly above or below it.

The quadratus lumborum originates on the twelfth rib and the transverse processes of L1 through L4. It inserts on the iliac crest. The quadratus elevates the pelvis.

Symptoms and signs Palpation of or pressure on a trigger point in the piriformis muscle in the sciatic notch refers pain to the posterior sacroiliac region, to the buttocks, and occasionally down to the posterior or posterolateral thigh. Pain is a deep ache that increases with exercise or with prolonged sitting while the hip is adducted,

Management PLAN

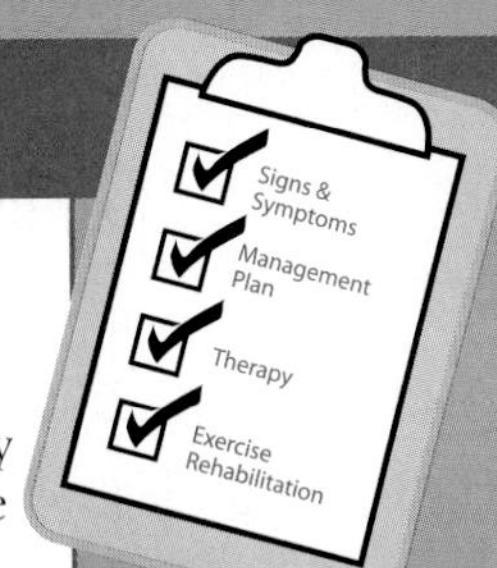

Lumbosacral Strain

Injury Situation A high school shot-putter came into the athletic training room complaining of a very sore back. He indicated that he woke up with the problem and was not sure how it occurred. Perhaps he had hurt it by doing dead lifts the day before or by throwing the shot incorrectly.

Symptoms and Signs The athlete complained of a constant dull ache and an inability to flex, extend, or rotate the trunk without increasing the pain. Inspection of the injury indicated the following:

1. The athlete had a pronounced lumbar lordosis.
2. There was an obvious muscle contraction of the right erector spinae.
3. There was severe point tenderness in the right lumbar region.
4. The right pelvis was elevated.
5. Passive movement did not cause pain; however, active and resistive movements produced severe pain.
6. Range of movement in all directions was restricted.
7. All tests for nerve root, hip joint, and sacroiliac joint were negative.
8. Leg length was measured, and the athlete had a functional shortening but no apparent structural shortening.
9. Both the left and right hamstring muscle groups and iliopsoas muscles were abnormally tight.
10. X-ray examination showed no pathological conditions of the lumbar vertebrae.

Based on the examination, it was concluded that the athlete had sustained a first- to second-degree strain of the lumbar muscles, primarily in the right erector spinae region.

Phase 1 *Acute Injury*

GOALS: to relieve muscle spasm and pain.
ESTIMATED LENGTH OF TIME (ELT): 2 or 3 days.

■ **Therapy** Ice pack (20 min) followed by exercise and then by TENS (15 to 20 min) 3 to 4 times daily.

■ **Exercise rehabilitation** Following cold application, gentle passive stretch of low back region and hamstring and iliopsoas muscles—all within pain tolerance levels—3 to 4 times daily, along with grade 1 and 2 mobilization of affected segments.

Phase 2 *Repair*

GOALS: to increase low back, hamstring, and iliopsoas rom to at least begin postural correction. 50% normal extensibility of the low back, hamstring, and iliopsoas muscles. Appropriate abdominal strength.
ELT: 4 to 12 days.

■ **Therapy** Ice massage followed by exercise 2 to 3 times daily. If still painful, TENS therapy should be used. Ultrasound 1 to 1.5 watts/cm^2 once daily.

■ **Exercise rehabilitation** Repeat Phase 1 exercise and begin PNF to hip and low back regions 2 to 3 times daily; or static low back, hamstring, and iliopsoas stretching (2 to 3 repetitions) and lower abdominal strengthening 2 to 3 times daily. Continue grade 1 and 2 mobilizations, progressing to grades 3 and 4 as tolerated. Practice realigning pelvis. General body maintenance exercises should be conducted (as long as they do not aggravate the injury) 3 times a week.

Phase 3 *Remodeling*

GOALS: To restore 90% of ROM, strength, and proper back alignment.

■ **Exercise rehabilitation** Return to weight training and shot put program 3 times a week. Athlete should be instructed about proper back alignment when throwing the shot. Athlete should avoid dead lifting and should wear a lifting belt while weight training. Athlete should begin a spinal stabilization program. Return to normal training 3 times a week. Gradual reentry into competition. Using an abdominal support belt is advisable during practice and competition.

Continued

Lumbosacral Strain—*continued*

Criteria for Return to Competitive Shot Put

1. The athlete's back must be pain free and spasm free.
2. The athlete must be near normal in hamstring, low back, and iliopsoas extensibility.
3. The athlete must be making good progress toward correcting lumbar lordosis.
4. The athlete must be able to perform the shot put with the spine and pelvis in good alignment.

flexed, and medially rotated. Isometric abduction and passive internal rotation will increase pain. Sciatic pain may also occur with diminished sensation in the leg.

A trigger point in the quadratus lumborum produces a sharp, aching pain in the lateral lower back or flank. Pain may be referred to the upper buttocks and posterior sacroiliac region and sometimes to the abdominal wall. Pain increases when the athlete stands for long periods, moves from sitting to standing, or coughs or sneezes. There will be muscle spasm with pain that is localized to one side. Pain increases when the athlete side bends toward the side of the trigger point.

25-8

***Critical Thinking* Exercise**

A swimmer complains of an area of tenderness in a tight band of muscle in the middle of her upper back. Palpation of the trigger point refers pain around the chest wall. Pain is increased by both passive and active stretching of the involved muscle. Pain is usually increased following a long training workout in the pool.

? What type of muscular problem frequently develops in the middle or low back of athletes who engage in repetitive motions that fatigue a muscle? How is this problem best managed?

Management Rehabilitation exercises should include both stretching and strengthening of the involved muscle. The key in treating myofascial pain is to stretch the muscle back to a normal resting length and thus relieve the irritation that created the trigger point.[23] The athlete should be placed in a comfortable position that also stretches the involved muscle. Active stretching should be mild and progressive. The use of electrical stimulation in combination with ultrasound is helpful in relieving the pain associated with a trigger point. A spray and stretch technique has also been used successfully (see Chapter 15). Progressive strengthening exercises should also be included.

Lumbar Sprains

Etiology Sprains may occur in any of the ligaments in the lumbar spine. The most common sprain involves lumbar facet joints. Facet joint sprain typically occurs when the athlete bends forward and twists while lifting or moving some object. A traumatic force overextends the spinal joints and causes a sudden onset of a deep, sharp pain. It can occur with a single episode or with chronic repetitive stress that causes a gradual onset that becomes progressively worse with activity.

Symptoms and signs The pain is localized and is located just lateral to the spinous process. Pain becomes sharper with certain movements or postures, and the athlete will limit movement in painful ranges. Passive anteroposterior or rotational movement of the vertebrae will increase pain. Pain can be reproduced with certain movements.

Management Like sprains to other joints in the body, the lumbar sprain will require some time to heal. Initial treatment should include RICE to reduce pain. Joint mobilizations that use anteroposterior and rotational glides can be used to help decrease pain. Strengthening exercises for abdominals and back extensors as well as stretches in all directions should be limited to a pain-free range. The athlete should be instructed in trunk stabilization exercises. A brace or support should be worn to limit movement during early return to activity. It is important to guard against the development of postural changes that may occur in response to pain.

Back Contusions

Etiology Back contusions rank second to strains and sprains in incidence. Because of its surface area, the back is quite vulnerable to bruises in sports. Football produces the greatest number of these injuries. A history that includes a significant impact to the back could indicate an extremely serious condition. Contusion of the back must be distinguished from a vertebral fracture. In some instances, this distinction is possible only through an X-ray examination.

Symptoms and signs The bruise causes local pain, muscle spasm, and point tenderness. A swollen, discolored area may be visible also.

Management Cold and pressure should be applied immediately for approximately seventy-two hours or longer, along with rest. Ice massage combined with gradual stretching benefits soft-tissue contusion in the region of the lower back. Recovery usually ranges from two days to two weeks. Ultrasound is effective in treating the deep muscles.

Sciatica

Etiology Sciatica is an inflammatory condition of the sciatic nerve that can accompany recurrent or chronic low back pain. The term *sciatica* has been incorrectly used as a general term to describe all low back pain without reference to exact causes. Sciatica is commonly associated with peripheral nerve root compression from intervertebral disk protrusion, structural irregularities within the intervertebral foramina, or tightness of the piriformis muscle. The sciatic nerve is particularly vulnerable to torsion or direct blows that tend to impose abnormal stretching and pressure on it as it emerges from the spine, thus effecting a traumatic condition.[34]

Symptoms and signs Sciatica may begin either abruptly or gradually. It produces a sharp shooting pain that follows the nerve pathway along the posterior and medial thigh. There may also be some tingling and numbness along its path. The nerve may be extremely sensitive to palpation. Straight leg raising usually intensifies the pain.

Management In the acute stage, rest is essential. The cause of the inflammation must be identified and treated. If there is a disk protrusion, lumbar traction may be appropriate. Stretching of a tight piriformis muscle may also decrease symptoms. Since recovery from sciatica usually occurs within two to three weeks, surgery should be delayed to see if symptoms resolve. Oral antiinflammatory medication may help reduce inflammation.

Herniated Lumbar Disk

Etiology The lumbar disks are subject to constant abnormal stresses that stem from faulty body mechanics, trauma, or both, which, over a period of time, can cause degeneration, tears, and cracks in the annulus fibrosus.[14] The disk most often injured lies between the L4–L5 vertebrae. The L5–S1 disk is the second most commonly affected.

A herniated lumbar disk can be prolapsed, extruded, or sequestrated.

In sports, the mechanism of a disk injury is the same as for the lumbosacral sprain—forward bending and twisting that places abnormal strain on the lumbar region. The movement that produces herniation or bulging of the nucleus pulposus may be minimal, and associated pain may be significant.[25] Besides injuring soft tissues, such a stress may herniate an already degenerated disk by causing the nucleus pulposus to protrude into or through the annulus fibrosis (Figure 25-49). A disk that progressively degenerates may develop into a *prolapsed disk,* in which the nucleus moves completely through the annulus. If the nucleus moves into the spinal canal and comes in contact with a nerve root, the result is an *extruded disk.* This protrusion of the nucleus pulposus may place pressure on the cord of spinal nerves and thus cause radiating pains similar to those of sciatica. A *sequestrated disk* occurs when the material of the nucleus separates from the disk and begins to migrate.

Pressure within the intervertebral disks changes with various positions or postures. Studies that used intervertebral pressure in the standing position as a constant found that pressure was decreased by 75 percent when the spine was in the supine position and by 25 percent when the spine was in the side-lying position. Pressure was increased by 33 percent while the athlete was sitting, by 33 percent while the athlete was standing slightly bent forward, by 45 percent while the athlete was sitting slightly

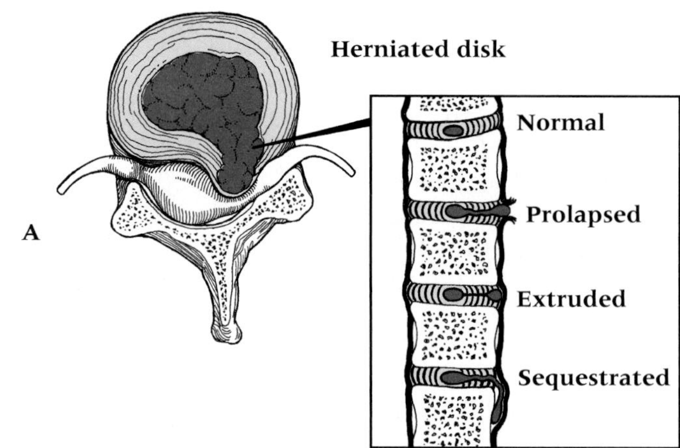

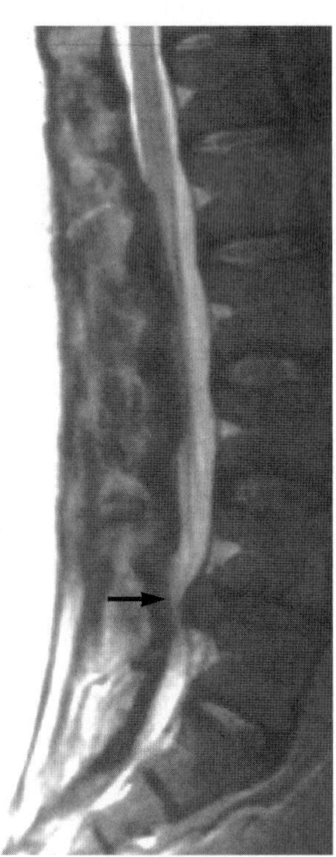

Figure 25-49

A herniated lumbar disk. **A,** Further degeneration can lead to a prolapsed disk, an extruded disk, or a sequestrated disk. **B,** MRI image of a lumbar herniated disk.

bent forward, 52 percent while the athlete was standing bent far forward, and 63 percent while the athlete was sitting bent well forward.

Symptoms and signs There is usually a sharp, centrally located pain that radiates unilaterally in a dermatomal pattern to the buttocks and down the back of the leg, or pain that spreads across the back. The athlete may describe weakness in the lower limb. Symptoms are worse in the morning with axial loading such as when the athlete gets out of bed. Onset may be sudden or gradual, and pain may increase after the athlete sits and then tries to resume activity. Forward bending and sitting increases pain. Backward bending reduces pain. The athlete's posture will exhibit a slight forward bend with side bending away from the side of pain. Side bending toward the side of pain is limited and increases pain. There is tenderness around the painful area. Straight leg raising to 30 degrees increases pain. Tendon reflexes may be diminished. Muscle testing may reveal weakness with bilateral differences. A Valsalva maneuver increases the pain (i.e., coughing, sneezing, etc.). The athlete has difficulty putting on shoes and socks.

Management Initial treatment should involve pain-reducing modalities such as ice or electrical stimulation. Manual traction combined with passive backward bending or extension makes the athlete more comfortable. The goal is to reduce the protrusion and restore normal posture. Thus, the athlete should be taught appropriate posture self-correction exercises. As pain and posture return to normal, back extensor and abdominal strengthening should be used.[18]

If the disk is extruded or sequestrated, all the athletic trainer can do is to modulate pain with electrical stimulation. Flexion exercises and lying supine in a flexed position may help with comfort. Sometimes the symptoms will resolve with time. But if there are signs of nerve damage, surgery may be required to eliminate pain and dysfunction.[87]

Spondylolysis and Spondylolisthesis

Etiology Spondylolysis refers to a degeneration of the vertebrae and, more commonly, a defect in the pars interarticularis of the articular processes of the vertebrae (Figure 25-50).[37] The condition is often attributed to a congenital weakness, and the defect occurs as a stress fracture.[45] It is more common among boys.[39] Spondylolysis may produce no symptoms unless a disk herniation occurs or there is sudden trauma such as hyperextension.[62] Sports movements that characteristically hyperextend the spine, such as the back arch in gymnastics, the lifting of weights, the football block, the tennis serve, the volleyball spike, and the butterfly stroke in swimming[49], are most likely to cause this condition.

Commonly, spondylolysis begins unilaterally. If it extends bilaterally, however, there may be some slipping of one vertebra on the one below it. This condition, called a

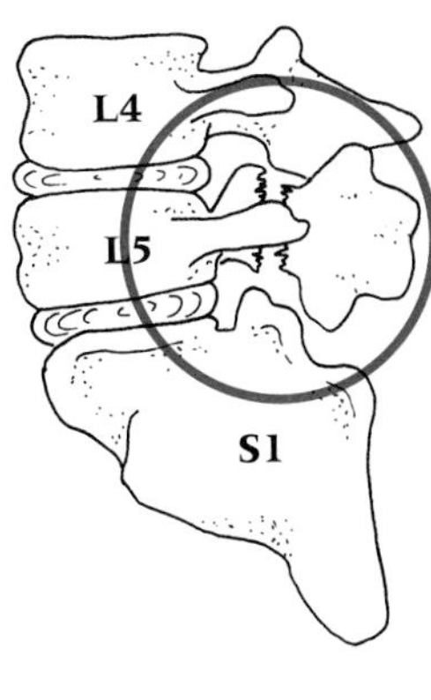

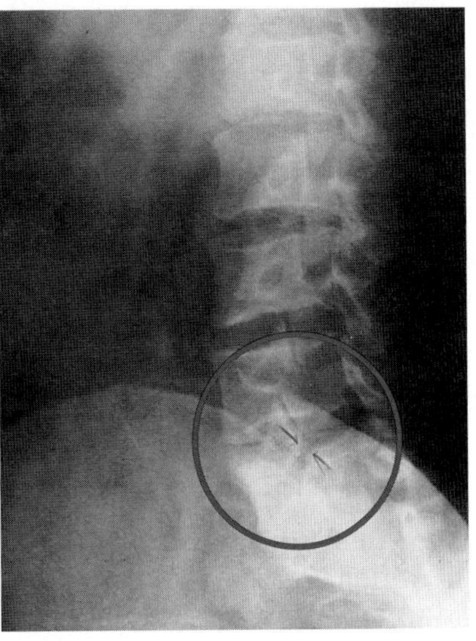

Figure 25-50

Spondylolysis of L5.

spondylolisthesis, is considered to be a complication of spondylolysis that often results in hypermobility of a vertebral segment, called a step deformity.[34] Spondylolisthesis's highest incidence is with L5 slipping on S1 (Figure 25-51).[72] Although pars interarticularis defects are more common among boys, the incidence of slippage is higher in girls. It is possible that a spondylolisthesis may be asymptomatic.[45] The athlete with this condition will usually have a lumbar hyperlordosis postural impairment. A direct blow or sudden twist or chronic low back strain may cause the defective vertebra to displace itself forward on the sacrum. A spondylolisthesis is easily detectable on X ray.

Spondylolisthesis is considered to be a complication of spondylolysis.

Symptoms and signs The athlete complains of persistent mild to moderate aching pain across the low back or a stiffness in the low back with increased pain after, but not usually during, physical activity. There is usually a complaint that the low back area feels tired and fatigues easily. The athlete feels the need to change positions frequently or to self-manipulate the low back to reduce the pain. Movements of the trunk are full range and painless with some hesitation in forward bending. At extreme ranges held for thirty seconds, an aching pain develops. The athlete feels weak when

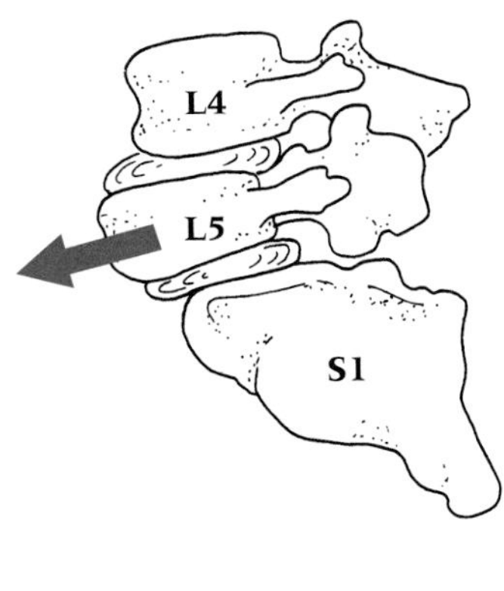

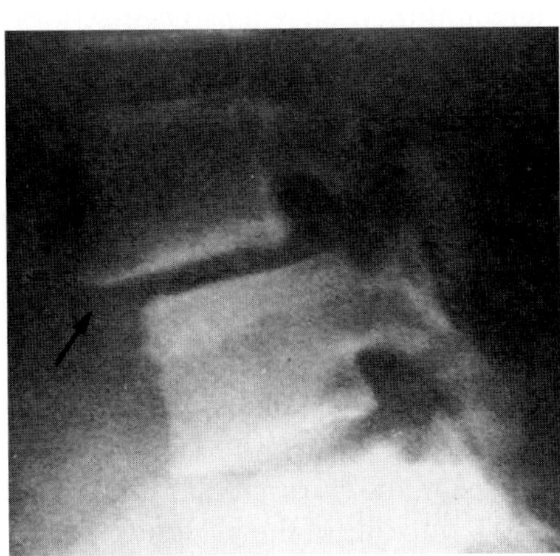

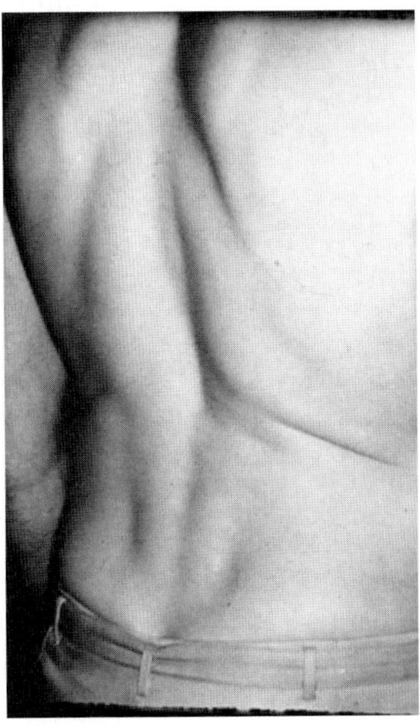

Figure 25-51

Spondylolisthesis.

25-9

Critical Thinking Exercise

A gymnast constantly hyperextends her low back. She complains of stiffness and persistent aching pain across the low back with increased pain after, but not usually during, practice. The athlete feels that she needs to change positions frequently or self-manipulate her low back to reduce the pain. She is beginning to develop pain in her buttock and some muscle weakness in her leg.

? What type of injury should the athletic trainer suspect the gymnast has, and what can be done about it?

straightening from forward bending. There may be tenderness localized to one segment. When applying posteroanterior pressure to the spinous process during palpation, the athletic trainer may note some segmental hypermobility. If displacement is great enough, there may be some neurological signs.

Management Bracing and, occasionally, bed rest for one to three days will help reduce pain. The major focus in rehabilitation should be directed toward exercises that control or stabilize the hypermobile segment. Progressive trunk strengthening exercises, especially through the midrange, should be incorporated. Dynamic core stabilization exercises that concentrate on abdominal muscles should also be used. Braces are most helpful during high-level activities. Hypermobility of a lumbar vertebra may make the athlete more susceptible to lumbar muscle strains and ligament sprains. Thus, it may be necessary for the athlete to avoid vigorous activity.[53]

Sacroiliac Joint Dysfunction

The sacroiliac is the junction formed by the ilium and the sacrum, and it is fortified by strong ligaments that allow little motion to take place. Because the sacroiliac joint is a synovial joint, disorders can include sprain, inflammation, hypermobility, and hypomobility.

Sacroiliac Sprain

Etiology A sprain of the sacroiliac joint may result when the athlete twists with both feet on the ground, stumbles forward, falls backward, steps too far down and lands heavily on one leg, or bends forward with the knees locked during lifting.[60] It may also occur from downhill running or repetitive unilateral activities like over- rotating a golf swing, dancing, punting, high jumping, hurdling, or gymnastics. Any of these mechanisms can produce irritation and stretching of the sacrotuberous or sacrospinous ligaments. These mechanisms may also cause either an anterior or posterior rotation of one side of the pelvis relative to the other. With rotation of the pelvis, there is hypomobility. As healing occurs, the joint on the injured side may become hypermobile, allowing that joint to sublux in either an anteriorly or posteriorly rotated position.[10,36] Stress fracture, although uncommon, can also occur in the sacrum with repetitive unilateral activities.[6]

Symptoms and signs With a sprain of the sacroiliac joint, there may be palpable pain and tenderness directly over the joint just inferior and medial to the PSIS with some associated muscle guarding. Occasionally, pain radiates to the posterior, lateral, or anterior thigh, and there may be a vaguely located groin pain without associated tenderness. Pain is increased or generated with unilateral stance on that leg and walking, with increased pain on up or downhill. Rolling over will often precipitate or increase the pain. Sitting is usually comfortable, but movement from sitting to standing will create pain. The athletic trainer may observe that the ASIS and/or PSIS may be asymmetrical when compared to the opposite side, which is caused by either anterior or posterior rotation of one side of the pelvis relative to the other (Figure 25-52). There may also be a measurable leg length difference. Forward bending reveals a block to normal movement, and the PSIS on the injured side moves sooner than the one on the normal side. Straight leg raising increases pain after 45 degrees. Side bending toward the painful side will increase pain.

Management Modalities can be used to reduce pain. A supportive brace is also helpful in an acute sprain. The sacroiliac joint should be mobilized to correct the existing asymmetry. If one side of the pelvis is posteriorly rotated, it should be mobilized in an anterior direction. Strengthening exercises should be incorporated to improve stability to a hypermobile joint.

Coccyx Injuries

Etiology Coccygeal injuries in sports are prevalent and occur primarily from direct impact, which may result from forcibly sitting down, falling, or being kicked by an op-

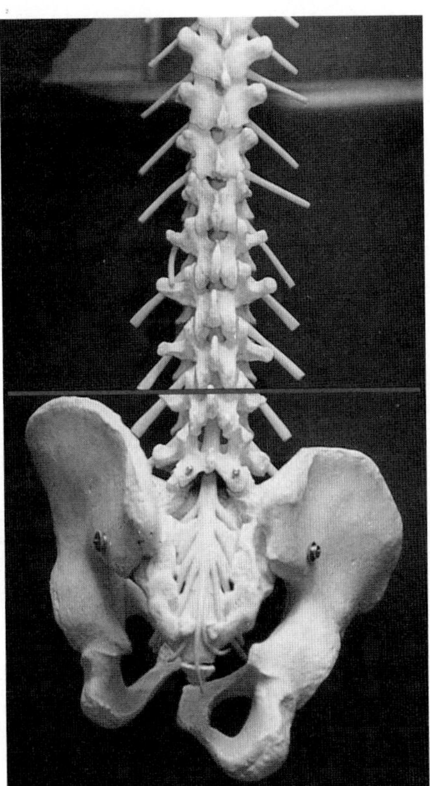

Figure 25-52

The right PSIS is anteriorly rotated relative to the left.

ponent. Injuries to the coccyx include sprains, subluxations, and fractures. With healing, the sacrococcygeal joint may become hypermobile and thus restrict passive motion.

Symptoms and signs Athletes with persistent coccyalgia should be referred to a physician for X rays and rectal examinations. Pain in the coccygeal region is often prolonged and at times chronic. Such conditions are identified by the term *coccygodynia* and occur as a result of an irritation to the coccygeal plexus.

Management Treatment consists of analgesics and a ring seat to relieve the pressure on the coccyx while sitting. Pain from a fractured coccyx may last for many months. Once a coccygeal injury has healed, the athlete should be protected against reinjury by appropriately applied padding.

REHABILITATION TECHNIQUES FOR THE NECK

Joint Mobilizations

Mobilization techniques for the cervical spine are extensively used in rehabilitating the injured neck. Mobilization can decrease pain, restore mobility, and increase range of motion.[15] The most common joint mobilization techniques for the cervical spine include (Figure 25-53):

1. Cervical flexion mobilizations, which increase forward bending and flexion
2. Cervical extension mobilizations, which increase backward bending and extension
3. Cervical rotation mobilizations, which treat pain or stiffness when there is some resistance in the same direction as the rotation
4. Cervical side bending mobilizations, which treat pain and stiffness when there is some resistance to side bending of the neck
5. Cervical traction, which is used to relieve discogenic pain or increase range of motion

Flexibility Exercises

The first consideration in neck rehabilitation should be restoration of the neck's normal range of motion. The athlete who had a prior restricted range of motion should

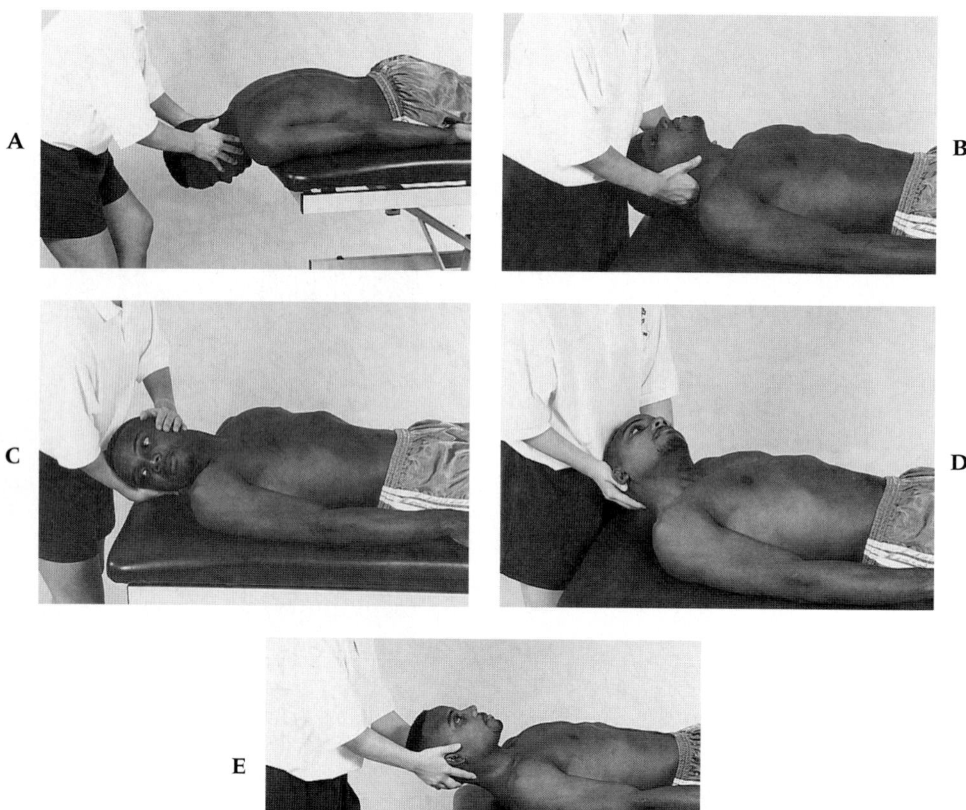

Figure 25-53

Cervical mobilizations.
A, Cervical flexion. **B,** Cervical extension. **C,** Cervical rotation. **D,** Cervical side bending. **E,** Cervical traction.

work on increasing it to a more normal range. A second goal is to strengthen the neck as much as possible. All mobility exercises should be performed pain free. Stretching exercises include passive and active movement.[67]

The athlete sits in a straight-backed chair while the athletic trainer applies a gentle passive stretch through a pain-free range. Extension, flexion, lateral flexion, and rotation in each direction is sustained for a count of six and repeated three times. Passive stretching should be conducted daily.

The athlete is also instructed to actively stretch the neck two to three times daily. Each exercise is performed for eight to ten repetitions, with each endpoint held for a count of six. All exercises are performed without force. Figure 25-54 shows forward flexion, extension, lateral flexion, and rotation.

Stretching can progress gradually to a more vigorous procedure, such as the Billig procedure. In this exercise, the athlete sits on a chair with one hand firmly grasping the seat of the chair. The other hand, over the top of the head, is placed on the ear on the side of the support hand. Keeping that hand in place, the athlete gently pulls the opposite side of the neck. The stretch should be held for six seconds (Figure 25-55). A rotary stretch in each direction can also be applied in the same manner by the athlete.

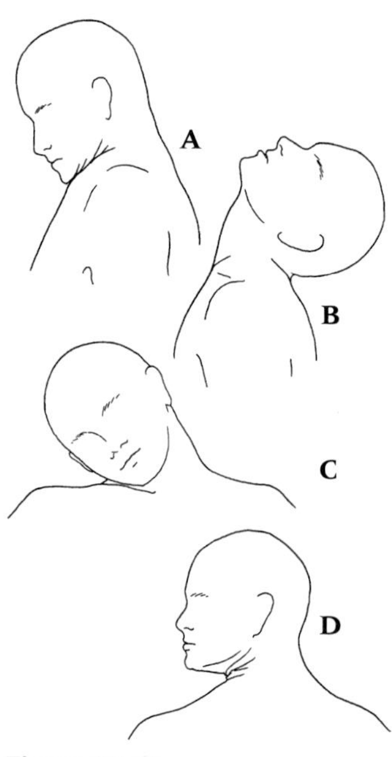

Figure 25-54

Active neck stretching is important in increasing neck mobility after injury.
A, Forward flexion. **B,** Extension. **C,** Lateral flexion. **D,** Rotation.

Strengthening Exercises

When the athlete has gained near-normal range of motion, a strength program should be instituted. All exercises should be conducted pain free. In the beginning, each exercise is performed with the head in an upright position facing straight forward. Exercises are performed isometrically; each resistance is held for a count of six. The athlete should start with five repetitions and progressing to ten repetitions (Figure 25-56).

1. Flexion—press forehead against palm of hand.
2. Extension—lace fingers behind head and press head back against hands.
3. Lateral flexion—place palm on side of head and press head into palm.

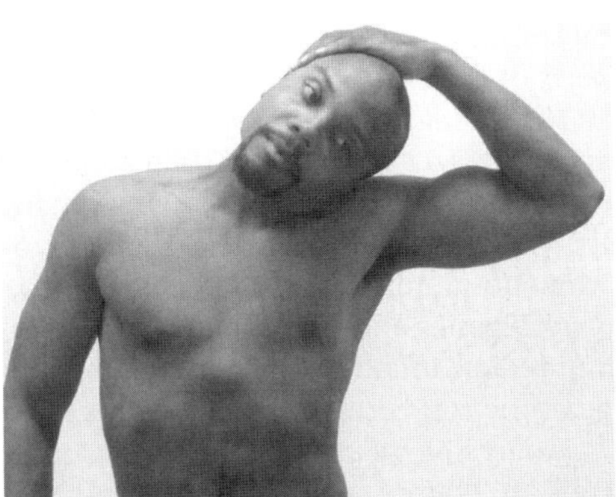

Figure 25-55

Stretching the lateral neck flexors by the Billig procedure.

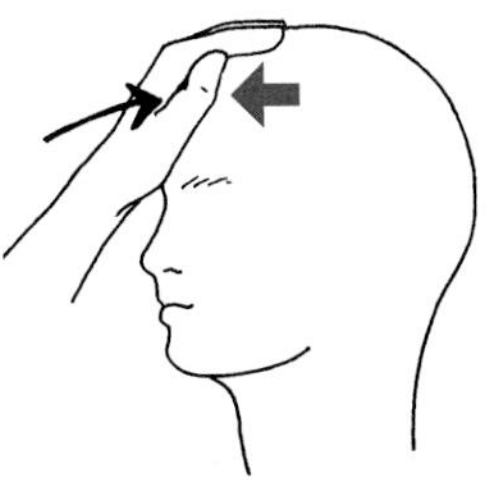

A. Flexion

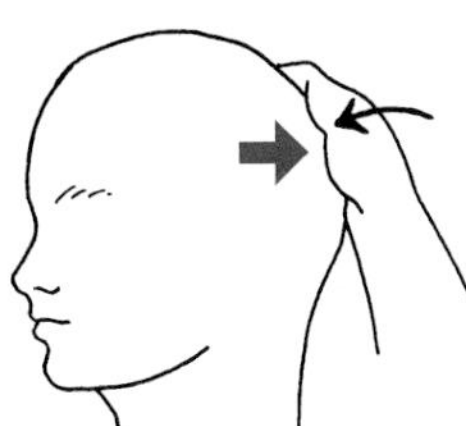

B. Extension

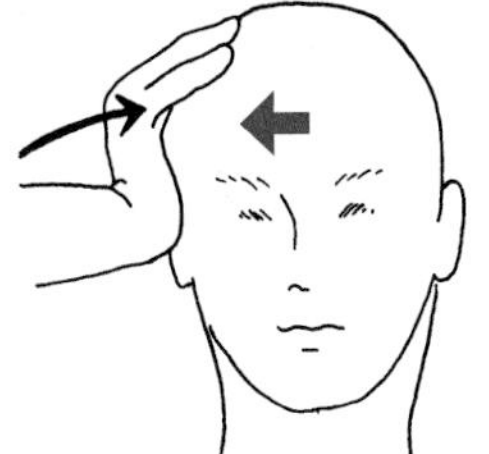

C. Lateral flexion

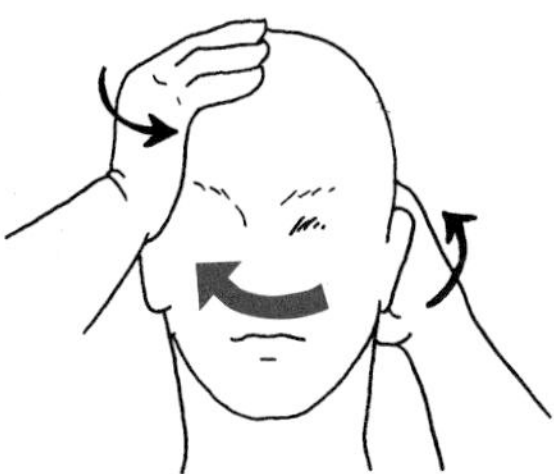

D. Rotation

Figure 25-56

Manual neck-strengthening exercises. **A,** Flexion. **B,** Extension. **C,** Lateral flexion. **D,** Rotation.

4. Rotation—put one palm on side of forehead and the other at back of the head. Push with each hand, attempting to rotate head. Change hands and reverse direction.

Strengthening progresses to isotonic exercises through a full range of motion using manual resistance, special equipment such as a towel, or weighted devices (Figure 25-57). Each exercise is performed for ten repetitions and two to three sets. NOTE: The athlete must be cautioned against overstressing the neck and must be encouraged to increase resistance gradually.

REHABILITATION TECHNIQUES FOR THE LOW BACK

Over the years many different techniques relative to the treatment and rehabilitation of low back pain have been recommended. Individuals such as Williams, McKenzie, Cyriax, Maitland, Paris, and Saal have proposed effective yet specific philosophical approaches for managing individuals with low back pain. In some instances, a particular approach tended to use the same exercises for all low back pain patients regardless of the existing etiology. Today the techniques for treating low back pain incorporate a

Figure 25-57

Neck strengthening using resistive devices. **A,** Towel. **B,** Free weight. **C,** Exercise machine.

A

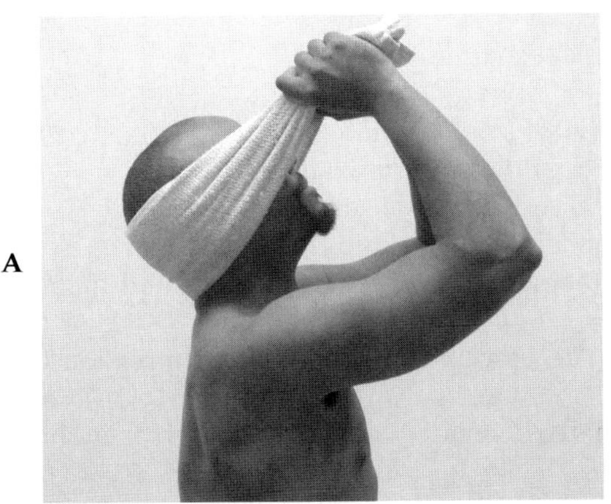

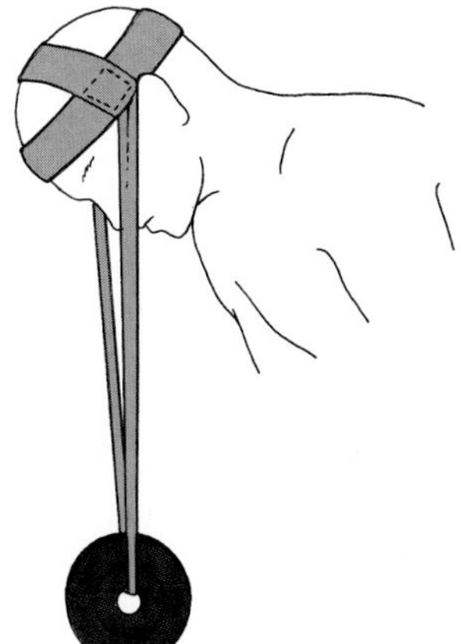

B

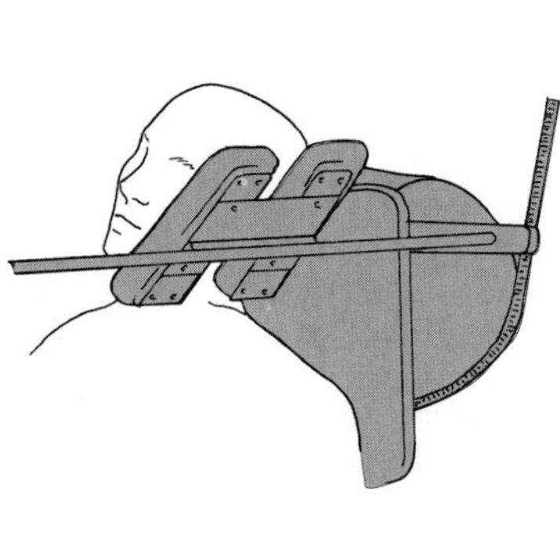

C

more eclectic approach and use a combination of the most applicable and useful aspects of each of the philosophic approaches.[3,71]

The initial treatment for low back pain should focus on modulating pain. Following acute injury, ice should be used along with electrical stimulating currents for analgesia. Rest is also helpful in allowing the injured structures to begin the healing process. It is essential that the athletic trainer avoid movements or positions that increase pain while positioning the athlete in a posture that minimizes pain and discomfort.

Analgesics and oral antiinflammatory agents are commonly given to inhibit pain and reduce inflammation in the athlete with a low back problem. If muscle spasm or guarding is severe, muscle relaxants may be prescribed.

Progressive relaxation techniques can also be useful in treating low back pain. With constant pain comes anxiety and increased muscular tension that compounds the low back problem. By systematically contracting and completely "letting go" of the body's major muscles, the athlete learns to recognize abnormal tension and to relax the muscles consciously. Various relaxation techniques are discussed in Chapter 11.

General Body Conditioning

The low back pain that athletes most often encounter is an acute, painful experience that rarely lasts longer than three weeks. In the initial stages of acute injury, however, there can be a great deal of pain and disability. In some of the conditions described in this chapter, any movement at all can produce incapacitating low back pain. Thus, athletes with certain conditions may find it difficult to maintain general body conditioning, particularly during the acute stage of healing. It may be necessary to eliminate any type of conditioning during the first several days. The athlete should resume conditioning activities as soon as the condition has resolved to the point that discomfort can be tolerated. The athlete may find it helpful to use aquatic exercise as a method for maintaining cardiorespiratory endurance, because the pain that often occurs with weight bearing may be minimized.

Joint Mobilizations

Joint mobilization of the lumbar spine may be used to improve joint mobility or to decrease joint pain by restoring to the joint accessory movements that will help the athlete achieve a full, nonrestricted, pain-free range of motion.[27] Vertebral joints in the lumbar region are capable of both anterior and posterior gliding or rotation, or some combination of the two; mobilization techniques should address all restricted joint motions. Grade 1 and 2 mobilizations may be incorporated early in the rehabilitation program for managing pain. Mobilization may progress to grades 3 and 4 once pain and muscle guarding are decreased. For best results, mobilization should be combined with manual traction techniques.

Joint mobilization techniques for the low back are indicated when

- Pain is centralized at a specific joint and increases with activity and decreases with rest.
- Active and passive range of motion is decreased.
- There is muscle tightness.
- Forward and backward bending deviates from the midline.
- Rotation and side bending produce asymmetrical movements.
- Accessory motion at individual spinal segments is decreased.

Specific mobilization techniques for the low back include (Figure 25-58):

1. Anterior/posterior lumbar vertebrae mobilizations to decrease pain and increase the mobility of individual vertebrae
2. Lumbar lateral distraction to reduce pain associated with some compression of a spinal nerve
3. Lumbar vertebral rotation mobilizations to decrease pain and increase the mobility of individual vertebrae

25-10

***Critical Thinking* Exercise**

During a back evaluation on a soccer player, the athletic trainer finds that backward bending is limited, yet the movement diminishes pain; straight leg raising is limited and painful; forward bending is extremely limited and increases pain; and back pain diminishes when the athlete is lying down but increases when he is sitting.

? What routine rehabilitative exercises should the athletic trainer recommend to the athlete?

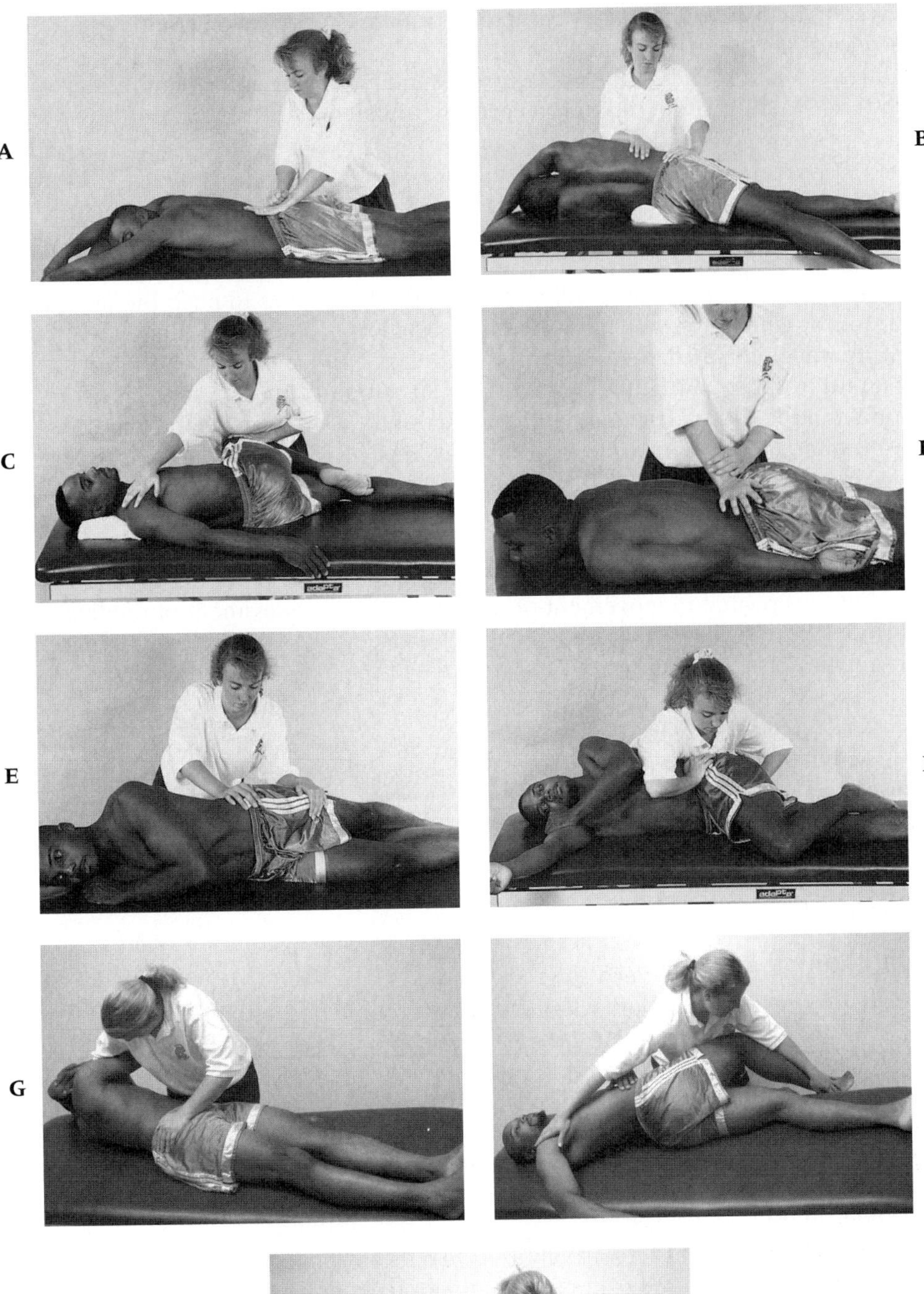

Figure 25-58

Low-back mobilizations. **A,** Anteroposterior lumbar vertabrae mobilization. **B,** Lumbar lateral distraction. **C,** Lumbar vertebral rotation. **D,** Anterior sacral mobilization. **E,** Anterior inominate rotation. **F,** Posterior inominate rotation mobilization. **G,** SI posterior rotation mobilization. **H,** SI anterior rotation mobilization. **I,** SI lateral rotation mobilization.

4. Anterior sacral mobilizations to reduce pain and muscle guarding around the sacroiliac joint
5. Anterior rotation mobilizations to correct a unilateral posterior rotation
6. Posterior rotation mobilizations to correct a unilateral anterior rotation

Traction

Traction is the treatment of choice when there is a small protrusion of the nucleus pulposus. Through traction, the lumbar vertebrae are distracted; a subatmospheric pressure is created, which tends to pull the protrusion to its original position; and there is tightening of the longitudinal ligament, which tends to push the protrusion toward its original position within the disk.[4] Traction may be done manually or with a traction machine. Sustained traction for at least thirty minutes with a force commensurate with body weight is preferred. An 80-pound (35-kilogram) force would be the minimum for a small woman, and a 180-pound (80-kilogram) force would be the minimum for a large man.[4] Traction is usually applied daily (five times per week) for two weeks.

25-11

Critical Thinking **Exercise**

An evaluation of a swimmer who is complaining of low back pain when swimming a freestyle stroke finds that back pain is diminished when the athlete is sitting and increased when lying down or standing; forward bending decreases the pain; the lordotic curve in the lumbar area does not reverse itself in forward bending; backward bending is painful, especially at the end range; and there is poor abdominal muscle strength.

? What type of exercises should the athletic trainer recommend?

Flexibility Exercises

Back pain may be caused by tightness or a lack of flexibility in a number of different muscle groups related to movement of the low back. An assessment of the flexibility of the muscle groups will indicate which ones are tight and need to be stretched. The following muscle groups may need to be stretched (Figure 25-59):

1. Low back extensors
2. Lumbar rotators
3. Hip abductors
4. Lumbar lateral flexors
5. Hip adductors
6. Hip rotators
7. Hip flexors
8. Hamstrings

Strengthening Exercises

Strengthening exercises should routinely be incorporated into the rehabilitation program to encourage the athlete to remain active and also to regain lumbar motion.[61] Strengthening exercises that reinforce pain-reducing movements and postures should be used, particularly in cases of low back pain. Any exercise or movement that causes pain to spread over a larger area should be avoided. Thus, selecting the correct strengthening exercises should centralize or diminish pain.

Flexion versus Extension Exercises

Extension exercises are used to strengthen the back extensors, to stretch the abdominals, and to reduce the pressure on the intervertebral disks.

Generally, strengthening exercises can involve either extension or flexion exercises.[66] Extension exercises are used to strengthen the back extensors, to stretch the abdominals, and to reduce the pressure on the intervertebral disks (Figure 25-60).[40,76] Athletes should engage in extension exercises when:

- Back pain diminishes when the athlete is lying down and increases when the athlete is sitting.
- Backward bending is limited, yet the movement diminishes pain.
- Forward bending is extremely limited and increases pain.
- Straight leg raising is limited and painful.

Flexion exercises are used to strengthen the abdominal muscles, to stretch the back extensors, and to take pressure off a nerve root by separating the lumbar facet joints and opening the intervertebral foramina (Figure 25-61). Athletes should engage in flexion exercises when:

- Back pain diminishes when the athlete is sitting and increases when the athlete is lying down or standing.
- Forward bending decreases the pain.

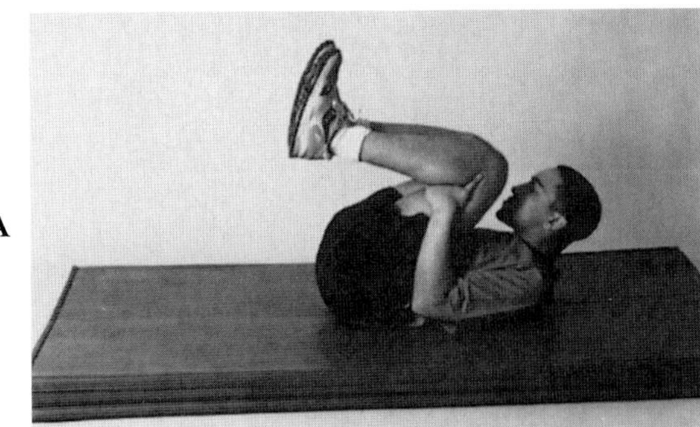

A

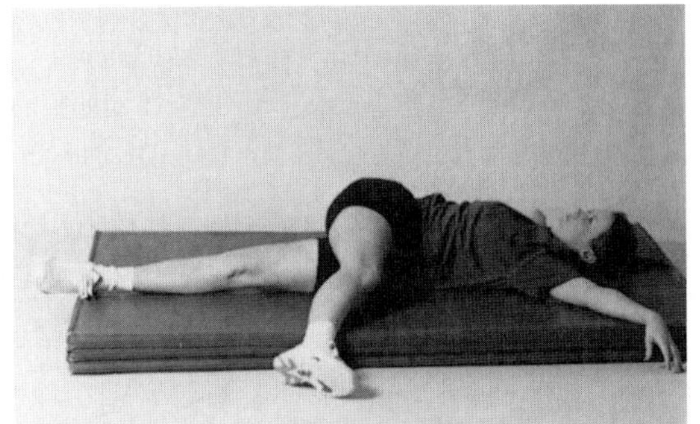

B

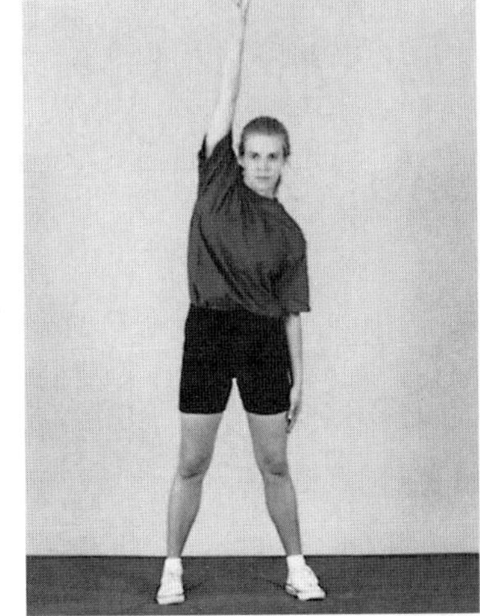

C

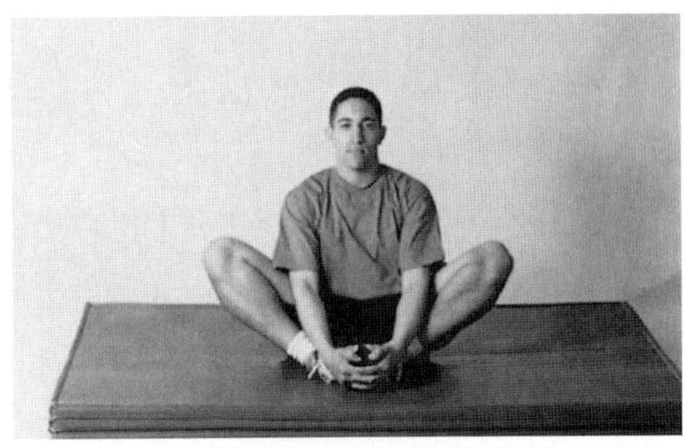

D

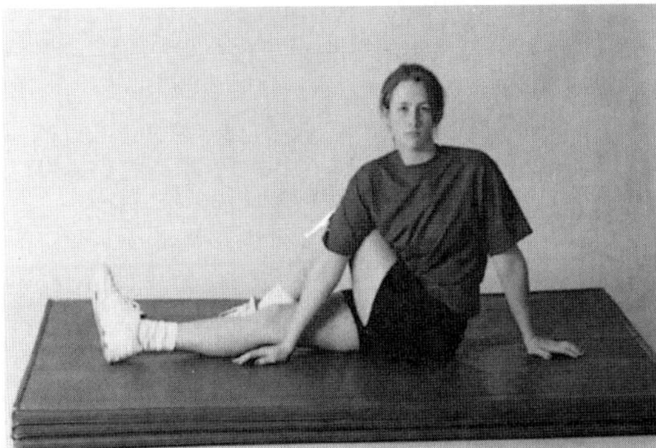

E

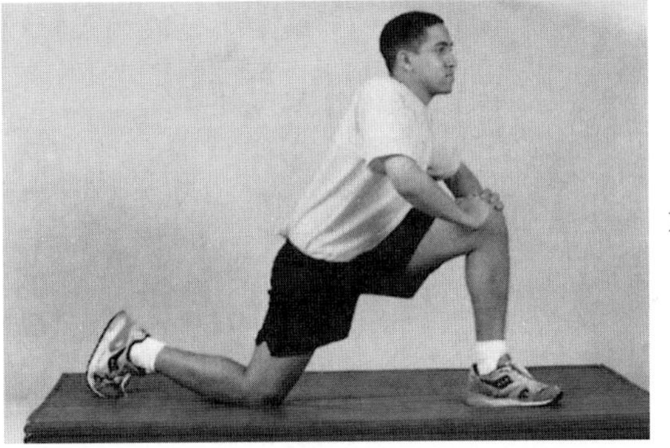

F

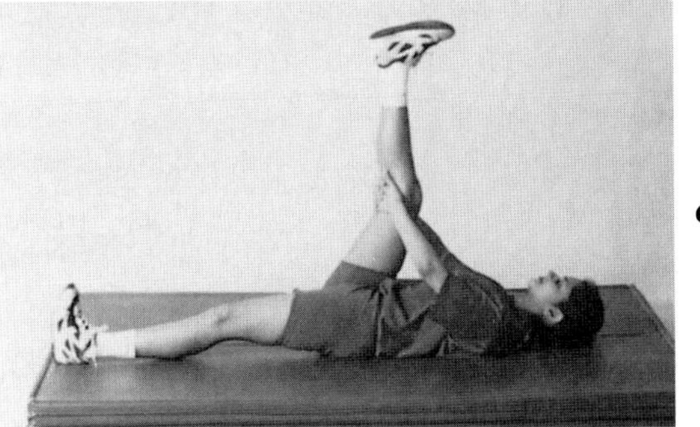

G

Figure 25-59

Low-back stretching exercises. **A,** Low back extensors. **B,** Lumbar rotators and hip abductors. **C,** Lumbar lateral flexors. **D,** Hip adductors. **E,** Hip rotators. **F,** Hip flexors. **G,** Hamstrings.

- The lordotic curve in the lumbar area does not reverse itself in forward bending.
- Backward bending is painful, especially at the end range.
- There is poor abdominal muscle strength.

PNF Exercises

PNF upper trunk chopping and lifting patterns may be used to strengthen the trunk musculature. Besides increasing strength, PNF exercises can help establish neuromuscular control and proprioception. Rhythmic stabilization, using isometric exercise, can facilitate the cocontraction of antagonistic muscle groups (see Chapter 16).

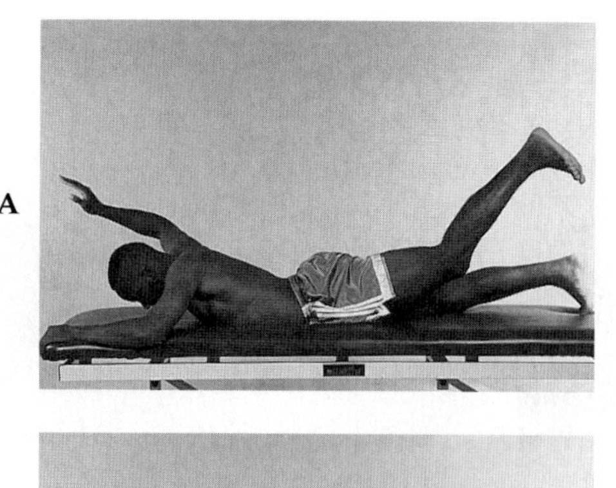

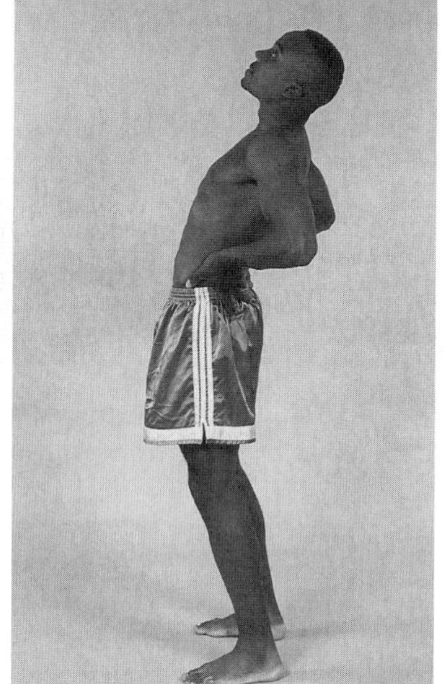

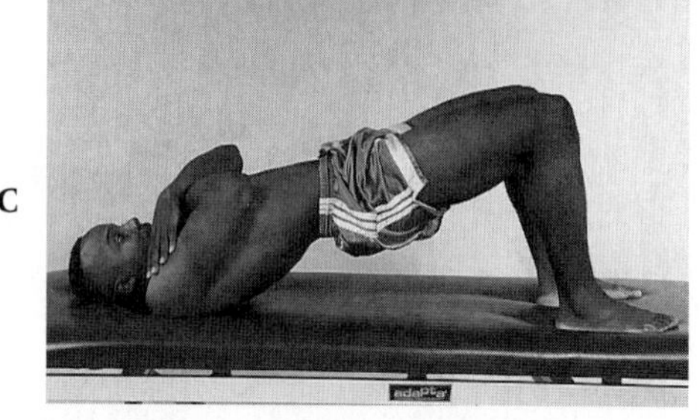

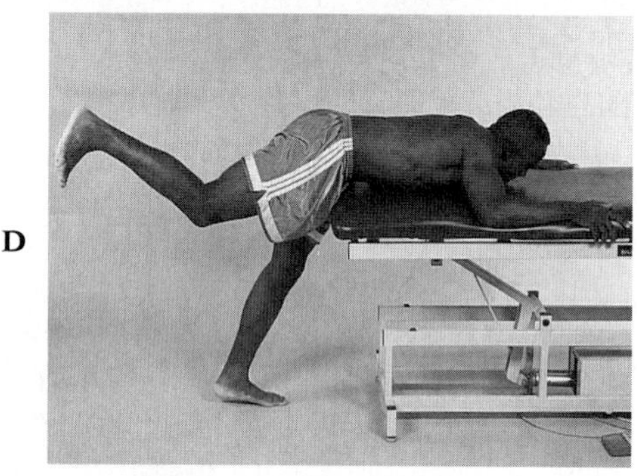

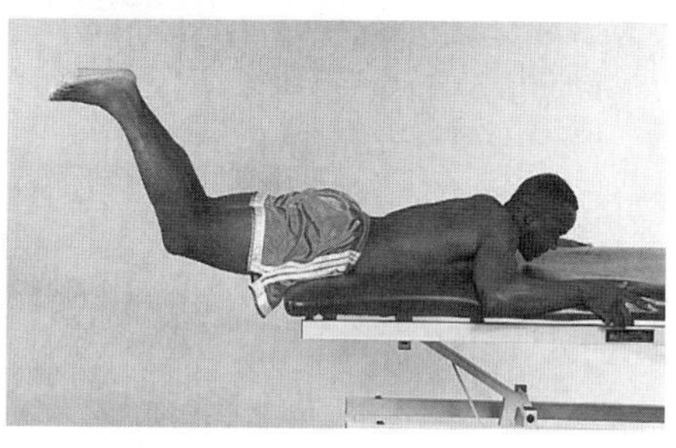

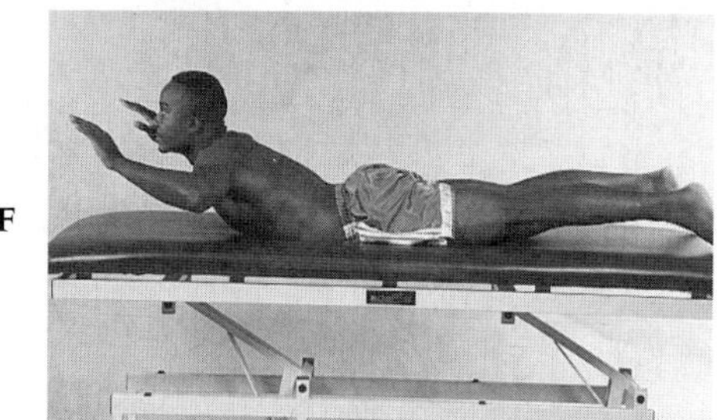

Figure 25-60

Extension strengthening exercises. **A,** Alternating leg extension. **B,** Standing extension. **C,** Supine hip extension. **D,** Prone single hip extension. **E,** Prone double-leg hip extension. **F,** Trunk extension.

Neuromuscular Control (Core Stabilization)

Despite the fact that the athlete may have adequate strength and flexibility, he or she may have difficulty controlling the spine if the athlete does not learn to contract the appropriate muscles in a desired sequence.[16] Stabilization, especially during complex functional movements, relies heavily on a learned response by the athlete to control the movement.[63] Stabilization exercises for the trunk and spine may help minimize the cumulative effects of repetitive microtrauma to the spine.[64] Spinal stabilization does not mean that the athlete maintains a static position. *Dynamic,* or *core, stabilization* involves the maintaining of a controlled range of motion that varies with the position and the activity being performed.[13] Core stabilization is achieved by

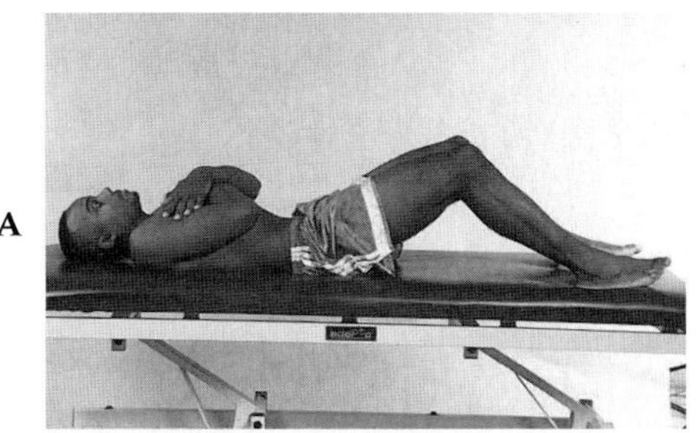
A

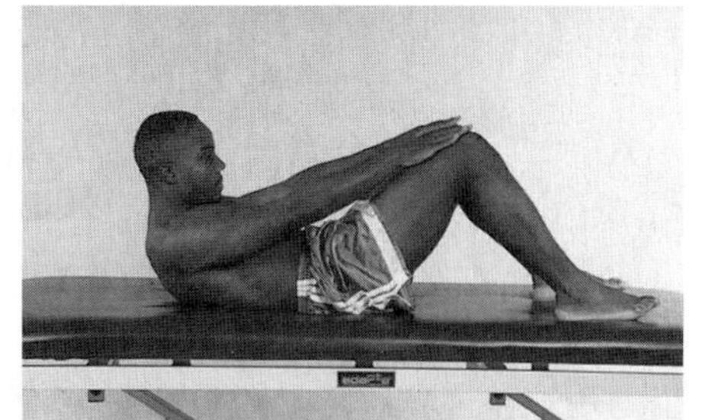
B

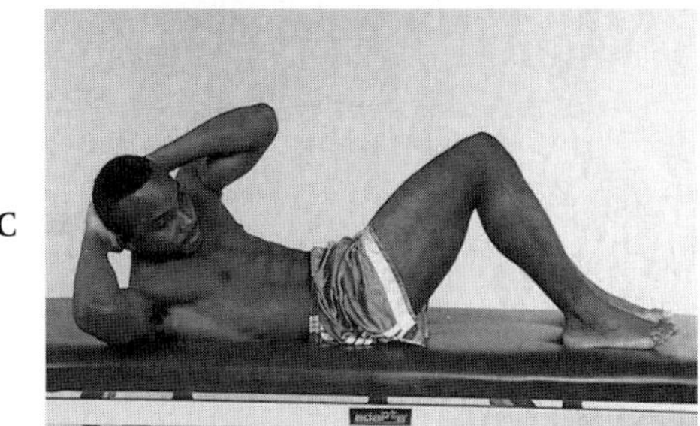
C

Figure 25-61

Flexion strengthening exercises. **A,** Posterior pelvic tilt. **B,** Partial sit-up. **C,** Partial sit-up with rotation.

conscious repetitive training that, over time, becomes an unconscious natural response.[85] Core stabilization techniques are widely used in rehabilitation programs for the low back.[36]

Dynamic stabilization involves maintaining a controlled range of motion that varies with the position and the activity being performed.

The first step in core stabilization is for the athlete to learn to control the pelvis in a neutral position.[85] A "drawing in" maneuver similar to a posterior tilt of the pelvis, which flattens the lumbar curve, is caused by a simultaneous cocontraction of the abdominal and gluteal muscles. Once the athlete has learned to simultaneously contract all muscles in the lumbo-pelvic-hip complex, then progressively more advanced activities should be incorporated that involve movements of both the spine and extremities while the pelvis is maintained in a neutral position (Figure 25-62).[12,36]

Abdominal muscle control is another key to stabilization of the low back.[21] Abdominal bracing exercises focus attention on motor control of the external oblique muscles in different positions. There should also be cocontraction of the abdominal muscles and lumbar extensors to maintain a "corset" control of the lumbar spine.[36] Core stabilization exercises may also be incorporated into aquatic therapy.[43]

Functional Progressions

The progression of stabilization exercises should be from supine activities, to prone activities, to kneeling activities, and eventually, to weight-bearing activities,[29] all performed while the athlete actively stabilizes the trunk. The athlete should be taught to perform a stabilization contraction before starting any movement. As the movement begins, he or she will become less aware of the stabilization contraction. The athlete may begin by incorporating stabilization into every movement performed in the strengthening exercises. Stabilization contractions can also be used in aerobic conditioning activities. The exercises should include those activities that replicate the demands of the athlete's individual sport. The various components of a sport activity should be broken down into separate activities or skills that allow the athlete to consciously practice the stabilization technique with each drill. Each athlete will differ in degree of control and in the speed at which the skills of dynamic core stabilization are acquired.[36]

25-12

***Critical Thinking* Exercise**

A basketball player has been told by his family physician that he has an unstable back. The physician referred him to a therapist who recommended that the athlete perform dynamic stabilization exercises. Unfortunately, the athlete had to leave home and return to college before he had a chance to learn the exercises.

? The athlete asks the athletic trainer to show him the appropriate dynamic stabilization exercises. What progression should the athletic trainer recommend?

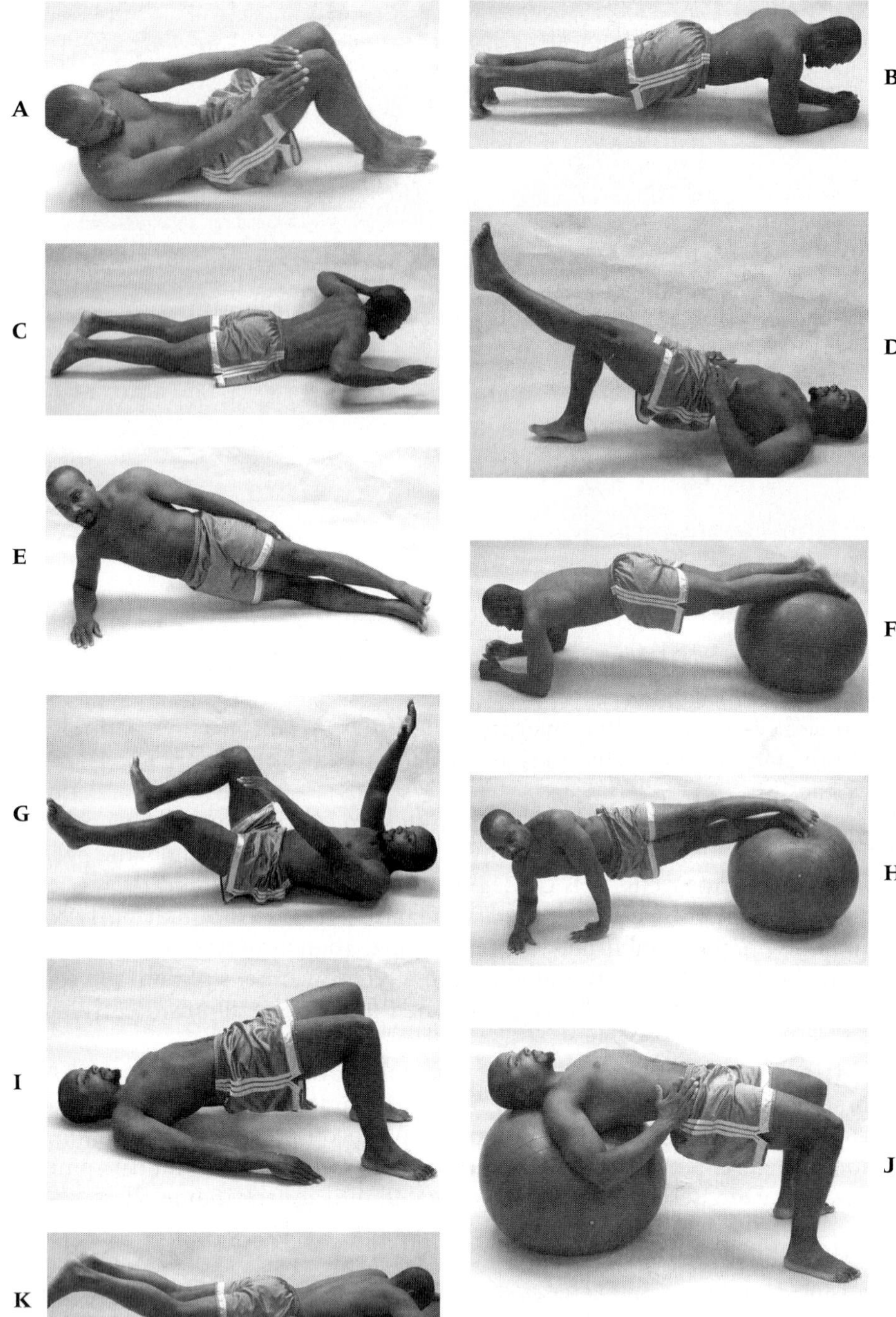

Figure 25-62

Core Stabilization Exercises. **A,** Three point crunches. **B,** Human arrow. **C,** Prone head and arm lift. **D,** Bridge with leg extension. **E,** Side lying hip lift. **F,** Human arrow on ball. **G,** Dead bug (alternate arm and leg). **H,** Side lying lift on ball. **I,** Abdominal bridge. **J,** Bridge on ball. **K,** Prone hip extension on table.

Continued

25-13

***Critical Thinking* Exercise**

A golfer is experiencing low back pain. Before beginning the round he does a lot of stretching exercises to help loosen his back. As the round progresses he reports that his back gets stiffer, and after twelve or thirteen holes, the pain is so bad that it is almost impossible for him to hit with his driver, fairway woods, or long irons. He says that he tries to keep stretching throughout the round to make his back feel better.

? What can the athletic trainer recommend that might help correct this problem?

Return to Activity

Most acute muscular strains or ligament sprains in the low back take as long to heal as acute strains and sprains in the extremities do. However, if the injury becomes recurrent or the problem becomes chronic, achieving full return to activity may be frustrating to both the athlete and the athletic trainer. Injuries to the low back can be incapacitating for anyone, but the physical demands of sports activity increase the likelihood of recurrent injury.[55] Thus, the athletic trainer must take whatever time is required to fully rehabilitate the athlete with a low back problem and must educate the athlete about the skills and techniques that can minimize additional injury.

L

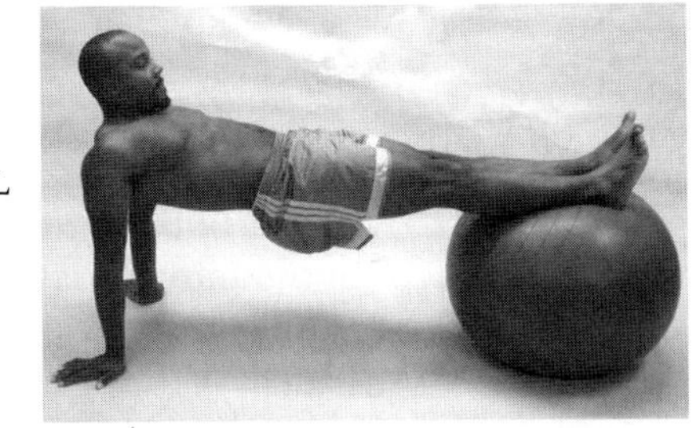

M

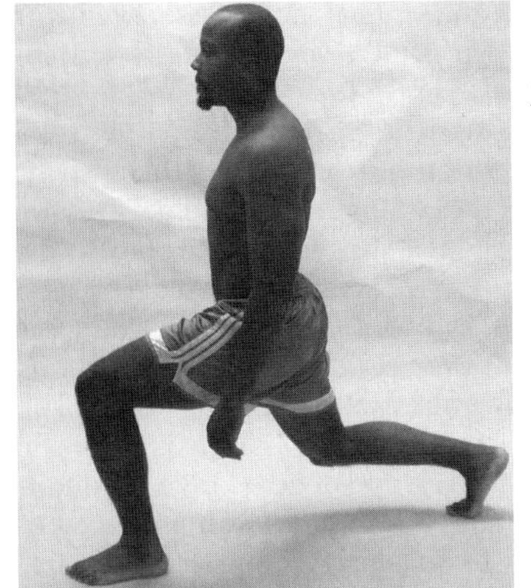

N

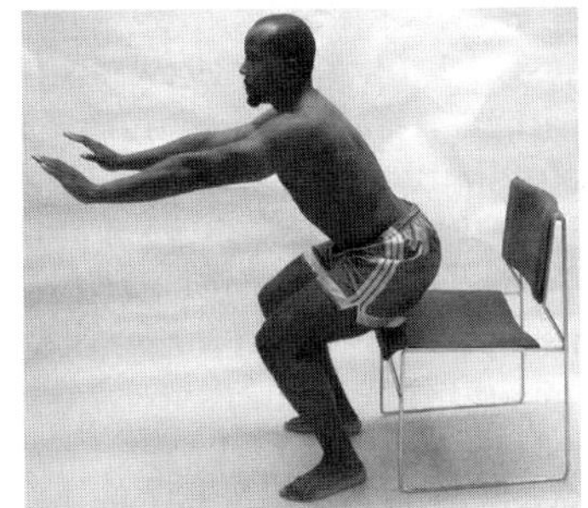

O

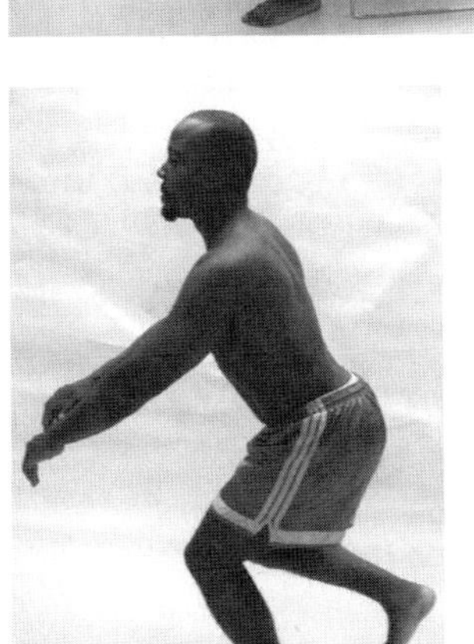

P

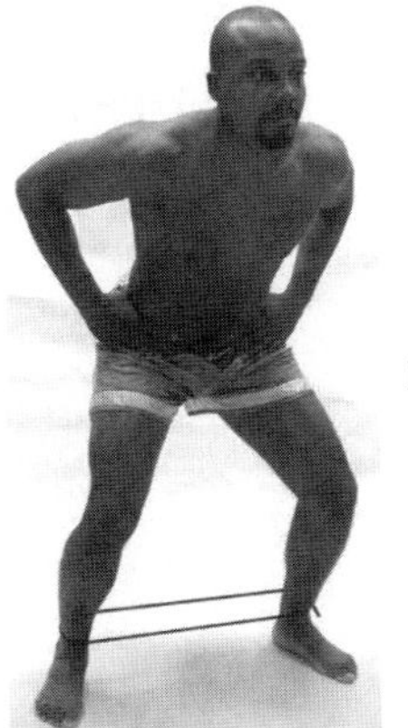

Q

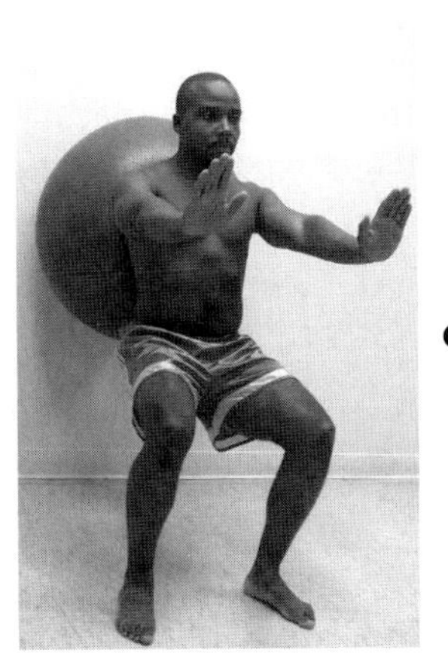

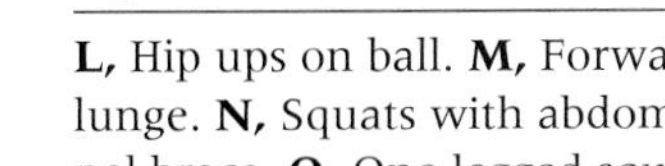

Figure 25-62—continued

L, Hip ups on ball. **M,** Forward lunge. **N,** Squats with abdominal brace. **O,** One legged squat. **P,** Lateral shuffle with tubing. **Q,** Wall slides with ball.

SUMMARY

- The spine, or vertebral column, is composed of thirty-three individual vertebrae. The design of the spine allows for flexion, extension, lateral flexion, and rotation. The movable vertebrae are separated by intervertebral disks, and their position is maintained by a series of muscular and ligamentous supports. The spine can be divided into three different regions: cervical, thoracic, and lumbar. The sacrum and coccyx are fused vertebrae within the vertebral column.
- The spinal cord is that portion of the central nervous system that is contained within the vertebral canal of the spinal column. Thirty-one pairs of spinal nerves extend from the sides of the spinal cord. The spinal nerve roots combine to form the peripheral nerves, which provide motor and sensory innervation. Each pair of spinal nerves has a specific area of cutaneous sensory distribution called a dermatome.
- Acute traumatic injuries to the spine can be potentially life threatening, particularly if the cervical region of the spinal cord is involved. Thus the athlete must do everything possible to minimize the possibility of injury. Strengthening the musculature of the neck is critical. In addition to strong muscles, the athlete's neck should have a full range of motion. Athletes involved in collision sports must be taught and required to use techniques that reduce the likelihood of cervical injury.
- Low back pain is one of the most common and disabling ailments known to humans. The athlete, like everyone else, can prevent low back pain by avoiding unnecessary

stresses and strains that are associated with standing, sitting, lying, working, or exercising. The athlete should take care to avoid postures and positions that can cause injuries.

- The most critical part of evaluating spine injuries is to rule out the possibility of spinal cord injury. Observing the posture and movement capabilities of the athlete during the evaluation can help clarify the nature and extent of the injury. Classic postural deviations include kyphosis, forward head posture, lordosis, flatback posture, swayback posture, and scoliosis. Special tests may be performed with the athlete in standing, sitting, supine, side-lying, and prone positions.
- Because the cervical and lumbar regions of the spine are so mobile, they are extremely vulnerable to a wide range of sports injuries including fractures, dislocations, strains, sprains, contusions, lesions of the intervertebral disks, injuries to spinal nerves, and degenerative conditions. Although relatively uncommon, severe sports injury to the neck can produce catastrophic impairment of the spinal cord.
- The first consideration in neck rehabilitation should be restoration of the neck's normal range of motion. When the athlete has gained near-normal range of motion, a strength program should be instituted. Mobilization techniques for the cervical spine are extensively used in rehabilitating the injured neck.
- Rehabilitation of low back pain focuses on teaching the athlete dynamic stabilization techniques that involve exercises for the trunk and spine to minimize the cumulative effects of repetitive microtrauma to the spine. Exercises are designed to strengthen or stretch specific muscles of spinal movement and are divided into extension and flexion exercises.

Websites

AAOS Online Service on Low Back Pain: www.orthoinfo.aaos.org/brochure/thr_report.cfm?Thread_ID=10&topcategory=Spine

Information on low back pain from the American Academy of Orthopedic Surgeons.

MEDLINEplus: Back Pain: www.nlm.nih.gov/medlineplus/backpain.html

Information on back pain from the Mayo Foundation for Medical Education and Research.

The Physician and Sportsmedicine: Low-Back Pain Relief: www.physsportsmed.com/issues/1997/01jan/back_pa.htm

Discusses causes and relief for low back pain.

Back Pain: www.orthopedics.about.com/cs/backpain/

Discusses the many causes of low back pain.

AAFP-Diagnosis and Management of Acute Low Back Pain: www.aafp.org/afp/20000315/1779.html

Information on managing low back pain from the American Academy of Family Practice

The Cleveland Clinic Foundation: Spinal Cord Trauma: http://www.clevelandclinic.org/health/health-info/docs/1300/1364.asp

Spine-Health: http://www.spine-health.com

Written and updated by a multispecialty team of medical professionals, this site provides a comprehensive overview of causes and treatments for low back pain, and a variety of services and in-depth features.

The Back Page: http://www.thebackpage.net

Comprehensive information on low back and neck pain.

The Cleveland Clinic Foundation: Spinal Cord Trauma: http://www.anes.ccf.org:8080/PILOT/NEURO/sci.htm

Spine-Health: http://www.spine-health.com

Written and updated by a multispecialty team of medical professionals, this site provides a comprehensive overview of causes and treatments for low back pain, and a variety of services and in-depth features.

The Back Page: http://www.thebackpage.net

This site comprehensive information on low back and neck pain.

Spinal Cord 101: http://www.goes.com/billr/html/_spinal_cord_101.html

This site gives basic information about spinal cord structure, function, and injury.

Solutions to Critical Thinking EXERCISES

25-1 The normal curves include the cervical, thoracic, lumbar, and sacrococcygeal curves. The cervical and lumbar curves are convex anteriorly, whereas the thoracic and sacrococcygeal curves are convex posteriorly. Lordotic posture is characterized by an increased curve in the lumbar spine with an increase in both anterior tilt of the pelvis and hip flexion. When combined with kyphosis and a forward head posture, this condition is referred to as a kypho-lordotic posture.

25-2 Left rotation is produced when the sternocleidomastoid, scalenes, semispinalis cervicis, and upper trapezius on the right side contract in addition to contractions of the left splenius capitus, splenius cervicis, and longissimus capitus.

25-3 The athletic trainer should look for symmetry of the ASIS, PSIS, and iliac crests. Sacroiliac compression and distraction tests and a positive Patrick, or FABER, test are all useful in determining a problem in the sacroiliac joint. In forward bending or flexion, the PSISs on each side should move together. If one moves further than the other, a motion restriction is likely present in the sacroiliac joint on the side that moves most. If they move at different times, the side that moves first usually has a restriction.

25-4 Pain present in forward bending and restriction in backward bending with radiating pain are usually associated with a disk problem. However, such pain may also be related to spondylolysis or spondylolisthesis.

25-5 Straight leg raising applies pressure to the sacroiliac joint and may indicate a problem in the sciatic nerve, sacroiliac joint, or lumbar spine. Pain at 30 degrees of straight leg raising indicates either a hip problem or an inflamed nerve. Pain from 30 to 60 degrees indicates some sciatic nerve involvement. Pain between 70 and 90 degrees is indicative of a sacroiliac joint problem. Pain on bilateral straight leg raising indicates some problem with the lumbar spine.

25-6 The athlete may have cervical spine stenosis, which involves a narrowing of the spinal canal in the cervical region that can impinge the spinal cord. The presence of cervical stenosis is determined by an X ray that measures the canal diameter and divides that by the anteroposterior width of the same vertebral body. The athlete should be advised of the potential risks of continued participation in football.

25-7 A stinger is a term to describe an injury to the brachial plexus resulting in transient neuropraxia. Common symptoms of a brachial plexus injury are burning, numbness and tingling, possible loss of function, and pain from the shoulder to the hand.

25-8 The athlete has most likely developed a myofascial trigger point. The key in treating myofascial pain is to stretch the muscle back to a normal resting length and thus relieve the irritation that created the trigger point. Active stretching should be mild and progressive. The use of electrical stimulation in combination with ultrasound is helpful in relieving the pain associated with a trigger point. Progressive strengthening exercises should also be included.

25-9 The gymnast likely has a spondylolisthesis that has resulted in hypermobility of a vertebral segment. Initially rest will help reduce pain. Rehabilitation should consist of exercises that control or stabilize the hypermobile segment and progressive trunk strengthening exercises, especially to the abdominal muscles through the midrange. A brace can be helpful during practice.

25-10 Given this set of existing conditions, the athletic trainer should have the athlete engage in extension exercises to strengthen the back extensors, to stretch the abdominals, and to reduce the pressure on the intervertebral disks.

25-11 It is likely that some pressure on the nerve root is causing this pain. The athletic trainer should recommend using flexion exercises to strengthen the abdominal muscles, to stretch the back extensors, and to take pressure off a nerve root by separating the lumbar facet joints and opening the intervertebral foramina.

25-12 The first step in core stabilization is for the athlete to learn to control the lumbo-pelvic-hip complex in a neutral position. Once the athlete has learned the "drawing in" maneuver, the athletic trainer should incorporate progressively more advanced activities that involve movements of both the spine and extremities while the pelvis is maintained in a neutral position. Abdominal muscle control is another key to stabilization of the low back. Stabilization exercises include weight shifting in kneeling, standing lunges, bridging on a ball, wall slides, and alternating arm and leg extensions.

25-13 It could be that the golfer should not be stretching for his back problem except during a warm-up before playing. Perhaps a better way to manage his back pain is to engage in a core stabilization training program to make his back more stable. It might also help to suggest that before hitting a golf shot, he perform the "drawing in" maneuver to stabilize the lumbo-pelvic-hip complex.

REVIEW QUESTIONS AND CLASS ACTIVITIES

1. Identify the various regions of the spine.
2. Describe the mechanisms of a catastrophic neck injury.
3. What is the relationship between the spinal cord, the nerve roots, and the peripheral nerves?
4. Describe the various postural abnormalities.
5. Describe the special tests used in evaluating the lumbar and sacroiliac portions of the spine.
6. Discuss the various considerations in the prevention of cervical injuries.
7. What are the mechanisms of injury to the spinal cord?
8. What can be done to minimize the incidence of low back pain?
9. Describe the various types of herniated disks.
10. How does a spondylolysis become a spondylolisthesis?
11. What is the usual mechanism for injury to the sacroiliac joint?
12. Explain when flexion exercises should be used and when extension exercises should be used in treating conditions of the low back.
13. Explain the rationale for using dynamic stabilization to rehabilitate low back pain.

REFERENCES

1. Anderson C: Neck injuries, backboard, bench, or return to play, *Physician Sportsmed* 21(8):23, 1993.
2. Ashmen KJ, Swanik CB, Lephart SM: Strength and flexibility characteristics of athletes with chronic low-back pain, *J Sport Rehabil* 5(4):275, 1996.
3. Beattie P: The use of an eclectic approach for the treatment of low back pain: a case study, *Phys Ther* 72(12):923, 1992.
4. Binkley J, Finch E, Hall J: Diagnostic classification of patients with low back pain: a survey of physical therapy experts, *Phys Ther* 73(3): 138, 1993.
5. Blanksby BA, Wearne FK, Elliott BC, Blitvich JD: Etiology and occurrence of diving injuries: a review of diving safety, *Sports Med* 23(4):228, 1997.
6. Boissonnault W, Thein-Nissenbaum J: Differential diagnosis of a sacral stress fracture, *J Orthop Sports Phys Ther* 32(12):613, 2002.
7. Brolinson PG: Practical approach to low back pain, *Sports Medicine in Primary Care* 3(4):30, 1997.
8. Cailliet R: *Low back pain*, ed 3, Philadelphia, 1995, FA Davis.

9. Cantu R: Functional cervical spinal stenosis: a contraindication to participation in contact sports, *Med Sci Sports Exerc* 25(3):316, 1993.
10. Cappaert T: The sacroiliac joint as a factor in low back pain: a review, *J Sport Rehabil* 9(2):169, 2000.
11. Carpenter DM, Nelson BW: Low back strengthening for the prevention and treatment of low back pain. *Med Sci Sports Exerc* 31(1):18, 1999.
12. Chen L, Bih L, Ho C: Endurance times for trunk-stabilization exercises in healthy women: comparing 3 kinds of trunk-flexor exercises, *J Sport Rehab* 12(3):199, 2003.
13. Cholewicki J, Greene H, Galloway M: Neuromuscular function in athletes following recovery from a recent acute low back injury, *J Orthop Sports Phys Ther* 32(11):568, 2002.
14. Cibulka M: The treatment of the sacroiliac joint component to low back pain, *Phys Ther* 72(12):917, 1992.
15. Coppieters M, Stappaerts K, Wouters L: The immediate effects of a cervical lateral glide treatment technique in patients with neurogenic cervicobrachial pain, *J Orthop Sports Phys Ther* 33(6):369, 2003.
16. Cottingham JT, Maitland J: A three-paradigm treatment model using soft-tissue mobilization and guided movement-awareness techniques for a patient with chronic low back pain, *J Orthop Sports Phys Ther* 26(3):155, 1997.
17. Cuppett M: The anatomy and pathomechanics of the sacroiliac joint. *Athletic Therapy Today* 6(4):6, 2001.
18. Cyriax J: Refresher course for general practitioners: the treatment of lumbar disk lesions, *J Orthop Sports Phys Ther* 12(4):163, 1990.
19. Del Rossi G: Management of cervical spine injuries, *Athletic Therapy Today* 7(2):46, 2002.
20. Denegar CR, Peppard A: Evaluation and treatment of persistent pain and myofascial pain syndrome, *Athletic Therapy Today* 2(4):40, 1997.
21. DeRosa C, Poterfield J: A physical therapy model for the treatment of low back pain, *Phys Ther* 72(4):261, 1992.
22. Drezner JA, Herring SA: Exercises in the treatment of low-back pain, *Physician Sportsmed* 29(8):67, 2001.
23. Fomby EW, Mellion MB: Identifying and treating myofascial pain syndrome, *Physician Sportsmed* 25(2):67, 1997.
24. Fourre M: On-site management of cervical spine injuries, *Physician Sportsmed* 19:4, 1991.
25. Fritz J: Lumbar intervertebral disk injuries in athletes, *Athletic Therapy Today* 4(2):27, 1998.
26. George S: Characteristics of patients with lower extremity symptoms treated with slump stretching: a case series, *J Orthop Sports Phys Ther* 32(8):391, 2002.
27. Haldeman S: Spinal manipulative therapy in sports medicine. In Spencer III CW: *Injuries to the spine: clinics in sports medicine,* vol 5, no 2, Philadelphia, 1986, Saunders.
28. Hall C: Differential diagnosis of lumbar spine injuries in athletes, *Athletic Therapy Today* 4(2):7, 1998.
29. Hammann L: Functional back rehabilitation, *Athletic Therapy Today* 5(2):22, 2000.
30. Haperin J: Whiplash, *Physician Sportsmed* 81(11):856, 2002.
31. Hartman C, Hartman D, Jones M: Back injuries in golfers: a simple preventive program, *Athletic Therapy Today* 3(4):44, 1998.
32. Haynes S: Systematic evaluation of brachial plexus injuries, *J Ath Train* 28(3):263, 1993.
33. Heck JF: A classification system for the assessment of lumbar pain in athletes, *J Ath Train* 35(2):204, 2000.
34. Herring S, Weinstein S: Assessment and neurological management of athletic low back injury. In Nicholas J, Herschman E: *The lower extremity and spine in sports medicine,* St Louis, 1995, Mosby.
35. Holland B, Sacco D: Imaging of the spine. In White A, Schofferman J: *Spine care: diagnosis and conservative treatment,* vol 1, St Louis, 1995, Mosby.
36. Hooker D, Prentice W: Back rehabilitation. In Prentice W: *Rehabilitation techniques in sports medicine and athletic training,* St Louis, 2004, WCB/McGraw-Hill.
37. Ikata T, Miyake R, Katoh S, Morita T, Murase M: Pathogenesis of sports-related spondylolisthesis in adolescents: radiographic and magnetic resonance imaging study, *Am J Sports Med* 24(1):94,1996.
38. Johnson EK, Chiarello CM: The slump test: the effects of head and lower extremity position on knee extension, *J Orthop Sports Phys Ther* 26(6):310, 1997.
39. Johnson R: Low back pain in sports: managing spondylolysis in young athletes, *Physician Sportsmed* 21(4):53, 1993.
40. Kuritzky L, White J: Low-back pain: consider extension education, *Physician Sportsmed* 25(1):56, 1997.
41. Markey K, Benedetto M, Curl W: Upper trunk and brachial plexopathy, *Am J Sports Med* 21(5):650, 1993.
42. Massie D, Haddox A: Influence of lower extremity biomechanics and muscle imbalances on the lumbar spine, *Athletic Therapy Today* 4(2):46, 1998.
43. Moss C: Aquatic core strengthening for preventing low back manifestations. *Athletic Therapy Today* 7(4):26, 2002.
44. Moss RI: Posture and pathology, *Athletic Therapy Today* 6(5):38, 2001.
45. Motley G et al: The pars interarticularis stress reaction, spondylolysis and spondylolisthesis progression, *J Ath Train* 33(4):351, 1998.
46. Nissen SJ, Laskowski ER, Rizzo TD: Burner syndrome: recognition and rehabilitation, *Physician Sportsmed* 24(6):57, 1996.
47. Nourbakhsh M, Arab A: Relationship between mechanical factors and incidence of low back pain, *J Orthop Sports Phys Ther* 32(9):447, 2002.
48. Nuber G, Bowen M, Schaffer M: Diagnosis and treatment of lumbar and thoracic spine injuries. In Nicholas J, Herschman E: *The lower extremity and spine in sports medicine,* St Louis, 1995, Mosby.
49. Nyska M: Spondylolysis as a cause of low back pain in swimmers, *Int J Sports Med* 21(5):375, 2000.
50. Oldridge NB, Stoll JE: Low back pain syndrome. In American College of Sports Medicine: *ACSM's exercise management for persons with chronic disease and disabilities,* Champaign, Ill, 2002, Human Kinetics.
51. Olson SL et al: Tender point sensitivity, range of motion, and perceived disability in subjects with neck pain, *J Orthop Sports Phys Ther* 30(1):13, 2000.
52. Perle SM: Myofascial trigger points, *Chiropractic Sports Medicine* (Baltimore, Md) 9(3):1, 1995.
53. Pezzullo D: Spondylolisthesis and spondylolysis in athletes, *Athletic Therapy Today* 4(2):36, 1998.
54. Rapport L, O'Leary P, Cammisa F: Diagnosis and treatment of cervical spine injuries. In Nicholas J, Herschman E: *The lower extremity and spine in sports medicine,* St Louis, 1995, Mosby.
55. Resnik L, Dobrzykowski E: Guide to outcomes measurement for patients with low back pain syndromes, *J Orthop Sports Phys Ther* 33(6):307, 2003.
56. Rimoldi RL: Cervical injuries. In Baker, CL et al, editors: *The Hughston Clinic sports medicine book,* Baltimore, Md, 1995, Williams & Wilkins.
57. Ritz S, Lorren T, Simpson S: Rehabilitation of degenerative diseases of the spine. In Hochschuler S, Cotler H, Guyer R: *Rehabilitation of the spine: science and practice,* St Louis, 1993, Mosby.
58. Rodriquez J: Clinical examination and documentation. In Hochschuler S, Cotler H, Guyer R: *Rehabilitation of the spine: science and practice,* St Louis, 1993, Mosby.
59. Ross M: Treating low back pain in a middle-age recreational athlete, *Athletic Therapy Today* 4(2):22, 1999.
60. Saunders D: *Evaluation, treatment, and prevention of musculoskeletal disorders,* Bloomington, Minn, 1994, Educational Opportunities.
61. Shiple B: Relieving low-back pain with exercise, *Physician Sportsmed* 25(8):67, 1997.

62. Standaert CJ, Herring SA: Spondylolysis: a critical review, *British Journal of Sports Medicine* 34(6):415, 2000.
63. Stevans J, Hall KG: Motor skill acquisition strategies for rehabilitation of low back pain, *J Orthop Sports Phys Ther* 28(3):165, 1998.
64. Stone JA: Back stabilization exercises, *Athletic Therapy Today* 4(3):23, 1999.
65. Storey MD: Anterior neck trauma, *Physician Sportsmed* 17(9):85, 1993.
66. Szajnuk TL: Low back pain in athletes: flexion or extension? *Athletic Therapy Today* 1(3):47, 1996.
67. Teitz CC: Rehabilitation of neck and low back injuries. In Harvey JS, editor: *Symposium on rehabilitation of the injured athlete. Clinics in sports medicine*, vol 4, no 3, Philadelphia, 1985, Saunders.
68. Tierney RT: Measuring isometric strength in the cervical spine, *Athletic Therapy Today* 8(3):56, 2003.
69. Tierney R, Maldjian C, Mattacola C: Cervical spine stenosis measures in normal subjects, *J Ath Train* 37(2):190, 2002.
70. Timm K: An algorithm for assessing lumbar spine injuries, *Athletic Therapy Today* 3(2):18, 1998.
71. Timm K: Therapeutic exercise guidelines for rehabilitating lumbar spine injuries in athletes, *Athletic Therapy Today* 4(2):17, 1998.
72. Tonks SM: Spondylolysis and spondylolisthesis, *Sports Medicine in Primary Care* 1(3):18, 1995.
73. Torg JS et al: The axial load teardrop fracture, *Am J Sports Med* 19(4):355, 1991.
74. Torg JS et al: The epidemiologic, pathologic, biomechanical, and cinematographic analysis of football-induced cervical spine trauma, *Am J Sports Med* 18(1):50, 1990.
75. Torg J, Fay C: Cervical spinal stenosis with cord neurapraxia and transcient quadriplegia. In Torg J: *Athletic injuries to the head, neck, and face*, St Louis, 1991, Mosby.
76. Udermann B, Mayer J, Graves J: Quantitative assessment of lumbar paraspinal muscle endurance, *J Ath Train* 38(3), 2003.
77. Vereschagin KS et al: Burners, *Physician Sportsmed* 1(9):96, 1991.
78. Wainner RS, Gill H: Diagnosis and nonoperative management of cervical radiculopathy, *J Orthop Sports Phys Ther* 30(12):728, 2000.
79. Watkins RG: Acute cervical spine injuries in the adult competitive athlete: football injuries (burners), *Sports Med Arthroscopy Review* 5(3):182, 1997.
80. Weber MD, Woodall WR: Spondylogenic disorders in gymnasts, *J Orthop Sports Phys Ther* 14(1):6, 1991.
81. Whalen R et al: EMG analysis of patients with unilateral neck pain, *J Sport Rehabil* 8(1):32, 1999.
82. Wiesenfarth J, Briner W: Neck injuries: urgent decisions and actions, *Physician Sportsmed* 24(1):35, 1996.
83. Wilkerson JE, Maroon JC: Cervical spine injuries in athletes, *Physician Sportsmed* 18(3):57, 1990.
84. Winkelstein BA, Myers BS: The biomechanics of cervical spine injury and implications for injury prevention, *Med Sci Sports Exerc* 29(7 suppl):S246, 1997.
85. Wisbey-Roth T: Dysfunctional muscle recruitment patterns affecting core stability: the theory of synergistic stabilizer retraining. Abstract from Australian Conference of Science and Medicine in Sport, National Convention Centre, Canberra, October 1996.
86. Wrisley DM et al: Cervicogenic dizziness: a review of diagnosis and treatment, *J Orthop Sports Phys Ther* 30(12):755, 2000.
87. Young JL, Press JM, Herring SA: The disk at risk in athletes: perspectives on operative and nonoperative care, *Med Sci Sports Exerc* 29(7 suppl):S222, 1997.

ANNOTATED BIBLIOGRAPHY

Braggins S: *Back care: a clinical approach*, Philadelphia, 2000, Churchill-Livingstone.

A comprehensive text that focuses on all aspects of treatment and rehabilitation of the spine.

Cailliet R: *Low back pain syndrome*, ed 3, Philadelphia, 1995, FA Davis.

This text presents the subject of low back pain in a clear, concise, and interesting manner.

Hochschuler S, Cotler H, Guyer R: *Rehabilitation of the spine: science and practice*, St Louis, 1993, Mosby.

This comprehensive text focuses on all aspects of treatment and rehabilitation of the spine. Injuries specific to individual sports are discussed.

McGill S, editor: *Low back disorders:* evidence-based prevention and rehabilitation, Champaign, Ill, 2002, Human Kinetics.

This book presents approaches to help professionals make clinical decisions for building prevention and rehabilitation programs.

McNab I, McCulloch J, Transfeldt E: *McNab's backache*, Baltimore, 1997, Lippincott, Williams & Wilkins.

This in-depth text is about the evaluation and treatment of back conditions.

Nicholas J, Herschman E: *The lower extremity and spine in sports medicine*, St Louis, 1995, Mosby.

This two-volume text discusses all aspects of injury to the extremities and the spine. The section on evaluation and treatment of spinal conditions is concise but thorough.

Saunders D: *Evaluation, treatment, and prevention of musculoskeletal disorders*, Bloomington, Minn, 1994, Educational Opportunities.

This text takes a manual therapy approach to treating and rehabilitating musculoskeletal injuries in general and injuries to the spine in particular.

Torg JS, editor: *Head and neck injuries. Clinics in sports medicine*, vol 6, no 1, Philadelphia, 1991, Saunders.

This text provides in-depth coverage of head and neck injuries stemming from sports activities.

White A, Schofferman J: *Spine care: diagnosis and conservative treatment*, St Louis, 1995, Mosby.

This two-volume set looks at both conservative and surgical management of back injuries.

Chapter 26 The Head, Face, Eyes, Ears, Nose, and Throat

When you finish this chapter you should be able to

- Propose a plan for helping to prevent or at least minimize the frequency of injuries to the head.
- Review the related anatomy of the head.
- Establish a systematic process for evaluating concussions and mild head injuries.
- Make an informed decision regarding the sideline and follow-up management of sport-related concussions based on a comprehensive presentation of the available options.
- Recognize the seriousness of a variety of injuries to the head and be aware of the length of time potentially needed for recovery.
- Discuss the value of neuropsychological tests in determining the state of recovery following concussion.
- Be able to correctly identify the various injuries that can occur to the face, eyes, ears, nose, and throat.

Injuries to the region of the head, face, eyes, ears, nose, and throat are common in sports. The severity of injuries to this region can vary from something as benign as a nosebleed to severe concussions of the cortex.

PREVENTION OF INJURIES TO THE HEAD, FACE, EYES, EARS, NOSE, AND THROAT

Although injuries to the head and face are more prevalent in collision and contact sports, the potential for head injuries exists in all sports (Table 26-1).[35] The use of helmets or protective headgear and, in some instances, face masks in sports like football, ice hockey, lacrosse, wrestling, and baseball has dramatically reduced the incidence of injuries to the head, face, eyes, ears, and nose. Some have argued that if the face mask were eliminated in a sport like football, the number of cervical spine and head injuries would be reduced, because the athlete would be less likely to use the head when making contact. It is certain, however, that the incidence of injuries to the face, eyes, ears, and nose would significantly increase. A helmet can do only so much in preventing injury to the brain. Manufacturers of protection headgear for soccer have made unsubstantiated claims about its ability to minimize concussions.[7] All football helmets have written warnings that discourage the use of the head as a weapon. The athletic

TABLE 26-1 Sports with a High Risk for Head Injury[35]

Boxing	Wrestling	Motorcycle racing
Football	Soccer	Diving
Ice hockey	Auto racing	Bicycling
Martial arts	Equestrian events	Snow skiing
Rugby		

trainer has a responsibility to make certain that coaches are teaching and athletes are using correct and safe techniques.

The single most important consideration in reducing injuries to this region involves educating the athlete in (1) proper techniques for initiating contact, and (2) the danger of concussive brain injury and the second impact syndrome.

THE HEAD

Anatomy of the Head

Bones

The skull is composed of twenty-two bones. With the single exception of the mandible, all the bones of the skull are joined together in immovable joints called sutures. The cranial vault, which houses the brain, is enclosed by the cranium, or skull, and is made up of the frontal, ethmoid, sphenoid, two parietal, two temporal, and occipital bones. The skull's thickness varies in different locations; it is thinner over the temporal regions (Figure 26-1).

Scalp

The scalp is the covering of the skull. It has five layers of soft tissue. The skin, connective tissue, and aponeurosis epicranalis are the three outermost tissue layers. They are fused and move as a single layer. The aponeurosis epicranalis is a thick connective tissue sheet that acts as an attachment for the occipitalis and frontalis muscles. Between the first three tissue layers and the periosteum lies a loose connective tissue layer.

Brain

The *brain*, or encephalon, is the part of the central nervous system that is contained within the bony cavity of the cranium (Figure 26-2). It is divided into four sections. The *cerebrum* is the largest part of the brain and is divided into two hemispheres that are separated by a deep longitudinal fissure. The cerebrum, also referred to as the *cortex*, coordinates all voluntary muscle activities and interprets sensory impulses in addition to controlling higher mental functions, including memory, reasoning, intelligence, learning, judgment, and emotions. The *cerebellum* controls synergistic movements of skeletal muscle and plays a critical role in the coordination of voluntary muscular movements. The *pons* controls sleep, posture, respiration, swallowing, and the bladder. The *medulla oblongata* is the lowest part of the brain stem and regulates heart rate, breathing, and blood pressure as well as coughing, sneezing, and vomiting.[74]

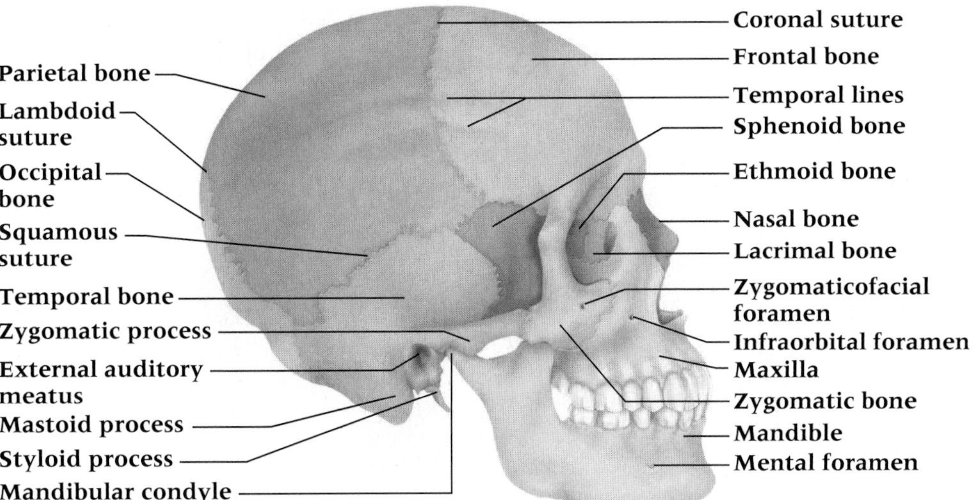

Figure 26-1

Bones of the skull and face.

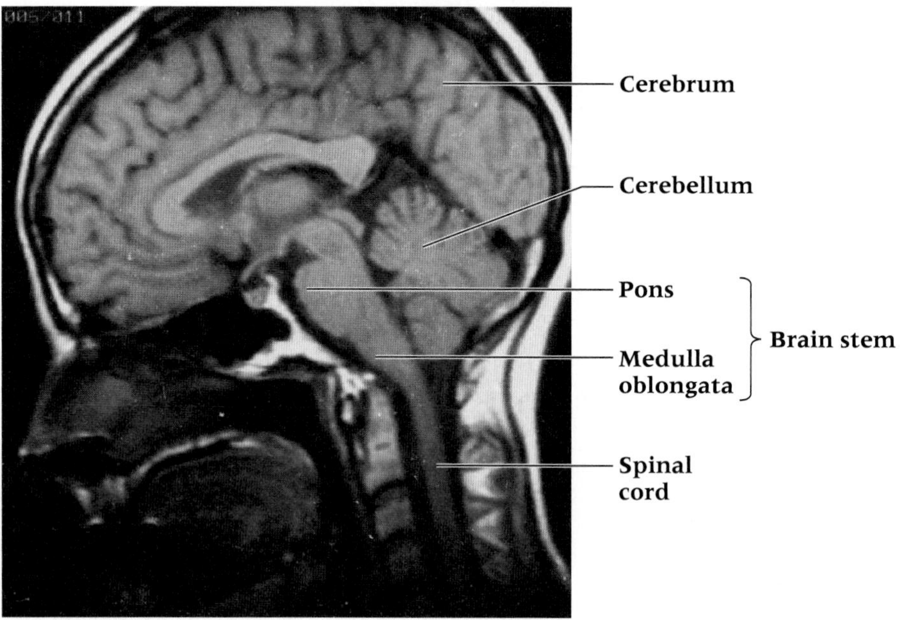

Figure 26-2

Major portions of the brain.

Meninges

Investing the spinal cord and the brain are the *meninges,* which are the three membranes that protect the brain and the spinal cord. Outermost is the dura mater, consisting of a dense, fibrous, and inelastic sheath that encloses the brain and cord. In some places it is attached directly to the vertebral canal, but for the most part, a layer of fat that contains the vital arteries separates this membrane from the bony wall and forms the epidural space. The arachnoid, an extremely delicate sheath, lines the dura mater and is attached directly to the spinal cord by many silklike tissue strands. The dura and arachnoid are separated by the *subdural space,* which contains the veins. The space between the arachnoid and the pia mater, the membrane that helps contain the spinal fluid, is called the *subarachnoid space.* The subarachnoid cavity projects upward and, running the full length of the spinal cord, connects with the ventricles of the brain. The pia mater is a thin, delicate, and highly vascularized membrane that adheres closely to the spinal cord and to the brain (Figure 26-3).[74]

Cerebrospinal fluid is contained between the arachnoid and the pia mater membrane and completely surrounds and suspends the brain. Its main function is to act as a cushion, helping diminish the transmission of shocking forces.

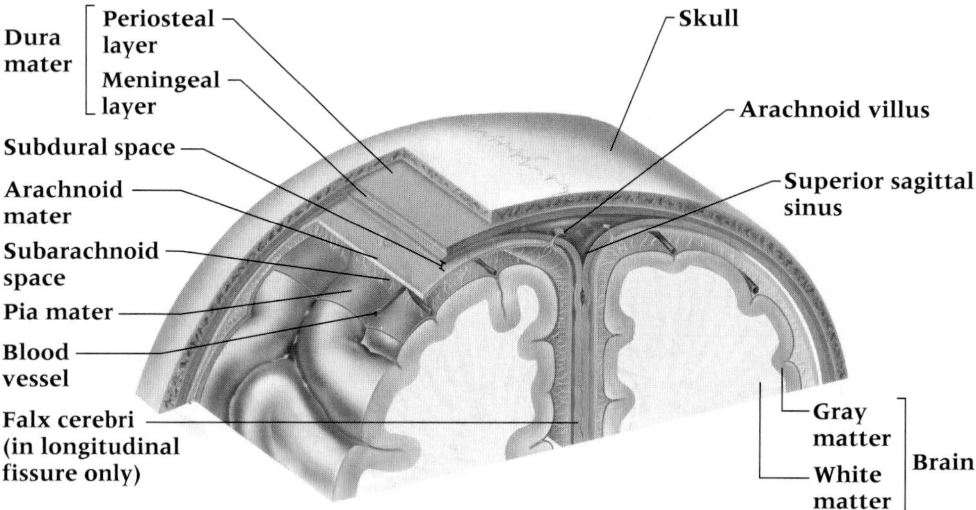

Figure 26-3

The meningeal membranes covering the brain.

Assessment of Head Injuries

Head trauma results in more fatalities than any other sports injury. The morbidity and mortality associated with traumatic brain injury have been labeled a silent epidemic. Traumatic brain injury is common in contact sports such as football, soccer, boxing, ice hockey, and wrestling. But head trauma has also been reported in noncontact sports such as track, baseball, gymnastics, softball, field hockey, volleyball, and cheerleading.[46]

An athlete who receives either a direct blow to the head or body contact that causes the head to snap forward, backward, or rotate to the side must be carefully evaluated for injury to the brain. Injuries to the brain may or may not result in unconsciousness; disorientation or amnesia; motor, coordination, or balance deficits; and cognitive deficits.

The majority of concussions sustained by athletes do not involve loss of consciousness. Nevertheless, the athletic trainer must be prepared to manage those injuries in which there is a loss of consciousness.

The majority of concussions do not involve loss of consciousness.

On-the-field management of the unconscious athlete was discussed in detail in Chapter 12. The athletic trainer must be adept at recognizing and interpreting the signs that an unconscious athlete presents. Priority first aid for any head injury must always deal with any life-threatening condition, but in particular with loss of breathing. When assessing an unconscious athlete, the athletic trainer must always suspect a cervical neck injury and manage the situation accordingly, as described in Chapter 12.[2] An athlete who has been unconscious should be removed from the field on a spine board.

If no life-threatening condition exists, the athletic trainer should note the length of time that the athlete is unconscious and should not move the athlete until he or she regains consciousness. Once the athlete regains consciousness, or if the athlete never lost consciousness, the athletic trainer should obtain a history from the athlete.

History

The two primary components of the history involve determining if the athlete lost consciousness and if he or she has sustained any amnesia.[31] This can be accomplished through a series of questions.

An athlete who has sustained a head injury may or may not be able to respond to questions about exactly what happened to cause the loss of consciousness. Nevertheless, the following questions should be asked:

- Do you know where you are?
- Can you tell me what happened to you?
- Can you remember the score or who we played last week? (This question will determine whether there is retrograde amnesia.)
- Can you remember walking off the field? (This question will determine whether there is antegrade amnesia.)
- Does your head hurt?
- Do you have any pain in your neck?
- Can you move your hands and feet?
- Can you remember if you have ever been knocked out before?

Observation

The athletic trainer who is usually around the athlete both on and off the field has the advantage of knowing what the athlete's affect is normally like and how he or she normally acts. The following observations should be made:

- Is the athlete disoriented and unable to tell where he or she is, what time it is, what date it is, who the opponent is?
- Does the athlete have a blank or vacant stare? Does he or she have difficulty keeping his or her eyes open?
- Does the athlete have slurred or incoherent speech?
- Does the athlete have delayed verbal and motor responses (slow to answer questions or follow instructions)?

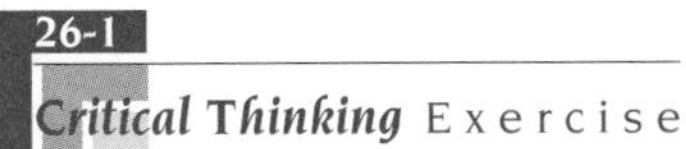

An athlete falls and hits her head, incurring a possible cerebral injury.

? Initially, what observational signs may indicate a cerebral injury?

26-2
Critical Thinking Exercise

A football player sustains a cerebral concussion during a game.

? How should the athletic trainer determine the athlete's level of orientation and memory?

- Does the athlete have a gross coordination disturbance (i.e., stumbling, inability to walk a straight line, can't touch finger to nose)?
- Is the athlete unable to focus attention, and is he or she easily distracted?
- Does the athlete appear to have a memory deficit exhibited by repeatedly asking the same questions or no knowledge of what happened?
- Does the athlete have normal cognitive function (serial sevens, assignment on a particular play)?
- Does the athlete elicit a normal emotional response?
- How long was the athlete's affect abnormal?
- Is the athlete's scalp swollen or bleeding?
- Does the athlete have a clear or straw-colored fluid in the ear canal (cerebrospinal fluid that would occur with skull fracture)?

Palpation

Palpation of both the neck and the skull should be performed in a systematic manner to identify areas of point tenderness or deformity. Deformity to either structure may indicate the presence of a fracture.

Special Tests

Neurologic exam In all cases of head injury, the athletic trainer should administer an on-the-field neurological exam. The neurological exam was discussed in detail in Chapter 13. It consists of six major areas: cerebral testing, which assesses cognitive function; cranial nerve testing; cerebellar testing, which assesses coordination and motor function; sensory testing; reflex testing; and motor testing.

Eye function Abnormal function of the eyes is often related to head injury. The following conditions should be tested:

Checking eye signs can yield crucial information about possible brain injury.

1. Pupils equal and reactive to light (PEARL).
   a. Dilated or irregular pupils. Checking pupil sizes may be particularly difficult at night and under artificial lights. To ensure accuracy, the athlete's pupil size should be compared with that of an official or another player present. However, some individuals normally have pupils that differ in size.[39]
   b. Inability of the pupils to accommodate rapidly to light variance. The athletic trainer can test eye accommodation by covering one of the athlete's eyes with a hand. The covered eye normally will dilate, whereas the uncovered pupil will remain the same. When the hand is removed, the previously covered pupil normally will accommodate readily to the light. A slow-accommodating pupil may indicate cerebral injury.[39]
2. Eyes track smoothly. The athlete is asked to hold the head in a neutral position with both eyes looking straight ahead. The athlete is then asked to follow the top of a pen or pencil, first up as far as possible, then down as far as possible. The eyes are observed for smooth movement and any signs of pain. Next, the tip of the pen or pencil is slowly moved from left to right to determine whether the eyes follow the tip smoothly across the midline of the face or whether they make involuntary movements. A constant involuntary back and forth, up and down, or rotary movement of the eyeball is called *nystagmus* and indicates possible lesion in the posterior fossa of the brain often involving the brain stem or cerebellum.[32]
3. Vision blurred. The athletic trainer can test for blurred vision by determining if the athlete has difficulty reading or is unable to read a game program or the scoreboard.

Balance tests

Romberg test In the past, if the athlete was capable of standing following head injury, a Romberg test was used to assess static balance. Originally, the test was to have the athlete shut the eyes and stand erect with the hands at the sides. Normally, a person can stand motionless in this position, but the tendency to sway or fall to one side is considered a positive Romberg sign indicating a loss of proprioception. A positive sign is one in which the athlete begins to sway, cannot keep the eyes closed, or obviously loses balance. Over the years there have been several variations and modifications to the original Romberg test, most involving changes in foot positions during static stance to alter the base of support. The most commonly used variations have involved a single leg stance and a tandem (heel to toe) stance. Recent evidence suggested that the best on-the-field balance test uses a tandem stance performed on a foam surface[61] or a single-limb (nondominant) stance on a foam surface (Figure 26-4). The standard Romberg test has, however, been criticized for its lack of sensitivity and objectivity. It is considered to be a rather qualitative assessment of static balance because a considerable amount of stress is required to make the subject sway enough for an observer to characterize the sway.

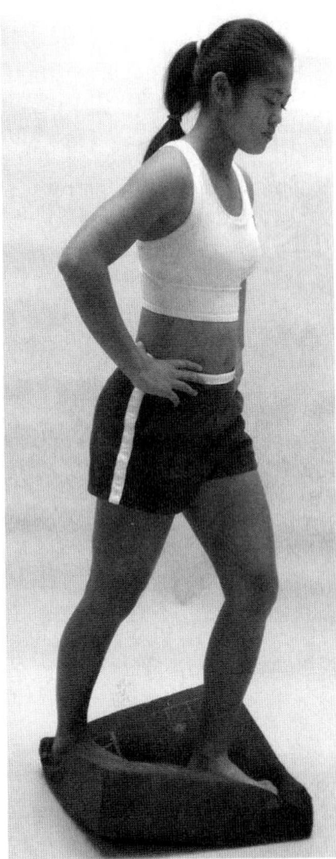

Figure 26-4

A tandem Romberg test standing on an unstable foam surface.

Balance Error Scoring System The use of a quantifiable clinical test battery called the *Balance Error Scoring System (BESS)* is recommended over the standard Romberg test.[31,54,61] Three different stances (double, single, and tandem) are completed twice, once while on a firm surface and once while on a 10-cm-thick piece of medium-density foam (45 cm by 13 cm thick, density 60 kg/m, load deflection 80 to 90) for a total of six trials (Figure 26-5). Athletes are asked to assume the required stance by placing their hands on the iliac crests and close their eyes for twenty seconds. During the single-leg stances, subjects are asked to maintain the contralateral limb in 20 to 30 degrees of hip flexion and 40 to 50 degrees of knee flexion. The athlete is also asked to stand quietly and as motionless as possible in the stance position, keeping the hands on the iliac crest, and eyes closed. The single-limb stance tests are performed on the nondominant foot. This same foot is placed toward the rear in the tandem stances. Subjects are told that upon losing their balance, they are to make any necessary adjustments and return to the testing position as quickly as possible. Performance is scored by adding one error point for each error committed (see *Focus Box:* "Balance Error Scoring System [BESS]"). Trials are considered to be incomplete if the athlete cannot sustain the stance position for longer than five seconds during the entire twenty-second testing period. These trials are assigned a standard maximum error score of 10. Balance test results during injury recovery are best compared to baseline measurements, and athletic trainers working with athletes or patients on a regular basis should try to attain baseline measurements when possible. The focus box provides a sheet for scoring the BESS. The results from this test have been shown to correlate strongly with the results from more sophisticated tests conducted on highly sensitive computerized force plate systems. There does appear to be a slight practice effect with repeated administration of the BESS.[78] It also appears that fatigue decreases performance on the BESS.[82] More sensitive testing can be done off the field with sophisticated balance systems such as those manufactured by Neurocom, Biodex, Chattex, and Breg.

Coordination tests A number of tests have been used to determine whether the head injury has affected coordination. These tests include the finger-to-nose test, heel-to-toe walking, and the standing heel to knee test. Inability to perform any of these tests may be indicative of injury to the cerebellum.

Cognitive tests The purpose of cognitive testing is to establish the effects of head trauma on various cognitive functions and to obtain an objective measure to assess the patient's status and improvement.[35] Cognitive tests may be performed as part of the on-the-field neurological exam. Among the more traditional commonly used on-the-field cognitive tests are serial sevens, in which the athlete counts backwards from 100 by 7; spelling a word backwards; and naming the months in reverse order. Tests of recent memory (the game score, who won last week, what was eaten at breakfast, three-word recall) have also been used.

Neuropsychological assessments Other cognitive tests also referred to as neuropsychological assessments have been developed for use in both on- and off-the-field

Figure 26-5

Balance Error Scoring System (BESS) performed with three different stances. **A,** Double leg. **B,** Single leg. **C,** Tandem on two different surfaces (firm, foam).

Firm

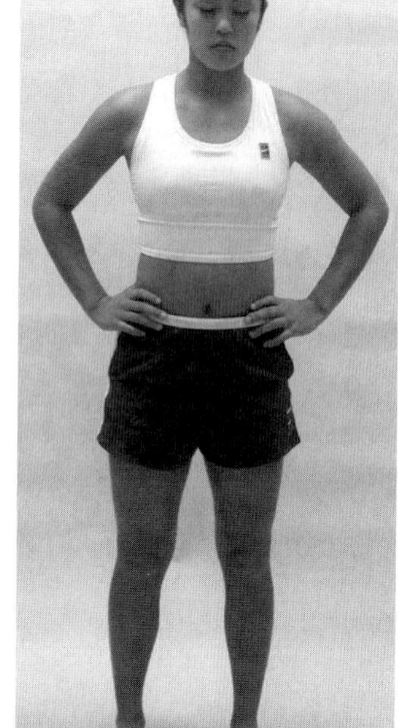

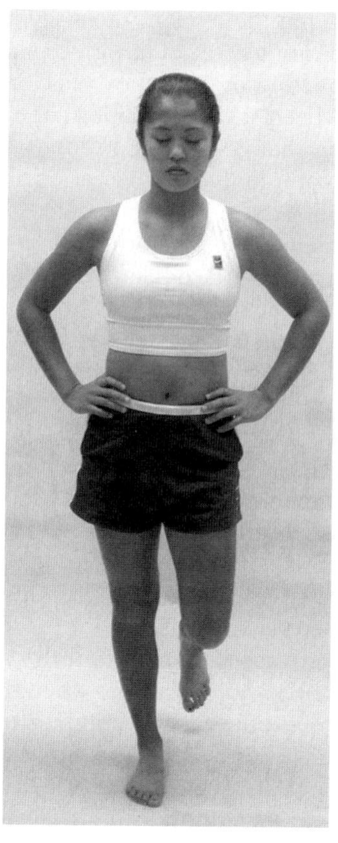

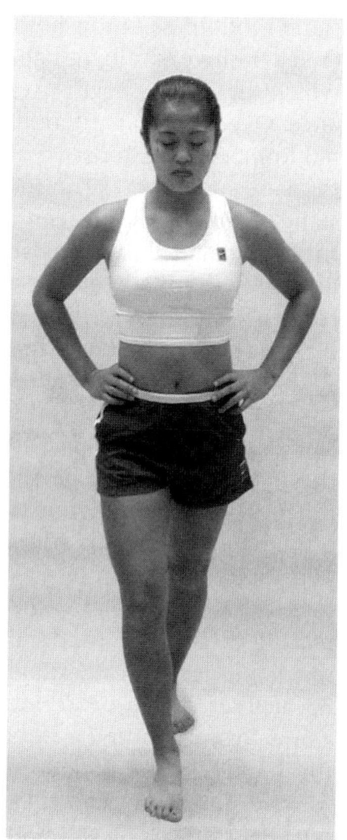

Foam

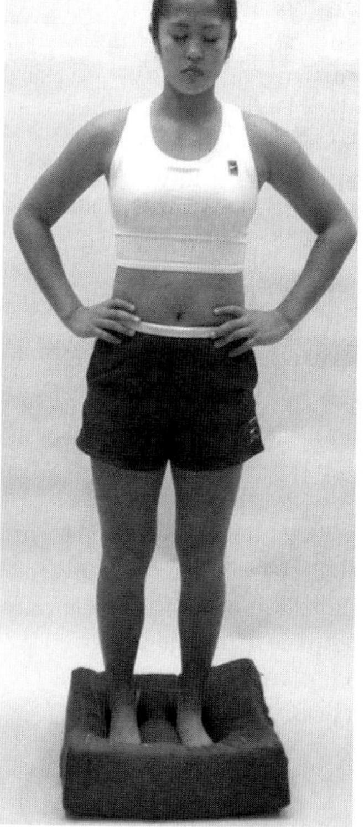

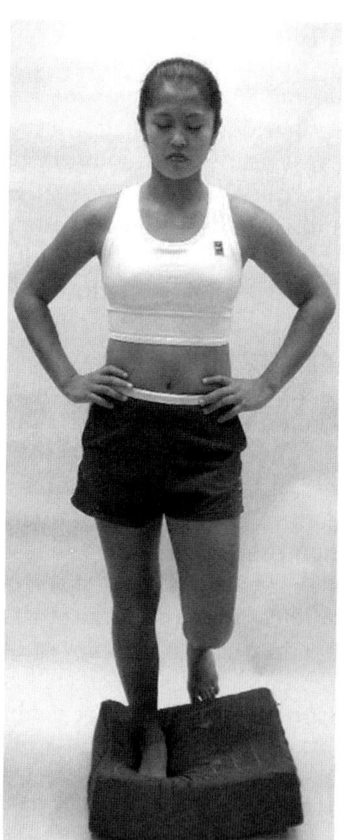

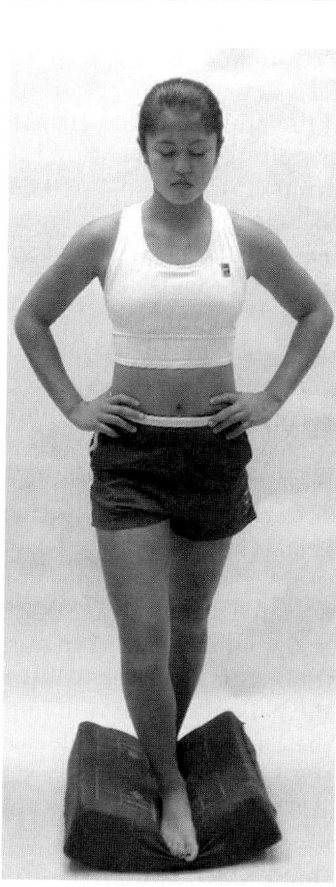

A **B** **C**

Focus

Balance Error Scoring System (BESS)

Balance Error Scoring System (BESS)

Balance Error Scoring System—Types of Errors
1. Hands lifted off iliac crest 2. Opening eyes 3. Step, stumble, or fall 4. Moving hip into > 30 degrees abduction 5. Lifting forefoot or heel 6. Remaining out of testing position > 5 seconds
The BESS is calculated by adding one error point for each error during the six 20-second tests.

SCORE CARD (# errors):	FIRM Surface	FOAM Surface
Double Leg Stance (narrow stance—feet together)		
Single Leg Stance (nondominant foot)		
Tandem Stance (nondominant foot in back)		
Total Scores:		

Total Score:	

evaluation.[20] The *Standardized Assessment of Concussion (SAC)* is an abbreviated neuropsychological test that was designed to provide athletic trainers and other medical personnel responsible for clinical decision making in the care of athletes with immediate objective data concerning the presence and severity of neurocognitive impairment associated with concussion.[43] The test has been designed to be used either on or off the field and includes measures of orientation, immediate memory recall, concentration, and delayed recall. *Focus Box:* "Standardized Assessment of Concussion (SAC) form" provides a form for administering the SAC.

A number of additional neuropsychological assessments focus on short-term memory, working memory, attention, concentration, visual spatial capacity, verbal learning, information processing speed, and/or reaction time. Paper-and-pencil tests have been available for several years and include the *Hopkins Verbal Learning Test, Trail-Making Test Parts A and B, Symbol Digit Modalities Test, Wechsler Digit Span Test—Forward and Backward, Stroop Test,* and the *Controlled Oral Word Association Test.*

More recently, computerized neuropsychological testing programs have been developed and are currently being validated in the athletic setting. The *Automated Neuropsychological Assessment Metrics (ANAM)* system has recently been employed in studies of mild traumatic brain injury, which demonstrated the instrument to be sensitive to measuring cognitive functions most susceptible to deficit after concussion. Other computerized systems include the *CogState,* the *Concussion Resolution Index (CRI),* and the *Immediate Post-Concussion Assessment and Cognitive Testing (ImPACT).* These software packages show great promise for eliminating some of the logistical challenges of baseline testing hundreds of athletes in a timely fashion. Computerized neuropsychological testing has the potential to make a significant contribution to the management of concussion, especially once the tests are validated in the sports medicine setting and their usefulness is better understood. Athletic trainers should be cautioned against trying to interpret the results of neuropsychological tests without the assistance of a licensed neuropsychologist. Neuropsychological assessment scores can be used as part of the decision for return to play following head injury.[21,51] *Focus Box:* "Commonly used neuropsychological tests for sport concussion" lists some of the more commonly used cognitive tests.[51]

TABLE 26-7 Guidelines for Returning to Play After Repeat or Recurrent Concussions[4]

Classification	Grade	First Concussion	Second Concussion	Third Concussion
Colorado Medical Society Guidelines[13]	1 (mild)	May return to play if without symptoms for at least 20 minutes	Terminate contest or practices; may return to play if without symptoms for at least 1 week	Terminate season or may return to play in 3 months if without symptoms
	2 (moderate)	Terminate contest or practice; my return to play if without symptoms for at least 1 week	Consider terminating season; may return to play in 1 month if without symptoms	Terminate season; may return to play next season if without symptoms
	3 (severe)	Terminate contest or practice and transport to hospital; may return to play in 1 month, after 2 consecutive weeks without symptoms	Terminate season; may return to play next season if without symptoms	Terminate season; strongly discourage return to contact or collision sports
Cantu Grading System[10]	1 (mild)	May return to play if asymptomatic* for 1 week; terminate season if CT or MRI abnormality	Return to play in 2 weeks if asymptomatic at the time for 1 week	Terminate season; may return to play next season if asymptomatic
	2 (moderate)	Return to play after asymptomatic* for 2 weeks; terminate season if CT or MRI abnormality	Minimum of 1 month; may return to play then if asymptomatic for 1 week; consider terminating season	Terminate season; may return to play next season if asymptomatic
	3 (severe)	Minimum of 1 month; may then return to play if asymptomatic* for 1 week	Terminate season; may return to play next season if asymptomatic	Consider no further contact sports
American Academy of Neurology Guidelines[36]	1 (mild)	Remove from contest; may return to play if abnormalities or symptoms clear within 15 minutes	Terminate contest; may return to play after 1 week without symptoms at rest and with exercise	
	2 (moderate)	Terminate contest; may return to play after 1 full asymptomatic week at rest and with exertion	Terminate contest; may return to play after at least 2 asymptomatic weeks at rest and with exertion; terminate season if any CT or MRI abnormality	
	3 (severe)	Terminate contest; transport to hospital if unconscious or neurologic abnormality; if concussion brief (seconds) may return in 1 week if no symptoms at rest and with exertion; if concussion prolonged (minutes) return in 2 weeks, no symptoms	Terminate contest; may return to play after minimum of 1 month asymptomatic; terminate season if any CT or MRI abnormalities	

*Asymptomatic in all cases means no postconcussive symptoms, including retrograde or anterograde amnesia at rest or with exertion.
Modified from Bailes JE, Hudson V: Classification of sport-related head trauma: a spectrum of mild to severe injury, *J Ath Train* 36(3):236, 2001.

decision to allow an athlete to return to play following an initial head injury must be carefully made based on the absence of postconcussive symptoms.

Cerebral Contusion

Etiology A contusion of the cerebrum is a focal injury to the brain that involves small hemorrhages or *intracerebral bleeding* within either the cortex, the brain stem, or the cerebellum (Figure 26-6).[23] Brain contusions usually result from an impact injury in which the head strikes a stationary, immovable object such as the floor.

Symptoms and signs Depending on the extent of trauma and the injury site, symptoms and signs may vary significantly. In most instances, the athlete experiences a loss of consciousness but subsequently becomes very alert and talkative. A neurological exam will be normal; however, symptoms such as headaches, dizziness, and nausea will persist.

Management Hospitalization and CT or MRI tests are standard for a cerebral contusion. Treatment varies according to the clinical status of the athlete.[23] A decision to return to play can only be made when the athlete is asymptomatic and a CT scan is normal.

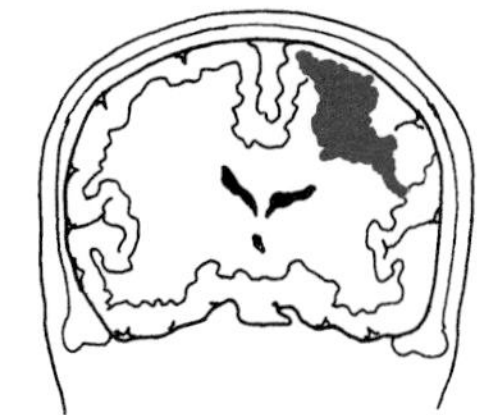

Figure 26-6

Intracerebral bleeding.

The three major types of intracranial hematomas:

- Epidural
- Subdural
- Intracerebral

Malignant Brain Edema Syndrome

Etiology This condition occurs in the young athletic population. In adults this syndrome occurs due to an intracranial clot. However in children there is diffuse brain swelling resulting from hyperemia or vascular engorgement with little or no injury to the brain. The serious or perhaps life-threatening consequences of this condition are due to raised intracranial pressure with herniation.[12]

Symptoms and signs There is rapid neurologic deterioration from a normal alert state that progresses to coma and occasionally death within minutes to several hours following head trauma.

Management This condition is a life-threatening situation that requires immediate recognition and subsequent rapid treatment in an emergency care facility.

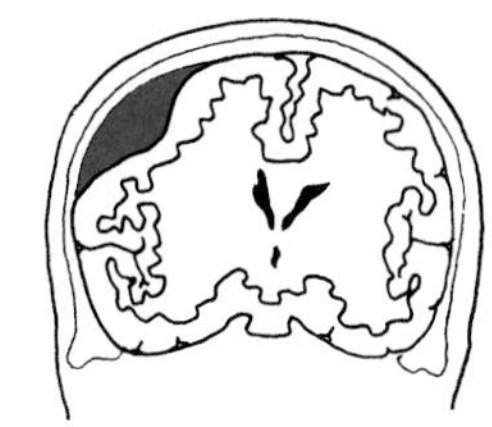

Figure 26-7

Epidural bleeding.

Epidural Hematoma

Etiology A blow to the head or a skull fracture can cause a tear of the meningeal arteries, which are imbedded in bony grooves in the skull (Figure 26-7). Because of arterial blood pressure, blood accumulation and the creation of a hematoma occur extremely quickly—usually within minutes to a few hours.[8]

Symptoms and signs In most cases, initially, there will be a loss of consciousness. In some cases, once the athlete regains consciousness, he or she may be lucid and show few or none of the symptoms of serious head injury. Gradually symptoms begin to worsen, and the athlete experiences severe head pains; dizziness; nausea; dilation of one pupil, usually on the same side as the injury; or sleepiness (see *Focus Box:* "Conditions indicating the possibility of increasing intracranial pressure"). Later stages of an epidural hematoma are characterized by deteriorating consciousness, neck rigidity, depression of pulse and respiration, and convulsions.[4] An epidural hematoma is a life-threatening situation that necessitates urgent neurosurgical care.[8]

Management A CT scan is necessary to diagnose an epidural hematoma. The pressure of an epidural hematoma must be surgically relieved as soon as possible to avoid the possibility of death or permanent disability.

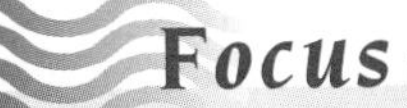

Conditions indicating the possibility of increasing intracranial pressure

- Headache
- Nausea and vomiting
- Unequal pupils
- Disorientation
- Progressive or sudden impairment in consciousness
- Gradual increase in blood pressure
- Decrease in pulse rate

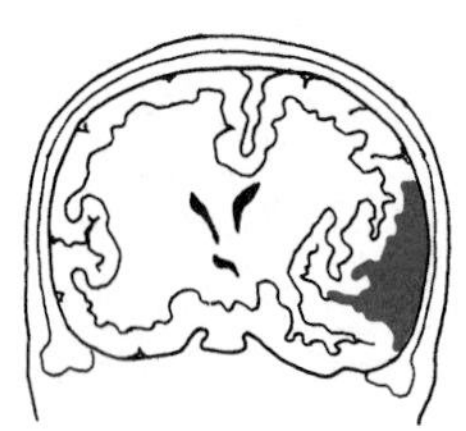

Figure 26-8

Subdural bleeding.

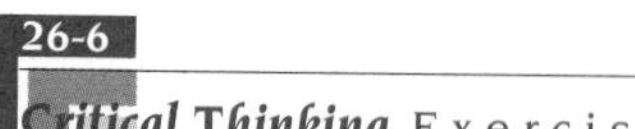

A football player sustains a subdural hematoma following a helmet hit during a game.

? How do the symptoms of a subdural hematoma compare to the symptoms of an epidural hematoma?

Subdural Hematoma

Etiology Acute subdural hematomas occur much more frequently than do epidural hematomas and are the most common cause of death in athletes.[41] Subdural hematomas result from acceleration/deceleration forces that tear vessels that bridge the dura mater and the brain (Figure 26-8).[4]

There are three kinds of subdural hematoma. One is an acute subdural hematoma which progresses rapidly and acts like an epidural hematoma. It occurs due to arterial bleeding. The second is the subdural hematoma seen in association with other brain (contusions) and skull injuries. The third is a chronic subdural hematoma, which occurs due to venous bleeding. If the bridging veins are torn, low pressure venous bleeding occurs into the subdural space, but because of the low pressure, the rising intracranial pressure tamponades the bleeding before serious intracranial pressure occurs. Most subdural hematomas that occur in athletes involve the acute rapidly progressing form. The acute subdural hematoma is also a common cause of death in boxers.

Symptoms and signs With a simple subdural hematoma, the athlete is not likely to be unconscious; the athlete with a complicated subdural hematoma would almost always be unconscious and would exhibit dilation of one pupil, usually on the same side as the injury. Both types would show signs of headache, dizziness, nausea, or sleepiness.

Management An acute subdural hematoma is a life-threatening situation that calls for immediate medical attention. A diagnostic CT scan or MRI is necessary to determine the extent and location of the hemorrhage.

Migraine Headaches

Etiology A migraine is a type of headache that usually happens in episodes or attacks that may last anywhere from four hours to as long as seventy-two hours. A migraine is now recognized as a distinct neurologic disorder. Migraines are more common in women than men. The exact cause of migraines is unknown, however it is thought to be an inherited problem. Many factors or triggers may cause a migraine. Triggers could include certain foods, medications, sensory stimuli (flickering/bright lights, bright sunlight, odors), or lifestyle changes (sleep patterns, eating habits, stress). Falling estrogen levels that occur just before menstruation can precipitate a migraine headache in many women.[56]

Symptoms and signs The pain of a migraine headache is generally moderate to severe and can disrupt normal activities. It may feel like it is throbbing or pulsating and may be located on one side of the head. It is not uncommon for the pain and other symptoms to be so severe that the person only wants to lie down in a dark room and go to sleep. The pain may be accompanied by nausea; vomiting; or sensitivity to light, sound, or smell. Some people experience an aura ten to thirty minutes before they have a migraine headache, which can include visual changes such as bright flashing lights or colored zigzag lines, blind spots, or loss of vision on one side. An aura also can include a tingling sensation or numbness in the arms or legs, or dizziness. The cause of this aura is still unknown.[75]

Management The best management of migraine is prevention. Prophylactic medications such as promethazine can help reduce the recurrence of migraines. For severe attacks, the administration of a prescription drug, such as ergotamine tartrate or sumatriptan succinate (Imitrex), has a high success rate.

Scalp Injuries

The scalp can receive lacerations, abrasions, contusions, and hematomas.

Etiology The cause of scalp injury is usually blunt or penetrating trauma. A scalp laceration could exist in conjunction with a serious skull or cerebral injury.

Symptoms and signs The athlete complains of being hit in the head. Bleeding is often extensive, making it difficult to pinpoint the exact site. Matted hair and dirt can also disguise the actual point of injury.

Management The treatment of a scalp laceration poses a special problem because of its general inaccessibility. (See *Focus Box:* "Care of scalp lacerations.")

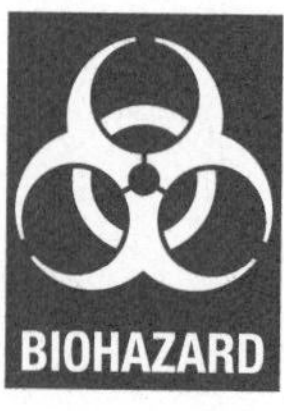

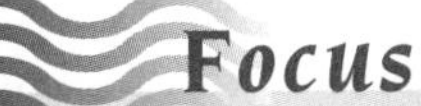

Care of scalp lacerations

Materials needed

Antiseptic soap, water, antiseptic, 4-inch (10-cm) gauze pads, sterile cotton, and hair clippers.

Position of the athlete

The athlete lies on the table with the wound upward.

Procedure

1. The entire area of bleeding is thoroughly cleansed with antiseptic soap and water. Washing the wound to remove dirt and debris is best done in lengthwise movements.
2. After the injury site is cleansed and dried, it is exposed and, if necessary, the hair is cut away. Enough scalp should be exposed so that a bandage and tape may be applied.
3. Firm pressure or an astringent can be used to reduce bleeding if necessary.
4. Wounds that are more than ½ inch (1.25 cm) in length and ⅛ inch (0.3 cm) in depth should be referred to a physician for treatment. In less severe wounds the bleeding should be controlled and an antiseptic applied, followed by the application of a protective coating such as collodion and a sterile gauze pad. A tape adherent is then painted over the skin area to ensure that the tape sticks to the skin.

THE FACE

Anatomy of the Face

The facial skin covers subcutaneous bone that has very little protective muscle, fascia, or fat. The supraorbital ridges house the frontal sinuses. In general, the facial skeleton is composed of dense bony buttresses combined with thin sheets of bone. The middle third of the face consists of the maxillary bone, which supports the nose and nasal passages. The lower aspect of the face consists of the lower jaw, or mandible. Besides supporting teeth, the mandible also supports the larynx, trachea, upper airway, and upper digestive tract (see Figure 26-1).

Temporomandibular Joint

The temporomandibular joint (TMJ) is the articulation between the mandibular condyle and the mandibular fossa of the temporal bone.[69] It moves in a hingelike manner when the mouth is opened and closed and glides forward, backward, and side to side when biting or chewing. The TMJ is surrounded by a joint capsule. Within the joint capsule lies a fibrocartilaginous meniscus that separates and cushions the bones and provides for a better fit between the articulating surfaces. The joint capsule is supported by sphenomandibular, temporomandibular, and stylomandibular ligaments (Figure 26-9).

Recognition and Management of Specific Facial Injuries

With any type of injury to the face, the athletic trainer should always suspect the possibility of an associated head injury.

Mandible Fracture

Etiology Fractures of the lower jaw, or mandible (Figure 26-10), occur most often in collision sports. They are second most common type of all facial fracture. Because it has relatively little padding and sharp contours, the lower jaw is prone to injury from a direct blow. The most frequently fractured area is near the jaw's frontal angle.

Symptoms and signs The main indications of a fractured mandible are deformity, loss of normal occlusion of the teeth, pain when biting down, bleeding around teeth, and lower lip anesthesia.[67]

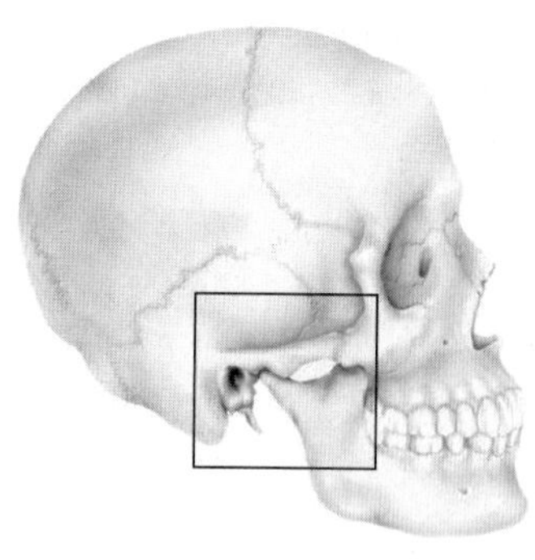

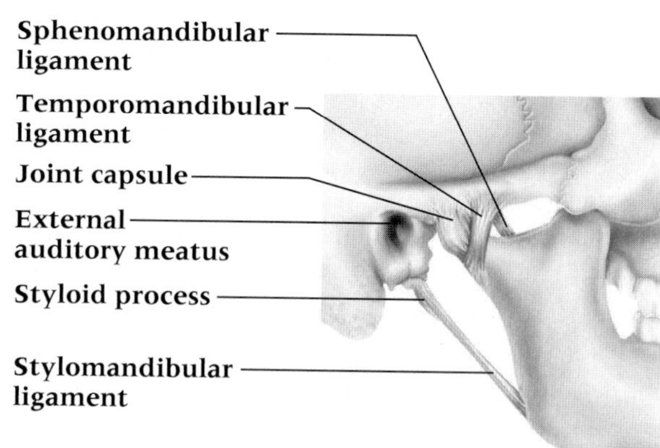

Figure 26-9

The temporomandibular joint (TMJ).

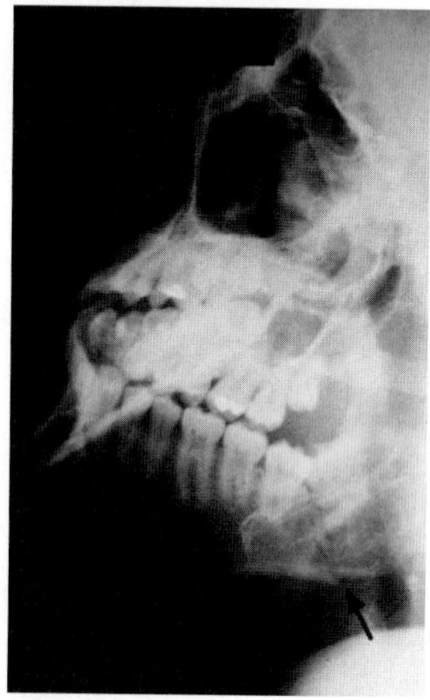

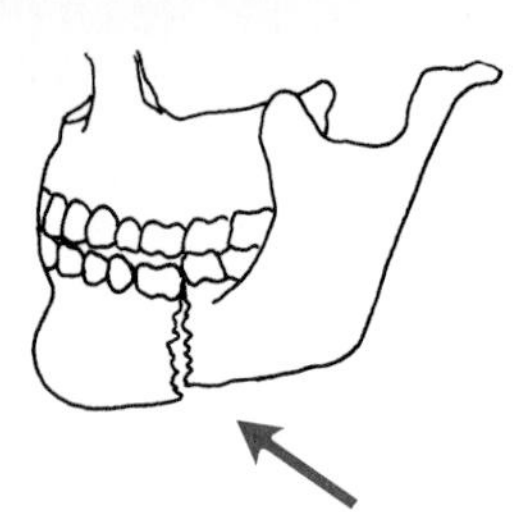

Figure 26-10

Mandibular fracture.

Management Fracture of the mandible requires temporary immobilization with an elastic bandage followed by reduction and fixation of the jaw by a physician. Mild repetitive activities can be carried out, such as light weight lifting, swimming, or cycling. Recovery time is from four to six weeks. Full activity is resumed in two to three months with appropriate special headgear and customized mouth guard.[67]

Mandibular Dislocation

Etiology A dislocation of the jaw, or *mandibular luxation,* involves the temporomandibular joint (see Figure 26-9). Because of its wide range of movement and the inequity of size between the mandibular condyle and the temporal fossa, the jaw is somewhat prone to dislocation. The mechanism of injury in dislocations is usually a side blow to the open mouth of the athlete, which forces the mandibular condyle forward out of the temporal fossa. This injury may occur as either a luxation (complete dislocation) or a subluxation (partial dislocation).

Symptoms and signs The major signs of the dislocated jaw are a locked-open position, with jaw movement being almost impossible, and an overriding malocclusion of the teeth.

Management Initially, cold is applied along with elastic bandage immobilization and reduction. Follow-up care includes a soft diet, NSAIDs, and analgesic when needed for one to two weeks. A gradual return to activity can begin seven to ten days after the acute period.[67] Complications of jaw dislocations are recurrent dislocation, malocclusion, and TMJ dysfunction.

Temporomandibular Joint Dysfunction

Etiology The TMJ is important for both communication and mastication, and it has a high degree of mobility. Because of this extreme mobility, the stability of the joint is compromised. The bony configuration of the joint does not limit its mobility, so the muscles and ligaments provide the primary stability.

The most common cause of TMJ dysfunction is a disk-condyle derangement in which the disk is positioned anteriorly with respect to the condyle when the jaw is closed. As the jaw opens and the condyle translates forward, the disk relocates over the condyle, producing an audible click. A second click may occur when the jaw is closed. This chronic derangement eventually leads to deterioration of the posterior stabilizing structures and, ultimately, anterior dislocation of the disk. This chronic derangement is most typically treated through the use of a custom-designed removable mouthpiece that repositions the condyles anteriorly.[69]

A dislocation of the TMJ occurs when one or occasionally both condyles are dislocated forward and prevent the jaw from closing.

Symptoms and signs TMJ dysfunction has been identified as a cause of various signs and symptoms within the head and neck, including headache, earache, vertigo, inflammation, and neck pain associated with trigger points and muscle guarding.

Problems in and about the TMJ are similar to those of other synovial joints in that TMJ dysfunction may result from inflammation of the synovial capsule, internal disk derangement, malocclusion, hypermobility or hypomobility, muscle dysfunction, or limited mandibular joint range of motion.[69]

Management Management of TMJ dysfunction should address the causes of the problem. Hypermobility can be corrected using strengthening exercises. Hypomobility may be corrected by using techniques of joint mobilization. Therapeutic modalities can be used to treat pain and to provide heat as needed. Often the use of a dental appliance is recommended. A custom-fitted mouth guard or even a manufactured mouth guard can be used to correct problems of occlusion. If these corrective measures fail, the athlete should be referred to a dentist for treatment.

Zygomatic Complex (Cheekbone) Fracture

Etiology A fracture of the zygoma represents the third most common facial fracture.[71] The mechanism of injury is a direct blow to the cheekbone. This can be classified as a LeFort fracture which refers to a fracture of one or more of the facial bones, including not only the zygoma but also potentially the maxillary, orbital, and nasal bones as well.

Symptoms and signs An obvious deformity occurs in the cheek region, or a bony discrepancy can be felt during palpation. There is usually a nosebleed **(epistaxis),** and the athlete commonly complains of seeing double **(diplopia).** There is also numbness of the cheek.

epistaxis (epp is **tax** is)
Nosebleed.

diplopia (dip **low** peeah)
Seeing double.

Management Care by the athletic trainer should usually involve cold application for the control of edema and immediate referral to a physician. Healing takes six to eight weeks. Proper protective gear must be worn when the athlete returns to activity.

Maxillary Fracture

Etiology A severe blow to the upper jaw, such as from a hockey puck or stick, can fracture the maxilla. This injury ranks as the fourth most common type of facial fracture.

Symptoms and signs After being struck a severe blow to the upper jaw, the athlete complains of pain while chewing, malocclusion, nosebleed, double vision, and numbness in the lip and cheek region.[67]

Management Because bleeding is usually profuse, airway passages must be maintained. A brain injury may also be associated with this condition, as with all injuries to the face. The athlete must be transported immediately to a hospital; the conscious athlete should be transported in an upright, forward-leaning position. This position allows external drainage of saliva and blood.[67] Fracture reduction, fixation, and immobilization are carried out as specific treatment.[66]

26-7
Critical Thinking Exercise

A lacrosse player sustains a severe blow to her cheek by a stick. The blow fractures her maxilla but does not knock her unconscious.

? How should the athlete be transported to the hospital and why?

Facial Lacerations

Etiology Facial lacerations are common in contact and collision sports. Lacerations about the face are caused by a direct impact to the face with a sharp object or by an indirect compressive force.

Symptoms and signs The athlete feels pain, and there is substantial bleeding and obvious tearing of the epidermis, dermis, and often the subcutaneous layer of skin (Figure 26-11).

Management The procedures for facial lacerations are presented in the section on wound care in Chapter 28. The athlete should be referred to a physician for definitive care, such as suturing. Athletic trainers should note that with *eyebrow lacerations,* they should not shave the eyebrow because it may not regrow, or if it does, it may do so in an irregular pattern.[16] Lip, oral, ear, cheek, and nasal lacerations, like all facial lacerations, are grossly contaminated and must be carefully cleaned before suturing to avoid infection. Systemic antibiotics and tetanus prophylaxis may be necessary.[16]

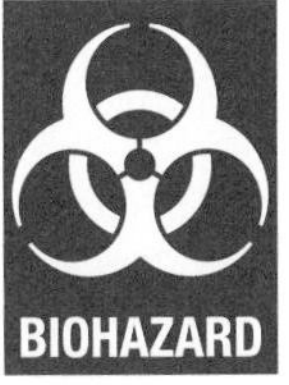

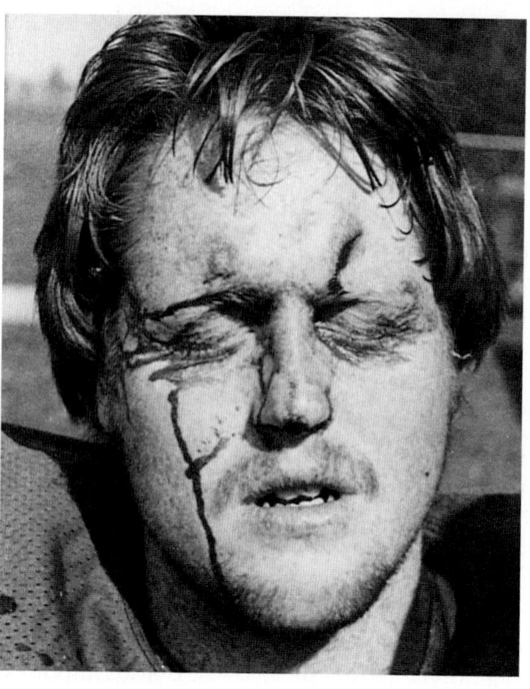

Figure 26-11

Facial lacerations can be a medical emergency.

DENTAL INJURIES

Anatomy of the Teeth

The tooth is a composite of mineral salts of which calcium and phosphorus are most abundant. The portion protruding from the gum, called the *crown,* is covered by the hardest substance within the body, the enamel. The portion that extends into the alveolar bone of the mouth is called the *root* and is covered by a thin, bony substance known as *cementum.* Underneath the enamel and cementum lies the bulk of the tooth, a hard material known as *dentin*. Within the dentin is a central canal and chamber containing the *pulp,* which is composed of nerves, lymphatics, and blood vessels that supply the entire tooth (Figure 26-12). With the use of face guards and properly fitting mouth guards, most dental injuries can be prevented (see Chapter 7).

Preventing Dental Injuries

There is universal agreement within the dental community that all athletes, but particularly those in contact/collision sports, should routinely wear mouth guards to prevent injuries to the teeth.[5] Chapter 7 includes a discussion of the different types of mouthguards available and the relative advantages and disadvantages of each. Without question, the mandatory use of mouth guards by both high school and collegiate football players has significantly reduced the incidence of oral injuries in those sports. However, there is still a high incidence of dental injuries in those sports that do not require mouth guards to be worn.[19]

Athletes should practice good dental hygiene that includes regular brushing, rinsing, and flossing. Like everyone else, athletes should have dental screenings at least once each year to prevent the development of dental caries (cavities), which is a gradual decay and degeneration of soft or bony tissue of a tooth. If this decay progresses, the tissue surrounding the tooth can become inflamed and an *abscess* forms from a bacterial infection of the tooth. Poor dental hygiene can also lead to *gingivitis,* which is an inflammation of the gums that causes swelling, redness, tenderness, and a tendency to bleed easily. Chronic gingivitis can lead to *periodontitis,* in which there is an inflammation and/or a degeneration of the dental periosteum, the surrounding bone, and the cementum; loosening of the teeth; recession of the gingiva; and infection.[60]

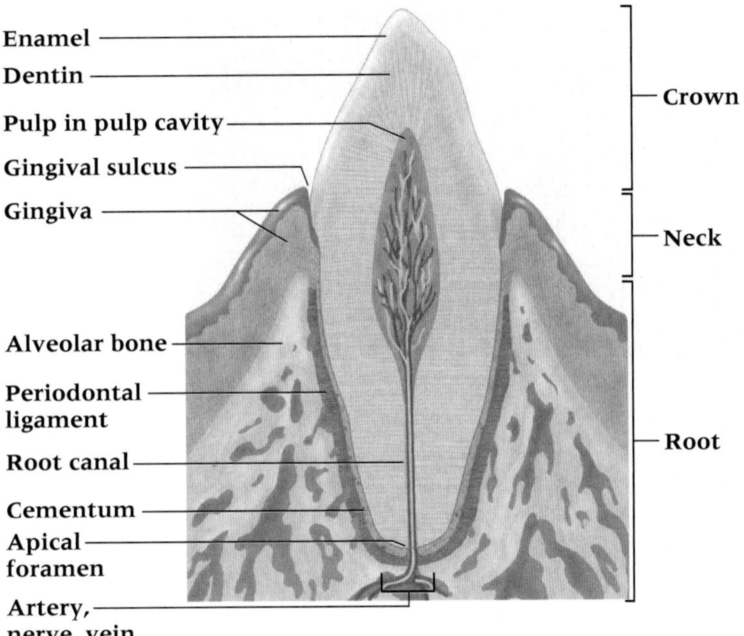

Figure 26-12

Anatomy of a tooth.

Recognition and Management of Specific Dental Injuries

Tooth Fractures

Etiology Any impact to the upper or lower jaw or direct trauma can potentially fracture the teeth.[63] Three types of fractures can occur to the teeth: an uncomplicated crown fracture, a complicated crown fracture, and a root fracture (Figure 26-13).

Symptoms and signs In an uncomplicated crown fracture, a small portion of the tooth is broken but there is no bleeding from the fracture and the pulp chamber is not exposed. In a complicated crown fracture, a portion of the tooth is broken and there is bleeding from the fracture. The pulp chamber is exposed, and there is a great deal of pain (Figure 26-14). A root fracture occurs below the gum line; therefore, diagnosis is difficult and may require an X ray. Root fractures account for only 10 percent to 15 percent of all dental fractures. The tooth may appear to be in the normal position, but there is bleeding from the gum around the tooth, and the crown of the tooth may be pushed back or loose.

Any impact great enough to cause a fracture of a tooth could also produce a fracture of the mandible or even a concussion.[63]

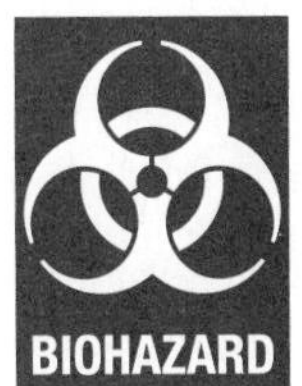

Management Neither uncomplicated nor complicated crown fractures require immediate treatment by a dentist. The fractured piece of tooth can simply be placed in a plastic bag, and if the fractured tooth is not extremely sensitive to air or cold, the athlete can continue to play and can see the dentist within twenty-four to forty-eight

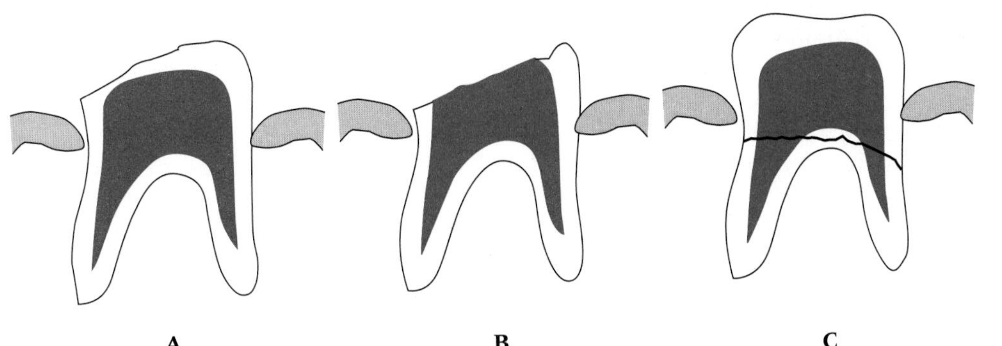

Figure 26-13

Tooth fractures. **A,** Uncomplicated crown fracture. **B,** Complicated crown fracture. **C,** Root fracture.

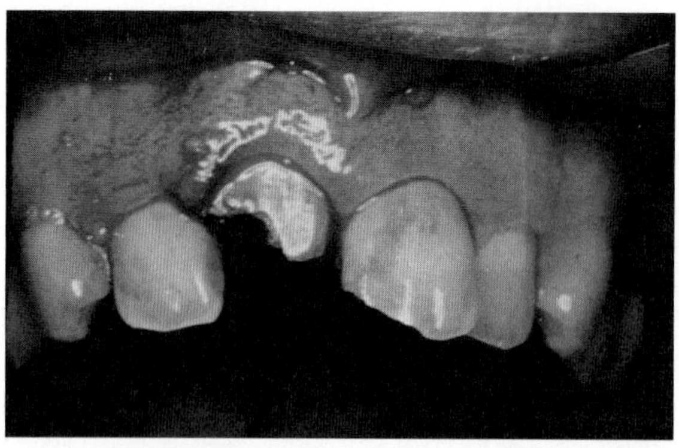

Figure 26-14

A fractured tooth.

26-8

***Critical Thinking* Exercise**

A basketball player is elbowed in the mouth while fighting for a rebound. He comes to the sidelines with blood in his mouth saying that he thinks he has chipped a tooth. Upon examination the athletic trainer determines that the blood is coming from a cut in the lip and that a small portion of one of his upper front teeth is broken but there is no bleeding from the fracture and it does not appear that the pulp chamber has been exposed.

? What type of tooth fracture does this athlete have, and how should this incident be managed?

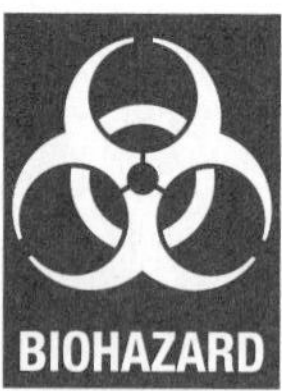

hours after the game. If there is bleeding, a piece of gauze can be placed over the fracture. For the sake of appearance, the fractured piece of tooth can be glued in place or the tooth can be capped with a synthetic composite material.

In the case of a root fracture, the athlete may continue to play but should see a dentist as soon as possible after the game. A tooth that is pushed back should not be forced forward because doing so is likely to make the fracture worse. The dentist will reposition the tooth and apply a brace to be worn for three to four months. The athlete should wear a mouth guard while competing.

Tooth Subluxation, Luxation, Avulsion

Etiology The same mechanisms that can cause a tooth fracture may also cause loosening or dislocation of the tooth.[63] Loosening of the tooth can result in concussion or subluxation, luxation, or avulsion.

Symptoms and signs A tooth may be slightly loosened or totally dislodged. In the case of a concussion or subluxation, the tooth is still in its normal place and is only slightly loose. The athlete feels little or no pain but indicates that the tooth just feels different. In a luxation, the tooth is not fractured but is very loose and has moved either forward to an extruded position or backward to an intruded position. In an avulsion, the tooth is knocked completely out of the mouth.

Management For a concussion or subluxation, no immediate treatment is required, and the athlete should be referred to a dentist within forty-eight hours for evaluation only. In a luxation, the tooth should be moved back into its normal position only if it is easy to move. The athlete should be referred to a dentist as soon as possible, especially if the tooth could not be moved back to its normal position. The athletic trainer should try to reimplant an avulsed tooth. The avulsed tooth can be rinsed off but should never be scraped or scrubbed to get dirt off. If the tooth cannot be reimplanted, it should be stored in a "Save a Tooth" kit, which contains Hank's Balanced Salt Solution (HBSS), or in milk or saline.[49] If the athlete is conscious and a Save a Tooth kit is not available the tooth can be placed between the cheek and gum while the athlete is transported to a dentist. The athlete should be referred to the dentist immediately. The sooner the tooth can be reimplanted, the better the prognosis.

NASAL INJURIES

Anatomy of the Nose

The nose functions to clean, warm, and humidify inhaled air. The external portion of the nose is formed by a combination of bone in the superior portion and fibrocartilage inferiorly that spreads laterally to form the ala. The nasal cavity extends from the nostrils posteriorly to the choanae. A nasal septum divides the nasal cavity into right and left chambers.

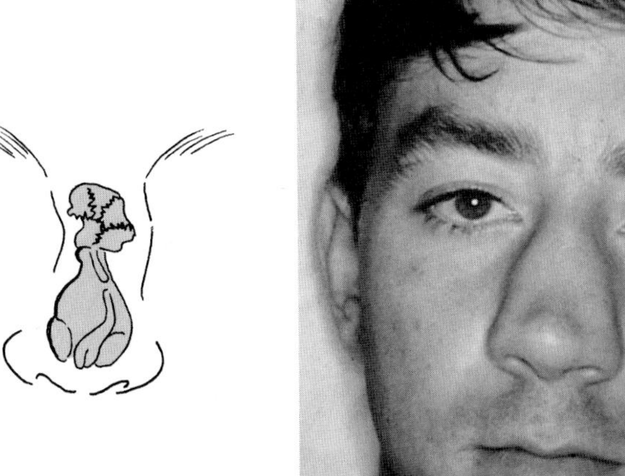

Figure 26-15

A nasal fracture may pose a serious medical problem.

Recognition and Management of Specific Nose Injuries

Nasal Fractures and Chondral Separation

Etiology A fracture of the nose is the most common fracture of the face. The force of the blow to the nose may come either from the side or from a straight frontal force. A lateral force causes greater deformity than a straight-on blow does.

Symptoms and signs The nasal fracture appears frequently as a separation of the frontal processes of the maxilla, a separation of the lateral cartilages, or a combination of the two (Figure 26-15).

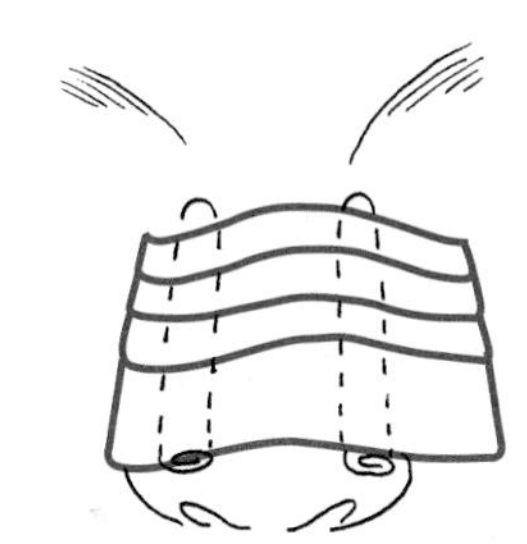

Figure 26-16

Splinting the nose fracture.

In nasal fractures, hemorrhage is profuse because of laceration of the mucous lining. Swelling is immediate. Deformity is usually present if the nose has received a lateral blow. Gentle palpation may reveal abnormal mobility and emit a grating sound (crepitus).

Management The athletic trainer should control the bleeding and then refer the athlete to a physician for X-ray examination and reduction of the fracture. Simple and uncomplicated fractures of the nose will not hinder the athlete or be unsafe, and he or she will be able to return to competition within a few days. Fracture deformity reduction must be performed by a trained person.[73] Adequate protection can be provided through splinting (see *Focus Box:* "Nose splinting" and Figure 26-16).

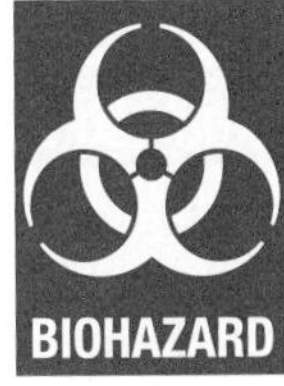

Deviated Septum

Etiology The mechanism of injury to the septum, like that to the nasal fracture, is compression or lateral trauma.

Symptoms and signs A careful evaluation of the nose must be made after the trauma. Injury commonly produces bleeding and, in some cases, a septal hematoma. The athlete complains of nasal pain.

Management Compression should be applied to the site at which a hematoma may occur. When a hematoma is present, it must be drained immediately via a surgical incision through the nasal septal mucosa. After surgical drainage, a small wick is inserted for continued drainage, and the nose is firmly packed to prevent the hematoma from re-forming. If a hematoma is neglected, an abscess will form, causing bone and cartilage loss and, ultimately, a difficult-to-correct deformity.

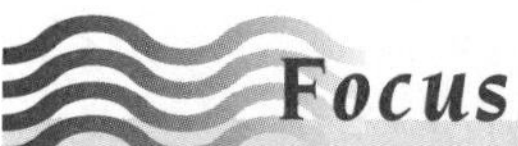

Nose splinting

The following procedure is used for nose splinting.

Materials needed

Two pieces of gauze, each 2 inches (5 cm) long and rolled to the size of a pencil; three strips of 1½-inch (3.8 cm) tape cut approximately 4 inches (10 cm) long; and clear tape adherent.

Position of the athlete

The athlete lies supine on the training table.

Procedure

1. The rolled pieces of gauze are placed on either side of the athlete's nose.
2. Gently but firmly, 4-inch (10 cm) lengths of tape are laid over the gauze rolls.

26-9

Critical Thinking **Exercise**

A wrestler is hit in the nose, which injures the lateral nasal wall and causes epistaxis.

? How should this nosebleed be managed?

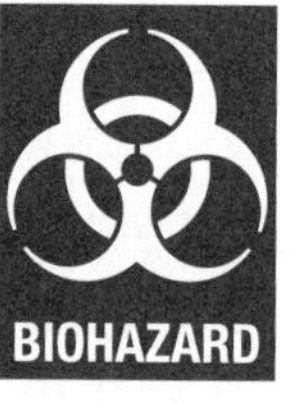

Nosebleed (Epistaxis)

Etiology Nosebleeds in sports are usually the result of direct blows that cause varying degrees of contusion to the septum. Epistaxis can be classified as either anterior or posterior. Anterior epistaxis originates from the nasal septum, and posterior epistaxis from the lateral wall. Anterior epistaxis is more common by far and may result from a direct blow, a sinus infection, high humidity, allergies, a foreign body lodged in the nose, or some other serious facial or head injury.[79]

Symptoms and signs Hemorrhages arise most often from the highly vascular anterior aspect of the nasal septum. In most situations, the nosebleed presents only a minor problem and stops spontaneously after a short period of time. However, there are persistent types that require medical attention and possibly cauterization. As always when blood is present, universal precautions must be used.

Management An athlete with an acute nosebleed should sit upright with a cold compress placed over both the nose and the ipsilateral carotid artery while finger pressure is applied to the affected nostril for five minutes. A piece of rolled-up gauze also may be placed between the upper lip and gum, which places direct pressure on the arteries that supply the nasal mucosa.[79]

If this procedure fails to stop the bleeding within five minutes, more extensive measures should be taken. The athletic trainer should use an applicator to paint the hemorrhage point with an astringent or a styptic such as tannic acid or epinephrine hydrochloride solution. The application of a gauze or cotton pledget will provide corking action and encourage blood clotting. If a pledget is used, the ends should protrude from the nostrils at least ½ inch (1.25 cm) to facilitate removal. After bleeding has ceased, the athlete may resume activity but should be reminded not to blow the nose under any circumstances for at least two hours after the initial insult.

EAR INJURIES

Anatomy of the Ear

The ear (Figure 26-17) is responsible for the sense of hearing and for equilibrium. It is composed of three parts: the external ear; the middle ear (tympanic membrane), lying just inside the skull; and the internal ear (labyrinth), which is formed in part by the temporal bone of the skull. The middle ear and internal ear are structured to transport auditory impulses to the brain. Aiding the organs of hearing and equalizing pressure between the middle and the internal ear is the eustachian tube, a canal that joins the nose and the middle ear.[65]

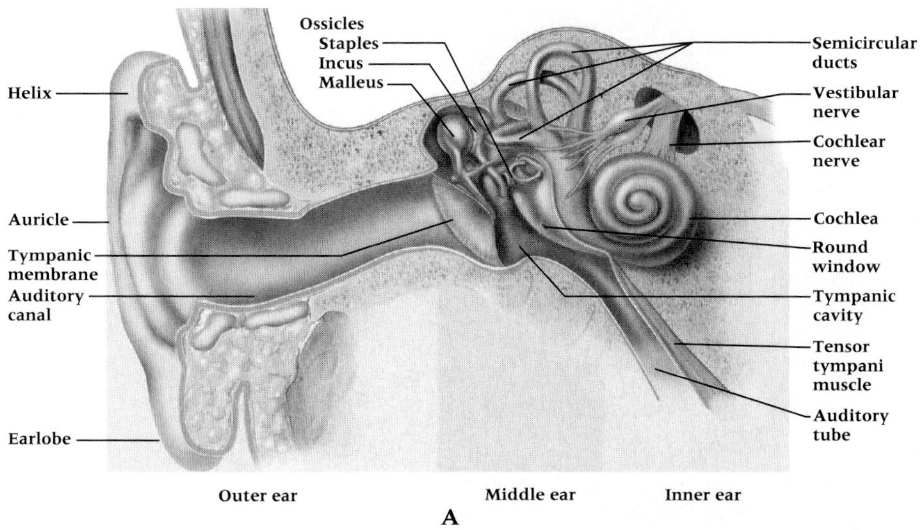

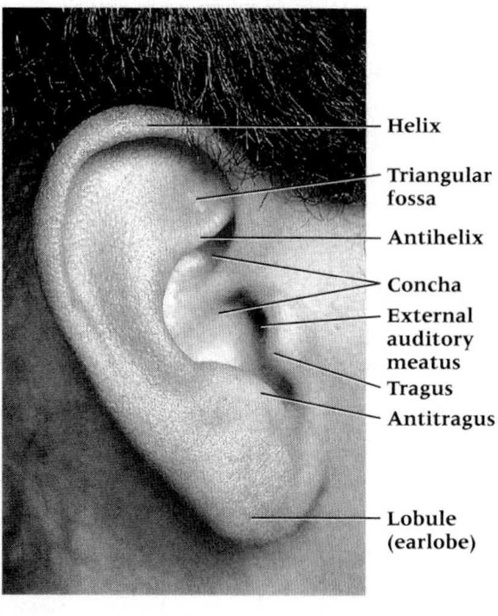

Figure 26-17

Anatomy of the ear.
A, Internal. **B,** Auricular.

Sports injuries to the ear occur most often to the external portion. The external ear is separated into the auricle (pinna) and the external auditory canal (meatus). The auricle, which is shaped like a shell, collects and directs sound waves into the auditory canal. It is composed of flexible yellow cartilage, muscles, and fat padding and is covered by a closely adhering, thin layer of skin. Most of the blood vessels and nerves of the auricle turn around its borders, with just a few penetrating the cartilage proper.

Recognition and Management of Specific Ear Injuries

Auricular (Pinna) Hematoma (Cauliflower Ear)

Etiology Hematomas of the ear are common in boxing, rugby, and wrestling. They are most common in athletes who do not wear protective headgear. This condition usually occurs either from compression or from a shearing injury (single or repeated) to the auricle that causes subcutaneous bleeding into the auricular cartilage.[17]

Symptoms and signs Trauma may tear the overlying tissue away from the cartilaginous plate, resulting in hemorrhage and fluid accumulation. A hematoma usually forms before the limited circulation can absorb the fluid. If the hematoma goes unattended, a sequence of coagulation, organization, and fibrosis results in a keloid that appears elevated, rounded, white, nodular, and firm, resembling a cauliflower (Figure 26-18). Often the keloid forms in the region of the helix fossa or concha; once developed, the keloid can be removed only through surgery.[17]

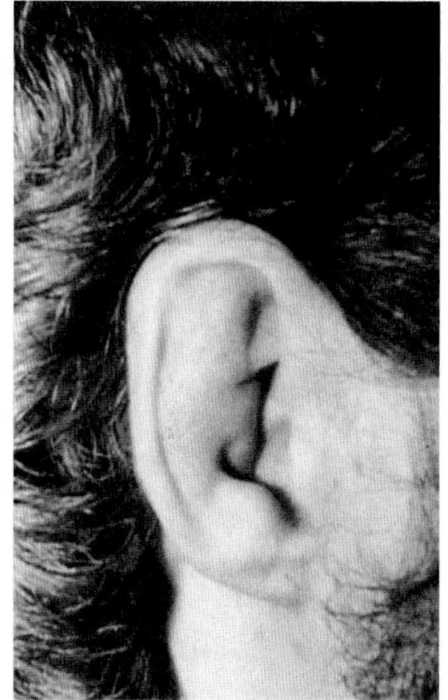

Figure 26-18

Hematoma of the auricle; also called cauliflower ear.

Management To prevent this disfiguring condition from arising, some friction-reducing agent such as petroleum jelly should be applied to the ears of athletes susceptible to this condition. These athletes should also routinely wear ear guards in practice and in competition.

If an ear becomes "hot" because of excessive rubbing or twisting, the immediate application of a cold pack to the affected spot will alleviate hemorrhage. Once swelling is present in the ear, special care should be taken to prevent the fluid from solidifying; a cold pack should be placed immediately over the ear and held tightly by an elastic bandage for at least twenty minutes. If the swelling is still present at the end of this time, aspiration by a physician is required.[17] After drainage, pressure is applied to the area to prevent return of the hematoma. The physician may suture dental rolls into position to ensure uniform pressure.[17] Instead of this procedure, a collodion pack may be opted for as follows:

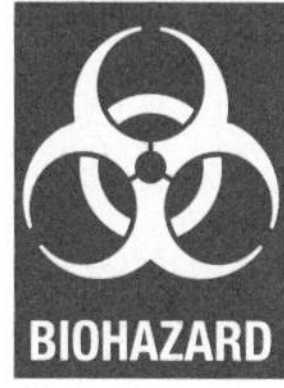

1. Cotton is packed into the ear canal.
2. The auricle is coated with collodion.
3. Small pieces of gauze also coated with collodion are inserted and packed into the auricle of the ear until it is completely filled.

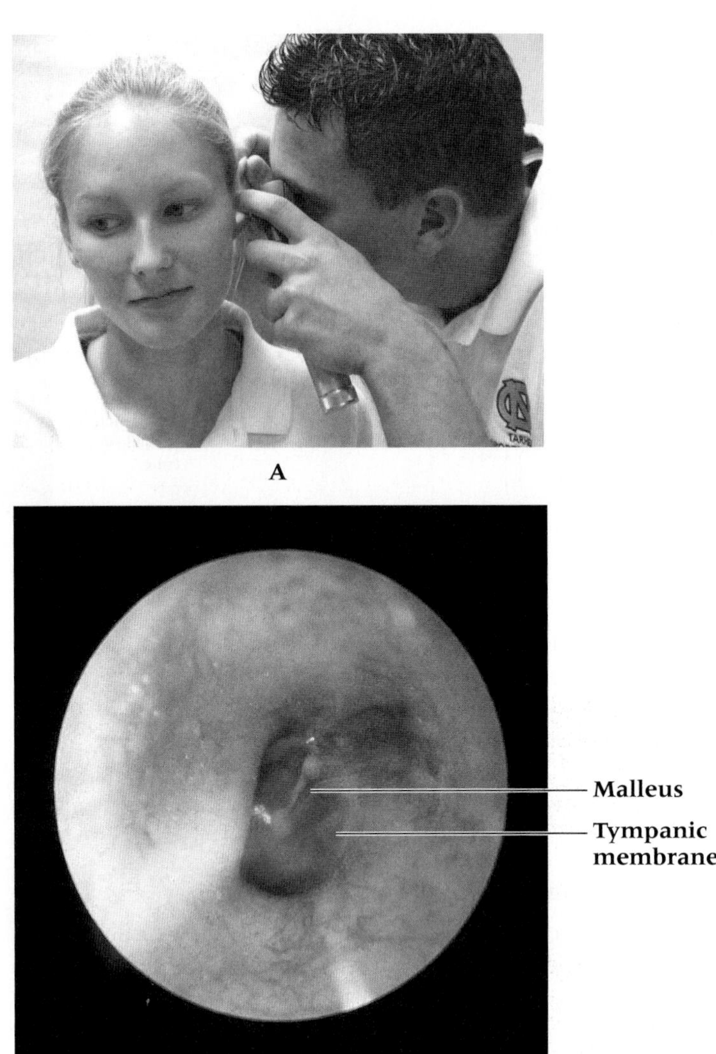

Figure 26-19

Examining the eye with an otoscope. **A,** The position of the examiner. **B,** The view of a normal ear through the otoscope.

4. A ¼-inch-thick (0.6 cm) felt piece is cut to fit and placed behind the ear.
5. A pressure wrap is placed completely around the head, kept in place for two days, and then removed.
6. The collodion pack is left in place until it can be easily removed.

Rupture of the Tympanic Membrane

Etiology Rupture of the tympanic membrane is commonly seen in contact and collision sports as well as in water polo and diving.[40] A fall or slap to the unprotected ear or sudden underwater variation can rupture the tympanic membrane.

Symptoms and signs The athlete complains of a loud pop followed by pain in the ear, nausea, vomiting, and dizziness.[40] The athlete demonstrates hearing loss and visible rupture of the tympanic membrane. An otoscope is an instrument used to visually examine the ear canal and the tympanic membrane (Figure 26-19). Tympanic membrane ruptures can be seen through the otoscope.

Management Small to moderate perforations of the tympanic membrane usually heal spontaneously in one to two weeks. Infection can occur and must be continually monitored.

Swimmer's Ear (Otitis Externa)

Etiology A common condition in athletes engaged in water sports is *swimmer's ear,* or external otitis. Swimmer's ear is a general term for infection of the ear canal caused by *Pseudomonas aeruginosa,* a type of gram-negative bacillus. Contrary to current thought among swimming coaches, swimmer's ear is not usually associated with a fungal infection. Water can become trapped in the ear canal as a result of obstructions created by cysts, bone growths, plugs of earwax, or swelling caused by allergies.[44]

Symptoms and signs The athlete complains of pain and dizziness and may also complain of itching, discharge, or even a partial hearing loss.

Management Athletes can best prevent ear infection by drying the ears thoroughly with a soft towel, using ear drops containing a mild acid (3% boric acid) and alcohol solution before and after each swim, and avoiding situations that can cause ear infections, such as overexposure to cold wind or sticking foreign objects into the ear.

When a swimmer displays symptoms of external otitis, he or she should be referred immediately to a physician. Tympanic membrane rupture should be ruled out. Treatment may include acidification through drops into the ear to make an inhospitable environment for the gram-negative bacteria. Antibiotics may be used in athletes with a mild ear infection.[18] In the event of a ruptured tympanic membrane, custom-made earplugs must be used.

Middle Ear Infection (Otitis Media)

Etiology Otitis media is an accumulation of fluid in the middle ear caused by local and systemic inflammation and infection.[18]

Symptoms and signs There will usually be intense pain in the ear, fluid draining from the ear canal, and a transient loss of hearing. In addition, the systemic infection may also cause fever, headache, irritability, loss of appetite, and nausea.[74]

Management A physician may choose to draw a small amount of fluid from the middle ear to determine the most appropriate antibiotic therapy. Analgesics can be used to help reduce pain. The problem will generally begin to resolve within twenty-four hours although pain may last for seventy-two hours.

Impacted Cerumen

Etiology Cerumen, or earwax, is secreted by glands in the outer portion of the ear canal. Occasionally, an excessive amount of earwax may accumulate, clogging the ear canal.

Symptoms and signs Impacted cerumen causes some degree of muffled hearing or hearing loss. However, there will generally be little or no pain because no infection is involved.[74]

Management Initially, an attempt can be made to remove excess cerumen by irrigation of the ear canal with warm water. The athlete should not attempt to remove the cerumen with a cotton tip applicator because that may increase the degree of impaction. If irrigation fails, the impacted cerumen must be physically removed by a physician using a curette.

EYE INJURIES

Eye injuries account for approximately 2 percent of all sports injuries.[45] In the United States, basketball, baseball, boxing, soccer, swimming, and racket sports have a high incidence of eye injuries (Table 26-8).[67]

TABLE 26-8 Percentage of Sports Eye Injuries in the United States

Sport	Percent (%)
Baseball	27
Racket sports	20
Basketball	20
Football and soccer	7
Ice hockey	4
Ball hockey	1

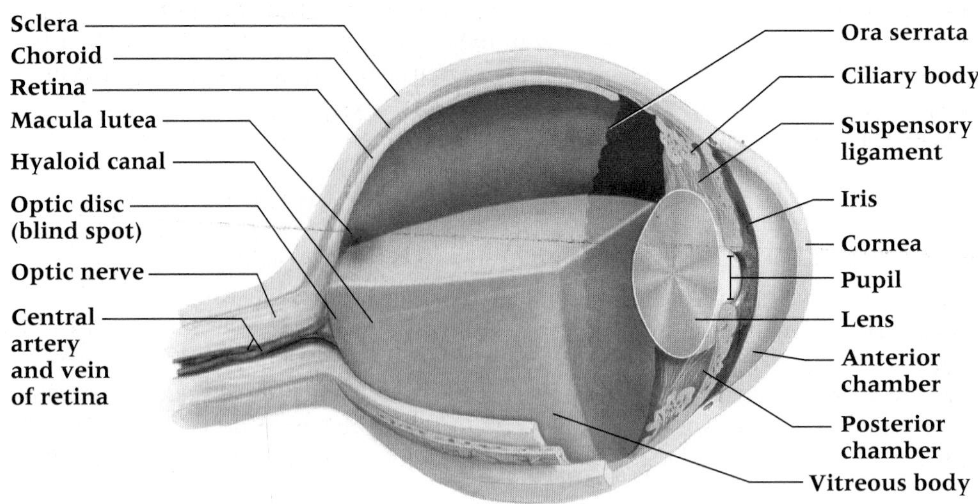

Figure 26-20

Anatomy of the eye.

Anatomy of the Eye

The eye has many anatomical protective features.[55] It is firmly retained within an oval socket formed by the bones of the head. A cushion of soft fatty tissue surrounds it, and a thin skin flap (the eyelid), which functions by reflex action, covers the eye for protection. Foreign particles are prevented from entering the eye by the lashes and eyebrows, which act as a filtering system. A soft mucous lining that covers the inner conjunctiva transports and spreads tears, which are secreted by many accessory lacrimal glands. A larger lubricating organ is located above the eye and secretes heavy quantities of fluid through the lacrimal duct to help wash away foreign particles. The eye proper is well protected by the sclera, a tough, white, outer layer possessing a transparent center portion called the *cornea.*

The cornea covers the pupil, which is the central opening of the eye. Light passes through the cornea, then through the anterior chamber past the iris and the lens, and finally through the vitreous body, all of which function collectively to focus an image on the retina, where it is detected by the optic nerve (Figure 26-20).

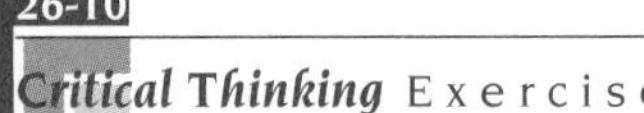

26-10 Critical Thinking Exercise

A wrestler gets a thumb pushed hard into the left eye.

? What symptoms indicate that this injury may be a serious eye injury?

Preventing Eye Injuries

The eye can be injured in a number of different ways. Shattered eyeglass or goggle lenses can lacerate; ski pole tips can penetrate; and fingers, racquetball balls, and larger projectiles can seriously compress and injure the eye. High-energy sports such as ice hockey, football, and lacrosse require full-face and helmet protection, whereas low-energy sports such as racquetball and tennis require eye guards that rest on the face.[67] Protective devices must provide protection from front and lateral blows.

Sport goggles can be made with highly impact-resistant polycarbonate lenses for refraction. The major problem with sport goggles is that they distort peripheral vision and tend to become fogged under certain weather conditions (see Chapter 7).

Assessment of the Eye

It has been said that "evaluating and managing eye injuries is no place for amateurs."[6] Thus, the athletic trainer must use extreme caution in evaluating eye injuries (Figure 26-21). If any of the following conditions are evident, the athlete should be immediately referred to an ophthalmologist:[56] retinal detachment, perforation of the globe, a foreign object embedded in the cornea, blood in the anterior chamber, decreased vision, loss of the visual field, poor pupillary adaptation, double vision, laceration, or impaired lid function.

Extreme care must be taken with any eye injury: Transport the athlete in a recumbent position; cover both eyes, but do not put pressure on the eye.

Ideally, the athlete with a serious eye injury should be transported to the hospital by ambulance in a recumbent position. Both eyes must be covered during transport. At no time should pressure be applied to the eye. In case of surrounding soft-tissue

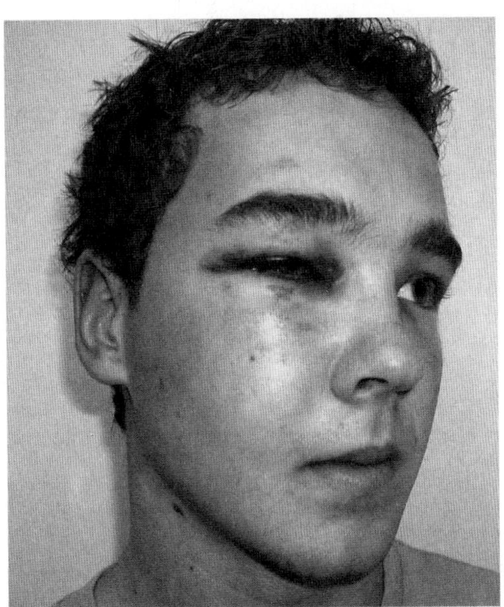

Figure 26-21

A serious eye injury should be treated as a medical emergency.

injury, a cold compress can be applied for thirty to sixty minutes to control hemorrhage. See also *Focus Box:* "Supplies for managing eye injuries."

The athletic trainer's first concerns are to understand the mechanism of injury and to determine if there is a related condition to the head, face, or neck.[44] The evaluation process should include the following steps.

History

- What was the mechanism of injury (sharp and penetrating or blunt)?
- Was loss of vision gradual or immediate?
- What was the visual status before injury?
- Was there loss of consciousness?

Observation

- Inspect the external ocular structures for swelling and discoloration, penetrating objects, deformities, and movement of the lid.
- Inspect the globe of the eye for lacerations, foreign bodies, hyphema, or deformities.
- Inspect the conjunctiva and sclera for foreign bodies, hemorrhage, or deformities.

Focus

Supplies for managing eye injuries

To make an appropriate eye injury assessment, the athletic trainer must have a properly equipped first aid kit. The following items should be available for use in the immediate care of eye injuries in sports:

- Vision card for testing visual acuity
- Penlight
- Cotton-tipped applicators
- Sterile ocular irrigating solution
- Sterile eye patches
- Plastic eye shields
- Fluorescein strips
- Plunger for removing contact lenses

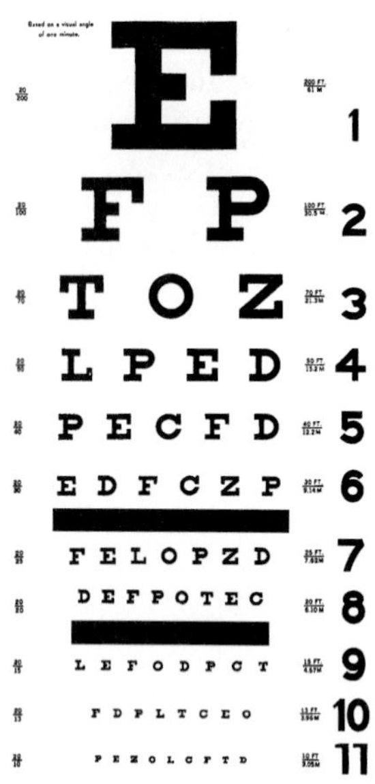

Figure 26-22

When using the Snellen eye chart to check visual acuity, one eye is covered at a time. The vision of each eye, as well as both eyes together, is recorded separately. In the Snellen fraction 20/20, the first number represents the test distance of 20 feet, while the second number represents the distance that the average eye can see the letters on a certain line of the eye chart. Thus 20/20 means that the person being tested can read a certain size letter when it is 20 feet away. If a person sees 20/40, at 20 feet from the chart that person can read letters that a person with 20/20 vision could read from 40 feet away.

Palpation

Palpate the orbital rim for point tenderness or bony deformity.

Special Tests

Pupillary response Tests to determine pupillary response were described in the section on the assessment of head injuries; they include pupil dilation and accommodation by covering the eye and then exposing it to light.

Visual acuity The evaluator determines visual acuity by asking the athlete to report what is seen when he or she looks at some object with the unaffected eye covered. A Snellen eye chart can be used to determine the extent of impairment (Figure 26-22). There may be blurring of vision, diplopia, floating black specks, or flashes of light, all of which indicate serious eye involvement.

Ophthalmoscope An ophthalmoscope is an instrument for observing the interior of the eye, especially the retina (Figure 26-23). An athletic trainer may occasionally use an ophthalmoscope to look into the eye. Obviously, special training is necessary to recognize the presence of specific conditions or injuries.

Recognition and Management of Specific Eye Injuries

Orbital Hematoma (Black Eye)

Etiology Although well protected, the eye may be bruised during sports activity. The severity of eye injuries varies from a mild bruise to an extremely serious condition affecting vision to the fracturing of the orbital cavity. Fortunately, most eye injuries sustained in sports are mild. A blow to the eye may initially injure the surrounding tissue and produce capillary bleeding into the tissue spaces. If the hemorrhage goes unchecked, the result may be a classic black eye.

Symptoms and signs The signs of a more serious contusion may be displayed as a subconjunctival hemorrhage or as faulty vision.

Management Care of an eye contusion requires cold application for at least half an hour, plus a twenty-four-hour rest period if the athlete has distorted vision. Under no circumstances should an athlete blow the nose after an acute eye injury. To do so might increase hemorrhaging.

Orbital Fractures

Etiology A fracture of the bony framework of the orbit surrounding the eye can occur when a blow to the eyeball forces it posteriorly, compressing the orbital fat until a blowout or rupture occurs to the floor of the orbit. Both fat and the inferior extraocular muscles can herniate through this fracture.[57]

Symptoms and signs The athlete with a fracture of the orbit will often exhibit diplopia, restricted movement of the eye, a downward displacement of the eye, and pain accompanied by soft-tissue swelling and hemorrhage. There may be numbness associated with injury to the infraorbital nerve on the floor of the orbit. An X ray must be taken to confirm the fracture.

Management A physician should administer antibiotics prophylactically to decrease the likelihood of infection. A fracture in the orbital floor allows communication with the maxillary sinus, which may contain potentially infectious bacteria. Most orbital fractures are treated surgically, although some physicians prefer to wait and see if the symptoms resolve on their own.

Foreign Body in the Eye

Etiology Foreign bodies in the eye are a frequent occurrence in sports and are potentially dangerous.

Symptoms and signs A foreign object produces considerable pain and disability. No attempt should be made to remove the body by rubbing or to remove it with the fingers.

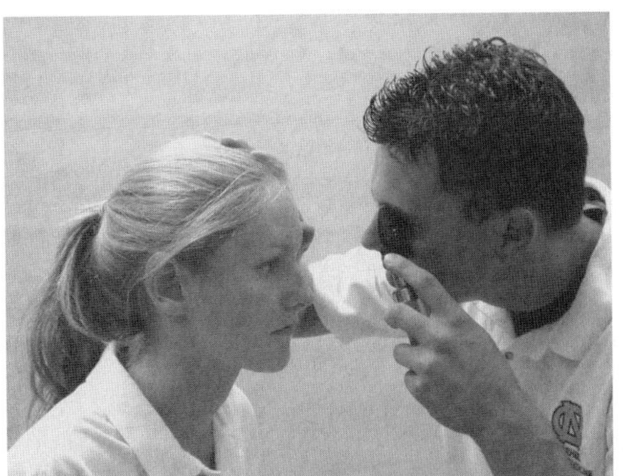

A

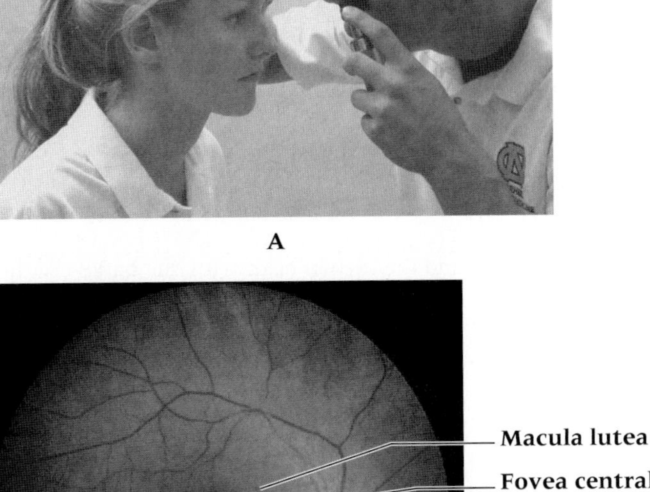

B

Figure 26-23

Examing the eye with an ophthalmoscope. **A,** Position of the examiner. **B,** The view of the normal eye through the ophthalmoscope.

Management The athletic trainer should instruct the athlete to close the eye until the initial pain has subsided and then attempt to determine if the object is in the vicinity of the upper or lower lid. Foreign bodies in the lower lid are relatively easy to remove by depressing the tissue and then wiping it with a sterile cotton applicator. Foreign bodies in the area of the upper lid are usually much more difficult to localize. Two methods may be used. The first technique is performed as follows: Gently pull the upper eyelid over the lower lid while the subject looks downward. This causes tears to be produced, which may flush the object down onto the lower lid. If this method is unsuccessful, the second technique should be used (see *Focus Box:* "Removing a foreign body from the eye" and Figure 26-24). After the foreign particle is removed, the affected eye should be washed with a saline solution. Often after removal of the foreign body there is a residual soreness, which may be alleviated by the application of petroleum jelly or some other mild ointment. If the athletic trainer encounters extreme difficulty in removing the foreign body, or if the foreign body has become embedded in the eye itself, the eye should be closed and patched with a gauze pad held in place by strips of tape. The athlete should be referred to a physician as soon as possible.[57]

Corneal Abrasions and Lacerations

Etiology An athlete who gets a foreign object in his or her eye will usually try to rub it away. In doing so, the cornea can become abraded or perhaps sustain a small laceration.

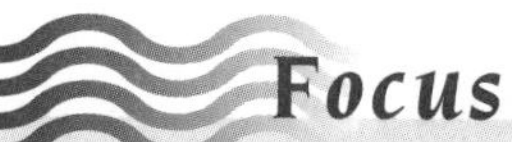

Removing a foreign body from the eye

Materials needed

Applicator stick, sterile cotton-tipped swab, eyecup, and eyewash (solution of boric acid).

Position of the athlete

The athlete lies supine on a table.

Procedure

1. Gently pull the eyelid down and place an applicator stick crosswise at its base.
2. Have the athlete look down; then grasp the lashes and turn the lid back over the stick.
3. Holding the lid and the stick in place with one hand, use the sterile cotton swab to lift out the foreign body.
4. Rinse with eyewash in an eye cup.

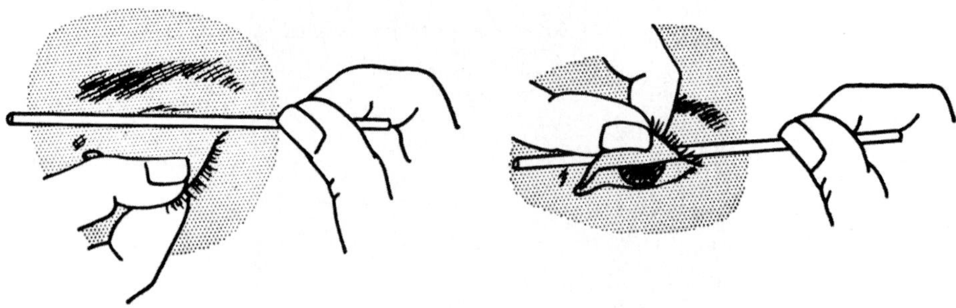

Figure 26-24

Removing a foreign body from the eye.

Symptoms and signs The athlete will complain of severe pain and watering of the eye, photophobia, and spasm of the orbicular muscle of the eyelid.

Management The eye should be patched, and the athlete should be sent to a physician. Corneal abrasion is diagnosed through the application of a fluorescein strip to the abraded area, which stains the abrasion a bright green. Once diagnosed, the eye is dilated for further assessment. Antibiotic ointment is applied with a semipressure patch placed over the closed eyelid.

Hyphema

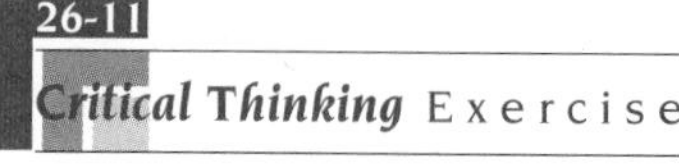

26-11 Critical Thinking Exercise

After receiving a blunt blow to her right eye, an athlete develops a collection of blood in the anterior chamber.

? What type of eye injury is this, and what complications may follow?

Etiology A blunt blow to the anterior aspect of the eye can produce a hyphema, which is a collection of blood within the anterior chamber.[72] This injury is often caused when an athlete is struck in the eye with a racquetball ball or squash ball when not wearing the appropriate protective eyewear.[72]

Symptoms and signs Initially there is a visible reddish tinge in the anterior chamber, and within the first two hours, the blood settles inferiorly or may fill the entire chamber. The blood may turn to a pea green color. Vision is partially or completely blocked. The athletic trainer must be aware that a hyphema is a major eye injury that can lead to serious problems of the lens, choroid, or retina.

Management An athlete with a hyphema should be immediately referred to a physician. Conventional treatment involves hospitalization and bed rest with the head elevated 30 degrees to 40 degrees, patching of both eyes, sedation, and medication to reduce pressure in the anterior chamber. The initial hemorrhage resorbs in a few days, although occasionally there is rebleeding. If not managed properly, irreversible vision damage can occur.

Rupture of the Globe

Etiology A blow to the eye by an object smaller than the eye orbit produces extreme pressure that can rupture the globe. A golf ball or racquetball fits this category. Larger objects such as a tennis ball or a fist will often fracture the bony orbit before the eye is overly compressed. Even if it does not cause rupture of the globe, such a force can cause internal injury that may ultimately lead to blindness.[57]

Symptoms and signs The athlete complains of severe pain, decreased visual acuity, and diplopia. Inspection reveals irregular pupils, increased intraocular pressure, and orbital leakage.

Management Treatment requires immediate rest, eye protection with a shield, and antiemetic medication to avoid increasing intraocular pressure. Immediate referral to an ophthalmologist must be made.

Retinal Detachment

Etiology A blow to the athlete's eye can partially or completely separate the retina from its underlying retinal pigment epithelium. Retinal detachment is more common among athletes who have myopia (nearsightedness).[74]

Symptoms and signs Detachment is painless; however, early signs include specks floating before the eye, flashes of light, or blurred vision. As the detachment progresses, the athlete complains of a "curtain" falling over the field of vision. Any athlete with symptoms of detachment must be immediately referred to an ophthalmologist.

Management Initially, there is bed rest with patches on both eyes. The athlete should immediately be referred to an ophthalmologist to determine if surgery is required.

Acute Conjunctivitis

Etiology The conjunctiva is the tissue that lines the back of the eyelid, moves into the space between the eyelid and eye globe, and spreads up over the sclera to the cornea.[56] Acute conjunctivitis is usually caused by various bacteria or allergens. It may begin with conjunctival irritation from wind, dust, smoke, or air pollution. It may also be associated with the common cold or other upper respiratory conditions.

Symptoms and signs The athlete complains of eyelid swelling, sometimes with a purulent discharge. Itching is associated with allergy. Eyes may burn or itch.

Management Acute conjunctivitis can be highly infectious. A 10 percent solution of sodium sulfacetamide is often the treatment of choice.

Hordeolum (Sty)

Etiology A sty is an infection of the eyelash follicle or the sebaceous gland at the edge of the eyelid. The infection is usually caused by a staphylococcal organism that has been spread by rubbing or by dust particles.

Symptoms and signs The condition starts as erythema of the eye. It localizes into a painful pustule within a few days.

Management Treatment consists of the application of hot, moist compresses and an ointment of 1 percent yellow oxide or mercury. Recurrent sties require the attention of an ophthalmologist.

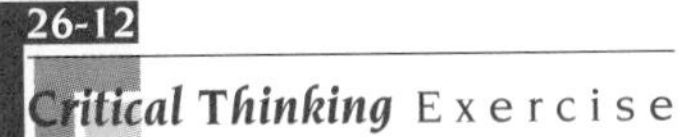

An athlete develops an eyelash follicle infection.

? What is the cause of this condition, and how should it be treated?

THROAT INJURIES

Contusions

Etiology Blows to the throat do not occur frequently in sports, but occasionally an athlete may receive a kick or blow to the throat. One type of trauma is known as clotheslining, in which the athlete is struck in the throat region by another player's outstretched arm. Such a force could conceivably injure the carotid artery, causing a clot to form that occludes the blood flow to the brain. This same clot could become dislodged and migrate to the brain. In either case, serious brain injury may result.

26-13

Critical Thinking Exercise

While carrying the ball, a football back is clotheslined and seriously injures his throat.

? What should the athletic trainer be concerned with in such an injury?

Symptoms and signs Immediately after throat trauma, the athlete may experience severe pain and spasmodic coughing, speak with a hoarse voice, and complain of difficulty in swallowing. The athlete may also have difficulty breathing, particularly if the vocal cords have been traumatized.[48]

Fracture of throat cartilages of the larynx is rare, but it is possible and may be indicated by an inability to breathe and by expectoration of frothy blood. Cyanosis may be present. Throat contusions are extremely uncomfortable and are often frightening to the athlete.

Management The most immediate concern is the integrity of the airway. The athlete who is experiencing difficulty breathing should be sent to an emergency care facility immediately. In most situations, cold should be applied intermittently to control superficial hemorrhage and swelling, and after a twenty-four-hour rest period, moist hot packs may be applied. For the most severe neck contusions, stabilization with a well-padded collar is beneficial.

Thyroid Gland Disorders

Etiology The thyroid gland is an endocrine system gland located in the base of the neck on both sides of the lower larynx and upper trachea. It produces two hormones, thyroxine and triiodothyronine. Two disorders related to the function of the thyroid gland are hyperthyroidism and hypothyroidism.[74]

Symptoms and signs Hyperthyroidism involves the overproduction of thyroxine and results in impaired glucose metabolism, increased metabolism, rapid fatigue during exercise, weight loss, and hyperthermia during exercise. Graves' disease is a form of hyperthyroidism that, in addition to the symptoms already mentioned, may lead to weakness, tremors, and difficulty swallowing and/or speaking. Hypothyroidism is a condition caused by deficient secretion of thyroid hormone that results in lowered metabolism, poor circulation, dry skin, low blood pressure, slow pulse, depressed muscle activity, intolerance to cold, increasing obesity, and potentially the development of a goiter, which is an enlargement of the thyroid gland.[74]

Management An athlete who shows signs of hyper- or hypothyroidism should be referred to a physician for diagnosis. The treatment for hyperthyroidism usually involves medication to slow the production of thyroxine or surgery to remove a part of the thyroid gland. Treatment of hypothyroidism most often involves hormone replacement therapy.

SUMMARY

- The skull is lined with the meninges, which collectively serve to protect the underlying cortex and midbrain from trauma.
- An athlete who receives either a direct blow to the head or body contact that causes the head to snap forward, backward, or rotate to the side must be carefully evaluated for injury to the brain. Injuries to the brain may or may not result in unconsciousness; disorientation or amnesia; motor coordination or balance deficits; and cognitive deficits.
- It is important to realize that in the athletic population, the majority of concussions do not involve loss of consciousness.
- Concussions usually occur as a result of a direct impact or through a combination of rotational and acceleration/deceleration forces.
- A variety of classification systems have been proposed for determining the severity of concussion. To date, none of these classification systems has been universally endorsed, and thus debate continues.
- Returning an athlete to competition following concussion often creates a difficult dilemma for the athletic trainer. There must be ongoing concern for postconcussion syndrome, second impact syndrome, and epidural and subdural hematomas.
- Injuries to the face could involve fractures of the mandible, maxilla, or zygoma; dislocations of the mandible; temporomandibular dysfunction; and facial lacerations.

- Impact to the upper or lower jaw or direct trauma to the teeth can result in one or more of three types of fractures to the teeth: an uncomplicated crown fracture, a complicated crown fracture, and a root fracture. A tooth may also be subluxated, luxated, or avulsed. The athletic trainer should know when to refer an athlete for dental care.
- Most injuries to the ear involve the auricle, with cauliflower ear being the most common injury. Rupture of the tympanic membrane, swimmer's ear, and middle ear infections are common in the athletic population.
- Injuries to the eye should be treated by physicians who are specifically trained. Even injuries as simple as a black eye, a sty, or a corneal abrasion have the potential to cause some irreversible damage to vision if not properly managed. An orbital fracture, a foreign body in the eye, a hyphema, a rupture of the globe, and a retinal detachment are all considered serious injuries to the eye.
- The most serious consequence of a throat contusion is airway interference.

Websites

American Academy of Neurology: www.aan.com

American Academy of Ophthalmology: www.aao.org

American Dental Association: www.ada.org

American Academy of Otolaryngology—Head and Neck Surgery: www.entnet.org

Solutions to Critical Thinking EXERCISES

26-1 The athlete's face color is pale, her skin moist, her pulse is rapid with shallow breathing, and her pupils may become dilated.

26-2 The athletic trainer should ask the athlete questions that are related to recently acquired information, such as the current date, the name of last week's opponent, who won that game, and who scored this game's last goal.

26-3 The athlete should be out of play for at least one month. After this period, he may return to play for one week if asymptomatic. The physician may consider terminating the athlete for the rest of the season.

26-4 This athlete is experiencing a postconcussion syndrome. The athlete cannot return completely to play until cleared by a thorough neurological examination.

26-5 In an athlete of this age, there should always be some concern about the possibility of second impact syndrome. From the athletic trainer's perspective, the decision to allow an athlete to return to play after an initial head injury must be carefully made based on the absence of postconcussive symptoms.

26-6 A subdural hematoma is due to venous bleeding and the symptoms appear gradually over hours or even days. However, an epidural hematoma results from arterial bleeding and therefore the symptoms appear rapidly.

26-7 The conscious athlete with a fractured maxilla is transported to the hospital in a forward-leaning position. This position allows external drainage of saliva and blood.

26-8 This appears to be an uncomplicated crown fracture, which does not require immediate treatment by a dentist. The fractured piece of tooth if found can be placed in a plastic bag. The athlete can finish the game and then should be seen by a dentist within twenty-four to forty-eight hours.

26-9 The athlete should sit up with a cold compress placed over the nose and ipsilateral carotid artery. Digital pressure should also be applied to the affected nostril for five minutes.

26-10 The symptoms that the athletic trainer should look for are blurred vision, a loss in the visual field, major pain, and double vision.

26-11 Blood in the anterior eye chamber is known as a hyphema, which could lead to major lens, choroid, or retina problems.

26-12 This sty is caused by a staphylococcal organism that is commonly spread by rubbing or by dust particle contamination. The condition should be managed with hot, moist compresses and a 1 percent yellow oxide or mercury ointment.

26-13 The compressive force of clotheslining could produce a blood clot in the carotid artery. A large enough force could fracture the larynx and cause a breathing crisis.

REVIEW QUESTIONS AND CLASS ACTIVITIES

1. What is the difference between the terms *concussion* and *mild head injury?*
2. What are the different classification systems for determining grades of concussion?
3. How are postconcussion syndrome and second impact syndrome related to concussion?
4. Demonstrate the following procedures in evaluating a concussion: testing eye signs, testing balance, testing coordination, testing cognition.
5. What immediate care procedures should be performed for athletes with facial lacerations?
6. Describe the immediate care procedures that should be performed when a tooth is fractured and when it is dislocated.
7. Describe the procedures that should be performed for an athlete with a nosebleed.

8. How can cauliflower ear be prevented?
9. How can eye injuries be prevented?

REFERENCES

1. Alexander M: Mild traumatic brain injury: pathophysiology, natural history, and clinical management, *Neurology* 45:1253, 1995.
2. Almquist J, Broshek D, Erlanger D: Assessment of mild head injuries, *Athletic Therapy Today* 6(1):13, 2001.
3. Aubry M, Cantu R, Dvorak J: Summary and agreement statement: recommendations for the improvement of safety and health of athletes who may suffer concussive injuries, *British Journal of Sports Medicine* 36(1):6, 2002.
4. Bailes JE, Hudson V: Classification of sport-related head trauma: a spectrum of mild to severe injury, *J Ath Train* 36(3):236, 2001.
5. Berry DC, Miller MG: Athletic mouth guards and their role in injury prevention, *Athletic Therapy Today* 6(5):52, 2001.
6. Biggers P: Personal communication, 1998.
7. Broglio SP: Soccer heading: are there risks involved? *Athletic Therapy Today* 6(1):28, 2001.
8. Bruzzone E, Cocito L, Pisani R: Intracranial delayed epidural hematoma in a soccer player: a case report, *Am J Sports Med* 28(6):901, 2000.
9. Cameron KL, Yunker CA, Austin MC: A standardization protocol for the initial evaluation and documentation of mild brain injury, *J Ath Train* 34(1):34, 1999.
10. Cantu RC: Posttraumatic retrograde and anterograde amnesia: pathophysiology and implications in grading and safe return to play, *J Ath Train* 36(3):244, 2001.
11. Cantu RC: Head and spine injuries in youth sports. In Michelle LJ, editor: *The young athlete. Clinics in sports medicine,* vol 14, no 3, Philadelphia, 1995, Saunders.
12. Cantu RC: Second impact syndrome. In Cantu RC: *Clinics in sports medicine,* 17(1):37, 1998.
13. Colorado Medical Society: The School Health and Sports Medicine Committee guidelines for the management of concussions in sport. In National Athletic Trainer's Association: *Proceedings of mild brain injury in sports summit,* 106, Dallas, 1994, NATA.
14. Cooper ER: Definitional problems in mild head injury epidemiology. *Athletic Therapy Today* 6(1):6, 2001.
15. Covassin T, Swanik C, Sachs M: Sex differences and the incidence of concussions among collegiate athletes, *J Ath Train* 38(3):238, 2003.
16. Crow RW: Sports-related lacerations, *Physician Sportsmed* 21(2):134, 1993.
17. Davidson TM, Neuman TR: Managing ear trauma, *Physician Sportsmed* 22(7):27, 1994.
18. Davidson TM, Neuman TR: Managing inflammatory ear conditions, *Physician Sportsmed* 22(8):56, 1994.
19. DeYoung A, Robinson E, Godwin W: Comparing comfort and wearability: custom-made vs. self-adapted mouth guards, *J Am Dental Assoc* 125:1112, 1994.
20. Erlanger D, Saliba E, Barth J: Monitoring resolution of post concussion symptoms in athletes: preliminary results of a web-based neuropsychological test protocol. *J Ath Train* 36(3):280, 2001.
21. Ferrara M, McCrea M, Peterson C: A survey of practice patterns in concussion assessment and management, *J Ath Train* 36(2):145, 2001.
22. Fick D: Management of concussion in collision sports, *Post Graduate Medicine* 97(2):53, 1995.
23. Gennarelli TA, Torg JS: Closed head injuries. In Torg JS, Shephard RJ, editors: *Current therapy in sports medicine,* St Louis, 1995, Mosby.
24. Guskiewicz K: Concussion in sport: The grading system dilemma. *Athletic Therapy Today* 6(1):18, 2001.
25. Guskiewicz K et al: National Athletic Trainers' Association position statement: Management of sport-related concussion. *J Ath Train* 39(3):280, 2004.
26. Guskiewicz K, Cantu R: The concussion puzzle: evaluation of sport-related concussion. *Am J Sports Med* 6:13, 2004.
27. Guskiewicz K, McCrea M, Marshall S: Cumulative effects of recurrent concussion in collegiate football players, *JAMA* 290:2549, 2003.
28. Guskiewicz K, Padua D, Weaver N: Incidence of mild head injury in high school and college football players, *Review Am J Sports Med,* 1999.
29. Guskiewicz K, Perrin D, Gansneader B: Effect of mild head injury on postural stability in athletes, *J Ath Train* 31(4):300, 1996.
30. Guskiewicz K, Riemann B, Perrin D, Nashner L: Alternative approaches to the assessment of mild head injury in athletes, *Med Sci Sports Exerc* 29(7):S213, 1997.
31. Guskiewicz KM, Ross SE, Marshall SE: Postural stability and neuropsychological deficits after concussion in collegiate athletes, *J Ath Train* 36(3):263, 2001.
32. Hamou D, Zagelbaum B: Incidence of sports related eye injuries, *Athletic Therapy Today* 4(5):27, 1999.
33. Henderson JM: Head injuries in sports, *Sports Med Digest* 15(9):1, 1993.
34. Hugenholtz H, Richard M: Return to athletic competition following concussion, *Canadian Medical Assoc J* 127:827, 1982.
35. Jordan B: Head injuries in sports. In Jordan B, Tsairis P, Warren R: *Sports neurology,* Philadelphia, 1998, Lippincott, Williams, and Wilkins.
36. Kelly JP: Loss of consciousness: pathophysiology and implications in grading and safe return to play, *J Ath Train* 36(3):249, 2001.
37. Kirkendall DT, Garret WE: Heading in soccer: integral skill or grounds for cognitive dysfunction? *J Ath Train* 36(3):328, 2001.
38. Kuland D: *The injured athlete,* Philadelphia, 1982, Lippeincott.
39. Laio J, Zagelbaum, BM: Eye injuries in sports, *Athletic Therapy Today* 4(5):36, 1999.
40. Lenker C: Traumatic tympanic membrane perforation in a collegiate football player, *Athletic Therapy Today* 5(1):43, 2000.
41. Logan S, Bell G, Leonard J: Acute subdural hematoma in a high school football player after 2 unreported episodes of head trauma: a case report, *J Ath Train* 36(4):433, 2001.
42. Maddocks DL: The assessment of orientation following concussion in athletes, *Cl J Sports Med* 5(1):32, 1995.
43. McCrea M: Standardized mental status testing on the sideline after sport-related concussion, *J Ath Train* 36(3):274, 2001.
44. Mellion MB et al: Medical problems in athletes. In Birrer RB, editor: *Sports medicine for the primary care physician,* ed 2, Boca Raton, Fla, 2004, CRC Press.
45. Moss, RI: Preventing postconcussion sequelae, *Athletic Therapy Today* 6(2):28, 2001.
46. Mueller FO: Catastrophic head injuries in high school and college sports, *J Ath Train* 36(3):312, 2001.
47. Nelson W, Jane J, Geick J: Minor head injury in sports: A new system of classification and management, *Physician Sportsmed* 12:103, 1984.
48. Newsham K, Klaben B: Paradoxical vocal cord dysfunction: management in athletes, *J Ath Train* 37(3):325, 2002.
49. Norwig J: Sideline assessment of mild head injuries, *Athletic Therapy Today* 3(6):35, 1998.
50. Oliaro SM, Anderson S, Hooker D: Management of cerebral concussion in sports: the athletic trainer's perspective, *J Ath Train* 36(3):257, 2001.
51. Oliaro S, Guskiewicz K, Prentice W: Establishment of normative data on cognitive tests for comparison with athletes sustaining mild head injury, *J Ath Training* 33(1):36, 1998.
52. Ommaya A, Gennarelli T: Cerebral concussion and traumatic unconsciousness: correlation of experimental and clinical observations on blunt head injuries, *Brain* 97:638, 1974.
53. Ommaya A, Salazar A: A spectrum of mild head injuries in sport. In National Athletic Trainers' Association: *Proceedings of mild brain injury in sports summit,* 72–80, Dallas, 1994, NATA.

54. Onate JA, Guskiewicz K, Riemann B, Prentice W: A comparison of sideline versus clinical cognitive test performance in collegiate athletes, *J Ath Train* 35(2):155, 2000.
55. Parver D: Anatomy of the eye, *Athletic Therapy Today* 4(5):13, 1999.
56. Parver D: Recognizing diseases and disorders of the eye, *Athletic Therapy Today* 4(5):22, 1999.
57. Pashby RC, Pashby TJ: Ocular injuries. In Torg JS, Shephard RJ, editors: *Current therapy in sports medicine,* St Louis, 1995, Mosby.
58. Piland S, Motl R, Ferrara M: Evidence for the factorial and construct validity of a self-report concussion symptoms scale, *J Ath Train* 38(2):104, 2003.
59. Powell JW: Cerebral concussion: causes, effects, and risks in sports, *J Ath Train* 36(3):307, 2001.
60. Practice parameter: the management of concussion in sports (summary statement). Report of the Quality Standards Subcommittee of the American Academy of Neurology. *Neurology,* 48:581, 1997.
61. Reimann B, Guskiewicz K, Shields E: Relationship between clinical and forceplate measures of postural stability, *J Orthop Sports Phys Ther,* 1999.
62. Randolph C: Implementation of neuropsychological testing models for the high school, collegiate, and professional sport settings, *J Ath Train* 36(3):280, 2001.
63. Roberts WO: Field care of the injured tooth, *Physician Sportsmed* 28(1):101, 2000.
64. Roberts WO: Who plays? Who sits? Managing concussions on the sidelines, *Physician Sportsmed* 20(6):66, 1992.
65. Robinson T, Birrer RB: Ear injuries. In Birrer RB, editor: *Sports medicine for the primary care physician,* ed 3, Boca Raton, Fla, 2004, CRC Press.
66. Robinson T, Greenberg MD: Nasal injuries. In Birrer RB, editor: *Sports medicine for the primary care physician,* ed 3, Boca Raton, Fla, 2004, CRC Press.
67. Robinson T et al: Head injuries. In Birrer RB, editor: *Sports medicine for the primary care physician,* ed 3, Boca Raton, Fla, 2004, CRC Press.
68. Saal JA: Common American football injuries, *Sports Med* 12(2):132, 1991.
69. Sailors ME: Evaluation of sports-related temporomandibular dysfunctions, *J Ath Train* 31(4):346, 1996.
70. Schuller DE, Mountain RE: Auricular injury. In Torg JS, Shephard RJ, editors: *Current therapy in sports medicine,* St Louis, 1995, Mosby.
71. Snouse S, Casterline M, Stephens B: Zygomatic arch fracture in women's ice hockey, *Athletic Therapy Today* 3(6):13, 1998.
72. Stilger VG, Alt JM, Robinson TW: Traumatic hyphema in an intercollegiate baseball player: a case report, *J Ath Train* 34(1):25, 1999.
73. Swenson EJ Jr: Sports medicine emergencies. In Birrer RB, editor: *Sports medicine for the primary care physician,* ed 3, Boca Raton, Fla, 2004, CRC Press.
74. *Taber's cyclopedic medical dictionary,* Philadelphia, 2001, FA Davis.
75. Taylor LP: Neurologic disorders. In Agostini R, editor: *Medical and orthopedic issues of active and athletic women,* Philadelphia, 1994, Hanley & Belfus.
76. Torg JS: *Athletic injuries to the head, neck, and face,* St Louis, 1991, Mosby.
77. Torg JS: Emergency management of head and cervical spine injuries. In Torg JS, Shephard RJ, editors: *Current therapy in sports medicine,* St Louis, 1995, Mosby.
78. Valovich T, Perrin D, Gansneder B: Repeat administration elicits a practice effect with the balance error scoring system but not with the standardized assessment of concussion in high school athletes, *J Ath Train* 38(1):51, 2003.
79. Weir J: Effective management of epistaxis in athletes, *J Ath Train* 32(3):254, 1997.
80. Whitney SL: Vestibular disorders in mild head injury. *Athletic Therapy Today* 6(1):33, 2001.
81. Wilberger JE, Maroon JC: Head injuries in athletes, *Clin Sports Med* 8:1, 1989.
82. Wilkins J, McCleod T, Perrin D: Performance on the balance error scoring system decreases after fatigue, *J Ath Train* 39(2):156, 2004.

ANNOTATED BIBLIOGRAPHY

Cantu RC: *Neurologic athletic head and neck injuries. Clinics in sports medicine,* vol 17, no 1, Philadelphia, 1998, Saunders.

This recent text looks at head and neck trauma that occurs specifically in the athletic population.

Cantu RI: *Neurologic athletic head and spine injuries,* Philadelphia, 2000, WB Saunders.

The text addresses topics related to neurologic athletic head and spine injuries such as injury epidemiology, prevention, on-the-field management, diagnosis, treatment, rehabilitation, and return-to-play decisions.

Currie D, Ritchie E, Scott S: *The management of head injuries,* London, 2000, Oxford University Press.

Chapters cover initial assessment, resuscitation, neurological deterioration, scalp and skull injuries, cervical spine injuries, children's injuries, and more.

National Athletic Trainers' Association Research and Education Foundation: *Proceedings: Mild brain injury in sports,* Dallas, TX, 1994, NATA.

This collection of papers, presented at a conference about mild brain injuries, provides a concise summary of information on this topic.

Special Issue: Sports vision: sports vision/the eye, *Athletic Therapy Today* 4(5): September 1999.

This issue focuses on articles that look at injuries to the eye.

Special Issue: Concussion in athletes, *Journal of Athletic Training* 36(3): July–September, 2001.

This issue contains a variety of data-based research articles dealing with sport-related concussion.

Zagelbaum BM: *Sports ophthalmology,* 1996, Blackwell Scientific Inc.

A reference on diagnosing and treating sports-related eye injuries for ophthalmologists, team doctors, athletic trainers, and primary care physicians.

Chapter 27 The Thorax and Abdomen

When you finish this chapter you should be able to

- Understand the anatomy of the thorax and abdomen.
- Identify the location and function of the heart and lungs.
- Be aware of the location and function of the abdominal viscera related to the urinary system, the digestive system, the reproductive system, and the lymphatic system.
- Be familiar with techniques for assessing thoracic and abdominal injuries.
- Recognize various injuries to the structures of the thorax.
- Review various injuries and conditions in structures of the abdomen.

This chapter deals with sports injuries to the thorax and abdomen. In an athletic environment, injuries to the thorax and abdomen have a lower incidence than do injuries to the extremities. However, unlike the musculoskeletal injuries to the extremities discussed to this point, injuries to the heart, lungs, and abdominal viscera can be potentially serious and even life threatening if not recognized and managed appropriately. It is imperative for the athletic trainer to be familiar with the anatomy and more common injuries seen in the abdomen and thorax (Figure 27-1).

ANATOMY OF THE THORAX

The thoracic cavity is that portion of the body commonly known as the chest, which lies between the base of the neck and the diaphragm. It consists of the thoracic vertebrae, the twelve pairs of ribs with their associated costal cartilages, and the sternum (Figure 27-2). Its main functions are to protect the vital respiratory and circulatory organs and to assist the lungs in inspiration and expiration during the breathing process. Within the thoracic cage lie the lungs, the heart, and the thymus.

The thoracic cage protects the heart and lungs.

Ribs, Costal Cartilage, and Sternum

The ribs are flat bones that are attached to the thoracic vertebrae in the back and to the sternum in the front. The upper seven ribs are called sternal, or true, ribs, and each rib is joined to the sternum by a separate costal cartilage. The eighth, ninth, and tenth ribs (false ribs) have a common cartilage that joins the seventh rib before attaching to the

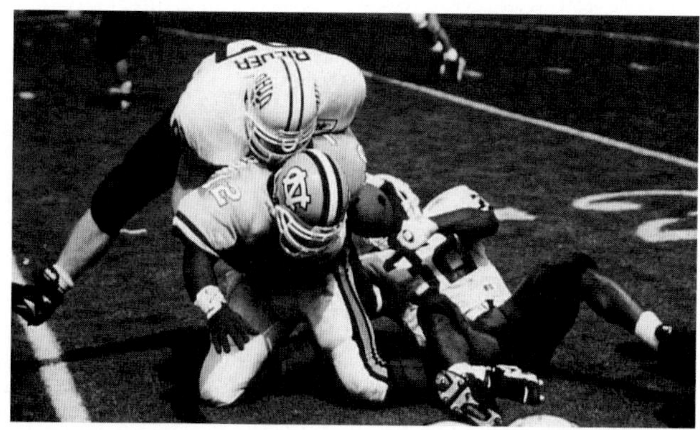

Figure 27-1

Collision sports can produce serious thoracic and abdominal injuries.

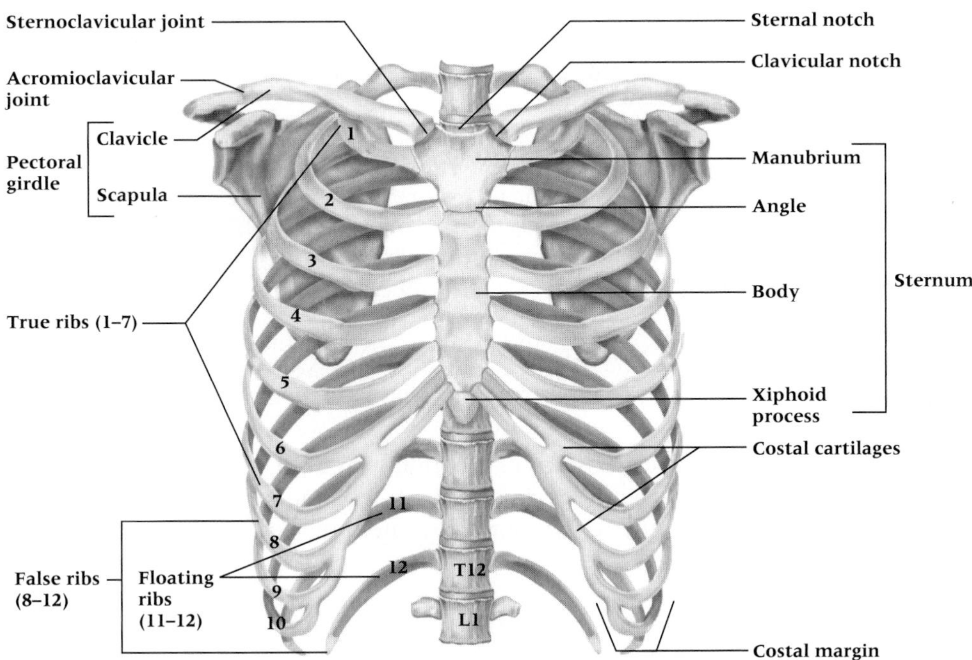

Figure 27-2

The thoracic cage.

sternum. The eleventh and twelfth ribs (floating ribs) remain unattached to the sternum but do have muscle attachments. The individual rib articulation produces a slight gliding action.

The inside of the thoracic cage is lined with the pleura, a thin double-layer membrane filled with pleural fluid that permits the lungs to slide along the thoracic cage.

Thoracic Muscles

There are eleven pairs of both external intercostal muscles and internal intercostal muscles between the ribs (Figure 27-3). They attach on the inferior border of the rib above and the superior border of the rib below. The external intercostals elevate the diaphragm during inspiration, whereas the internal intercostals depress the rib cage to assist with expiration. The intercostal muscles are innervated by the intercostal nerves (Table 27-1).

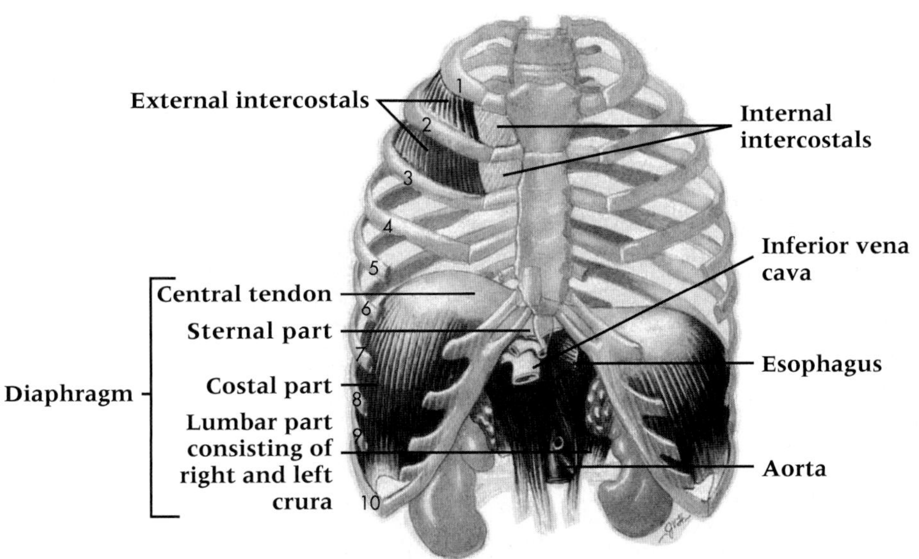

Figure 27-3

Anatomy of the thoracic muscles.

TABLE 27-1 Muscles of the Thorax

Muscle	Origin	Insertion	Muscle Action	Innervation
External intercostals	Inferior border of the ribs and the costal cartilages	Superior border of the rib below the rib of origin	Elevates the ribs, aiding in inspiration	Intercostal
Internal intercostals	Inner surface of the ribs and the costal cartilages	Superior border of the rib below the rib of origin	Draws ribs together, aiding in expiration	Intercostal
Diaphragm	Inferior border of the rib cage; the xiphoid process; the costal cartilages; and the lumbar vertebrae	Central tendon of the diaphragm	Pulls central tendon downward, increasing the size of the thoracic cavity, and therefore causing inspiration	Phrenic

The pectoralis minor, trapezius, serratus anterior, serratus posterior, levator scapula, and rhomboids are muscles that originate on the thorax and were discussed in Chapter 22. Their primary function is controlling movement of the scapula.

Lungs

The trachea, or windpipe, branches into right and left primary bronchi, which branch into smaller divisions and ultimately terminate in clusters of air sacs called alveoli within the lungs (Figure 27-4). Alveoli facilitate the exchange of oxygen and carbon dioxide with the capillaries. The lungs are elastic and expand and constrict in response to contraction of the diaphragm muscle.

Respiratory Muscles

The diaphragm is a large, dome-shaped muscle that separates the thoracic cavity from the abdominal cavity. When the diaphragm contracts, the dome flattens, which in-

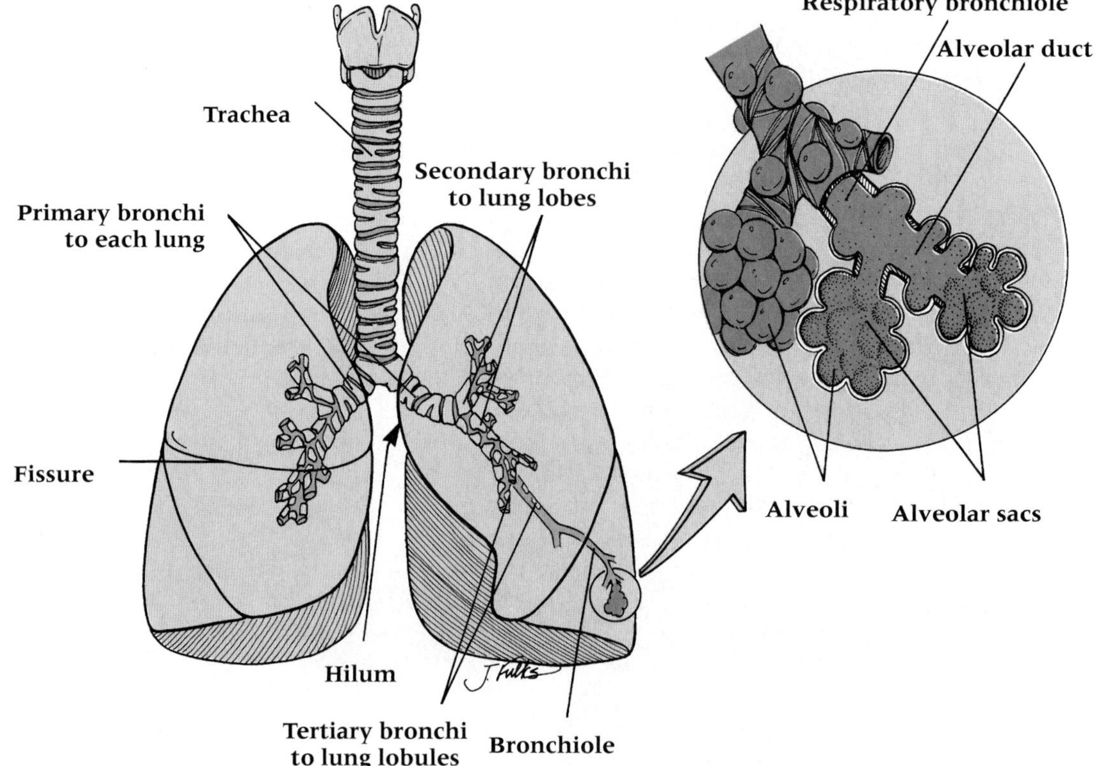

Figure 27-4

Anatomy of the trachea, lungs, and alveoli.

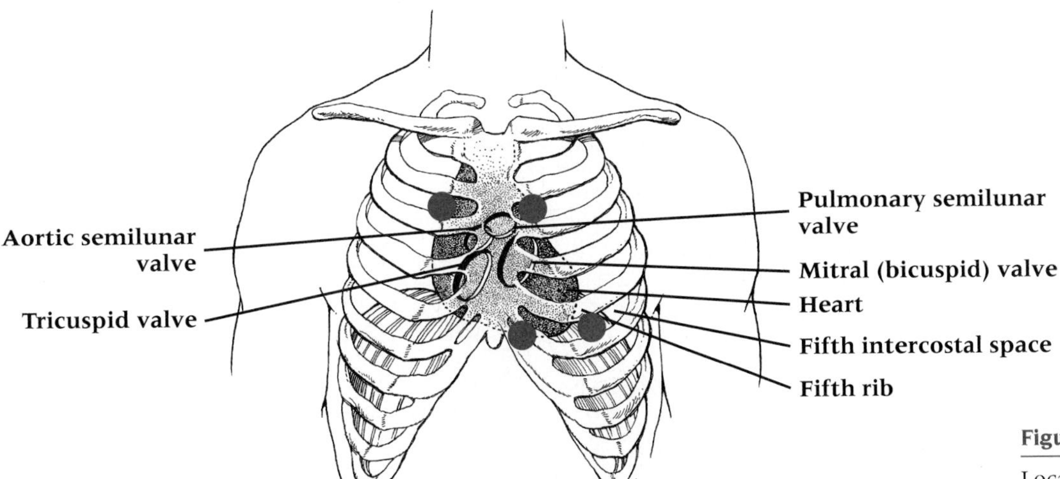

Figure 27-5

Location of the heart in the thorax. (The colored dots indicate the points for auscultation of heart sounds through a stethoscope.)

creases the volume of the thorax and results in inspiration of air. Expiration occurs when the diaphragm relaxes and the elastic components of the lungs and thoracic cage passively decrease thoracic volume.

Blood Supply

Blood flows to the lungs through the pulmonary arteries to the alveoli, where it is oxygenated and returns to the heart through the pulmonary veins. The bronchi are supplied with oxygenated blood through the bronchial arteries that branch from the aorta. Deoxygenated blood returns to the heart from the bronchi via both the bronchial and pulmonary veins.

Heart

The heart is the main pumping mechanism; it circulates oxygenated blood throughout the body to the working tissues. The transport of oxygen involves the coordinated function of the heart, the blood vessels, the blood, and the lungs.

The adult heart lies under the sternum, slightly to the left, between the lungs, and in front of the vertebral column (Figure 27-5). It is about the size of a clenched fist. It extends from the first rib to the space between the fifth and sixth ribs.

The heart muscle consists of four chambers: the right and left atria and the right and left ventricles (Figure 27-6). Deoxygenated blood returns from all parts of the body through the venous system to the right atrium and passes through the tricuspid valve to the right ventricle. The right ventricle pumps the blood through the pulmonary valve to the pulmonary artery and into the lungs, where it is oxygenated. Blood returns from the lungs via the pulmonary vein to the left atrium and passes through the mitral valve into the left ventricle. Blood is ejected past the aortic valve into the aorta, which supplies the entire body through the arterial system.

A single heartbeat consists of a contraction of both atria followed immediately by a contraction of both ventricles. Contraction of the chambers is referred to as systole, and relaxation as diastole.

Blood Supply

The heart is supplied by right and left coronary arteries branching from the aorta. Cardiac veins drain into the right atrium.

Thymus

The thymus is located in the thorax just anterior to and above the heart. The function of the thymus is to produce lymphocytes, which migrate to other lymphatic tissues to

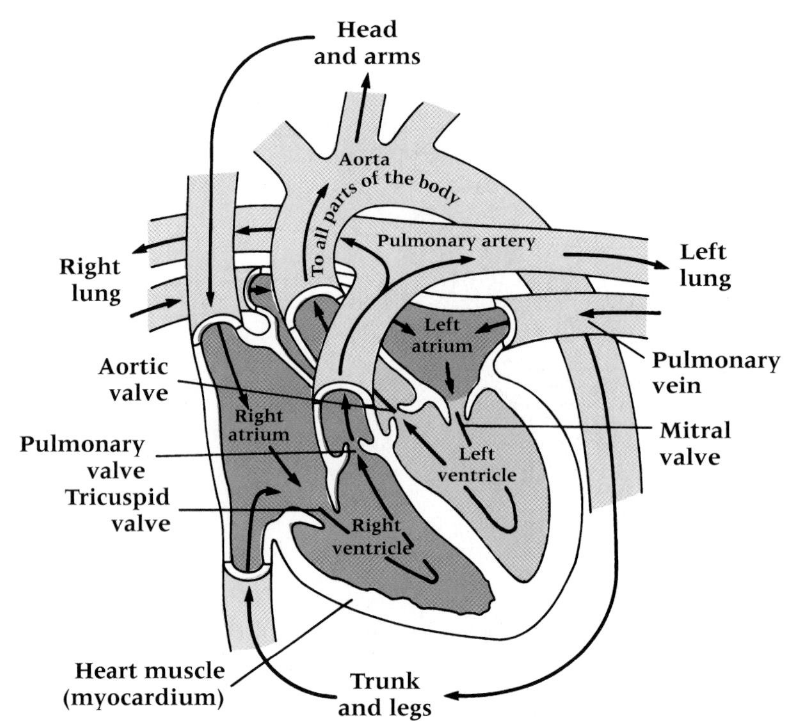

Figure 27-6

Anatomy of the heart and blood flow.

respond to foreign substances. The thymus is relatively large in the infant and after puberty gradually decreases in size.[59]

ANATOMY OF THE ABDOMEN

The abdominal cavity lies between the diaphragm and the bones of the pelvis and is bounded by the margin of the lower ribs, the abdominal muscles, and the vertebral column. The abdominal cavity is sometimes called the abdominopelvic cavity, although there is no physical separation between the abdominal and pelvic cavities.

Abdominal Muscles

The abdominal muscles are the rectus abdominis, the external oblique, the internal oblique, and the transversus abdominis (Figure 27-7). They are invested with both superficial and deep fasciae (Table 27-2).

The rectus abdominis muscle, a trunk flexor, is attached to the rib cage above and to the pubis below. It is divided into three segments by transverse tendinous inscriptions; longitudinally it is divided by the linea alba. It functions in trunk flexion, rotation, and lateral flexion and in compression of the abdominal cavity. A heavy fascial sheath encloses the rectus abdominis muscle, holding it in its position but in no way restricting its motion. The inguinal ring, which serves as a passageway for the spermatic cord, is formed by the abdominal fascia.

The external oblique muscle is a broad, thin muscle that arises from slips attached to the borders of the lower eight ribs. It runs obliquely forward and downward and inserts on the anterior two-thirds of the crest of the ilium, the pubic crest, and the fascia of the rectus abdominis and the linea alba at their lower front. Its principal functions are trunk flexion, rotation, lateral flexion, and compression.

The internal oblique muscle forms the anterior and lateral aspects of the abdominal wall. Its fibers arise from the iliac crest, the upper half of the inguinal ligament, and the lumbar fascia. It runs principally in an obliquely upward direction to the cartilages of the tenth, eleventh, and twelfth ribs on each side. The main functions of the internal oblique are trunk flexion, lateral flexion, and rotation.

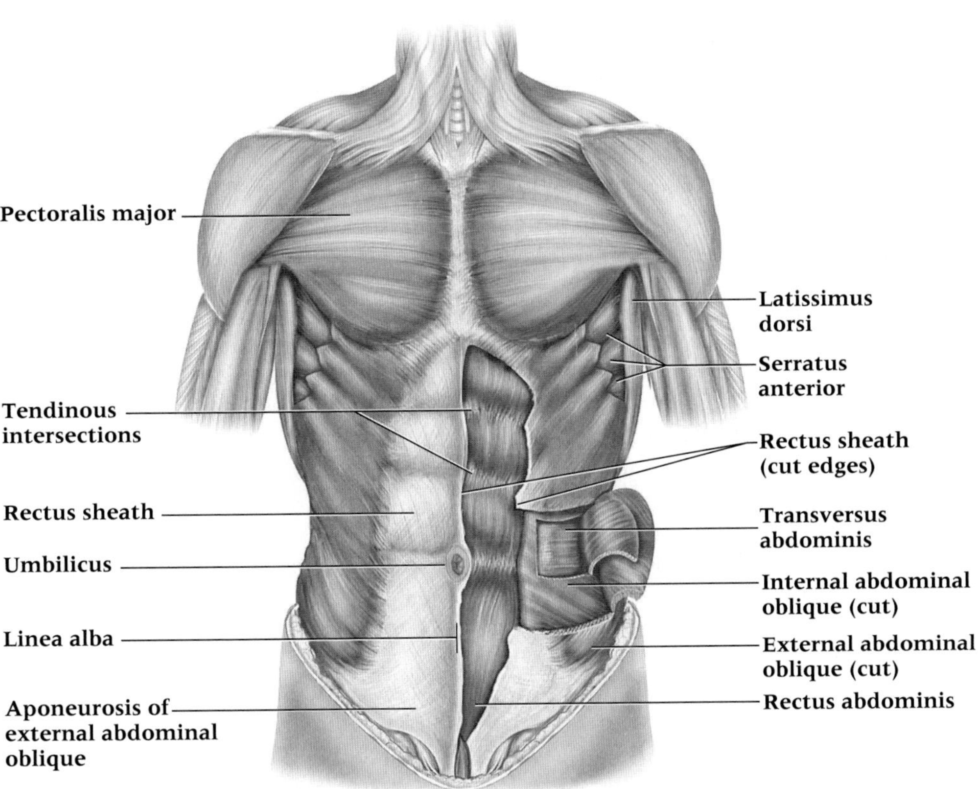

Figure 27-7

Abdominal muscles.

TABLE 27-2 Muscles of the Abdominal Wall

Muscle	Origin	Insertion	Muscle Action	Innervation
External abdominal oblique	External surface of the lower eight ribs	Linea alba and the anterior half of the iliac crest	Compresses the abdominopelvic cavity; assists in flexing and rotating the vertebral column	Intercostals, iliohypogastric, and ilioinguinal
Internal abdominal oblique	Inguinal ligament, the iliac crest, and the lumbodorsal fascia	Linea alba, the pubic crest, and the lower four ribs	Compresses the abdominopelvic cavity; assists in flexing and rotating the vertebral column	Intercostals, iliohypogastric, and ilioinguinal
Transversus abdominis	Inguinal ligament, the iliac crest, the lumbodorsal fascia, and the costal cartilages of the last six ribs	Linea alba and the pubic crest	Compresses the abdominopelvic cavity	Intercostals, iliohypogastric, and ilioinguinal
Rectus abdominis	Pubic crest	Xiphoid process and the costal cartilages of the fifth through the seventh ribs	Compresses the abdominopelvic cavity; flexes the vertebral column	Intercostals
Quadratus lumborum	Iliac crest, and the iliolumbar ligament	Lower border of the twelfth ribs; the transverse processes of the upper lumbar vertebrae	Pulls the thoracic cage toward the pelvis; abducts the vertebral column toward the side that is being contracted	Twelfth thoracic and first lumbar

The transversus abdominis is the deepest of the abdominal muscles. Its fibers run transversely across the abdominal cavity, arising from the outer third of the inguinal ligament, the iliac crest, the lumbar fascia of the back, and the lower six ribs. It inserts into the linea alba and the front half of the iliac crest. The main functions of the transversus abdominis are to hold the abdominal contents in place and to aid in forced expiration. All the abdominal muscles work together in performing defecation, micturition, and forced expiration.

Abdominal Viscera

Abdominal viscera are part of the urinary, digestive, reproductive, and lymphatic systems.

The abdominal viscera are composed of both hollow and solid organs. The solid organs are the kidneys, spleen, liver, pancreas, and adrenal glands. The hollow organs include vessels, tubes, and receptacles such as the stomach, intestines, gallbladder, and urinary bladder (Figure 27-8). Organs in the abdominal cavity may be classified as being part of the urinary system, the digestive system, the reproductive system, or the lymphatic system.

27-1 Critical Thinking Exercise

A soccer player is kicked in the abdomen above the umbilicus. Initially, she had the wind knocked out of her. Now she is complaining of pain and her abdomen is tight on palpation.

? What should the athletic trainer be most concerned about and what organs may potentially be involved?

Urinary System Organs

The kidneys, the ureters, and the urinary bladder are the urinary system organs.

Kidneys The kidneys are situated on each side of the spine, approximately in the center of the back. They are bean shaped, approximately 4½ inches (11.25 cm) long, 2 inches (5 cm) wide, and 1 inch (2.5 cm) thick. The right kidney is usually slightly lower than the left because of the pressure of the liver. The uppermost surfaces of the kidneys are connected to the diaphragm by strong, ligamentous fibers. As breathing occurs, the kidneys move up and down as much as ½ inch (1.25 cm). The inferior aspect is positioned 1 to 2 inches (2.5 to 5 cm) above the iliac crest. Resting anterior to the left kidney are the stomach, spleen, pancreas, and small and large intestines. Organs that are situated anterior to the right kidney are the liver and the intestines. The kidneys lie posterior to the abdominal cavity. Their primary function is to filter metabolic wastes, ions, or drugs from blood and expel them from the body via urination.[57]

Adrenal glands Although part of the endocrine system rather than the urinary system, the adrenal glands, also called the suprarenal glands, are located on top of each kidney. They secrete the hormones epinephrine, norepinephrine, cortisol, estrogen, aldosterone, and androgen, which have a variety of physiologic functions throughout the body.[63]

Ureters and urinary bladder The ureters are small tubes that extend inferiorly from the kidney to the urinary bladder, which stores urine. The bladder is a hollow container that lies posterior to the pubic symphysis. In the male, the bladder is anterior to the rectum, and in the female, it is anterior to the vagina and inferior to the uterus.

Digestive System Organs

The liver, gallbladder, pancreas, stomach, small intestine, and large intestine are digestive system organs.

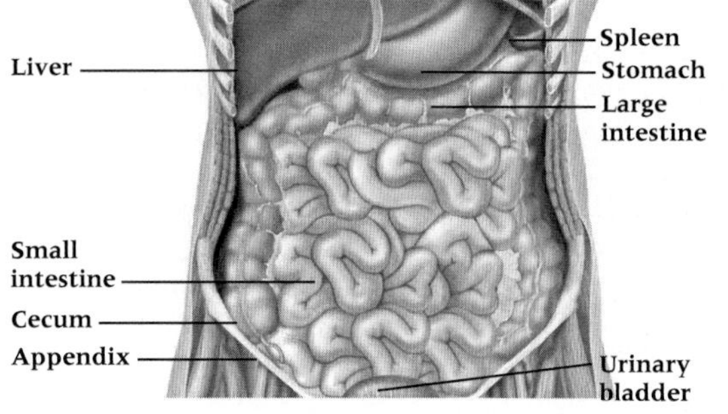

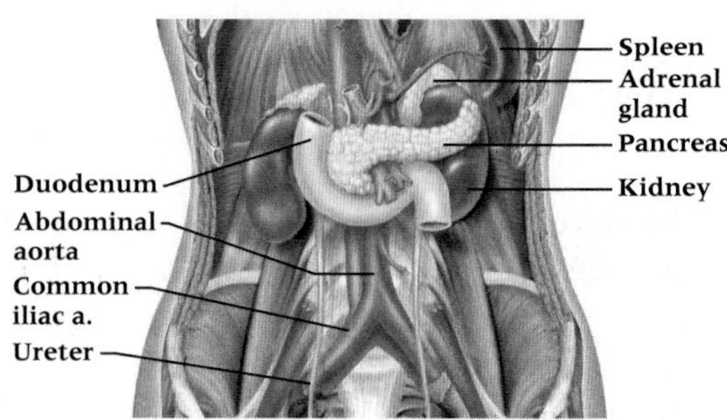

Figure 27-8

A, Anterior abdominal viscera. **B,** Posterior abdominal viscera.

Liver The liver is the largest internal organ of the body. It lies in the upper right quadrant of the body against the inferior surface of the diaphragm and weighs about three pounds. It consists of two major right and left lobes. The liver performs digestive and excretory functions; absorbs and stores excessive glucose; processes nutrients; and detoxifies harmful chemicals. It secretes bile, which is essential in neutralizing and diluting stomach acid and for digesting fat in the small intestine during the digestive process.[50]

Hepatitis is an inflammation of the liver caused by viral infection or alcohol consumption. If it is not corrected, the cells in the liver may die and be replaced by scar tissue, which can lead to cirrhosis or impaired liver function.[57] Cirrhosis is a progressive disease of the liver that results in diffuse scarring and fibrosis and disruption of hepatic blood flow that can eventually result in liver failure. Cirrhosis can have many causes but it is most often associated with chronic alcoholism.[63]

Gallbladder The gallbladder is a pear-shaped, saclike structure located on the inferior surface of the liver. It serves as a storage reservoir for bile secreted from the liver. Shortly after a meal, the gallbladder secrets the stored bile into the small intestine. Cholesterol, which is secreted by the liver, may cause the gallbladder to produce a gallstone, which can potentially block the release of bile. The gallstone interferes with digestion and must usually be removed surgically.[63]

Pancreas The pancreas is located between the small intestine and the spleen. It secretes pancreatic juice, which is critical in the digestion of fats, carbohydrates, and proteins. It also produces insulin and glucagon, which are hormones that control the amount of glucose and amino acids in the blood.

Stomach The stomach is found primarily in the upper left quadrant between the esophagus and the small intestine. It functions mainly as a storage and mixing chamber for food that has been ingested. Some digestion and absorption occur in the stomach. Gastric secretions assist in the partial digestion of protein and the absorption of alcohol and caffeine. Ingested food is mixed with secretions from the stomach glands to form a semifluid material called chyme, which passes from the stomach into the small intestine.[57]

Small intestine The small intestine is connected to the stomach via a series of tubelike folds. The small intestine has three portions: the duodenum, the jejunum, and the ileum. In total, it is approximately 20 feet (6 m) in length. Secretions from the liver and pancreas mix with secretions from the small intestine, which are essential to the process of digestion. Mucus is secreted in large amounts to lubricate and protect the wall of the intestine as a mixture of chyme and the digestive enzymes is propelled through the small intestine by a series of peristaltic contractions. Chyme moves through the small intestine over a period of three to five hours. Most of the digestion and absorption of food occurs in the small intestine.[56]

Large intestine The large intestine is that portion of the digestive tract that extends from the small intestine to the anus and is approximately 6½ feet (2 m) in length. It has three divisions: the cecum, the colon, and the rectum. The vermiform appendix extends from the cecum. In the colon, chyme is converted to feces through the absorption of water, secretion of mucus, and activity of microorganisms. Feces remain in the colon and rectum until the time of defecation.

Lymphatic System Organs

The spleen and the thymus, which is discussed in the section on the thoracic cavity, are organs of the lymphatic system.

Spleen The spleen is the largest lymphatic organ in the body. It weighs approximately 6 ounces (170 grams) and is approximately 5 inches (12.5 cm) long. It lies under the diaphragm on the left side and behind the ninth, tenth, and eleventh ribs. It is surrounded by a fibrous capsule that is firmly invested by the peritoneum. The spleen's main functions are to serve as a reservoir of red blood cells; to regulate the number of red blood cells in the general circulation, to destroy ineffective red cells, to produce antibodies for immunological function, and to produce lymphocytes.[63]

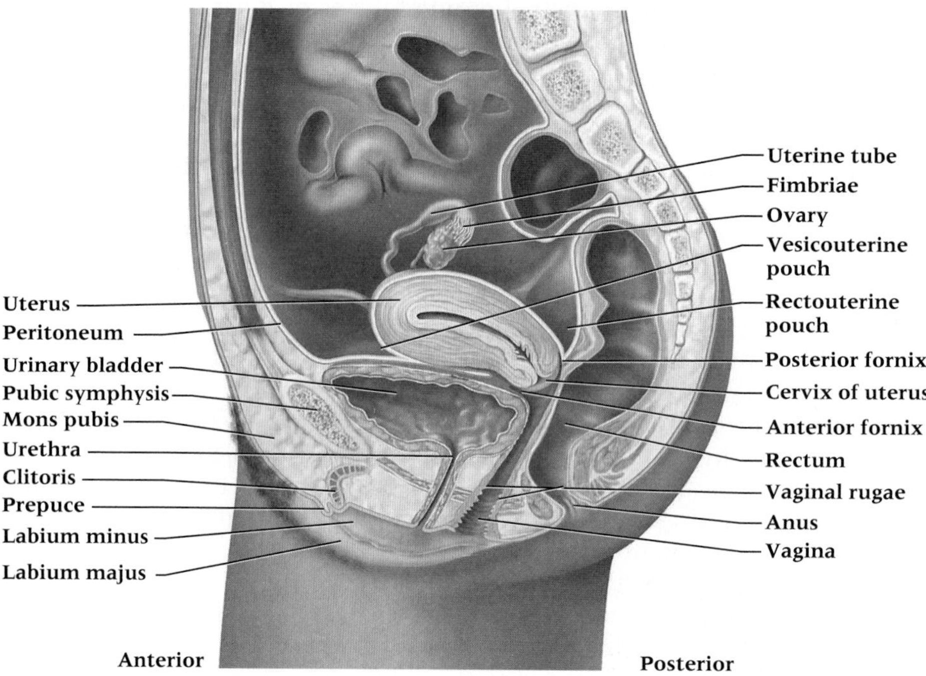

Figure 27-9

Female reproductive organs.

Reproductive System Organs

Unlike the other organ systems discussed to this point, the reproductive system differs considerably between males and females. The female reproductive organs include the ovaries, uterus, uterine tubes (fallopian tubes), and vagina. The male reproductive organs include the seminal vesicles, prostate gland, testes, vas deferens, epididymis, urethra, and penis.

Female reproductive organs The reproductive organs in the female are between the urinary bladder and the rectum; the uterus and vagina are in the midline, and the uterine tubes and ovaries extend to either side (Figure 27-9). Their position is maintained by a group of ligaments, the primary one being the broad ligament. The vagina is a receptacle for sperm, which swim upward into the uterus to fertilize the egg.

The ovaries produce and store the female eggs (ova) which are released one at a time each month into the uterine tubes. The uterine tubes transport the ovum to the uterus, where a fertilized ovum attaches to the uterine wall and becomes a developing embryo. If the ovum is not fertilized, the process of menstruation begins.

The reproductive organs in the female are well protected by the pelvis. Thus, traumatic injury to these structures is rare in the athletic population.

Male reproductive organs The reproductive organs in the male are found both inside and outside the abdominal cavity (Figure 27-10). The prostate is dorsal to the pubic symphysis and inferior to the bladder. The urethra and the ejaculatory ducts pass through the prostate. The prostate is made of both glandular and muscular tissue and is similar in size to a walnut. The prostate secretes a milky fluid that is discharged by twenty to thirty ducts into the prostatic portion of the urethra as a component of semen. The seminal vesicles are also glandular structures found posterior and superior to the prostate gland under the bladder. The seminal vesicles contribute the majority of the fluid to the semen through the ejaculatory ducts.

The remainder of the male reproductive organs are exposed outside the abdominal cavity and are more susceptible to injury. The testes are the primary male sex organs. They are located within the scrotum and produce spermatozoa and testosterone. The epididymis is a comma-shaped structure connected to the posterior surface of the testis in which the sperm are stored until mature. The vas deferens is a duct running

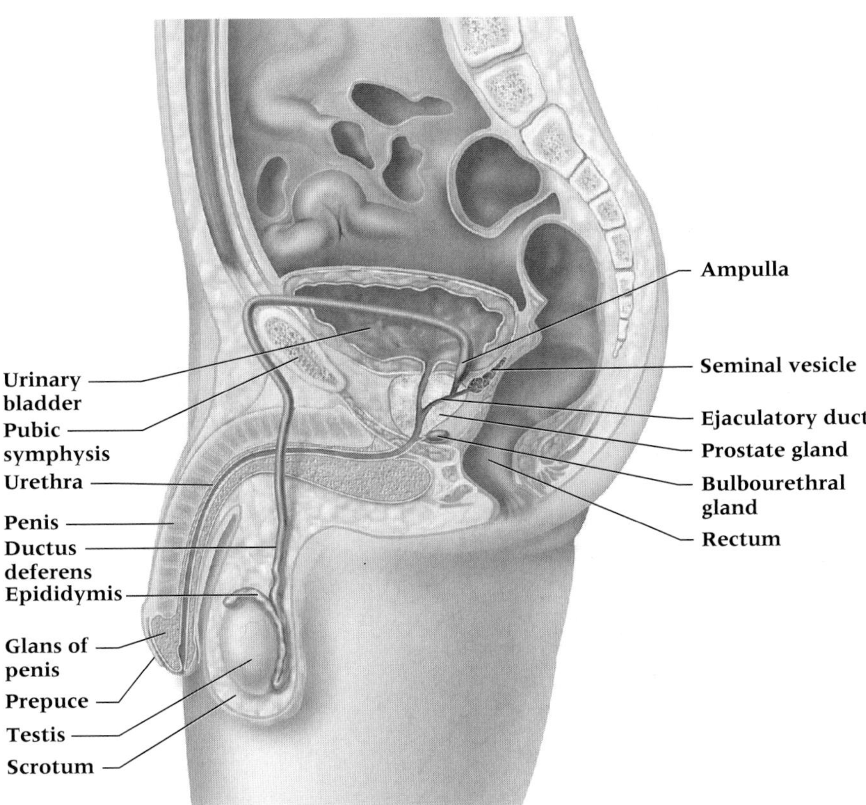

Figure 27-10

Male reproductive organs.

from the epididymis to the ejaculatory duct. The urethra runs from the bladder to the tip of the penis and serves as a pathway through which both urine and semen are ejected through the penis. The penis consists of three layers of erectile tissue, which, when engorged with blood, cause an erection.

PREVENTION OF INJURIES TO THE THORAX AND ABDOMEN

Injuries to the thorax may be prevented by appropriate protective equipment, particularly in collision sport activities. In football, for example, shoulder pads are usually designed to extend to at least below the level of the sternum. Rib protectors may be worn to cover the entire thoracic cage if necessary.

The muscles of the abdomen should be strengthened to provide protection to the underlying viscera. A consistent regimen of core stabilization exercises done in various positions can markedly increase the strength and size of the abdominal musculature (see Figure 25-62).

Making sure that the hollow organs, in particular the stomach and bladder, are emptied prior to competition can reduce the chance of injury to those structures. Meals should be eaten at least three to four hours before competition to allow foods to clear the stomach. Urination immediately before stepping onto the field or court will protect the bladder from injury.

ASSESSMENT OF THE THORAX AND ABDOMEN

Injuries to the thorax and abdomen can produce potentially life-threatening situations.[54] An injury that may seem to be relatively insignificant at first may rapidly develop into one that requires immediate and appropriate medical attention.[4] Thus, the athletic trainer's primary survey should focus on those signs and symptoms that indicate some life-threatening condition. The injured athlete should be continually monitored by the athletic trainer to identify any disruption of normal breathing or circulation or any indication of internal hemorrhage that could precipitate shock.

History

The questions that the athletic trainer should asked to determine a history for thoracic and abdominal injuries are somewhat different than the questions that are pertinent to musculoskeletal injuries of the extremities.[51] The primary mechanism of injury should be determined first.

- What happened to cause this injury?
- Was there direct contact or a direct blow?
- What position were you in?
- What type of pain is there (sharp, dull, localized, etc)?
- Was the pain immediate or gradual?
- Do you feel any pain other than in the area where the injury occurred?
- Have you had any difficulty breathing?
- Are certain positions more comfortable than others?
- Do you feel faint, light-headed, or nauseous?
- Do you feel any pain in your chest?
- Did you hear or feel a pop or crack in your chest?
- Have you had any muscle spasms?
- Have you noticed any blood in your urine?
- Have you had any difficulty or pain in urinating?
- Was the bladder full or empty?
- How long has it been since you have eaten?
- Is there a personal or family history of any heart problems, any abdominal problems, or any other diseases involving the thorax and abdomen?

Observation

The athletic trainer should observe the athlete immediately following injury to check for normal breathing and respiratory patterns.

- Most importantly, is the athlete breathing at all?
- Is the athlete having difficulty breathing deeply, or is he or she catching the breath?
- Does breathing cause pain?
- Is the athlete holding the chest wall?
- Is there symmetry in movement of the chest during breathing?
- If the athlete's wind was knocked out, is normal breathing returning rapidly or is there prolonged difficulty? Prolonged difficulty may indicate a more severe injury.

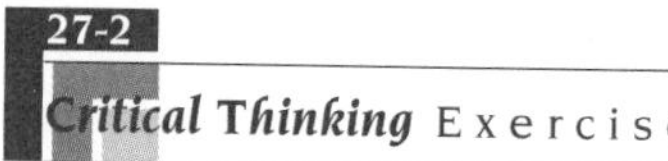

A basketball player goes for a rebound and is accidentally hit in the abdomen by an opponent's elbow. He is lying on the court on his side with his legs drawn up. The athletic trainer decides to remove him from the court on a stretcher and evaluate him in the training room. On palpation, the abdomen feels extremely tight.

? How can the athletic trainer differentiate between muscle guarding, rigidity, and rebound tenderness in the athlete who has sustained an abdominal injury?

The body position of the athlete should be observed. An athlete who has sustained some type of thoracic injury will often be leaning toward the side that is injured, holding or splinting the area with the opposite hand (Figure 27-11A). In the case of an abdominal injury, the athlete will typically lie on his or her side with the knees pulled up toward the chest (Figure 27-11B).[63] The male who has sustained an injury to the external genitalia will be lying on his side holding the scrotum (Figure 27-11C).

The athletic trainer should check for areas of discoloration, swelling, or deformities that may produce asymmetries. Discoloration or ecchymosis around the umbilicus is indicative of intraabdominal bleeding, whereas ecchymosis on the flanks may indicate swelling outside the abdomen.

- Is there protrusion or swelling of any portion of the abdomen? Such swelling may indicate internal bleeding.
- Does the thorax appear to be symmetrical? Rib fractures can cause one side to appear different.
- Are the abdominal muscles tight and guarding?
- Is the athlete holding or splinting a specific part of the abdomen?

Other observable signs and symptoms may indicate the nature of a thoracic or abdominal injury. Bright red blood being coughed up indicates some injury to the lungs.

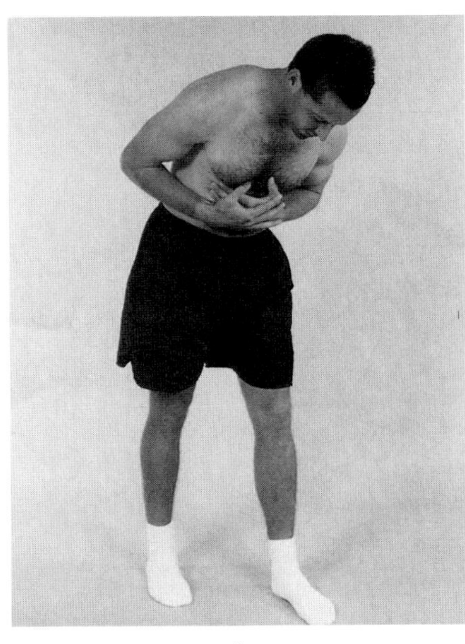

A

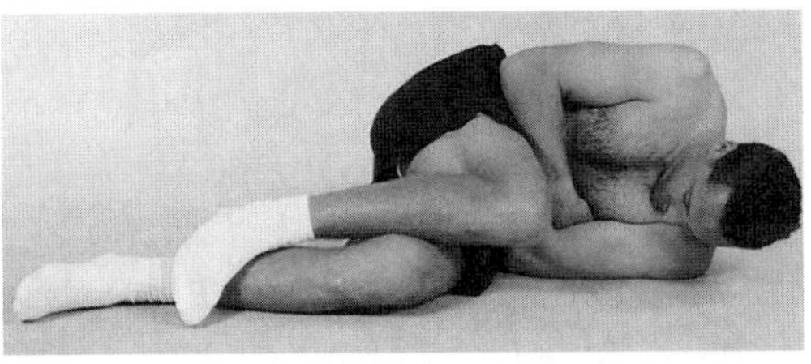

B

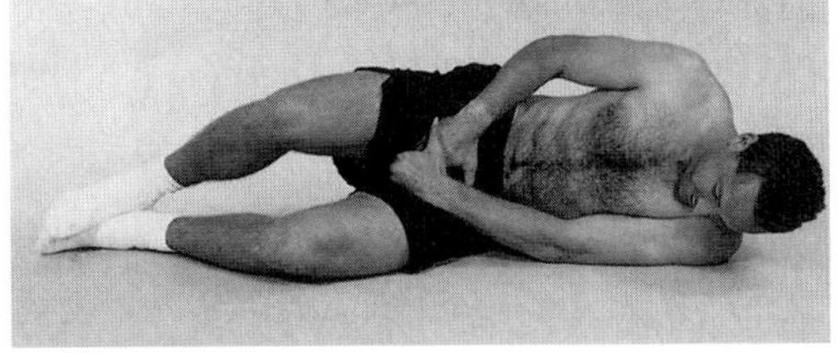

C

Figure 27-11

Typical body positions after injury. **A,** Thoracic injury. **B,** Abdominal injury. **C,** External genitalia injury.

Bright red frothy blood being vomited may indicate injury to the esophagus or stomach, although the blood may also be swallowed from the mouth or nose and then vomited. Cyanosis generally indicates some respiratory difficulty, whereas pale, cool, clammy skin indicates lowered blood pressure.

It is important to monitor vital signs, including pulse, respirations, and blood pressure (see Chapter 12). A rapid, weak pulse and/or a significant drop in blood pressure is an indication of some potentially serious internal injury that very often involves loss of blood.

Palpation

Thorax

The athletic trainer should first place his or her hands on either side of the chest wall to check for symmetry in chest wall movement during deep inspiration and expiration and to begin to isolate areas of tenderness (Figure 27-12).[32] Once a tender area is identified, the athletic trainer should palpate along the ribs in the intercostal space between the ribs, and at the costochondral junction to locate a specific point of tenderness. Applying anterioposterior compression to the thoracic cage is done to identify potential rib fractures (Figure 27-13A). Transverse compression applied laterally identifies costochondral injuries (Figure 27-13B). If the athlete is having difficulty breathing, it may be helpful to use a semireclining position for these tests.

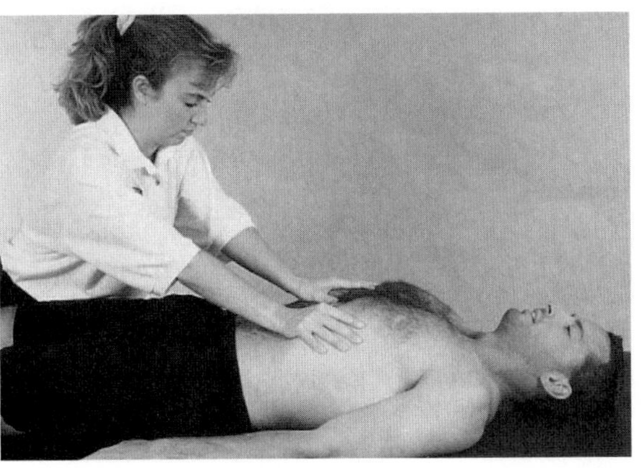

Figure 27-12

Checking asymmetry of the chest wall during breathing.

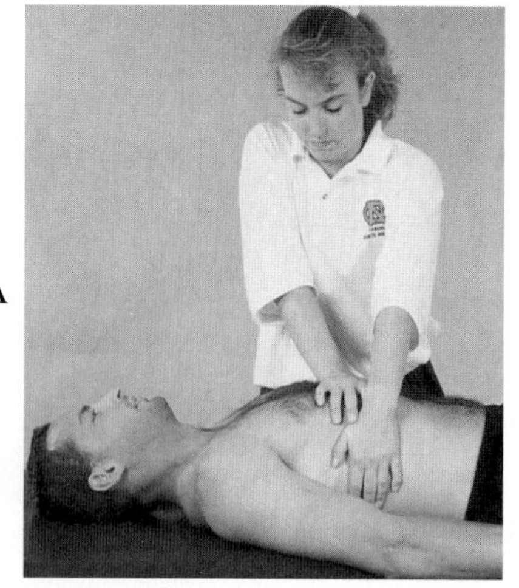
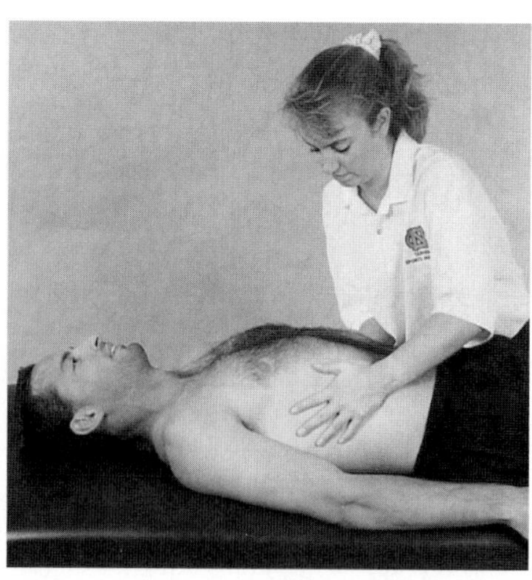

Figure 27-13

A, Checking for rib fractures.
B, Checking for costochondral injuries.

Abdomen

For abdominal palpation, the athlete should be supine with the arms at the side and with the hips and knees flexed to relax the abdominal muscles. Palpation should occur in a systematic manner using the four abdominopelvic quadrants that were discussed in Chapter 13 (see Figure 13-3). Palpation should begin in the right upper quadrant and move clockwise to the left upper quadrant, the left lower quadrant, and finally, the right lower quadrant (appendix). The athletic trainer should begin palpating uninjured areas first, using the tips of the fingers to feel for any tightness or rigidity (Figure 27-14).[49] An athlete with an abdominal injury will voluntarily contract the abdominal muscles to guard or protect the tender area. If there is bleeding or irritation inside the abdominal cavity, the abdomen will exhibit boardlike rigidity and cannot be voluntarily relaxed. Rebound tenderness may also accompany intraabdominal bleeding. The evaluator can produce rebound tenderness by pressing firmly on the abdomen and then quickly releasing pressure, which causes intense pain. If the athlete is exhibiting only voluntary guarding, the evaluator can palpate over the liver, gallbladder, spleen, stomach, small intestine, large intestine, vermiform appendix, and bladder while searching for tenderness, swelling, or enlargement. The kidneys should be palpated with the athlete in a prone position.

Pressure on the abdominal organs may elicit referred pain in predictable patterns away from the source.[52] Figure 27-15 identifies patterns of referred pain.

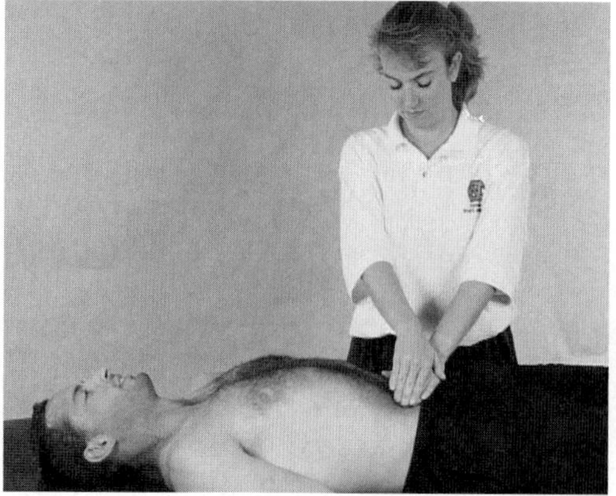

Figure 27-14

Palpating the abdomen for guarding or rigidity.

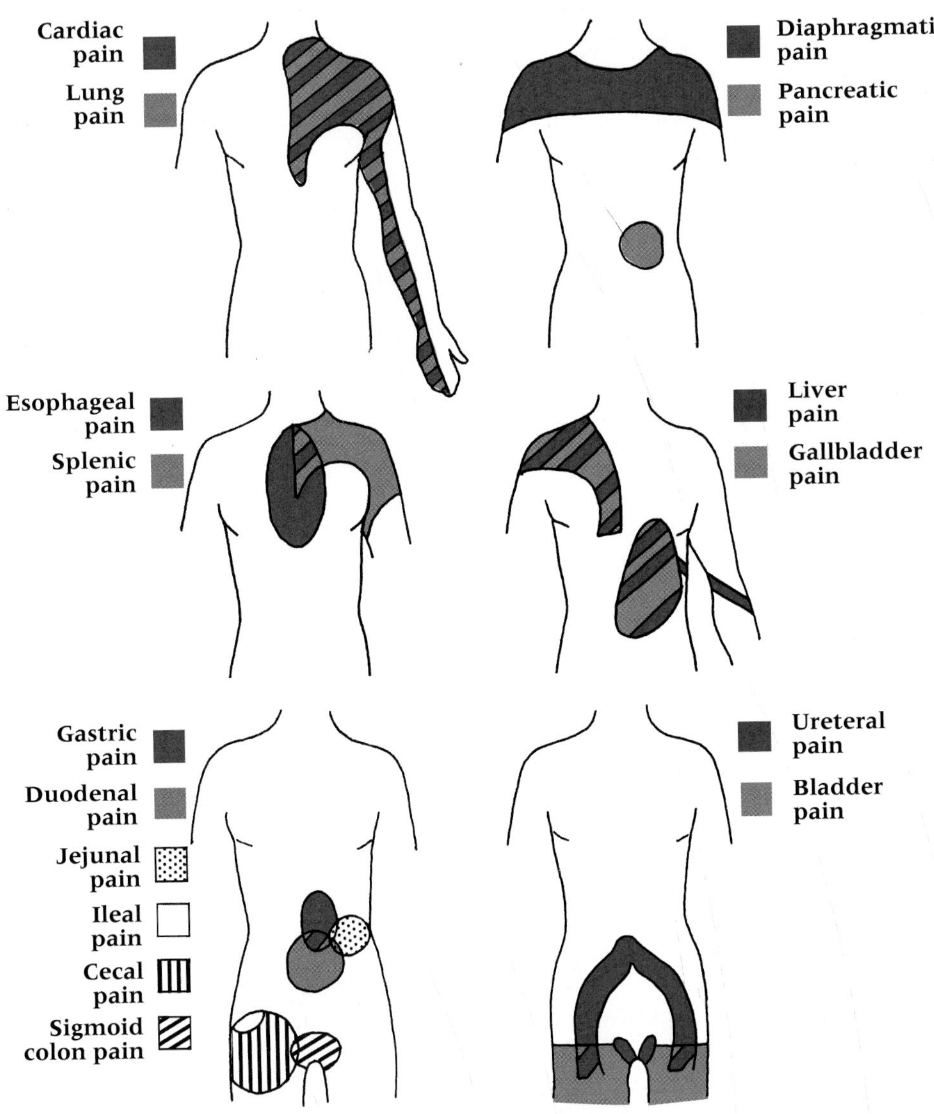

Figure 27-15

Patterns of referred pain.
Continued

Auscultation

Auscultation involves listening to body sounds through a stethoscope.[37] Auscultation is often used to listen to heart sounds, breathing sounds, or bowel sounds (Figure 27-16A).

Heart sounds A normal cardiac cycle includes two sounds, often called "lubb-dupp," which are caused by the turbulence of the blood as the valves close. In children, it is not unusual to hear a third sound.[56] An abnormal periodic sound that occurs in auscultation of the heart is called a murmur. A murmur often occurs because of some defect in one of the valves within the heart. Murmurs can sound soft and blowing or loud and booming. A murmur does not necessarily mean that some pathogenic condition exists in the heart. A murmur that exists in the absence of any organic disease in the heart is called a *functional murmur.*[63] Figure 27-5 shows the positions for auscultation of the heart with a stethoscope.

Breath sounds The rate of breathing patterns should be even and consistent. Abnormal breathing patterns include *Cheyne-Stokes* breathing, in which the rate speeds up and then slows down over a one- to three-minute period; *Biot's* breathing, in which a series of breaths at the normal rate are followed by complete cessation of breathing; *apneustic* breathing, in which there are pauses in the respiratory cycle at full

27-3 Critical Thinking Exercise

A crew athlete complains that when she takes a deep breath she feels some funny crackling sensations in her lungs. The athletic trainer wants to listen to the athlete's chest with a stethoscope.

? What sounds should the athletic trainer listen for?

Figure 27-15—continued

Patterns of referred pain.

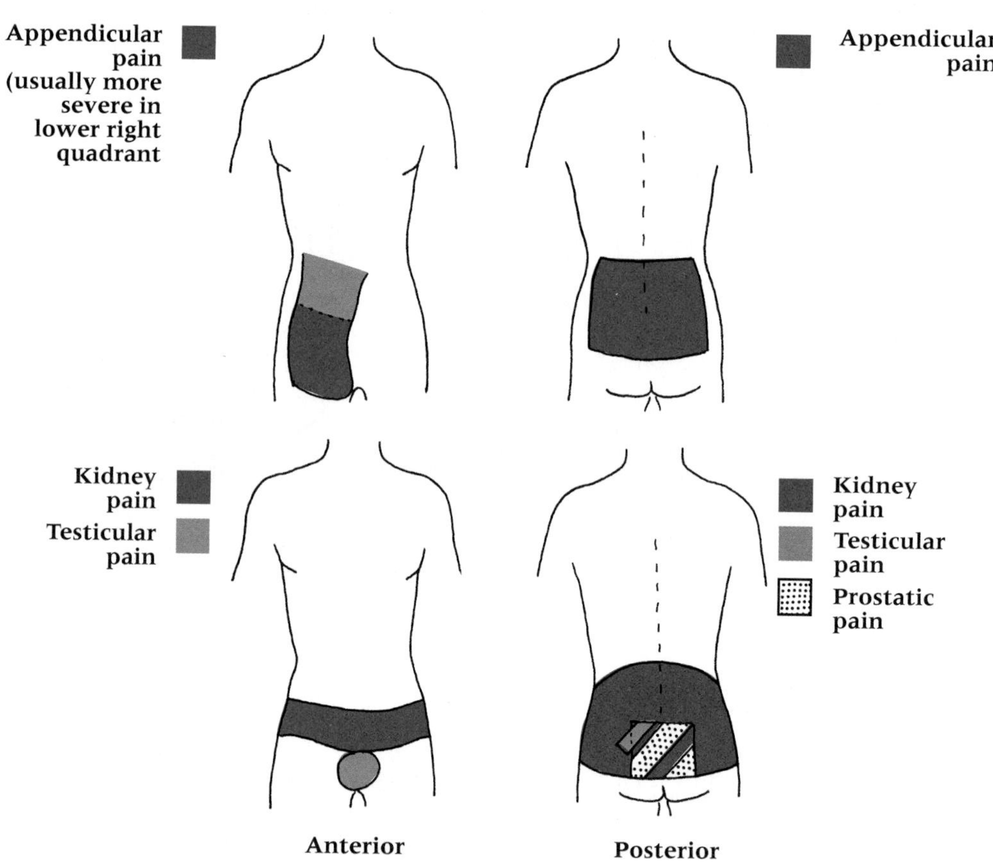

inspiration; and *thoracic breathing,* which occurs without diaphragmatic breathing. Abnormal breathing sounds are often superimposed on normal breathing sounds. Adventitious breath sounds are those that are not normally heard and may be either continuous musiclike sounds with a high pitch, called *wheezes* or *rhonchi,* or crackling or bubbling sounds, called *rales.* Positions for auscultation should be over the apex, centrally, and at the base of each lung, both anteriorly and posteriorly.[59]

Bowel sounds Normal bowel sounds are liquidlike gurgling sounds created by normal peristaltic actions that propel intestinal contents through the lower gastrointestinal tract. Following abdominal injury, bowel signs may be absent or diminished, which may indicate paralytic ilieus or peritonitis. High-pitched tinkling sounds are as-

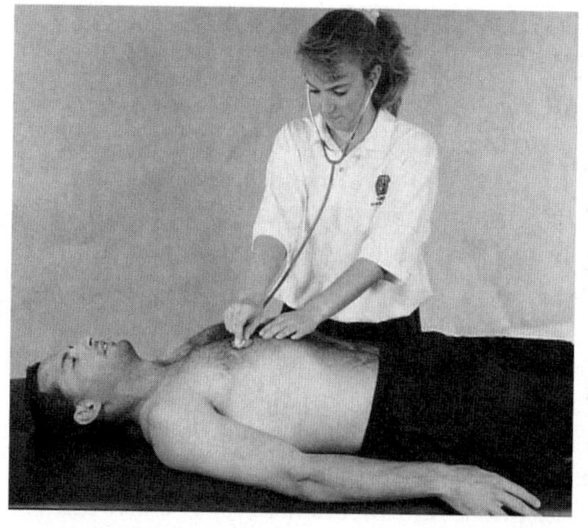

A

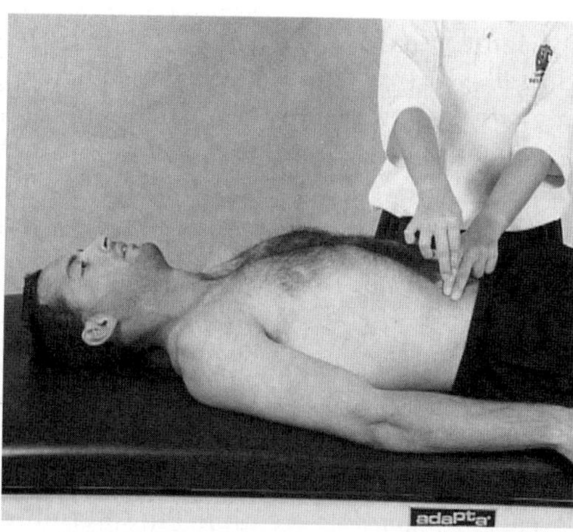

B

Figure 27-16

A, Auscultation.
B, Percussion.

sociated with intestinal obstruction.[63] Auscultation may provide valuable diagnostic information. The stethoscope can be placed in multiple positions anywhere over the lower abdomen.[59]

Percussion

The athletic trainer performs percussion by placing a finger of one hand over an organ and then using one or two fingers from the other hand to strike that finger (Figure 27-16B). The resulting sound may provide some indication as to the status of the organ being percussed. A solid organ such as the liver will produce a dull sound, whereas a hollow organ like a lung will produce a tympanic or resonant sound.

Some special training is required to know exactly what to listen for in auscultation and percussion. The athletic trainer should know what sounds are normal and be able to determine when something sounds abnormal. The physician is certainly better qualified to make diagnostic decisions based on auscultation and percussion.

RECOGITION AND MANAGEMENT OF SPECIFIC INJURIES AND CONDITIONS OF THE THORACIC REGION

The thorax is vulnerable to a variety of injuries to the ribs, the costochondral junction, and the muscles. Injuries to the lungs and heart are more serious and require special attention.[69]

Rib Contusions

Etiology A blow to the rib cage can contuse intercostal muscles or, if severe enough, produce a fracture. Because the intercostal muscles are essential for the breathing mechanism, both expiration and inspiration become very painful when they are bruised.

Symptoms and signs Characteristically the pain is sharp during breathing, there is point tenderness, and pain is elicited when the rib cage is compressed. X-ray examination should be routine in such an injury.

Management RICE and antiinflammatory agents are commonly used. Like most rib injuries, contusions to the thorax are self-limiting; they respond best to rest and to the cessation of sports activities.

Rib Fractures

Etiology Rib fractures (Figure 27-17) are not uncommon in sports and have their highest incidence in collision sports, particularly wrestling and football. Fractures can be caused by either direct or indirect traumas and can, infrequently, be the result of violent muscular contractions.[19] A direct injury is caused by a kick or a well-placed block, with the fracture developing at the site of force application. An indirect fracture

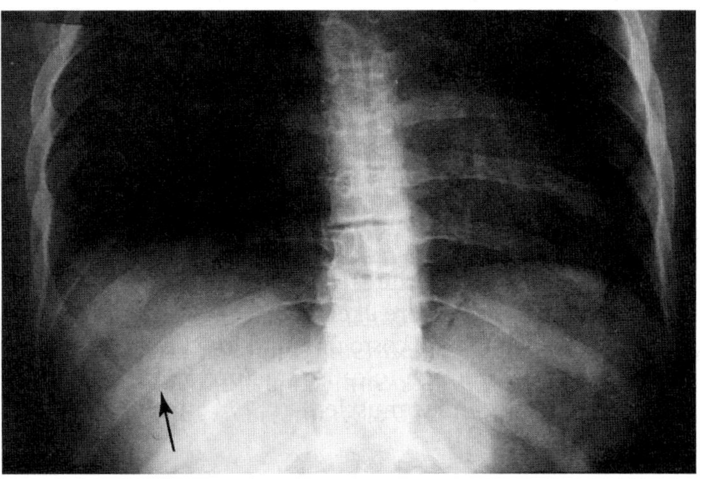

Figure 27-17

A rib fracture.

TENSION PNEUMOTHORAX A tension pneumothorax occurs when the pleural sac on one side fills with air and displaces the lung and the heart toward the opposite side, which compresses the opposite lung (Figure 27-20B).[67] There will be shortness of breath and chest pain on the side of the injury. There may be absence of breath sounds, cyanosis, and distention of neck veins. The trachea may deviate away from the side of injury. A total collapse of the opposite lung is possible; therefore, medical attention is required immediately.[25]

HEMOTHORAX Hemothorax is the presence of blood within the pleural cavity (Figure 27-20C). It results from the tearing or puncturing of the lung or pleural tissue, which involves the blood vessels in the area. Like pneumothorax, hemothorax produces pain, difficulty in breathing, and cyanosis.

A violent blow or compression of the chest without an accompanying rib fracture may cause a lung hemorrhage. This condition results in severe pain during breathing, dyspnea (difficult breathing), coughing up of frothy blood, and signs of shock. If these signs are observed, the athlete should be treated for shock and immediately referred to a physician.

TRAUMATIC ASPHYXIA Traumatic asphyxia occurs as the result of a violent blow to or a compression of the rib cage that causes a cessation of breathing.[33] Signs include purple discoloration of the upper trunk and head, and the conjunctivas of the eyes display a bright red color. A condition of this type demands immediate mouth-to-mouth resuscitation and medical attention.

Management Each of these conditions is a medical emergency that requires immediate physician attention.[5,10] The athlete must be transported to a hospital emergency room as quickly as possible.

27-5 Critical Thinking Exercise

A lacrosse player is hit in the thorax with an opponent's stick. He has immediate localized pain over his ribs and within minutes begins to develop some respiratory difficulty. The athletic trainer suspects that the player has likely fractured a rib and is extremely concerned that the fracture has damaged the lungs.

? What lung injuries are possible, and how should this injury be managed?

Hyperventilation

Etiology An athlete who has an excessively rapid rate of ventilation usually due to anxiety-induced stress or asthma gradually develops a decreased amount of carbon dioxide in the blood (hypocapnia).[62]

Symptoms and signs The athlete appears to be having great difficulty in getting air and seems to be struggling to breathe. He or she is in somewhat of a panic state. There may also be some gasping and wheezing. While it appears that the athlete is not getting enough oxygen, the problem is that the levels of carbon dioxide are too low relative to the amount of oxygen.

Management The immediate treatment consists of decreasing the rate of carbon dioxide loss. This is accomplished by first having the athlete slow the rate of respiration and concentrate on breathing in through the nose and exhaling through the mouth. A second technique would be to have the athlete inhale and exhale through one nostril with the other pinched closed and the mouth also closed. A third technique involves having the athlete breathe slowly into a paper or plastic bag. All of these techniques should help to rapidly increase the level of carbon dioxide. Typically

27-6 Critical Thinking Exercise

A football player is running sixty-yard sprints during a conditioning workout with the rest of the team. Even before beginning the first practice, the athlete knew that he was not very fit and was worried about how he would do. On the fifth sprint he called for the athletic trainer and said that he felt as if he could not breathe. He appeared to be gasping for air.

? What might the athletic trainer suspect is wrong with this athlete and what is the immediate treatment?

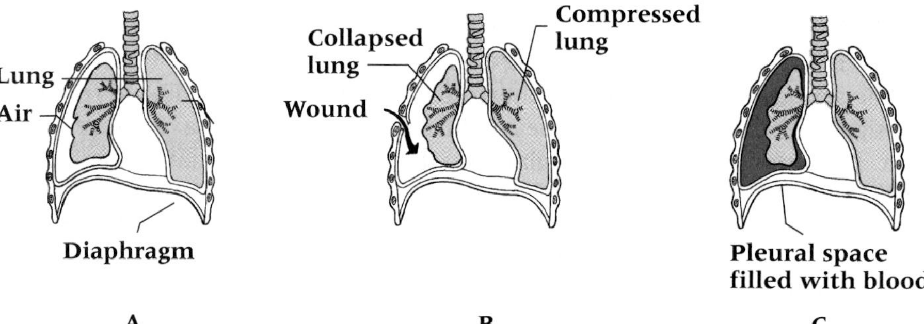

Figure 27-20

A, Pneumothorax. **B,** Tension pneumothorax. **C,** Hemothorax.

within a minute or two the athlete has returned to a normal respiratory pattern. After the acute phase of hyperventilation has been treated, it is necessary to determine the underlying cause and take appropriate treatment measures.

Heart Contusion

Etiology A heart contusion may occur when the heart is compressed between the sternum and the spine by a strong outside force. Examples are if an athlete is hit by a pitched ball or bounces a barbell off the chest in a bench press. The right ventricle is most often injured. The most severe consequence of a violent impact to the heart would be a rupture of the aorta, which would be immediately life threatening.[70]

Symptoms and signs This injury produces severe shock and heart pain. The heart may exhibit certain arrhythmias that cause a decrease in cardiac output, which is followed by death if medical attention is not administered immediately.[35]

Management The athlete should be taken immediately to a hospital emergency room. The athletic trainer should be prepared to administer CPR and treat the athlete for shock (see Chapter 12).

Sudden Death Syndrome in Athletes

Etiology It is indeed catastrophic when a young athlete dies suddenly for no apparent reason. It is estimated that 1 in 280,000 men under age thirty experience sudden death each year.[13] More than twenty different causes have been identified.[29] In athletes thirty-five years and younger, the most common cause of exercise-induced sudden death is some congenital cardiovascular abnormality.[66] The three most prevalent conditions are hypertrophic cardiomyopathy, anomalous origin of the coronary artery, and Marfan's syndrome.[17]

The most common causes of sudden death syndrome include hypertrophic cardiomyopathy, anomalous origin of the coronary artery, and Marfan's syndrome.

Hypertrophic cardiomyopathy (HCM) is a condition in which there is thickened cardiac muscle, with no evidence of chamber enlargement, and extensive myocardial scarring. With this condition, there is an increased frequency of ventricular arrhythmia.[34] In an anomalous origin of the coronary artery, one of the two coronary vessels originates in a different site than normal, which compromises or obstructs that artery because of its unusual course. People with Marfan's syndrome have an abnormality of the connective tissue that results in a weakening of the structure of the aorta and cardiac valves, which can lead to a rupture of either a valve or the aorta itself.[66] Mitral valve prolapse has been associated with both HCM and Marfan's syndrome.[66]

Other potential cardiac causes of sudden death in athletes include coronary artery disease (CAD), which results from atherosclerosis, in which there is a narrowing of the coronary arteries that is usually due to hypercholesterolemia in the young athlete; right ventricular dysplasia, in which enlargement of the right ventricle causes a potentially lethal disturbance in heartbeat; cardiac conduction system abnormalities, which can result from abnormalities of the sinus or atrioventricular nodes; aortic stenosis, which is usually associated with a heart murmur that can cause a fall in blood pressure and cardiac collapse during exercise; Wolff-Parkinson-White syndrome, in which an abnormality in cardiac rhythm manifests itself as ventricular tachycardia; and myocarditis, an inflammation of the heart associated with a viral condition.[2,13,15,42,43,53,65]

Noncardiac causes of sudden death have been attributed to the use of certain drugs, including alcohol, cocaine, amphetamines, and erythropoietin (stimulates red blood cell production). A vascular event—bleeding in the brain caused by a cerebral aneurysm, for example, or head trauma that causes intracranial bleeding—may also result in sudden death. Obstructive respiratory diseases such as asthma can result in sudden death because of drug toxicity or undertreatment.[13]

Symptoms and signs Most afflicted athletes have no symptoms before death.[29] Common symptoms and signs associated with cardiac causes of sudden death include chest

27-7

Critical Thinking Exercise

A basketball player collapses during a practice session when running sprints. The player is conscious and complains of chest pain, heart palpitations or flutters, syncope, nausea, profuse sweating, shortness of breath, and general malaise. The athletic trainer suspects some cardiac-related problem, yet the player has no history of such a condition.

? What can cause these symptoms, and how can the athletic trainer provide the most appropriate and immediate care for this athlete?

pain or discomfort during exertion, heart palpitations or flutters, syncope, nausea, profuse sweating, heart murmurs, shortness of breath, general malaise, and fever.[46,60]

Occasionally the symptoms and signs of athletic heart syndrome raise concern when there is no disease present.[3] Athletic heart syndrome is normal for any individual who is exercising. Like skeletal muscle, cardiac muscle will hypertrophy in response to exercise. It is characterized by a heart enlargement, a systolic heart murmur, slow heart rate, and electrocardiogram changes.

Prevention It has been suggested that a major number of deaths could be avoided by counseling, screening, and early identification of preventable causes of sudden death.[23,24] The use of diagnostic tests to screen for cardiovascular abnormalities has proven to be ineffective.[38] It appears that currently, a history and physical exam in accordance with American Heart Association guidelines is the most effective method of preparticipation screening.[29] Initial screening should include the following questions:

- Has a physician ever told you that you have a heart murmur?
- Have you had chest pain during exercise?
- Have you fainted during exercise?
- Has anyone in your family under age thirty-five ever died suddenly?
- Has anyone in your family been diagnosed with a thickened heart?
- Does anyone in your family have Marfan's syndrome?

If the answer to any of these questions is yes, a more in-depth medical examination should be performed. Resting and exercise electrocardiograms and echocardiograms may be necessary to determine existing pathology.[11]

Commotio Cordis

Etiology Commotio cordis is a syndrome resulting in cardiac arrest that occurs from some traumatic blunt impact to the chest. It occurs in healthy young athletes and is primarily the result of the unfortunate timing of the blow during a narrow window within the repolarization phase of the cardiac cycle, 15 to 30 msec prior to the peak of the T wave. Young athletes are especially at risk because of the pliability of their chest walls. Since 1998, 130 cases have been documented in baseball, lacrosse, hockey, softball, football, basketball, cricket, martial arts, and boxing. The true number of deaths is unknown because of underreporting and misclassification.

Symptoms and signs Ventricular fibrillation is the most common associated arrhythmia. In most cases the blow occurs to the precordial area, but cases of left lateral chest trauma have also been reported. Immediate death occurs in about half of the cases, while in others there is a brief period of consciousness before collapse.

Management Resuscitation of the victims of commotio cordis is seldom successful. Time is a critical factor after the onset of the event. Early cardiopulmonary resuscitation, and especially early defibrillation with an AED, is essential. The NATA has issued an official statement on commotio cordis which appears in Appendix J.

RECOGNITION AND MANAGEMENT OF SPECIFIC INJURIES AND CONDITIONS OF THE ABDOMEN

Although abdominal injuries comprise only about 10 percent of sports injuries, they can require long recovery periods and can be life threatening.[14,20] The abdominal area is particularly vulnerable to injury in all contact sports. A blow can produce superficial or even deep internal injuries, depending on its location and intensity.[22] In internal injuries of the abdomen that occur in sports, the solid organs are most often affected. Strong abdominal muscles give good protection when they are tensed, but when relaxed, they are easily damaged. It is very important to protect the trunk region properly against the traumatic forces of collision sports. Good conditioning is essential, as is the use of proper protective equipment and the application of safety rules.

Injuries and Conditions Related to the Urinary System

Kidney Contusion

Etiology The kidneys are seemingly well protected within the abdominal cavity. However, on occasion, contusions and even ruptures of these organs occur. The kidney may be susceptible to injury because of its normal distention by blood. An external force, usually one applied to the back of the athlete, will cause abnormal extension of an engorged kidney, resulting in injury. The degree of renal injury depends on the extent of the distention and the angle and force of the blow.[16]

Symptoms and signs An athlete who has received a contusion of the kidney may display signs of shock, nausea, vomiting, rigidity of the back muscles, and hematuria (blood in the urine).[47] Like injuries to other internal organs, kidney injuries may cause referred pain to the outside of the body. Pain may be felt high in the costovertebral angle posteriorly and may radiate forward around the trunk into the lower abdominal region. Any athlete who reports having received a severe blow to the abdomen or back region should be instructed to urinate two or three times and to look for the appearance of blood in the urine. If there is any sign of hematuria, the athlete must be referred to a physician immediately.[63]

Kidney and bladder contusions can cause hematuria.

Management Medical care of the contused kidney usually consists of a twenty-four-hour hospital observation and a gradual increase of fluid intake. If the hemorrhage fails to stop, surgery may be indicated. Controllable contusions usually require two weeks of bed rest and close surveillance after activity is resumed. In questionable cases, complete withdrawal from one active playing season may be required.

27-8

Critical Thinking Exercise

A football receiver jumps to catch a high pass thrown over the middle. A defensive back hits the receiver in the low back. The athlete does not seem to have a specific injury. After the game, the player notices blood in the urine and gets really worried.

? Is blood in the urine a cause for concern? What should the athletic trainer do to manage this condition?

Kidney Stones

A kidney stone, or calculus, is usually composed of crystalline mineral salts (calcium, phosphate, uric acid) that form in the urinary tract.[9] The cause of kidney stones is unknown. Kidney stones eventually pass through the urethra and are excreted. Passing a kidney stone is an extremely painful process.[63]

Contusion of the Ureters, Bladder, and Urethra

Etiology On rare occasions, a blunt force to the lower abdominal region may avulse a ureter or contuse or rupture the urinary bladder. Injury to the urinary bladder usually occurs only if it is distended by urine. Hematuria is often associated with contusion of the bladder during running and has been referred to as a runner's bladder.[71] Abnormal concentrations of protein in urine is referred to as proteinuria. Injury to the urethra is more common in men, because the male's urethra is longer and more exposed than is the female's. Injury may produce severe perineal pain and swelling.

Symptoms and signs After a severe blow to the pelvic region, the athlete may display the following recognizable signs: pain and discomfort in the lower abdomen; abdominal rigidity; nausea, vomiting, and signs of shock; blood coming from the urethra; and the passing of a great quantity of bloody urine, which indicates possible injury to the kidney. With a bladder contusion, the athlete will be able to urinate. With a bladder rupture, the athlete will be unable to urinate. Bladder injury commonly causes referred pain to the lower trunk, including the upper thigh anteriorly and suprapubically.

Prevention With any impact to the abdominal region, the possibility of internal damage must be considered; after such trauma, the athlete should be instructed to check periodically for blood in the urine. To lessen the possibility of rupture, the athlete must always empty the bladder before practice or game time. The bladder can also be irritated by intraabdominal pressures during long-distance running. In this situation, repeated impacts to the bladder's base are produced by the jarring of the abdominal contents, resulting in hemorrhage and blood in the urine.

Cystitis

Cystitis is an inflammation of the bladder that most often occurs because of some urinary tract infection. The kidney, prostate, and urethra may also be involved. Acute cystitis causes frequent painful urination, chills, and fever. Antibiotics are used to treat cystitis.[59]

Urinary Tract Infections

Urinary tract infections (UTI) are usually caused by staphylococcus bacteria or chlamydia. They are much more likely to occur in females. UTI causes frequent, burning, painful urination and is treated with antibiotics. Athletes may prevent UTI by increasing fluid intake, practicing sanitary bowel and bladder habits, washing the genital area before intercourse, emptying the bladder after intercourse, and immediately removing contraceptive diaphragms and sponges following intercourse.[63]

Urethritis

Urethritis is an inflammation of the urethra that is most often caused by gonorrhea or occasionally by other, nongonococcal organisms. The symptoms include pain on urination along with a urethral discharge. Urethritis is treated by antibiotic therapy.[63]

Injuries and Conditions Related to the Digestive System

Like any other individual, the athlete may develop various complaints of the digestive system. The athlete may display various disorders of the gastrointestinal tract as a result of poor eating habits or the stress engendered from competition. The athletic trainer should recognize the more severe conditions and cases so that early referrals to a physician can be made.

Gastrointestinal Bleeding

Gastrointestinal bleeding that is reflected in bloody stools occurs in a variety of athletes. Distance runners often have blood in their stools during and following a race. The causes of gastrointestinal bleeding can vary. Possible reasons are gastritis, iron-deficiency anemia, ingestion of aspirin or other antiinflammatory agents, stress, bowel irritation, and colitis. Colitis is an inflammation of the colon, usually caused by an ulceration of the mucosal lining of the colon. Signs of colitis include abdominal pain with colic, watery stools that contain pus, dehydration, intermittent fever, and possible hemorrhage and perforation. Athletes displaying gastrointestinal bleeding must be referred immediately to a physician.[51]

Liver Contusion

Etiology Compared to other organ injuries from blunt trauma, injuries to the liver are the second most common.[63] In sports activities, however, liver injury is relatively infrequent. A hard blow to the right side of the rib cage can tear or seriously contuse the liver, especially if it has been enlarged as a result of some disease, such as hepatitis. Hepatitis is an inflammation of the liver caused by either viral infection or alcohol consumption. If not corrected, hepatitis can lead to cirrhosis of the liver, in which liver function is impaired because liver cells die and are replaced by scar tissue.

Hepatitis can cause enlargement of the liver.

Symptoms and signs Liver injury can cause hemorrhage and shock, requiring immediate surgical intervention. Liver injury commonly produces a referred pain that is just below the right scapula, right shoulder, and substernal area and, on occasion, a referred pain located in the anterior left side of the chest.

Management A liver contusion requires immediate referral to a physician for diagnosis and treatment.

Pancreatitis

Etiology Inflammation of the pancreas may be acute or chronic and is often related to obstruction of the pancreatic duct. An acute inflammation leads to necrosis, suppuration, gangrene, and hemorrhage. Chronic inflammation results in the formation of scar tissue that causes malfunction of the pancreas; inflammation may occur gradually from chronic alcoholism.[63]

Symptoms and signs Acute epigastric pain causes vomiting, belching, constipation, and potentially, shock. There may also be tenderness and rigidity to palpation. Chronic pancreatitis causes jaundice, diarrhea, and mild to moderate pain that radiates to the back.

Management Acute pancreatitis requires rehydration, pain reduction, treatment of shock, reduction of pancreatic secretions using medication, and prevention of secondary infection. Surgery would be indicated only if the pancreatic duct is blocked. Treatment of chronic pancreatitis is difficult and requires large doses of analgesics, the administration of pancreatic enzymes, and a low-fat diet.

Indigestion (Dyspepsia)

Etiology Some athletes have certain food idiosyncrasies that cause them considerable distress after eating. Others develop reactions when eating before competition. The term given to digestive upset is *indigestion* (dyspepsia). Indigestion can be caused by any number of conditions. The most common in sports are emotional stress, esophageal and stomach spasms, and/or inflammation of the mucous lining of the esophagus and stomach.[8]

Indigestion, vomiting, diarrhea, and constipation are common problems in the athlete.

Symptoms and signs Dyspepsia causes an increased secretion of hydrochloric acid (sour stomach), nausea, and flatulence (gas).

Management Care of acute dyspepsia involves eliminating irritating foods from the diet, developing regular eating habits, and avoiding anxieties that may lead to gastric distress.

Constant irritation of the stomach may lead to more chronic and serious disorders, such as gastritis, an inflammation of the stomach wall, or ulcerations of the gastrointestinal mucosa. Athletes who appear nervous and high-strung and suffer from dyspepsia should be examined by the sports physician.

Vomiting

Etiology Vomiting results from some type of irritation, most often in the stomach. This irritation stimulates the vomiting center in the brain to cause a series of forceful contractions of the diaphragm and abdominal muscles, thus compressing the stomach and forcefully expelling the contents.[57]

Management Antinausea medications should be administered (see Chapter 17). Fluids to prevent dehydration should be administered by mouth if possible. If vomiting persists, fluids and electrolytes must be administered intravenously.

Food Poisoning (Gastroenteritis)

Etiology Food poisoning, which may range from mild to severe, results from infectious organisms (bacteria of the salmonella group, certain staphylococci, streptococci, or dysentery bacilli) that enter the body in either food or drink. Foods become contaminated, especially during warm weather, when improper food refrigeration permits the organisms to multiply rapidly. Contamination can also occur if the food is handled by an infected food handler.

Symptoms and signs Infection results in nausea, vomiting, cramps, diarrhea, and anorexia. The symptoms of staphylococcal infections usually subside in three to six hours. Salmonella infection symptoms may last from twenty-four to forty-eight hours or more.

Management Management requires the rapid replacement of lost fluids and electrolytes, which, in severe cases, may need to be replaced intravenously. Bed rest is desirable in all but mild cases; as long as the nausea and vomiting continue, nothing should be given by mouth. If tolerated, light fluids or foods such as clear, strained broth, bouillon with a small amount of added salt, soft-cooked eggs, or bland cereals may be given.

Peptic Ulcer

Etiology A peptic ulcer is a condition in which the acids secreted in the stomach destroy the mucous lining either in the stomach or the small intestine. Peptic ulcers most often occur in people who experience severe anxiety for long periods of time.[57]

Symptoms and signs A gnawing pain, localized in the epigastric region, usually appears between one and three hours following a meal. Other symptoms include dyspepsia, heartburn, nausea, or vomiting. Pain usually lasts for minutes rather than hours.[63]

Management Occasionally, symptoms may disappear without the aid of medication. Antacids may be helpful in neutralizing gastric secretions. Altering the diet has not proven to be effective in managing the peptic ulcer. If hemorrhaging or perforation occur, surgery may be necessary.

Gastroesophageal Reflux

Etiology This condition occurs when there is a reflux or backward flow of the acidic gastric contents into the esophagus that usually occurs due to some malfunction of the lower esophageal sphincter. It can also occur as a result of a hiatal hernia. The incidence is increased with exercise. If this occurs repeatedly, the lower esophagus can become inflamed, and this condition is referred to as *esophagitis*.[59]

Symptoms and signs There is heartburnlike retrosternal pain that can progress to a gripping chest pain that would be similar to angina pectoris. There is a burning feeling with a sour liquid taste in the throat. The athlete also may have difficulty swallowing.

Management Usually this regurgitation can be controlled by medication. However, if the medication does not stop the reflux, surgery may be needed.

Diarrhea

Etiology Diarrhea is abnormal stool looseness or passage of a fluid, unformed stool and is categorized as acute or chronic, according to the type present. Diarrhea can be caused by problems in the diet, inflammation of the intestinal lining, gastrointestinal infection, the ingestion of certain drugs, and psychogenic factors.[57]

Symptoms and signs Diarrhea is characterized by abdominal cramps, nausea, and possibly vomiting, coupled with frequent elimination of stools, ranging from three to twenty a day. The infected person often has a loss of appetite and a light brown or gray, foul-smelling stool. Extreme weakness caused by fluid dehydration is usually present.

Management The cause of diarrhea is often difficult to establish. The loose stool may be caused by any irritant, including an infestation of parasitic organisms or an emotional upset. Management of diarrhea requires a knowledge of its cause. The athletic trainer can care for less severe cases by having the athlete omit foods that cause irritation, drink boiled milk, eat bland food until symptoms have ceased, and use pectins two or three times daily for the absorption of excess fluid.[9]

Constipation

Etiology Some athletes are subject to constipation, which is the failure of the bowels to evacuate feces.[9] There are numerous causes of constipation, the most common of which are lack of abdominal muscle tone; insufficient moisture in the feces, causing it to be hard and dry; lack of a sufficient proportion of roughage and bulk in the diet to stimulate peristalsis; poor bowel habits; nervousness and anxiety; and overuse of laxatives and enemas.[63]

Symptoms and signs Constipation results in a feeling of fullness, with occasional cramping and pain in the lower abdomen. When the athlete strains hard to defecate, some vessels may be ruptured in the rectum and bleeding from the anus may occur.

Management The best means of overcoming constipation is to regulate eating patterns to include foods that will encourage normal defecation. Cereals, fruits, vegetables, and fats stimulate bowel movement, whereas sugars and carbohydrates tend to inhibit it. Some persons become constipated as the result of psychological factors. In such cases, the athletic trainer may try to determine the causes of stress and, if needed, refer the athlete to a physician or school psychologist for counseling. Above all, laxatives or enemas should be avoided unless their use has been prescribed by a physician.

Irritable Bowel Syndrome

Etiology Irritable bowel syndrome (IBS) is a group of disorders related to the gastrointestinal tract that present themselves differently depending on the individual. The causes of these variations in symptoms are related to the different causes of IBS. IBS is thought to occur in 10 to 20 percent of the adult population and is slightly more common in women than men. No psychological factors have been identified as a cause of IBS, but psychological factors often determine how the individual experiences and handles the condition.

Symptoms and signs The individual with IBS experiences abdominal pain that is relieved with defecation. There is an irregular pattern of defecation at least 25 percent of the time. In addition there may be some alteration in stool frequency, stool form, stool passage, the passage of mucus, and abdominal bloating and distension.

Management The athlete should be referred for long-term physician management. Initially, treatment should include modifying diet to eliminate those foods that seem to cause a problem. Most often dairy foods and gas-forming foods are the cause. Antidiarrheal or antispasmodic medications may help to reduce symptoms. Some psychological counseling intervention may also prove helpful. The long-term prognosis for this condition is positive.

Appendicitis

Etiology Inflammation of the vermiform appendix can be chronic or acute. It is caused by a variety of conditions, such as a fecal obstruction, lymph swelling, or even a carcinoid tumor. Its highest incidence is in males between the ages of fifteen and twenty-five. Appendicitis can be mistaken for a common gastric complaint. In early stages, the appendix becomes red and swollen; in later stages, it may become gangrenous, rupturing into the bowels or peritoneal cavity and causing peritonitis.[63] Bacterial infection is a complication of rupture of the inflamed appendix.

Appendicitis is often mistaken for a common gastric problem.

Symptoms and signs The athlete may complain of a mild-to-severe pain in the lower abdomen, associated with nausea, vomiting, and a low-grade fever ranging from 99° to 100° F (37° to 38° C). Later, the cramps may localize into a pain in the right side, and palpation may reveal abdominal rigidity and tenderness at a point (McBurney's point) between the anterior superior spine of the ilium and the umbilicus, about 1 to 2 inches (2.5 to 5 cm) above the latter.[63]

A strain of the psoas muscle or an abcess in the sheath of the psoas can sometimes be mistaken for appendicitis.

Management Surgical removal of the appendix is often necessary. If the bowel is not obstructed, there is no need to rush surgery. However, an obstructed bowel with an acute rupture is a life-threatening condition.

27-9

Critical Thinking **Exercise**

Immediately after finishing a meal, a fencer begins to complain of a mild-to-severe pain in the lower abdomen. She has nausea, vomiting, and a low-grade fever. The athletic trainer suspects that she may have indigestion; in about an hour, however, the cramps begin to localize into a pain in the right side, and palpation reveals abdominal rigidity and tenderness at McBurney's point.

? What should the athletic trainer suspect is wrong with this athlete, and how should this injury be managed?

Hemorrhoids (Piles)

Etiology Hemorrhoids are varicosities of the hemorrhoidal venous plexus of the anus. There are both internal and external anal veins. Chronic constipation or straining at the stool may stretch the anal veins, resulting in either a protrusion (prolapse) and bleeding of the internal or external veins or a thrombus in the external veins.

Symptoms and signs Hemorrhoids are painful nodular swellings near the sphincter of the anus. They may cause slight bleeding and itching. The majority of hemorrhoids are self-limiting and spontaneously heal within two to three weeks.

Management The management of hemorrhoids is mostly palliative and serves to eliminate discomfort until healing takes place. The following measures can be suggested: use of proper bowel habits, ingestion of one tablespoon of mineral oil daily to assist in lubricating dry stool, application of an astringent suppository (tannic acid), and application of a local anesthetic to control pain and itching (dibucaine). If palliative measures are unsuccessful, surgery may be required.

Injuries and Conditions Related to the Reproductive Organs

Injuries to the reproductive organs in sports are much more likely to occur in the male because the genitalia is more exposed.

Injuries to the reproductive organs in sports are much more likely to occur in the male because the genitalia are more exposed.

Scrotal Contusion

Etiology As the result of its considerable sensitivity and particular vulnerability, the scrotum may sustain a contusion that causes a very painful, nauseating, and disabling condition.

Symptoms and signs Like any other contusion or bruise, the scrotal contusion causes hemorrhage, fluid effusion, and muscle spasm, the degree of which depends on the intensity of the impact to the tissue.

Management Immediately following a scrotal contusion, the athlete must be put at ease and testicular spasms must be reduced. Several techniques have been proposed to help reduce testicular pain following contusion. The most commonly used technique is to place the athlete in a sitting position, lift him a few inches, and drop him to the ground (Figure 27-21). Two other techniques are less commonly used. The first of these techniques is to place the athlete in a kneeling position and have him or her bounce up and down. The second technique is to place the athlete supine with knees and hips flexed to 90 degrees and have him or her perform a Valsalva maneuver. These maneuvers will aid in reducing discomfort and relaxing the muscle spasm. After the

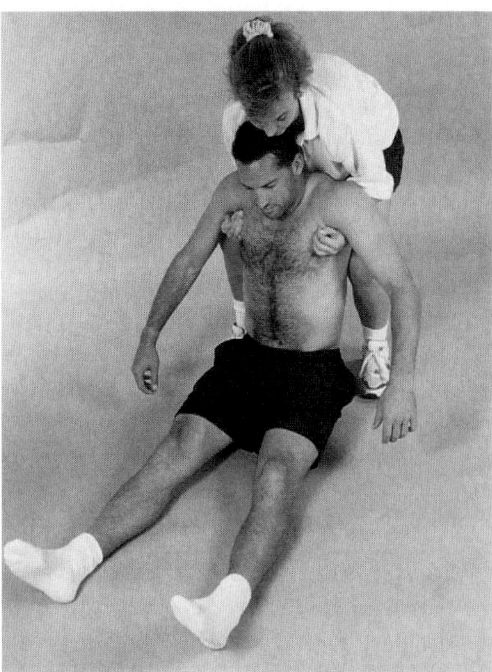

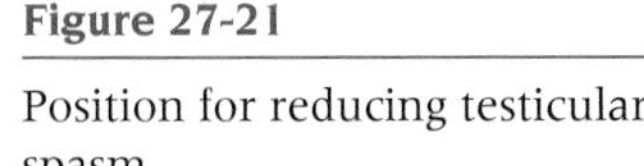

Figure 27-21

Position for reducing testicular spasm.

pain has diminished, the athlete is helped from the playing area, and a cold pack is applied to the scrotum. Increasing or unresolved pain after fifteen to twenty minutes requires prompt referral to a physician for evaluation.

Spermatic Cord Torsion

Etiology Torsion of the spermatic cord results from the testicle's revolving in the scrotum after a direct blow to the area or as a result of coughing or vomiting.

Symptoms and signs Cord torsion produces acute testicular pain, nausea, vomiting, and inflammation in the area.

Management In this case, the athlete must receive immediate medical attention to prevent irreparable complications. Twisting of the spermatic cord may present the appearance of a cluster of swollen veins and may cause a dull pain combined with a heavy, dragging feeling in the scrotum. This condition may eventually lead to atrophy of the testicle. A physician should be consulted when this condition is suspected.

Traumatic Hydrocele of the Tunica Vaginalis

Etiology Traumatic hydrocele of the tunica vaginalis is an excess fluid accumulation caused by a severe blow to the testicular region. The venous plexus on the posterior aspect of the testicle can become engorged, creating a varicocele. A rupture of this plexus results in a rapid accumulation of blood in the scrotum called a hematocele.

Symptoms and signs After trauma, the athlete complains of pain. Swelling in the scrotum can significantly increase the size of the sac.

Management Cold packs should be applied to the scrotum, and the athlete should be referred to a physician. Irreversible damage can occur to the testicle if medical treatment is delayed.

27-10

Critical Thinking Exercise

A male soccer player receives a blow to the genitalia. Shortly after the hit, the athlete is in significant pain and begins vomiting.

? How should this injury be managed?

Vaginitis

Etiology Vaginitis is an inflammation of the vagina that may be caused by a variety of microorganisms, many of which are associated with sexually transmitted infections (STIs) (discussed in Chapter 29). Other non-STI causes may exist, however, including bacterial infection, strong chemicals from douching, irritation from a tampon, and poor hygiene habits.[55]

Symptoms and signs There will be purulent (filled with pus) and, occasionally, bloody vaginal discharge. There may also be a strong odor with vaginal itching. Urination is frequent and painful. The vagina is red and painful to touch.

Management For vaginitis caused by an STI, appropriate antibiotic or antifungal medications should be given. The athlete should also be instructed in correct bowel and bladder hygiene and cleanliness and should be counseled regarding sexual behavior.

27-11

Critical Thinking Exercise

A baseball player is hit with a pitch in the left upper quadrant. Initially he appears to be all right, but toward the end of the game, he becomes nauseous and starts to vomit. He complains of pain in the left upper quadrant and also pain in his left shoulder extending down his arm. The athletic trainer palpates the abdomen and detects rigidity. Within a matter of minutes, the player begins to develop shock-like symptoms.

? What should the athletic trainer suspect has happened to this athlete, and how should the injury be treated?

Contusion of the Female Genitalia

The female reproductive organs have a low incidence of injury in sports. By far the most common gynecologic injury in the female athlete involves a contusion to the external genitalia, or vulva, which includes the labia, clitoris, and the vestibule of the vagina. A hematoma results from the contusion, which most often occurs with a direct impact to this area. A contusion of this area may also injure the pubic symphysis, producing osteitis pubis (discussed in Chapter 21).

Injury to Lymphatic Organs

Injury of the Spleen

Etiology Injuries to the spleen are relatively uncommon. If injury does occur, it is most often due to a fall or a direct blow to the left upper quadrant of the abdomen (see Figure 13-3) when some existing medical condition has caused splenomegaly (enlargement of the spleen).[18] Infectious mononucleosis is the most likely cause of spleen enlargement. Athletes with mononucleosis should not engage in any activity

Infectious mononucleosis can cause spleen enlargement.

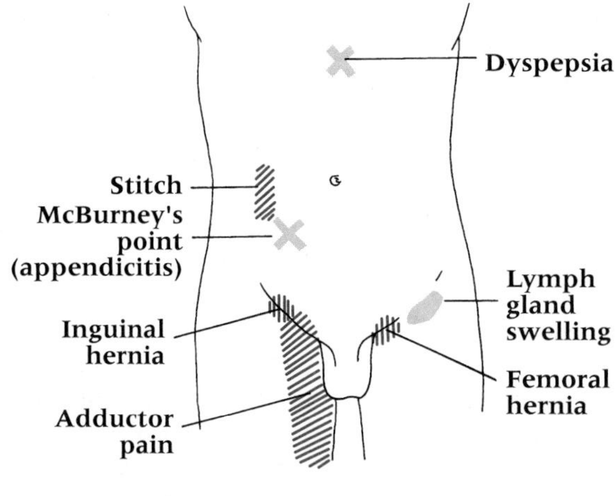

Figure 27-22

Common sites of abdominal pain.

for three weeks because approximately 50 percent of sufferers exhibit splenomegaly, which is difficult to diagnose clinically (see Chapter 29).

Symptoms and signs The gross indications of a ruptured spleen must be recognized so that an immediate medical referral can be made. Indications include a history of a severe blow to the abdomen and possibly signs of shock, abdominal rigidity, nausea, and vomiting. There may be a reflex pain occurring approximately thirty minutes after injury, called Kehr's sign, which radiates to the left shoulder and one-third of the way down the left arm.

Athletes who complain of external pain in the shoulders, trunk, or pelvis after a severe blow to the abdomen or back may be describing referred pain from an injury to an internal organ.

Complications The great danger with a ruptured spleen lies in its ability to splint itself and then produce a delayed hemorrhage. Splinting of the spleen is effected by a loose hematoma formation and the constitution of the supporting and surrounding structures. Any slight strain may disrupt the splinting effect and allow the spleen to hemorrhage profusely into the abdominal cavity, causing the athlete to die of internal bleeding days or weeks after the injury.[1]

Management Conservative, nonoperative treatment is recommended initially with a week of hospitalization.[41] At three weeks, the athlete can engage in light conditioning activities, and at four weeks, the athlete can return to full activity as long as no symptoms appear. If surgical repair is necessary, the athlete will require three months to recover, whereas removal of the spleen will require six months before the athlete can return to activity.[64]

Injuries to the Abdominal Wall

A number of other abdominal pain sites can be disabling to the athlete. The athletic trainer should be able to discern the pain sites that are potentially more serious and refer the athlete accordingly.[39] Figure 27-22 shows some of the pain sites in the abdomen.

Abdominal Muscle Strains

Sudden twisting of the trunk or reaching overhead can tear an abdominal muscle. These injuries can be very incapacitating, with severe pain and hematoma formation. The rectus abdominis is the most commonly strained abdominal muscle. Initially, ice and an elastic compression wrap should be used. Treatment should be conservative, with exercise staying within pain-free limits.

Contusions of the Abdominal Wall

Etiology Compressive forces that injure the abdominal wall are not common in sports. When they do happen, they are more likely to occur in collision sports such as football or ice hockey; however, any sports implements or high-velocity projectiles can injure. Hockey goalies and baseball catchers would be very vulnerable to injury without their protective torso pads. Contusion may occur superficially to the abdominal skin or subcutaneous tissue or much deeper to the musculature. The extent and type of injury vary, depending on whether the force is blunt or penetrating.

Symptoms and signs A contusion of the rectus abdominis muscle can be very disabling. A severe blow may cause a hematoma that develops under the fascial tissue surrounding this muscle. The pressure that results from hemorrhage causes pain and tightness in the region of the injury.

Management A cold pack and a compression elastic wrap should be applied immediately after injury. The athletic trainer must look for signs of possible internal injury.

Hernia

Etiology The term *hernia* refers to the protrusion of abdominal viscera through a portion of the abdominal wall. Hernias may be congenital or acquired.[27] A congenital hernial sac is developed before birth, and an acquired hernia develops after birth. Structurally, a hernia has a mouth, a neck, and a body. The mouth, or hernial ring, is the opening from the abdominal cavity into the hernial protusion; the neck is the portion of the sac that joins the hernial ring and the body. The body is the sac that protrudes outside the abdominal cavity and contains portions of the abdominal organs.[36]

Inguinal hernias usually occur in males; femoral hernias usually occur in females.

Hernias resulting from sports most often occur in the groin area. Inguinal hernias (Figure 27-23A), which occur in men (more than 75%), and femoral hernias (Figure 27-23B), most often occurring in women, are the most prevalent types. Externally, the inguinal and femoral hernias appear similar because of the groin protrusion, but a considerable difference is indicated internally. The inguinal hernia results from an abnormal enlargement of the opening of the inguinal canal, through which the vessels and nerves of the male reproductive system pass. In contrast, the femoral hernia arises in the canal that transports the vessels and nerves that go to the thigh and lower limb.[36]

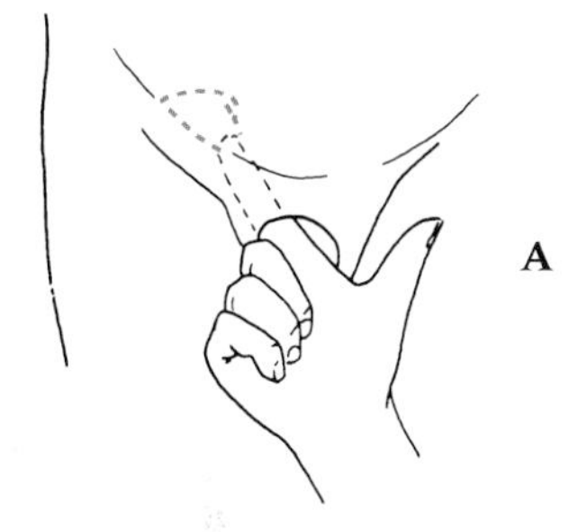

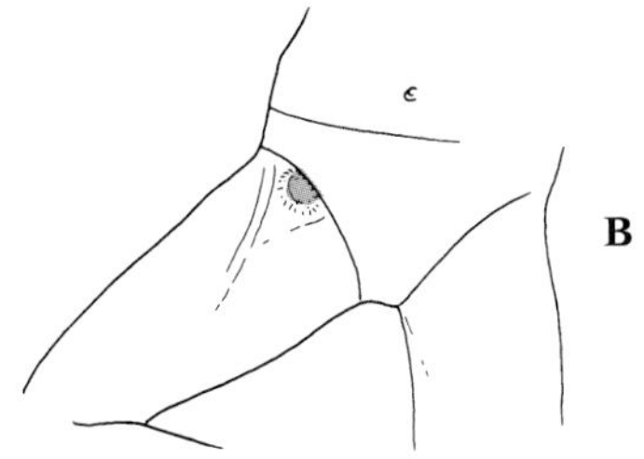

Figure 27-23

A, Inguinal hernia. **B,** Femoral hernia.

Under normal circumstances, the inguinal and femoral canals are protected by muscle control against abnormal opening. When intraabdominal tension affects these areas, muscles produce contractions around these canal openings. If the muscles fail to react or if they prove inadequate in their shutter action, abdominal contents may be pushed through the opening. Repeated protrusions serve to stretch and increase the size of the opening. Most physicians think that any athlete who has a hernia should be prohibited from engaging in hard physical activity until surgical repair has been made.

One danger of a hernia in an athlete is the possibility that it may become irritated by falls or blows. Besides the hernial aggravations caused by trauma, another concern that athletic trainers need to be aware of is the development of a strangulated hernia, in which the inguinal ring constricts the protruding sac and occludes normal blood circulation. If the strangulated hernia is not surgically repaired immediately, gangrene and death may ensue.

Symptoms and signs The acquired hernia occurs when a natural weakness is further aggravated by either a strain or a direct blow. Athletes may develop this condition as the result of violent activity. An acquired hernia may be recognized by the following signs: previous history of a blow or strain to the groin area that has produced pain and prolonged discomfort, superficial protrusion in the groin area that is increased by coughing, or reported feeling of weakness and pulling sensation in the groin area.

Management The treatment preferred by most physicians is surgery.[31] Mechanical devices, which prevent hernial protrusion, are for the most part unsuitable in sports because of the friction and irritation they produce. Exercise has been thought by many to be beneficial to a mild hernia, but such is not the case. Exercise will not affect the stretched inguinal or femoral canals positively.

Blow to the Solar Plexus

Etiology A blow to the sympathetic celiac plexus (solar plexus) produces a transitory paralysis of the diaphragm ("wind knocked out").

Symptoms and signs Paralysis of the diaphragm stops respiration and leads to anoxia. When the athlete is unable to inhale, hysteria because of fear may result. These symptoms are usually transitory. It is necessary to allay such fears and instill confidence in the athlete.

A blow to the solar plexus can lead to transitory paralysis of the diaphragm and to unconsciousness.

Management In dealing with an athlete who has had the wind knocked out of him or her, the athletic trainer should adhere to the following procedures: help the athlete overcome apprehension by talking in a confident manner, loosen the athlete's belt and the clothing around the abdomen, have the athlete bend the knees, and encourage the athlete to relax by initiating short inspirations and long expirations.

Because of the fear of not being able to breathe, the athlete may hyperventilate. Hyperventilation is an increased rate of ventilation that results in a lowered carbon dioxide level. It causes a variety of physical reactions, such as dizziness, a lump in the throat, pounding heart, and fainting.

The athletic trainer should always be concerned that a blow hard enough to knock out the wind could also cause internal organ injury.

Stitch in the Side

Etiology A "stitch in the side" is the name given to an idiopathic condition that occurs in some athletes. The cause is obscure, although several hypotheses have been advanced. Among these possible causes are the following: constipation, intestinal gas, overeating, diaphragmatic spasm as a result of poor conditioning, lack of visceral support because of weak abdominal muscles, distended spleen, breathing techniques that lead to a lack of oxygen in the diaphragm, ischemia of either the diaphragm or the intercostal muscles, and a fluid-engorged gut that tugs on visceral ligaments.

Signs and symptoms A stitch in the side is a cramplike pain that develops on either the left or right costal angle during hard physical activity. Sports that involve running apparently produce this condition.

Management Immediate care of a stitch in the side demands relaxation of the spasm, for which two methods have proved beneficial. First, the athlete is instructed to stretch the arm on the affected side as high as possible. If this method is inadequate, flexing the trunk forward on the thighs while tightening the abdominal muscles may prove of some benefit.[48]

Athletes with recurrent abdominal spasms may need special study. The identification of poor eating habits, poor elimination habits, or an inadequate athletic training program may explain the athlete's particular problem. A stitch in the side, although not considered serious, may require further evaluation by a physician if abdominal pains persist.

27-12
Critical Thinking Exercise

A wrestler is engaged in a strenuous off-season weightlifting program. Recently he has begun to experience pain in his groin. It seems that whenever he strains hard to lift a weight and especially if he holds his breath, the pain appears. He is concerned that he has developed a hernia.

? What symptoms and signs should the athletic trainer look for that would indicate that the athlete does in fact have a hernia?

27-13
Critical Thinking Exercise

A cross-country runner complains of a recurring stitch in the side. She has a cramplike pain that develops on the left costal angle during a hard run. She indicates that when she stops running, the cramp disappears, but it comes back when she starts to run again.

? What can the athletic trainer recommend that might help this runner alleviate this problem?

SUMMARY

- Injuries to the heart, lungs, and abdominal viscera can be potentially serious and even life threatening if not recognized and managed appropriately.
- The thorax is that portion of the body commonly known as the chest, which lies between the base of the neck and the diaphragm. Its main functions are to protect the vital respiratory and circulatory organs and to assist the lungs in inspiration and expiration during the breathing process. Within the thoracic cage lie the lungs, the heart, and the thymus.
- The abdominal cavity lies between the diaphragm and the bones of the pelvis and is bounded by the margin of the lower ribs, the abdominal muscles, and the vertebral column. The abdominal viscera are composed of both hollow and solid organs. Organs in the abdominal cavity may be classified as being part of the urinary system, the digestive system, the reproductive system, or the lymphatic system.
- The primary survey by the athletic trainer who is evaluating an injury to the abdomen or thorax should focus on those signs and symptoms that indicate some life-threatening condition. Asking pertinent questions, observing body positioning, and palpating the injured structures are critical in assessing the nature of the injury.

- Rib fractures and contusions, costochondral junction separations, sternum fractures, muscle strains, and breast injuries are all common injuries to the chest wall.
- Injuries involving the lungs include pneumothorax, tension pneumothorax, hemothorax, and traumatic asphyxia.
- The most common cause of exercise-induced sudden death is some congenital cardiovascular abnormality. The three most prevalent conditions are hypertrophic cardiomyopathy, anomalous origin of the coronary artery, and Marfan's syndrome.
- With any injury to the abdominal region, internal injury to the abdominal viscera must be considered. Injuries to the liver, spleen, and kidneys are among the more common injuries to the abdominal viscera associated with athletics.
- A number of conditions of the digestive system, such as diarrhea, constipation, and gastroenteritis, commonly affect the athletic population.
- Injuries to the reproductive organs in sports are much more likely to occur in the male because the genitalia are more exposed.
- Injuries to the abdominal wall include muscle strains, getting the wind knocked out, and developing an inguinal or femoral hernia.

Websites

Acute Appendicitis: www.emedicine.com/emerg/topic41.htm

Anatomy of the Human Body: http://www.bartleby.com/107/

Sports Injury Clinic: abdominal injuries www.sportsinjuryclinic.net/ cybertherapist/front/stomach.htm

American Society of Abdominal Surgeons: www.abdominalsurg.org

The Society of Thoracic Surgeons: www.sts.org

Chest Trauma: http://www.madsci.com/manu/trau_che. htm#30

A description of myocardial contusion, flail chest, hemothorax, and pneumothorax are included in this site.

National Heart, Lung, and Blood Institute: http://www.nhlbi.nih.gov

Trauma.Org: http://www.trauma.org/

American Thoracic Society—About ATS: http://www.thoracic.org/

Solutions to Critical Thinking EXERCISES

27-1 The athletic trainer should be concerned about the possibility of injury to an organ that can potentially lead to internal blood loss and eventually result in shock. It is possible that the spleen, liver, stomach, small intestine, pancreas, or gallbladder may all be injured. It is also possible that there may be a contusion to the muscles of the abdominal wall that is causing muscle guarding.

27-2 To palpate the abdominal structures, the athlete should be supine with the hips and knees flexed. An athlete with an abdominal injury will voluntarily contract the abdominal muscles to guard or protect the tender area. If there is bleeding or irritation inside the abdominal cavity, the abdomen will exhibit boardlike rigidity and cannot be voluntarily relaxed. The athletic trainer can produce rebound tenderness by pressing firmly on the abdomen and then quickly releasing pressure, which causes intense pain.

27-3 The athletic trainer should know what sounds are normal and be able to determine when something sounds abnormal. Abnormal breathing sounds are often superimposed on normal breathing sounds. Adventitious breath sounds are those that are not normally heard and may be either continuous music-like sounds with a high pitch, called wheezes or rhonchi, or crackling or bubbling sounds, called rales.

27-4 The athletic trainer should palpate along the rib, in the intercostal space between the ribs, and at the costochondral junction to locate a specific point of tenderness. The athletic trainer should also apply anterioposterior compression to the thoracic cage to identify potential rib fractures. If the athlete complains of increased pain or tenderness on transverse compression applied laterally to the rib cage, a costochondral injury is more likely.

27-5 Injuries severe enough to cause a rib fracture might also result in pneumothorax, tension pneumothorax, hemothorax, or traumatic asphyxia. Any of these conditions should be considered life threatening, and the athletic trainer should access the rescue squad immediately. The trainer should also be prepared to initiate CPR if indicated.

27-6 It is most likely that the athlete is hyperventilating. This was likely caused by the anxiety that existed over having to do these sprints. The athletic trainer needs to increase the level of carbon dioxide in the lung and can do this by having the athlete either breathe slowly through one nostril or breathe into a paper bag.

27-7 Potential causes could include myocardial infarction, hypertrophic cardiomyopathy, Marfan's syndrome, coronary artery disease resulting from atherosclerosis, right ventricular dysplagia, cardiac conduction system abnormalities, aortic stenosis, or myocarditis. All these causes have been attributed to sudden death syndrome in athletes. The athletic trainer is dealing with a life-threatening situation and must seek emergency medical care as soon as possible.

27-8 Anytime blood appears in the urine, there is cause for concern. In this case it is likely that the kidneys have been contused, and the blood that appears in the urine will usually disappear over the next couple of days. Nevertheless, the athlete should be referred to the team physician for diagnosis.

27-9 It is possible that the athlete has an inflamed vermiform appendix. Most often, surgical removal of the appendix is necessary. Occasionally, an inflamed appendix results from an obstructed bowel. A rupture of the appendix because of bowel obstruction becomes a life-threatening emergency.

27-10 This athlete may have spermatic cord torsion and needs to be evaluated by a physician immediately to avoid permanent damage.

27-11 The athlete is exhibiting the symptoms and signs of a ruptured spleen. The spleen has the ability to splint itself and stop hemorrhage. However, because of the potential of shock, the athletic trainer should treat this injury as life threatening. Usually, treatment will be conservative and involve brief hospitalization, but surgical management is necessary when the spleen has ruptured and is hemorrhaging.

27-12 Most often the athlete will have some previous history of a blow or strain to the groin area that has produced pain and prolonged discomfort. There may be a superficial protrusion in the groin area that is increased when the athlete coughs, or the athlete may experience a feeling of weakness and a pulling sensation in the groin area. An inguinal hernia results from an abnormal enlargement of the opening of the inguinal canal through which the abdominal contents may be pushed.

27-13 The athletic trainer should try to modify the athlete's eating habits, which might produce constipation or gas. Cramps can be caused by improper breathing techniques, which may cause a lack of oxygen in the diaphragm and ischemia of either the diaphragm or the intercostal muscles. Cramps may also be caused by diaphragmatic spasm that results from poor conditioning or by a lack of visceral support because of weak abdominal muscles. Athletes with recurrent abdominal spasms should have further evaluation by a physician if abdominal pains persist.

REVIEW QUESTIONS AND CLASS ACTIVITIES

1. Describe the anatomy of the thorax.
2. Differentiate among rib contusions, rib fractures, and costochondral separations.
3. Compare the signs of pneumothorax, tension pneumothorax, hemothorax, and traumatic asphyxia.
4. Identify the possible causes of sudden death syndrome among athletes.
5. List the abdominal viscera and other structures associated with the urinary system, the digestive system, the lymphatic system, and the reproductive system.
6. What muscles protect the abdominal viscera?
7. What conditions of the abdominal viscera produce pain in the abdominal region?
8. Contrast the signs of a ruptured spleen with the signs of a severely contused kidney.
9. What are the most common sports injuries and conditions related to the digestive system?
10. How should an athlete who has had his or her wind knocked out be managed?
11. Distinguish an inguinal hernia or a femoral hernia from a groin strain.
12. Describe the signs of a stitch in the side.

REFERENCES

1. Affleck TP: Severe sports-related spleen injury: Not all patients require surgery, *Physician Sportsmed* 20(9):109, 1992.
2. Allison T: Counseling athletes at risk for sudden death, *Physician Sportsmed* 20(6):140, 1992.
3. Alpert J, Pape L, Ward A: Athletic heart syndrome, *Physician Sportsmed* 17(7):103, 1989.
4. Bergman RT: Assessing acute abdominal pain: a team physician's challenge, *Physician Sportsmed* 26(4):72, 1996.
5. Ciocca M: Pneumothorax in a weight lifter: the importance of vigilance, *Physician Sportsmed* 28(4):97, 2000.
6. Curtin SM, Tucker AM, Gens DR: Pneumothorax in sports: issues in recognition and follow-up care, *Physician Sportsmed* 28(8):23, 2000.
7. Cvengros RD, Lazor JA: Pneumothorax—a medical emergency, *J Ath Train* 31(2):167, 1996.
8. Eichner ER: Throw no stones: how to prevent kidney stones. *Sports Med Digest* 24(2):22, 2002.
9. Eichner ER: Gut reactions: athletes' gastrointestinal problems, *Sports Med Digest* 21(10):111, 1999.
10. Erickson SM, Rich BS: Pulmonary and chest wall emergencies: Onsite treatment of potentially fatal conditions, *Physician Sportsmed* 23(11):95, 1995.
11. Evan C, Cassady S: Sudden cardiac death in athletes: what sport-rehabilitation specialists need to know, *J Sport Rehab* 12(3):259, 2003.
12. Fait PE: Third-degree spleen laceration in a male varsity athlete. *Athletic Therapy Today* 8(3):32, 2003.
13. Falsetti H: Sudden death syndrome, *Training and Conditioning* 5(3): 26, 1995.
14. Fillion DT: Abdominal injuries: subtle symptoms may indicate a serious condition, *Sports Med Update* 12(3):12, 1997.
15. Franklin BA, Fletcher GF, Gordon NF: Cardiovascular evaluation of the athlete: issues regarding performance, screening, and sudden cardiac death, *Sports Med* 26(2):97, 1997.
16. Freitas JE: Renal imaging following blunt trauma, *Physician Sportsmed* 17(12):59, 1989.
17. Futterman LG, Myerburg R: Sudden death in athletes: an update, *Sports Med* 26(5):335, 1998.
18. Getz B: Spleen injuries in athletes, *Hughston Health Alert* 13(2): 7, 2001.
19. Hammond S: Chest injuries in the trauma patient, *Nurs Clin N Amer* 25(1):35, 1990.
20. Haycock CE: Abdominal injuries. In Fu FH, Stone DA, editors: *Sports injuries: mechanisms, prevention, and treatment,* Philadelphia, 2001, Lippincott, Williams & Wilkins.
21. Haycock CE: How I manage breast problems in athletes, *Physician Sportsmed* 15(3):89, 1987.
22. Haycock CE: How I manage abdominal injuries, *Physician Sportsmed* 14(6):86, 1986.
23. Herbert DL: Preparticipation cardiovascular screening: toward a national standard, *Physician Sportsmed* 25(3):112, 1997.
24. Hosey RG: Sudden cardiac death. *Clin Sports Med* 22(1):51, 2003.
25. Johnson MB, Haines M, Barry B: Recognizing pneumothorax—a case study, *Athletic Therapy Today* 1(6):42, 1996.
26. Jones H, McBride G, Murphy R: Sternal fractures associate with spinal injury, *J Trauma* 29(3):360, 1989.
27. Kemp S, Batt ME: The "sports hernia": a common cause of groin pain, *Physician Sportsmed* 26(1):3, 1998.
28. Kersey RD: Primary spontaneous pneumothorax in a collegiate soccer player, *Athletic Therapy Today* 5(2):48, 2000.

29. Koester MC: A review of sudden cardiac death in young athletes and strategies for preparticipation cardiovascular screening, *J Ath Train* 36(2):197, 2001.
30. Konrad P, Schmitz K, Denner A: Neuromuscular evaluation of trunk-training exercises, *J Ath Train* 36(2):109, 2001.
31. Lacroix VJ: Acomplete approach to groin pain, *Physician Sportsmed* 28(1):66, 2000.
32. Leaver-Dunn D, Robinson J, Laubenthal J: Assessment of respiratory conditions in athletes, *Athletic Therapy Today* 5(6):14, 2000.
33. Lee M, Wong S, Chu J: Traumatic asphyxia, *Ann Thoracic Surg* 51(1):86, 1991.
34. Maron B: Hypertrophic cardiomyopathy in athletes: catching a killer, *Physician Sportsmed* 21(9):83, 1993.
35. Maron B, Liviu C, Kaplan J, Mueller F: Blunt trauma to the chest leading to sudden death from cardiac arrest during sports activities, *N Engl J Med* 333(6):337, 1995.
36. McCarthy P: Hernias in athletes: what you need to know, *Physician Sportsmed* 18(5):115, 1990.
37. McChesney J: Auscultation of the chest and abdomen by athletic trainers, *J Ath Train* 36(2):190, 2001.
38. Merrick MA: Cardiovascular pathologies: to screen or not to screen? *Athletic Therapy Today* 6(4):28, 2001.
39. Meyers WC, Foley DP, Garrett WE: Management of severe lower abdominal or inguinal pain in high-performance athletes, *Am J Sports Med* 28(1):2, 2000.
40. Miles J, Barrett G: Rib fractures in athletes, *Sports Med* 12(1):66, 1991.
41. Morden R, Berman B, Nagle C: Spleen injury in sports: avoiding splenectomy, *Physician Sportsmed,* 20(4):126, 1992.
42. Newsham KR: Exertional chest pain in an intercollegiate athlete, *J Ath Train* 32(1):59, 1997.
43. Norris R, Kovan J: Assessment of cardiovascular conditions in the athlete, *Athletic Therapy Today* 5(6):11, 2000.
44. O'Kane J, O'Kane E, Marquet J: Delayed complication of a rib fracture, *Physician Sportsmed* 26(4):69, 1998.
45. Page KA, Steele JR: Breast motion and sports brassiere design: implications for future research, *Sports Med* 27(4): 205, 1999.
46. Perron AD: Chest pain in athletes. *Clin Sports Med* 22(1):37, 2003.
47. Piccininni JP: Kidney laceration in a university football player. *Athletic Therapy Today* 7(5):42, 2002.
48. Plunkett BT, Hopkins WG: Investigation of the side pain "stitch" induced by running after fluid ingestion, *Med Sci Sports Exerc* 31(8): 1169, 1999.
49. Putukian M: Assessment of abdominal conditions in athletes, *Athletic Therapy Today* 5(6):20, 2000.
50. Ray R, Lemire JE: Liver laceration in an intercollegiate football player, *J Ath Train* 30(4):326, 1995.
51. Reid D: *Sports injury assessment,* New York, 1992, Churchill & Livingstone.
52. Reut R, Bach B, Johnson C: Pectoralis major rupture, *Physician Sportsmed* 19(3):89, 1991.
53. Rink LD: Cardiac problems and sudden death in athletes. In Baker CL et. al, editors: *The Hughston Clinic sports medicine book,* Baltimore, 1995, Williams & Wilkins.
54. Ryan JM: Abdominal injuries and sport, *British Journal of Sports Medicine* 33(3):155, 1999.
55. Ryan SW: Managing urinary tract and vaginal infections, *Physician Sportsmed* 24(7):101, 1996.
56. Saladin K: Anatomy and physiology: the unity of form and function, New York, 2001, McGraw-Hill.
57. Seeley R, Stephens T, Tate P: *Anatomy and physiology,* ed 4, New York, 2003, McGraw-Hill.
58. Simoneauz S, Murphy B, Tehranzadeh J: Spontaneous pneumothorax in a weight lifter, *Am J Sports Med* 18(6):647, 1990.
59. *Stedman's concise medical dictionary for the health professions,* Baltimore, 2003, Lippincott, Williams & Wilkins.
60. Steine H: Chest pain and shortness of breath in a collegiate basketball player: case report and literature review, *Med Sci Sports Exerc* 26:504, 1992.
61. Stopka CB, Zambito KL: Referred visceral pain: what every sports medicine professional needs to know, *Athletic Therapy Today* 4(1):29, 1999.
62. Suman OE, Beck KC, Babcock MA: Airway obstruction during exercise and isocapnic hyperventilation in asthmatic subjects, *Journal App Physiol* 87(3):1107, 1999.
63. *Taber's cyclopedic medical dictionary,* Philadelphia, 2001, FA Davis.
64. Terrell, TR: Management of splenic rupture and return-to-play decisions in a college football player. *Clin Sports Med* 12(6):400, 2002.
65. Van Camp S: Sudden death. In Puffer J, editor: *Clinics in sports medicine,* Philadelphia, 1992, Saunders.
66. Van Camp S, Bloor C, Mueller F: Nontraumatic sports death in high school and college athletes, *Med Sci Sports Exerc* 27(9):641, 1995.
67. Volk CP, McFarland EG, Horsmon G: Pneumothorax: on-field recognition, *Physician Sportsmed* 23(10):43, 1995.
68. Wagner R, Sidhu G, Radcliffe W: Pulmonary contusion in contact sports, *Physician Sportsmed* 20(2): 126, 1992.
69. Widner PE: Thoracic injuries: mechanisms, characteristics, management, *Ath Train* 23(2):148, 1988.
70. Yates M, Aldrete V: Blunt trauma causing aortic rupture, *Physician Sportsmed* 19(11):96, 1991.
71. York J: Bladder trauma from jogging, *Physician Sportsmed* 18(9):116, 1990.

ANNOTATED BIBLIOGRAPHY

Taber's cyclopedic medical dictionary, Philadelphia, 2001, FA Davis.

Despite the dictionary format, this guide is excellent for the athletic trainer who is searching for clear, concise descriptions of various injuries and illnesses accompanied by brief recommendations for management and treatment.

Seeley R, Stephens T, Tate P: *Anatomy and physiology,* ed 4, New York, 2003, McGraw-Hill.

This anatomy text helps clarify anatomy of the various systems of the abdomen and thorax and also provides clinical correlations for specific injuries and illnesses.

Chapter 28 Skin Disorders

When you finish this chapter you should be able to

- Explain the structure and function of the skin and identify the lesions that result from skin abnormalities.
- Describe in detail how skin trauma occurs, how it may be prevented, and how it may be managed.
- Identify bacterial skin infections that are potentially contagious.
- Describe the correct hygiene practices to use to avoid fungal infections.
- Identify potentially threatening viral infections.
- Contrast allergic, thermal, and chemical reactions of the skin.
- Identify infestations and insect bites and contrast them with other skin infections.

It is essential that athletic trainers understand conditions that adversely affect the skin and mucous membranes, especially highly contagious conditions.[15]

SKIN ANATOMY AND FUNCTION

The skin is the largest organ of the human body. The average adult skin varies in total weight from 6 to 7½ pounds and is from 1/32 to 1/8 inch thick. It is composed of three layers: the epidermis, dermis, and subcutis (Figure 28-1; Table 28-1).[21]

Epidermis

The epidermis acts as a barrier against invading microorganisms, foreign particles from dirt and debris, chemicals, and ultraviolet rays and also helps contain the body's water and electrolytes. The epidermis is the outermost layer of the skin and itself is composed of several layers identified as the stratum corneum, stratum granulosum, stratum spinosum, and stratum basale. The stratified nature of the epidermal cell layers results from the migration of keratinocytes, the epidermal epithelial cells, from the basal layer outward to the stratum corneum. During this migration process, the cells undergo a well-described change in shape from round basal cells to flat elongated cells. In the final stage of differentiation, the flattened keratinocytes secrete a variety of substances into the extracellular space and then lose their nuclei to form the horny layer known as the stratum corneum. The stratum corneum acts as a permeability barrier, allowing only small molecules to diffuse into the lower regions of the epidermis, and thus it protects against environmental irritants, toxins, and pathogens. Other cells, including melanocytes and Langerhans cells, are also found in the epidermis. Melanocytes synthesize and transfer to keratinocytes the pigment melanin, which blocks harmful solar radiation. Langerhans cells aid in immunologic surveillance by collecting and presenting to lymphocytes foreign substances, such as bacterial proteins.

Dermis

The dermis is beneath the epidermis and is composed of connective tissue. The dermis provides mechanical support to the epidermis and also contains blood vessels, nerves, sweat glands, hair follicles, and sebaceous glands. The dermis forms a series of finger-like projections, the dermal papilla, that reach into the epidermis. This creates an

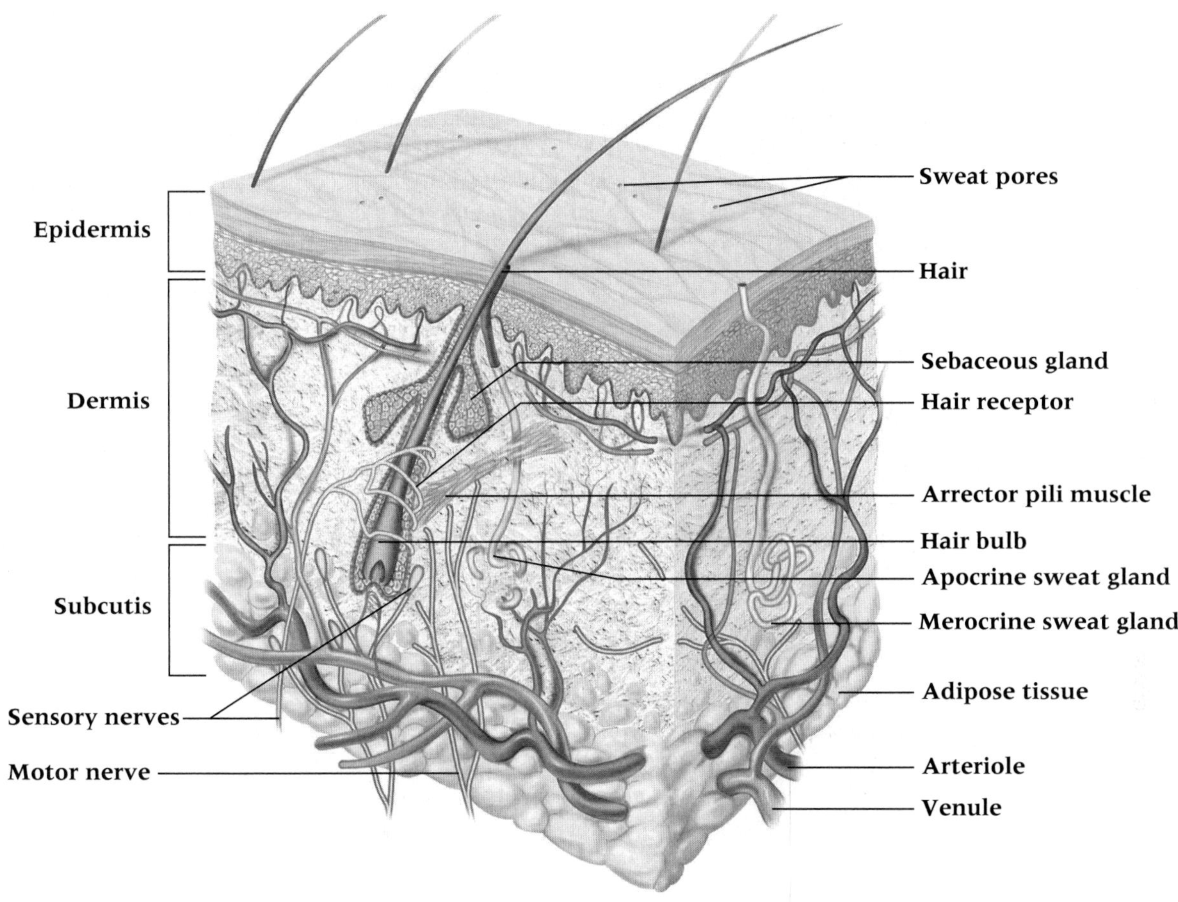

Figure 28-1

Cross section of the skin.

interlocking arrangement that increases the surface area of dermal-epidermal contact and thereby prevents the epidermis from slipping off the dermis.

Adnexal Structures: Hair, Sebaceous Glands, and Eccrine Glands

Hair grows from hair follicles in the skin. It extends into the dermis, where it is nourished by the blood capillaries. Small muscles called arrectores pilorum connect to the hair and, when contracted by stimuli such as cold or fear, pull the hair into a vertical position, creating a "standing-on-end" effect, or goose bumps. This increases the insulating effect of hair and protects the body from cold.

TABLE 28-1 Outline of the Skin's Structure and Function

Layer	Subregion	Function
Epidermis	Stratum corneum	Prevents intrusion of microorganisms, debris, chemicals, ultraviolet radiation Prevents loss of water and electrolytes Performs heat regulation for conduction, radiation, convection
	Melanin (pigmentation)	Prevents intrusion of ultraviolet radiation
Dermis		Protects against physical trauma Contains sensory nerve endings Holds water and electrolytes
	Appendages	Contains eccrine and apocrine sweat glands, hair, nails, sebaceous glands
Subcutis		Stores fat, regulates heat

The sebaceous glands, which surround the hair, secrete sebum, an oily substance, which is extruded into the hair follicles. Sebaceous glands can become enlarged, a condition known as sebaceous hyperplasia. This is a benign condition; however, the appearance of the enlarged glands can sometimes be confused with basal cell carcinoma, a form of skin cancer. The term **sebaceous cyst** is a misnomer, since it is not derived from the sebaceous glands, but is an epithelial lined space originating from the upper portion of the hair follicle. Enlargement of this cyst results from the accumulation of keratin, the major skin protein, into the cavity of the cyst. The more correct term, *epithelial inclusion cyst,* should be used to describe this common and benign skin lesion.

sebaceous cyst
A cyst filled with sebum; usually found in the scalp.

Sweat Glands

Sweat glands are necessary for cooling the surface of the body and the internal organs. Patients with anhidrotic ectodermal dysplasia, a rare inherited disease, do not make functional sweat glands and are susceptible to significant overheating with physical exertion. There are two main types of glands: the eccrine glands, which are present at birth and are generally present throughout the skin, and the apocrine glands, which are much larger than the eccrine glands and mature during adolescence in conjunction with the axillary and pubic hair. Sweat gland secretions contain antibacterial agents that aid in controlling infection.

Nails

The nails are special horny cell structures that come from the phalanges. The nail matrix, located beneath the proximal nail fold and visible as a white semicircular structure beneath the proximal nail plate, synthesizes the hard, keratinaceous nail plate. The nails grow approximately ½ inch in four months.

Sensory Nerve Endings

Besides its many other functions, the dermis contains sensory nerve endings. These peripheral nerves provide tactile sensation and detect temperature changes and pain.

Subcutis

The subcutis contains fat. Subcutaneous fat has a role in temperature regulation/insulation and energy storage, and it increases the mobility of the skin over the underlying tissues.

SKIN LESIONS DEFINED

Skin that is healthy has a smooth, soft appearance. Different amounts of the skin pigment melanin are responsible for ethnic variations in skin color. Areas of increased melanin can result in pale brown areas of skin and are referred to as café au lait spots or macules. These are common in infancy and disappear with age. They can sometimes be markers for systemic disease. Additional and sometimes transient changes in skin color are due to anatomic, physiologic, or pathophysiologic changes in skin blood flow. Increased blood flow to the skin capillaries results in a red-colored skin, whereas, decreased blood flow to the skin causes pallor.[1]

The normal appearance of the skin can be altered by external and internal factors. Some changes may be signs of other involvements. The different intensities of paleness or redness of the skin, which is related to the extent of superficial circulation, may be hereditary. Pigment variation may result from an increase of sun exposure or from organic disease; a yellowish discoloration, for example, may be indicative of jaundice. **Cellulitis,** the infectious inflammation of deep skin structures, is characterized by a reddening of the skin called erythema and by increased warmth.

cellulitis
An inflammation of cells and connective tissue that extends deep into the tissues.

Skin abnormalities may be divided into primary and secondary lesions. Primary lesions include macules, papules, plaques, nodules, turmors, cysts, wheals, vesicles, bullae, and pustules (Figure 28-2; Table 28-2). Secondary lesions, such as excoriations, result from primary lesions that have been manipulated (Figure 28-3; Table 28-3).

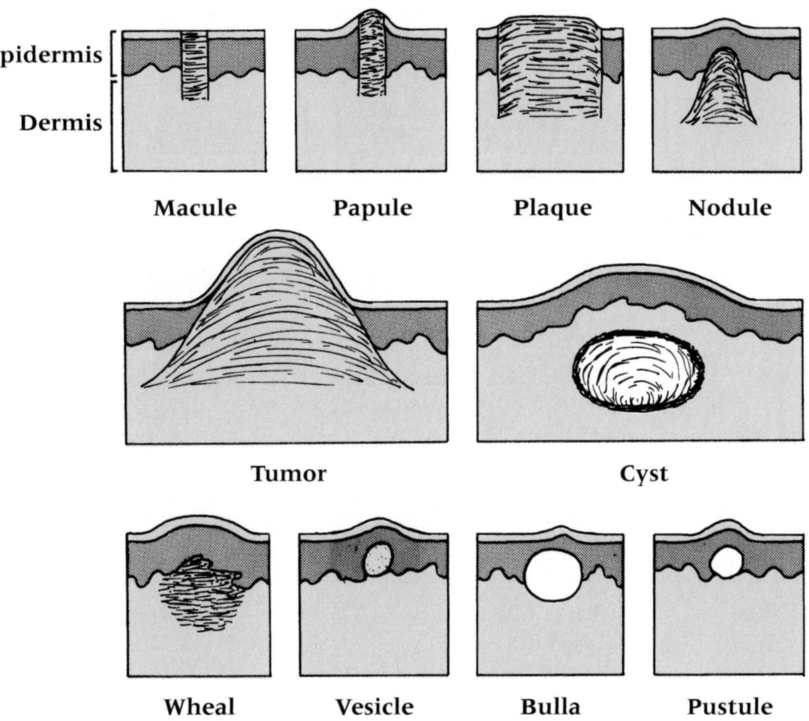

Figure 28-2

Typical primary skin lesions.

TABLE 28-2 Primary Skin Lesions

Type	Description	Example
Macule	A small, flat, circular discoloration smaller than 1 cm in diameter	Freckle or flat nevus café au lait macules (spots)
Papule	A solid elevation less than 1 cm in diameter	Wart
Plaque or patch	May be a macule or papule larger than 1 cm in diameter	Vitiligo patch (patches of depigmentation)
Nodule	A solid mass less than 1 cm, deeper into the dermis than a papule	Dermatofibroma fibrosis
Tumor	Solid mass larger than 1 cm	Cavernous hemangioma (tumor filled with blood vessels)
Cyst	Encapsulated, fluid filled, in dermis or subcutis	Epidermoid cyst
Wheal	A papule or plaque caused by serum collection into the dermis, allergic reactions	Urticaria (hives)
Vesicle	Fluid-filled elevation less than 1 cm, just below epidermis	Smallpox, chicken pox
Bulla	Like a vesicle but larger	Second-degree burn, friction blister
Pustule	Like vesicle or bulla but contains pus	Acne

SKIN TRAUMA

Sports participation can place a great deal of mechanical force on the skin. Mechanical forces that can apply to the skin include friction, compression, shearing, stretching, scraping, tearing, avulsing, and puncturing, all of which can lead to painful and serious injuries.[34,35]

Friction and Pressure Problems

Excessive rubbing back and forth over the skin, along with abnormal pressure, can cause thickening of the stratum corneum, or horny layer, of the epidermis, especially

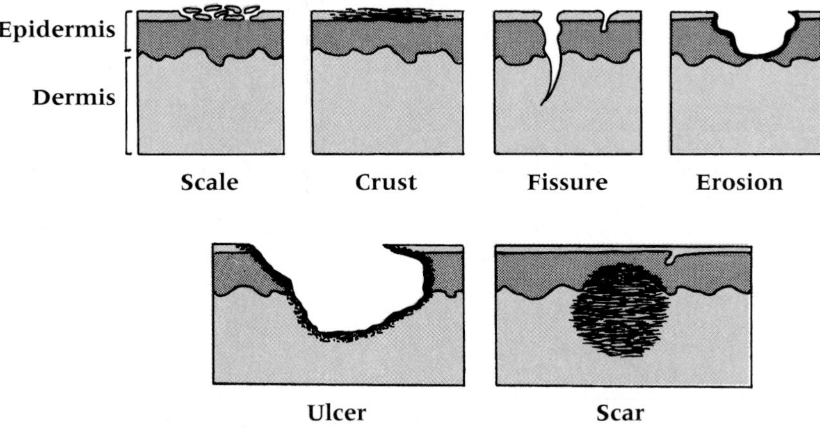

Figure 28-3
Typical secondary skin lesions.

TABLE 28-3 Secondary Skin Lesions

Type	Description	Example
Scales	Flakes of skin	Psoriasis
Crust	Dried fluid or exudates on skin	Impetigo
Fissure	Skin crack	Chapping
Excoriation	Superficial scrape	Abrasion
Erosion	Loss of superficial epidermis	Scratches (superficial)
Ulcer	Destruction of entire epidermis	Pressure sore
Scar	Healing of dermis	Vaccination, laceration

hyperkeratosis Excessive growth of the horny tissue layer.

on the soles of the feet and the palms of the hands. This causes **hyperkeratosis** that is characteristic of callus formation. Pressure, shearing, and frictional forces can also produce corns and blisters.

Hyperkeratosis of the Feet and Hands

Skin, typically the epidermal skin layer, increases in thickness when constant friction and pressure are applied externally. Excessive callus accumulation may occur over bony protuberances.

Etiology Foot calluses may become excessive on an athlete who wears shoes that are too narrow or short. As with the foot, hand calluses can become painful when the subcutaneous fatty layer loses its elasticity, which is an important cushioning effect. The callus moves as a mass when pressure and a shearing force are applied. Hyperkeratotic skin is less pliable, and mechanical stress on hyperkeratotic skin, as occurs with movement, can result in tears or cracks in the epidermis that are painful and that also facilitate the entry of infectious organisms.

Prevention Athletes whose shoes are properly fitted but who still develop heavy calluses commonly have foot mechanics problems that may require special orthotics.

Special cushioning devices such as wedges, doughnuts, and arch supports may help distribute the weight on the feet more evenly and thus reduce skin stress. Excessive callus accumulation can be prevented by wearing two pairs of socks, a thin cotton or nylon pair next to the skin and a heavy athletic pair over the cotton pair, or a single doubleknit sock; wearing shoes that are the correct size and are in good condition; routinely applying materials such as lubricants to reduce friction; and shaving the callus with a scalpel, using extreme caution. Hand calluses also can be controlled by using a special glove for direct protection such as is used in batting, or by applying elastic tape or moleskin. In sports such as gymnastics, athletic trainers and athletes go to great lengths to protect the athlete's hands against tearing calluses. Grip is a protective device that has a special type of hand covering that may include a wood dowel placed across the grip portion of the hand.

Symptoms and signs The callus appears as a circumscribed thickening and hypertrophy of the horny layer of the skin. It may be ovular, elongated, brownish, and/or slightly elevated. Calluses may not be painful when pressure is applied.

Management Because callus formation represents a protective response to frictional and shearing forces applied to the skin, exposure to such forces should be minimized. The use of emery files or pumice stones should be discouraged since their use results in frictional forces that stimulate the skin to produce additional callus. Athletes who are prone to excess calluses should be encouraged to use moisturizers and keratolytic agents. Massaging small amounts of lanolin into calluses twice a day may help maintain some tissue elasticity. A keratolytic agent, such as 25 percent urea (Ultramide), lactic acid (Lachydrin) or salicylic acid (3 percent salicylic acid in petrolatum) may be applied. Additional formulations of salicylic acid, such as 5 percent to 10 percent in a flexible collodion, can be applied at night and peeled off in the morning. Before applying a keratolytic ointment, the athletic trainer might manually decrease the calluses' thickness by carefully paring it with a sharp scalpel. Great care should be taken not to remove the callus totally and the protection it affords a pressure point. A donut pad may be cut to size and placed on a pressure point to prevent pain.

Blisters

Like calluses, blisters are often a major problem in sports participation, especially early in the season. Shearing forces produce a raised area that contains a collection of fluid below or within the epidermis.

Etiology Blisters are particularly associated with rowing, pole vaulting, basketball, football, and weight events in track and field, such as the shot put and discus. Such activities commonly cause the skin to be subjected to horizontal shearing, which produces a friction blister.

Prevention Soft feet and hands, coupled with shearing skin stress, can produce severe blisters. A dusting of talcum powder or applying petroleum jelly can protect the skin against abnormal friction. Wearing tubular socks or two pairs of socks to prevent calluses is also desirable, particularly for athletes who have sensitive feet or feet that perspire excessively. Wearing the correct-size shoe is essential. The shoes must be broken in before they are worn for long periods of time. If, however, a friction area ("hot spot") does arise, the athlete has several options. The athlete can cover the irritated skin with a friction-reducing material such as "second skin" or cover it with a piece of moleskin. Another method that has proved effective against blisters is applying ice over skin areas that have developed abnormal friction.

Symptoms and signs The athlete normally will feel a hot spot, a sharp, burning sensation as the blister is formed. The area of sensation should be examined immediately. The blister may be superficial, containing clear liquid. On the other hand, a blood blister may form in which deeper tissue is disrupted, causing blood vessels to rupture. Pain is caused by the pressure of the fluid.

Management As stated previously, blister prevention is of paramount importance. Once developed, blisters can be a serious problem for the athlete, as well as for the athletic trainer. *Focus Box:* "Managing blisters" presents general rules for managing a blister (OSHA standards must be followed; see Chapter 14).

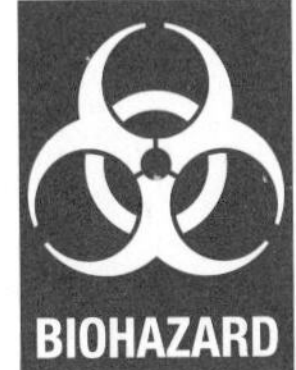

Soft Corns and Hard Corns

Soft corns and hard corns are other examples of hyperkeratosis caused by abnormal skin pressure and friction.

Etiology A hard corn (clavus durus) is the most serious type of corn. It is caused by the pressure of improperly fitting shoes and other anatomical abnormalities—the same mechanisms that cause calluses. Hammertoes are usually associated with the

Focus

Managing blisters

The intact blister:

1. Leave the blister intact for the first twenty-four hours. Often during that time, many of the symptoms will lessen.
2. If the blister is large and in a place on the skin that will be continually irritated, clean it thoroughly with antiseptic soap.
3. With a sterile scalpel, cut a small incision one-eighth to one-quarter inch long in the blister along the periphery of the raised tissue. The hole should be large enough that it will not become sealed. NOTE: In some states this procedure could be considered a surgical technique and thus would be a violation of certain practice acts.
4. Disperse the fluid by applying a pressure pad, keeping the pad in place to prevent refilling.
5. Once the fluid has been removed, clean the area again with an antiseptic such as providone-iodine (Betadine) and cover it with an antibiotic ointment such as Polysporin.
6. Place a doughnut pad around the dressed blister to avoid further irritation.
7. Monitor the blistered area daily for the possibility of infection. If infection occurs, refer the athlete to a physician immediately.
8. Replace the dressing if it becomes wet from fluid seepage. A wet environment encourages the growth of bacteria and therefore infection.
9. If there is necrotic skin, debridement can be done when the tenderness is completely gone. Debridement should not be attempted if any tenderness persists.

The open (torn) blister:

1. Keep the open blister clean to avoid infection. In the beginning of management, carefully and thoroughly wash it with soap and water. Once it is cleaned, apply hydrogen peroxide or benzalkonium chloride. If the blister site is torn along less than one-half of its diameter, apply a liquid antiseptic and allow it to dry, then apply an antibiotic ointment.
2. Lay the flap of skin back over the treated tissue, then apply a sterile, nonadhering dressing and a doughnut pad.
3. As when managing the intact blister, monitor the open blister daily for the possibility of infection.

The completely denuded blister:

1. If the blister is torn one-half inch or more, completely remove the flap of skin, using sterile scissors.
2. Completely clean the exposed tissue with soap and water. Apply an antiseptic liquid such as benzalkonium with occlusive dressing.[15]
3. If the athlete has completed his or her activity, apply the "second-skin" dressing by Spenco (Spenco Medical Corporation, Waco, Texas) to the raw area. When applied, this gel ensures healing through the night.

28-1 Critical Thinking Exercise

A basketball player wearing new shoes during a game sustains a completely denuded blister on the back of the heel.

? How should this condition be managed during and after the game?

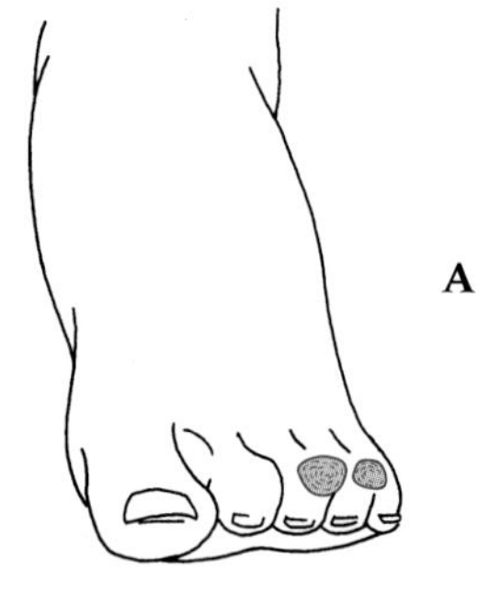

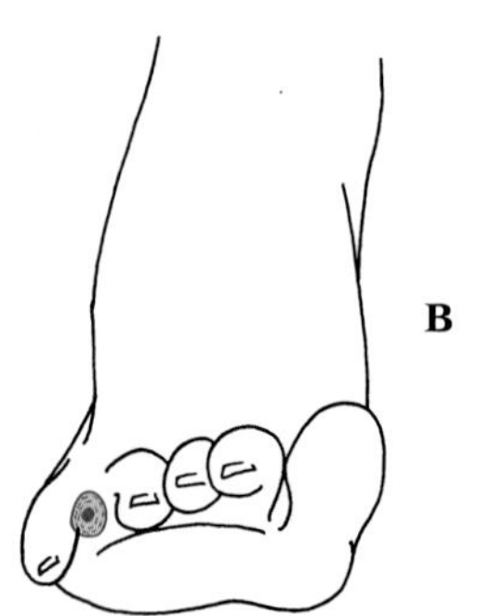

Figure 28-4

A, Hard corn (clavus durus).
B, Soft corn (clavus mollis).

hard corns that form on the tops of deformed toes (Figure 28-4A). Symptoms are local pain and disability, with inflammation and thickening of soft tissue. Because of the chronic nature of this condition, it requires a physician's care.

A soft corn (clavus mollis) is the result of the combination of wearing narrow shoes and having excessive foot perspiration. It is also associated with an exostosis. Because of the pressure of the shoe coupled with the exudation of moisture, the corn usually forms between the fourth and fifth toes (Figure 28-4B). A circular area of thickened, white, macerated skin appears between the toes at the base of the proximal head of the phalanges. Both pain and inflammation are likely to be present.[4]

Prevention The primary way to prevent a soft or hard corn is to wear properly fitted shoes. Soft corns can be avoided by wearing shoes that are wide enough. Conversely, hard corns can be avoided by wearing shoes that are long enough.

Symptoms and signs With a soft corn, the athlete complains of pain laterally on the fifth toe. During inspection, the soft corn appears as a circular piece of thickened, white, **macerated skin** on the lateral side of the fifth toe at the base of the proximal head of the phalanges. In contrast, hard corns are on the tops of hammertoes. The bony prominence of the toe is forced up, and it presses on the inner top of the shoe, causing the corn to form. It appears hard and dry, with a callus that is sharply demarcated.

macerated skin
Skin softened by exposure to wetting.

Management The corn is difficult to manage. If pain and imflammation are major, referral to a podiatrist for surgical removal may be advisable. The athletic trainer may ameliorate the condition by having the athlete wear properly fitting shoes and socks and may alleviate further irritation of the corn by protecting it with a small felt pad or sponge pad, which can act as a buffer between the shoe and the toe. In caring for a soft corn the best procedure is to have the athlete wear properly fitting shoes, keep the skin between the toes clean and dry, decrease pressure by keeping the toes separated with cotton or lamb's wool, and apply a keratolytic agent such as 25 percent urea (Ultramide) or 40 percent salicylic acid in liquid or plasters.

Excessive Perspiration (Hyperhidrosis)

Excessive perspiration can be a cause of serious skin irritation.

Etiology Excessive perspiration (hyperhidrosis) occurs in a small segment of the population. This problem can make the handling of sports objects difficult, causing both performance and safety problems. Emotional excitement often makes the situation worse. Hyperhidrotic perspiration from palms is syruplike in appearance and extremely high in sodium chloride. This problem also increases the possibility of skin irritations and often makes the adherence of bandages difficult, especially where adhesive tape is necessary. The condition makes callus development, blisters, and intertrigo (chafing) much more likely to occur.

Management Treatment of excessive perspiration should include using an astringent such as alcohol or an absorbent powder (see *Focus Box:* "Foot hygiene for excessive perspiration and odor"). Aluminum chloride (Drysol) applied topically or electric current (iontophoresis) are also used to control hyperhidrosis.

Chafing of the Skin

Chafing of the skin is another condition that stems from friction or from rubbing the skin unduly.

28-2 *Critical Thinking* Exercise

A heavy-limbed shotputter complains of a skin irritation in his groin region. The area appears red and macerated. Some of the tissue is cracked, and there are oozing sores.

? How could this chafing have been prevented?

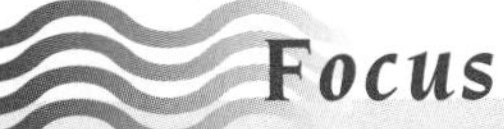

Foot hygiene for excessive perspiration and odor

Before practice

1. Apply an astringent such as 20 percent aluminum chloride in anhydrous ethyl alcohol (Drysol) to the skin and allow it to air dry.
2. Liberally apply a powder such as talcum, alum, or boric acid to the skin, socks, and sports footwear.

After practice

1. Thoroughly wash and dry the feet, then follow the before-practice procedure. Apply an astringent to the skin and an absorbent powder to street socks and shoes.
2. Change footwear frequently.
3. Liberally powder sports footwear after practice to absorb moisture during storage. Ideally, a different pair of shoes should be worn daily.

Etiology Chafing occurs particularly in athletes who are obese or heavy limbed. It results from friction and maceration (softening) of the skin in a climate of heat and moisture.

Symptoms and signs Repeated skin rubbing, as in the groin and axilla, can separate the keratin from the granular layer of the epidermis. This separation causes oozing wounds that develop into crusting and cracking lesions.

Prevention To prevent chafing, keep the skin dry, clean, and friction free. For groin conditions the athlete should wear loose, soft, cotton underwear. A male athlete should wear his supporter over a pair of loose cotton boxer shorts.

Management The chafed area should be cleansed once daily with mild soap and lukewarm water. Treatment of a chafed area includes wet packs, using a medicated solution such as Burrows for fifteen to twenty minutes, three times daily. This is followed by applying a 1 percent hydrocortisone cream.

Xerotic (Dry) Skin

Dry skin is a condition that athletes commonly experience during the winter months.[26]

Etiology Athletes who are exposed to weather and bathe often commonly develop dry or chapped skin. The drying cold of winter tends to dehydrate the stratum corneum. Some athletes naturally may have fewer skins lipids, which increases the tendency to lose water.[26] A decrease in humidity along with cold winds causes the skin to lose water.

Symptoms and signs The skin appears dry with variable redness and scaling. It occurs first on the shins, forearms, backs of the hands, and face. There may be itching. The skin may crack and develop fissures.

Management The major goals in treatment are to prevent water loss and to replace lost water.[11] The following treatment procedures should be followed:

- Bathe in tepid water and shower one time per day.
- Use moisturizing soaps such as Dove or Aveeno. Avoid soaping dry areas. Restrict washing to genitalia, underarms, hands, feet, and face.
- Use emollient lotions, which hydrate the skin. Apply them after each washing.
- When the condition is more severe, the athlete should be referred to a physician for antipruritics, alpha-hydroxy acids, and perhaps topical corticosteroids.[26]

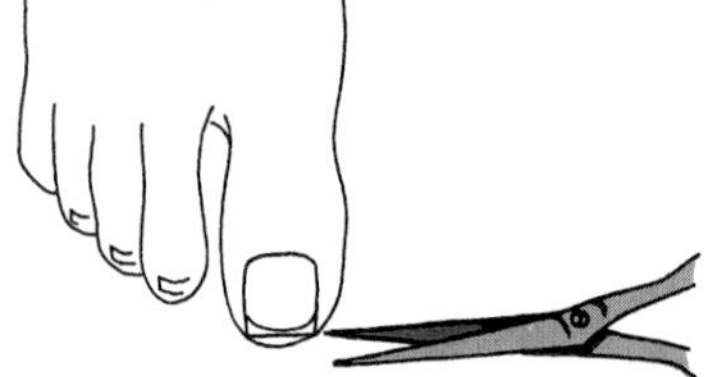

Figure 28-5

Preventing an ingrown toenail requires proper trimming.

Ingrown Toenails

An ingrown toenail is a common condition among athletes. The large toe is the most often affected. The nail grows into the lateral nail fold and enters the skin.[12]

Etiology In general, the ingrown nail results from the lateral pressure of poorly fitting shoes, improper toenail trimming, or trauma such as repeated pressure from sliding to the front of the shoe (Color Plate, Figure A).

Prevention Because of the handicapping nature of this condition, prevention of ingrown toenails is much preferred over management. Properly fitted shoes and socks are essential. The toenails should be trimmed weekly by cutting straight across, avoiding rounding so that the margins do not penetrate the tissue on the sides (Figure 28-5). The nail should be left sufficiently long so that it is clear of the underlying skin, but it should be cut short enough so as to not irritate the skin by pushing against shoes or socks.

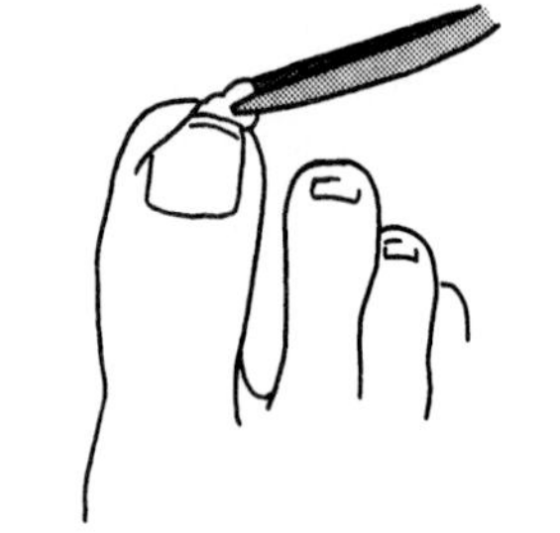

Figure 28-6

Application of a wisp of cotton under the ingrown side.

Symptoms and signs The first indications of an ingrown toenail are pain and swelling. If not treated early, the penetrated skin becomes severely inflamed and purulent. The lateral nail fold becomes swollen and irritated.

Management There are a number of ways to manage the ingrown toenail. If it is in the first stages of inflammation, a more conservative approach can be taken.

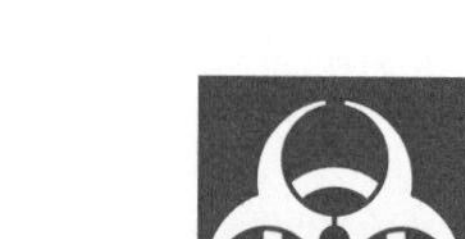

- Soak the inflamed toe in warm water (105° to 110° F) for approximately twenty minutes.
- After soaking, the nail will be soft and pliable and may be pried out of the skin. Using sterile forceps or scissors, lift the nail from the soft tissue and insert a piece of cotton to keep the nail out of the skin (Figure 28-6). This also relieves the

pain. Perform this procedure daily until the corner of the nail has grown past the irritated tissue.

If the condition becomes chronically irritated, a more aggressive approach is likely to be taken by a physician.

- After applying an anesthetic (e.g., 1 percent or 2 percent lidocaine), slip the nail-splitting scissor under the ingrown nail.[21]
- With the scissor inserted to the point of resistance, cut away and remove the wedge-shaped nail. Keep a moist antiseptic compress in place until the inflammation has subsided.

Athletes with recurrent ingrown nails may require the use of phenol for permanent destruction of the lateral portion of the nail.

Signs of wound infection, which appear two to seven days after injury:

- Red, swollen, hot, and tender wound
- Swollen and painful lymph glands near the area of infection (groin, axilla, or neck)
- Mild fever and headache

Wounds

Traumatic skin lesions, commonly called wounds, are extremely prevalent in sports; abrasions, lacerations, incisions, punctures, and bruises are daily occurrences[25] (Figure 28-7).[16]

Abrasions

Abrasions are common and occur when the skin is scraped against a rough surface. The top layer of skin is worn away, thus exposing numerous blood capillaries. This general exposure, with dirt and foreign materials scraping and penetrating the skin,

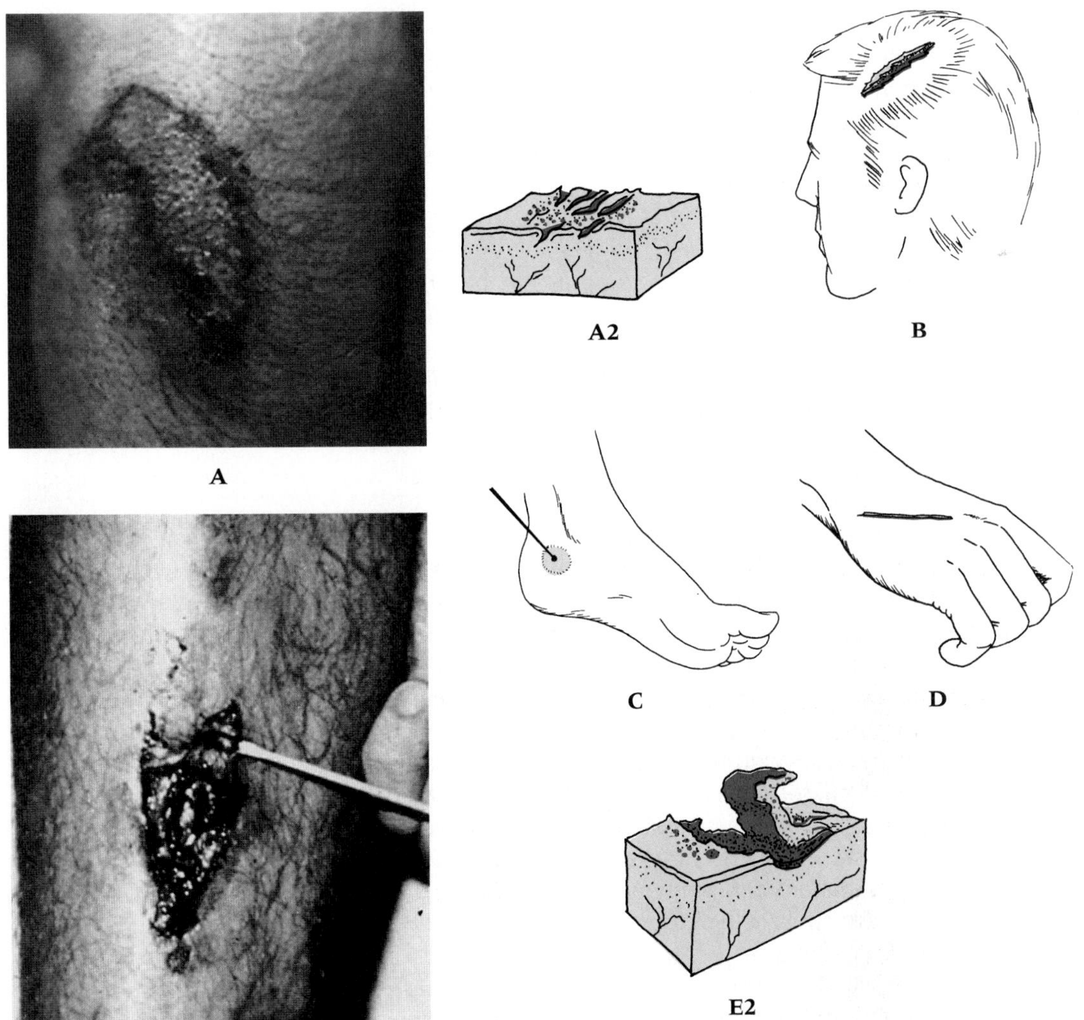

Figure 28-7

Wounds occurring in sports can present a serious problem of infection. **A1 & A2,** Abrasion. **B,** Laceration. **C,** Puncture. **D,** Incision. **E1 & E2,** Avulsion.

28-3
Critical Thinking Exercise

A baseball player slides into second base and sustains a serious slide burn on the left side.

? What are the major concerns with this type of injury, and how should it be managed?

28-4
Critical Thinking Exercise

A baseball player is hit with an elbow just above her eyebrow. There is a laceration with a good deal of bleeding. Upon closer inspection the athletic trainer realizes that despite the large amount of bleeding, the laceration is not that long, but it is fairly deep.

? Should this laceration be closed with steri-strips or a butterfly band-aid or should it be sutured by the team physician?

increases the probability of infection unless the wound is properly debrided and cleansed.

Punctures

Puncture wounds can easily occur during physical activities and have a high potential for infection. Direct penetration of tissues by a pointed object such as a track shoe spike can introduce the tetanus bacillus into the bloodstream. All puncture wounds and severe lacerations should be referred immediately to a physician.[36]

Lacerations

Lacerations are also common in sports and occur when a sharp or pointed object tears the tissues, giving the wound the appearance of a jagged-edged cavity.[20] Also, blunt trauma over a sharp bone can cause a wound that is similar in appearance to a laceration. As with abrasions, lacerations present an environment conducive to severe infection.[19] The same mechanism that causes a laceration can also cause a skin avulsion, in which a piece of skin is completely ripped from its source.

Skin Incisions

Incisions are similar to lacerations, but the cut is smooth as opposed to jagged as would occur with a knife or piece of glass. Incision wounds in sports often occur where a blow has been delivered over a sharp bone or over a bone that is poorly padded.

Skin Avulsions

Avulsion wounds occur when skin is torn from the body; they are often associated with major bleeding. The avulsed tissue should be placed on moist gauze that is preferably saturated with saline solution. The tissue and gauze are put into a plastic bag that is then immersed in cold water and taken, along with the athlete, to the hospital for possible reattachment.

Skin Bruises

The consequence of a sudden compressive, blunt force to the skin is a bruise. The skin is not broken, but the soft tissue is traumatized. A bruise (ecchymosis) results from the disruption of superficial blood vessels and results in black and blue discoloration. A great force affects the underlying structures, producing a bone or muscle contusion. Rest, ice, compression, and elevation (RICE) is the treatment of choice to control the hemorrhage that may occur.

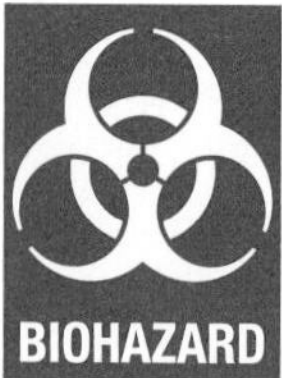

Wound Management

All open wounds should be cared for immediately (Table 28-4). All wounds, even those that are relatively superficial, must be considered contaminated by microorganisms and therefore must be cleansed, medicated (when called for), and dressed. Athletic trainers who perform wound management must pay strict attention to universal precautions.[16] In caring for wounds that involve bleeding and other body fluids, the athletic trainer must be concerned with the chance of becoming infected by the human immunodeficiency virus (HIV), hepatitis B, and hepatitis C (see Chapter 14).

In general all wounds must be cleansed with soap and water to minimize the chances of microorganism contamination.[7] After a thorough cleansing, a **dressing** containing an antiseptic should be applied. However, if the wound is to be examined by a physician, no medication should be added to the dressing.

dressing
Covering, protective or supportive, that is applied to an injury or wound.

Most lacerations and puncture wounds should be treated by a physician. Uninfected abrasions are not usually referred to a physician. They are managed by debridement and thorough cleansing with soap and water, followed by the application of an occlusive dressing.[18] Occlusive dressings are widely used by athletic trainers in wound care management.[32] There are three main types of occlusive dressings: semipermeable films, hydrogels, and hydrocolloids.[11] All have been shown to be more effective than conventional dressings in wound healing. Several explanations as to their effectiveness have

TABLE 28-4 Care of Open Wounds

Type of Wound	Action of Coach or Athletic Trainer	Initial Care	Follow-Up Care
Abrasion	Provide initial care. Wound seldom requires medical attention unless infected.	Cleanse abraded area with mild soap and water; debride with brush. Apply solution of hydrogen peroxide over abraded area; continue until foaming has subsided. Follow with povidone-iodine. Apply antibiotic ointment to keep abraded surface moist—in sports, it is not desirable for abrasions to acquire a scab. Place an occlusive dressing over the antibiotic.	Change dressing daily; look for signs of infection.
Laceration	Cleanse around wound; avoid wiping more contaminating agents into the area. Apply dry, sterile compress pad; refer to physician.	Complete cleansing and suturing are performed by physician; injections of tetanus toxoid are given, if needed.	Change dressing daily; look for signs of infection.
Puncture	Cleanse around wound; avoid wiping more contaminating agents into the area. Apply dry, sterile compress pad; refer to physician.	Complete cleansing and injections of tetanus toxoid are performed by physician, if needed.	Change dressing daily; look for signs of infection.
Incision	Clean around wound. Apply dry, sterile compress pad to control bleeding; refer to physician.	Cleanse wound. Suturing and injection of tetanus toxoid are performed by physician, if needed.	Change dressing daily; look for signs of infection.
Avulsion	Clean around wound; save avulsed tissue. Apply dry, sterile compress pad to control bleeding; refer to physician.	Wound is cleansed thoroughly; avulsed skin is replaced and sutured by a physician; tetanus toxoid injection is administered, if needed.	Change dressing daily; look for signs of infection.

been proposed: scab formation is minimized, perceived pain from exposed nerve endings is lowered; they are cost and time effective; they provide a barrier against bacteria; and, they make wound care easier.[11] Using a topical antibiotic ointment prevents secondary infection. If a wound is discharging fluid (serum), the dressing should be changed often to minimize bacterial growth.[27] After drainage has stopped, there is no need for a dressing. When changing the dressing, wounds may be cleansed with hydrogen peroxide or Betadine, which has been shown to be effective against bacteria yet not harmful to fibroblasts.[29] Antibacterial ointments should be reapplied to limit surface bacterial growth and to prevent the dressing from sticking to the wound. Good wound care will minimize the inflammatory response, speed healing and minimize scarring.

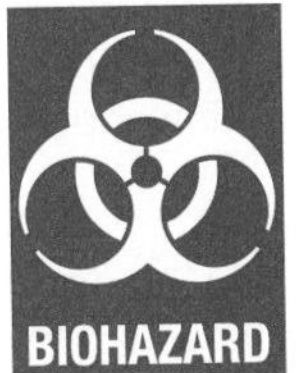

Are Sutures Necessary? Deeper lacerations, incisions, or occasionally puncture wounds may require some sort of manual closure using sutures.[20] If an athlete has a wound that appears to be severe, the athlete should be sent to the physician who will make a decision as to whether it is necessary to use sutures to close the wound. Sutures should be put in as soon as possible but certainly within a maximum of twelve hours following injury. In relatively simple wounds, the edges may be brought in close approximation by the use of sutures to minimize scar formation. Before closing a wound with a suture, the doctor will usually anesthetize the local area with a short acting anesthetic. Fine suture material and minimal tightening limit any additional tissue damage, inflammation and scarring. Wounds in areas that heal slower (areas that are less vascularized) or are in high stress areas require larger suture material and that the stitches be left in longer. Sometimes sutures may be removed after only a few days to minimize scarring.

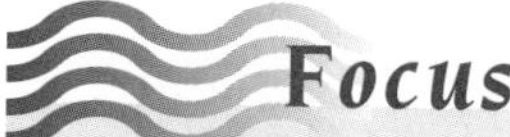

Wound care

1. Make sure all instruments such as scissors, tweezers, and swabs are sterilized.
2. Clean hands thoroughly and put on latex gloves.
3. Clean in and around a skin lesion thoroughly.
4. Place a nonmedicated dressing over a lesion if the athlete is to be sent for medical attention.
5. Avoid touching any part of a sterile dressing that may come in contact with a wound.
6. Place medication on a pad rather than directly on a lesion.
7. Secure the dressing with tape or a wrap; always avoid placing pressure directly over a lesion.

The physician may decide that the wound does not require sutures and that the torn tissues may be approximated using steri-strips or butterfly bandages. Generally lacerations, incisions, and puncture wounds require an innoculation with tetanus toxoid if a booster has not been given within ten years.

Athletic Training Room Practices in Wound Care *Focus Box:* "Wound care" suggests procedures to use in the athletic training room to cut down the possibility of wound infections. See Table 28-4 for more specific suggestions regarding the care of external wounds.

Athletes with bacterial infections associated with pus may pass the infection onto other athletes through direct contact.

BACTERIAL INFECTIONS

Bacteria are single-celled microorganisms that can be seen only with a microscope after they are stained with specific dyes. They are of three major shapes: spherical (cocci), which occur in clumps; doublets, or chains, and rods (bacilli); and spirochetes, which are corkscrew shaped.

Staphylococcus Genus of gram-positive bacteria normally present on the skin and in the upper respiratory tract and prevalent in localized infections.

Staphylococcus is a genus of gram-positive bacteria that commonly appear in clumps on the skin and in the upper respiratory tract. It is a common cause of skin infection.

Streptococcus Genus of gram-positive bacteria found in the throat, respiratory tract, and intestinal tract.

Streptococcus is also a genus of gram-positive bacteria, but unlike staphylococci, it appears in long chains. Most species are harmless, but some are among the most dangerous bacteria affecting humans. They can be associated with serious systemic diseases such as scarlet fever and, along with staphylococci, are common causes of skin infections.

Bacillus is a genus of bacteria belonging to the family Bacillaceae. They are spore forming, aerobic, gram-positive, and some are mobile. Most bacilli are not pathological; those that are can cause major systemic damage.

Impetigo Contagiosa

Impetigo contagiosa is an extremely common skin disease, primarily observed in children, with the greatest number of cases occurring in late summer and early fall.

Etiology *Impetigo contagiosa* is caused by group A beta-hemolytic streptococci, *S. aureus,* or a combination of these two bacteria. It is spread rapidly when athletes are in close contact with one another. Wrestling presents a particular risk for spreading this disease.[33]

28-5 Critical Thinking Exercise

A wrestler first experiences a mild itching and soreness in his left axillary region. Later, small pustules form that develop into yellow crusts.

? How should the athletic trainer handle this problem?

Symptoms and signs *Impetigo contagiosa* is first characterized by mild itching and soreness, which are followed by the eruption of small vesicles and/or pustules that rupture to form honey-colored crusts (Color Plate, Figure B). Up to 20 percent of people carry *Staphylococcus aureus* in and about their nostrils. In general, impetigo develops in body folds that are subject to friction.[37]

Management Impetigo usually responds rapidly to proper treatment. This treatment consists of thorough cleansing of the crusted area, followed by the application of

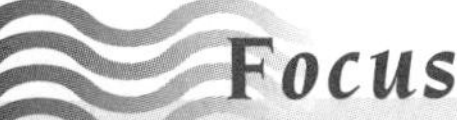

Management of impetigo

1. Wash vigorously four or five times daily, using a medicated cleansing agent and hot water to remove all the crustations.
2. After cleansing, dry the area by patting gently.
3. When completely dried, apply an antibiotic or prescribed medicated ointment.
4. Every precaution should be taken to make sure that the athlete uses isolated gym clothing and towels to prevent the spread of the disease.

a topical antibacterial agent such as Bactroban (see *Focus Box:* "Management of impetigo"). Systemic antibiotics also are used.

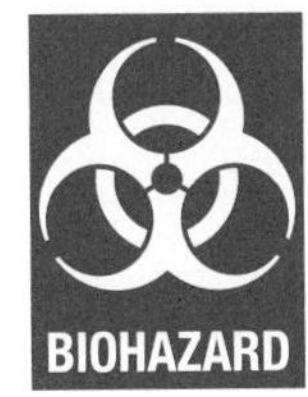

Furunculosis (Boils)

Furuncles (boils) are common among athletes.

Etiology Furuncles and carbuncles are infections of the hair follicle that usually result in pustule formation. Staphylococci are usually the responsible organism.

Symptoms and signs The areas of the body most affected are the back of the neck, the face, and the buttocks. The pustule becomes enlarged, reddened, and hard from internal pressure. As pressure increases, extreme pain and tenderness develop (Color Plate, Figure C). Most furuncles will mature and rupture spontaneously, emitting the contained pus. NOTE: Furuncles should not be squeezed, because squeezing forces the infection into adjacent tissue or extends it to other skin areas.[22] Furuncles on the face can be dangerous, particularly if they drain into veins that lead to venous sinuses of the brain. Such conditions should immediately be referred to a physician.

Management Care of the furuncle involves protecting it from additional irritation, referring the athlete to a physician for antibiotic treatment, and keeping the athlete from contact with other team members while the boil is draining. The common practice of hot dressings or special drawing salves is not beneficial to the maturation of the boil.

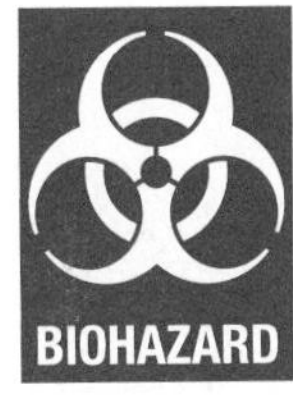

Carbuncles

Etiology Carbuncles are similar to furuncles in their early stages, having also developed from staphylococci.

Symptoms and signs The principle difference between it and a furuncle is that the carbuncle is larger and deeper and usually has several openings in the skin. It may produce fever and elevation of the white cell count. A carbuncle starts as a painful node that is covered by tight, reddish skin that later becomes very thin. The site of greatest occurrence is the back of the neck, where it appears early as a dark red, hard area and then in a few days emerges into a lesion that discharges yellowish-red pus from a number of places.

One must be aware of the dangers inherent in carbuncles—they may result in the athlete's developing an internal infection or may spread to adjacent tissue or to other athletes.

Management The most common treatment is surgical drainage combined with the administration of antibiotics. A warm compress is applied to promote circulation to the area.

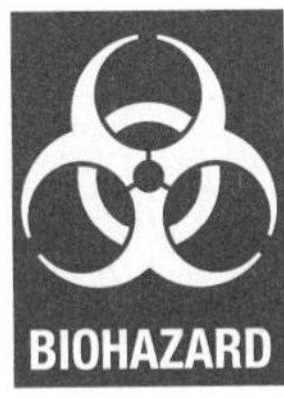

Folliculitis

Folliculitis is an inflammatory condition of the hair follicle. It is common in the hair follicles of the beard, scalp, groin and buttocks (Color Plate, Figure D); however, it can occur anywhere that hair exists on the body.

Etiology Folliculitis can be caused by either noninfectious or infectious agents. Occlusive folliculitis is a common form of noninfectious folliculitis in athletes. Moist, warm environments and mechanical occlusion contribute to create a primary irritant folliculitis. This is often seen in bicyclists who wear tight biking shorts. Pseudofolliculitis barbae (PFB) is common in African Americans and is due to penetration of the epidermis by curved hair; this creates a foreign body reaction in the skin that can mimic the appearance of folliculitis. PFB occurs most often in areas in which hair is shaved or rubs against clothing, such as the neck, face, buttocks, or thigh.[18] Infectious folliculitis can be due to bacteria (*Staphylococcus* or *Pseudomonas*), yeast (*Pityrosporum*), or mites (*Demodex follicularum*).

Symptoms and signs Folliculitis starts with redness around the hair follicle and is followed by the development of a papule or pustule at the hair follicle opening. This may be followed by the development of a crust that can later slough off along with the hair. A deeper infection may cause scarring and permanent baldness (alopecia) in that area. The most common microorganism associated with this condition is *Staphylococcus*.

Management The management of acute folliculitis is similar to that of impetigo. Moist heat is applied intermittently to increase local circulation. Antibiotic medication may be applied locally, as well as systemically, depending on the scope of the condition.

Hidradenitis Suppurativa

Hidradenitis suppurativa is a chronic inflammatory condition of the apocrine glands or large sweat glands commonly found in the axilla, scrotum, labia majora, and nipples.

Etiology The exact cause of this condition is unclear. Some authorities have suggested that a primary inflammatory event in the hair follicle results in secondary blockage and inflammation of the apocrine gland. The role of bacteria is not exactly known.

Symptoms and signs The condition begins as a small papule and grows to the size of a small tumor that is filled with purulent material. Deep dermal inflammation can occur, resulting in large abscesses that result in bands of scar tissue.[12]

Management Treatment of this problem includes avoiding the use of antiperspirants, deodorants, and shaving creams; using medicated soaps such as those containing chlorhexidine or povidone-iodine (Betadine); and applying a prescribed antibiotic lotion. Systemic antibiotics such as tetracycline and mincocyline are used for their antiinflammatory effects. In severe cases, surgical excision of skin containing the involved aprocrine glands can be curative.

Acne Vulgaris

Acne vulgaris is an inflammatory disease that involves the hair follicles and the sebaceous glands. It occurs near puberty and usually is less active after adolescence. Acne is characterized by closed comedones (whiteheads), open comedones (blackheads), papules, pustules, and cysts.

Etiology Although most adolescents experience some form of acne, only a few develop an extremely disfiguring case (Color Plate, Figure E). Its cause is not definitely known, but it has been suggested that sex hormones may contribute to the development of the acne. The hair follicles of acne patients have increased numbers of the anaerobic bacterium *Propionobacterium acnes*. *P. acnes* breaks down sebaceous gland triglycerides into free fatty acids, which contributes to the inflammatory reaction by attracting inflammatory cells to the follicle.

Symptoms and signs Acne can present with different types of lesions, including whiteheads, blackheads, flesh- or red-colored papules, pustules, or cysts. Commonly affected areas are the face, neck, and back. The superficial lesions usually heal spontaneously, whereas the deeper ones may become chronic and form disfiguring scars.[12]

The athlete with a serious case of acne vulgaris has a scarring disease and because of it may have serious emotional problems. The individual may become nervous, shy, and even antisocial, with feelings of inferiority in interpersonal relations with peer groups. The athletic trainer's major responsibility in aiding athletes with acne is to help the athlete follow the physician's directions and to give constructive guidance and counseling.[12]

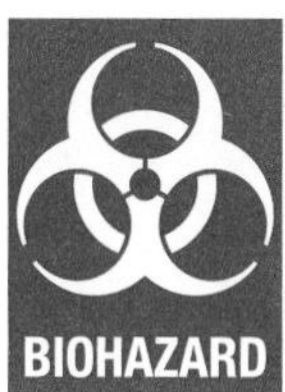

Management A variety of topical and systemic agents are used to treat acne. Over-the-counter preparations containing benzoyl peroxide formulated as washes or creams are helpful in mild cases. Topical antibiotics such as clindamycin (Cleocin) or erythromycin in combination with a topical retinoid such as Retin-A are useful for moderate acne. Treatment of more severe or inflammatory acne involves the use of the systemic antibiotics tetracycline, doxycycline, or mincocycline, which are used for their antiinflammatory effect. Severe, cystic acne is treated with the systemic retinoid Accutane. Accutane can cause profound birth defects, and its use is absolutely contraindicated in pregnant women. Women using Accutane are strongly advised to employ methods of birth control. Other therapeutic modalities include the manipulation of endogenous hormone levels with the use of certain formulations of oral contraceptives. Acne is not a result of having dirty skin, and excessive washing or the use of drying agents such as ethanol or isopropanol should be avoided, as these irritate the skin and cause excessive redness. Mild soaps and cleansers are recommended. Acne sufferers wishing to use cosmetics are advised to look for products listed as "non-comedogenic"; non-comedogenic products have been formulated to lessen the likelihood that they will block the hair follicles.

Paronychia and Onychia

Fingernails and toenails are continually subject to injury and infection in sports. A common infection is paronychia, which is a purulent infection of the proximal and/or lateral nail folds (the skin surrounding the nail; Color Plate, Figure F).

Etiology Paronychia and onychia develop from staphylococci, streptococci, and fungal organisms that accompany the contamination of open wounds or hangnails.[37] Infections are common in football linemen, who regularly stick their fingers in dirt. Loss of or damage to the cuticle, which forms a water-tight seal between the nail folds and the nail plate, is a risk factor for the development of paronychial infections.

Symptoms and signs Acute paronychia has a rapid onset, with painful, bright red swelling of the proximal and lateral nail fold. An accumulation of purulent material occurs within the nail fold.[12] The infection may spread and cause onychia and inflammation of the nail bed.

Management The athletic trainer should recognize paronychia early and have the athlete soak the affected finger or toe in a hot solution of Epsom salts or boric acid three times daily. Topical antibiotics are often used between soakings. Severe bacterial paronychia may require systemic antibiotics. The yeast *Candida albicans,* a common cause of nonbacterial paronychia in individuals whose hands are immersed in water for prolonged periods, can be treated with topical thymol in ethanol. The infected nail must be protected while the athlete is competing. Uncontrollable paronychia may require medical intervention, consisting of pus removal through a skin incision or the removal of a portion of the infected nail.

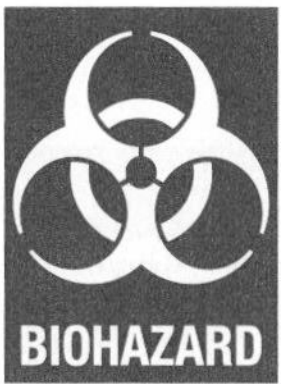

Tetanus Infection

Etiology **Tetanus (lockjaw)** is an acute infection of the central nervous system caused by the tetanus bacillus. The bacteria can enter the blood through an open wound.

tetanus (lockjaw) An acute, sometimes fatal condition characterized by tonic muscular spasm, hyperreflexia, and lockjaw.

Symptoms and signs The first sign of a tetanus infection is stiffness of the jaw and muscles of the neck. The muscles of facial expression produce contortion and become painful. The muscles of the back and extremities become tetanic. Fever becomes markedly elevated. Tetanus can be fatal.

Management The patient with an acute tetanus infection should be treated in an intensive care unit. Initial childhood immunization by tetanus toxoid is usually completed by the time a child reaches six years of age. Boosters should be given every five to ten years. An athlete not immunized should receive an injection of tetanus immune globulin (Hyper-Tet) immediately after injury.

FUNGAL INFECTIONS

Fungi are a group of organisms that include yeasts and molds. Fungal infections of the skin, hair, and nails are relatively common in athletes. Athlete's foot and jock itch are fungal infections of the foot and groin that are so named because of their prevalence in athletes.

Infection with superficial fungi takes place within the superficial keratinized tissue found in hair, nails, and the stratum corneum of the epidermis. These organisms are given the common name of ringworm (tinea) and are classified according to the area of the body infected. The contagious spores of these fungi may be spread by direct contact, contaminated clothing, or dirty locker rooms and showers. Diagnosis of a fungal infection can be made by microscopic examination of skin scrapings in which the keratinaceous material has been hydrolyzed by the addition of the base potassium hydroxide. Fungal cell walls are resistant to potassium hydroxide, and using this technique, an experienced observer can readily visualize the branching hyphae of dermatophytes or the pseudohyphae of candida.

Dermatophytes (Ringworm Fungi)

Etiology Dermatophytes, also known as ringworm fungi, are the cause of most skin, nail, and hair fungal infections. They belong to three genera: *Microsporum, Trichophyton,* and *Epidermophyton.*[24]

Tinea of the Scalp (Tinea Capitis)

tinea (ringworm) Common name given to many superficial fungal infections of the skin.

Symptoms and signs **Tinea (ringworm)** of the scalp *(tinea capitis),* beginning as a small papule of the scalp and spreading peripherally, is most common among children. The lesions appear as small, grayish scales, resulting in scattered bald patches. The primary sources of tinea capitis infection are contaminated animals, barber clippers, hairbrushes, and combs. This infection is easily spread among individuals with close physical contact.

Management Topical creams and shampoos cannot penetrate the hair shaft and are ineffective at eradicating tinea capitis infection. Systemic griseofulvin had been the treatment of choice; however, increased resistance to this medication has been observed, resulting in higher doses and more extended treatment. Because of increased resistance, the newer systemic antifungals itraconazole and terbenafine are replacing griseofulvin in the treatment of tinea capitis. Shampoos containing the antifungal ketoconazole may be used adjunctively to help prevent the spread of the disease.

Tinea of the Body (Tinea Corporis)

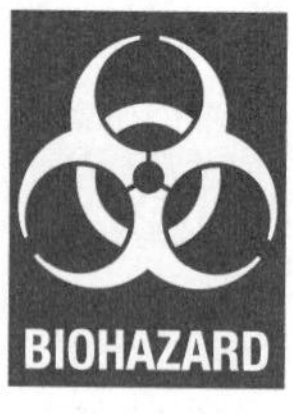

Symptoms and signs Tinea of the body *(tinea corporis)* commonly involve the extremities and trunk and present as an itchy, red-brown, scaling, annular ("ring-shaped") plaque that expands peripherally and clears centrally (Color Plate, Figure G). Excessive perspiration and friction increase susceptibility to the condition.[23]

Management Treatment usually consists of a topical antifungal cream such as 2 percent miconazole, 1 percent clotrimazole, or 1 percent econazole nitrate, applied once to twice a day.

Tinea of the Nail (Tinea Unguium/Onychomycosis)

Symptoms and signs Tinea of the nail *(tinea unguium)* is a fungal infection of the toenails and/or fingernails. It is often seen among athletes who are involved in water sports or who have chronic athlete's foot. Trauma predisposes the athlete to infection.[40] Many different organisms, including the dermatophyte species *Trichophyton* and *Epidermophtyon,* the molds *Scopulariopsis* and *Aspergillus,* and the yeast *Candida,* can infect the nail plate. Culture of the infected nail plate is helpful in identifying the causative agent. When infected, the nail becomes thickened, brittle, and separated from its bed.

Management The treatment of *tinea unguium* can be difficult. In general, topical creams or lotions do not penetrate the nail; however, a recent topical antifungal (Penlac) has been formulated and shown to clear infections in 12 percent of patients. The systemic medications itraconazole (Sporanox) and terbenafine (Lamisil) are the most effective drugs for onychomycosis, but they must be used for at least three months if the infection is to be cleared. Surgical removal of the nail may have to be performed on the athlete with extremely infected nails.[31]

Tinea of the Groin (Tinea Cruris)

Etiology Tinea of the groin *(tinea cruris)*, more commonly called jock itch, appears as a bilateral and often symmetric red-brown scaling plaque with a serpiginous (snakelike) border. Tinea cruris may resemble the outline of a butterfly in the groin area. Erythrasma, a bacterial infection, can often mimic the appearance of tinea cruris, but it is characterized by the absence of scale.

Symptoms and signs The athlete complains of mild to moderate itching, resulting in scratching and the possibility of a secondary bacterial infection (Color Plate, Figure H).

Management The athletic trainer must be able to identify lesions of tinea cruris and handle them accordingly. Conditions of this type must be treated until cured. Most ringworm infections will respond to many of the nonprescription medications that are available as aerosol sprays, liquids, powders, or ointments. Ointments are perhaps the most commonly used medication. Medications that are irritating or tend to mask the symptoms of a groin infection, such as the topical corticosteriod hydrocortisone, should be avoided. The failure to respond to normal management may suggest a nonfungal skin problem such as the bacterial infection erythrasma or a primary inflammatory dermatoses, and the athlete should be referred to the team physician.

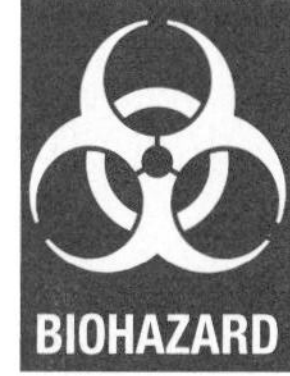

Atypical or complicated groin infection must receive medical attention. Secondary bacterial infection is not an uncommon problem and will not respond to topical antifungals. Superficial fungal infections in immunocompromised individuals may not respond to topical over-the-counter medications. Additional topical and oral prescription medications are available and effective in treating these patients.

Athlete's Foot (Tinea Pedis)

Etiology Dermatophyte infection of the foot, *tinea pedis* or athlete's foot, is the most common form of superficial fungal infection. *Tricophyton* species, particularly *T. rubrum*, are the most common cause of athlete's foot. *T. rubrum* causes a moccasin style *tinea pedis* characterized by an itchy, dry, scaling infection of the sole of the foot. Web space infections located between the toes are often caused by *T. mentagrophytes*. Toe webs that become macerated and infected may result from a mixed infection with the yeast *Candida* and gram-negative rods, in addition to or replacing the original dermatophyte.[38] The athlete wearing shoes that are enclosed will perspire, encouraging fungal growth. However, contagion is based mainly on the athlete's individual susceptibility. There are other conditions that may also be thought to be athlete's foot, such as allergic contact or eczematous dermatitis (Color Plate, Figure I).

Symptoms and signs Athlete's foot can present in many ways but appears most often as an extreme itching on the soles of the feet and between and on top of the toes. It appears as a dry, scaling patch or inflammatory, scaling red papules that may coalesce to form larger plaques. More inflammatory, blistering variants of athlete's foot are due to zoophilic dermatophytes, fungi such as *Microsporum canis* that normally infect animals. Scratching can cause the tissue to become inflamed and secondarily infected with bacteria.[9]

Management Topical antifungals as discussed previously for *tinea corporis* are effective in the treatment of *tinea pedis*. Of major importance is good foot hygiene (see *Focus Box:* "Basic care of athlete's foot").[26]

28-6

Critical Thinking **Exercise**

Fungal infections are commonly found among athletes. Fungi grow best in unsanitary conditions combined with an environment of warmth, moisture, and darkness.

? What are the symptoms and signs of the fungal infection *tinea pedis*?

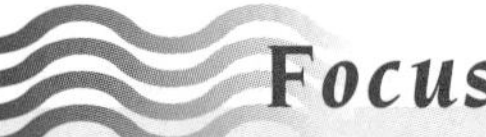

Basic care of athlete's foot

- Keep the feet as dry as possible through frequent use of talcum powder.
- Wear clean white socks to avoid reinfection, and change them daily.
- Use a standard fungicide for specific medication. Over-the-counter medications such as Desenex and Tinactin are useful in the early stages of the infection. For stubborn cases see the team physician; a dermatologist may need to make a culture from foot scrapings to determine the best combatant to be used.

The best cure for the problem of athlete's foot is prevention. To keep the condition from spreading to other athletes, the following steps should be faithfully followed by individuals in the sports program:

- All athletes should powder their feet daily.
- All athletes should dry their feet thoroughly, especially between and under the toes, after every shower.
- All athletes should keep sports shoes and street shoes dry by dusting them with powder daily.
- All athletes should wear clean sports socks and street socks daily.
- The shower and dressing rooms should be cleaned and disinfected daily.

Candidiasis (Moniliasis)

Candidiasis is a yeastlike fungus that can produce skin, mucous membrane, and internal infections.

Etiology *Candidiasis* is caused by the yeastlike fungus *Candida albicans* and some other species. It will attack the skin, as well as other structures, if the environment is right. Weather that is hot and humid, tight clothing that rubs, and poor hygiene provide the ideal environment for fungal growth.

Symptoms and signs Among athletes, candidiasis commonly causes candidal intertrigo, a skin infection of body folds such as the axilla and groin. Noninfectious interigo, a dermatitis of the same body folds that may be precipitated by occlusion, heat, and moisture, can predispose an individual to develop secondary candidal intertrigo. Both candidal and noncandidal intertrigo present as beefy red patches, but *candidal intertrigo* can be distinguished from noncandidal variants by the additional presence of satellite pustules.[21] In cases in which it occurs where the skin is folded, a white, macerated border may surround the red area. Later, deep, painful fissures may develop where the skin creases.

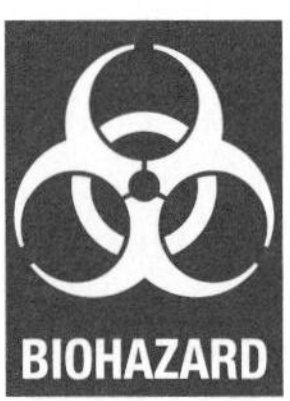

Management The first concern in treatment is to maintain a dry area. Antifungal creams containing miconazole, ketoconazole, or econazole applied twice daily will clear the infection. (NOTE: Genital candidiasis is discussed in Chapter 29 in the section on sexually transmitted diseases.)

Tinea Versicolor

Tinea versicolor is a common fungal infection of young adults.

Etiology *Tinea versicolor* is caused by the yeast *Malassezia furfur* (synonyms *Pityrosporum ovale, P. orbiculare, M. ovalis*). *M. furfur* is a normal part of the skin's flora, appearing commonly in areas in which sebaceous glands actively secrete body oils (Color Plate, Figure J).

Symptoms and signs The fungus characteristically produces multiple, small, circular macules that are pink, brown, or white. They commonly occur on the abdomen, neck, and chest. The lesions do not tan when exposed to the sun and are usually asymptomatic.

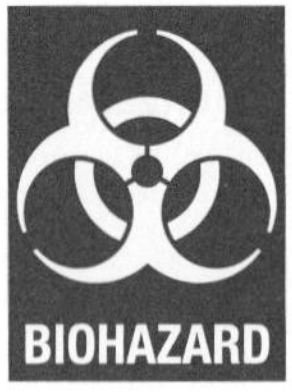

Management Treatment of *tinea versicolor* is straightforward; however, recurrences are common. Treatment options include selenium sulfide (Selsun shampoo) applied topically for ten minutes each day for one to two weeks, topical econazole nitrate or ketoconazole, or systemic ketoconazole. Once the microorganism has been eradicated, repigmentation of the affected areas will occur, but may take up to several months.

VIRAL INFECTIONS

Viruses are ultramicroscopic organisms that require host cells to complete their life cycle. Entering a tissue cell, the virus exists as nucleic acid. Inside, the virus may stimulate the cell chemically to produce more virus until the host cell dies or the virus is ejected to infect additional cells. Instead of killing the cell, a budlike growth may occur, with harm to the cell, or the virus may remain within a cell without ever causing an infection. A number of skin infections are caused by viruses.

Common viruses that attack the skin of athletes:

- Herpes virus
- Verruca
- Poxvirus (molluscum contagiosum)

Herpes Simplex Labialis, Gladiatorum, and Herpes Zoster

Herpes simplex is a strain of virus that is associated with skin and mucous membrane infection. Types 1 and 2 cause cutaneous lesions and are indistinguishable from one another (Color Plate, Figures K and Y); however, type 1 is found, for the most part, extragenitally and type 2 genitally. However, both can be found anywhere on the skin or mucous membrane.

Etiology *Herpes simplex* is highly contagious and is usually transmitted directly through a lesion in the skin or mucous membrane. After the initial outbreak, it is thought to move down a sensory nerve's neurilemmal sheath to reside in a resting state in a local ganglion. Recurrent attacks can be triggered by sunlight, emotional disturbances, illness, fatigue, infection, or other situations that may stress the organism.[8] However, sunlight does not adversely affect the reactivation rate if a sunscreen of sun protection factor (SPF) 15 is used.

Symptoms and signs Not all individuals infected with the virus develop overt symptoms.[8] An early indication that a herpes infection is about to erupt is a tingling or hypersensitivity in the infected area twenty-four hours before the appearance of lesions. Local swelling occurs, followed by the appearance of vesicles. The athlete may feel generally ill with a headache and sore throat, lymph gland swelling, and pain in the area of lesions. The vesicles generally rupture in one to three days, spilling out a serous material that will form into a yellowish crust. The lesions will normally heal in ten to fourteen days.

Genital herpes is discussed in Chapter 29. Of the two areas of the body most often affected, *herpes labialis* (cold sore) is usually the less symptomatic, *Herpes simplex* gladiatorum is the more serious, with lesions commonly on the side of the face, neck, or shoulders, which occurs quite often in wrestlers. *Herpes simplex* infection is so highly contagious that it may run rampant through an entire team in a short time. Wrestlers having any signs of a herpes infection should be disqualified from body contact until these lesions have crusted and dried. *Herpes zoster* appears in a specific pattern on the body in an area that is innervated by a specific nerve root. It may appear on the face or anywhere on the trunk. It is the chicken pox virus that has remained dormant for many years (Color Plate, Figure L).

28-7 Critical Thinking Exercise

An athlete comes into the training room concerned about multiple, small, white, circular macules on the abdomen, neck, and chest.

? What possible infection could cause these symptoms?

28-8 Critical Thinking Exercise

An athlete experiences a tingling and sometimes painful sensation in the upper lip region. Twenty-four hours later, swelling occurs followed by the formation of vesicles. The athlete also experiences a mild headache, sore throat, and lymph gland swelling.

? What condition does this scenario describe, and how could the later symptoms have been prevented?

Management *Herpes simplex* lesions are self-limiting. Therapy usually is directed toward reducing pain and promoting early healing. Antiviral drugs such as acyclovir are used to shorten the course and reduce the recurrence of herpes outbreaks.[3,4] Quite often acyclovir is administered prophylactically.

Complications *Herpes simplex,* if not carefully managed, can lead to secondary infection. A major problem is keratoconjunctivitis, an inflammation of the cornea and conjunctiva that could lead to loss of vision and that must be considered a medical emergency.

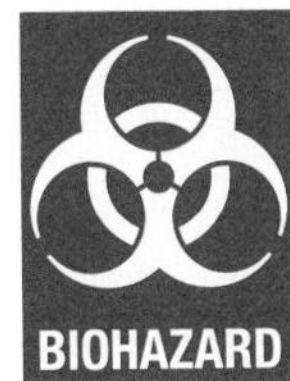

Verruca Virus and Warts

Numerous forms of verruca exist, including the *verruca plana* (flat wart), *verracu plantaris* (plantar wart), and the *condyloma acuminatum* (venereal wart) (Color Plate, Figure Z). Different isotypes of human papilloma virus have been identified. The human papillomavirus uses the skin's epidermal layer for reproduction and growth. The verruca wart enters the skin through a lesion that has been exposed to contaminated fields, floors, or clothing. Contamination can also occur from exposure to other warts.

Common Wart

Etiology *Verruca vulgaris* and plana are prevalent on the hands of children (Color Plate, Figure M).

Symptoms and signs This wart appears as a small, round, elevated lesion with rough, dry surfaces. It may be painful if pressure is applied. These warts are subject to secondary bacterial infection, particularly if they are located on the hands or feet, where they may be constantly irritated.

Management Vulnerable warts must be protected until they can be treated by a physician. The application of a topical salicylic acid preparation or liquid nitrogen and electrocautery are the most common ways of managing this condition.

Plantar Warts

28-9 Critical Thinking Exercise

A tennis player complains to the athletic trainer that she has a sharp pain in the ball of her right foot. She says that it feels as though she stepped on a piece of glass. On inspection, the athletic trainer observes excessive callus formation on the ball of the foot that is dotted with a cluster of black specks.

? What is this condition, and how should it be managed?

Etiology Plantar warts are found on the sole of the foot, on or adjacent to areas of abnormal weight bearing. The papillomavirus can be spread to the hands and other body parts.

Symptoms and signs Plantar warts are seen as areas with excessive epidermal thickening and cornification (Color Plate, Figure N). They produce general discomfort and point tenderness in the areas of excessive callus formation. Commonly the athlete complains that the condition feels as though he or she has stepped on broken glass. A major characteristic of the plantar wart is hemorrhagic puncta, which look like clusters of small black seeds.

Management There are many different approaches to the treatment of warts. In general, while the athlete is competing, a conservative approach is taken. Concern is to protect the wart against infection and to keep the growth of the warts under control. A common approach to controlling plantar warts is the careful paring away of accumulated callous tissue and the application of a keratolytic such as 40 percent salicylic acid plaster. When the competitive season is over, the physician may decide to remove the wart by freezing it with liquid nitrogen or by electrodessication. Until its removal, a wart should be protected by a doughnut pad. A plantar wart may also be treated using salicylate iontophoresis.[39]

Molluscum Contagiosum

Etilogy *Molluscum contagiosum* is a poxvirus infection. It is more contagious than warts, particularly during direct body contact activities such as wrestling (Color Plate, Figure O).

Symptoms and signs *Molluscum contagiosum* appear as small, flesh- or red- colored, smooth-domed papules with a central umbilication. When this condition is identified, it must be referred immediately to a physician.

Management Treatment often consists of cleansing thoroughly and using a destructive procedure. Destructive procedures include the use of a powerful counterirritant such as cantharidin (Cantharone), surgical removal of the lesion, or cryosurgery, using liquid nitrogen.

ALLERGIC, THERMAL, AND CHEMICAL SKIN REACTIONS

Skin reactions to allergy:
- Reddening
- Elevated patches
- Eczema

The skin can react adversely to a variety of nonpathogenic influences. Among the most common affecting athletes are allergies, temperature extremes, and chemical irritants.[9]

Allergic Reactions

The skin displays allergic reactions in various ways (Color Plate, Figures P and Q). An allergy is an immunologically mediated reaction to molecules such as a dye or protein (termed allergens) against which the body's immune system has been previously sensitized. Allergens may be foods, drugs, clothing, dusts, pollens, plants, animals, heat, cold, or light. The skin may reflect an allergy in several ways, such as reddening and swelling

COMMON BACTERIAL INFECTIONS

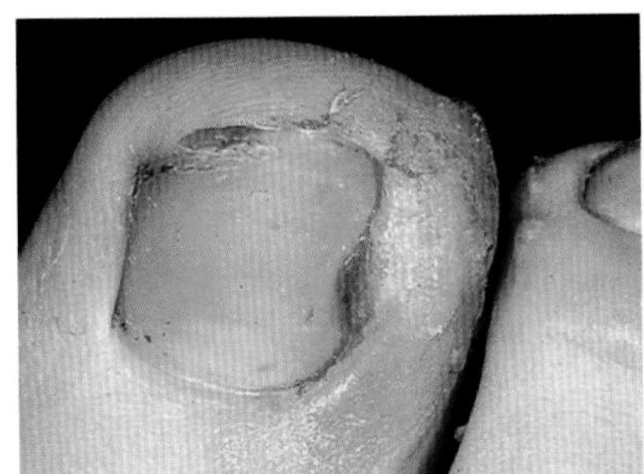

Figure A

Ingrown toenail.

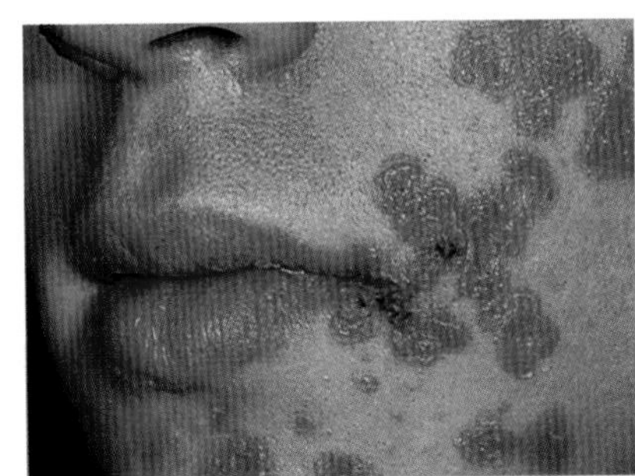

Figure B

Impetigo contagiosa.

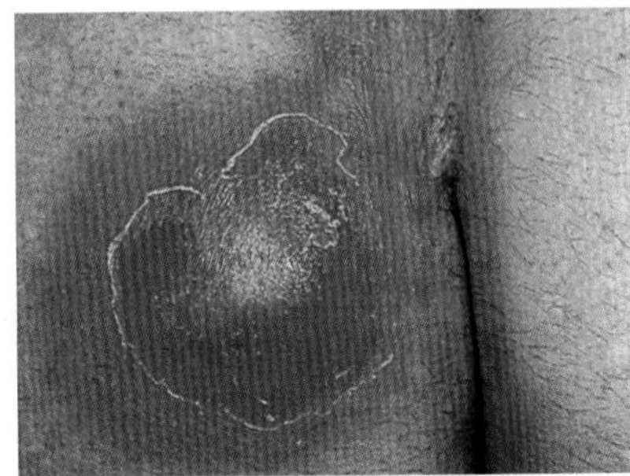

Figure C

Furuncle.

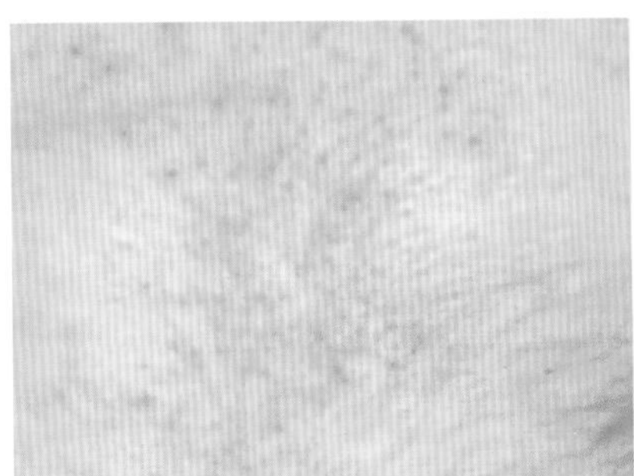

Figure D

Folliculitis.

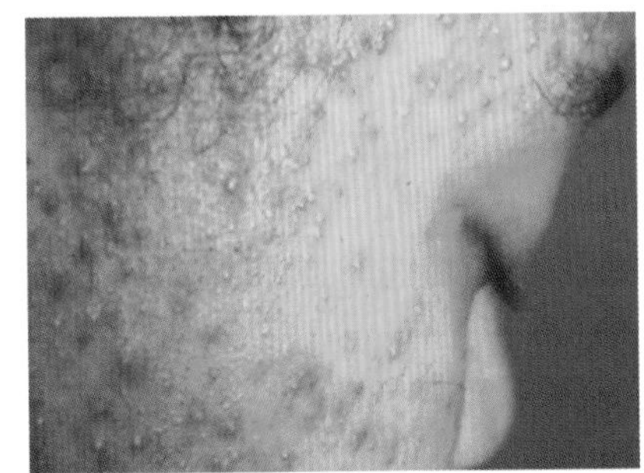

Figure E

Acne vulgaris.

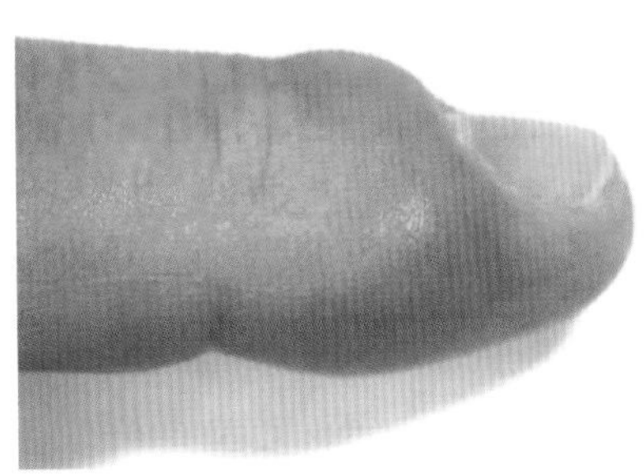

Figure F

Paronychia.

COMMON SEXUALLY TRANSMITTED INFECTIONS

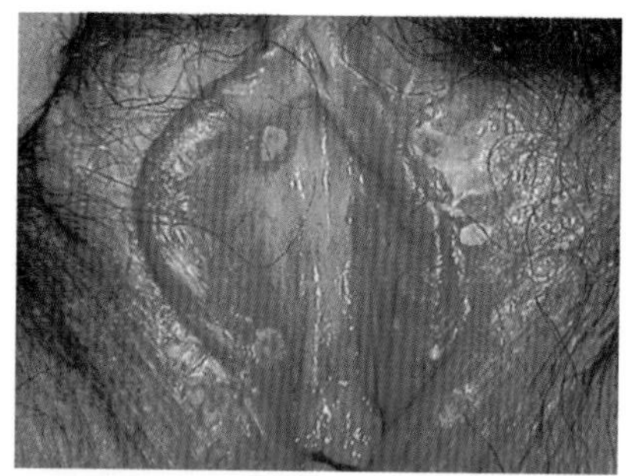

Figure Y

Genital herpes simplex (Type 2).

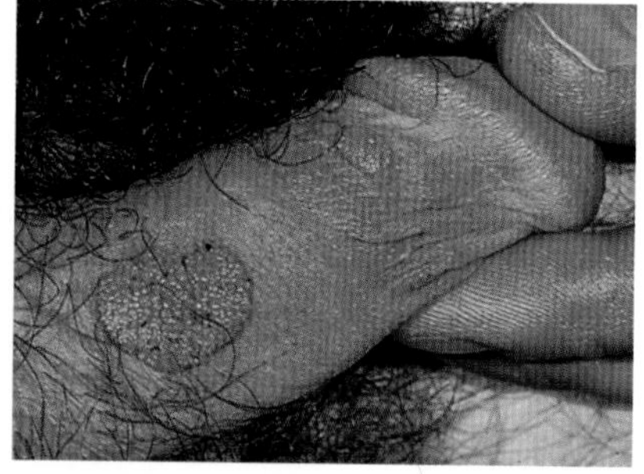

Figure Z

Genital warts.

of the tissue, which may occur either locally or generally from an increased dilation of blood capillaries. Different clinical patterns of allergy are reflective of the causative immunologic mechanism. For example, immediate hypersensitivity reactions manifest as *urticaria* or *hives*, which appear as red edematous elevations (wheal, papule, or plaque) of the skin, characterized by a burning or an itching sensation. Delayed-type hypersensitivity reactions can manifest as acute dermatitis, which appears as intensely pruritic erythematous papules, plaques, and vesicles. *Eczema* is a term commonly used to describe an acute inflammatory dermatosis characterized by redness, edema, papules and/or vesicles or a chronic inflammatory dermatosis characterized by erythema, lichenification (thickening of the skin that exaggerates the skin lines), and scale.

Urticaria = Hives

The athletic trainer should be able to recognize gross signs of allergic reactions and should then refer the athlete to the physician. Treatment usually includes avoidance of the sensitizing agents and the use of a topical or systemic antipruritic agent (such as calamine lotion and antihistamines, respectively) and/or topical or systemic corticosteroids.

Contact Dermatitis (Allergic and Irritant)

There are many substances in the sports environment to which the athlete may be allergic, causing a skin reaction. Allergic contact dermatitis represents an immunologically mediated reaction to a foreign substance, whereas irritant contact dermatitis represents a nonimmunologic reaction to a chemical irritant.

Etiology The most common plants that cause allergic contact dermatitis are poison ivy, poison oak, sumac, ragweed, and primrose.[19] Over time the athlete may become allergic to topical medications such as antibiotics, antihistamines, anesthetics, or antiseptics. Chemicals such as fragrances and preservatives commonly found in soaps, detergents, and deodorants can create an allergic reaction; detergents and soaps themselves are more likely to cause an irritant contact dermatitis, which is not a hypersensitivity reaction, but rather represents a primary chemical irritant. Some athletes are allergic to materials in the adhesive used in athletic tape. Also, the countless chemicals used in the manufacture of shoes, clothing, and other materials have been known to produce allergic contact dermatitis.

Symptoms and signs The period of onset from the time of initial exposure may range from one day to one week. The skin reacts with redness, swelling, and the formation of vesicles that ooze fluid and form a crust. A constant itch develops that is increased with heat and made worse by rubbing. Secondary infection is a common result of scratching (Color Plate, Figure R). Over time, the morphology may change from the redness and blistering of acute contact dermatitis to the erythematous, scaling, lichenified papules and plaques characteristic of chronic contact dermatitis.

Management The most obvious treatment approach is to determine the allergic contactant or irritant and avoid it. This may not always be simple and may require extensive testing. In the acute phase, tap water compresses or soaks soothe and dry the vesicles. Topical corticosteroids may be beneficial.[19]

28-10
Critical Thinking **Exercise**

Actinic dermatitis, or sunburn, occurs from overexposure to the sun's rays.

? What should an athlete be told about the sun's rays?

Miliaria (Prickly Heat)

Prickly heat is common in sports and occurs most often during the hot season of the year in those athletes who perspire profusely and who wear heavy clothing.

Etiology Continued exposure to heat and moisture causes retention of perspiration by the sweat glands and subsequent miliaria.

Symptoms and signs Miliaria results in itching and burning vesicles and pustules.[3] It occurs most often on the arms, trunk, and bending areas of the body.

Management Care of prickly heat requires avoidance of overheating, frequent bathing with a nonirritating soap, wearing loose-fitting clothing, and the use of antipruritic lotions.

Chilblains (Pernio)

Etiology Chilblains is a common type of dermatitis caused by excessive exposure to cold.

Symptoms and signs The tissue does not freeze but reacts with edema, reddening, possibly blistering, and a sensation of burning and itching after exposure to cold. The parts of the body most often affected are the ears, face, hands, and feet.

Management Treatment consists of exercise and a gradual warming of the part. Massage and the application of heat are contraindicated in cases of chilblains. The systemic drug nifedipine can be used for more severe cases. (See Chapter 6 for more information about reactions to cold.)

Burns

Burns can result from excessive exposure to thermal, chemical, electrical, or radiation sources. In a sports environment, the athlete is certainly most susceptible to radiation burns from exposure to sunlight.

Sunburn

Serious skin damage can occur from overexposure to the sun's rays. Sunburn represents an inflammatory response to ultraviolet radiation–induced skin damage.

Etiology Sunburn is an inflammatory response to injury caused by ultraviolet solar radiation that varies in intensity from a mild erythema (pink color) to a severe blistering reaction. Every protection should be given to athletes who have thin, white skin. Their skin tends to absorb a greater amount of ultraviolet radiation than more pigmented individuals. Individuals who may be taking photosensitizing drugs such as thiazide diuretics, some tetracyclines, and phenothiazine are also sensitive. The chemical psoralen in oil of limes, parsnips, and celery, as well as other foods, can produce a severe adverse reaction in some individuals who expose themselves to sunlight.

Symptoms and signs If a large area of the skin is sunburned, the athlete may display all the symptoms of severe inflammation accompanied by shock. A sunburn can cause malfunctioning of the organs within the skin, which in turn may result in the infection of structures such as hair follicles and sweat glands.

Sunburn appears two to eight hours after exposure. Symptoms become most extreme in approximately twelve hours and dissipate in seventy-two to ninety-six hours. After once receiving a severe sunburn, the skin is more susceptible to burning.[13] The skin remains injured for months after a severe sunburn has been sustained. Prevention of sunburn should be accomplished by the judicial use of sunscreens that filter ultraviolet light. Products containing chemical blocks such as parsol 1789 or physical blocks such as titanium dioxide are very effective sunscreens. The amount of protection provided by sunscreens is determined by the sun protection factor (SPF).[13] An SPF of 15 means that it would require 15 times longer to sustain the same amount of UV radiation with the sunscreen than without. Water-resistant or waterproof sunscreens are recommended for athletics, since nonwaterproof sunscreens are easily washed away by perspiration. Constant overexposure to the sun can lead to chronic skin thickening, damage, and the development of skin cancers.[5]

Management A sunburn is treated according to the degree of inflammation present. Mild burns are best treated using cool water in a shower or bath. Aloe-based compounds have also proved beneficial. Moderate and severe burns can be relieved by a tub bath in which a pound of cornstarch is used; a vinegar solution will also help. Severe sunburn may be treated by a physician with corticosteroids and other anti-inflammatory drugs.

Ultraviolet radiation is damaging—it can prematurely age the skin and can increase the chances of skin cancers. Basal cell and squamous cell carcinomas are the most common cancers.[38]

Psoriasis

Etiology This is a relatively common chronic disease of the skin that causes itching. The exact cause of psoriasis is not known, but there is some genetic factor present. Certain conditions such as infection, smoking, some drugs, climate, and maybe hormonal factors may cause an outbreak.

Symptoms and signs The lesions begin as reddish papules that collectively form plaques with distinctive borders. As the condition progresses, the lesions develop a yellowish-white, scaly appearance (Color Plate, Figure S). The lesions may occur anywhere but are most likely to appear on the elbows, knees, scalp, genitalia, and trunk, particularly around the umbilicus. Trauma causes new lesions to appear.

Management Treatment involves teaching the patient how to self-manage this condition. Topical glucocorticoids in combination with a kerolytic agent to remove the scales are used, thus enhancing penetration of the glucocorticoids. Calciportriene ointment is used to inhibit the proliferation of keratinocytes. In severe cases that are resistant to treatment, long-term oral medications may be warranted. Counseling may be required to help the individual deal with the psychological aspects of managing these lesions.

INFESTATION AND BITES

Certain parasites cause dermatoses or skin irritations when they suck blood, inject venom, and even lay their eggs under the skin. Athletes who come in contact with these organisms may develop various symptoms such as itching, allergic skin reactions, and secondary infections from insult or scratching. The more common parasitic infestations and bites in sports are caused by mites, crab lice, fleas, ticks, mosquitoes, and stinging insects such as bees, wasps, hornets, and yellow jackets.

Depending on the part of the country in which the athlete resides, parasites such as mites, crab lice, fleas, ticks, mosquitoes, and stinging insects can cause serious discomfort and infection.

Scabies

Etiology Scabies is a skin disease caused by the mite *Sarcoptes scabiei,* which produces extreme nocturnal itching (Color Plate, Figure T). The parasitic itch mite is small, with the female causing the greatest irritation. The mite burrows a tunnel approximately one-quarter to one-half inch (1.25 cm) long into the skin to deposit its eggs.

Symptoms and signs The mite's burrows appear as dark lines between the fingers, toes, body flexures, nipples, and genitalia. Excoriations, pustules, and papules caused by the resulting scratching frequently hide the true nature of the disease. The young mite matures in a few days and returns to the skin surface to repeat the cycle. The skin often develops a hypersensitivity to the mite, which produces extreme itching.

Management Permethrin 5 percent cream (Elimite) is the treatment of choice for individuals over two months of age. It should be applied topically from the neck down overnight. Affected family members should be similarly treated and bedding and clothing should be thoroughly washed in hot, soapy water. Gamma benzene hexachloride (Lindane) is no longer the treatment of choice because it is absorbed systemically through the skin and causes central nervous system toxicity. Resistant cases can be treated with the systemic agent Ivermectin. Because of the athlete's itching and scratching, secondary infections are common and must also be treated (see *Focus Box: "Treatment of scabies"*). After treatment with a scabecide, itching can be controlled with a topical corticosteroid cream.

28-11

Critical Thinking **Exercise**

A cross-country runner complains to the athletic trainer of extreme nocturnal itching. Observation of the athlete's skin reveals dark lines in the area of the finger and toes.

? What insect infestation does this scenario describe?

Focus

Treatment of scabies

- The entire body should be thoroughly cleansed, with attention to skin lesions.
- Bedding and clothing should be disinfected.
- The coating of gamma benzene hexachloride (Lindane) should be applied on the lesions for three nights.
- All individuals who have come in contact with the infected athlete should be examined by the physician.
- Locker and game equipment must be disinfected.

Lice (Pediculosis)

Etiology Pediculosis is an infestation by the louse, of which three types are parasitic to humans. The *Pediculus humanus capitis* (head louse) infests the head, where its eggs (nits) attach to the base of the hair shaft (Color Plate, Figure U). The *Phthirus pubis* (crab louse) lives in the hair of the pubic region and lays its eggs at the hair base. The *Pediculus humanus corporis* (body louse) lives and lays its eggs in the seams of clothing.

Symptoms and signs The louse is a carrier of many diseases; its bite causes an itching dermatitis, which, through subsequent scratching, provokes pustules and excoriations.

Management Cure is rapid with the use of any of a number of agents. NIX is a synthetic pyrethroid permethrin that is available over the counter and is very effective in treating head and pubic lice. NIX shampoo should be lathered into the affected area, allowed to sit for ten minutes, and then rinsed away. The area should be re-treated after seven to ten days. Body lice can be treated by overnight application of 5 percent permethrin cream. To prevent reinfestation, all clothing and bedding should be washed in hot, soapy water or discarded.

Fleas

Etiology Fleas are small, wingless insects that suck blood. Singly, their bites cause only minor discomfort to the recipient. Certain species of fleas can transmit the systemic diseases bubonic plague and endemic typhus.

Symptom and signs When there are a large number of biting fleas, a great deal of discomfort can occur. After attaching themselves to a moving object such as a dog or a human, most fleas bite in patterns of three. Fleas seem to concentrate their bites on the ankle and lower leg.

Management Once the flea bite has been incurred, the main concern is to prevent itching with an antipruritic lotion such as calamine or a topical corticosteroid. Scratching the bite should be avoided to prevent a secondary infection. Areas in which fleas abound can be sprayed with selected insecticides containing malathion or some other effective insecticide.

28-12

Critical Thinking Exercise

The lacrosse team takes a team retreat hiking in the woods. One of the players returns from the trip and finds a tick on his leg.

? What signs and symptoms should the athlete look for as a warning sign of a disease transmission?

Ticks

Etiology Ticks are parasitic insects that have an affinity for the blood of many animals, including humans. They are carriers of a variety of microorganisms that can cause Rocky Mountain spotted fever or Lyme disease.[14] Because ticks are commonly found on grass and bushes, they can easily become attached to the athlete who brushes against them.

Symptoms and signs Rocky Mountain spotted fever (RMSF) and Lyme disease are characterized by constitutional symptoms, including headache, fever, malaise, myalgia, and rash. Petechiae and purpura (small dark spots that retain their color when pressure is applied) localized to the distal arms, legs, hands, and feet characterize the skin manifestations of RMSF. Erythema chronicum migrans, an enlarging annular red ring with or without a central red papule, is the typical rash of Lyme disease (Color Plate, Figure V).

Management To remove a tick, mineral oil or fingernail polish is applied to its body, at which time it will withdraw its head. Grasping or pulling the tick by its head is an acceptable method for removal. RMSF and Lyme disease are serious illnesses with significant morbidity and mortality that require systemic antibiotic treatment by a physician.

Mosquitoes

Etiology Unless it is the carrier of a disease, the mosquito, as a blood sucker, produces a bite that causes only mild discomfort. Generally mosquitoes are attracted to lights, dark clothing, and warm, moist skin.

Symptoms and signs The mosquito bite produces a small reddish papule. Multiple bites may lead to a great deal of itching.

Management Itching is most often relieved by the application of a topical medication such as calamine lotion or topical corticosteroids. In climates where mosquitoes are prevalent, repellents should be used directly on the skin.

Stinging Insects

Etiology Bees, wasps, hornets, and yellow jackets inflict a venomous sting that is temporarily painful for most individuals; however, some hypersensitive individuals may respond with an allergic reaction that may be fatal. Stings to the head, face, and neck are particularly dangerous to the athlete. Athletes having a history of allergic reactions from stings must be carefully monitored after a sting for an anaphylactic reaction. To avoid stings, the athlete should not wear scented lotions or shampoos; should not wear brightly colored clothes; should not wear jewelry, suede, or leather; and should not go barefoot. Athletes predisposed to anaphylactic reactions from stings should be provided with and instructed in the use of an EpiPen.[5]

Symptoms and signs The allergic athlete may respond with an increase in heart rate, fast breathing, chest tightness, dizziness, sweating, and even loss of consciousness.

Management In uncomplicated sting cases, the stinging apparatus must be carefully removed with tweezers, followed by the application of a soothing medication. Detergent soap applied directly on the sting often produces an immediate lessening of symptoms. In severe reactions to a sting, the athlete must be treated for anaphylactic shock and referred immediately to a physician.[28] Sensitive athletes who perform outdoors should avoid using scented cosmetics, scented soap, colognes, or aftershave lotions and colorful, floral, or dark-colored clothing.

28-13

***Critical Thinking* Exercise**

An athlete who is allergic to bee stings is stung.

? What physical reactions should the athlete be expected to have?

Spider Bite

Etiology Most spiders are not dangerous to humans, although all spiders have some amount of venom with varying degrees of potency. Bite marks from most spiders are usually too small to easily be seen. Frequently the patient will not recall being bitten. Spiders rarely bite more than once. The two spiders most likely to cause significant problems are the black widow and the brown recluse. The black widow spider is a shiny black spider with red to orange-colored markings, usually in the shape of an hourglass found on the underside of the belly. The brown recluse has a violin-shaped body with long legs.

Symptoms and signs Most spider bites will result in pain, small puncture wounds, redness, itching and swelling that lasts a couple of days (Color Plate, Figure W). The wound will have a center blister surrounded by a red ring and then a white ring. The blister breaks open, leaving an ulcer that scabs over. A bite from a black widow or a brown recluse may result in severe muscle pain and cramps in the back, shoulders, abdomen and thighs within the first two hours. Other symptoms include weakness, sweating, headache, anxiety, itching, nausea, vomiting, difficult breathing, and increased blood pressure.

Management Treatment consists of washing the wound and applying an antibiotic ointment. The victim should seek medical attention if there are signs of an infection; an ulcer that does not heal; or a bite accompanied by nausea, vomiting, fever or a rash. If muscle cramps develop, the victim should be taken to the nearest emergency facility.

OTHER SKIN CONDITIONS

Pityriasis rosea

Etiology This is an acute inflammatory skin rash of unknown origin that occurs most commonly in people between the ages of ten and thirty-five, but may occur at any age. It may occur at anytime of year, but it is most common in the spring and fall. It is not a sign of any internal disease, nor is it caused by a fungus, a bacteria, or an allergy.

There is recent evidence suggesting that it may be caused by a virus since the rash resembles certain viral illnesses, and occasionally a person feels slightly ill for a short while just before the rash appears. However, this has not been proven. It does not seem to spread from person to person and it usually occurs only once in a lifetime.

Symptoms and signs Pityriasis rosea is characterized initially by a single pinkish-red patch called a "herald patch" that appears somewhere on the chest or back and over several days enlarges to a few centimeters. Within two days to three weeks a secondary macular eruption occurs on the trunk over the ribs and on the upper extremities. The lesions are red and scaly with a clearing in the center (Color Plate, Figure X). They appear in a symmetrical distribution over the trunk and extremities. Usually there are no permanent marks as a result of this condition, although some darker-skinned persons may develop long-lasting flat brown spots that eventually fade.

Management Most cases usually do not need treatment and fortunately, even the most severe cases eventually go away. The rash gradually disappears over a two- to ten-week period. Local application of antipruretics may help to relieve itching. Occasionally, anti-inflammatory medications such as corticosteroid may be necessary to stop itching or make the rash go away.

SUMMARY

- The skin is the largest organ of the human body. It is composed of three layers: the epidermis, the dermis, and the subcutis. The outermost layer, the epidermis, acts as protection against infections from a variety of sources. The dermis contains sweat glands, sebaceous glands, and hair follicles. The subcutis layer is the major area for fat storage and temperature regulation.
- Primary skin lesions include macules, papules, plaques, nodules, tumors, cysts, wheals, vesicles, bulla, and pustules. Secondary skin lesions include scales, crusts, fissures, erosions, ulcers, and scars.
- Microorganisms, trauma, allergies, temperature variations, chemicals, infestations, and insect bites can cause skin lesions.
- Sports participation can place a great deal of mechanical force on the skin, which can lead to many different problems. Abnormal friction causes hyperkeratosis, blisters, and intertrigo. Hyperhidrosis adds to the problems of skin friction and infections. A tearing force can lacerate or avulse skin. Compression can bruise, scraping abrades, and a pointed object can puncture.
- Providing immediate proper care is essential to avoid skin infections. Streptococcal and staphylococcal bacteria are associated with wound contamination, and the tetanus bacillus can cause lockjaw.
- *Impetigo contagiosa* is a highly infectious disease among athletes and is associated with both the staphylococcal and streptococcal bacteria. Furuncles, carbuncles, and folliculitis are staphylococcal-caused afflictions and can be spread by direct contact.
- The sports environment, which is often one of excessive moisture, warmth, and darkness, is conducive to fungal growth. An extremely common fungus, ringworm, is under the general heading of dermatophytes. Under the right conditions, these fungi can attack a wide variety of body tissues.
- *Herpes simplex* is a virus associated with *herpes labialis* and *herpes gladiatorum*. Human papillomavirus causes a variety of warts such as the plantar wart *verruca plantaris* or the common wart *verruca vulgaris*. The poxvirus causes *molluscum contagiosum*, a highly contagious wart spread by direct contact.
- Athletes are also subject to many other causes of skin conditions, including allergies, extremes of heat or cold, and chemical irritations.
- One major problem that produces an insidious destruction of the skin is prolonged overexposure to sunlight.
- Different parts of the country have problems with insect infestations and bites. Two of these problems are scabies (caused by mites) and pediculosis (from lice), and there are others that may be produced by fleas, ticks, mosquitoes, and stinging insects.

Websites

American Academy of Dermatology: www.aad.com

American Society for Dermatologic Surgery: http://www.asds_net.org

American Society of Dermatology: http://www.asd.org

Canadian Dermatology Association: http://dermatologie.ca

Dermatology Foundation: http://www.dermatologyfoundation.org

UWEC Student Health Service Dermatology Information: http://www.uwec.edu/Admin/HlthSvs/derm.htm

Solutions to Critical Thinking EXERCISES

28-1 Initially, the skin flap should be completely removed. The area should be cleaned with soap and water, and the antiseptic liquid benzalkonium should be applied along with an occlusive dressing. After the game, a second-skin dressing should be applied to the raw area.

28-2 To prevent intertrigo, the skin should be kept dry, clean, and friction free. The athlete who is prone to this problem should wear loose cotton underwear. Males should wear a supporter over underwear.

28-3 A major concern for this abrasion is infection. The abraded area should be cleaned with mild soap and debrided with a brush. The injury should be covered with an antibiotic ointment to prevent scabbing, and a nonocclusive dressing should be applied.

28-4 Because this laceration is on the face, the best advice is to have this wound sutured by a qualified physician as soon as the contest has ended.

28-5 This skin condition is the highly contagious disease *impetigo contagiosa*. The athlete must not have physical contact with other athletes until the disease is resolved. It is managed with daily thorough cleansing of crusted material followed by an application of an antibiotic salve or oral medication.

28-6 With *tinea pedis,* there is severe itching on the top of and between the toes and on the soles of the feet. A rash occurs with blisters that secrete a yellow serum. Scratching can cause an infection. A red, white, or grayish scaling may also be present.

28-7 It is likely that the athlete has *tinea versicolor.* Treatment of this condition is difficult and recurrences are common. Perhaps the most effective treatment is to use selenium sulfide. Pigment changes occur slowly even after the microorganism has been eradicated.

28-8 This condition is a herpes simplex viral infection. Once the herpes virus is contracted it is impossible to get rid of it. When symptoms begin to appear the athlete should be referred immediately to a physician for a prescription drug called acyclovir, which can minimize symptoms.

28-9 The black specks are plantar warts. The accumulated callus should be pared down and a 40 percent salicylic acid plaster should be applied. A doughnut pad should be used to protect the area.

28-10 Athletes should be cautioned to use sunscreen routinely to prevent the damaging effects of overexposure to sunlight.

28-11 This scenario describes infestation by the mite Sarcoptes scabiei. Another name for this condition is scabies. The mite burrows a tunnel under the skin to deposit her eggs. The eggs hatch, and the young mites return to the skin surface to repeat the cycle. A hypersensitivity develops that causes extreme itching at night.

28-12 Headache, fever, malaise, myalgia, and a rash are symptoms of both Rocky Mountain spotted fever and Lyme disease. Any small dark spots or an enlarging red ring also may indicate that the athlete may have contracted a disease from the tick.

28-13 The athlete may experience an anaphylactic reaction with an increase in heart rate, fast breathing, chest tightness, dizziness, sweating, and possibly a loss of consciousness. This condition is a medical emergency.

REVIEW QUESTIONS AND CLASS ACTIVITIES

1. Describe the skin's anatomy and functions. Describe lesions that are indicative of infection.
2. Contrast the microorganisms that are related to skin infections.
3. Relate the mechanical forces of friction, compression, shearing, stretching, scraping, tearing, avulsing, and puncturing to specific skin injuries.
4. List the steps to take in managing major skin traumas.
5. How should wounds be managed to avoid serious infections?
6. Characterize the different viruses that are associated with common skin infections that occur in sports.
7. What bacterial skin infections are commonly seen in athletes?
8. Tinea (ringworm) is a fungus that can be present on different parts of the body. Name the body parts.
9. How may skin infections related to microorganisms be avoided?
10. Why is candidiasis considered one of the most serious fungal infections in sports?
11. What allergic, thermal, and chemical skin reactions could an athlete sustain in the typical sports environment?
12. Different parts of the United States have their own problems with insects that infect the skin of humans. Identify the insects in your area that can cause problems to athletes. How may they be avoided?

REFERENCES

1. Allen AC: Skin. In Damjanou I, editor: *Anderson's pathology,* ed 10, Philadelphia, 1996, Elsevier Science.
2. American Academy of Orthopaedic Surgeons: *Athletic training and sports medicine,* ed 2, Park Ridge, Ill, 1991, American Academy of Orthopaedic Surgeons.
3. Anderson BJ: Herpes gladiatorum: anti-viral therapy. In *Proceedings, National Athletic Trainers' Association 51st Annual Meeting and Clinical Symposia,* Champaign, Ill, 2000, Human Kinetics.
4. Anderson BJ: The effectiveness of valacyclovir in preventing reactivation of herpes gladiatorum in wrestlers, *Clin J Sports Med* 9(2):86, 1999.
5. Arntizen KR: Dermatologic issues. In Agostini R, editor: *Medical and Orthopaedic Issues of Active and Athletic Women,* Philadelphia, 1994, Hanley & Belfus.
6. Basler RSW, Garcia MA: Acing common skin problems in tennis players, *Physician Sportsmed* 26(12):37, 1998.
7. Baxter DE: *The foot and ankle in sport,* St Louis, 1995, Mosby.
8. Bergfeld WF, Munnings F: How to manage herpes in active patients, *Physician Sportsmed* 22(9):71, 1994.
9. Brooks CD: Cutaneous allergic reactions induced by sporting activities. *Sports Med* 33(9):699, 2003.
10. Burkhart CG: Skin disorders of the foot in active patients, *Physician Sportsmed* 27(2):88, 1999.

11. Claus EE, Fusco CF, Ingram T, Ingersoll CD, Edwards JE, Melham TJ: Comparison of the effects of selected dressings on the healing of standardized abrasions, *J Ath Train* 33(2):145, 1998.
12. Conklin RJ: Acne vulgaris in the athlete, *Physician Sportsmed* 16(10): 65, 1988.
13. Davis JL: Sun and active patients: preventing acute and cumulative skin damage, *Physician Sportsmed* 28(7):79, 2000.
14. Dodds WN: Ticks: danger lurking in the long grass, *British Journal of Sports Medicine* 32(2):235, 1998.
15. Dougherty TM: Sports dermatology: what certified athletic trainers and therapists need to know. *Athletic Therapy Today* 8(3):46, 2003.
16. Fincher LA: Wound care management, *Athletic Therapy Today* 4(1):11, 1999.
17. Fletcher SB et al: Medicated compress for blister treatment, *J Ath Train* 28(1):81, 1993.
18. Foster DT et al: Management of wounds, *J Ath Train* 30(2):135, 1995.
19. Garner LA: Poison ivy, oak, and sumac dermatitis: identification, treatment, and prevention, *Physician Sportsmed* 27(5):33, 1999.
20. Glazer JL: Laceration care. *Physician Sportsmed* 30(7):50, 2002.
21. Habif TP: *Clinical dermatology,* Philadelphia, 2003, Elsevier Science.
22. Hamann BP: *Disease: identification, prevention, and control,* St Louis, 2001, McGraw-Hill.
23. Hand JW, Wroble RR: Prevention of tinea corporis in collegiate wrestlers, *J Ath Train* 34(4):350, 1999.
24. Kohl TD et al: Wrestling mats: are they a source of ringworm infections? *J Ath Train* 35(4):427, 2000.
25. Leski MJ: Common dermatological conditions in sports: a review of environmental, traumatic, and infectious causes. *Athletic Therapy Today* 7(3):8, 2002.
26. Mackey S: Relieving winter skin discomfort, *Physician Sportsmed* 23(1):53, 1995.
27. Martin M: Problematic external wound healing after ACL-reconstructive surgery. *Athletic Therapy Today* 7(3):36, 2002.
28. Norris RL: Managing arthropod bites and stings, *Physician Sportsmed* 26(7):47, 1998.
29. Rabenberg V, Ingersoll C, Sandrey M: The bactericidal and cytotoxic effects of antimicrobial wound cleansers, *J Ath Train* 37(1):51, 2002.
30. Ramsey ML: Clearing up fungal infections of the nail plate, *Physician Sportsmed* 21(2):70, 1993.
31. Rheinecker SB: Wound management: the occlusive dressing, *J Ath Train* 30(2):143, 1995.
32. Riemann BL: Use of occlusive dressings in wound management, *Athletic Therapy Today* 2(1):42, 1997.
33. Rubin A: Managing abrasions and lacerations, *Physician Sportsmed* 26(5):45, 1998.
34. Rush S: Sports dermatology. *ACSM's Health & Fitness Journal* 6(4):24, 2002.
35. Sammarco GJ: Soft tissue injuries. In Torg JS, editor: *Current therapy in sports medicine,* ed 3, St Louis, 1995, Mosby.
36. Scheinberg RS: Exercise-related skin infection, *Physician Sportsmed* 22(6):47, 1994.
37. Scheinberg RS: Stopping skin assailants: fungi, yeasts, and viruses, *Physician Sportsmed* 22(7):33, 1994.
38. Simandl G: Alterations in skin function and integrity. In Porth CM, editor: *Pathophysiology: Concepts of Altered Health States,* Philadelphia, 2004, Lippincott, Williams & Wilkins.
39. Soroko YT, Repking MC, Clemment JA, et al: Treatment of plantar verrucae using 2% sodium salicylate iontophoresis. *Phys Ther* 82:1184, 2002.
40. Tanzi EL, Scher RK: Managing common nail disorders in active patients and athletes, *Physician Sportsmed* 27(9):35, 1999.
41. Thibodeau GA, Patton KT: *Anatomy and physiology,* ed 5, Philadelphia, 2002, Elsevier Science.
42. Williams JGP: *Color atlas of injuries in sports,* Chicago, 1990, Year Book.

ANNOTATED BIBLIOGRAPHY

Bolognia J, Jorizzo J, Rapini R: *Dermatology,* Philadelphia, 2003, Elsevier Science.

Featuring over 3,000 full-color photographs and line drawings, this text focuses on the clinical aspects of dermatology and only includes "need-to-know" basic science.

Douglas LG: Facial injuries. In Torg JS, Welsh RP, Shephard RJ, editors: *Current therapy in sports medicine,* vol 2, Philadelphia, 1990, Decker.

This text contains an excellent overview of the major open skin wounds that occur among athletes.

Fitzpatrick TB, Wolff K, Suurmond D, Johnson RA: *Color atlas and synopsis of clinical dermatology,* New York, 2000, McGraw-Hill.

*This text presents an outstanding and varied array of skin conditions, from the most common to those that are life-threatening.*Habif T: *Clinical dermatology: a color guide to diagnosis and therapy,* Philadelphia, 2003, Elsevier Science.

This illustrated guide to the diagnosis and treatment of skin abnormalities and diseases covers various topical therapies as well as specific skin diseases such as dermatitis, warts, and tumors.

Habif T: *Clinical dermatology: a color guide to diagnosis and therapy,* Philadelphia, 2003, Elsevier Science.

This illustrated guide to the diagnosis and treatment of skin abnormalities and diseases covers various topical therapies as well as specific skin diseases such as dermatitis, warts, and tumors.

McCulloch JM, Kloth L: *Wound healing: alternatives in management,* ed 3, Philadelphia, 2002, FA Davis.

Originally intended for physical therapists, this text is appropriate for any health professional involved in the management of wounds.

Additional General Medical Conditions

Chapter 29

When you finish this chapter you should be able to

- Analyze the role of the immune system in preventing disease.
- Differentiate different viral infections that may affect the athlete.
- Identify symptoms and signs of respiratory infections.
- Categorize disorders of the muscular system.
- Examine disorders associated with the nervous system.
- Recognize disorders of the vascular and lymphatic systems.
- Explain diabetes mellitus, and contrast diabetic coma and insulin shock.
- Indicate the causes of epilepsy and explain how to perform the appropriate action when a seizure occurs.
- Explain what causes hypertension and how it may be controlled.
- Describe the classic signs and symptoms of cancer.
- Compare and contrast the signs and symptoms of the most common sexually transmitted infections.
- Explain menstrual irregularities and their effect on the athlete.
- Review female reproduction and pregnancy as they relate to the athlete.

In addition to the many injuries that have been discussed in previous chapters, a variety of additional medical conditions can potentially affect the athlete. Like everyone else, athletes inevitably become ill. When illnesses occur, it is the athletic trainer's responsibility to recognize these conditions and to follow up with appropriate care. Appropriate care for the illnesses and conditions discussed in this chapter often means referring the athlete to a physician to provide medical care that is well beyond the scope of the athletic trainer. The information provided in this chapter serves as a reference for the athletic trainer in making appropriate decisions regarding care of the sick athlete.

THE ROLE OF THE IMMUNE SYSTEM

The immune system is not an organ system but is instead a collection of disease-fighting cells that recognize the presence of foreign substances in the body and act to neutralize or destroy them.[40] Illness results when the immune system fails to neutralize or destroy the invading offender. Immunity means being protected from a disease by having been previously exposed to an invading agent, called an *antigen*. Immunity may be acquired *actively* as a result of a natural infection or invasion of antigens, or *passively* from inoculation.[39]

An immune response disposes of the antigen and thus prevents damage. The immune response may be *cell-mediated,* in which lymphocytes (T cells) are produced by the thymus in response to the antigen exposure. There may also be a *humoral immune response* in which plasma lymphocytes (B cells) are produced with subsequent formation of *antibodies*. A *nonspecific immune response,* or inflammation, is the reaction of the tissues to injury from trauma, chemicals, or ischemia. These immune responses are all positive responses that collectively act to destroy or neutralize an antigen.[43]

An autoimmune response directed against an individual's own tissues causes damage. Autoimmune diseases include, among others, diabetes mellitus, rheumatoid arthritis, multiple sclerosis, hemolytic anemia, myasthenia gravis, and HIV.

VIRAL INFECTIONS

Athletes, like everyone else, are highly susceptible to viral infection. Among the more common viral infections are rhinovirus (common cold), influenza (flu), infectious mononucleosis, rubella (German measles), rubeola (measles), mumps, and varicella-zoster (chicken pox).

Rhinovirus (Common Cold)

The common cold (coryza) is the most prevalent of all communicable diseases. It is referred to as an upper respiratory infection.

Etiology More than 100 different rhinoviruses cause colds. Colds are transmitted by either direct or indirect contact. They are spread by droplets expelled by a person with a cold who sneezes, coughs, or speaks. One method of infection is by touching a contaminated article and then rubbing the eyes.[15]

Symptoms and signs Frequently the cold begins with a scratchy or sore throat, watery discharge or stopped-up nose, and sneezing. Not all colds follow the same pattern. In some instances, a secondary bacterial infection occurs, which produces a thickened yellowish nasal discharge, watering eyes, mild fever, sore throat, headache, **malaise,** myalgia, and dry cough. In addition to the secondary infection can be laryngitis (hoarseness), tracheitis (irritation of the trachea), acute bronchitis, sinusitis, and even an inflammation of the middle ear (otitis media).

malaise
Discomfort and uneasiness caused by an illness.

Management Treatment of the common cold is symptomatic. Most colds last for five to ten days regardless of treatment. Nonprescription cold medications may help ease some symptoms. To avoid colds, athletes should stay out of crowds, wash their hands frequently, avoid sharing personal items, eat a balanced diet, and drink at least eight 8-ounce glasses of water per day. Emotional stress and extreme fatigue should be avoided as much as possible.[52] Late in 2001, medical researchers developed the first medicine proven to reduce the length and severity of the common cold. The drug called *pleconaril* seems to cause symptoms to clear up sooner than normal. It is thought that the medication attacks the rhinovirus.

Recently the use of Breathe Right nasal strips has been recommended as a drug-free alternative for managing nasal congestion due to colds and allergies. When adhered to the nose, the nasal strips have two springlike pieces that pull upwards, mechanically "lifting" open the nasal passages.[36] Many athletes routinely use these nasal strips to facilitate breathing (Figure 29-1).

Influenza (Flu)

Influenza, commonly known as the flu, is one of the most persistent and debilitating diseases. It usually occurs in various forms as an annual epidemic that causes severe illness among the population.[42]

Etiology Influenza is caused by myoviruses classified as types A, B, and C. Type A influenza is the most common and causes serious and widespread epidemics. The virus enters the cell through its genetic material. The virus multiplies and is released from the cell by a budding process, to be spread throughout the body. Not all athletes need influenza vaccines; however, athletes engaging in winter sports, basketball, wrestling, and swimming may require them.[35]

Symptoms and signs The athlete with the flu will have the following symptoms: fever, cough, headache, malaise, and inflamed respiratory mucous membranes with **coryza.** Certain viruses can increase the body's core temperature. Flu generally has an incubation period of forty-eight hours and comes on suddenly, accompanied by chills

coryza (core **eez** ah)
Profuse nasal discharge.

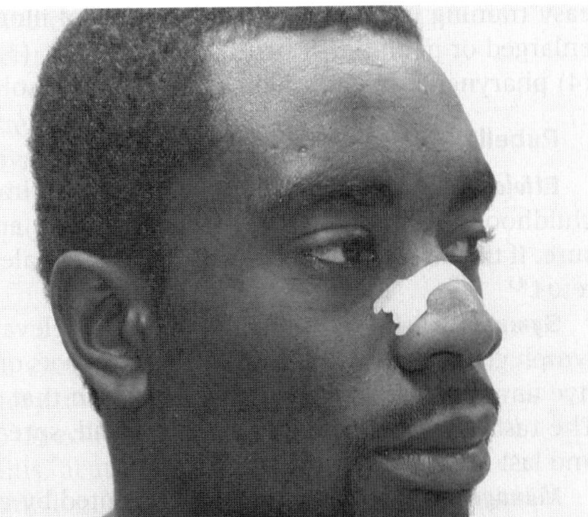

Figure 29-1

Nasal strips mechanically lift open the nasal passages.

and a fever of 102° to 103° F (39° to 39.5° C), which develops over a twenty-four-hour period. The athlete complains of a headache and general aches and pains—mainly in the back and legs. The headache increases in intensity, and the athlete may develop **photophobia** and an aching at the back of the skull. There is often sore throat, burning in the chest, and in the beginning, a nonproductive cough, which later may develop into bronchitis. The skin is flushed, and the eyes are inflamed and watery. The acute stage of the disease usually lasts up to five days. Weakness, sweating, and fatigue may persist for many days. Flu prevention includes avoiding infected persons and maintaining good resistance through healthy living. Vaccines, including prevalent strains, may be recommended to individuals to decrease the incidence or severity of illness.

photophobia
Unusual intolerance to light.

Management If the flu is uncomplicated, its management consists of bed rest and supportive care. During the acute stage, the temperature often returns to normal. Symptomatic care such as aspirin should be avoided for all individuals under eighteen years of age because of Reye's syndrome. Amantadine and Relenza are medications that may be used for influenza A for individuals at risk. They are also beneficial for fever and respiratory symptoms.[4] Steam inhalation, cough medicines, and gargles may be given.

29-1 Critical Thinking Exercise

A high school swimmer complains of a fever, cough, headache, malaise, aching in the back of the head, and a sore throat along with light sensitivity.

? What condition is this scenario describing, and how could it be managed?

Infectious Mononucleosis

Infectious mononucleosis is an acute viral disease that affects mainly young adults and children.

Etiology Infectious mononucleosis, commonly called mono, is caused by the Epstein-Barr virus (EBV), a member of the herpes group.[21] It has major significance to athletes because it can produce severe fatigue and raise the risk of splenic rupture.[35] Incubation is four to six weeks. The EBV is carried in the throat and transmitted to another person through saliva. It has been called the kissing disease.[15]

Symptoms and signs The EBV syndrome usually starts with a three- to five-day prodrome of headache, fatigue, loss of appetite, and myalgia. From days 5 to 15, there is fever, swollen lymph glands, and a sore throat.[15] By the second week 50 percent to 70 percent of those infected with EBV will have an enlarged spleen, 10 percent to 15 percent will have jaundice, and 5 percent to 15 percent will have a skin rash, a pinkish flush to the cheeks, and puffy eyelids.[35] A blood test will reveal an elevated white blood cell count. Complications include ruptured spleen, meningitis, encephalitis, hepatitis, and anemia.[15]

29-2 Critical Thinking Exercise

A lacrosse player comes to the training room complaining that for the past three days he has had a headache, fatigue, loss of appetite, muscle aches, swollen lymph glands, and a sore throat. He also complains of mild tenderness in the left upper quadrant of the abdomen.

? What illness is likely to cause these symptoms?

Management Treatment is supportive and symptomatic. Acetaminophen is often given for headache, fever, and malaise. Mellion indicates that "athletes may resume

Management The throat should be cultured to look for streptoccocal bacteria, and if the culture is positive, antibiotics should be used for ten days. Gargling with warm saline solution, a liquid diet, and antipyretic medication should all be recommended. Frequent bouts of tonsillitis may eventually necessitate surgical removal of the tonsils.[45]

Seasonal Atopic (Allergic) Rhinitis (Hay Fever)

Hay fever, or pollinosis, is an acute seasonal allergic condition that results from airborne pollens.

Etiology Hay fever can occur during the spring as a reaction to pollens from trees such as oak, elm, maple, alder, birch, and cottonwood. During the summer, grass and weed pollens can be the culprits. In the fall, ragweed pollen is the prevalent cause. Airborne fungal spores also have been known to cause hay fever. These substances act as allergens and cause an allergic reaction in susceptible people. The body's immune system produces allergic antibodies that release the chemical histamine, which produces the symptoms of hay fever.[10]

Symptoms and signs In the early stages, the athlete's eyes, throat, mouth, and nose begin to itch; these symptoms are followed by watering of the eyes, sneezing, and a clear, watery, nasal discharge. The athlete may complain of a sinus-type headache, emotional irritability, difficulty sleeping, red and swollen eyes and nasal mucous membranes, and a wheezing cough.[4] Other adverse allergic conditions are asthma, anaphylaxis, urticaria, angioedema, and rhinitis.[5,44]

Management Most athletes obtain relief from hay fever through oral antihistamines. However, antihistamines may cause a sedating effect that the athlete must be aware of. The use of decongestants can cause a stimulating effect.

Acute Bronchitis

An inflammation of the mucous membranes of the bronchial tubes is called bronchitis. It occurs in both acute and chronic forms. If it occurs in an athlete, bronchitis is more likely to be in the acute form.

Etiology Acute bronchitis usually occurs as an infectious winter disease that follows a common cold or other viral infection of the nasopharynx, throat, or tracheobronchial tree. Secondary to this inflammation is a bacterial infection that may follow overexposure to air pollution. Fatigue, malnutrition, or becoming chilled could be predisposing factors.

Symptoms and signs The symptoms of an athlete with acute bronchitis usually start with an upper respiratory infection, nasal inflammation and profuse discharge, slight fever, sore throat, and back and muscle pains. A cough signals the beginning of bronchitis. In the beginning, the cough is dry, but in a few hours or days, a clear mucus secretion begins, which becomes yellowish, indicating an infection. In most cases, the fever lasts three to five days, and the cough lasts two to three weeks or longer. The athlete may wheeze, and rales may be present when auscultation of the chest is performed. Pneumonia could complicate bronchitis. To avoid bronchitis, an athlete should not sleep in an area that is extremely cold or exercise in extremely cold air without wearing a face mask to warm inhaled air.

Management Management of acute bronchitis requires that the athlete rest until fever subsides, drink 3 to 4 quarts (3 to 4 liters) of water per day, and ingest an antipyretic analgesic, a cough suppressant, and an antibiotic (when severe lung infection is present) on a daily basis.

Pneumonia

Etiology Pneumonia is an infection of the alveoli and bronchioles that may be caused by viral, bacterial, or fungal microorganisms. It may also be caused by irritation from chemicals, aspiration of vomitus, or other agents.[35] The alveolar spaces become filled with exudate, inflammatory cells, and fibrin.

Symptoms and signs If the cause of pneumonia is bacterial, there will be a rapid onset. High fever with chills, pain on inspiration, decreased breath sounds and

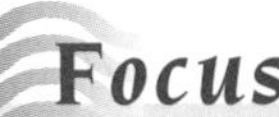

Focus

Management of the acute asthmatic attack

Athletes who have a history of asthma usually know how to care for themselves when attack occurs. However, the athletic trainer must be aware of what to look for and what to do if called on.

Early symptoms and signs

- Anxious appearance
- Sweating and paleness
- Flared nostrils
- Breathing with pursed lips
- Fast breathing
- Vomiting
- Hunched-over body posture
- Physical fatigue unrelated to activity
- Indentation in the notch below the Adam's apple
- Sinking in of rib spaces as the athlete inhales
- Coughing for no apparent reason
- Excess throat clearing
- Irregular, labored breathing or wheezing

Actions to take

- Attempt to relax and reassure the athlete.
- If medication has been cleared by the team physician, have the athlete use it.
- Encourage the athlete to drink water.
- Have the athlete perform controlled breathing along with relaxation exercises.
- If an environmental factor triggering the attack is known, remove it or the athlete from the area.
- If these procedures do not help, immediate medical attention may be necessary.

rhonchi on auscultation, and the coughing up of purulent, yellowish-colored sputum are all associated with bacterial pneumonia.

Management Bacterial pneumonia must be treated with antibiotics. Deep breathing exercises and removal of sputum through a productive cough are helpful. Analgesics and antipyretics may also be useful for controlling pain and fever.[43]

Bronchial Asthma

Etiology One of the most common respiratory diseases, bronchial asthma can be produced from a number of stressors, such as a viral respiratory tract infection, emotional upset, changes in barometric pressure or temperature, exercise, inhalation of a noxious odor, or exposure to a specific allergen.

Symptoms and signs Bronchial asthma is characterized by a spasm of the bronchial smooth muscles, edema, and inflammation of the mucous membrane. In addition to asthma's narrowing of the airway, copious amounts of mucus are produced. Difficulty breathing may cause the athlete to hyperventilate, resulting in dizziness. The attack may begin with coughing, wheezing, shortness of breath, and fatigue (see *Focus Box:* "Management of the acute asthmatic attack").

Exercise-Induced Bronchial Obstruction (Asthma)

Exercise-induced bronchial obstruction is also known as exercise-induced asthma[51] (EIA). EIA is a form of asthma, and it may present itself exclusive of other asthma precipitators[25] (i.e., it may be the only asthma condition the patient has).

Etiology An exercise-induced asthmatic attack can be stimulated by exercise in some individuals; in others, the attack may be provoked, only on rare occasions, during moderate exercise. The exact cause of EIA is not clear. Metabolic acidosis, postexertional hypocapnia, stimulation of tracheal irritant receptors, adrenergic abnormalities such as a defective catecholamine metabolism, and psychological factors have been suggested as possible causes. Loss of heat and water causes the greatest loss of airway reactivity. Sinusitis can also trigger an attack in an individual with chronic asthma.

Symptoms and signs The athlete with EIA often displays an airway narrowing caused by bronchial-wall spasm and excess production of mucus. Athletes who have a chronic inflammatory asthmatic condition (bronchiectasis) characteristically have a constant dilation of the bronchi or bronchioles. There is chest tightness, breathlessness, coughing, and wheezing.[33] The athlete with EIA may show signs of nausea, hypertension, fatigue,[33] respiratory stridor (high-pitched noise on respiration), headaches, and redness of the skin. Symptoms may occur within three to eight minutes of strenuous activity.[2]

Management Swimming produces the fewest bronchospasms, which may be a result of the moist, warm air environment. A regular exercise program can benefit asthmatics.[20] Conditioning and running longer distances reduce EIA bouts.[22] The athlete should engage in gradual warm-ups and cooldowns.[9] The duration of exercise should build slowly to thirty to forty minutes, four or five times a week. Exercise intensity and loading also should be graduated slowly, for example, ten to thirty seconds of work followed by thirty to ninety seconds of rest. (Many athletes with chronic or exercise-induced asthma use the inhaled bronchodilator. Exercise is best performed in warm, humid conditions. A mask or scarf may be beneficial in avoiding cold, dry air. Slow nasal breathing is suggested, and athletes should avoid exercising in areas with high levels of air pollution or high pollen counts.[22] (See Chapter 17.) The most commonly prescribed B_2 agonist for EIA is albuterol, which acts for about two hours. Salmeterol provides a prophylaxis for up to twelve hours. Albuterol should be administered fifteen minutes before exercise, and salmeterol, thirty to sixty minutes before exercise. Cromolyn sodium should be inhaled thirty minutes before exercise. Metered-dose inhalers are preferred for administration.[33] It has also been found that prophylactic use of the bronchodilator fifteen minutes before exercise delays the symptoms by two to four hours.[4] Asthmatic athletes who receive medication for their condition should make sure that what they take is legal for competition.[20]

> **29-3**
> ***Critical Thinking*** Exercise
>
> A soccer player has a history of exercise-induced asthma (EIA).
>
> ? How should the athlete avoid incidences of EIA?

Cystic Fibrosis

Etiology Cystic fibrosis is a genetic disorder that can affect many different body systems; it can manifest itself as a type of chronic obstructive pulmonary disease, as pancreatic deficiency, as urogenital dysfunction, and as increased electrolytes in sweat.[34] It usually begins in infancy and is a major cause of severe chronic lung disease in children. Maximum life expectancy is about thirty years.

Symptoms and signs A number of physical symptoms may exist, including bronchitis, pneumonia, respiratory failure, gallbladder diseases, pancreatitis diabetes, and nutritional deficiencies. There is an abnormally high production of mucus secretions in the lungs.

Management Drug therapy, including ibuprofen, can help slow the progress of the disease. Antibiotics are used to control pulmonary disease. The patient must undergo consistent postural drainage, using a cupping or hacking massage technique followed by deep breathing and coughing to help mobilize secretions. High fluid intake to thin secretions and the breathing of humidified air is also recommended.[45]

MUSCULAR SYSTEM DISORDERS

The muscular system suffers from fewer disorders than other systems do. Two serious muscular disorders are muscular dystrophy and myasthenia gravis.

Duchenne Muscular Dystrophy

Etiology Duchenne muscular dystrophy is a hereditary disease in which there is degeneration of skeletal muscle with an associated loss in strength. Muscle tissue is gradually replaced by adipose and fibrous connective tissue. This connective tissue impedes circulation, which accelerates the degenerative process. Onset is usually in early childhood, between the ages of two and ten years.[40]

Symptoms and signs The problem begins to appear as the child learns to walk; he or she takes frequent falls and has difficulty standing up. The progressive degeneration first affects the hips, then the legs, and finally, the abdominal and spinal musculature. Muscles tend to shorten as they atrophy, which causes scoliosis and other postural abnormalities.[40]

Management Muscular dystrophy cannot be cured; however, consistent exercise can be used to retard atrophy. Individuals may ambulate with braces for a while before they are confined to a wheelchair. Death usually occurs before the age of twenty.

Myasthenia Gravis

Etiology Myasthenia gravis is an autoimmune disease in which antibodies attack the synaptic junctions between nerves and muscles. A deficiency in aceytlcholine (a neurotransmitter) creates an abnormality that produces early fatigue of skeletal muscle.[45] Myasthenia gravis occurs most often in females between the ages of twenty and forty years.

Symptoms and signs One of the first signs is a drooping of the upper eyelid and double vision due to weakness in the extraocular muscles. Following the initial symptoms, there may be difficulty in chewing and swallowing, weakness of the extremities, and a general decrease in muscular endurance.[40]

Management The disease may be treated with drugs that inhibit the breakdown of aceytlcholine, enabling it to stimulate the muscle for longer periods. Corticosteroids may also be used to suppress the immune system and thus reduce the production of antibodies that destroy acetylcholine receptors.[40]

NERVOUS SYSTEM DISORDERS

Disorders that can affect the nervous system include meningitis, multiple sclerosis, and amyotrophic lateral sclerosis.

Meningitis

Etiology Meningitis is an inflammation of the meninges, or membranes, that surround the spinal cord and brain that is caused by infection, usually from the meningococcus bacteria. Bacteria may enter the central nervous system through the nose or throat following infections of the ear, throat, or respiratory tract. The bacteria get into the arachnoid or pia mater, and inflammation spreads to the adjacent nervous tissue, causing swelling of the brain, enlargement of the ventricles, and hemorrhage of the brain stem.[40] Meningitis is a serious disease in children; it usually occurs between the ages of three months and two years.

Symptoms and signs Symptoms include a high fever, stiff neck, intense headache, and sensitivity to light and sound, and they progress to vomiting, convulsions, and coma.

Management The cerebrospinal fluid (CSF) must be analyzed for bacteria and the presence of white blood cells. CSF is taken through a puncture in the lumbar area, or spinal tap. If meningococcus bacteria are identified, isolation is necessary for at least twenty-four hours due to the highly contagious nature of the condition. Intravenous antibiotics must begin immediately. Because of the severity of this condition, the patient should be monitored and treated in an intensive care unit.

Multiple Sclerosis

Etiology Multiple sclerosis (MS) is an autoimmune inflammatory disease of the central nervous system that causes deterioration and permanent damage to the myelin sheath that surrounds a nerve cell axon. Nerve conduction is disrupted, causing diverse symptoms. MS most often affects individuals between the ages of twenty and forty years. The exact cause of MS is uncertain, but there is currently no cure.[43]

Symptoms and signs Specific signs depend on the part of the nervous system that is affected, and damage may occur in several different locations. Blurred vision with blind spots, speech defects, tremors, and muscle weakness and numbness in the extremities are common. Some people experience tremor, spasticity, and neurotic behavior that involves mood swings. The disease may progress steadily, or there may be acute attacks followed by partial or complete temporary remission of symptoms.[45]

Management Management involves dealing with the symptoms as they appear and disappear. The individual should avoid overexertion and fatigue, exposure to extreme temperatures, and stressful situations. A regular plan for daily activity and exercise should be established. Several new drugs, including interferon, appear to slow the progression of the disease.[45]

Amyotrophic Lateral Sclerosis

Etiology Amyotrophic lateral sclerosis (ALS), also known as Lou Gehrig's disease, involves a sclerosis of the lateral regions of the spinal cord along with degeneration of motor neurons and significant atrophy of muscles.

Symptoms and signs Symptoms include difficulty in speaking, swallowing, and use of the hands. However, sensory and intellectual function remain intact. There is rapid progression of muscle atrophy, usually resulting in paralysis and confinement to a wheelchair.[35]

Management Although there is no cure for this devastating disease, the individual who is totally incapacitated still has normal intellectual function but simply is unable to communicate feelings and ideas.[40]

Reflex Sympathetic Dystrophy

29-4

***Critical Thinking* Exercise**

A gymnast has been casted for a radial styloid fracture from falling off the balance beam. She comes into the training room concerned about her hand, which looks swollen, red, and is extremely sensitive to the touch.

? What should the athletic trainer be concerned about?

Etiology Reflex sympathetic dystrophy (RSD) is an abnormal and excessive response of the sympathetic portion of the autonomic nervous system that occurs following injury.[48] Most commonly it is seen in the hand or the foot resulting from the immobilization of an injured part due to pain. It has been associated with injuries to bone, soft tissue, nerve, or blood vessels.

Symptoms and signs There is a series of changes mediated by the sympathetic nervous system that progressively result in extreme hypersensitivity to touch, redness, sweating, burning/aching type pain, swelling with palpable tightness and shining of the skin, and atrophy. Symptoms may persist for months and even as long as a year. With ongoing chronic pain there is certainly the potential for psychologic depression to occur.

Management Early recognition and intervention are essential for a good prognosis. Treatment should be directed at disrupting the abnormal sympathetic response. A sympathetic ganglion nerve block administered by a physician is critical to treatment. Active range of motion exercise through a pain-free range along with the use of various therapeutic modalities for managing pain and reducing swelling also have been recommended. In cases where symptoms persist for months, antidepressant medication may be necessary.

BLOOD AND LYMPH DISORDERS

Diseases that can affect the vascular and lymphatic systems include anemias, hemophilia, and lymphangitis.

Iron-Deficiency Anemia

Iron deficiency is the most common form of true anemia among athletes. Stores of iron are depleted before clinical signs occur. Iron is mainly stored in hemoglobin (64%) and bone marrow (27%).[17] Iron-deficiency anemia is most prevalent among menstruating women and males eleven to fourteen years old.[16]

Etiology Three conditions occur during anemia: erythrocytes (red blood cells) are too small, hemoglobin is decreased, and ferritin concentration is low. Ferritin is an iron-phosphorous-protein complex that normally contains 23 percent iron. There are many ways that athletes can be iron deficient. Gastrointestinal (GI) losses are common in runners because of bowel ischemia. Aspirin or NSAIDs may cause GI blood loss. Runners absorb 16 percent of iron from the GI tract compared with 30 percent in nonathletes who are iron deficient. Menstrual losses account for most iron loss in female athletes. Average menstrual iron loss is 0.6 to 1.5 mg per day. Inadequate dietary intake of iron is the primary cause of iron deficiency. The recommended daily allowance (RDA) is 15 mg per day for females and 10 mg per day for males. The average diet contains 5 to 7 mg of iron per 100 kcal. Because female athletes often eat less than they need, they also fail to consume enough iron. Athletes who are vegetarians might lack iron.

Symptoms and signs In the first stages of iron deficiency, the athlete's performance begins to decline. The athlete may complain of burning thighs and nausea from becoming anaerobic. Ice craving is also common. Athletes with mild iron-deficiency anemia may display some mild impairment in their maximum performance. Determining serum ferritin is the most accurate test of iron status. Two factors must be checked by the physician: the athlete's mean corpuscular volume (MCV), which is the average volume of individual cells in a cubic micron, and the relative sizes of the erythrocytes.

Management Athletes can manage iron deficiency in the following ways: eat a proper diet, including more red meat or dark poultry; avoid coffee and tea, which hamper iron absorption from grains; ingest vitamin C sources, which enhance iron absorption; and take an iron supplement (dosage depends on the degree of anemia).

29-5

***Critical Thinking* Exercise**

A female athlete complains of burning thighs and nausea when she exercises. The athlete also craves ice.

? What should the athletic trainer expect from this scenario, and how should it be handled?

Runners' Anemia

Runners' anemia, or **hemolysis,** is the second most prevalent cause of iron deficiency in athletes.

hemolysis
Destruction of red blood cells.

Etiology The cause of runners' anemia, as its name implies, is the impact of the foot as it strikes the surface. Impact forces destroy normal erythrocytes within the vascular system.

Symptoms and signs Hemolysis is characterized by mildly enlarged red cells, an increase in circulatory reticulocytes, and a decrease in the concentration of haptoglobin, which is a glycoprotein bound to hemoglobin and released into the plasma. Even if the athlete wears a well-designed and well-constructed running shoe, this condition can occur. Runners' anemia varies according to the amount of running performed.

Management Athletes can manage runners' anemia by running on soft surfaces, wearing well-cushioned shoes and insoles, and running "light on the feet."

Sickle-Cell Anemia

Sickle-cell anemia is a chronic hereditary hemolytic anemia. The frequency of the genetic defect responsible for this chronic anemia disorder is highest in the African American, Native American, and Mediterranean populations.[45] In these populations, 8 percent to 13 percent are not anemic but carry this trait in their genes. If both parents carry the defective gene, the child will have sickle-cell anemia; if only one parent carries the gene, the child will not have sickle-cell trait.[15] The person with sickle-cell anemia or trait can have sicklemia. The person with the sickle-cell trait may participate in sports and never encounter problems until symptoms are brought on by some unusual circumstance.

Etiology Individuals with sickle-cell anemia have red cells that are sickle, or crescent, shaped. Within the red cells, an abnormal type of hemoglobin exists. It has been speculated that the sickling of the red blood cells results from an adaptation to malaria, which is prevalent in Africa.

The sickle cell has less potential for transporting oxygen and is fragile when compared with normal cells. A sickle cell's life span is 15 to 25 days, compared with the 120 days of a normal red cell; the short life of the sickle cell can produce severe anemia in individuals with acute sickle-cell anemia. The cell's distorted shape inhibits its

thrombi
Plural of thrombus; blood clots that block small blood vessels or a cavity of the heart.

embolus
A mass of undissolved matter.

passage through the small blood vessels and can cause clustering of the cells and, consequently, clogging of the blood vessels. This clogging produces **thrombi,** which block circulation. For individuals having this condition, death can occur (in the severest cases of sickle-cell anemia) from a stroke, heart disease, or an **embolus** in the lungs. Conversely, persons with sickle-cell trait may never experience any problems. Four factors of exercise can cause sickling: acidosis; hyperthermia; dehydration of red blood cells, which increases hemoglobin concentration; and severe hypoxemia.

Symptoms and signs An athlete may never experience any complications from having the sickle-cell trait. However, a sickle-cell crisis can be brought on by exposure to high altitudes or by overheating of the skin, as is the case with a high fever. Crisis symptoms include fever, severe fatigue, skin pallor, muscle weakness, and severe pain in the limbs and abdomen. Abdominal pain in the right upper quadrant may indicate a splenic syndrome in which there is an infarction.[11] This syndrome is especially characteristic of a crisis triggered by a decrease in ambient oxygen while the athlete is flying at high altitudes. The athlete may also experience headache and convulsions.

Management Treatment of a sickle-cell crisis is usually symptomatic. The physician may elect to give anticoagulants and analgesics for pain.

Hemophilia

Etiology Hemophilia is a hereditary disease characterized by a deficiency in any one of a number of clotting factors in the blood. Consequently, there is prolonged coagulation time, failure of the blood to clot, and abnormal bleeding.[45] Hemophilia occurs predominantly in males.

Symptoms and signs In hemophiliacs, physical exertion can cause bleeding into muscles and joints, which can be extremely painful. Eventually joints may become immobilized.[40]

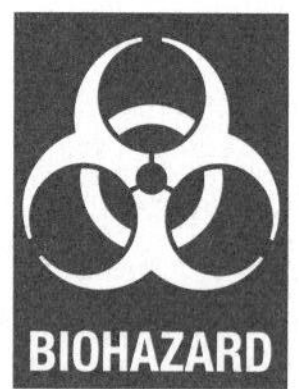

Management A hemophiliac who begins bleeding should be taken to an emergency medical care facility immediately. Unfortunately, there is no cure for hemophilia, but concentrated clotting factors have been developed that can control the bleeding for several days. Patients may be taught to self-administer these clotting factors should bleeding occur. The hemophiliac should avoid trauma and should wear a medical alert bracelet to alert care providers to his or her condition.[12,13]

Lymphangitis

bacteremia (back ter ee-**me** ah)
Bacterial infection in the blood.

Etiology Lymphangitis is an inflammation of the lymphatic channels that is most often caused by streptococcal bacteria.[40] Bacterial infection may also occur in the blood, which is referred to as **bacteremia.**

Symptoms and signs Lymphangitis usually occurs in the extremities. There is a deep reddening of the skin, warmth, lymphandentitis, and a raised border over the affected area, particularly in cases of infection. The condition is accompanied by an onset of chills and high fever with moderate pain and swelling. In lay terms, lymphangitis is sometimes called blood poisoning.[40]

Management The patient should be hospitalized and vital signs should be closely monitored. The affected extremity should be elevated and warm, moist compresses applied. Antibiotics should be administered, and fluid intake is encouraged to restore fluid balance.

DIABETES

Diabetes Mellitus

Diabetic athletes engaging in vigorous physical activity should eat before exercising and, if the exercise is protracted, should have hourly glucose supplementation. As a rule, the insulin dosage is not changed, but food intake is increased. The response of diabetics varies among individuals and depends on many variables. Although there are some hazards, with proper medical evaluation and planning by a professional, diabetics can feel free to engage in most physical activities. The most common types of diabetes are type

I, insulin-dependent diabetes mellitus (IDDM), and type II, non–insulin-dependent diabetes mellitus (NIDDM).[49] Insulin-dependent diabetes is found primarily in individuals under thirty-five years of age and represents between 5 percent and 10 percent of all cases. Non–insulin-dependent diabetes is most commonly detected after age thirty or forty, represents 80 percent of all cases, and is associated with obesity.[46]

Etiology Diabetes is a syndrome that results from an interaction of physical and environmental factors. Its etiology is not distinct. There is a complete or partial decrease in the secretion of insulin by the pancreas.

Symptoms and signs IDDM is most commonly seen in childhood. It may occur suddenly; symptoms include frequent urination, constant thirst, weight loss, constant hunger, tiredness and weakness, itchy dry skin, and blurred vision. NIDDM occurs later in life, when the patient is forty years old or older. It is usually associated with being overweight. The pancreas does not produce enough insulin, or the body resists the insulin that is produced. Like IDDM, NIDDM can be a threat to the heart, kidneys, blood vessels, and eyes.

Management It is essential that blood glucose levels be controlled to acceptable levels. This control includes a balanced diet and, when needed, daily doses of insulin. Regular vigorous exercise can be effective in increasing peripheral insulin action to enhance glucose tolerance. Exercise, in general, improves the diabetic person's quality of life. It helps increase type I insulin sensitivity and use and may reduce long-term complications. In persons with type II diabetes, exercise decreases insulin resistance, improves glycemia control, and reduces or eliminates the need for insulin.[22] The athletic trainer should be aware that the diabetic athlete can adversely respond to extreme temperature variations or to an unpredictable level of activity duration or intensity and may require rapid-acting carbohydrates.

Diabetic Coma and Insulin Shock

It is important that athletic trainers who work with athletes who have diabetes mellitus be aware of the major symptoms of diabetic coma and insulin shock and the proper actions to take when either one occurs.[46]

Diabetic Coma If diabetes is not treated adequately through proper diet or too little insulin is produced, the diabetic athlete can develop acidosis.

Etiology A loss of sodium, potassium, and ketone bodies through excessive urination produces ketoacidosis, which can lead to coma.

Symptoms and signs Symptoms and signs include labored breathing or gasping for air, fruity-smelling breath caused by acetone, nausea and vomiting, thirst, dry mucous membrane of the mouth, flushed skin, and mental confusion or unconsciousness followed by coma.

Management Because of the life-threatening nature of diabetic coma, early detection of ketoacidosis is essential. The injection of insulin into the athlete may in part help to prevent coma.

Insulin Shock

Etiology Unlike diabetic coma, insulin shock occurs when the body has too much insulin and too little blood sugar, and hypoglycemia results.

Symptoms and signs The athlete complains of tingling in the mouth, hands, or other body parts; physical weakness; headaches; and abdominal pain. It may be observed that the athlete has normal or shallow respirations, rapid heartbeat, and tremors along with irritability and drowsiness.

Management The diabetic athlete who engages in intense exercise and metabolizes large amounts of glycogen could inadvertently take too much insulin and thus have a severe reaction.[7] To avoid this problem, the athlete must adhere to a carefully planned diet that includes a snack before exercise. The snack should contain a combination of a complex carbohydrate and protein, such as cheese and crackers. Activities that last for more than thirty to forty minutes should be accompanied by snacks of simple carbohydrates. Some diabetics carry with them a lump of sugar or have candy or orange juice readily available in the event that an insulin reaction seems imminent.[37]

29-6

Critical Thinking **Exercise**

A diabetic field hockey player appears irritable and weak during practice. In the middle of a scrimmage, the player is unable to continue playing and has shallow respirations and a rapid heartbeat.

? What is this athlete experiencing, and how should it be treated?

SEIZURE DISORDERS

Berkow defines seizure disorders as "a recurrent paroxysmal disorder of cerebral function characterized by sudden, brief attacks of altered consciousness, motor activity, sensory phenomena, or inappropriate behavior caused by an abnormal excessive discharge of cerebral neurons."[4]

Epilepsy

epilepsy
Recurrent paroxysmal disorder characterized by sudden attacks of altered consciousness, motor activity, sensory phenomena, or inappropriate behavior.

Any recurrent seizure pattern is termed **epilepsy.** Epilepsy is not a disease but is a symptom that can be caused by a large number of underlying disorders.

Etiology For some types of epilepsy, there is a genetic predisposition and a low threshold to having seizures. In others, altered brain metabolism or a history of injury may be the cause. A seizure can range from extremely brief episodes that last five to fifteen seconds (petit mal seizures) to major episodes (grand mal seizures) that last a few minutes and include unconsciousness and uncontrolled tonic-clonic muscle contractions. There are approximately 1 million epileptics in the United States, most of whom can participate in some form of physical activity.[18] Sports-related injuries are not increased in the epileptic, nor is the sudden death syndrome linked to strenuous activity by the epileptic.[22]

Individuals who have major daily or weekly seizures may need to avoid collision sports.

Symptoms and signs Each person with epilepsy must be considered individually as to whether he or she should engage in competitive sports. If an individual has daily or even weekly major seizures, collision sports should be prohibited. This prohibition is not because a hit on the head will necessarily trigger a seizure, but because a blow during participation that causes unconsciousness could result in a serious injury. If the seizures are properly controlled by medication or occur only during sleep, little if any sports restriction should be imposed except for scuba diving, swimming alone, or participating in activities that occur at a great height.[22,45]

Management The athlete commonly takes an anticonvulsant medication that is specific for the type and degree of seizures that occur. On occasion, the athlete may experience some undesirable side effects from drug therapy, such as drowsiness, restlessness, nystagmus, nausea, vomiting, problems with balance, skin rash, or other adverse reactions.

When an athlete with epilepsy becomes aware of an impending seizure, he or she should take measures to avoid injury, such as immediately sitting or lying down. When a seizure occurs without warning, the athletic trainer should follow the steps outlined in *Focus Box:* "Management during a seizure."

HIGH BLOOD PRESSURE

Excessive pressure applied against arterial walls while blood circulates is known as hypertension, or high blood pressure (HBP). A normal resting blood pressure is 120/80 mm Hg (systolic/diastolic).

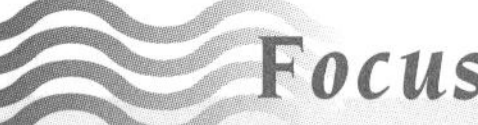

Management during a seizure

- Be emotionally composed.
- If possible, cushion the athlete's fall.
- Keep the athlete away from injury-producing objects.
- Loosen restrictive clothing.
- Prevent the athlete from biting the mouth by placing a soft cloth between the teeth.
- Allow the athlete to awaken normally after the seizure.
- Do not restrain the athlete during the seizure.

Hypertension

Hypertension may be a factor that excludes players from sports participation.

Etiology Hypertension is classified as primary, or essential, and secondary.[32] Primary hypertension accounts for 90 percent of all cases and has no disease associated with it. Secondary hypertension is related to a specific underlying cause, such as kidney disorder, overactive adrenal glands (increased blood volume), hormone-producing tumor, narrowing of the aorta, pregnancy, and medications (oral contraceptives, cold remedies, etc.). The presence of prolonged high blood pressure increases the chances of premature mortality and morbidity due to such causes as coronary artery disease, congestive heart failure, and stroke.[1]

Symptoms and signs Primary hypertension is usually asymptomatic until complications occur.[4] High blood pressure may cause dizziness, flushed appearance, headache, fatigue, epistaxis, and nervousness.

Management The upper range of normal blood pressure is a systolic pressure of 120 mm/Hg and a diastolic pressure of 80 mm/Hg. The risk of death from heart disease and stroke begins to rise at blood pressures as low as 115 over 75, and it doubles for each 20 over 10 mm/Hg increase. Blood pressure is classified as follows: normal—less than 120/less than 80 mm/Hg; prehypertension—120–139/80–89 mm/Hg; stage 1 hypertension—140–159/90–99 mm/Hg; stage 2 hypertension—at or greater than 160/at or greater than 100 mm/Hg (Table 29-1). Medication is not recommended for those with prehypertension unless it is required by another condition, such as diabetes or chronic kidney disease. However, those with prehypertension should make any needed lifestyle changes, including losing excess weight, becoming physically active, limiting alcoholic beverages, quitting smoking, and following a heart-healthy eating plan. It is recommended that those who have Stage 1 or 2 hypertension should also be on medication.

CANCER

Etiology Cancer is the second leading cause of death in adults, behind coronary artery disease. It is estimated that about 30 percent of all Americans will get cancer during their lifetime, and one of five will eventually die from it.[40] Cancer is a condition in which cellular behavior becomes abnormal. The cells no longer perform their normal functions. In general, cancer cells do not multiply at an increased rate. Instead, whatever causes cancer alters the cell's genetic makeup and changes the way it functions. This abnormal cell then divides, forming additional cancer cells, and over a period of time, this tumor or collection of abnormal cells tends to invade and ultimately take over normal tissue.

TUMORS Tumors may be either benign or malignant. Benign tumors typically pose only a small threat to a tissue and tend to remain confined in a limited space. Malignant tumors, though, are cancerous; they grow out of control and spread within a specific tissue. Unfortunately, malignancies can invade surrounding tissues and can spread via the blood and lymphatic systems (metastasize) to the entire body, making it difficult to control the cancer.[40]

TABLE 29-1 Classifying Blood Pressure

Blood Pressure Classification	Systolic (mm/Hg)		Diastolic (mm/Hg)
Normal	less than 120	and	less than 80
Prehypertension	120–139	or	80–89
High			
Stage 1	140–159	or	90–99
Stage 2	160 or higher	or	100 or higher

Malignancies are classified according to the type of tissues in which they occur and according to the rate at which they affect the tissue. Although different types of cancer cells share similar characteristics, each is separate and distinct. Some types are relatively easy to cure, whereas others are difficult to cure and are even life threatening. Skin cancer is the most common type and, fortunately, one of the easiest to detect and cure. Males and females have a different incidence of other types of cancers. In males, the highest incidence of cancer is in the prostate, followed closely by lung, colon/rectal, urinary, and leukemias/lymphomas. In females, the highest incidence is found in the breast, followed by colon/rectal, lung, uterus, and leukemias/lymphomas.

CAUSES OF CANCER The precise causes of cancer are not easily identified. Researchers have identified more than 100 types of cancer with genetic origins. Certain cancers appear to run along family lines. The onset of most cancer has also been attributed to certain environmental factors, including viruses; exposure to ultraviolet light, radiation, and certain chemicals such as tobacco; and alcohol use. A fatty diet has been linked to cancer. It is likely that a combination of hereditary and environmental factors is responsible for the development of cancer.[40]

Warning signs of cancer:

- A change in bowel and bladder habits
- A sore throat that does not heal
- Unusual bleeding or discharge
- Thickening or a lump in the breast or elsewhere
- Indigestion or difficulty swallowing
- Obvious change in a wart or mole
- A nagging cough or hoarseness

Symptoms and signs Specific signs of cancer can vary tremendously, depending on the type of cancer.[8] The American Cancer Society has identified the classic warning signs of cancer: a change in bowel and bladder habits, a sore throat that does not heal, unusual bleeding or discharge, thickening or a lump in the breast or elsewhere, indigestion or difficulty swallowing, obvious change in a wart or mole, and a nagging cough or hoarseness. The presence of any of these signs warrants immediate attention by a physician.

Management Unquestionably, early detection and treatment of cancer markedly improves the patient's chances of beating the disease. The most effective forms of treatment involve three traditional techniques: surgery, radiation, and chemotherapy.

SEXUALLY TRANSMITTED INFECTIONS (STIs)

Sexually transmitted infections are of major concern in sports because many athletes are at an age during which they are more sexually active than they will be at any other time in their lives. The venereal diseases with the highest incidence among the relatively young are chlamydia, genital herpes, trichomoniasis, genital candidiasis, *condyloma acuminata,* gonorrhea, and syphilis. HIV and hepatitis B were discussed in Chapter 14.

Chlamydia Trachomatis

Chlamydia trachomatis
A microorganism that can cause a wide variety of diseases in humans, one of which is venereal and causes nonspecific urethritis.

Chlamydia trachomatis is considered by many to be the most common STI in the United States. It is more common than gonorrhea.[4]

Etiology In females, chlamydia may result in pelvic inflammatory disease and is an important cause of infertility and ectopic pregnancy.

Symptoms and signs In the male, inflammation occurs, along with a purulent discharge, seven to twenty-eight days after intercourse.[2] On occasion, painful urination and traces of blood in the urine occur. Most females with this infection are asymptomatic, but some may experience a vaginal discharge, painful urination, pelvic pain, and pain and inflammation in other sites.

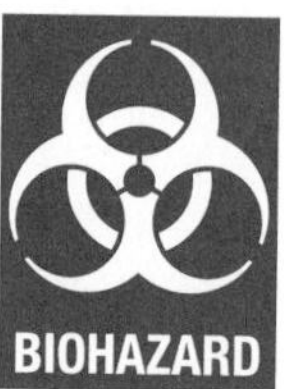

Management A bacteriological examination is given to determine the exact organisms present. Once identified, the infection must be treated promptly to prevent complications. Organism identification and treatment must take place immediately in women who are pregnant. Chlamydial ophthalmia neonatorum can cause conjunctivitis and pneumonia in the newborn from an infected mother.[2] Uncomplicated cases are usually treated with antibiotics. Approximately 20 percent of the sufferers have one or more relapses.

Genital Herpes

Genital herpes is a venereal infection that is currently widespread.

Etiology Type 2 herpes simplex virus is associated with genital herpes infection, which is now the most prevalent cause of genital ulcerations. Signs of the disease appear approximately four to seven days after sexual contact. Primary genital herpes crusts in fourteen to seventeen days, and secondary cases crust in ten days.

Symptoms and signs The first signs in the male are itching and soreness, but women may be asymptomatic in the vagina and cervix. It is estimated that 50 percent to 60 percent of individuals who have had one attack of herpes genitalis will have no further episodes, or if they do, the lesions are few and insignificant. Like the lesions in herpes labialis and gladiatorum, the lesions that develop in herpes genitalis eventually become ulcerated with a red areola. Ulcerations crust and heal in approximately ten days, leaving a scar (Color Plate, Figure Y). Of major importance to a pregnant woman with a history of genital herpes is whether there is an active infection when she is nearing delivery. Herpes simplex can be fatal to a newborn child. There may be some relationship between a higher incidence of cervical cancer and the incidence of genital herpes.[4]

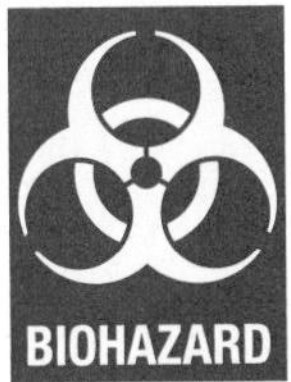

Management At this time, there is no cure for genital herpes. Systemic medications, specifically antiviral medications such as acycloguanosine or acyclovir (Zovirax) and vidarabine (Vira-A), are being used to lessen the early symptoms of the disease.[4]

Trichomoniasis

Trichomoniasis is an infection that affects 20 percent of all females during their reproductive years and 5 percent to 10 percent of males.

Trichomoniasis affects 20 percent of all females and 5 percent to 10 percent of all males.

Etiology Trichomoniasis is caused by the flagellate protozoan *Trichomonas vaginalis.*

Symptoms and signs The female with trichomoniasis typically has a vaginal discharge that is greenish yellow and frothy. The disease causes irritation of the vulva, perineum, and thighs. The female may also experience painful urination. Males are usually asymptomatic, although some may experience a frothy, purulent urethral discharge.

Management Two grams of metronidazole in one dose, usually the drug of choice in the treatment of trichomoniasis, cures up to 95 percent of women. Men, in contrast, should be treated with 500 milligrams twice a day for seven days. The sexual partner should be treated concurrently. Complete cure is required before the individual can again engage in sexual intercourse.

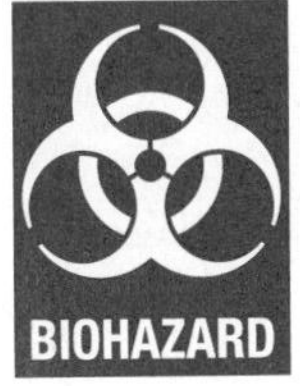

Genital Candidiasis

As discussed in Chapter 27, *Candida* (a genus of yeastlike fungi) is commonly part of the normal flora of the mouth, skin, intestinal tract, and vagina.

Etiology The *Candida* organism is one of the most common causes of vaginitis in women of reproductive age. The infection may be transmitted sexually, but there can be numerous other causes.

Symptoms and signs The symptoms and signs are similar to other, related conditions. The female complains of vulval irritation that begins with redness, severe pain, and a vaginal discharge (scanty). The male is usually asymptomatic but could develop some irritation and soreness of the glans penis, especially after intercourse. Rarely, a slight urethral discharge may occur.

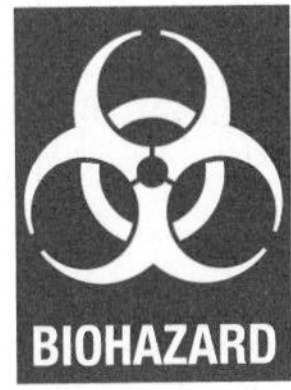

Management Because of the highly infectious nature of this disease, all sexual contact should cease until the completion of treatment. An antifungal cream should be applied to the vagina, labia, perineum, and perianal region for three days.

Condyloma Acuminata (Venereal Warts)

Another sexually transmitted disease that should be recognized and referred to a physician is *condyloma acuminata,* or venereal warts (Color Plate, Figure Z in Chapter 28).

Etiology These warts are transmitted through sexual activity. They appear on the glans penis, vulva, or anus.

Symptoms and signs This form of wart virus produces nodules that can have a cauliflower-like lesion or can be singular. In their early stage, the nodules are soft, moist, pink or red swellings that rapidly develop a stem with a flowerlike head. They may be mistaken for secondary syphilis or carcinoma (Color Plate, Figure Z).

Management Moist condylomas are often carefully treated by the physician with a solution containing 20 percent to 25 percent podophyllin. Dry warts may be treated with a freezing process such as liquid nitrogen.

Gonorrhea

Gonorrhea, commonly called clap, is an acute venereal disease that can infect the urethra, cervix, and rectum.

Etiology The organism of infection is the gonococcal bacteria *Neisseria gonorrhoea,* which is usually spread through sexual intercourse.

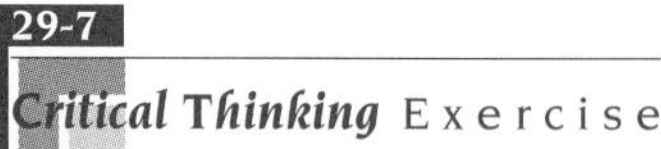

A male college basketball player confides in the athletic trainer about a greenish-yellow urethral discharge and painful urination.

? How should this situation be managed by the athletic trainer?

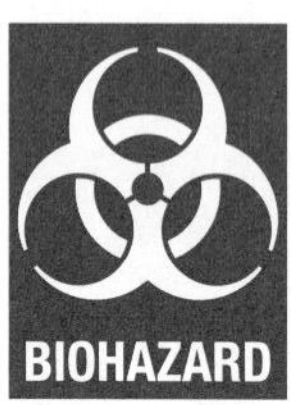

Symptoms and signs In men, the incubation period is two to ten days. The onset of the disease is marked by a tingling sensation in the urethra, followed in two or three hours by a greenish-yellow discharge of pus and by painful urination. Sixty percent of infected women are asymptomatic. For those who have symptoms, onset is between seven and twenty-one days. In these cases, symptoms are mild, with some vaginal discharge. Gonorrheal infection of the throat and rectum are also possible.

Management Because of embarrassment, some individuals fail to secure proper medical help for the treatment of gonorrhea, and although the initial symptoms will disappear, such an individual is not cured and can still spread the infection. Untreated gonorrhea becomes latent and will manifest itself in later years, usually causing sterility or arthritis. Treatment consists of large amounts of penicillin or other antibiotics. Recent experimental evidence suggests an increasing resistance of the gonococci to penicillin. The athletic trainer who sees evidence of any of the symptoms should immediately remand the individual to a physician for testing and treatment. *All sexual contact must be avoided* until it has been medically established that the disease is no longer active. Because of the latent residual effects, including sterility and arthritis, that are the end result of several diseases in this group, immediate medical treatment is mandatory. Although outward signs may disappear, the disease is still insidiously present in the body. Additionally, such treatment will alleviate the discomfort that accompanies the initial stages of the disease.[45]

Syphilis

A sexually transmitted infection that is on an increase is syphilis. Reasons for this increase are high-risk sexual behavior, drug usage, and lack of knowledge about preventing infection.[11]

Etiology *Treponema pallidum,* a spirochete bacteria, is the organism related to syphilis. It enters the body through mucous membranes or skin lesions.[4]

Symptoms and signs Untreated syphilis may have a course of four stages within the body: primary, secondary, latent, and late, or tertiary. The incubation period of syphilis is normally three to four weeks but can range anywhere from one to thirteen weeks. A painless chancre, or ulceration, develops and heals within four to eight weeks. Syphilis during this primary stage is highly contagious. Ulcerations can occur on the penis, urethra, vagina, cervix, mouth, hand, or foot or around the eye.

The secondary stage of syphilis occurs within six to twelve weeks after the initial infection. It is characterized by a skin rash, lymph swelling, body aches, and mild flulike symptoms. Hair may fall out in patches.

Latent syphilis follows the secondary stage and is characterized by no or few symptoms. If untreated, approximately one-third of persons with latent syphilis will develop late, or tertiary, syphilis.

The late stage of syphilis is characterized by a deep penetration of spirochetes that damage skin, bone, and the cardiovascular and nervous systems. Tertiary syphilis can develop within three to ten years of infection. Neurosyphilis can progress into severe muscle weakness, paralysis, and various types of psychoses.

Management Penicillin is currently the appropriate antibiotic for all stages of syphilis. Those patients allergic to penicillin may be treated with erythromycin. Because *T. pallidum* can exist only in body fluids, air drying and cleaning with soap and water will destroy it. Because of the rise of penicillin resistance, ceftriaxone may be the drug of choice.

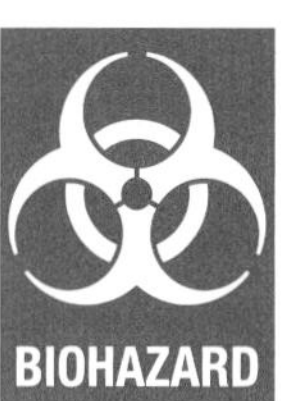

MENSTRUAL IRREGULARITIES AND THE FEMALE REPRODUCTIVE SYSTEM

There are special menstrual and reproductive concerns related to the female who engages in intense physical activity. This section addresses some of the more prevalent issues.

Physiology of the Menstrual Cycle

Menstruation refers to the periodic discharge of bloody fluid from the uterus, usually at regular intervals, during the life of a woman from the age of puberty to menopause.

Menarche

Menarche—the onset of the menses—and puberty normally occur between ages nine and seventeen, with the majority of girls usually entering puberty between ages thirteen and fifteen. Puberty is that period of life in which either sex becomes able to reproduce. There is indication that strenuous sports training and competition will delay the onset of menarche. The greatest delay is related to the higher-caliber competition. In itself, a delay in the first menses does not appear to pose any significant danger to the young female athlete. Delayed menarche, or primary amenorrhea, is defined as menstruation not occurring by age sixteen or a failure to develop secondary sexual characteristics by age fourteen. The late-maturing girl commonly has longer legs, narrower hips, and less adiposity and body weight for her height, all of which are more conducive to sports.

During the prepubertal period, girls are equal to, and often superior to, boys of the same age in activities that require speed, strength, and endurance.

The onset of menarche may be delayed by strenuous training and competition.

Menstruation

The effects of sustained and strenuous training and competition on the menstrual cycle and the effects of menstruation on performance still cannot be fully explained with any degree of certainty.

The classic twenty-eight-day cycle consists of the follicular and luteal phases, each of which is approximately fourteen days long. The menses vary from three to seven days, with an average of four to seven days. The majority of women tend to show some variation in the length of their cycles; these differences occur principally because of differences in the duration of the preovulatory phase rather than the premenstrual phase.

With the onset of menarche, a cyclic hormone pattern commences, which establishes the menstrual cycle. These hormonal changes result from complex feedback mechanisms and specifically controlled interactions that occur between the hypothalamus, ovaries, and pituitary gland. Two gonadotropins induce the release of the egg from the mature follicle at midcycle (ovulation): follicle-stimulating hormone (FSH), which stimulates the maturation of an ovarian follicle, and luteinizing hormone (LH), which stimulates the development of the corpus luteum and the endocrine structure that secretes progesterone and estrogens. The control and eventual inhibition of the production of FSH when the follicle reaches maturity is brought about by the estrogenic steroids produced by the ovaries. Progesterone, a steroid hormone produced within the corpus luteum—a small body that develops within a ruptured ovarian follicle after ovulation—eventually inhibits the production of LH. Estrogen is secreted principally by the luteal cells. Before the onset of a new menstrual period, FSH levels are already rising, probably to initiate the maturation of new follicles to reinstitute the next cycle.

of endocrine changes are strong candidates for bone loss. Low bone mass leads to bone fragility and increased susceptibility to stress fractures in female athletes with premature osteoporosis, especially athletes with late menarche.[24] There is evidence that estrogen receptors on bone cells have a direct relation to growth and bone function.[19] Calcium nutrition is also needed; a recommended daily allowance for adolescents through age twenty-four is 1,200 milligrams daily.[29]

An athlete experiencing loss of periods with low bone mass should decrease training intensity and volume, increase total calories, and ingest 1,500 milligrams of calcium daily. A program of resistance training designed for both muscle mass and strength may enhance the skeletal profile and protect against muscle injury. Estrogen replacement therapy may be warranted if other means fail.[24]

Contraceptives and Reproduction

Female athletes have been known to take extra oral contraceptive pills to delay menstruation during competition. This practice is not recommended. Such practices can cause nausea, vomiting, fluid retention, amenorrhea, hypertension, double vision, and thrombophlebitis.[14] Some oral contraceptives make women hypersensitive to the sun. Any use of oral contraceptives related to physical performance should be under the express direction and control of a physician. However, oral contraceptive use is acceptable for females with no medical problems. The new low-dose preparations, containing less than fifty milligrams of estrogen, add negligible risks to the healthy woman.

In general, athletes who wear intrauterine devices are free of such problems. However, intrauterine devices are not recommended for adolescents who are nulliparous (have never borne a viable child) because of the associated risk of pelvic inflammatory disease. On occasion the athlete may complain of a lower-abdominal cramp while being active. In such cases, the athlete should be referred to a physician.

Pregnancy

Generally, an athlete can participate in physical activity and even competition well into the third month of pregnancy, unless bleeding or cramps are present, and she can frequently continue such activity until the seventh month if no handicapping or physiological complications arise.[28] Such activity may make pregnancy, childbirth, and postparturition less stressful. Many women athletes do not continue beyond the third month because of a drop in their performance. This decline may result from a number of causes, some related to the pregnancy, others perhaps psychological. It is during the first three months of pregnancy that the dangers of disturbing the pregnancy are greatest.[30] After that period, there is less danger to the mother and fetus because the pregnancy is stabilized.

Exercise and Pregnancy

In general, childbirth is not adversely affected by a history of hard physical exercise.

There is no indication that mild to moderate exercise during pregnancy is harmful to fetal growth and development or causes reduced fetal mass, increased perinatal or neonatal mortality, or physical or mental retardation.[6] It has been found, however, that extreme exercise may lower birth weight (see *Focus Box:* "American College of Obstetricians and Gynecologists guidelines for exercise during pregnancy and postpartum"). Many athletes compete during pregnancy with no ill effects. Most physicians, although advocating moderate activity during this period, believe that especially vigorous performance, particularly in activities with severe body contact or heavy jarring or falls, should be avoided.[26] Contraindications to exercise include the following:

- Pregnancy-induced hypertension
- Preterm rupture of membranes
- Preterm labor during the prior or current pregnancy or both
- Incompetent cervix or cerclage
- Persistent second- or third-trimester bleeding
- Intrauterine growth retardation

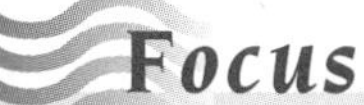

American College of Obstetricians and Gynecologists guidelines for exercise during pregnancy and postpartum[39]

1. During pregnancy, women can continue to exercise and derive health benefits even from a mild to moderate exercise routine. Regular exercise (at least three times per week) is preferable to intermittent activity.
2. Women should avoid exercise in the supine position after the first trimester. Such a position is associated with decreased cardiac output in most pregnant women; because the remaining cardiac output will be preferentially distributed away from splanchnic beds (including the uterus) during vigorous exercise, such regimens are best avoided during pregnancy. Prolonged periods of motionless standing should also be avoided.
3. Women should be aware of the decreased amount of oxygen available for aerobic exercise during pregnancy. They should be encouraged to modify the intensity of their exercise according to maternal symptoms. Pregnant women should stop exercising when fatigued and not exercise to exhaustion. Weight-bearing exercises may under some circumstances be continued throughout pregnancy at intensities similar to those before pregnancy. Non–weight bearing exercise such as cycling or swimming will minimize the risk of injury and facilitate the continuation of exercise during pregnancy.
4. Morphological changes in pregnancy should serve as relative contraindications to types of exercise in which loss of balance could be detrimental to maternal or fetal well-being, especially in the third trimester. Any type of exercise involving the potential for even mild abdominal trauma should be avoided.
5. Pregnancy requires an additional 300 kcal per day to maintain metabolic homeostasis. Thus women who exercise during pregnancy should be particularly careful to ensure an adequate diet.
6. Pregnant women who exercise in the first trimester should augment heat dissipation by ensuring adequate hydration, appropriate clothing, and optimal environmental surroundings during exercise.
7. Many of the physiological and morphological changes of pregnancy persist four to six weeks postpartum. Thus the woman's prepregnancy exercise routine should be resumed gradually based on her physical capability.

Ectopic Pregnancy

In ectopic pregnancy, the fertilized egg is implanted outside the uterine cavity because of some inflammation of the fallopian tubes or some mechanical blockage to the normal downward movement of the ovum. The symptoms include amenorrhea, tenderness, soreness and pain on the affected side, referred pain in the shoulders, pallor, and potentially, signs of shock and hemorrhage. Operative treatment is necessary to terminate the nonviable pregnancy and to control the hemorrhage if a rupture of the tube has occurred.

SUMMARY

- The immune system is not an organ system but is instead a collection of disease-fighting cells that recognize the presence of foreign substances in the body and act to neutralize or destroy them.
- Among the more common viral infections are rhinovirus (common cold), influenza (flu), infectious mononucleosis, rubella (German measles), rubeola (measles), mumps, and varicella-zoster (chicken pox).
- Conditions that affect the respiratory system include sinusitis, pharyngitis, tonsillitis, seasonal rhinitis, acute bronchitis, pneumonia, bronchial asthma, exercise-induced bronchial obstruction, and cystic fibrosis.

- The muscular system suffers from fewer disorders than do other systems. Two serious muscular disorders are muscular dystrophy and myasthenia gravis.
- Disorders that can affect the nervous system include meningitis, multiple sclerosis, and amyotrophic lateral sclerosis.
- Diseases that can affect the vascular and lymphatic systems include anemias, hemophilia, and lymphangitis.
- Diabetes mellitus is a complex hereditary or developmental disease. Diabetics must be extremely cautious about the possibility of going into diabetic coma or insulin shock.
- Some athletes have a history of epilepsy that could lead to an alteration of consciousness. Epilepsy is not a disease, and each person with epilepsy must be considered individually.
- The athlete with high blood pressure may have to be carefully monitored by a physician. Hypertension may require the avoidance of heavy resistive activities.
- Cancer is a condition in which cellular behavior becomes abnormal. Malignant tumors are cancerous; they grow out of control and spread within a specific tissue. Skin cancer is the most common type. In males, the highest incidence of cancer is in the prostate, followed closely by lung, colon/rectal, urinary, and leukemias/ lymphomas. In females the highest incidence is found in the breast, followed by colon/rectal, lung, uterus, and leukemias/lymphomas.
- The sexually transmitted infections with the highest incidence among the young athletic population are chlamydia, genital herpes, trichomoniasis, genital candidiasis, *condyloma acuminata,* gonorrhea, and syphilis.
- The highly active female may have menstrual irregularities, including dysmenorrhea, amenorrhea, or oligomenorrhea. Menstrual irregularities could lead to a thinning of bone and subsequent fractures.
- Many female athletes compete during pregnancy with no ill effects. There is no indication that mild to moderate exercise during pregnancy is harmful to fetal development.

Websites

Asthma and Allergy Foundation of America (AAFA): http://www.aafa.org/

Asthma and Allergy Foundation of America (AAFA) is dedicated to helping people with asthma and allergic diseases through education and support for research.

American Gastroenterological Association: http://www.gastro.org/

This site includes information for physicians and the public about digestive disease symptoms, treatments, and research.

American Diabetes Association: http://www.diabetes.org/

This site offers the latest information on diabetes and living with the disease.

American Epilepsy Society: http://www.aesnet.org/

The American Epilepsy Society promotes research and education for professionals dedicated to the prevention, treatment, and cure of epilepsy.

Hypertension Network: BloodPressure.com:http://www.bloodpressure.com/

This site provides information for the consumer on hypertension (high blood pressure).

Sexually Transmitted Infections: Index: http://www.plannedparenthood.org/STI-SAFESEX/stifacts.htm

American Board of Obstetrics and Gynecology: http://www.abog.org/

Solutions to Critical Thinking EXERCISES

29-1 This scenario describes flu symptoms. There should be symptomatic care and aspirin should be avoided.

29-2 It is possible that this athlete has infectious mononucleosis. Treatment should be supportive and symptomatic. Acetaminophen is often given for headache, fever, and malaise. The athlete may resume easy training in about three weeks after the onset of illness if: (1) the spleen is not markedly enlarged or painful, (2) he or she is afebrile, (3) liver function tests are normal, and (4) pharyngitis and any complication have resolved.

29-3 The athlete should maintain a high level of conditioning, including running of longer distances, and should always warm up and cool down gradually. All exercise intensity and loading should be graduated slowly. A bronchodilator may be employed. A mask or scarf should be used in cold, dry air. The athlete should avoid exercising in areas with high levels of air pollution or when there is a high pollen count.

29-4 It is possible that the gymnast has reflex sympathetic dystrophy. Her concern is justified, since this problem could persist for months. The physician will likely do a sympathetic ganglion nerve block. The athletic trainer should have the athlete do active range of motion exercises in a pain-free range.

29-5 The athlete appears to have iron-deficiency anemia. After verification by a physician, the athlete should eat a diet rich in iron, avoid coffee and tea, eat foods high in vitamin C, and take a daily iron supplement.

29-6 This athlete is experiencing insulin shock as a result of too much insulin and not enough blood sugar. Glucose should be administered to this patient as soon as possible in the form of sugar, candy, orange juice, or a glucose solution.

29-7 This situation must be handled with the strictest confidentiality. Because this condition could be gonorrhea, immediate medical referral must be made. All sexual contact must be avoided until this condition has been resolved.

29-8 These medical disorders make up the female athlete triad. Osteoporosis is the softening and increased porosity of bones with subsequent fracturing. Athletes who have anorexia nervosa or bulimia to establish a perceived body image are at risk. Athletes who train so hard that they stop menstruating also stop their estrogen production, which results in a loss of calcium in the bones.

REVIEW QUESTIONS AND CLASS ACTIVITIES

1. Contrast the symptoms and signs of the following respiratory tract conditions: the common cold, influenza, and allergic rhinitis.
2. Discuss mononucleosis in detail, including prevention and etiology.
3. Discuss and contrast bronchial obstructive diseases such as bronchitis and asthma. How do you care for an athlete having an acute asthmatic attack?
4. Describe the most common gastrointestinal complaints. How are the conditions that produce them acquired and managed?
5. What is diabetes mellitus? What value might exercise have for the person with diabetes mellitus? How are diabetic coma and insulin shock managed?
6. In a sports setting, what are some major indications that an athlete has a contagious disease?
7. What is epilepsy? How should a grand mal seizure be managed?
8. Define hypertension. What dangers does it present to the athlete?
9. Describe the anemias that most often affect the athlete. How should each be managed?
10. What are the classic warning signs for cancer according to the American Cancer Society?
11. Discuss the etiology, symptoms and signs, and management of the most common sexually transmitted infections. How can they be prevented?
12. Discuss menstrual irregularities that occur in highly active athletes. Why do they occur? How should they be managed? How do they relate to reproduction?
13. What are the implications of pregnancy for extensive physical activity?

REFERENCES

1. American College of Sports Medicine: Position stand: physical activity, physical fitness, and hypertension, *Med Sci Sports Exerc* 25(10):1, 1993.
2. Bartimole J: Exercise-induced asthma: pre-treating for prevention, *NATA News* 4, 1995.
3. Benson MT, editor: *2001–02 NCAA sports medicine handbook: menstrual-cycle dysfunction,* Indianapolis, Ind, 2001, National Collegiate Athletic Association.
4. Berkow R, editor: *The Merck manual,* Rahway, NJ, 1999, Merck.
5. Blumenthal MN: Sports-aggravated allergies, *Physician Sportsmed* 18(12):70, 1990.
6. Clapp JF III: A clinical approach to exercise during pregnancy. In Agostini R, editor: *The athletic woman. Clinics in sports medicine,* vol 13, no 2, Philadelphia, 1994, Saunders.
7. Colberg SR, Swain, DP: Exercise and diabetes control: a winning combination, *Physician Sportsmed* 28(4):63, 2000.
8. DeWald LL: Cancer education and prevention in the athletic training center. *Athletic Therapy Today* 7(1):16, 2002.
9. Dishuck J: Educating the asthmatic athlete. *Athletic Therapy Today* 6(5):26, 2001.
10. Dishuck J, Harrelson GL: Management and treatment of allergic rhinitis and sinusitis, *Athletic Therapy Today* 6(5):6, 2001.
11. Eichner ER: Sickle-cell trait, heroic exercise, and fatal collapse, *Physician Sportsmed* 21(7):51, 1993.
12. Fiala K, Hoffman S, Ritenour D: A survey of team physicians on the participation status of hemophilic athletes in National Collegiate Athletic Association Division I athletics, *J Ath Train* 38(3), 2003.
13. Fiala K, Hoffman S, Ritenour D: Traumatic hemarthrosis of the knee secondary to hemophilia A in a collegiate soccer player: a case report, *J Ath Train* 37(3):315, 2002.
14. Frankovich RJ, Lebrun CM: Menstrual cycle, contraception, and performance, *Clin Sports Med* 19(2):251, 2000.
15. Hamann B: *Disease: identification, prevention, and control,* St Louis, 2000, Mosby.
16. Harris SS: Exercise-related anemias. In Agostini R, editor: *Medical and orthopedic issues of active and athletic women,* St Louis, 1994, Mosby.
17. Harris SS: Helping active women avoid anemia, *Physician Sportsmed* 23(5):34, 1995.
18. Harter-Snow C: Athletic amenorrhea and bone health. In Agostini R, editor: *Medical and orthopedic issues of active and athletic women,* St Louis, 1994, Mosby.
19. Harter-Snow CM: Bone health and prevention of osteoporosis in active and athletic women. In Agostini R, editor: *The athletic woman. Clinics in sports medicine,* vol 13, no 2, Philadelphia, 1994, Saunders.
20. Houglum JE: The basics of asthma therapy for athletes, *Athletic Therapy Today* 6(5):16, 2001.
21. Horodyski M, Fiolkowski P, Stopka C: Returning to athletics after mononucleosis, *Athletic Therapy Today* 6(4):47, 2001.
22. Howe WB: The athlete with chronic illness. In Birrer RB, editor: *Sports medicine for the primary care physician,* ed 2, Boca Raton, Fla, 1994, CRC Press.
23. Jong EC: Infections. In Agostini R, editor: *Medical and orthopedic issues of active and athletic women,* St Louis, 1994, Mosby.
24. Karpalcka J et al: Recurrent stress fracture in a female athlete with primary amenorrhea, *Cl J Sports Med* 4(2):136, 1994.
25. Kovan JR, Mackowiak TJ: Exercise-induced asthma, *Athletic Therapy Today* 6(5):22, 2001.
26. Kulpa P: Exercise during pregnancy and post partum. In Agostini R, editor: *Medical and orthopedic issues of active and athletic women,* St Louis, 1994, Mosby.
27. Leaver-Dunn D, Robinson JB, Laubenthal J: Assessment of respiratory conditions in athletes, *Athletic Therapy Today* 5(6):14, 2000.
28. LeBrun CM: Effects of the menstrual cycle and birth control pills on athletic performance. In Agostini R, editor: *Medical and orthopedic issues of active athletic women,* St Louis, 1994, Mosby.
29. Lemcke DP: Osteoporosis and menopause. In Agostini R, editor: *Medical and orthopedic issues of active and athletic women,* St Louis, 1994, Mosby.
30. Lively MW: Sports participation and pregnancy. *Athletic Therapy Today* 7(1):11, 2002.
31. Locke RJ, Warren MP: Exercise and primary dysmenorrhoea, *British Journal of Medicine* 33(4):227, 1999.
32. MacKnight JM: Hypertension in athletes and active patients: tailoring treatment to the patient, *Physician Sportsmed* 27(4):35, 1999.
33. Mahler DA: Exercise-induced asthma, *Med Sci Sports Exerc* 25(5):554, 1993.

34. Marshall LA: Clinical evaluation of amenorrhea. In Agostini R, editor: *Medical and orthopedic issues of active and athletic women,* St Louis, 1994, Mosby.
35. Mellion MB et al: Medical problems in athletes. In Birrer RB, editor: *Sports medicine for the primary care physician,* Boca Raton, Fla, 1994, CRC Press.
36. Merrick MA: Do nasal dilator strips help athletes? *Athletic Therapy Today* 6(2):42, 2001.
37. Merrick MA: Managing Type-1 diabetes in athletes, *Athletic Therapy Today* 6(5):40, 2001.
38. Nattiv A et al: The female athletic triad. In Agostini R, editor: *Medical and orthopedic issues of active and athletic women,* St Louis, 1994, Mosby.
39. *PACOG Technical Bulletin 189. Exercise during pregnancy and postpartum period,* Washington, DC, 1994, The American College of Obstetricians and Gynecologists.
40. Saladin K: Anatomy and physiology: the unity of form and function, New York, 2001, McGraw-Hill.
41. Sanborn CF, Horea M, Siemers BJ, Dieringer KI: Disordered eating and the female athlete triad, *Clin Sports Med* 19(2):199, 2000.
42. Schnirring L: New drugs should help fight influenza this winter, *Physician Sportsmed* 27(12):15, 1999.
43. *Stedman's concise medical dictionary for the health professions,* Baltimore, 2001, Lippincott, Williams & Wilkins.
44. Swann E: Emergency management of allergic reactions. *Athletic Therapy Today* 6(5):11, 2001.
45. *Taber's cyclopedic medical dictionary,* Philadelphia, 1997, FA Davis.
46. Taunton JE, McCargarl EL: Staying active with diabetes, *Physician Sportsmed* 23(3):55, 1995.
47. Vantu RV: Epilepsy and athletics, *Clin Sports Med* 17(1):61, 1998.
48. Velasquez BJ: Reflex sympathetic dystrophy syndrome in a female recreational athlete, *Athletic Therapy Today* 6(2):36, 2001.
49. Vinci DM: Athletes and type 1 diabetes mellitus. *Athletic Therapy Today* 7(6):48, 2002.
50. Vinci DM: The female athlete triad: amenorrhea and osteoporosis, *Athletic Therapy Today* 4(5):34, 1999.
51. Weaver J, Denegar CR, Hertel J: Exercise-induced asthma, *Athletic Therapy Today* 5(3):38, 2000.
52. Weidner TG: Preventing the common cold and associated secondary problems in athletes, *Athletic Therapy Today* 6(4):44, 2001.

ANNOTATED BIBLIOGRAPHY

Berkow R, Beers M, Fletcher A, editors: *The Merck manual of medical information: home edition,* New York, 1999, Pocket Books.

This book is one of the classic medicine references available to health care professionals. It covers most medical conditions.

Colbert S, editor: *The diabetic athlete,* Champaign, Ill, 2001, Human Kinetics.

This text describes the effects different sports and activities have on blood sugar and the body. It also provides tables and advice on how to manage glucose levels depending on the sport and type of insulin being used.

Fields KB, Fricker PA, Delaney MJ: *Medical problems in athletes,* London, 1997, Blackwell Scientific Inc.

This is a book about how exercise and disease interact. Divided into three sections, it covers infectious problems in athletes; cardiologic and other regional medical conditions and chronic illnesses; and special medical problems in the athlete, from hypothermia to exercise during pregnancy.

Hamann B: *Diseases, identification, prevention, and control,* St. Louis, 2000, Mosby.

This is an excellent reference guide for the health professional on the most common human diseases.

Tabor's cyclopedic medical dictionary, Philadelphia, 2001, FA Davis.

Despite the fact that this text appears in dictionary format, it contains a wealth of valuable information on various health conditions.

Appendix A

NATA Code of Ethics*

PREAMBLE

The Code of Ethics of the National Athletic Trainers' Association (NATA) has been written to make the membership aware of the principles of ethical behavior that should be followed in the practice of athletic training. The primary goal of the Code is the assurance of high quality health care. The Code presents aspirational standards of behavior that all members should strive to achieve.

The principles cannot be expected to cover all specific situations that may be encountered by the practicing athletic trainer, but should be considered representative of the spirit with which athletic trainers should make decisions. The principles are written generally and the circumstances of a situation will determine the interpretation and application of a given principle and of the Code as a whole. Whenever there is a conflict between the Code and legality, the laws prevail. The guidelines set forth in this Code are subject to continual review and revision as the athletic training profession develops and changes.

PRINCIPLE 1:

Members shall respect the rights, welfare, and dignity of all individuals.

1.1 Members shall not discriminate against any legally protected class.

1.2 Members shall be committed to providing competent care consistent with both the requirements and the limitations of their profession.

1.3 Members shall preserve the confidentiality of privileged information and shall not release such information to a third party not involved in the patient's care unless the person consents to such release or release is permitted or required by law.

PRINCIPLE 2:

Members shall comply with the laws and regulations governing the practice of athletic training.

2.1 Members shall comply with applicable local, state, and federal laws and institutional guidelines.

2.2 Members shall be familiar with and adhere to all National Athletic Trainers' Association guidelines and ethical standards.

2.3 Members are encouraged to report illegal or unethical practice pertaining to athletic training to the appropriate person or authority.

2.4 Members shall avoid substance abuse and, when necessary, seek rehabilitation for chemical dependency.

PRINCIPLE 3:

Members shall accept responsibility for the exercise of sound judgment.

3.1 Members shall not misrepresent in any manner, either directly or indirectly, their skills, training, professional credentials, identity, or services.

3.2 Members shall provide only those services for which they are qualified via education and/or experience and by pertinent legal regulatory process.

3.3 Members shall provide services, make referrals, and seek compensation only for those services that are necessary.

PRINCIPLE 4:

Members shall maintain and promote high standards in the provision of services.

4.1 Members shall recognize the need for continuing education and participate in various types of educational activities that enhance their skills and knowledge.

*From www.nata.org

4.2 Members who have the responsibility for employing and evaluating the performance of other staff members shall fulfill such responsibility in a fair, considerate, and equitable manner, on the basis of clearly enunciated criteria.

4.3 Members who have the responsibility for evaluating the performance of employees, supervisees, or students, are encouraged to share evaluations with them and allow them the opportunity to respond to those evaluations.

4.4 Members shall educate those whom they supervise in the practice of athletic training with regard to the Code of Ethics and encourage their adherence to it.

4.5 Whenever possible, members are encouraged to participate and support others in the conduct and communication of research and educational activities that may contribute knowledge for improved patient care, patient or student education, and the growth of athletic training as a profession.

4.6 When members are researchers or educators, they are responsible for maintaining and promoting ethical conduct in research and educational activities.

PRINCIPLE 5:

Members shall not engage in any form of conduct that constitutes a conflict of interest or that adversely reflects on the profession.

5.1 The private conduct of the member is a personal matter to the same degree as is any other person's except when such conduct compromises the fulfillment of professional responsibilities.

5.2 Members of the National Athletic Trainers' Association and others serving on the Association's committees or acting as consultants shall not use, directly or by implication, the Association's name or logo or their affiliation with the Association in the endorsement of products or services.

5.3 Members shall not place financial gain above the welfare of the patient being treated and shall not participate in any arrangement that exploits the patient.

5.4 Members may seek remuneration for their services that is commensurate with their services and in compliance with applicable law.

Appendix B

Canada's Food Guide to Healthy Eating

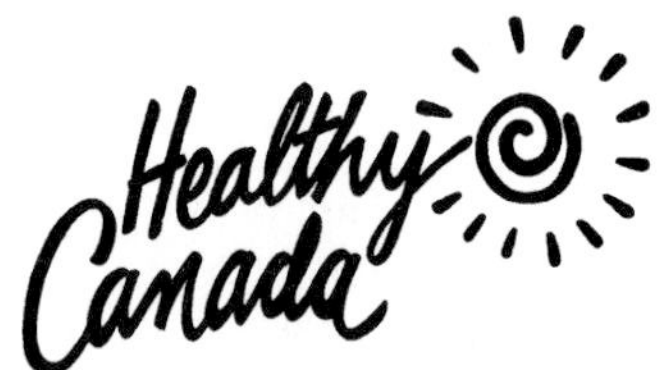

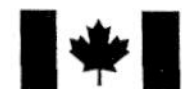

Health and Welfare Canada

Santé et Bien-être social Canada

CANADA'S

Food Guide

TO HEALTHY EATING

Enjoy a variety of foods from each group every day.

Choose lower-fat foods more often.

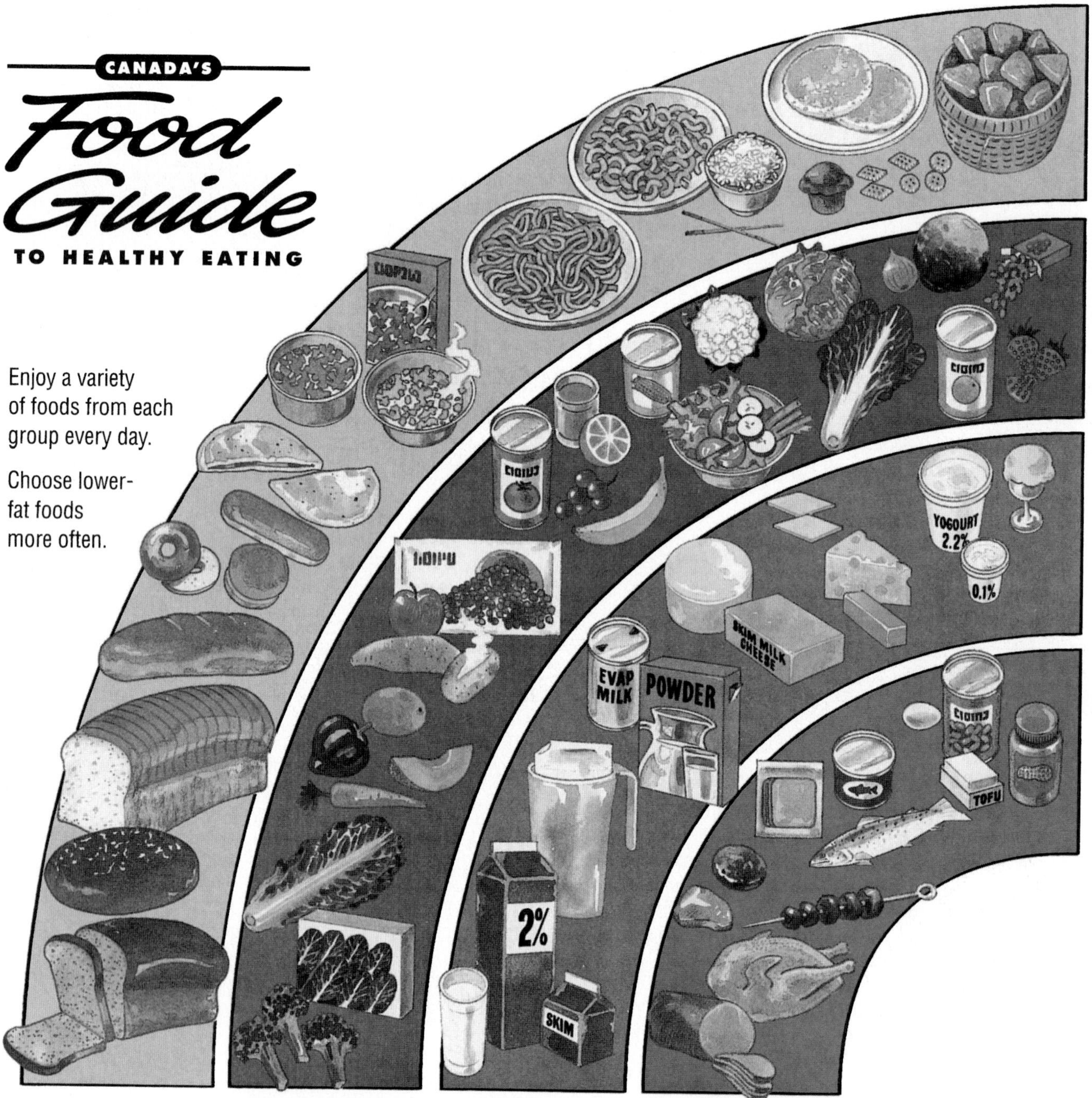

Grain Products
Choose whole grain and enriched products more often.

Vegetables & Fruit
Choose dark green and orange vegetables and orange fruit more often.

Milk Products
Choose lower-fat milk products more often.

Meat & Alternatives
Choose leaner meats, poultry and fish, as well as dried peas, beans and lentils more often.

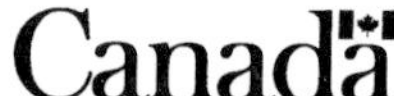

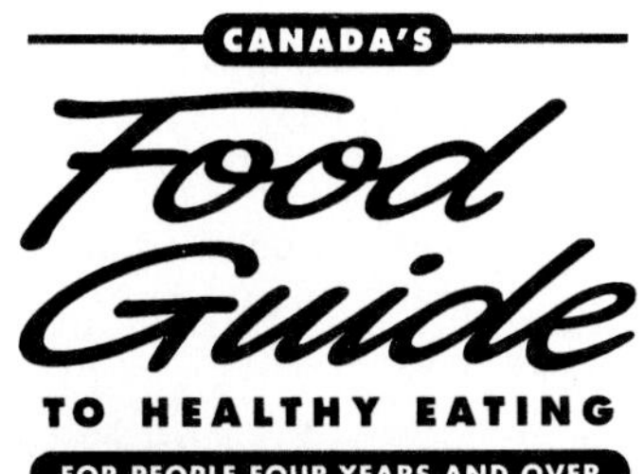
CANADA'S
Food Guide
TO HEALTHY EATING
FOR PEOPLE FOUR YEARS AND OVER

Different People Need Different Amounts of Food

The amount of food you need every day from the 4 food groups and other foods depends on your age, body size, activity level, whether you are male or female and if you are pregnant or breast-feeding. That's why the Food Guide gives a lower and higher number of servings for each food group. For example, young children can choose the lower number of servings, while male teenagers can go to the higher number. Most other people can choose servings somewhere in between.

Grain Products
5–12
SERVINGS PER DAY

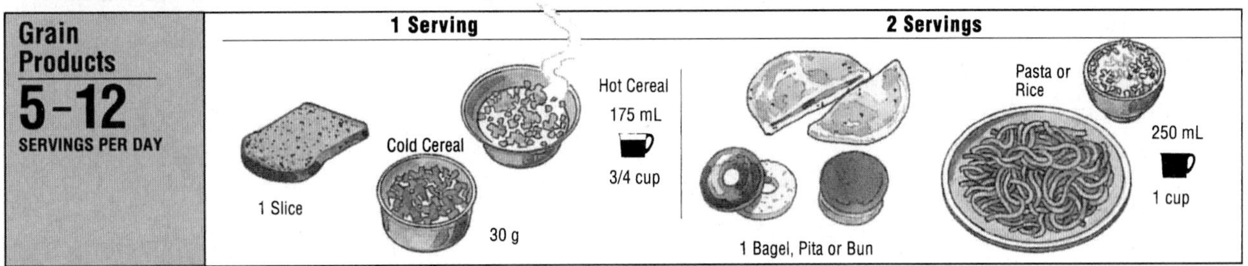

Vegetables & Fruit
5–10
SERVINGS PER DAY

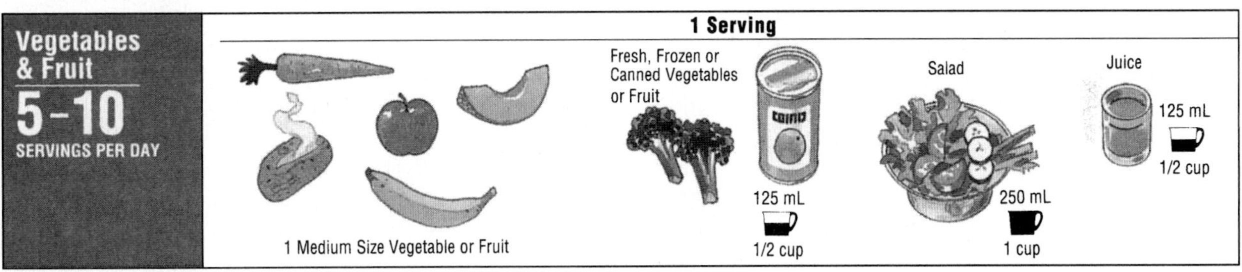
1 Serving
1 Medium Size Vegetable or Fruit
Fresh, Frozen or Canned Vegetables or Fruit
125 mL
1/2 cup
Salad
250 mL
1 cup
Juice
125 mL
1/2 cup

Milk Products
SERVINGS PER DAY
Children 4–9 years: 2–3
Youth 10–16 years: 3–4
Adults: 2–4
Pregnant & Breast-feeding Women: 3–4

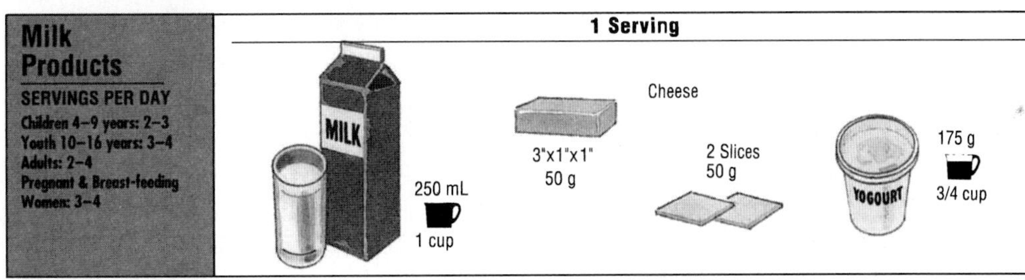

Meat & Alternatives
2–3
SERVINGS PER DAY

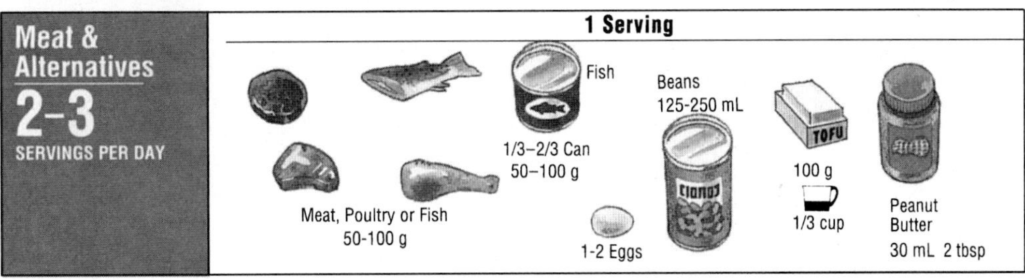

Other Foods

Taste and enjoyment can also come from other foods and beverages that are not part of the 4 food groups. Some of these foods are higher in fat or Calories, so use these foods in moderation.

Enjoy eating well, being active and feeling good about yourself. That's VITALITÉ®

 ISBN 0-662-19648-1

Nutrient Recommendations for Canadians

		Recommended Nutrient Intake													
Age	Sex	Weight (kg)	Protein (g)	Vit. A (RE[a])	Vit. D (μg)	Vit. E (mg)	Vit. C (mg)	Folate (μg)	Vit. B_{12} (μg)	Calcium (mg)	Phosphorus (mg)	Magnesium (mg)	Iron (mg)	Iodine (μg)	Zinc (mg)
Months															
0–4	Both	6.0	12[b]	400	10	3	20	25	0.3	250[c]	150	20	0.3[d]	30	2[d]
5–10	Both	9.0	12	400	10	3	20	40	0.4	400	200	32	7	40	3
Years															
1	Both	11	13	400	10	3	20	40	0.5	500	300	40	6	55	4
2–3	Both	14	16	400	5	4	20	50	0.6	550	350	50	6	65	4
4–6	Both	18	19	500	5	5	25	70	0.8	600	400	65	8	85	5
7–9	M	25	26	700	2.5	7	25	90	1.0	700	500	100	8	110	7
	F	25	26	700	2.5	6	25	90	1.0	700	500	100	8	95	7
10–12	M	34	34	800	2.5	8	25	120	1.0	900	700	130	8	125	9
	F	36	36	800	2.5	7	25	130	1.0	1100	800	135	8	110	9
13–15	M	50	49	900	2.5	9	30	175	1.0	1100	900	185	10	160	12
	F	48	46	800	2.5	7	30	170	1.0	1000	850	180	13	160	9
16–18	M	62	58	1000	2.5	10	40[e]	220	1.0	900	1000	230	10	160	12
	F	53	47	800	2.5	7	30[e]	190	1.0	700	850	200	12	160	9
19–24	M	71	61	1000	2.5	10	40[e]	220	1.0	800	1000	240	9	160	12
	F	58	50	800	2.5	7	30[e]	180	1.0	700	850	200	13	160	9
25–49	M	74	64	1000	2.5	9	40[e]	230	1.0	800	1000	250	9	160	12
	F	59	51	800	2.5	6	30[e]	185	1.0	700	850	200	13	160	9
50–74	M	73	63	1000	5	7	40[e]	230	1.0	800	1000	250	9	160	12
	F	63	54	800	5	6	30[e]	195	1.0	800	850	210	8	160	9
75+	M	69	59	1000	5	6	40[e]	215	1.0	800	1000	230	9	160	12
	F	64	55	800	5	5	30[e]	200	1.0	800	850	210	8	160	9
Pregnancy (additional)															
1st Trimester			5	0	2.5	2	0	200	0.2	500	200	15	0	25	6
2nd Trimester			20	0	2.5	2	10	200	0.2	500	200	45	5	25	6
3rd Trimester			24	0	2.5	2	10	200	0.2	500	200	45	10	25	6
Lactation (additional)			20	400	2.5	3	25	100	0.2	500	200	65	0	50	6

[a]Retinol equivalents.

[b]Protein is assumed to be from breast milk and must be adjusted for infant formula.

[c]Infant formula with high phosphorus should contain 375 mg calcium.

[d]Breast milk is assumed to be the source of the mineral.

[e]Smokers should increase vitamin C by 50%.

SOURCE: Scientific Review Committee. *Nutrition Recommendations,* Ottawa, Canada: Health and Welfare, 1990. Reproduced with permission of the Minister of Supply and Services Canada, 1996.

Continued

Nutrient Recommendations for Canadians—continued

		Energy Expressed as Daily Rates					
Age	Sex	Energy (Cal)	Thiamin (mg)	Riboflavin (mg)	Niacin (NE[b])	n-3 PUFA[d] (g)	n-6 PUFA (g)
Months							
0–4	Both	600	0.3	0.3	4	0.5	3
5–12	Both	900	0.4	0.5	7	0.5	3
Years							
1	Both	1100	0.5	0.6	8	0.6	4
2–3	Both	1300	0.6	0.7	9	0.7	4
4–6	Both	1800	0.7	0.9	13	1.0	6
7–9	M	2200	0.9	1.1	16	1.2	7
	F	1900	0.8	1.0	14	1.0	6
10–12	M	2500	1.0	1.3	18	1.4	8
	F	2200	0.9	1.1	16	1.2	7
13–15	M	2800	1.1	1.4	20	1.5	9
	F	2200	0.9	1.1	16	1.2	7
16–18	M	3200	1.3	1.6	23	1.8	11
	F	2100	0.8	1.1	15	1.2	7
19–24	M	3000	1.2	1.5	22	1.6	10
	F	2100	0.8	1.1	15	1.2	7
25–49	M	2700	1.1	1.4	19	1.5	9
	F	1900	0.8	1.0	14	1.1	7
50–74	M	2300	0.9	1.2	16	1.3	8
	F	1800	0.8[c]	1.0[c]	14[c]	1.1[c]	7[c]
75+	M	2000	0.8	1.0	14	1.1	7
	F[d]	1700	0.8[c]	1.0[c]	14[c]	1.1[c]	7[c]
Pregnancy (additional)							
1st Trimester		100	0.1	0.1	1	0.05	0.3
2nd Trimester		300	0.1	0.3	2	0.16	0.9
3rd Trimester		300	0.1	0.3	2	0.16	0.9
Lactation (additional)		450	0.2	0.4	3	0.25	1.5

[a]PUFA, polyunsaturated fatty acids.
[b]Niacin equivalents.
[c]Level below which intake should not fall.
[d]Assumes moderate physical activity.
SOURCE: Scientific Review Committee. *Nutrition Recommendations,* Ottawa, Canada: Health and Welfare, 1990.
Reproduced with permission of the Minister of Supply and Services Canada, 1996.

NATA Position Statement: Exertional Heat Illnesses*

BACKGROUND

Certified athletic trainers evaluate and treat heat-related injuries during athletic activity in "safe" and high-risk environments. While the recognition of heat illness has improved, the subtle signs and symptoms associated with heat illness are often overlooked, resulting in more serious problems for affected athletes. The recommendations presented here provide athletic trainers and allied health providers with an integrated scientific and practical approach to the prevention, recognition, and treatment of heat illnesses. These recommendations can be modified based on the environmental conditions of the site, the specific sport, and individual considerations to maximize safety and performance. Certified athletic trainers and other allied health providers should use these recommendations to establish on-site emergency plans for their venues and athletes. The primary goal of athlete safety is addressed through the prevention and recognition of heat-related illnesses and a well-developed plan to evaluate and treat affected athletes. Even with a heat-illness prevention plan that includes medical screening, acclimatization, conditioning, environmental monitoring, and suitable practice adjustments, heat illness can and does occur. Athletic trainers and other allied health providers must be prepared to respond in an expedient manner to alleviate symptoms and minimize morbidity and mortality.

RECOMMENDATIONS

1. Ensure that appropriate medical care is available and the rescue personnel are familiar with exertional heat illness prevention, recognition, and treatment.
2. Conduct a thorough, physician-supervised, preparticipation medical screening before the season starts to identify athletes predisposed to heat illness on the basis of risk factors and those who have a history of exertional heat illness.
3. Adapt athletes to exercise in the heat (acclimatization) gradually over 10 to 14 days. Progressively increase the intensity and duration of work in the heat with a combination of strenuous interval training and continuous exercise.
4. Educate athletes and coaches regarding the prevention, recognition, and treatment of heat illnesses and the risks associated with exercising in hot, humid environmental conditions.
5. Educate athletes to match fluid intake with sweat and urine losses to maintain adequate hydration. Instruct athletes to drink sodium-containing fluids to keep their urine clear to light yellow to improve hydration and to replace fluids between practices on the same day and on successive days to maintain less than 2% body-weight change.
6. Encourage athletes to sleep at least 6 to 8 hours at night in a cool environment, to eat a well-balanced diet that follows the Food Guide Pyramid and United States Dietary Guidelines, and maintain proper hydration status.
7. Develop event and practice guidelines for hot, humid weather that anticipate potential problems encountered based on the wet-bulb globe temperature or heat and humidity as measured by a sling psychrometer. Modify activity under high-risk conditions to prevent exertional heat illnesses. Identify individuals who are susceptible to

*From Binkley H, Beckett J, Casa D, Kleiner D, Plummer P: National Athletic Trainers Association position statement: exertional heat illnesses. *J Ath Train* 37(3):329, 2002.

heat illnesses. In some athletes, the prodromal signs and symptoms of heat illnesses are not evident before collapse, but in many cases, adept medical supervision will allow early intervention.

8. Check the environmental conditions before and during the activity, and adjust the practice schedule accordingly. Schedule training sessions to avoid the hottest part of the day (10 AM to 5 PM) and to avoid radiant heating from direct sunlight, especially in the acclimatization during the first few days of practice sessions.

9. Plan rest breaks to match the environmental conditions and the intensity of the activity.

10. Implement rest periods at mealtime by allowing 2 to 3 hours for food, fluids, nutrients, and electrolytes (sodium and potassium) to move into the small intestine and bloodstream before the next practice.

11. Provide and adequate supply of proper fluids (water or sport drinks) to maintain hydration and institute a hydration protocol that allows the maintenance of hydration status.

12. Weigh high-risk athletes (in high-risk conditions, weigh all athletes) before and after practice to estimate the amount of body water lost during practice and to ensure a return to prepractice weight before the next practice.

13. Minimize the amount of equipment and clothing worn by the athlete in hot or humid (or both) conditions.

14. Minimize warm-up time when feasible, and conduct warm-up sessions in the shade when possible to minimize the radiant heat load.

15. Allow athletes to practice in shaded areas and use electric or cooling fans to circulate air whenever feasible.

16. Include the following supplies on the field, in the locker room, and at various other stations: a supply of water or sport drinks; ice for active cooling; rectal thermometer to assess body-core temperature; telephone or 2-way radio; tub, wading pool, or whirlpool for ice immersion.

17. Notify local hospital and emergency personnel before mass participation events to inform them of the event and the increased possibility of heat-related illnesses.

18. Mandate a check of hydration status at weigh-in to ensure athletes in sports requiring weight classes (eg, wrestling, judo, rowing) are not dehydrated.

19. An athlete showing signs or symptoms including dehydration, thirst, sweating, transient muscle cramps, and fatigue is likely experiencing exercise-associated muscle (heat) cramps. To relieve muscle spasms, the athlete should stop activity, replace lost fluids with sodium-containing fluids, and begin mild stretching with massage of the muscle spasm. Fluid absorption is enhanced with sport drinks that contain sodium. A high-sodium sport product may be added to the rehydration beverage to prevent or relieve cramping in athletes who lose large amounts of sodium in their sweat.

20. If an athlete experiences a brief episode of fainting associated with dizziness, tunnel vision, pale or sweaty skin, and a decreased pulse rate but has a normal rectal temperature then heat syncope is most likely the cause. Move the athlete to a shaded area, monitor vital signs, elevate the legs above the level of the head, and rehydrate.

21. With exercise (heat) exhaustion, if feasible, measure body-core temperature (rectal temperature) and assess cognitive function and vital signs. Rectal temperature is the most accurate method possible in the field to monitor body-core temperature. If temperature is elevated, remove the athlete's excess clothing; cool the athlete with fans, ice towels, or ice bags; remove the athlete to a cool or shaded environment; start fluid replacement: and, transfer care to a physician if intravenous fluids are needed.

22. In exertional heat stroke, measure the rectal temperature if feasible to differentiate between heat exhaustion and heat stroke (rectal temperature > 104 degrees); assess cognitive function, which is markedly altered; lower the body-core temperature as quickly as possible by removing clothes and equipment and immersing the body into a pool or tub of cold water (35°F to 59°F). If a physician is not present, aggressive

first-aid cooling should be initiated on site and continued during emergency medical system transport and at the hospital. First-aid emergency procedures for heat stroke may include airway management.

23. In exertional hyponatremia the plasma sodium level is less than 130 mEq/L and is characterized by increasing headache, significant mental compromise, altered consciousness, seizures, lethargy, and swelling in the extremities. The athlete may be dehydrated, normally hydrated, or overhydrated. If hyponatremia is suspected, immediate transfer to an emergency medical center via the emergency medical system is indicated. An intravenous line should be placed to administer medication as needed to increase sodium levels, induce diuresis, and control seizures.

24. Prior to returning to activity in cases of exercise-associated muscle (heat) cramps or heat syncope, the ATC should discuss the athlete's case with the supervising physician. The cases of athletes with heat exhaustion who were not transferred to the physician's care should also be discussed with the physician. After exertional heat stroke or exertional hyponatremia, the athlete must be cleared by a physician before returning to athletic participation. The return to full activity should be gradual and monitored.

NATA Position Statement: Fluid Replacement for Athletes*

RECOMMENDATIONS

The National Athletic Trainers' Association (NATA) recommends the following practices regarding fluid replacement for athletic participation:

1. Establish a hydration protocol for athletes, including a rehydration strategy that considers the athlete's sweat rate, sport dynamics (eg, rest breaks, fluid access), environmental factors, acclimatization state, exercise duration, exercise intensity, and individual preferences.

2. A proper hydration protocol considers each sport's unique features. If rehydration opportunities are frequent (eg, baseball, football, track and field), the athlete can consume smaller volumes at a convenient pace based on sweat rate and environmental conditions. If rehydration must occur at specific times (eg, soccer, lacrosse, distance running), the athlete must consume fluids to maximize hydration within the sport's confines and rules.

3. Fluid-replacement beverages should be easily accessible in individual fluid containers and flavored to the athlete's preference. Individual containers permit easier monitoring of fluid intake. Clear water bottles marked in 100-mL (3.4-fl oz) increments provide visual reminders to athletes to drink beyond thirst satiation or the typical few gulps. Carrying water bottles or other hydration systems, when practical, during exercise encourages greater fluid volume ingestion.

4. Athletes should begin all exercise sessions well hydrated. Hydration status can be approximated by athletes and athletic trainers in several ways. Assuming proper hydration, pre-exercise body weight should be relatively consistent across exercise sessions. Determine the percentage difference between the current body weight and the hydrated baseline body weight. Remember that body weight is dynamic. Frequent exercise sessions can induce nonfluid-related weight loss influenced by timing of meals and defecation, time of day, and calories expended in exercise. The simplest method is comparison of urine color (from a sample in a container) with a urine color chart. Measuring urine specific gravity (USG) with a refractometer (available for less than $150) is less subjective than comparing urine color and also simple to use. Urine volume is another indicator of hydration status but inconvenient to collect and measure. For color analysis or specific gravity, use midstream urine collection for consistency and accuracy. Remember that body weight changes during exercise give the best indication of hydration status. Because of urine and body weight dynamics, measure urine before exercise and check body weight (percentage of body weight change) before, during, and after exercise sessions to estimate fluid balance.

5. To ensure proper pre-exercise hydration, the athlete should consume approximately 500 to 600 mL (17 to 20 fl oz) of water or a sports drink 2 to 3 hours before exercise and 200 to 300 mL (7 to 10 fl oz) of water or a sports drink 10 to 20 minutes before exercise.

6. Fluid replacement should approximate sweat and urine losses and at least maintain hydration at less than 2% body weight reduction. This generally requires 200 to 300 mL (7 to 10 fl oz) every 10 to 20 minutes. Specific individual recommendations are calculated based on sweat rates, sport dynamics, and individual tolerance. Maintaining hydration status in athletes with high sweat rates, in sports with limited fluid

*From Casa DJ, Armstrong LE, Hillman S: National Athletic Trainer's Association position statement: fluid replacement for athletes, *J Ath Train* 35(2):212, 2000.

access, and during high-intensity exercise can be difficult, and special efforts should be made to minimize dehydration. Dangerous hyperhydration is also a risk if athletes drink based on published recommendations and not according to individual needs.

7. Postexercise hydration should aim to correct any fluid loss accumulated during the practice or event. Ideally completed within 2 hours, rehydration should contain water to restore hydration status, carbohydrates to replenish glycogen stores, and electrolytes to speed rehydration. The primary goal is the immediate return of physiologic function (especially if an exercise bout will follow). When rehydration must be rapid, the athlete should compensate for obligatory urine losses incurred during the rehydration process and drink about 25% to 50% more than sweat losses to assure optimal hydration 4 to 6 hours after the event.

8. Fluid temperature influences the amount consumed. While individual differences exist, a cool beverage of 10° to 15°C (50° to 59°F) is recommended.

9. The Wet Bulb Globe Temperature (WBGT) should be ascertained in hot environments. Very high relative humidity limits evaporative cooling; the air is nearly saturated with water vapor, and evaporation is minimized. Thus, dehydration associated with high sweat losses can induce a rapid core temperature increase due to the inability to dissipate heat. Measuring core temperature rectally allows the athlete's thermal status to be accurately determined. See the NATA position statement on heat illnesses for expanded information on this topic.

10. In many situations, athletes benefit from including carbohydrates (CHOs) in their rehydration protocols. Consuming CHOs during the pre-exercise hydration session (2 to 3 hours pre-exercise), as in item 5, along with a normal daily diet increases glycogen stores. If exercise is intense, then consuming CHOs about 30 minutes pre-exercise may also be beneficial. Include CHOs in the rehydration beverage during exercise if the session lasts longer than 45 to 50 minutes or is intense. An ingestion rate of about 1 g/min (0.04 oz/min) maintains optimal carbohydrate metabolism: for example, 1 L of a 6% CHO drink per hour of exercise. CHO concentrations greater than 8% increase the rate of CHO delivery to the body but compromise the rate of fluid emptying from the stomach and absorbed from the intestine. Fruit juices, CHO gels, sodas, and some sports drinks have CHO concentrations greater than 8% and are not recommended *during* an exercise session as the sole beverage. Athletes should consume CHOs at least 30 minutes before the normal onset of fatigue and earlier if the environmental conditions are unusually extreme, although this may not apply for very intense, short-term exercise, which may require earlier intake of CHOs. Most CHO forms (ie, glucose, sucrose, glucose polymers) are suitable, and the absorption rate is maximized when multiple forms are consumed simultaneously. Substances to be limited include fructose (which may cause gastrointestinal distress); those to be avoided include caffeine, alcohol (which may increase urine output and reduce fluid retention), and carbonated beverages (which may reduce voluntary fluid intake due to stomach fullness).

11. Those supervising athletes should be able to recognize the basic signs and symptoms of dehydration: thirst, irritability, and general discomfort, followed by headache, weakness, dizziness, cramps, chills, vomiting, nausea, head or neck heat sensations, and decreased performance. Early diagnosis of dehydration decreases the occurrence and severity of heat illness. A conscious, cognizant, dehydrated athlete without gastrointestinal distress can aggressively rehydrate orally, while one with mental compromise from dehydration or gastrointestinal distress should be transported to a medical facility for intravenous rehydration. For a complete description of heat illnesses and issues related to hyperthermia, see the NATA position statement on heat illnesses.

12. Inclusion of sodium chloride in fluid-replacement beverages should be considered under the following conditions: inadequate access to meals or meals not eaten; physical activity exceeding 4 hours in duration; or during the initial days of hot

weather. Under these conditions, adding modest amounts of salt (0.3 to 0.7 g/L) can offset salt loss in sweat and minimize medical events associated with electrolyte imbalances (eg, muscle cramps, hyponatremia). Adding a modest amount of salt (0.3 to 0.7 g/L) to all hydration beverages would be acceptable to stimulate thirst, increase voluntary fluid intake, and decrease the risk of hyponatremia and should cause no harm.

13. Calculate each athlete's sweat rate (sweating rate = pre-exercise body weight − postexercise body weight + fluid intake − urine volume/exercise time in hours) for a representative range of environmental conditions, practices, and competitions (Table 3). This time-consuming task can be made easier by weighing a large number of athletes before an intense 1-hour practice session and then reweighing them at the end of the 1-hour practice. Sweat rate can now be easily calculated (do not allow rehydration or urination during this 1 hour when sweat rate is being determined to make the task even easier). This calculation is the most fundamental consideration when establishing a rehydration protocol. Average sweat rates from the scientific literature or other athletes can vary from 0.5 L/h to more than 2.5 L/h (0.50 to 2.50 kg/h) and are not ideal to use.

14. Heat acclimatization induces physiologic changes that may alter individual fluid-replacement considerations. First, sweat rate generally increases after 10 to 14 days of heat exposure, requiring a greater fluid intake for a similar bout of exercise. An athlete's sweat rate should be reassessed after acclimatization. Second, moving from a cool environment to a warm environment increases the overall sweat rate for a bout of exercise. The athlete's hydration status must be closely monitored for the first week of exercise in a warm environment. Third, increased sodium intake may be warranted during the first 3 to 5 days of heat exposure, since the increased thermal strain and associated increased sweat rate increases the sodium lost in sweat. Adequate sodium intake optimizes fluid palatability and absorption during the first few days and may decrease exercise-associated muscle cramping. After 5 to 10 days, the sodium concentration of sweat decreases, and normal sodium intake suffices.

15. All sports requiring weight classes (ie, wrestling, judo, rowing) should mandate a check of hydration status at weigh-in to ensure that the athlete is not dehydrated. A USG less than or equal to 1.020 or urine color less than or equal to 4 should be the upper range of acceptable on weigh-in. Any procedures used to induce dramatic dehydration (eg, diuretics, rubber suits, exercising in a sauna) are strictly prohibited.

16. Hyperhydration by ingesting a pre-exercise glycerol and water beverage has equivocal support from well-controlled studies. At this time, evidence is insufficient to endorse the practice of hyperhydration via glycerol. Also, a risk of side effects such as headaches and gastrointestinal distress exists when glycerol is consumed.

17. Consider modifications when working with prepubescent and adolescent athletes who exercise intensely in the heat and may not fully comprehend the medical and performance consequences of dehydration. Focus special attention on schedules and event modification to minimize environmental stress and maximize time for fluid replacement. Make available the most palatable beverage possible. Educate parents and coaches about rehydration and the signs of dehydration. Monitor and remove a child from activity promptly if signs or symptoms of dehydration occur.

18. Large-scale event management (eg, tournaments, camps) requires advance planning. Ample fluid and cups should be conveniently available. With successive practice sessions during a day or over multiple days (as in most summer sport camps), check hydration status daily before allowing continued participation. Be aware of unhealthy behaviors, such as eating disorders and dehydration in weight-class sports. Use extra caution with novice and unconditioned athletes, and remember, many athletes are not supervised on a daily basis. If the WBGT dictates, modify events (change game times or cancel) or change game dynamics (insert nonroutine water breaks, shorten game times). Recruit help from fellow athletic trainers in local schools, student athletic

trainers, and athletes from other sports to ensure that hydration is maintained at all venues (ie, along a road race course, on different fields during a tournament). Be sure all assistants can communicate with the supervising athletic trainer at a central location. For successive-day events, provide educational materials on rehydration principles to inform athletes and parents of this critical component of athletic performance.

19. Implementing a hydration protocol for athletes will only succeed if athletes, coaches, athletic trainers, and team physicians realize the importance of maintaining proper hydration status and the steps required to accomplish this goal. Here are the most critical components of hydration education:

- Educate athletes on the effects of dehydration on physical performance.
- Inform athletes on how to monitor hydration status.
- Convince athletes to participate in their own hydration protocols based on sweat rate, drinking preferences, and personal responses to different fluid quantities.
- Encourage coaches to mandate rehydration during practices and competitions, just as they require other drills and conditioning activities.
- Have a scale accessible to assist athletes in monitoring weight before, during, and after activity.
- Provide the optimal oral rehydration solution (water, CHOs, electrolytes) before, during, and after exercise.
- Implement the hydration protocol during all practices and games, and adapt it as needed.
- Finally, encourage event scheduling and rule modifications to minimize the risks associated with exercise in the heat.

NATA Position Statement: Lightning Safety for Athletics and Recreation*

The guidelines presented in this article govern all outdoor activities, as well as indoor swimming-pool activities. The purpose of this position statement is to recommend lightning-safety policy guidelines and strategies and to educate athletic trainers and others involved with athletic or recreation activities about the hazards of lightning.

RECOMMENDATIONS

1. Formalize and implement a comprehensive, proactive lightning-safety policy or emergency action plan specific to lightning safety. The components of this policy should include the following:
   - An established chain of command that identifies who is to make the call to remove individuals from the field or an activity.
   - A designated weather watcher (ie, a person who actively looks for the signs of threatening weather and notifies the chain of command if severe weather becomes dangerous).
   - A means of monitoring local weather forecasts and warnings.
   - A listing of specific safe locations (for each field or site) from the lightning hazard.
   - The use of specific criteria for suspension and resumption of activities (refer to recommendations 4, 5, and 6).
   - The use of the recommended lightning-safety strategies (refer to recommendations 7, 8, and 9).
2. The primary choice for a safe location from the lightning hazard is any substantial, frequently inhabited building. The electric and telephone wiring and plumbing pathways aid in grounding a building, which is why buildings are safer than remaining outdoors during thunderstorms. It is important not to be connected to these pathways while inside the structure during ongoing thunderstorms.
3. The secondary choice for a safer location from the lightning hazard is a fully enclosed vehicle with a metal roof and the windows closed. Convertible cars and golf carts do not provide protection from lightning danger. It is important not to touch any part of the metal framework of the vehicle while inside it during ongoing thunderstorms.
4. Seeking a safe structure or location at the first sign of lightning or thunder activity is highly recommended. By the time the flash-to-bang count approaches 30 seconds (or is less than 30 seconds), all individuals should already be inside or should immediately seek a safe structure or location. To use the flash-to-bang method, the observer begins counting when a lightning flash is sighted. Counting is stopped when the associated bang (thunder) is heard. Divide this count by 5 to determine the distance to the lightning flash (in miles). For example, a flash-to-bang count of 30 seconds equates to a distance of 6 miles (9.66 km).
5. Postpone or suspend activity if a thunderstorm appears imminent before or during an activity or contest (regardless of whether lightning is seen or thunder heard) until the hazard has passed. Signs of imminent thunderstorm activity are darkening clouds, high winds, and thunder or lightning activity.

*From Walsh K, Bennett B, Cooper M: National Athletic Trainer's Association position statement: lightning safety for athletics and recreation. *J Ath Train* 35(4):471, 2000.

6. Once activities have been suspended, wait at least 30 minutes after the last sound of thunder or lightning flash before resuming an activity or returning outdoors. A message should be read over the public address system and lightning-safety tips should be placed in game programs alerting spectators and competitors about what to do and where to go to find a safer location during thunderstorm activity.

7. Extremely large athletic events are of particular concern with regard to lightning safety. Consider using a multidisciplinary approach to lessen lightning danger, such as integrating weather forecasts, real-time thunderstorm data, a weather watcher, and the flash-to-bang count to aid in decision making.

8. Avoid being in contact with, or in proximity to, the highest point of an open field or on the open water. Do not take shelter under or near trees, flag poles, or light poles.

9. Avoid taking showers and using plumbing facilities (including indoor and outdoor pools) and land-line telephones during thunderstorm activity. Cordless or cellular telephones are safer to use when emergency help is needed.

10. Individuals who feel their hair stand on end or skin tingle or hear crackling noises should assume the lightning-safe position (ie, crouched on the ground, weight on the balls of the feet, feet together, head lowered, and ears covered). Do not lie flat on the ground.

11. Observe the following basic first-aid procedures, in order, to manage victims of lightning strike.

- Survey the scene for safety. Ongoing thunderstorms may still pose a threat to emergency personnel responding to the situation.
- Activate the local emergency management system.
- Move the victim carefully to a safer location, if needed.
- Evaluate and treat for apnea and asystole.
- Evaluate and treat for hypothermia and shock.
- Evaluate and treat for fractures.
- Evaluate and treat for burns.

12. All persons should maintain current cardiopulmonary resuscitation (CPR) and first-aid certification.

13. All individuals should have the right to leave an athletic site or activity, without fear of repercussion or penalty, in order to seek a safe structure or location if they feel they are in danger from impending lightning activity.

Appendix F

NATA Position Statement: Emergency Planning in Athletics*

Although most injuries that occur in athletics are relatively minor, limb-threatening or life-threatening injuries are unpredictable and can occur without warning. Because of the relatively low incidence rate of catastrophic injuries, athletic program personnel may develop a false sense of security over time in the absence of such injuries. However, these injuries can occur during any physical activity and at any level of participation. Of additional concern is the heightened public awareness associated with the nature and management of such injuries. Medico legal interests can lead to questions about the qualifications of the personnel involved, the preparedness of the organization for handling these situations, and the actions taken by program personnel.

Proper emergency management of limb- or life-threatening injuries is critical and should be handled by trained medical and allied health personnel. Preparation for response to emergencies includes education and training, maintenance of emergency equipment and supplies, appropriate use of personnel, and the formation and implementation of an emergency plan. The emergency plan should be thought of as a blueprint for handling emergencies. A sound emergency plan is easily understood and establishes accountability for the management of emergencies. Furthermore, failure to have an emergency plan can be considered negligence.

POSITION STATEMENT

Based on an extensive survey of the literature and expert review, the following is the position of the National Athletic Trainers' Association (NATA):

1. Each institution or organization that sponsors athletic activities must have a written emergency plan. The emergency plan should be comprehensive and practical, yet flexible enough to adapt to any emergency situation.
2. Emergency plans must be written documents and should be distributed to certified athletic trainers, team and attending physicians, athletic training students, institutional and organizational safety personnel, institutional and organizational administrators, and coaches. The emergency plan should be developed in consultation with local emergency medical services department.
3. An emergency plan for athletics identifies the personnel involved in carrying out the emergency plan and outlines the qualifications of those executing the plan. Sports medicine professionals, officials, and coaches should be trained in automatic external defibrillation cardiopulmonary resuscitation, first aid, and prevention of disease transmission.
4. The emergency plan should specify the equipment needed to carry out the tasks required in the event of an emergency. In addition, the emergency plan should outline the location of the emergency equipment. Further, the equipment available should be appropriate to the level of training of the personnel involved.
5. Establishment of a clear mechanism for communication to appropriate emergency care service providers and identification of the mode of transportation for the injured participant are critical elements of an emergency plan.
6. The emergency plan should be specific to the activity venue. That is, each activity site should have a defined emergency plan that is derived from the overall institutional or organizational policies on emergency planning.

*From Anderson, JC, Courson, RW, Kleinert, DM: National Athletic Trainers' Association position statement: emergency planning in athletics, *J Ath Train*, 37(1):99, 2002.

7. Emergency plans should incorporate the emergency care facilities to which the injured physically active individual will be taken. Emergency receiving facilities should be notified in advance of scheduled events and contests. Personnel from the emergency receiving facilities should be included in the development of the emergency plan for the institution or organization.

8. The emergency plan specifies the necessary documentation supporting the implementation and evaluation of the emergency plan. This documentation should identify responsibility for documenting actions taken during the emergency, evaluation of the emergency response and institutional personnel training.

9. The emergency plan should be reviewed and rehearsed annually, although more frequent review and rehearsal may be necessary. The results of these reviews and rehearsals should be documented and should indicate whether the emergency plan was modified with further documentation reflecting how the plan was changed.

10. All personnel involved with the organization and sponsorship of athletic activities share a professional responsibility to provide for the emergency care of an injured participant, including the development and implementation of an emergency plan.

11. All personnel involved with the organization and sponsorship of athletic activities share a legal duty to develop, implement, and evaluate an emergency plan for all sponsored athletic activities.

12. The emergency plan should be reviewed by the administration and legal counsel of the sponsoring organization or institution.

Sample Venue-Specific Emergency Protocol*

__________ University Sports Medicine Football Emergency Protocol

1. Call 911 or other emergency number consistent with organizational policies
2. Instruct emergency medical services (EMS) personnel to "report to __________ and meet __________ at __________ that we have an injured student-athlete in need of emergency medical treatment."

   University Football Practice Complex: __________ st. entrance (gate across street from __________) cross street __________ street

   University Stadium: Gates __________ entrance off __________ Road
3. Provide necessary information to EMS personnel:
   - Name, address, telephone number of caller
   - Number of victims; condition of victims
   - First-aid treatment initiated
   - Specific directions as needed to locate scene
   - Other information as requested by dispatcher
4. Provide appropriate emergency care unit arrival of EMS personnel: on arrival of EMS personnel, provide pertinent information (method of injury, vital signs, treatment rendered, medical history) and assist with emergency care as needed

NOTE:

- Sports medicine staff member should accompany student-athlete to hospital
- Notify other sports medicine staff immediately
- Parents should be contacted by sports medicine staff
- Inform coach(es) and administration
- Obtain medical history and insurance information
- Appropriate injury reports should be completed

Emergency Telephone Numbers

__________ Hospital	__________ - __________
__________ Emergency Department	__________ - __________
University Health Center	__________ - __________
Campus Police	__________ - __________

Emergency Signals

Physician arm extended overhead with clenched fist
Paramedics point to location in end zone by home locker room and wave onto field
Spine board: arms held horizontally
Stretcher: supinated hands in front of body or waist level
Splints: hand to lower leg or thigh

SUMMARY

The purpose of this statement is to present the position of the NATA on emergency planning in athletics. Specifically, professional and legal requirements mandate that organizations or institutions sponsoring athletic activities have a written emergency plan. A well-thought-out emergency plan consists of a number of factors, including, but not necessarily limited to personnel, equipment, communication, transportation, and documentation. Finally, all sports medicine professionals, coaches, and organizational administrators share professional and legal duties to develop, implement, and evaluate emergency plans for sponsored athletic activities.

NATA Helmet Removal Guidelines (1998)*

The National Athletic Trainers' Association has adopted the following guidelines with regard to the on-site removal of the athletic helmet.

Removing helmets from athletes with potential cervical spine injuries may worsen existing injuries or cause new ones. Removal of athletic helmets should, therefore, be avoided unless individual circumstances dictate otherwise.

Before removing the helmet from an injured athlete, appropriate alternatives such as the following should be considered:

- Most injuries can be visualized with the helmet in place.
- Neurological tests can be performed with the helmet in place. The eyes may be examined for reactivity, the nose and ears checked for fluid, and the level of consciousness determined.
- The athlete can be immobilized on a spine board with the helmet in place.
- The helmet and shoulder pads elevate the supine athlete. Removal of helmet and shoulder pads, if required, should be coordinated to avoid cervical hyperextension.
- Removal of the face mask allows full airway access to be achieved. Plastic clips securing the face mask can be cut using special tools, permitting rapid removal.

In all cases, individual circumstances must dictate appropriate actions.

*From www.nata.org

Appendix H

NATA Blood Borne Pathogens Guidelines for Athletic Trainers

The NATA recognizes that blood borne pathogens such as HIV, HBV, and HCV present many complex issues for athletic trainers, athletic administrators, and others involved with the care and training of athletes. As the primary health care professional involved with the physically active, it is important for athletic trainers to be aware of these issues. The NATA therefore offers the following guidelines and information concerning the management of blood borne pathogen–related issues in the context of athletics and settings in which the physically active are involved.

It is essential to remember, however, that the medical, legal and professional knowledge, standards and requirements concerning blood borne pathogens are changing and evolving constantly, and vary, in addition, from place to place and from setting to setting. The guidance provided in these guidelines must not, therefore, be taken to represent national standards applicable to members of the NATA. Rather, the guidance here is intended to highlight issues, problems, and potential approaches to (or management of) those problems that NATA members can consider when developing their own policies with respect to management of these issues.

ATHLETIC PARTICIPATION

Decisions regarding the participation of athletes infected with blood borne pathogens in athletic competitions should be made on an individual basis. Such decisions should be made following the standard or appropriate procedures generally followed with respect to health-related participation questions, and taking into account only those factors that are directly relevant to the health and rights of the athlete, the other participants in the competition, and the other constituencies with interests in the competition; the athletic program, the athletes, and the sponsoring schools and organizations.

The following are examples of factors that are appropriate in many settings to the decision-making process:

- The current health of the athlete
- The nature and intensity of the athlete's training
- The physiological effects of the athletic competition
- The potential risks of the infection being transmitted
- The desires of the athlete
- The administrative and legal needs of the competitive program

EDUCATION OF THE PHYSICALLY ACTIVE

In a rapidly changing medical, social, and legal environment, educational information concerning blood borne pathogens is of particular importance. The athletic trainer should play a role with respect to the creation and dissemination of educational information that is appropriate to and particularized with respect to that athletic trainer's position and responsibilities.

Athletic trainers who are responsible for developing educational programs with respect to blood borne pathogens should provide appropriate information concerning:

- The risk of transmission or infection during competition
- The risk of transmission or infection generally
- The availability of HIV testing
- The availability of HBV testing and vaccinations

Athletic trainers who have educational program responsibility should extend educational efforts to include those, such as the athletes' families and communities, who are directly or indirectly affected by the presence of blood borne pathogens in athletic competitions.

All educational activities should, of course, be limited to those within athletic trainers' scope of practice and competence, be within their job descriptions or other relevant roles, and be undertaken with the cooperation and/or consent of appropriate personnel, such as team physicians, coaches, athletic directors, school or institutional counsel, and school and community leaders.

THE ATHLETIC TRAINER AND BLOOD BORNE PATHOGENS AT ATHLETIC EVENTS

The risk of blood borne pathogen transmission at athletic events is directly associated with contact with blood or other body fluids. Athletic trainers who have responsibility for overseeing events at which such contact is possible should use appropriate preventative measures and be prepared to administer appropriate treatment, consistent with the requirements and restrictions of their job, and local, state, and federal law.

In most cases, these measures will include:

- Pre-event care and covering of existing wounds, cuts, and abrasions
- Provision of the necessary or usual equipment and supplies for compliance with universal precautions, including, for example, latex gloves, biohazard containers, disinfectants, bleach solutions, antiseptics, and sharps containers
- Early recognition and control of a bleeding athlete, including measures such as appropriate cleaning and covering procedures, or changing of blood-saturated clothes
- Requiring all athletes to report all wounds immediately
- Insistence that universal precaution guidelines be followed at all times in the management of acute blood exposure
- Appropriate cleaning and disposal policies and procedures for contaminated areas or equipment
- Appropriate policies with respect to the delivery of life-saving techniques in the absence of protective equipment
- Post-event management including, as appropriate, re-evaluation, coverage of wounds, cuts, and abrasions
- Appropriate policy development, including incorporation, with necessary legal and administrative assistance, of existing OSHA and other legal guidelines and conference or school rules and regulations

STUDENT ATHLETIC TRAINER EDUCATION

NATA encourages appropriate education of and involvement of the student athletic trainer in educational efforts involving blood borne pathogens. These efforts and programs will vary significantly based on local needs, requirements, resources, and policies.

At the secondary school level, educational efforts should include items such as the following:

- Education and training in the use of universal precautions and first aid for wounds
- Education regarding the risks of transmission/infection from the participants that they care for
- Education on the availability of HIV testing
- Education on the availability of HBV vaccinations and testing
- Education of parents or guardians regarding the students' risk of infection

At the college or university level, education efforts should include items such as those listed above, and, additionally, as appropriate, the following:

- Education in basic and clinical science of blood borne pathogens

- Discussions regarding the ethical and social issues related to blood borne pathogens
- The importance of prevention programs
- Education concerning the signs and symptoms of HBV and HIV, as consistent with the scope of practice of the athletic profession and state and local law

UNIVERSAL PRECAUTIONS AND OSHA REGULATIONS

Athletic trainers should, consistent with their job descriptions and the time and legal requirements and limitations of their jobs and professions, inform themselves and other affected and interested parties of the relevant legal guidance and requirements affecting the handling and treatment of blood borne pathogens.

Athletic trainers cannot be expected to practice law or medicine, and efforts with respect to compliance with these guidelines and requirements must be commensurate with the athletic trainer's profession and professional requirements. It may be appropriate for athletic trainers to keep copies of the Center for Disease Control regulations and OSHA regulations and guidelines available for their own and others' use.

MEDICAL RECORDS AND CONFIDENTIALITY

The security, record-keeping, and confidentiality requirements and concerns that relate to athletes' medical records generally apply equally to those portions of athletes' medical records that concern blood borne pathogens.

Since social stigma is sometimes attached to individuals infected with blood borne pathogens, athletic trainers should pay particular care to the security, record-keeping, and confidentiality requirements that govern the medical records for which they have a professional obligation to see, use, keep, interpret, record, update, or otherwise handle.

Security, record-keeping, and confidentiality procedures should be maintained with respect to the records of other athletic trainers, employees, student athletic trainers, and athletes, to the extent that the athletic trainer has responsibility for these records.

THE INFECTED ATHLETIC TRAINER

An athletic trainer infected with a blood borne pathogen should practice the profession of athletic training taking into account all professionally, medically, and legally relevant issues raised by the infection. Depending on individual circumstances, the infected athletic trainer will or may wish to:

- Seek medical care and ongoing evaluation
- Take reasonable steps to avoid potential and identifiable risks to his or her own health and the health of his or her patients
- Inform, as or when appropriate, relevant patients, administrators, or medical personnel

HIV AND HBV TESTING

Athletic trainers should follow federal, state, local, and institutional laws, regulations, and guidelines concerning HIV and HBV testing. Athletic trainers should, in appropriate practice settings and situations, find it advisable to educate or assist athletes with respect to the availability of testing.

HBV VACCINATIONS

Consistent with professional requirements and restrictions, athletic trainers should encourage HBV vaccinations for all employees at risk, in accordance with OSHA guidelines.

WITHHOLDING OF CARE AND DISCRIMINATION

NATA's policies and its Code of Ethics make it unethical to discriminate on the basis of medical conditions.

REFERENCES

American Academy of Pediatrics. Human immunodeficiency virus [acquired immunodeficiency syndrome (AIDS) virus] in the athletic setting. *Pediatrics.* 1991;88:640–641.

American Medical Association, Department of HIV, Division of Health Science. Digest of HIV/AIDS Policy. Chicago, IL: Department of HIV, American Medical Association; 1993:1–15.

American Medical Society for Sports Medicine and American Academy of Sports Medicine. Human immunodeficiency virus (HIV) and other blood-borne pathogens in sports. *American Journal of Sports Medicine.* In Press.

Benson MT, ed. Guideline 2H: blood-borne pathogens and intercollegiate athletics. NCAA Sports Medicine Handbook. 1993;24–28.

Michigan Department of Public Health. Michigan recommendations on HBV and/or HIV infected health care workers. *Triad.* 1992;4:32–34.

NATA Position Statement: Management of Sport-Related Concussion*

RECOMMENDATIONS

The NATA recommends the following practices regarding management of sport-related concussion:

1. The ATC should develop a high sensitivity for the various mechanisms and presentations of traumatic brain inury (TBI), including mild, moderate, and severe cerebal concussion, as well as the severe but less common head injuries that can cause damage to the brain stem and other vital centers of the brain.

2. The colloquial term "ding" should not be used to describe a sport-related concussion. This stunned confusional state is a concussion most often reflected by the athlete's initial confusion, which may disappear within minutes, leaving no outward observable signs and symptoms. Use of the term "ding" generally carries a connotation that diminishes the seriousness of the injury. If an athlete shows concussion-like signs and reports symptoms after a contact to the head, the athlete has, *at the very least,* sustained a mild concussion and should be treated for a concussion.

3. To detect deteriorating signs and symptoms that may indicate a more serious head injury, the ATC should be able to recognize both the obvious signs (fluctuating levels of consciousness, balance problems, memory and concentration difficulties, etc.) and common self-reported symptoms (headache, ringing in the ears, nausea, etc.)

4. The ATC should play an active role in educating athletes, coaches, and parents about the signs and symptoms associated with concussion, as well as the potential risks of playing while still symptomatic.

5. The ATC should document all pertinent information surrounding the concussive injury, including, but not limited to a) mechanism of injury, b) initial signs and symptoms, c) state of consciousness, d) findings on serial testing of symptoms, neuropsychological function, and postural stability (noting any deficits compared with baseline), e) instructions given to the athlete and/or parent, f) recommendations provided by the physician, g) date and time of the athlete's return to participation, and h) relevant information on the player's history of prior concussion and associated recovery pattern(s).

6. ATCs and team physicians working together should agree on a philosophy for managing sport-related concussion before the start of the athletic season. The ATC-physician team should be consistent in its use regardless of the athlete, sport, or circumstances surrounding the injury.

7. For athletes playing sports with a high risk of concussion, baseline cognitive and postural-stability testing should be considered. In addition to the concussion injury assessment, the evaluation should also include an assessment of the cervical spine and cranial nerves to identify any cervical spine or vascular intracerebal injuries.

8. The ATC should record the time of the initial injury and document serial assessments of the injured athlete, noting the presence or absence of signs and symptoms of injury. The ATC should monitor vital signs and level of consciousness every 5 minutes

*From Guskiewicz K, et al: National Athletic Trainers' Association position statement: management of sport-related concussion, *J Ath Train* 39:280, 2004.

after a concussion until the athlete's condition improves. The athlete should also be monitored over the next few days after the injury for the presence of delayed signs and symptoms and to assess recovery.

9. Concussion severity should be determined by paying close attention to the severity and persistence of *all* signs and symptoms, including the presence of amnesia (retrograde and anterograde) and loss of consciousness (LOC), as well as headache, concentration problems, dizziness, blurred vision, etc. It is recommended that ATC and physicians consistently use a symptom checklist.

10. In addition to a thorough clinical evaluation, formal cognitive and postural-stability testing is recommended to assist in objectively determining injury severity and readiness to return to play (RTP). No one test should be used solely to determine recovery or return to play, as concussion presents in many different ways.

11. Once symptom-free or asymptomatic, the athlete should be reassessed to establish that cognition and postural stability have returned to normal for that player, preferably by comparison with preinjury baseline test results. The RTP decision should be made after an incremental increase in activity with an initial cardiovascular challenge, followed by sport-specific activities that do not place the athlete at risk for concussion. The athlete can be released to full participation as long no recurrent signs or symptoms are present.

12. Baseline testing on concussion-assessment measures is recommended to establish the individual athlete's "normal" preinjury performance and to provide the most reliable benchmark against which to measure postinjury recovery. Baseline testing also controls for extraneous variables (attention deficit disorder, learning disabilities, age, education, etc.) and for the effects of earlier concussion, while also evaluating the possible cumulative effects of recurrent concussions.

13. The use of objective concussion-assessment tools will help ATCs in more accurately identifying deficits caused by injury and postinjury recovery and protect players from the potential risks associated with prematurely returning to competition and sustaining a repeat concussion. The concussion-assessment battery should include a combination of tests for cognition, postural stability, and self-reported symptoms known to be affected by concussion.

14. A combination of brief screening tools appropriate for use on the sideline (eg, Standardized Assessment of Concussion [SAC], Balance Error Scoring System [BESS], symptom checklist) and more extensive measures (eg, neuropsychological testing, computerized balance testing) to more precisely evaluate recovery later after injury is recommended.

15. Before instituting a concussion neuropsychological testing battery, the ATC should understand the test's user requirements, copyright restrictions, and standardized instructions for administration and scoring. All evaluators should be appropriately trained in the standardized instructions for test administration and scoring before embarking on testing or adopting an instrument for clinical use. Ideally, the sports medicine team should include a neuropsychologist, but in reality, many ATCs may not have access to a neuropsychologist for interpretation and consultation, nor the financial resources to support a neuropsychological testing program. In this case, it is recommended that the ATC use screening instruments (SAC, BESS, symptoms checklist) that have been developed specifically for use by sports medicine clinicians without extensive training in psychometric or standardized testing and that do not require a special license to administer or interpret.

16. Athletic trainers should adopt for clinical use only, those neuropsychological and postural stability measures with population-specific normative data, test-retest reliability, clinical validity, and sufficient sensitivity and specificity established in the peer-reviewed literature. These standards provide the basis for how well the test can distinguish between those with and without cerebral dysfunction in order to reduce the possibility of making false-positive and false-negative errors which could lead to clinical decision-making errors.

17. As is the case with all clinical instruments, results from assessment measures to evaluate concussion should be integrated with all aspects of the injury evaluation (eg, physical examination, neurologic evaluation, neuroimaging, player's history, etc) for the most effective approach to injury management and RTP decision making. Decisions about an athlete's return to play should never be based solely on the use of any *one* test.

18. The ATC or team physician should monitor an athlete with a concussion at 5-minute intervals from the time of the injury until the athlete's condition completely clears or the athlete is referred for further care. Coaches should be informed that in situations when a concussion is suspected but an ATC or physician is not available, their primary role is to ensure that the athlete is immediately seen by an ATC or physician.

19. An athlete with a concussion should be referred to a physician on the day of injury if he or she lost consciousness or experienced amnesia lasting longer than 15 minutes.

20. A team approach for the assessment of concussion should be used to include a variety of medical specialties. In addition to family practice or general medicine physician referrals, the ATC should secure other specialist referral sources within the community. For example, neurologist are trained to assist in the management of patients experiencing persistent signs and symptoms, including sleep disturbances. Similarly, a neuropsychologist should be identified as part of the sports medicine team for assisting athletes who require more extensive neuropsychological testing and for interpreting the results of neuropsychological tests.

21. A team approach should be used in making RTP decision after concussion. This approach should involve input from the ATC, physician, athlete, and any referral sources. The assessment of all information including the physical examination, imaging studies, objective tests, and exertional efforts should be considered prior to making a RTP decision.

22. Athletes who are symptomatic at rest and after exertion for a least 20 minutes should be disqualified from returning to participation on the day of the injury. Exertional exercises should include sideline jogging followed by sprinting, sit-ups, push-ups, and any sport-specific, noncontact activities (or positions or stances) the athlete might need to perform upon returning to participation. Athletes who return on the same day because symptoms resolved quickly (<20 minutes) should be monitored closely after they return to play. They should be repeatedly reevaluated on the sidelines, after the practice or game, and again at 24 and 48 hours postinjury to identify any delayed onset of symptoms.

23. Athletes who experience LOC or amnesia should be disqualified from participating on the day of the injury.

24. The decision to disqualify from further participation on the day of a concussion should be based on a comprehensive physical examination, assessment of self-reported post concussion signs and symptoms, functional impairments, and the athlete's past history of concussions. If assessment tools such as the SAC, BESS, neuropsychological test battery, and symptom checklist are not used, a 7-day symptom-free waiting period before returning to participation is recommended. Some circumstances, however, will warrant even more conservative treatment.

25. Athletic trainers should be more conservative with athletes who have a history of concussion. Athletes with a history of concussion are at increased risk for sustaining subsequent injuries, as well as for slowed recovery of self-reported post concussion signs and symptoms, cognitive dysfunction, and postural instability after subsequent injuries. Disqualification (either temporary or permanent) from contact sports may be warranted for these athletes, especially those athletes with a history of three or more concussions experiencing slowed recovery.

26. Athletic trainers working with younger (pediatric) athletes should be aware that recovery may take longer than in older athletes. Additionally, these younger

athletes are maturing at a relatively fast rate and will likely require more frequent updates of baseline measures compared with older athletes.

27. Many young athletes experience sport-related concussion. Athletic trainers should play an active role in helping to educate young athletes, their parents and coaches and about the dangers of repeated concussions. Continued research into the epidemiology of sport-related concussion in young athletes and prospective investigations to determine the acute and long-term effects of recurrent concussion in younger athletes are warranted.

28. Because damage to the maturing brain of a young athlete can be catastrophic (i.e., almost all reported cases of second-impact syndrome are in young athletes), younger athletes (under age 18 years) should be managed more conservatively, using stricter RTP guidelines than those used to manage concussion in the more mature athlete.

29. An athlete with a concussion should be instructed to avoid taking medications except acetaminophen after the injury. Acetaminophen and other medications should only be given at the recommendation of a physician. Additionally, the athlete should be instructed to avoid ingesting alcohol, illicit drugs, or other substances that might interfere with cognitive function and neurologic recovery.

30. Any athlete with a concussion should be instructed to rest, but complete bed rest is not recommended. The athlete should resume normal activities of daily living as tolerated, while avoiding activities that potentially increase symptoms. Once he or she is asymptomatic, the athlete may resume a graded program of physical and mental exertion, without contact or risk of concussion, up to the point at which postconcussion signs and symptoms recur. If symptoms appear, the exertion level should be scaled back to allow maximal activity without triggering symptoms.

31. An athlete with a concussion should be instructed to eat a well-balanced diet that is nutritious in both quality and quantity.

32. An athlete should be awakened during the night to check on deteriorating signs and symptoms only if he or she experienced LOC, had prolonged periods of amnesia, or was still experiencing significant symptoms at bedtime. The purpose of the wake-ups is to check for deteriorating signs and symptoms, such as decreased levels of consciousness or increasing headache, which could indicate a more serious head injury or a late-onset complication such as an intracranial bleed.

33. Oral and written instructions for home care should be given to the athlete and to a responsible adult (eg, parents or roommate) who will observe and supervise the athlete during the acute phase of the concussion while at home or in the dormitory. The ATC and physician should agree on standard concussion home-instruction form and it should be used consistently for all concussions.

34. The ATC should enforce the standard use of helmets for protecting against catastrophic head injuries and reducing the severity of cerebral concussions. In sports that require helmet protection (football, lacrosse, ice hockey, baseball/softball, etc.) the ATC should ensure that all equipment meets either National Operating Committee on Standards for Athletic Equipment (NOCSAE) or American Society for Testing and Materials (ASTM) standards.

35. The ATC should enforce the standard use of mouthguards for protection against dental injuries, even though the scientific evidence supporting their use for reducing concussive injury is not yet convincing.

36. At this time, the ATC should neither endorse nor discourage the use of soccer headgear for protecting against concussion or the consequences of cumulative, subconcussive impacts to the head. Currently, no scientific evidence supports the use of headgear in soccer for reducing concussive injury to the head.

NATA Position Statement: Commotio Cordis*

According to the U.S. Commotio Cordis Registry, since 1998, 130 athletes have died from blunt force injury to the heart (commotio cordis). Of those, 70 were children ages four to eighteen, according to the Heart Center at Tufts New England Medical Center.

In an effort to educate the public about the potential risk physically active youth can face, the National Athletic Trainers' Association (NATA) Age-Specific Task Force recommends that parents and coaches take the proactive steps to protect their athletes against commotio cordis.

Commotio cordis is caused by a blow to the chest (directly over the heart) that occurs between heart contractions. The blunt force causes a lethal abnormal heart rhythm.

The following suggestions can help prevent commotio cordis and keep young athletes safe.

- Encourage all coaches and officials to become trained in cardiopulmonary resuscitation (CPR), automatic external defibrillator (AED) use, and first aid.
- Establish an emergency action plan at all athletic venues. Parents, coaches, and officials should be involved in these plans. (NATA's Position Statement on Emergency Planning in Athletics—http://www.nata.org/publicinformation/files/emergencyplanning.pdf—is a useful resource.)
- Use all-purpose sport chest protectors during practices and games. *(Note: NATA recommends continued research in this area because current information is limited. However, use of properly fitted, quality chest protectors are recommended to reduce the risk of injury to the athlete.)*
- Ensure all protective equipment fits properly and is used as intended by the manufacturer.
- Teach athletes how to protect themselves against chest injuries.
- Maintain an even and clean playing surface.

*From www.nata.org

Sample Resume

Joseph Q. Doe, A.T.C.
jqdoe@email.unc.edu
100 Lexington Highway
Chapel Hill, NC 27514
(919) 555-1234

EDUCATION

UNIVERSITY OF NORTH CAROLINA AT CHAPEL HILL
Graduation: Masters of Arts, May 2002
Major: Exercise and Sports Science
Specialization: Athletic Training (NATA Accredited Program)

UNIVERSITY OF NORTH CAROLINA AT CHAPEL HILL
Graduation: Bachelor of Arts, May 21, 2000 with Highest Honors
Major: Exercise and Sports Science GPA: 3.456, Major: 3.644
Specialization: Athletic Training (CAAHEP Accredited Program)

ATHLETIC TRAINING EXPERIENCE

Graduate Assistant Athletic Trainer
University of North Carolina Chapel Hill, NC August 2000–Present
Responsible for evaluation, treatment and rehabilitation of injuries.
Coverage of practices and meets, record keeping, and updating coaches and medical staff for football, men's lacrosse, and fencing.
Advanced Clinical Instructor for undergraduate student athletic trainers
Supervising undergraduate athletic trainers
Head Trainer for the University of North Carolina's Junior Varsity Football Team

Student Athletic Trainer
University of North Carolina Chapel Hill, NC August 1998–2000
Responsible for evaluation, treatment, and rehabilitation of injuries.
Coverage of practices and meets, record keeping, and updating coaches and medical staff for wrestling, women's lacrosse and women's volleyball

University of North Carolina Summer Camp Athletic Training
Served as Camp Coordinator for wrestling camp; in charge of ordering medical supplies and overseeing the athletic training staff.
Served as an athletic trainer at various camps, including men's and women's lacrosse, cheerleading, and soccer.

TEACHING EXPERIENCE

Instructor
- Golf
- Bowling
- Racquetball
- Self-defense

Teaching Assistant
- Emergency Care class
- Gross Anatomy labs
- Guess lecture in Personal Health class

CERTIFICATIONS AND MEMBERSHIPS

- Certified Athletic Trainer
- Responding to Emergency Instructor
- First Aid and Community CPR Instructor
- Automatic External Defibrilator Instructor
- Epi-Pen Certified
- NATA member
- UNC Student Athletic Trainer member
- USS Swimming and YMCA Stroke and Turn Official certified

OTHER WORK EXPERIENCE	**Security Officer** Falconer and Sons LTD, 1 W47st NYC, NY 1990–1992 In charge of safety policy for the store, arranging schedules of other security personal, jewelry delivery, and store security
VOLUNTEER EXPERIENCES	**Coaching** • Chapel Hill-Carrboro YMCA, Basketball Coach, 1999–2000 • Carrboro Park and Recs., Baseball Coach, 1995–2000 • Rainbow Soccer, Soccer Coach, 1992–1995 • Staten Island Boys Football League, Football Coach, 1989–1992 • Blessed Sacrament Titan League, Baseball Coach, 1987–1989
REFERENCES	**Available on Request**

Glossary

A

abduction Movement of a body part away from the midline of the body.

accident An act that occurrs by chance or without intention.

active range of motion (AROM) Joint motion that occurs because of muscle contraction.

acute injury An injury with sudden onset and short duration.

adduction Movement of a body part toward the midline of the body.

adipose cell Stores triglyceride.

afferent nerves Nerves that transport messages toward the brain.

agonist muscles Muscles directly engaged in contraction as related to muscles that relax at the same time.

ambient Environmental (e.g., temperature or air that invests one's immediate environment).

ambulation Move or walk from place to place.

ameboid action Cellular action like that of an amoeba, using protoplasmic pseudopod.

amenorrhea Absence or suppression of menstruation.

ampere Volume or amount of electrical energy.

analgesia Pain inhibition.

analgesic Agent that relieves pain without causing a complete loss of sensation.

anaphylaxis Increased susceptibility or sensitivity to a foreign protein or toxin as the result of previous exposure to it.

androgen Any substance that aids the development and controls the appearance of male characteristics.

anemia Lack of iron.

anesthesia Partial or complete loss of sensation.

anomaly Deviation from the normal.

anorexia Lack or loss of appetite; aversion to food.

anorexia nervosa Eating disorder characterized by a distorted body image.

anoxia Lack of oxygen.

antagonist muscles Muscles that counteract the action of the agonist muscles.

anterior Before or in front of.

anteroposterior Refers to the position of front to back.

anteversion Tipping forward of a part as a whole, without bending.

antipyretic Agent that relieves or reduces fever.

anxiety A feeling of uncertainty or apprehension.

apnea Temporary cessation of breathing.

apophysis Bony outgrowth to which muscles attach.

apophysitis Inflammation of an apophysis.

arrhythmical movement Irregular movement.

arthrogram Radiopaque material injected into a joint to facilitate the taking of an X ray.

arthrokinematics Physiological and accessory movements of the joint.

arthroscopic examination Viewing the inside of a joint through an arthroscope, which uses a small camera lens.

assumption of risk An individual, through express or implied agreement, assumes that some risk or danger will be involved in a particular undertaking; a person takes his or her own chances.

asymmetry (body) Lack of symmetry of sides of the body.

ATC Certified Athletic Trainer.

atrophy Wasting away of tissue or of an organ; decrease in the size of a body part or muscle.

attenuation Decrease in intensity as ultrasound enters deeper into tissues.

aura Preepileptic phenomenon, involving visual sensation of fire or glow, along with other possible sensory hallucinations and dreamlike states.

autogenic inhibition The relaxation of the antagonist muscle during contractions.

automatism Automatic behavior before consciousness or full awareness has been achieved after a brain concussion.

avascular Devoid of blood circulation.

avascular necrosis Death of tissue caused by the lack of blood supply.

avulsion Forcible tearing away of a part or a structure.

axilla Armpit.

B

bacteremia Bacterial infection in the blood.

bacteria Morphologically, the simplest group of nongreen vegetable organisms, various species of which are involved in fermentation and putrefaction, the production of disease, and the fixing of atmospheric nitrogen; a schizomycete.

bacteriostatic Halting the growth of bacteria.

ballistic stretching Older stretching technique that uses repetitive bouncing motions.

bandage Strip of cloth or other material used to cover a wound or hold a dressing in place.

beam nonuniformity ratio (BNR) Amount of variability in intensity of the ultrasound beam.

bending Force on a horizontal beam or bone that places stresses within the structure, causing it to bend or strain.

beta-endorphin Chemical substance produced in the brain.

bioavailability How completely a particular drug is absorbed by the system.

bioequivalence Having a similar biological effect.

biomechanics Branch of study that applies the laws of mechanics to living organisms and biological tissues.

biotransformation Transforming a drug so it can be metabolized.

bipedal Having two feet or moving on two feet.

BMR Basal metabolic rate.

body composition Percent body fat plus lean body weight.

bradykinin Peptide chemical that causes pain in an injured area.

bradypnea Slow breathing.

buccal Pertaining to the cheek or mouth.

bulimia Binge-purge eating disorder.

bursitis Inflammation of bursa at sites of bony prominences between muscle and tendon such as those of the shoulder and knee.

C

calcific tendinitis Deposition of calcium in a chronically inflamed tendon, especially the tendons of the shoulder.

calisthenic Exercise involving free movement without the aid of equipment.

calorie (large) Amount of heat required to raise 1 kg of water 1° C; used to express the fuel or energy value of food or the heat output of the organism; the amount of heat required to heat 1 lb of water to 4° F.

cardiorespiratory endurance Ability to perform activities for extended periods of time.

catastrophic injury Relates to a permanent injury of the spinal cord that leaves the athlete quadriplegic or paraplegic.

catecholamine Active amines, epinephrine and norepinephrine, that affect the nervous and cardiovascular systems.

cellulitis An inflammation of cells and connective tissue that extends deep into the tissues.

cerebrovascular accident Stroke.

chafing Superficial inflammation that develops when skin is subjected to friction.

chemical mediator A chemical that causes or produces a specific physiological response.

chemotaxis Response to influence of chemical stimulation.

chiropractor One who practices a method for restoring normal condition by adjusting the segments of the spinal column.

Chlamydia trachomatis A microorganism that can cause a wide variety of diseases in humans, one of which is venereal and causes nonspecific urethritis.

chondromalacia Abnormal softening of cartilage.

chronic injury Injury with long onset and long duration.

cicatrix Scar or mark formed by fibrous connective tissue; left by a wound or sore.

circadian rhythm Biological time clock by which the body functions.

circuit training Exercise stations that consist of various combinations of weight training, flexibility, calisthenics, and aerobic exercises.

circumduct Act of moving a limb such as the arm or hip in a circular manner.

clonic muscle contraction Alternating involuntary muscle contraction and relaxation in quick succession.
coenzymes Enzyme activators.
collagen Main organic constituent of connective tissue.
collision sport Sport in which athletes use their bodies to deter or punish opponents.
colloid Liquid or gelatinous substance that retains particles of another substance in a state of suspension.
commission (legal liability) Person commits an act that is not legally his or hers to perform.
communicable disease Disease that may be transmitted directly or indirectly from one individual to another.
compression Force that crushes tissue.
concentric (positive) contraction The muscle shortens while contracting against resistance.
conduction Heating through direct contact with a hot medium.
conjunctiva Mucous membrane that lines the eyes.
contact sport Sport in which athletes do make physical contact but not with the intent to produce bodily injury.
contrast bath procedure Technique that uses immersion in ice slush, followed by immersion in tepid water.
contrecoup brain injury After head is struck, brain continues to move within the skull, resulting in injury to the side opposite the force.
convection Heating indirectly through another medium such as air or liquid.
conversion Heating through other forms of energy (e.g., electricity).
convulsions Paroxysms of involuntary muscular contractions and relaxations.
core temperature Internal, or deep, body temperature monitored by cells in the hypothalamus, as opposed to shell, or peripheral, temperature, which is registered by that layer of insulation provided by the skin, subcutaneous tissues, and superficial portions of the muscle masses.
corticosteroid Steroid produced by the adrenal cortex.
coryza Profuse nasal discharge.
counterirritant Agent that produces mild inflammation and acts, in turn, as an analgesic when applied locally to the skin (e.g., liniment).
coupling medium Used to facilitate the transmission of ultrasound into the tissues.
crepitation Crackling sound heard during the movement of ends of a broken bone.
cryokinetics Cold application combined with exercise.
cryotherapy Cold therapy.
cubital fossa Triangular area on the anterior aspect of the forearm directly opposite the elbow joint (the bend of the elbow).
cyanosis Slightly bluish, grayish, slatelike, or dark purple discoloration of the skin caused by a reduced amount of blood hemoglobin.

D

DAPRE Daily adjustable progressive resistance exercise.
debride Removal of dirt and dead tissue from a wound.
deconditioning State in which the athlete's body loses its competitive fitness.
degeneration Deterioration of tissue.
dermatome Segmental skin area innervated by various spinal cord segments.
diagnosis Identification of a specific condition.
diapedesis Passage of blood cells, via ameboid action, through the intact capillary wall.
diarthrodial joint Ball-and-socket joint.
diastolic blood pressure The residual pressure when the heart is between beats.
DIP Distal interphalangeal joint.
diplopia Seeing double.
distal Farthest from a center, from the midline, or from the trunk.
DNA Deoxyribonucleic acid.
doping The administration of a drug that is designed to improve the competitor's performance.
dorsiflexion Bending toward the dorsum or rear; opposite of plantar flexion.
dorsum The back of a body part.
dressing Covering, protective or supportive, that is applied to an injury or wound.
drug A chemical agent used in the prevention, treatment, or diagnosis of disease.
drug vehicle The substance in which a drug is transported.
dyspnea Difficult breathing.
dysrhythmia Irregular heartbeats.

E

eccentric (negative) contraction The muscle lengthens while contracting against resistance.
ecchymosis Black-and-blue skin discoloration caused by hemorrhage.
ectopic Located in a place different from normal.
edema Swelling as a result of the collection of fluid in connective tissue.
effective radiating area Portion of the transducer that produces sound energy.
efficacy A drug's capability of producing a specific therapeutic effect.
effleurage Stroking.
electrolyte Solution that is a conductor of electricity.
embolus A mass of undisolved matter.
emetic Agent that induces vomiting.
endurance Body's ability to engage in prolonged physical activity.
enthesitis Group of conditions characterized by inflammation, fibrosis, and calcification around tendons, ligaments, and muscle insertions.
enzyme An organic catalyst that can cause chemical changes in other substances without being changed itself.
epidemiological approach Study of sports injuries that involves the relationship of as many factors as possible.
epilepsy Recurrent paroxysmal disorder characterized by sudden attacks of altered consciousness, motor activity, sensory phenomena, or inappropriate behavior.
epiphysis Cartilaginous growth region of a bone.
epistaxis Nosebleed.
ethics Principles of morality.
etiology Science dealing with causes of disease.
eversion of the foot To turn the foot outward.
excoriation Removal of a piece or strip of skin.
exostoses Benign bony outgrowths, usually capped by cartilage, that protrude from the surface of a bone.
extraoral mouth guard Protective device that fits outside the mouth.
extracellular matrix Collagen, elastin, ground substance, proteoglycans, and glycosaminoglycans.
extravasation Escape of a fluid from its vessels into the surrounding tissues.
exudate Accumulation of fluid in an area.

F

facilitation To assist the progress of.
fascia Fibrous membrane that covers, supports, and separates muscles.
fasciitis Inflammation of fascia.
fibrinogen Blood plasma protein that is converted into a fibrin clot.
fibroblast Any cell component from which fibers are developed.
fibrocartilage Type of cartilage (e.g., intervertebral disks) in which the matrix contains thick bundles of collaginous fibers.
fibroplasia Period of scar formation.
fibrosis Development of excessive fibrous connective tissue; fibroid degeneration.
first intention Normal healing of a wound where new cells are formed to take the place of damaged cells leaving little or no scar.
flash-to-bang Number of seconds from lightning flash until the sound of thunder divided by five.
foot pronation Combined foot movements of plantar flexion, adduction, and eversion.
foot supination Combined foot movements of dorsiflexion and inversion.
force couple Depressor action by the subscapularis, infraspinatus, and teres minor muscles to stabilize the head of the humerus and to counteract the upward force exerted by the deltoid muscle during abduction of the arm.
frequency Measured in hertz (Hz), cycles per second (CPS), or pulses per second (PPS).
friction Heat producing.
FSH Follicle-stimulating hormone.

G

GAS theory General adaptation syndrome.
genitourinary Pertaining to the reproductive and urinary organs.
genu recurvatum Hyperextension at the knee joint.
genu valgum Knock-knee.
genu varum Bowleg.
GH Growth hormone.
glycogen supercompensation High-carbohydrate diet.
glycosuria Abnormally high proportion of sugar in the urine.
Good Samaritan law Provides limited protection against legal liability to any

individual who voluntarily chooses to provide first aid.
granulation tissue Fibroblasts, collagen, and capillaries.

H

half-life Rate at which a drug disappears from the body through metabolism, excretion, or both.
hemarthrosis Blood in a joint cavity.
hematolytic Pertaining to the degeneration and disintegration of the blood.
hematoma Blood tumor.
hematuria Blood in the urine.
hemoglobin Coloring substance of the red blood cells.
hemoglobinuria Hemoglobin in the urine.
hemolysis Destruction of red blood cells.
hemophilia Hereditary blood disease in which coagulation is greatly prolonged.
hemopoietic Forming blood cells.
hemorrhage Discharge of blood.
hemothorax Bloody fluid in the pleural cavity.
hertz (Hz) Number of sound waves per second.
hirsutism Excessive hair growth or the presence of hair in unusual places.
homeostasis Maintenance of a steady state in the body's internal environment.
HOPS Evaluation scheme that includes history, observation, palpation, and special tests.
hunting response Causes a slight temperature increase during cooling.
hyperemia Unusual amount of blood in a body part.
hyperextension Extreme stretching of a body part.
hyperflexibility Flexibility beyond a joint's normal range.
hyperhidrosis Excessive sweating; excessive foot perspiration.
hyperkeratosis Excessive growth of the horny tissue layer.
hypermobility Extreme mobility of a joint.
hyperpnea Hyperventilation; increased minute volume of breathing; exaggerated deep breathing.
hypertension High blood pressure; abnormally high tension.
hyperthermia Elevated body temperature.
hypertonic Having a higher osmotic pressure than a compared solution.
hypertrophy Enlargement of a body part or muscle caused by an increase in the size of its cells.
hyperventilation Labored breathing.
hypoallergenic Low allergy producing.
hypoxia Lack of an adequate amount of oxygen.

I

idiopathic Cause of a condition is unknown.
iliotibial band friction syndrome Runner's knee.
injury An act that damages or hurts.
innervation Nerve stimulation of a muscle.
interosseous membrane Connective tissue membrane between bones.
intertrigo Chafing of the skin.
interval training Alternating periods of work with active recovery.
inunctions Oily or medicated substances (e.g., liniments) that are rubbed into the skin to produce a local or systemic effect.
inversion of the foot To turn the foot inward; inner border of the foot lifts.
ions Electrically charged atoms.
ipsilateral Situated on the same side.
ischemia Lack of blood supply to a body part.
isokinetic exercise Resistance is given at a fixed velocity of movement with accommodating resistance.
isokinetic muscle resistance Accommodating and variable resistance.
isometric exercise Contracts the muscle statically without changing its length.
isotonic exercise Shortens and lengthens the muscle through a complete range of motion.

J

joint capsule Saclike structure that encloses the ends of bones in a diarthrodial joint.
joint play Movement that is not voluntary but accessory.

K

keratolytic Loosening of the horny skin layer.
keratosis Excessive growth of the horny tissue layer.
kilocalorie Amount of heat required to raise 1 kg of water 1° C.
kinesthesia; kinesthesis Sensation or feeling of movement; the awareness one has of the spatial relationships of one's body and its parts.
kyphosis Exaggeration of the normal curve of the thoracic spine.

L

labile Unsteady; not fixed and easily changed.
lactase deficiency Difficulty digesting dairy products.
laser Light amplification by stimulated emission of radiation.
leukocytes Consist of two types—granulocytes (e.g., basophils and neutrophils) and agranulocytes (e.g., monocytes and lymphocytes).
LH Luteinizing hormone.
liability The state of being legally responsible for the harm one causes another person.
load Outside force or forces acting on tissue.
lordosis Abnormal lumbar vertebral convexity.
luxation Complete joint dislocation.
lymphocytes Cells that are the primary means of providing the body with immune capabilities.
lysis To break down.

M

macerated skin Skin that has been softened by exposure to wetting.
macrophage A phagocytic cell of the immune system.
macrotear Soft tissue damage generally caused by acute trauma.
malaise Discomfort and uneasiness caused by an illness.
malfeasance (or act of commission) When an individual commits an act that is not legally his or hers to perform.
margination Accumulation of leukocytes on blood vessel walls at the site of injury during early stages of inflammation.
mast cells Connective tissue cells that contain heparin and histamine.
MCP Metacarpophalangeal joint.
mechanical failure Elastic limits of tissue are exceeded, causing tissue to break.
mechanism Mechanical description of the cause.
menarche Onset of menstrual function.
metabolism Changing a drug into a water-soluble compound that can be excreted.
metatarsalgia A general term to describe pain in the ball of the foot.
microtear Minor soft tissue damage associated with overuse.
microtrauma Microscopic lesion or injury.
misfeasance When an individual improperly does something that he or she has the legal right to do.
muscle contracture Permanent contraction of a muscle as a result of spasm or paralysis.
muscular endurance The ability to perform repetitive muscular contractions against some resistance.
muscular strength The maximal force that can be applied by a muscle during a single maximum contraction.
myocarditis Inflammation of the heart muscle.
myoglobin Respiratory protein in muscle tissue that is an oxygen carrier.
myositis Inflammation of muscle.
myositis ossificans Myositis marked by ossification of muscles.

N

necrosin Chemical substance that stems from inflamed tissue, causing changes in normal tissue.
negative resistance Slow, eccentric muscle contraction against a resistance.
negligence The failure to use ordinary or reasonable care.
nerve entrapment Nerve compressed between bone or soft tissue.
neuritis Inflammation of a nerve.
neuroma A bulging that emanates from a nerve.
nociceptor Receptor of pain.
noncontact sport Sport in which athletes are not involved in any physical contact.
nonfeasance (or an act of omission) When an individual fails to perform a legal duty.
nystagmus Constant involuntary back and forth, up and down, or rotary movement of the eyeball.

O

obesity Excessive amount of body fat.
obstructed Blocked airway caused by either partial or complete obstruction.
ohm Resistance.
omission (legal) Person fails to perform a legal duty.

orthopedic surgeon One who corrects deformities of the musculoskeletal system.
orthosis Used in sports as an appliance or apparatus to support, align, prevent, or correct deformities or to improve function of a movable body part.
orthotics Field of knowledge relating to orthoses and their use.
OSHA Occupational Safety and Health Administration.
osteoarthritis Chronic disease involving joints in which there is destruction of articular or hyaline cartilage and bony overgrowth.
osteoblasts Bone-producing cells.
osteochondral Refers to relationship of bone and cartilage.
osteochondritis Inflammation of bone and cartilage.
osteochondritis dissecans Fragment of cartilage and underlying bone is detached from the articular surface.
osteochondrosis Disease state of a bone and its articular cartilage.
osteoclasts Cells that resorb bone.
osteoporosis A decrease in bone density.

P

palpation Feeling an injury with the fingers.
paraplegia Paralysis of lower portion of the body and of both legs.
paresis Slight or incomplete paralysis.
paresthesia Abnormal or morbid sensation such as itching or prickling.
passive range of motion Movement that is performed completely by the examiner.
pathogenic Disease producing.
pathology Science of the structural and functional manifestations of disease.
pathomechanics Mechanical forces that are applied to a living organism and adversely change the body's structure and function.
pediatrician Specialist in the treatment of children's diseases.
pes anserinus tendinitis Cyclist's knee.
permeable Permitting the passage of a substance through a vessel wall.
petrissage Kneading.
phagocytosis Destruction of injurious cells or particles by phagocytes (white blood cells).
phalanges Bones of the fingers and toes.
phalanx Any one of the bones of the fingers and toes.
pharmacokinetics The method by which drugs are absorbed, distributed, metabolized, and eliminated.
pharmacology The study of drugs and their origin, nature, properties, and effects on living organisms.
phonophoresis Introduction of ions of soluble salt into the body through ultrasound.
photophobia Unusual intolerance to light.
piezoelectric effect Electrical current produced by applying pressure to certain crystals.
PIP Proximal interphalangeal joint.
plyometric exercise Type of exercise that maximizes the myotatic, or stretch, reflex.
pneumothorax Collapse of a lung as a result of air in the pleural cavity.
podiatrist Practitioner who specializes in the study and care of the foot.
point tenderness Pain produced when an injury site is palpated.
posterior Toward the rear or back.
potency The dose of a drug that is required to produce a desired therapeutic effect.
primary assessment Initial first aid evaluation.
primary survey An evaluation used to determine the existence of life-threatening, emergent conditions or illnesses.
prognosis Prediction as to probable result of a disease or injury.
prophylaxis Guarding against injury or disease.
proprioception The ability to determine the position of a joint in space.
proprioceptive neuromuscular facilitation (PNF) Stretching techniques that involve combinations of alternating contractions and stretches.
proprioceptor One of several receptors, each of which responds to stimuli elicited from within the body itself (e.g., the muscle spindles that invoke the myotatic, or stretch, reflex).
prostaglandin Acidic lipid widely distributed in the body; in musculoskeletal conditions it is concerned with vasodilation, a histamine-like effect; it is inhibited by aspirin.
prosthesis Replacement of an absent body part with an artificial part; the artificial part.
prothrombin Interacts with calcium to produce thrombin.
proximal Nearest to the point of reference.
psychogenic Of psychic origin; that which originates in the mind.
purulent Consisting of or containing pus.

Q

quadriplegia Paralysis affecting all four limbs.

R

radiation Transfer of heat through space from one object to another.
Raynaud's phenomenon Condition in which cold exposure causes vasospasm of digital arteries.
referred pain Pain that is felt somewhere other than its origin.
regeneration Repair, regrowth, or restoration of a part such as tissue.
residual That which remains; often used to describe a permanent condition resulting from injury or disease (e.g., a limp or a paralysis).
resorption Act of removal by absorption.
retroversion Tilting or turning backward of a part.
retrovirus A virus that enters a host cell and changes its RNA to a proviral DNA replica.
revascularize Restoration of blood circulation to an injured area.
RICE Rest, ice, compression, and elevation.
ringworm (tinea) Common name given to many superficial fungal infections of the skin.
RNA Ribonucleic acid.
rotation Turning around an axis in an angular motion.
rubefacients Agents that redden the skin by increasing local circulation through the dilation of blood vessels.

S

SAID principle Specific adaptation to imposed demands.
scoliosis Lateral rotary curve of the spine.
sebaceous cyst A cyst filled with sebum; usually found in the scalp.
secondary assessment Follow-up; a more detailed examination.
secondary survey An evaluation of existing signs and symptoms performed after the presence of life-threatening conditions has been ruled out.
second intention Healing where granulation tissue replaces damaged cells creating increased scar tissue and delays the healing process.
seizure Sudden attack.
septic shock Shock caused by bacteria, especially gram-negative bacteria commonly seen in systemic infections.
sequela Pathological condition that occurs as a consequence of another condition or event.
serotonin Hormone and neurotransmitter.
shearing Force that moves across the parallel organization of the tissue.
sign Objective evidence of an abnormal situation within the body.
sovereign immunity States that neither the government or any individual who is employed by the government can be held liable for negligence.
SPF Sun protection factor.
spica A figure-eight bandage with one of the two loops larger than the other.
stance phase Portion of the gait cycle from initial contact to toe-off.
Staphylococcus Genus of gram-positive bacteria normally present on the skin and in the upper respiratory tract and prevalent in localized infections.
stasis Blockage or stoppage of circulation.
static stretching Passively stretching an antagonist muscle by placing it in a maximal stretch and holding it there.
steady-state When the amount of the drug taken is equal to the amount that is excreted.
strain Extent of deformation of tissue under loading.
stretching Force which pulls beyond the yield point leading to rupturing of soft tissue or fracturing of a bone.
Streptococcus Genus of gram-positive bacteria found in the throat, respiratory tract, and intestinal tract.
stress The internal reaction or resistance to an external load.
stressor Anything that affects the body's physiological or psychological condition, upsetting the homeostatic balance.
subluxation Partial or incomplete dislocation of an articulation.
swing phase Portion of gait cycle that is a period of non–weight bearing.
symptom Subjective evidence of an abnormal situation within the body.

syndrome Group of typical symptoms or conditions that characterize a deficiency or disease.
synergy To work in cooperation with.
synovitis Inflammation of the synovium.
synthesis To build up.
systolic blood pressure The pressure caused by the heart's pumping.

T

tachypnea Rapid breathing.
tapotement Percussion.
tenosynovitis Inflammation of a tendon synovial sheath.
tension Force which pulls or stretches tissue.
tetanus (lockjaw) An acute, often fatal condition characterized by tonic muscular spasm, hyperreflexia, and lockjaw.
tetanus toxoid Tetanus toxin modified to produce active immunity against *Clostridium tetani.*
thermotherapy Heat therapy.
thrombi Plural of thrombus; blood clots that block small blood vessels or a cavity of the heart.
tinea (ringworm) Superficial fungal infections of the skin.
tonic muscle spasm Rigid muscle contraction that lasts over a period of time.
torsion Act or state of being twisted.
torts Legal wrongs committed against a person.
training effect Stroke volume increases while heart rate is reduced at a given exercise load.
transitory paralysis Temporary paralysis.
translation Refers to anterior gliding of tibial plateau.
trauma (*pl* traumas or **traumata)** A physical injury or wound sustained in sport and produced by an external or internal force.
traumatic Pertaining to an injury or wound.
trigger points Small hyperirritable areas within a muscle.

V

valgus Position of a body part that is bent outward.
varus Position of a body part that is bent inward.
vasoconstriction Decrease in the diameter of a blood vessel.
vasodilation Increase in the diameter of a blood vessel.
vasospasm Blood vessel spasm.
vehicle The substance in which a drug is transported.
verruca Wart caused by a virus.
vibration Rapid shaking.
viscoelastic Any material whose mechanical properties vary depending on rate of load.
viscosity Resistance to flow.
volar Referring to the palm or the sole.
voltage Force.
volume of distribution The volume of plasma in which a drug is dissolved.

W

Watt Power.

Y

yield point Elastic limit of tissue.

Credits

Chapter **1** *Focus boxes, pp. 4–8, 11, 13, 36, 37,* Courtesy, The National Athletic Trainers' Association; *Figure 1-2, p. 3,* From Prentice, WE and Arnheim, DD: *Essentials of athletic training,* ed. 6, St. Louis: McGraw-Hill Higher Education, 2005.

Chapter **2** *Figure 2-1A, p. 52,* Adapted from Myers, GC and Garrick, JG: The preseason examination of school and college athletes. In Strauss, RH (ed.): *Sports medicine,* Philadelphia: WB Saunders, 1984; *Figure 2-1B, p. 53,* From Prentice, WE and Arnheim, DD: *Essentials of athletic training,* ed. 6, St. Louis: McGraw-Hill Higher Education, 2005; *Figures 2-3, 2-4, pp. 59, 60,* Used with permission from *The Physician and Sportsmedicine; Figure 2-5, p. 61,* Adapted from Tanner, M: *Growth of adolescence,* Oxford, England: Blackwell Scientific Publications, 1962; *Figure 2-7, p. 63,* Courtesy, The University of North Carolina at Chapel Hill; *Figure 2-8, p. 64,* Modified from Health Style: A Self Test, U.S. Department of Health and Human Services, Public Health Service, National Clearing House, Washington, DC; *Table 2-2, pp. 65,* From Committee on Sports Medicine: *Pediatrics* 81: 738, 1988, Used with permission; *Figure 2-9, p. 66,* Courtesy, D. Bailey, California State University at Long Beach.

Chapter **3** *Focus box, pp. 79–80,* Source: DeCarlo, M: Reimbursement for health care services. In Kronin, J: *Clinical athletic training,* Thorofare, NJ: Slack, 1997.

Chapter **4** *Figure 4-12G, p. 109,* From Prentice, WE: *Get fit stay fit,* St. Louis: Mosby, 1996; *Focus box, p. 122,* From White, T: The wellness guide to lifelong fitness, *The University of California at Berkeley Wellness Letter,* New York: Random House, 1993.

Chapter **5** *Tables 5-1, 5-2, Figures 5-1, 5-4, pp. 133, 135, 139, 152,* From Prentice, WE: *Get fit stay fit,* ed. 3, St. Louis: McGraw-Hill Higher Education, 2004; *Table 5-3, pp. 127, 128,* Modified from *Recommended dietary allowances,* copyright 1998 by the National Academy of Sciences, National Academy Press, Washington, DC; *Figure 5-2, p. 140,* U.S. Department of Agriculture/U.S. Department of Health and Human Services, August, 1992; *Figure 5-3, p. 147,* From Prentice, WE: *Fitness for college and life,* ed. 6, Dubuque, IA: WCB/McGraw-Hill Higher Education, 1999; *Table 5-4, p. 148,* Source: Wardlaw, GM: *Perspectives in Nutrition,* ed. 5, Dubuque, IA: McGraw-Hill Higher Education, 2002.

Chapter **6** *Table 6-3, p. 166,* Modified from Berkow, R: *The Merck manual of diagnosis and therapy,* ed. 14, Rahway, NJ: Merck & Co, 1982; *Focus box p. 173,* Courtesy, ER Buskirk and WC Grasley, Human Performance Laboratory, The Athletic Institute, The Pennsylvania State University.

Chapter **7** *Figures 7-1 A&B, 7-25, 7-26, 7-27, pp. 190, 206, 207,* From Prentice, WE and Arnheim, DD: Essentials of athletic training, ed. 6, St. Louis: McGraw-Hill Higher Education, 2005; *Figures 7-1C, 7-5, 7-12, 7-13, 7-19, 7-20, 7-21, 7-22, 7-23, 7-27, pp. 190, 192, 197, 201, 202, 204,* Courtesy SportsAuthority (www.thesportsauthority.com); *Figures 7-15 & 7-16, pp. 199, 200,* From Nicholas, JA, and Hershman, EB: *The upper extremity in sports medicine,* ed. 2, St. Louis: Mosby, 1995; *Figure 7-18 A–C, p. 201,* Courtesy Title 9 Sports (www.title9sports.com); *Figure 7-18D, p. 201,* Courtesy TKO; *Figures 7-28, 7-29A & E, pp. 208, 209,* Courtesy, Mueller Sports Medicine; *Figures 7-33, 7-34, 7-35, pp. 211, 212,* From Nicholas, JA and Hershman, EB: *The lower extremity and spine in sports medicine,* ed. 2, St. Louis: Mosby, 1995.

Chapter **8** *Figures 8-2, 8-6, 8-10, 8-22, 8-25, 8-29, 8-32, 8-42, 8-43, pp. 219, 221, 223, 230, 232, 234, 236, 241, 242,* From Prentice, WE and Arnheim, DD, *Essentials of athletic training,* ed. 6 St. Louis: McGraw-Hill Higher Education, 2005; *Figures 8-26, 8-37, 8-38, 8-39, pp. 233, 240,* art by Donald O'Connor.

Chapter **9** *Figures 9-2, 9-3, 9-4, pp. 247, 248,* art by Donald O'Connor; *Figures 9-5, 9-10, 9-13, pp. 249, 254, 261,* From Saladin, KS: *Anatomy and physiology,* ed. 2, Dubuque, IA: McGraw-Hill Higher Education, 2001, *Figure 9-7, p. 251,* From Prentice, WE: *Rehabilitation techniques in sports medicine,* ed. 4, St. Louis: McGraw-Hill Higher Education, 2004.

Chapter **10** *Figure 10-2, 10-8, 10-9, 10-10, pp. 273, 274, 289, 290,* From Prentice, WE: *Therapeutic modalities in sports medicine,* ed. 4, Dubuque, IA: WCB/McGraw-Hill, 1999; *Figure 10-3, p. 281,* From Van De Graaff, K: *Human anatomy,* ed. 6, Dubuque, IA: McGraw-Hill Higher Education, 2002; *Figure 10-4, p. 283,* From Saladin, KS: *Anatomy and physiology,* ed. 2, Dubuque, IA: McGraw-Hill Higher Education, 2001.

Chapter **11** *Figure 11-1, p. 295,* Courtesy Ken Bartlett, California State University at Long Beach; *Figure 11-2, p. 296,* From Prentice, WE: *Rehabilitation techniques in sports medicine,* ed. 4, St. Louis: McGraw-Hill Higher Education, 2004.

Chapter **12** *Table 12-1, p. 324,* Modified from *International medical guide for ships,* Geneva: World Health Organization; *Figure 12-2, p. 326,* From Prentice, WE and Arnheim, DD, *Essentials of athletic training,* ed. 6, St. Louis: McGraw-Hill Higher Education, 2005.

Chapter **13** *Table 13-1, p. 363,* Adapted from Post, M: *Physical examination of the musculoskeletal system,* Chicago: Yearbook Medical Publishers, 1987; *Table 13-2, p. 370,* Modified from Veterans Administration Standard Form A, Washington, DC: U.S. Government Printing Office; *Figure 13-8, p. 381,* From Nicholas, JA and Hershman, EB: *The lower extremity and spine in sports medicine,* ed. 2, St. Louis: Mosby, 1995.

Chapter **14** *Figure 14-2, p. 388,* art by Donald O'Connor; *Focus box, p. 392,* From Hahn, DB and Payne, WA: *Focus on health,* ed. 5, Dubuque, IA: McGraw-Hill Higher Education, 2001; *Figures 14-3, 14-5, pp. 395, 396,* From Prentice, WE and Arnheim, DD, *Essentials of athletic training,* ed. 6, St. Louis: McGraw-Hill Higher Education, 2005.

Chapter **15** *Figure 15-6, p. 411,* Courtesy, Hygenic Corp, Akron, OH; *Figure 15-8, p. 412,* Courtesy, Maxxim Medical, Sugarland, TX; *Figures 15-12, 15-13, 15-14, pp. 418, 420,* From Prentice, WE: *Therapeutic modalities in sports medicine,* ed. 5, St. Louis: McGraw-Hill Higher Education, 2003; *Figure 15-23, p. 427,* Chattanooga Corp, Hickson, TN; *Figure 15-25, p. 428,* Courtesy, Country Technologies, Inc., Gay Mills, WI; *Figure 15-27, p. 430,* From Prentice, WE and Arnheim, DD, *Essentials of athletic training,* ed. 6, St. Louis: McGraw-Hill Higher Education, 2005; *Figure 15-28, p. 431,* Courtesy, International Medical Electronics, Kansas City, MO.

Chapter **16** *Figure 16-3B, p. 447,* Courtesy, BREG, Inc., Vista, CA; *Figure 16-3C, p. 447,* Courtesy, Biodex Medical Systems, Inc., Shirley, NY; *Figure 16-5, 16-11, 16-12, 16-14, 16-15B, pp. 448, 460, 461, 463, 464,* From Prentice, WE: *Rehabilitation techniques in sports medicine,* ed. 4, St. Louis: McGraw-Hill Higher Education, 2004; *Figures 16-6G, 16-10, pp. 453, 458,* From Prentice, WE: *Get fit stay fit,* ed. 3, St. Louis: McGraw-Hill Higher Education, 2004; *Figure 16-6H, p. 453,* Courtesy, Contemporary Design, Glacier, WA; *Figure 16-6I, p. 453,* Courtesy, Fitter International, Calgary, Alberta; *Figure 16-8, p. 455,* Aqua Jogger courtesy Excel Sport Science, Inc., Eugene, OR; *Figure 16-13, p. 463,* Source: Maitland, G: *Extremity manipulation,* London: Butterworth, 1977, and Maitland, G: *Vertebral manipulation,* London: Butterworth, 1978.

Chapter **17** *Table 17-2, p. 476,* From Huff, P: Drug distribution in the training room, *Clinics in Sports Medicine* 17(2): 214, 1998; *Focus box, pp. 496–503,* Adapted from Lombardo, JA: *Drugs in sports.* In Krakurer, LJ: *The yearbook of sports medicine,* Chicago: Yearbook Medical Publishers, 1986.

Chapter **18** *Figure 18-1, p. 520,* From Van De Graaff, K: *Human anatomy,* ed. 6, Dubuque, IA: McGraw-Hill Higher Education, 2002; *Figures 18-6, 18-7, pp. 524, 525,* From Saladin, KS: *Anatomy and physiology,* ed. 2, Dubuque, IA: McGraw-Hill Higher Education, 2001; *Figures 18-20, 18-32, pp. 539, 548,* From Williams, JPG: *Color atlas of injury in sport,* ed. 2, Chicago: Yearbook Medical Publishers, 1990; *Figures 18-25, 18-33, 18-35, pp. 545, 549, 550,* From

Prentice, WE and Arnheim, DD: *Essentials of athletic training, ed.* 6, St. Louis: McGraw-Hill Higher Education, 2005.

Chapter **19** *Figures 19-2, 19-3, 19-4, 19-5, 19-6, pp. 561, 562, 564, 565,* From Saladin, KS: *Anatomy and physiology,* ed. 2, Dubuque, IA: McGraw-Hill Higher Education, 2001; *Table 19-3, p. 574,* Adapted from Singer, KM and Jones, DC: Ligament injuries of the ankle and foot. In Nicholas, JA and Hershman, EB (eds): *The lower extremity and spine in sports medicine,* vol. 1, ed. 2, St. Louis: Mosby, 1995; *Figures 19-22 (left), 19-24, 19-31, pp. 578, 582, 589,* From Williams, JPG: *Color atlas of injury in sport,* ed. 2, Chicago: Yearbook Medical Publishers, 1990; *Figure 19-23 (left), p. 580,* Courtesy, Cramer Products, Gardner, KS; *Figures 19-27, p. 584,* From Prentice, WE and Arnheim, DD: *Essentials of athletic training,* ed. 6, St. Louis: McGraw-Hill Higher Education, 2005; *Figure 19-29 (left), p. 586,* From Nicholas, JA and Hershman, EB: *The lower extremity and spine in sports medicine,* vol. 2, ed. 2, St. Louis: Mosby, 1995.

Chapter **20** *Figures 20-1, 20-4A&B, 20-5, 20-6, pp. 602, 604, 606, 607,* From Saladin, KS: *Anatomy and physiology,* ed. 2, Dubuque, IA: McGraw-Hill Higher Education, 2001; *Figures 20-3, 20-28, 20-44, pp. 603, 624, 635,* art by Donald O'Connor; *Figures 20-4C, 20-46, pp. 571, 638,* From Van De Graaff, K: *Human anatomy,* ed. 6, Dubuque, IA: McGraw-Hill Higher Education, 2002; *Figure 20-21, p. 620,* Courtesy, Medmetric Corp., San Diego, CA; *Figure 20-53, p. 648,* Courtesy, Thera-Kinetics and JACE Systems, Mount Laurel, NJ.

Chapter **21** *Figures 21-1, 21-2, 21-10, 21-11, 21-12, 21-13, pp. 657, 659, 668, 670, 641,* From Saladin, KS: *Anatomy and physiology,* ed. 2, Dubuque, IA: McGraw-Hill Higher Education, 2001; *Figures 21-4, 21-7B and C, pp. 662, 681,* Courtesy Ken Bartlett, California State University at Long Beach; *Figures 21-6, 21-34 (right), pp. 664, 688,* From Williams, JPG: *Color atlas of injury in sport,* ed. 2, Chicago: Yearbook Medical Publishers; *Table 21-3, p. 666,* From Boland, AL and Hosea, JM: *Hip and back pain in runners,* Postgraduate Advances in Sports Medicine I–XII, Pennington, NJ: Forum Medicus, 1986; *Figure 21-29, p. 682,* Courtesy, BRACE International, Phoenix, AZ.

Chapterr **22** *Figures 22-2, 22-3, 22-4, 22-6, 22-7, pp. 701, 702, 704, 706, 707,* From Saladin, KS: *Anatomy and physiology,* ed. 2, Dubuque, IA: McGraw-Hill Higher Education, 2001; *Figures 22-8, 22-29, pp. 707, 728,* art by Donald O'Connor; *Figure 22-26, p. 721,* From Rockwood, C and Masten, F: *The shoulder,* Philadelphia: WB Saunders, 1990; *Figures 22-31, p. 734,* From Nicholas, JA and Hershman, EB: *The upper extremity in sports medicine,* ed. 2, St. Louis: Mosby, 1995; *Figure 22-37, p. 738,* Courtesy, PrePak Products, Carlsbad, CA; *Figure 22-43, p. 742,* Courtesy, Healthsouth Rehabilitation Program, Birmingham, AL.

Chapter **23** *Figures 23-1, 23-2, 23-3, pp. 749, 750, 751,* From Saladin, KS: *Anatomy and physiology,* ed. 2, Dubuque, IA: McGraw-Hill Higher Education, 2001; *Figures 23-7, 23-21, pp. 753, 764,* From Nicholas, JA and Hershman, EB: *The upper extremity in sports medicine,* ed. 2, St. Louis: Mosby, 1995; *Figures 23-8, 23-14, 23-15, 23-16, 23-18, pp. 754, 757, 760,* Courtesy Ken Bartlett, California State University at Long Beach; *Figure 23-26, p. 768,* From Prentice, WE: *Rehabilitation techniques in sports medicine,* ed. 4, St. Louis: McGraw-Hill Higher Education, 2004.

Chapter **24** *Figures 24-1, 24-2, 24-5, 24-8, 24-9, pp. 773, 774, 779, 782, 783,* From Saladin, KS: *Anatomy and physiology,* ed. 2, Dubuque, IA: McGraw-Hill Higher Education, 2001; *Figure 24-7, p. 780,* From Van De Graaff, K: *Human anatomy,* ed. 6, Dubuque, IA: McGraw-Hill Higher Education, 2002; *Figure 24-28 (left), 24-29 (left), 24-30B, 24-33, 24-34, 24-35 (left), 24-49, pp. 794, 795, 797, 798, 805,* From Nicholas, JA and Hershman, EB: *The upper extremity in sports medicine,* ed. 2, St. Louis: Mosby, 1995; *Figure 24-30 A&C, p. 795,* From Prentice, WE and Arnheim, DD: *Essentials of athletic training,* ed. 6, St. Louis: McGraw-Hill Higher Education, 2005; *Figure 24-37, 24-38, 24-39, 24-42, 24-43, 24-47, 24-48, pp. 800, 801, 802, 804, 805,* From Prentice, WE: *Rehabilitation techniques in sports medicine,* ed. 4, St. Louis: McGraw-Hill Higher Education, 2004; *Figure 24-41, p. 801,* Courtesy Ken Bartlett, California State University at Long Beach.

Chapter **25** *Figures 25-1, 25-5, pp. 810, 811, 813,* From Saladin, KS: *Anatomy and physiology,* ed. 2, Dubuque, IA: McGraw-Hill Higher Education, 2001; *Figures 25-3, 25-11, 25-49A, pp. 812, 824, 854,* art by Donald O'Connor; *Figure 25-6, p. 815,* From Seeley, RR, Stephens, TD, and Tate, P: *Anatomy and physiology,* ed. 3, St. Louis: Mosby, 1995; *Tables 25-2, 25-3, pp. 817–819,* From Seeley, RR, Stephens, TD, and Tate, P: *Anatomy and physiology,* St. Louis: Mosby, 1989; *Figure 25-47, p. 849,* From Nicholas, JA and Hershman, EB: *The lower extremity and spine in sports medicine,* vol. 2, ed. 2, St. Louis: Mosby, 1995; *Figure 25-51 (middle & right), p. 855,* From Williams, JPG: *Color atlas of injury in sport,* ed. 2, Chicago: Yearbook Medical Publishers, 1990; *Figure 25-59, p. 863,* From Prentice, WE: *Get fit stay fit,* ed. 3, St. Louis: McGraw-Hill Higher Education, 2004.

Chapter **26** *Figures 26-1, 26-3, 26-9, 26-12, 26-17, 26-20, pp. 873, 874, 894, 897, 901, 904,* From Saladin, KS: *Anatomy and Physiology,* ed. 2, Dubuque, IA: McGraw-Hill Higher Education, 2001; *Figures 26-2, 26-19B, 26-23B, pp. 874, 902, 907,* From Van De Graaff, K: *Human anatomy,* ed. 6, Dubuque, IA: McGraw-Hill Higher Education, 2002; *Figure 26-2, p. 874,* Courtesy Kent Van de Graff; *Figure 26-19B, p. 902,* © Southern Illinois University; *Figure 26-23B, p. 907,* © Al Blum/Visuals Unlimited; *Focus box, p. 891,* Adapted from Vegso, JJ and Lehman, RC: *Field evaluation and management of head and neck injuries.* In Torg, JS (ed.): *Head and neck injuries,* Clinics in Sports Medicine, vol. 6, no. 1, Philadelphia: WB Saunders, 1987; *Figure 26-14, p. 898,* From Prentice, WE and Arnheim DD: *Essentials of athletic training,* ed. 6, St. Louis: McGraw-Hill Higher Education, 2005; *Figures 26-15, 26-18, pp. 899, 901,* From Williams, JPG: *Color atlas of injury in sport, ed.* 2, Chicago: Yearbook Medical Publishers, 1990; *Table 26-8, p. 903,* Adapted from Pashby, RC and Pashby, TJ: *Ocular injuries in sport.* In Welsh, PR and Shepard, RJ (eds.): *Current therapy in sports medicine, 1985–1986,* Philadelphia: BC Decker, 1985.

Chapter **27** *Figure 27-2, 27-8, 27-9, 27-10, pp. 915, 920, 922, 923,* From Saladin, KS: *Anatomy and Physiology,* ed. 2, Dubuque, IA: McGraw-Hill Higher Education, 2001; *Figures 27-3, 27-4, 27-5, pp. 915, 916, 917,* From Seeley, RR, Stephens, TD, and Tate, P: *Anatomy and physiology,* ed. 3, St. Louis: Mosby, 1995. Art by John V. Hagen (Figure 27-3), Jody L. Fulks (Figure 27-4), Rusty Jones (Figure 27-5); *Figure 27-6, p. 918,* From Prentice, WE: *Fitness for college and life,* ed. 6, Dubuque, IA: WCB/McGraw-Hill, 1999; *Figure 27-15, pp. 927–928,* From Boyd, CE: Referred visceral pain in athletics, *Ath Train* 15:20, 1980.

Chapter **28** *Figure 28-1, p. 949,* From Saladin, KS: *Anatomy and Physiology,* ed. 2, Dubuque, IA: McGraw-Hill Higher Education, 2001; *Figure 28-7 (top left), p. 957,* From Booher, JM and Thibodeau, GA: *Athletic training assessment,* Dubuque, IA: McGraw-Hill, 2000; *Figure 28-7 (bottom left), p. 957,* Courtesy, Dr. James Garrick. ***Color plates A, B, C, G, H, I, K, M, N, P, Q, R,*** From Habif, TP: *Clinical dermatology,* ed. 3, St. Louis: Mosby, 1996; ***Color plate D:*** From Stewart, WD, Danto, JL, and Madden, S: *Dermatology: diagnosis and treatment of cutaneous disorders,* ed. 4, St. Louis: The CV Mosby Co., 1978.

Index

Index note: page references with an A-prefix indicate pages in the Appendices.

A

B

C

D

E

F

Q

R

S

U

V

W

X

Y

Z